T0325352

5TH EDITION

VIRULENCE MECHANISMS OF BACTERIAL PATHOGENS

5TH EDITION

VIRULENCE MECHANISMS OF BACTERIAL PATHOGENS

Edited by

Indira T. Kudva
National Animal Disease Center
Agricultural Research Service
U.S. Department of Agriculture
Ames, IA 50010

Nancy A. Cornick
Department of Veterinary Microbiology and
Preventive Medicine
College of Veterinary Medicine
Iowa State University
Ames, IA 50011

Paul J. Plummer
Department of Veterinary Diagnostic and
Production Animal Medicine
College of Veterinary Medicine
Iowa State University
Ames, IA 50011

Qijing Zhang
Department of Veterinary Microbiology and
Preventive Medicine
College of Veterinary Medicine
Iowa State University
Ames, IA 50011

Tracy L. Nicholson
National Animal Disease Center
Agricultural Research Service
U.S. Department of Agriculture
Ames, IA 50010

John P. Bannantine
National Animal Disease Center
Agricultural Research Service
U.S. Department of Agriculture
Ames, IA 50010

Bryan H. Bellaire
Department of Veterinary Microbiology
and Preventive Medicine
College of Veterinary Medicine
Iowa State University
Ames, IA 50011

ASM PRESS

Washington, DC

Library of Congress Cataloging-in-Publication Data

Names: Kudva, Indira T., editor.
Title: Virulence mechanisms of bacterial pathogens / edited by Indira T. Kudva [and six others].
Description: Fifth edition. | Washington, DC: ASM Press, [2016] | Includes bibliographical references and index.
Identifiers: LCCN 2016014513 (print) | LCCN 2016016980 (ebook) | ISBN 9781555819279 (hardcover) | ISBN 9781555819286 ()
Subjects: LCSH: Virulence (Microbiology) | Pathogenic bacteria. | Host-bacteria relationships.
Classification: LCC QR175 .V57 2016 (print) | LCC QR175 (ebook) | DDC 616.9/201--dc23
LC record available at https://lccn.loc.gov/2016014513

All Rights Reserved
Printed in the United States of America

10 9 8 7 6 5 4 3 2 1

Address editorial correspondence to
ASM Press, 1752 N St., N.W.,
Washington, DC 20036-2904, USA

Send orders to ASM Press, P.O. Box 605, Herndon, VA 20172, USA
Phone: 800-546-2416; 703-661-1593
Fax: 703-661-1501
E-mail: books@asmusa.org
Online: http://www.asmscience.org

Cover: *Neisseria gonorrhoeae* bacteria, TEM. Credit: Dr Linda Stannard, UCT/Science Photo Library.

Contents

Contributors

Devon L. Allison
Graduate Program in Life Sciences, Molecular Microbiology and Immunology, University of Maryland-Baltimore; Department of Microbial Pathogenesis, University of Maryland-Baltimore, Dental School, Baltimore, MD 21201

Christopher J. Alteri
Department of Microbiology and Immunology, University of Michigan Medical School, Ann Arbor, MI 48109

Cesar A. Arias
Department of Internal Medicine, Division of Infectious Diseases, University of Texas Medical School at Houston, Houston, TX 77030; International Center for Microbial Genomics; Molecular Genetics and Antimicrobial Resistance Unit, Universidad El Bosque, Bogota, Colombia

Louis S. Ates
Department of Medical Microbiology and Infection Control, VU University Medical Center, Amsterdam, The Netherlands

Yossef Av-Gay
Division of Infectious Diseases, Department of Medicine, University of British Columbia, Vancouver, BC V6H 3Z6 Canada

Troy Bankhead
Department of Veterinary Microbiology and Pathology, Paul G. Allen School for Global Animal Health, Washington State University, Pullman, WA 99164

Jorge L. Benach
Department of Molecular Genetics and Microbiology, Stony Brook University, Center for Infectious Diseases at the Center for Molecular Medicine, Stony Brook, NY 11794

Minny Bhatty
Department of Microbiology and Molecular Genetics, University of Texas Medical School at Houston, Houston, TX 77030

Wilbert Bitter
Department of Medical Microbiology and Infection Control, VU University Medical Center; Section Molecular Microbiology, Amsterdam Institute of Molecules, Medicine and Systems, Vrije Universiteit Amsterdam, 1081 BT Amsterdam, The Netherlands

Kimberly A. Bliven
Department of Microbiology and Immunology, F. Edward Hébert School of Medicine, Uniformed Services University of the Health Sciences, Bethesda, MD 20814

Grant W. Booker
Department of Molecular and Cellular Biology, School of Biological Science; Center for Molecular Pathology, The University of Adelaide, North Terrace Campus, Adelaide, South Australia 5005, Australia

Vincent M. Bruno
The Institute for Genomic Sciences; Department of Microbiology and Immunology, School of Medicine, University of Maryland-Baltimore, Baltimore, MD 21201

James Butcher
Ottawa Institute of Systems Biology, Department of Biochemistry, Microbiology and Immunology, Faculty of Medicine, University of Ottawa, Ottawa, Ontario, Canada K1H 8M5

Mariana X. Byndloss
Department of Medical Microbiology and Immunology, School of Medicine, University of California at Davis, Davis, CA 95616

Elizabeth Di Russo Case
Department of Microbial Pathogenesis and Immunology, College of Medicine, Texas A&M Health Sciences Center, Bryan, TX 77807

Marie-Eve Charbonneau
Department of Microbiology and Immunology, University of Michigan Medical School, Ann Arbor, MI 48109

Nandini Chauhan
Department of Biosciences, University of Oslo, Blindern, 0316 Oslo, Norway

Peter J. Christie
Department of Microbiology and Molecular Genetics, University of Texas Medical School at Houston, Houston, TX 77030

Jason N. Cole
Department of Pediatrics, University of California San Diego, La Jolla, CA 92093; School of Chemistry and Molecular Biosciences, Australian Infectious Diseases Research Center, University of Queensland, St Lucia, Queensland 4072, Australia

Jenna G. Conner
Microbiology and Environmental Toxicology, University of California Santa Cruz, Santa Cruz, CA 95064

Zachary T. Cusumano
Department of Molecular Microbiology, Washington University School of Medicine, St. Louis, MO 63110

Adam Driks
Loyola University Chicago, Stritch School of Medicine, Maywood, IL 60153

Enguo Fan
Institute of Biochemistry and Molecular Biology, University of Freiburg, Freiburg D-79104, Germany

Annika Flint
Ottawa Institute of Systems Biology, Department of Biochemistry, Microbiology and Immunology, Faculty of Medicine, University of Ottawa, Ottawa, Ontario, Canada K1H 8M5

Christian Gonzalez-Rivera
Department of Microbiology and Molecular Genetics, University of Texas Medical School at Houston, Houston, TX 77030

Erin R. Green
Program in Molecular Microbiology, Sackler School of Graduate Biomedical Sciences, Tufts University, Boston, MA 02111

David E. Heinrichs
Department of Microbiology and Immunology, University of Western Ontario, London, Ontario, Canada N6A 5C1

Alexander R. Horswill
Department of Microbiology, Roy J. and Lucille A. Carver College of Medicine, University of Iowa, Iowa City, IA 52242

Edith N. G. Houben
Section Molecular Microbiology, Amsterdam Institute of Molecules, Medicine and Systems, Vrije Universiteit Amsterdam, 1081 BT Amsterdam, The Netherlands

Scott J. Hultgren
Department of Molecular Microbiology, Washington University School of Medicine, St. Louis, MO 63110

Kevin Hybiske
Division of Allergy and Infectious Diseases, Department of Medicine, University of Washington, Seattle, WA 98195

J.A.M.S. Jayatilake
Department of Oral Medicine and Periodontology, Faculty of Dental Sciences, University of Peradeniya, Sri Lanka

Albert E. Jergens
Department of Veterinary Clinical Sciences, College of Veterinary Medicine, Iowa State University, Ames, IA 50010

Christopher J. Jones
Microbiology and Environmental Toxicology, University of California Santa Cruz, Santa Cruz, CA 95064

Roger D. Klein
Department of Molecular Microbiology, Washington University School
of Medicine, St. Louis, MO 63110

Theresa M. Koehler
University of Texas Medical School at Houston, Houston, TX 77030

Holly A. Laakso
Department of Microbiology and Immunology, University of Western Ontario,
London, Ontario, Canada N6A 5C1

Jack C. Leo
Department of Biosciences, University of Oslo, Blindern, 0316 Oslo, Norway

Dirk Linke
Department of Biosciences, University of Oslo, Blindern, 0316 Oslo, Norway

Mark Lyte
Department of Veterinary Microbiology and Preventive Medicine,
College of Veterinary Medicine, Iowa State University, Ames, IA 50011

Sarah E. Maddocks
Department of Biomedical Sciences, Cardiff School of Health Sciences,
Cardiff Metropolitan University, Western Avenue, Llandaff, Wales, CF5 2YB

Anthony T. Maurelli
Department of Microbiology and Immunology, F. Edward Hébert School of
Medicine, Uniformed Services University of the Health Sciences, Bethesda,
MD 20814

Joan Mecsas
Program in Molecular Microbiology, Sackler School of Graduate Biomedical
Sciences; Department of Molecular Biology and Microbiology, Tufts University
School of Medicine, Boston, MA 02111

Harry L.T. Mobley
Department of Microbiology and Immunology, University of Michigan Medical
School, Ann Arbor, MI 48109

Jose M. Munita
Department of Internal Medicine, Division of Infectious Diseases, University of
Texas Medical School at Houston, Houston, TX 77030; International Center for
Microbial Genomics; Clinica Alemana de Santiago, Universidad del Desarrollo
School of Medicine, Santiago, Chile

Victor Nizet
Department of Pediatrics; Skaggs School of Pharmacy and Pharmaceutical
Sciences; Center for Immunity, Infection & Inflammation, University of
California San Diego, La Jolla, CA 92093

Ryan Q. Notti
Laboratory of Structural Microbiology, Rockefeller University, New York,
NY 10065; Tri-Institutional Medical Scientist Training Program, Weill Cornell
Medical College, New York, NY 10021

Mary X.D. O'Riordan
Department of Microbiology and Immunology, University of Michigan Medical School, Ann Arbor, MI 48109

Alexandra E. Paharik
Department of Microbiology, Roy J. and Lucille A. Carver College of Medicine, University of Iowa, Iowa City, IA 52242

Guy H. Palmer
Department of Veterinary Microbiology and Pathology, Paul G. Allen School for Global Animal Health, Washington State University, Pullman, WA 99164

Karla D. Passalacqua
Department of Microbiology and Immunology, University of Michigan Medical School, Ann Arbor, MI 48109

Brian M. Peters
Department of Clinical Pharmacy, University of Tennessee Health Science Center, Memphis, TN 38103

Valérie Poirier
Division of Infectious Diseases, Department of Medicine, University of British Columbia, Vancouver, BC V6H 3Z6

Steven W. Polyak
Department of Molecular and Cellular Biology, School of Biological Science; Center for Molecular Pathology, The University of Adelaide, North Terrace Campus, Adelaide, South Australia 5005, Australia

Wanisa Salaemae
Department of Molecular and Cellular Biology, School of Biological Science, The University of Adelaide, North Terrace Campus, Adelaide, South Australia 5005, Australia

James E. Samuel
Department of Microbial Pathogenesis and Immunology, College of Medicine, Texas A&M Health Sciences Center, Bryan, TX 77807

H. Steven Seifert
Department of Microbiology-Immunology, Feinberg School of Medicine, Northwestern University, Chicago, IL 60611

Cynthia M. Sharma
Research Center for Infectious Diseases (ZINF) University of Würzburg, Würzburg, Germany 97080

Jessica R. Sheldon
Department of Microbiology and Immunology, University of Western Ontario, London, Ontario, Canada N6A 5C1

Mark E. Shirtliff
Department of Microbial Pathogenesis, University of Maryland-Baltimore, Dental School; The Institute for Genomic Sciences, School of Medicine, University of Maryland-Baltimore, Baltimore, MD 21201

C. Erec Stebbins
Laboratory of Structural Microbiology, Rockefeller University, New York, NY 10065

Richard Stephens
Program in Infectious Diseases, School of Public Health, University of California, Berkeley, Berkeley, CA 94720

Alain Stintzi
Ottawa Institute of Systems Biology, Department of Biochemistry, Microbiology and Immunology, Faculty of Medicine, University of Ottawa, Ottawa, Ontario, Canada K1H 8M5

Jan S. Suchodolski
Gastrointestinal Laboratory, Department of Small Animal Clinical Sciences, College of Veterinary Medicine and Biomedical Sciences, Texas A&M University, College Station, TX 77845

Sarah L. Svensson
Research Center for Infectious Diseases (ZINF) University of Würzburg, Würzburg, Germany 97080

Michelle C. Swick
University of Texas Medical School at Houston, Houston, TX 77030

Jennifer K. Teschler
Microbiology and Environmental Toxicology, University of California Santa Cruz, Santa Cruz, CA 95064

Alvaro Toledo
Department of Molecular Genetics and Microbiology, Stony Brook University, Center for Infectious Diseases at the Center for Molecular Medicine, Stony Brook, NY 11794

Renee M. Tsolis
Department of Medical Microbiology and Immunology, School of Medicine, University of California at Davis, Davis, CA 95616

D. B. R. K. Gupta Udatha
Department of Biosciences, University of Oslo, Blindern, 0316 Oslo, Norway

Hubertine M. E. Willems
Department of Clinical Pharmacy, University of Tennessee Health Science Center, Memphis, TN 38103

Joao B. Xavier
Program for Computational Biology, Memorial Sloan Kettering Cancer Center, New York, NY 10065

Fitnat H. Yildiz
Microbiology and Environmental Toxicology, University of California Santa Cruz, Santa Cruz, CA 95064

Preface

"Generation of new ideas and refinement or extension of established concepts are the essence of advances in knowledge": Dr. Carlton Gyles, Preface, Virulence Mechanisms of Bacterial Pathogens, 1st Edition, 1988, ASM Press. This was the driving force behind the current fifth edition of this monograph, which essentially is a compilation of bacterial virulence strategies and cutting-edge therapies (targeting these strategies) that have been unraveled in recent years and/or provide new insights into established dogmas.

Previous editions of this book always provided interesting and timely information on topics not always covered in textbooks making them reliable reference sources. Traditionally these were published as follow-up to a series of International Symposia on Virulence Mechanisms of Bacterial Pathogens, held in Ames, Iowa in 1987, 1994, 1999, and 2006. Hence, the last edition was published in 2007. With all the scientific advancements made in the area of bacterial pathogenesis since then, there was a pressing need for a more recent, updated version of this book. To make up for the lapsed time and the inevitable financial constraints, a general consensus was reached to initiate the publication sans a symposium. This turned out to be quite an insightful decision as it enabled the editors and all contributors to provide their undivided attention to weaving together a harmonious and comprehensive monograph.

Sections in this edition have been organized in a systematic manner keeping in sync with the journey a pathogen undertakes in its host. Therefore, these sections discuss, key events occurring at the bacterial-host interface (section I) that enable colonization, bacterial reliance on communication (section II) and secretion (section III) to initiate/enhance virulence, bacterial defense (section IV), persistence (section V), and host-exploitation strategies (section VI) that allow for extended survival in the host. The concluding section (section VII) discusses novel therapeutic approaches being developed to target some of these virulence mechanisms.

It was our intent to deliver the science through this monograph and allow our savvy readers the luxury of philosophizing. As such, we sought contributions from distinguished experts, whether as authors or reviewers, making this monograph a one-stop learning tool for recent advances made in the field of bacterial virulence while stepping away from being just another "textbook". The contents were selected to be beneficial to diverse readership (students, faculty, scientists in academic, clinical, corporate and/or government settings) while promoting discussion, extrapolation, exploration and multi-dimensional thinking.

Indira T. Kudva
Executive Editor

Acknowledgments

The Section Editors acknowledge the timely contributions made by all the authors and the tremendous support provided by:
ASM Press
Editors, *Microbiology Spectrum*
Reviewers:

Keith M. Derbyshire, PhD
Director, Division of Genetics,
Center for Medical Science, Wadsworth Center
Professor, Biomedical Sciences, University at Albany
NYSDOH
Albany, NY 12201

Cammie Lesser, MD, PhD
Associate Professor Medicine (Microbiology and Immunobiology)
Massachusetts General Hospital/Harvard Medical School
Cambridge, MA 02139

Joseph D. Mougous, PhD
Associate Professor
Department of Microbiology
University of Washington
Seattle, WA 98195

Joseph P. Vogel, PhD
Associate Professor
Department of Molecular Microbiology
Washington University
St. Louis, MO 63110

Timothy L. Yahr, PhD
Director of Graduate Studies
Professor of Microbiology
University of Iowa, Carver College of Medicine
Iowa City, IA 52242

BACTERIAL-HOST INTERFACE

Evolution of Bacterial Pathogens Within the Human Host

1

KIMBERLY A. BLIVEN[1] and ANTHONY T. MAURELLI[1]

INTRODUCTION

The success or failure of a pathogen is entirely dependent on its ability to survive, reproduce, and spread to a new host or environment. Host immune systems, predators, microbial competitors, parasites, and environmental resource limitations all exert selective pressures that shape the genomes of microbial populations (1). Host fitness, meanwhile, is determined by the ability of the host to survive and reproduce; the host must therefore effectively curtail diseases that impair either of these abilities.

Dawkins and Krebs suggest that the conflicting drives between host and pathogen have led to an evolutionary "arms race," where an asymmetric "attack-defense" strategy has come into play (2). At the basic level, this concept suggests that when the host evolves new defenses to thwart the pathogen's attack, the pathogen is forced to adapt a more effective attack strategy to penetrate the heightened defenses. In response, the host must once again evolve to cope with the new attack mechanism, and the cycle continues. Evolutionarily fit pathogens, which are able to survive, replicate, and spread effectively within the host, have the most likely chance

[1]Department of Microbiology and Immunology, F. Edward Hébert School of Medicine, Uniformed Services University of the Health Sciences, Bethesda, MD 20814.

Virulence Mechanisms of Bacterial Pathogens, 5th edition
Edited by Indira T. Kudva, Nancy A. Cornick, Paul J. Plummer, Qijing Zhang, Tracy L. Nicholson, John P. Bannantine, and Bryan H. Bellaire
© 2016 American Society for Microbiology, Washington, DC
doi:10.1128/microbiolspec.VMBF-0017-2015

of passing their genes on to the next generation. Similarly, host genotypes are more likely to persist within the population if those particular individuals are more capable of controlling or resisting infection. Evolution, therefore, is driven by positive directional selection in the arms race model; eventually, the most beneficial alleles will become fixed in a population. Another model favors frequency-dependent (balancing) selection, a process that maintains rare alleles and therefore preserves polymorphic diversity within a population (3). Simply put, allele fixation is prevented in certain instances because different bacterial alleles confer distinct advantages to the pathogen in the presence of different host alleles (i.e., different environments). Supporting evidence for both directional and frequency-dependent selection can be found within nature, and both types probably occur in bacterial populations.

In this chapter, we explore the host-pathogen interface and offer examples of pathogen adaptation in response to common host selective pressures (Table 1). Although we will focus exclusively on bacterial pathogens within the human host, many of the concepts discussed in this review are readily applicable to other organisms, such as viruses, parasites, and fungi, which can infect a wide range of hosts including plants, animals, and amoeba (4–6).

As a final note, much of the evidence presented here to support presumed evolutionary events is either speculation based on what is currently known or suspected about host and microbial biology or is the result of artificial laboratory-induced evolution during serial passaging of bacterial strains. Due to the sheer enormity of evolutionary timescales, defining the precise origins of and factors driving natural evolutionary events is often a difficult undertaking.

ANTAGONISTIC PLEIOTROPY AND THE FITNESS COST-BENEFIT ANALYSIS

At the most basic level, the theory of natural selection stipulates that within a bacterial population, beneficial traits will be conserved (selected for) and deleterious traits eventually discarded (selected against). The actual evolutionary process is considerably more complex, however, due to the existence of genetic drift (the change in genetic diversity of a population due to random chance) and antagonistic pleiotropy.

Antagonistic pleiotropy is the concept that a single gene may control more than one phenotype, some of which may be beneficial to the organism and some deleterious (7). Therefore, a gene may confer a selective advantage within one particular environment, but its expression could be detrimental within a different environment. Conservation of this gene ultimately is determined by the overall necessity of the gene to the organism's fitness and the timing of selection. Bacterial pathogens may evolve mechanisms to neutralize the deleterious effects arising

TABLE 1 Examples of pathogenic mechanisms to evade or overcome selective pressures within the human host

Selective pressures	Pathogenic mechanisms to evade or overcome these pressures
Physical barriers in host (i.e., mucosal epithelium)	Mucinases Enterotoxins Exfoliative toxins Transcytosis through M cells
Host complement	Complement inhibitor protein C3 protease
Sequestration of host resources (e.g., iron)	Enterobactin/aerobactin systems
Host B and T cell lymphocytes	Cytotoxins T3SS-mediated apoptosis
Antibiotics, antimicrobial peptides	Efflux pumps Mutations in antimicrobial targets Enzymes to inactivate antibiotics (e.g., beta-lactamases)
Bacterial colicins	Colicin immunity proteins
Bacterial T6SSs	T6S immunity proteins

from antagonistic pleiotropy, while at the same time conserving the beneficial ones. Temporal regulation is a powerful tool to ensure that specific genes are only turned on when required and are turned off to prevent detrimental expression within a particular environment. Certain outer membrane proteins or systems are temporally regulated within the host, because they may provide a marker for recognition by the host immune system. Flagellar expression, for example, is downregulated by *Salmonella enterica* serovar Typhi *in vivo* to prevent activation of the host inflammatory response; however, outside the host, motility is likely important for the bacterium to seek out and scavenge nutrients from the environment (8).

Other bacteria avoid the deleterious effects of a gene through gene inactivation; mutants that lose functionality of the gene once it becomes deleterious can out-compete the wild-type parent strain, and eventually these mutants will dominate the population. *Pseudomonas aeruginosa*, an opportunistic pathogen of cystic fibrosis patients, often switches to a mucoid phenotype *in vivo* as a result of overproduction of the exopolysaccharide alginate, which allows for the production of a bacterial biofilm in the lung (9, 10). MucA is a *P. aeruginosa* transmembrane protein that binds to and represses the sigma factor AlgU, which acts as the transcriptional activator of the alginate synthesis operon. AlgU activates AlgR, a suppressor of type III secretion system (T3SS) expression; when *mucA* is expressed, therefore, so are the T3SS genes. During acute infection, the T3SS plays an essential role in establishment of the bacterium within the respiratory tract. Once infection has been established, however, chronic infection appears to favor loss of T3SS and a switch to biofilm production (11). Both of these phenotypes are at least partially driven by various mutations in *mucA* which lead to derepression of AlgU, subsequent production of alginate, and suppression of the T3SS (9). Hauser speculates that loss of the T3SS protects the bacterium from eventual recognition

by the host, because patients infected with *P. aeruginosa* develop antibodies against T3SS effector proteins; conversely, biofilm production likely allows for the persistence of the organism in the respiratory tract (11).

Finally, certain bacteria simply tolerate deleterious fitness costs if the benefits of expressing the gene outweigh the negative effects. Antibiotic-resistance mutations that allow bacteria to survive exposure to antimicrobials often come with a significant fitness disadvantage, for example, and secondary compensatory mutations in these strains may eventually arise to restore fitness rather than lose resistance (12).

THE IMPACT OF HOST-PATHOGEN INTERACTIONS ON MICROBIAL EVOLUTION

Inside the host, a successful pathogen will pilfer resources to survive, replicate, and eventually escape; concomitantly, the host will attempt to recognize and subsequently rid the body of the intruder. Coevolution between host and pathogen naturally occurs as a result of these interactions (13). For practical purposes, we restrict our discussion to bacterial adaptation within the human host, but it is important to recognize that many of these concepts are applicable to pathogens of other hosts as well, such as plants and amoeba (14–16). As novel genetic variants within the human population emerge which prove more successful at preventing or overcoming infection, only pathogen variants that allow the bacteria to surmount or avoid this new response will be successful. Within the last century, these natural host defenses, which take much longer to evolve than their microbial counterparts, have been supplemented by man-made developments, such as antibiotics and modern medical interventions, which place added pressures on microbes to adapt (17). Host innate and adaptive immune responses and modern medical interventions are all selective pressures that contribute to pathogen evolution within the human host. Furthermore, microbial competition, against either other pathogens or commensal bacteria, also shapes pathogen genomes.

Bacteria have several advantages over the human host when it comes to evolution: first, their generation times are significantly shorter, leading to more rapid selection within a population. In conjunction with a shorter generation time, bacterial populations are typically larger, which may allow for greater genetic diversity from which to select. Lastly, many bacteria utilize horizontal gene transfer (HGT), which accounts for the rapid spread of advantageous alleles between strains or even species (18). Virulence genes are commonly located on transferred pathogenicity islands (PAIs), which are segments of the genome associated with mobility elements, such as integrase genes or transposons. PAIs can often be distinguished from the remainder of the genome by a disparate G+C content (19).

Host Selective Pressures: The Innate and Adaptive Immune Systems

The innate immune system is one of the first challenges encountered by the incoming pathogen following host contact. These diverse host defenses include physical barriers such as the mucosal epithelium, activation of the complement cascade, circulating antimicrobial peptides and cytokines, leukocytes, activation of the adaptive immune system, and sequestration of host nutrients away from pathogenic bacteria. In addition to effective evasion of innate immune mechanisms, bacteria must also prevent or avoid adaptive immune responses, which include B cell antibody production and T cell–mediated cytotoxicity. Pathogenic bacteria have evolved different approaches to overcome these host defenses.

In the human colon alone, intestinal microbiota concentrations average 10^{11} microorganisms per gram gut content, while 3×10^{8}

prokaryotes are thought to colonize the entire skin surface of the human adult (20). Consequently, bacteria that exploit more hostile and less frequently occupied niches may gain a selective edge in survival by avoiding sites of high competition. Natural structural barriers, however, typically prevent pathogens from engaging deeper host tissues. Physical blocks to infection include the intestinal and respiratory mucosa, the blood-brain barrier, the blood–cerebral spinal fluid barrier, and the placental barrier (21). Most of these structures consist of a single layer of epithelial or endothelial cells bound closely together by tight junctions, adherens junctions, and desmosomes, which preclude bacteria from passively crossing (21, 22). Gastric and respiratory epithelia support an additional protective coating of mucus, which consists primarily of mucin glycoproteins and antimicrobial molecules (23). Mucin glycoproteins, produced by epithelial goblet cells and submucosal glands, can either remain cell-associated or undergo secretion into the mucosa, where they contribute to the viscous layer of mucus that can effectively trap microbes (24). Additionally, nonspecific antimicrobials, such as defensins and lysozymes, and specific antimicrobials, such as IgG and secretory IgA, also limit the growth of microbes within the mucosa (23). Bacterial pathogens have developed numerous mechanisms to counteract these defenses.

The mucosal barrier can be broken down by mucinases such as the Pic enzyme of *Shigella* and enteroaggregative *Escherichia coli* (EAEC) (25, 26). The *pic* gene is located on a chromosomal pathogenicity island in *Shigella* and flanked by insertion-like elements in EAEC, indicating a history of horizontal gene transfer in these pathogens (26). This potential gene transfer is intriguing because mucin degradation is also important for certain gastrointestinal commensals, which metabolize mucin glycoproteins for energy (27). It is tempting to speculate that these enzymes first evolved within human commensal bacteria as a means of nutrient acquisition and only later spread to emerging pathogens to confer passage through the mucosal surface. Such a concept would support the hypothesis proposed by Rasko et al., who suggest that commensal *E. coli* acts as a "genetic sink" for pathogenic *E. coli* isolates (28). Other pathogens, such as *Yersinia enterocolitica* and *Vibrio cholerae*, avoid the thickest layers of the mucosal layer by targeting microfold cells within the small intestine for uptake (23, 29). These specialized epithelial cells sample microorganisms residing in the intestinal lumen and present them to immune cells in the underlying lymphoid tissue. Microfold cells are situated in the region of the epithelium known as the dome, which lacks mucin-secreting goblet cells (23).

Next, to breach the epithelial/endothelial barrier, pathogens must either actively cross using microbial-mediated processes or opportunistically cross following disruption of barrier integrity. Some pathogens, such as *Bacteroides fragilis* and *Staphylococcus aureus*, directly break cell-cell junctions (30, 31). *B. fragilis*, an opportunistic pathogen, encodes a zinc-dependent metalloprotease toxin, BFT (*B. fragilis* enterotoxin), which cleaves the extracellular domain of E-cadherin, a host zonula adherens protein (30). Like the *pic* genes of *Shigella* and EAEC, the *bft* gene is carried on a PAI present in all enterotoxigenic *B. fragilis* strains (32). *S. aureus* induces bullous impetigo and staphylococcal scalded skin syndrome through the actions of three exfoliative toxins (ETs): ETA, ETB, and ETD (31). The ETs act as serine proteases which cleave human desmoglein 1, a transmembrane protein of desmosomes. The genes encoding these toxins are carried on different mobile genetic elements: the ETA gene is carried by a family of Sa1int phages; the ETB gene is plasmid-encoded; and the ETD gene localizes to a 9-kB PAI (33, 34). Other pathogens, such as *Shigella*, *Salmonella*, and *Listeria*, transcytose through microfold cells in the gut to gain access to the basolateral surface of the intestinal epithelium (35). Because these specialized host cells overlay Peyer's patches

(or gut-associated lymphoid tissue), enteric bacteria transcytosed through microfold cells must then contend with macrophages, T lymphocytes, B lymphocytes, and dendritic cells.

As a putative example of counterevolution, the human host may have developed mechanisms to avoid bacterial-mediated adhesion processes. *Helicobacter pylori* binds to the adhesion decoy Muc1, a mucin expressed on the surface of epithelial cells in the gastrointestinal tract (36). Muc1 is subsequently shed from the epithelial surface along with coupled bacteria, precluding long-term adhesion. Consequently, wild type mice have a 5-fold lower *H. pylori* colonization burden than *Muc1*$^{-/-}$ mice. Furthermore, human epidemiological studies have linked shorter Muc1 alleles to a higher probability of chronic gastritis progression, indicating that longer Muc1 alleles may confer a protective advantage to the host (37). Polymorphisms between human Muc1 alleles are largely restricted to the extracellular domain, which consists of a region of 30 to 90 tandem repeat units rich in serine and threonine. A study by Costa et al., demonstrated a significant positive association between the number of Muc1 tandem repeats and bacterial adherence for two strains of *H. pylori in vitro* (38). Longer Muc1 alleles probably evolved from shorter alleles via duplication events and may have emerged to protect against pathogens such as *H. pylori* (39).

Complement cascade activation via the classical, lectin, and alternative pathways precedes the cleavage of C3 convertase into C3a, an anaphylatoxin, and C3b, which binds to the surface of microbes (otherwise known as opsonization) to promote the eventual clearance of bacteria through phagocytosis. Additionally, C3 convertase may convert to the lytic C5 convertase through addition of a C3b molecule. Pathogens have evolved mechanisms to evade or block these processes (40). The *S. aureus* staphylococcal complement inhibitor protein stabilizes C3 convertase, preventing its cleavage into the active C3a and

C3b fragments and attenuating anaphylatoxin activity and bacterial opsonization (41). Like many of the previously described pathogenicity factors, the gene encoding staphylococcal complement inhibitor (*scn*) is located on a PAI (42). Rather than preventing C3 cleavage, the *Neisseria meningitidis* serine protease NalP splits C3 at a unique site, generating shorter C3a-like and longer C3b-like fragments (43). The C3b-like fragments are capable of binding *N. meningitidis* but are rapidly degraded by host complement factors H (fH) and I (fI). Although the activity of the C3a-like fragment has not been determined, this fragment lacks the conserved C-terminal arginine residue found in wild type C3a that is essential for activity, and therefore this truncated version is likely inactive.

A final example of an innate host selective pressure is the sequestration of host resources or nutrients away from colonizing bacteria. Iron, an essential nutrient, is in short supply within the host, either sequestered away in host cells or stored as a complex in hemoglobin, which is inaccessible to most microbes (44). Correspondingly, pathogens have been forced to develop numerous mechanisms to scavenge host iron. Predictably, these systems are often iron-regulated, and their genes are expressed following bacterial exposure to the low-iron environment of the human host. Certain surface-bound receptors can recognize iron-bound complexes, such as heme, transferrin, or lactoferrin. Additionally, secreted bacterial siderophores (aerobactin and enterobactin) steal iron away from host transferrin and lactoferrin. *E. coli* strains can encode for both of these systems (45). Another putative example of arms race coevolution is the mammalian neutrophil gelatinase-associated lipoprotein (NGAL). NGAL directly binds the catecholate-type ferric siderophore complexed to iron, preventing bacterial iron sequestration and eventually exerting a bacteriostatic effect upon microbial populations (46). Some bacteria can even bypass this defense mechanism, however.

Uropathogenic *E. coli* strains express the siderophore salmochelin, a glycosylated form of enterobactin resistant to the effects of NGAL (47).

Finally, if a pathogen manages to evade the innate immune system and can successfully compete with commensal bacteria, it must then elude host adaptive immune responses, including B- and T-cell lymphocytes (48). One bacterial strategy employed in this evasion process inhibits lymphocyte proliferation. The VacA cytotoxin of *H. pylori* blocks the activity of host calcineurin, leading to downstream attenuation of interleukin-2 (IL-2) transcription, a key mediator of T cell proliferation (49). Alternatively, bacteria can avoid the adaptive immune response altogether by mediating lymphocyte cell death. For example, *Shigella* induces B-cell apoptosis through the actions of its T3SS (50).

Host Selective Pressures: Antibiotic Resistance

The rise of adaptive antibiotic resistance in bacteria is perhaps one of the most intensely studied examples of pathogen evolution in response to a specific selective pressure(s) (51). Blair et al. separated adaptive resistance mechanisms into three primary categories: reduced drug permeability through alterations in the bacterial membrane or the development of efflux pumps that quickly expel antimicrobials; prevention of binding through mutation of antimicrobial targets; and the direct inactivation of antimicrobial agents by specific enzymes (51). Well-characterized efflux pumps include the multidrug exporters discovered in the common food-borne pathogens *E. coli* (ArcAB-TolC), *S. enterica* (EmrAB), and *S. aureus* (QacA/B, NorA) (52). Linezolid, an oxazolidinone class antibiotic, binds the 23S rRNA subunit and blocks tRNA interactions with the A site to prevent peptide bond formation (53). Unsurprisingly, linezolid resistance in a number of bacterial species has been linked to a G2576T mutation in the 23S rRNA gene, precluding linezolid binding at this site and providing an example of Blair's second category of adaptive drug resistance (54, 55). Finally, inactivating enzymes such as beta-lactamases, aminoglycoside acyltransferases, and monooxygenases are responsible for the hydrolysis, group transfer, or oxidation of their respective antibiotics (56, 57).

The rapid spread of antimicrobial resistance, and the rise of multidrug resistance, is often linked to the HGT dissemination of genes encoding these enzymes, because many PAIs and plasmids have been shown to carry one or more drug-resistance genes (58). Resistance adaptations often come with a fitness cost, however, which has been demonstrated both *in vivo* and *in vitro* (59).

Microbial Competition

Competition between microbes undoubtedly plays a role in driving pathogen evolution, although this aspect of microbial evolution has not been widely studied and, except for a few examples, is still only very poorly understood. Bacteria can directly eliminate potential rivals through use of toxic peptides (bacteriocins) or through the utilization of type six secretion systems (T6SSs) (60, 61).

Bacteriocins are toxic peptides produced by bacteria that can target and kill neighboring microbes. Colicins, the most well-known members of this category, are produced by strains of *E. coli*, although bacteriocins have been described in a wide variety of bacteria, including *S. aureus*, *Pseudomonas pyogenes*, *Yersinia pestis*, and *Serratia marcescens* (61, 62). In *E. coli*, colicins exhibit a number of different modes of action. Pore-forming colicins, such as colicin A, can insert into the inner membranes of susceptible bacteria to create ion channels (63). Nuclease colicins, such as colicins E9 and E3, translocate across the outer and inner membranes of a susceptible bacterium to the cytoplasm, where they function as DNases (E9) or RNases (E3)

(64, 65). Lastly, colicin M, a unique member of the colicin family, blocks peptidoglycan biosynthesis by degrading undecaprenyl phosphate-linked peptidoglycan precursors. These lipid-anchored intermediates are critical for the transport of peptidoglycan subunits across the cytoplasmic membrane (66, 67). To protect their own population against the harmful effects of these toxic peptides, the producers of colicins must concomitantly express immunity proteins, which block the action of their respective colicins. Immunity proteins of pore-forming colicins sit in the inner membrane and block colicin insertion. Nuclease colicin immunity proteins bind to DNase or RNase colicins to prevent their enzymatic activity, and the immunity protein Cmi binds colicin M to render it catalytically inactive (61, 68). Competing bacteria can acquire these immunity proteins via HGT, providing protection against *E. coli* colicin toxicity. For example, *Shigella*, which does not produce the pore-forming colicin V, nevertheless encodes an immunity protein on its SHI-2 PAI, which protects against colicin V produced by strains of *E. coli* (69, 70).

The recently discovered T6SSs of Gram-negative bacteria are responsible for the direct delivery of effector proteins into neighboring eukaryotic or bacterial cells, resulting in the death of host cells or the lysis of potential microbial competitors (71). VgrG1, an ADP-ribosyltransferase, is secreted from the *Aeromonas hydrophila* T6SS into host cells, where it disrupts the actin cytoskeleton and induces host cell apoptosis (72). Most of the described T6SS effectors, however, have been shown to target other microbes. The T6SS-exported proteins 1 and 3 (Tse1 and Tse3) of *P. aeruginosa* exhibit amidase and muramidase activity, respectively, against bacterial peptidoglycan (73). *P. aeruginosa* also encodes type VI lipase effector (Tle) proteins, which degrade the bacterial phospholipid phosphatidylethanolamine (74). In *Dickeya dadantii*, the Rhs (rearrangement hotspots) proteins RhsA and RhsB are secreted through the T6SS and function as toxic endonucleases in susceptible bacteria. While *D. dadantii* is a plant pathogen, the human pathogen *S. marcescens* also expresses a T6SS-secreted Rhs-family protein, although its function is unknown (75, 76). Similar to the colicin proteins, pathogens which encode a T6SS must also express immunity proteins to prevent self-killing. *P. aeruginosa* encodes T6SS immunity 1 and 3 (Tsi1 and Tsi3) proteins, which interact with and inactivate Tse1 and Tse3 through mechanisms that are not yet understood (73).

Intriguingly, T6SSs may also be effective tools for gene acquisition via HGT. In *V. cholerae*, the T6SS is coregulated with competence genes by the regulator TfoX, and transformation events are dependent upon the presence of an active T6SS (77). Borgeaud et al., suggest that following activation of TfoX, both competence and T6SS systems are expressed and assembled. After T6SS-mediated lysis of neighboring cells, DNA is released to the extracellular space, where it can then transform the competent bacterium (77).

CONCLUDING REMARKS

Bacterial pathogens within the human host are exposed to a vast variety of selective pressures which shape bacterial genomes and drive the evolution of novel virulence factors. Concomitantly, human genomes also evolve as a result of these interactions, leading to a genetic arms race between pathogens and their hosts. In bacteria, HGT can enhance this process by allowing for the rapid dissemination of potentially beneficial alleles across strains or even species.

ACKNOWLEDGMENTS

This work was supported by National Institutes of Health grants RO1 AI024656-23 and RO1 AI044033-12.

CITATION

Bliven KA, Maurelli AT. 2016. Evolution of bacterial pathogens within the human host. Microbiol Spectrum 4(1):VMBF-0017-2015.

REFERENCES

1. **Toft C, Andersson SG.** 2010. Evolutionary microbial genomics: insights into bacterial host adaptation. *Nat Rev Genet* **11:**465–475.
2. **Dawkins R, Krebs JR.** 1979. Arms races between and within species. *Proc R Soc London B Biol Sci* **205:**489–511.
3. **Woolhouse ME, Webster JP, Domingo E, Charlesworth B, Levin BR.** 2002. Biological and biomedical implications of the coevolution of pathogens and their hosts. *Nat Genet* **32:**569–577.
4. **Taubenberger JK, Kash JC.** 2010. Influenza virus evolution, host adaptation, and pandemic formation. *Cell Host Microbe* **7:**440–551.
5. **Mideo N.** 2009. Parasite adaptations to within-host competition. *Trends Parasitol* **25:**261–268.
6. **Cooney NM, Klein BS.** 2008. Fungal adaptation to the mammalian host: it is a new world, after all. *Curr Opin Microbiol* **11:**511–516.
7. **Williams GC.** 1957. Pleiotropy, natural selection, and the evolution of senescence. *Evolution* **11:**398–411.
8. **Salazar-Gonzalez RM, Srinivasan A, Griffin A, Muralimohan G, Ertelt JM, Ravindran R, Vella AT, McSorley SJ.** 2007. *Salmonella* flagellin induces bystander activation of splenic dendritic cells and hinders bacterial replication *in vivo. J Immunol* **179:**6169–6175.
9. **Wu W, Badrane H, Arora S, Baker HV, Jin S.** 2004. MucA-mediated coordination of type III secretion and alginate synthesis in *Pseudomonas aeruginosa. J Bacteriol* **186:**7575–7585.
10. **Boucher JC, Yu H, Mudd MH, Deretic V.** 1997. Mucoid *Pseudomonas aeruginosa* in cystic fibrosis: characterization of *muc* mutations in clinical isolates and analysis of clearance in a mouse model of respiratory infection. *Infect Immun* **65:**3838–3846.
11. **Hauser AR.** 2009. The type III secretion system of *Pseudomonas aeruginosa*: infection by injection. *Nat Rev Microbiol* **7:**654–665.
12. **Schulz zur Wiesch P, Engelstadter J, Bonhoeffer S.** 2010. Compensation of fitness costs and reversibility of antibiotic resistance mutations. *Antimicrob Agents Chemother* **54:**2085–2095.
13. **Morgan AD, Koskella B.** 2011. Coevolution of host and pathogen, p 147–171. *In* Tibayreng M

(ed), *Genetics and Evolution of Infectious Diseases*. Elsevier, Burlington, MA.

14. **Langridge GC, Fookes M, Connor TR, Feltwell T, Feasey N, Parsons BN, Seth-Smith HM, Barquist L, Stedman A, Humphrey T, Wigley P, Peters SE, Maskell DJ, Corander J, Chabalgoity JA, Barrow P, Parkhill J, Dougan G, Thomson NR.** 2015. Patterns of genome evolution that have accompanied host adaptation in *Salmonella*. *Proc Natl Acad Sci USA* **112:** 863–868.

15. **Kemen AC, Agler MT, Kemen E.** 2015. Host-microbe and microbe-microbe interactions in the evolution of obligate plant parasitism. *New Phytol* **206:**1207–1228.

16. **Price CT, Richards AM, Von Dwingelo JE, Samara HA, Abu Kwaik Y.** 2014. Amoeba host-*Legionella* synchronization of amino acid auxotrophy and its role in bacterial adaptation and pathogenic evolution. *Environ Microbiol* **16:**350–358.

17. **Davies J, Davies D.** 2010. Origins and evolution of antibiotic resistance. *Microbiol Mol Biol Rev* **74:**417–433.

18. **Wiedenbeck J, Cohan FM.** 2011. Origins of bacterial diversity through horizontal genetic transfer and adaptation to new ecological niches. *FEMS Microbiol Rev* **35:**957–976.

19. **Houchhut B, Dobrindt U, Hacker J.** 2006. The contribution of pathogenicity islands to the evolution of bacterial pathogens, p 83–107. *In* Seifert HS, DiRita V (ed), *The Evolution of Microbial Pathogens*. ASM Press, Washington, DC.

20. **Whitman WB, Coleman DC, Wiebe WJ.** 1998. Prokaryotes: the unseen majority. *Proc Natl Acad Sci USA* **95:**6578–6583.

21. **Doran KS, Banerjee A, Disson O, Lecuit M.** 2013. Concepts and mechanisms: crossing host barriers. *Cold Spring Harbor Perspect Med* **3:** a010090. doi:10.1101/cshperspect.a010090

22. **Tsukita S, Yamazaki Y, Katsuno T, Tamura A, Tsukita S.** 2008. Tight junction-based epithelial microenvironment and cell proliferation. *Oncogene* **27:**6930–6938.

23. **McGuckin MA, Linden SK, Sutton P, Florin TH.** 2011. Mucin dynamics and enteric pathogens. *Nat Rev Microbiol* **9:**265–278.

24. **Linden SK, Sutton P, Karlsson NG, Korolik V, McGuckin MA.** 2008. Mucins in the mucosal barrier to infection. *Mucosal Immunol* **1:**183–197.

25. **Gutierrez-Jimenez J, Arciniega I, Navarro-Garcia F.** 2008. The serine protease motif of Pic mediates a dose-dependent mucolytic activity after binding to sugar constituents of the mucin substrate. *Microb Pathog* **45:**115–123.

26. **Henderson IR, Czeczulin J, Eslava C, Noriega F, Nataro JP.** 1999. Characterization of *pic*, a secreted protease of *Shigella flexneri* and enteroaggregative *Escherichia coli*. *Infect Immun* **67:**5587–5596.

27. **Sonnenburg JL, Xu J, Leip DD, Chen CH, Westover BP, Weatherford J, Buhler JD, Gordon JI.** 2005. Glycan foraging *in vivo* by an intestine-adapted bacterial symbiont. *Science* **307:**1955–1959.

28. **Rasko DA, Rosovitz MJ, Myers GS, Mongodin EF, Fricke WF, Gajer P, Crabtree J, Sebaihia M, Thomson NR, Chaudhuri R, Henderson IR, Sperandio V, Ravel J.** 2008. The pangenome structure of *Escherichia coli*: comparative genomic analysis of *E. coli* commensal and pathogenic isolates. *J Bacteriol* **190:**6881–6893.

29. **Jones B, Pascopella L, Falkow S.** 1995. Entry of microbes into the host: using M cells to break the mucosal barrier. *Curr Opin Immunol* **7:**474–478.

30. **Wu S, Lim KC, Huang J, Saidi RF, Sears CL.** 1998. *Bacteroides fragilis* enterotoxin cleaves the zonula adherens protein, E-cadherin. *Proc Natl Acad Sci USA* **95:**14979–14984.

31. **Hanakawa Y, Schechter NM, Lin C, Garza L, Li H, Yamaguchi T, Fudaba Y, Nishifuji K, Sugai M, Amagai M, Stanley JR.** 2002. Molecular mechanisms of blister formation in bullous impetigo and staphylococcal scalded skin syndrome. *J Clin Invest* **110:**53–60.

32. **Franco AA, Cheng RK, Chung GT, Wu S, Oh HB, Sears CL.** 1999. Molecular evolution of the pathogenicity island of enterotoxigenic *Bacteroides fragilis* strains. *J Bacteriol* **181:** 6623–6633.

33. **Yamaguchi T, Nishifuji K, Sasaki M, Fudaba Y, Aepfelbacher M, Takata T, Ohara M, Komatsuzawa H, Amagai M, Sugai M.** 2002. Identification of the *Staphylococcus aureus etd* pathogenicity island which encodes a novel exfoliative toxin, ETD, and EDIN-B. *Infect Immun* **70:**5835–5845.

34. **Jackson MP, Iandolo JJ.** 1986. Cloning and expression of the exfoliative toxin B gene from *Staphylococcus aureus*. *J Bacteriol* **166:**574–580.

35. **Jensen VB, Harty JT, Jones BD.** Interactions of the invasive pathogens *Salmonella typhimurium*, *Listeria monocytogenes*, and *Shigella flexneri* with M cells and murine Peyer's patches. *Infect Immun* **66:**3758–3766.

36. **McGuckin MA, Every AL, Skene CD, Linden SK, Chionh YT, Swierczak A, McAuley J, Harbour S, Kaparakis M, Ferrero R, Sutton P.** 2007. Muc1 mucin limits both *Helicobacter*

pylori colonization of the murine gastric mucosa and associated gastritis. *Gastroenterology* **133:**1210–1218.

37. **Vinall LE, King M, Novelli M, Green CA, Daniels G, Hilkens J, Sarner M, Swallow DM.** 2002. Altered expression and allelic association of the hypervariable membrane mucin MUC1 in *Helicobacter pylori* gastritis. *Gastroenterology* **123:**41–49.

38. **Costa NR, Mendes N, Marcos NT, Reis CA, Caffrey T, Hollingsworth MA, Santos-Silva F.** 2008. Relevance of MUC1 mucin variable number of tandem repeats polymorphism in *H pylori* adhesion to gastric epithelial cells. *World J Gastroenterol* **14:**1411–1414.

39. **Vos HL, de Vries Y, Hilkens J.** 1991. The mouse episialin (Muc1) gene and its promoter: rapid evolution of the repetitive domain in the protein. *Biochem Biophys Res Commun* **181:** 121–130.

40. **Lambris JD, Ricklin D, Geisbrecht BV.** 2008. Complement evasion by human pathogens. *Nat Rev Microbiol* **6:**132–142.

41. **Rooijakkers SH, Ruyken M, Roos A, Daha MR, Presanis JS, Sim RB, van Wamel WJ, van Kessel KP, van Strijp JA.** 2005. Immune evasion by a staphylococcal complement inhibitor that acts on C3 convertases. *Nature Immunol* **6:**920–927.

42. **Rooijakkers SH, van Wamel WJ, Ruyken M, van Kessel KP, van Strijp JA.** 2005. Antiopsonic properties of staphylokinase. *Microbes Infect* **7:**476–484.

43. **Del Tordello E, Vacca I, Ram S, Rappuoli R, Serruto D.** 2014. *Neisseria meningitidis* NalP cleaves human complement C3, facilitating degradation of C3b and survival in human serum. *Proc Natl Acad Sci USA* **111:**427–432.

44. **Skaar EP.** 2010. The battle for iron between bacterial pathogens and their vertebrate hosts. *PLoS Pathog* **6:**e1000949.

45. **Rogers HJ.** 1973. Iron-binding catechols and virulence in *Escherichia coli*. *Infect Immun* **7:**445–456.

46. **Goetz DH, Holmes MA, Borregaard N, Bluhm ME, Raymond KN, Strong RK.** 2002. The neutrophil lipocalin NGAL is a bacteriostatic agent that interferes with siderophore-mediated iron acquisition. *Mol Cell* **10:** 1033–1043.

47. **Fischbach MA, Lin H, Zhou L, Yu Y, Abergel RJ, Liu DR, Raymond KN, Wanner BL, Strong RK, Walsh CT, Aderem A, Smith KD.** 2006. The pathogen-associated *iroA* gene cluster mediates bacterial evasion of lipocalin 2. *Proc Natl Acad Sci USA* **103:** 16502–16507.

48. **Hornef MW, Wick MJ, Rhen M, Normark S.** 2002. Bacterial strategies for overcoming host innate and adaptive immune responses. *Nat Immunol.* **3:**1033–1040.

49. **Gebert B, Fischer W, Weiss E, Hoffmann R, Haas R.** 2003. *Helicobacter pylori* vacuolating cytotoxin inhibits T lymphocyte activation. *Science* **301:**1099–1102.

50. **Nothelfer K, Arena ET, Pinaud L, Neunlist M, Mozeleski B, Belotserkovsky I, Parsot C, Dinadayala P, Burger-Kentischer A, Raqib R, Sansonetti PJ, Phalipon A.** 2014. B lymphocytes undergo TLR2-dependent apoptosis upon *Shigella* infection. *J Exp Med* **211:**1215–1229.

51. **Blair JM, Webber MA, Baylay AJ, Ogbolu DO, Piddock LJ.** 2015. Molecular mechanisms of antibiotic resistance. *Nat Rev Microbiol* **13:**42–51.

52. **Andersen JL, He GX, Kakarla P, K CR, Kumar S, Lakra WS, Mukherjee MM, Ranaweera I, Shrestha U, Tran T, Varela MF.** 2015. Multidrug efflux pumps from *Enterobacteriaceae*, *Vibrio cholerae* and *Staphylococcus aureus* bacterial food pathogens. *Int J Environ Res Public Health* **12:**1487–1547.

53. **Wilson DN, Schluenzen F, Harms JM, Starosta AL, Connell SR, Fucini P.** 2008. The oxazolidinone antibiotics perturb the ribosomal peptidyl-transferase center and effect tRNA positioning. *Proc Natl Acad Sci USA* **105:**13339–13344.

54. **Feng J, Lupien A, Gingras H, Wasserscheid J, Dewar K, Legare D, Ouellette M.** 2009. Genome sequencing of linezolid-resistant *Streptococcus pneumoniae* mutants reveals novel mechanisms of resistance. *Genome Res* **19:**1214–1223.

55. **Meka VG, Gold HS.** 2004. Antimicrobial resistance to linezolid. *Clin Infect Dis* **39:** 1010–1015.

56. **Frere JM.** 1995. Beta-lactamases and bacterial resistance to antibiotics. *Mol Microbiol* **16:** 385–395.

57. **Wright GD.** 2005. Bacterial resistance to antibiotics: enzymatic degradation and modification. *Adv Drug Deliv Rev* **57:**1451–1470.

58. **Ochman H, Lawrence JG, Groisman EA.** 2000. Lateral gene transfer and the nature of bacterial innovation. *Nature* **405:**299–304.

59. **Andersson DI, Hughes D.** 2010. Antibiotic resistance and its cost: is it possible to reverse resistance? *Nat Rev Microbiol* **8:**260–271.

60. **Pukatzki S, Ma AT, Sturtevant D, Krastins B, Sarracino D, Nelson WC, Heidelberg JF, Mekalanos JJ.** 2006. Identification of a conserved bacterial protein secretion system in

Vibrio cholerae using the *Dictyostelium* host model system. *Proc Natl Acad Sci USA* **103:** 1528–1533.

61. **Cascales E, Buchanan SK, Duche D, Kleanthous C, Lloubes R, Postle K, Riley M, Slatin S, Cavard D.** 2007. Colicin biology. *Microbiol Mol Biol Rev* **71:**158–229.

62. **Gagliano VJ, Hinsdill RD.** 1970. Characterization of a *Staphylococcus aureus* bacteriocin. *J Bacteriol* **104:**117–125.

63. **Duche D, Parker MW, Gonzalez-Manas JM, Pattus F, Baty D.** 1994. Uncoupled steps of the colicin A pore formation demonstrated by disulfide bond engineering. *J Biol Chem* **269:** 6332–6339.

64. **Vankemmelbeke M, Healy B, Moore GR, Kleanthous C, Penfold CN, James R.** 2005. Rapid detection of colicin E9-induced DNA damage using *Escherichia coli* cells carrying SOS promoter-lux fusions. *J Bacteriol* **187:** 4900–4907.

65. **Boon T.** 1972. Inactivation of ribosomes *in vitro* by colicin E3 and its mechanism of action. *Proc Natl Acad Sci USA* **69:**549–552.

66. **Harkness RE, Braun V.** 1989. Colicin M inhibits peptidoglycan biosynthesis by interfering with lipid carrier recycling. *J Biol Chem* **264:**6177–6182.

67. **El Ghachi M, Bouhss A, Barreteau H, Touze T, Auger G, Blanot D, Mengin-Lecreulx D.** 2006. Colicin M exerts its bacteriolytic effect via enzymatic degradation of undecaprenyl phosphate-linked peptidoglycan precursors. *J Biol Chem* **281:**22761–22772.

68. **Olschlager T, Turba A, Braun V.** 1991. Binding of the immunity protein inactivates colicin M. *Mol Microbiol* **5:**1105–1111.

69. **Moss JE, Cardozo TJ, Zychlinsky A, Groisman EA.** 1999. The *selC*-associated SHI-2 pathogenicity island of *Shigella flexneri*. *Mol Microbiol* **33:**74–83.

70. **Gerard F, Pradel N, Wu LF.** 2005. Bactericidal activity of colicin V is mediated by an inner membrane protein, SdaC, of *Escherichia coli. J Bacteriol* **187:**1945–1950.

71. **Russell AB, Peterson SB, Mougous JD.** 2014. Type VI secretion system effectors: poisons with a purpose. *Nat Rev Microbiol* **12:**137–148.

72. **Suarez G, Sierra JC, Erova TE, Sha J, Horneman AJ, Chopra AK.** 2010. A type VI secretion system effector protein, VgrG1, from *Aeromonas hydrophila* that induces host cell toxicity by ADP ribosylation of actin. *J Bacteriol* **192:**155–168.

73. **Russell AB, Hood RD, Bui NK, LeRoux M, Vollmer W, Mougous JD.** 2011. Type VI secretion delivers bacteriolytic effectors to target cells. *Nature* **475:**343–347.

74. **Russell AB, LeRoux M, Hathazi K, Agnello DM, Ishikawa T, Wiggins PA, Wai SN, Mougous JD.** 2013. Diverse type VI secretion phospholipases are functionally plastic antibacterial effectors. *Nature* **496:**508–512.

75. **Koskiniemi S, Lamoureux JG, Nikolakakis KC, t'Kint de Roodenbeke C, Kaplan MD, Low DA, Hayes CS.** 2013. Rhs proteins from diverse bacteria mediate intercellular competition. *Proc Natl Acad Sci USA* **110:**7032–7037.

76. **Fritsch MJ, Trunk K, Diniz JA, Guo M, Trost M, Coulthurst SJ.** 2013. Proteomic identification of novel secreted antibacterial toxins of the *Serratia marcescens* type VI secretion system. *Mol Cell Proteomics* **12:** 2735–2749.

77. **Borgeaud S, Metzger LC, Scrignari T, Blokesch M.** 2015. The type VI secretion system of *Vibrio cholerae* fosters horizontal gene transfer. *Science* **347:**63–67.

Bacterial Metabolism Shapes the Host–Pathogen Interface

2

KARLA D. PASSALACQUA,[1] MARIE-EVE CHARBONNEAU,[1] and MARY X.D. O'RIORDAN[1]

THE INTERFACE BETWEEN TWO ORGANISMS IS SHAPED BY METABOLIC INTERACTIONS

Why do organisms "eat"? This core question drives the study of biochemistry—specifically metabolism. The short answer to this seemingly simple question is 2-fold: first, eating provides cells with the physical building blocks for the generation of cellular components (i.e., growth of the physical cell; something must come from something); second, eating is the way to extract energy to do cellular work (i.e., powering the process of growth; work is never done for free). These two processes—catabolism and anabolism—are inextricably linked. The pathways of catabolism, such as glycolysis and the tricarboxylic acid (TCA) cycle, which break down molecules for energy metabolism, also branch off into anabolic pathways that generate building blocks for the cell. Bacterial metabolism is dynamic and flexible, with different bacterial species encoding different metabolic capacities within their genomes. Thus, the canonical TCA cycle may function fully in one bacterial species, while another bacterium, missing a key enzyme of the cycle now uses the other TCA enzymes in branched oxidative and reductive pathways. Moreover, depending on the availability of carbon sources or oxygen, even if a bacterium encodes all of the

[1]Department of Microbiology and Immunology, University of Michigan Medical School, Ann Arbor, MI 48109.
Virulence Mechanisms of Bacterial Pathogens, 5th edition
Edited by Indira T. Kudva, Nancy A. Cornick, Paul J. Plummer, Qijing Zhang, Tracy L. Nicholson, John P. Bannantine, and Bryan H. Bellaire
© 2016 American Society for Microbiology, Washington, DC
doi:10.1128/microbiolspec.VMBF-0027-2015

enzymes for respiration, with its high-energy yield, the less energy-efficient but faster process of fermentation may predominate. Thus, the flexible metabolic space of rapidly evolving bacterial genomes enables many different ways for bacteria to take advantage of nutrients in complex environments for robust replication.

The essential infrastructure of metabolism is made more complex during bacterial infection when one organism thrives by drawing nutrients from the other. From a bacterial perspective, the mammalian host is a vast ecosystem, with some regions such as the intestine heavily populated with competitors, while other niches are wide open for exploitation. To appreciate how bacterial metabolism shapes infection, it is important to consider the localized host environment where the bacteria replicate, as well as the metabolic capacity of the pathogen. The host environment is not simply a source of food for bacteria. Rather, host cells are constantly controlling their own metabolic function, using available nutrients and removing waste products. In addition, host organisms actively survey their inner spaces for invading microorganisms. Thus, bacterial pathogens must overcome constant pressure from the predatory immune system of the host. These defining aspects of the host–pathogen interaction are drivers of disease, whether it is acute or chronic, inflammatory or silent, mild or deadly.

In this article, we consider three aspects of metabolism in the host–pathogen interaction: first, how bacteria within a host employ specific modules of central metabolism to generate energy, second, how bacterial pathogens exploit the host for critical nutrients required for proliferation, and lastly, how these bacterial invaders use metabolic tricks to sense their environment and to evade host immunity.

BACTERIAL ENERGY METABOLISM DURING INFECTION

This section focuses primarily on recent research that is revealing how bacterial path-ogens maintain energy metabolism within the host environment; in other words, how do bacterial pathogens uniquely go about the business of eating inside a host to meet their energy demands (1)? First, a brief note on energy: it is worth noting that energy is not a thing but, rather, a potential, and that the energy all cells work to acquire is the energy that "lives" within the chemical bonds of what the cell eats. Ultimately, for cells to do work, chemical bond energy from some food source must be moved to a molecule that can be used directly to fuel cellular tasks—the predominant, but not exclusive, form being adenosine triphosphate (ATP). The idea that phosphate bond energy transfer is the way cells power most cellular work stands as a monumental paradigm shift in the natural sciences (2, 3), ushering in the full elucidation of "central metabolism," the foundational energy yielding pathways for all cellular life. A more intimate way of viewing central metabolism is as the process that best illustrates the close kinship of all cellular life. Glycolysis shows us how we are related to *Escherichia coli*. The TCA cycle unites us with our cousins, the fungi. And no matter what the genetic content, there is a common need for ATP.

Thus, when considering the specific role of energy-yielding metabolism during bacterial infection, it is good to remember that both the pathogen and the infected host are engaging in nonstop, regulated central metabolic activity, often competing for the same resources and usually trying to influence the behavior of the other. Here, we start by exploring how some bacterial pathogens conduct energy metabolism during infection.

What's for Dinner Inside the Host?

Depending on where in the host an invading bacterium takes up residence, the food sources available within that niche will determine whether that microbe can successfully establish itself. Some pathogens, such as invasive streptococci, *Salmonella enterica*, and *Brucella abortus,* can feed their "sweet tooth" during infection by acquiring specific carbohydrates, whereas the "low-carb" pathogen *Mycobacterium tuberculosis* prefers to fuel itself with energy-rich fatty acids during a chronic infection that can last for many decades. Recent research has revealed some unique ways in which pathogens go about feeding themselves during host colonization.

Pathogenic streptococci are a group of Gram-positive bacteria that cause a range of disease from mild (dental caries) to severe (pneumonia and sepsis). These bacteria establish themselves on extracellular surfaces of the host, such as on the tissues of the human naso-pharynx or in dental biofilms. Here, they are positioned to be fed directly by the host as the host feeds him- or herself or to acquire nutrients from the extracellular surfaces of host tissues. *Streptococcus mutans,* a major cause of dental caries, sets itself apart from the resident, nonpathogenic oral microbiota by having a large and flexible metabolic range with regard to nutrient acquisition. As the human diet has changed over time to become richer in carbohydrates (especially sucrose), so has the physiological capability of *S. mutans* evolved (4, 5). A study that compared ancient and modern bacterial communities of dental plaque suggests that pathogenic *S. mutans* has become a more common resident of the human oral cavity as a result of this change in diet, especially in modern, postindustrial times (4). One of the reasons for this coevolutionary success has been the expansion of the *S. mutans* genome to contain a wide range of genes involved in carbohydrate uptake, especially the EII permeases of the phosphoenolpyruvate–sugar phosphotransferase system (PTS), the multi-enzyme pathway of carbohydrate uptake present in most bacteria. Also, the carbohydrate catabolite repression system, which allows bacteria to regulate which carbohydrates to use for energy catabolism by sensing intracellular nutrient content, also appears to be unique in *S. mutans* in that it has more levels of carbohydrate catabolite repression

flexibility than other Gram-positive bacteria (5, 6).

The phosphoenolpyruvate–sugar phosphotransferase and carbohydrate catabolite repression systems also have expanded roles in the more serious and invasive *Streptococcus* pathogens, *Streptococcus pneumoniae* and *Streptococcus pyogenes,* by being involved in controlling levels of virulence gene expression, such as the toxin streptolysin S (7–9). Also, *S. pneumoniae* is able to use a wider range of carbon sources for energy catabolism compared to other Gram-positive organisms (10) and has the ability to obtain and use complex carbohydrates that it is able to remove from host extracellular surfaces with specialized enzymes (11–13). A comprehensive review of streptococcal carbohydrate utilization during pathogenesis can be found elsewhere; these brief examples introduce and highlight the themes that (i) the ability of pathogens to exploit the host niche and obtain preferred food sources for energy catabolism is an important aspect of bacterial virulence, (ii) pathogens often set themselves apart from nonpathogens by having an expanded and flexible capability for obtaining preferred energy sources within the site of infection, and (iii) virulence gene expression is often intimately linked to the pathways of carbon acquisition and energy metabolism.

Focusing in more closely on central metabolism, it is essential to emphasize the key role played by glucose in energy-yielding catabolism. When considering energy metabolism via respiration, where glycolysis and the TCA cycle are both utilized, it is the simple sugar glucose that gives a fast and efficient energy yield in the form of ATP for host and pathogen alike. Thus, these pathways are important for many bacterial pathogens, such as *Salmonella* and *Brucella,* which have evolved to be able to feed their energy-yielding pathways during infection, specifically with glucose "stolen" from the host (Fig. 1).

The pathogenic streptococci previously mentioned reside at the surface of cell tissues

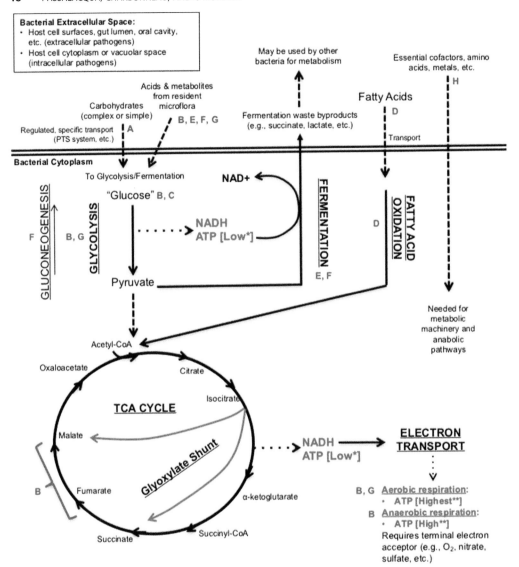

FIGURE 1 A simplified view of catabolic energy-yielding pathways in bacteria and points of relevance for the indicated bacterial pathogens. The figure shows a simplified outline of some of the different pathways for utilizing carbohydrates or fatty acids for the generation of ATP. These catabolic pathways and the anabolic pathways that they feed are under extremely complex levels of control, which have been studied mainly in noninfectious organisms (126). However, the unique metabolic strategies employed by infectious bacteria are becoming more appreciated as important aspects of bacterial pathogenesis (1). *ATP generated by substrate level phosphorylation; **ATP generated by oxidative phosphorylation; solid lines, metabolic pathway; dashed lines, substrates that feed into catabolic pathways and products generated by bacteria as a result of metabolism or required for metabolism; dotted lines, main energy-yielding metabolites generated from pathways. Blue letters indicate specific points of importance for the energy-yielding metabolism of select pathogens listed as follows (see Table 1 for summary): (A) Pathogenic streptococci (*Streptococcus mutans, Streptococcus pyogenes, Streptococcus pneumoniae*); (B) *Salmonella enterica* serovar Typhimurium; (C) *Brucella abortus*; (D) *Mycobacterium tuberculosis*; (E) *Clostridium difficile*; (F) Enterohemorrhagic *Escherichia coli*; (G) *Aggregatibacter actinomycetemcomitans*; (H) *Listeria monocytogenes*.

TABLE 1 **Summary points of energy-yielding metabolism for select pathogenic bacteria**

Label	Bacterium	Points of interest for metabolism during infection	Select references
A	Pathogenic streptococci *Streptococcus mutans* *Streptococcus pyogenes* *Streptococcus pneumoniae*	Extracellular pathogens Relies on simple and complex carbohydrates from host diet or from host cell surfaces Genomes have expanded sugar uptake systems for dietary flexibility Can express enzymes that cleave host glycans for use in energy-yielding metabolism Sugar uptake and control is tightly linked with expression of classic virulence factors	1–13
B	*Salmonella enterica* serovar Typhimurium	Can infect both intracellularly and extracellularly Intracellular infection requires glucose, glycolysis, and the TCA cycle Intracellular bacteria can influence host cell gene expression to favor glucose availability Specific TCA cycle reactions that generate malate are required for intracellular infection Bacteria that establish extracellular infection in the gut can engage in anaerobic respiration using resident metabolites generated by the host during inflammation and by the resident microbiota	14, 15, 19, 23, 44–47
C	*Brucella abortus*	Intracellular pathogen Requires glucose for intracellular infection Passively benefits from host cell metabolism for glucose	21
D	*Mycobacterium tuberculosis*	Intracellular pathogen Utilizes fatty acid oxidation for energy metabolism Associates with lipid bodies in specialized cells where they can acquire fatty acids Glyoxylate cycle required for replenishment of TCA cycle metabolites in the absence of glycolysis	24, 27–29
E	*Clostridium difficile*	Extracellular pathogen and obligate anaerobe Fermentation is main energy-yielding pathway May outcompete the resident microbiota by engaging in succinate to butyrate fermentation after antibiotic treatment by taking advantage of a rise in succinate generated by the gut microbiota	33
F	Enterohemorrhagic *Escherichia coli* (EHEC)	Extracellular pathogen that can form "attaching and effacing" lesions in the host gut May take advantage of colocalization with species of the resident microbiota in the carbohydrate-poor intestinal mucosal layer Metabolites produced by colocalized microbiota may induce shift from glycolysis to gluconeogenesis, increasing virulence gene expression	34–36
G	*Aggregatibacter actinomycetemcomitans*	Extracellular pathogen of the oral cavity Switches to L-lactate catabolism when colocalized with resident microbiota generating L-lactate Catabolic shift may favor bacterial expansion and increased host damage	38
H	*Listeria monocytogenes*	Intracellular pathogen Specifically scavenges the essential cofactor lipoate from host lipoyl-peptides Host-derived lipoate essential for catabolic enzymes	40, 41

where glucose concentration is low (12) but where many other carbohydrates, both simple and complex, are vastly abundant. *S. enterica* and *B. abortus*, on the other hand, are intracellular pathogens and must go about feeding themselves from the inside of host cells where the range and concentration of available carbon sources are very limited. Therefore, rather than evolve an expanded ability to utilize a range of carbohydrates, these bacteria are able to more efficiently steal the fewer carbon sources available to them from within the host cell—primarily, glucose or glucose phosphate. Using a mouse model and a series of bacterial metabolic deletion mutants, it has been shown that *S. enterica* serovar Typhimurium (*S.* Typhimurium) has a major dependence upon glucose, glycolysis, and the TCA cycle both in tissue culture and during infection in mice (14, 15). The *S.* Typhimurium mouse model has been used to elucidate the molecular mechanism of infection for the human pathogen *S. enterica* serovar Typhi, which causes typhoid fever (16, 17). In their intracellular niche within host macrophages (phagocytic cells of the innate immune system), *S.* Typhimurium resides within a *Salmonella*-containing vacuole, where it is protected from host defenses but where it nonetheless is able to obtain the nutrients needed for intracellular replication (18). Bacteria lacking both homologs of phosphofructokinase, a key enzyme unique to the glycolysis pathway, are unable to replicate within macrophage culture and are severely attenuated during infection of BALB/c mice (14), showing a major dependence on this pathway during intracellular infection.

Also in this study, extensive use of 15 different metabolic mutants of *S.* Typhimurium showed that glucose, specifically, is the preferred carbon source within macrophages and in the mouse host (14). Importantly, the key triple knockout strain from this study lacked genes for both glucose uptake (two phosphoenolpyruvate–sugar phosphotransferase systems) and glucose catabolism (glu-

cokinase), resulting in a total glucose catabolic mutant. However, although this strain was highly attenuated in tissue culture and *in vivo*, it was still able to replicate at low levels, suggesting that although glucose is the predominant energy source in this model, there likely exists another, less preferred carbon source available within the host.

At this point, it is important to emphasize how fundamental a role the glycolysis pathway plays within the metabolic infrastructure of the cell. This one central pathway participates in a variety of activities which include (i) providing the molecule pyruvate to the TCA cycle during aerobic or anaerobic respiration, (ii) being a sole anaerobic energy-yielding pathway called "fermentation," which has a lower energy yield than respiration, and (iii) providing most of the enzymes for gluconeogenesis, which is a glucose-generating pathway that is basically glycolysis in reverse. So considering the previous finding that glycolysis and glucose are of primary importance to intracellular *Salmonellae*, one might ask what role the glycolysis pathway serves for the bacterium. Again, using a systematic series of metabolic knockout strains, it has been shown that *S.* Typhimurium requires a fully intact TCA cycle within its host, in this case the BALB/c mouse, for full virulence (15). Just as importantly, this work revealed that certain metabolic pathways, including gluconeogenesis, fatty acid metabolism, and the glyoxylate bypass, are not essential for *S.* Typhimurium during infection (15). More recent refinement of this work has identified the specific steps in the TCA cycle that are the most important for full virulence, including the conversion of fumarate to malate and the conversion of malate to oxaloacetate and pyruvate (19) (Fig. 1).

But what makes this work both complex and confusing is that different metabolic mutants show a range of virulence phenotypes, from totally avirulent to attenuated to fully virulent. This observation along with the wide range of metabolic flexibility and redundancy in bacterial genomes highlights the difficulty of pinpointing the precise modes of metabolism during microbe–host interactions. Regardless, this example illustrates the modularity of metabolic pathways and the presence of key vulnerable chokepoints that may be unique to each organism. In this case, the vulnerability of infectious *S.* Typhimurium for running a complete TCA cycle is its need for malate to generate pyruvate and oxaloacetate to replenish the cycle. Ablating enzymatic steps upstream of the two essential reactions for generating malate results in only slight attenuation, suggesting that the microbe is able to use molecules potentially scavenged from the host to generate the key malate precursor, succinate, outside of those two steps. The authors intriguingly hypothesize that succinate, ornithine, or arginine scavenged from host cells may be used by the bacterium for malate generation; however, this idea needs further investigation.

This last point brings into focus the dynamic tension that exists between host cells and infecting microbes. To complete the discussion of the need for glucose, the following describes pathogens that rely on host cell behavior to provide adequate glucose needed for basic energy metabolism. Both *S.* Typhimurium and *B. abortus* infect and replicate within host cell macrophages, which are immune cells that can adopt a range of behaviors depending on which of their many jobs they are performing. Both pathogens are able to establish a persistent, chronic infection within macrophages that are in the "M2" state, a noninflammatory phenotype characterized by a certain repertoire of gene expression (20, 21), in particular, the regulatory proteins of the peroxisome proliferator-activated receptors (PPAR) (22). Each pathogen relies on host expression of a different PPAR protein to promote an intracellular environment with available glucose for bacterial metabolism. For *S.* Typhimurium, host expression of PPAR-delta is important for persistent infection, since the bacteria are

not able to establish a persistent infection in *Ppar*-delta$^{-/-}$ cells or mice (23). Host expression of PPAR-delta is not necessary for other intracellular pathogens such as *Listeria monocytogenes*, *Francisella tularensis*, and *M. tuberculosis*, illustrating the diversity in survival strategies of different pathogens. In general, PPAR-delta controls host cell metabolism, moving the macrophage away from glucose metabolism and promoting fatty-acid oxidation, putatively freeing up intracellular glucose that *S.* Typhimurium can then use. Testing whether increased glucose availability in the PPAR-delta-expressing, fat-metabolizing macrophage was permitting *S.* Typhimurium to replicate, the authors observed that a bacterial mutant deficient in glucose transport was unable to replicate within the macrophage. Additionally, the authors saw that wild type bacteria were able to acquire a fluorescent glucose analog from the macrophages and also replicated to higher levels when wild type host cells were treated with a PPAR-delta agonist (23). Together, these data provide strong evidence that the metabolic capacity of bacterial pathogens is strongly influenced by host metabolic function.

During chronic *B. abortus* infection in mice, M2 type macrophages in the spleen harbor replicating bacterial cells and express the gene for the PPAR-gamma regulator (21), another PPAR protein that tilts macrophage metabolism away from glucose usage and toward fatty acid oxidation. A PPAR-gamma agonist increased macrophage intracellular glucose concentration and also supported increased bacterial colonization, whereas blocking PPAR-gamma activity with a specific inhibitor decreased splenic colonization of *B. abortus* in mice. As in the previous study, mutant *B. abortus* deficient in glucose transport was greatly attenuated for growth in cell culture and in mice, strongly suggesting that glucose availability is key for this microbe to establish chronic infection. Two important observations comparing these two studies are that (i) both studies elucidated bacterial metabolism during persistent, chronic bacterial infections, suggesting that pathogens likely implement different metabolic strategies over the lifetime of an infection, and (ii) whereas *S.* Typhimurium may actively induce increased expression of PPAR-delta in the host since infected macrophages upregulate this gene in the absence of cytokine stimulation, it appears that *B. abortus* does not directly cause macrophages to increase PPAR-gamma. Thus, bacterial pathogens may actively or passively take advantage of host cell metabolic capacity. These studies then raise the question as to why these two pathogens benefit from host expression of different PPAR proteins, since both homologs have similar roles in the macrophage. Lastly, the dependence on glycolytic metabolism in these two bacteria and their ability to obtain host glucose demonstrate that central metabolism is a key determinant in virulence and infectious persistence.

Glucose is not the only molecule that can be oxidized by cells for energy metabolism. In fact, fatty acids harbor much more potential energy than glucose, and oxidation of fatty acids can provide a greater yield of ATP (Fig. 1). However, bacteria can only establish infection if they are able to acquire usable food sources. A landmark study revealed that the major pathogen *M. tuberculosis* prefers to metabolize fatty acids rather than glucose during persistent infection (24). The genomic era has expanded our view of *M. tuberculosis* metabolism by identifying the range of metabolic genes that this organism harbors, in particular, a high degree of redundancy in genes for fatty acid beta-oxidation enzymes (25). A large-scale genetic screen has shown that several *M. tuberculosis* glycolysis enzymes are not needed for growth in mice (26). More recent work has refined how this pathogen makes its energetic living during infection, answering key questions as to where in the host the microbes acquire their preferred food source and what pathogen-specific pathways/proteins are key for metabolism during infection.

The *M. tuberculosis* bacillus establishes a particularly resilient, chronic infection in the host lung by persisting in a dormant state within granulomas, conglomerations of host immune cells putatively working to wall off the spread of infection but inadvertently serving as a stable reservoir for bacilli. Recent work has shown that oxygenated mycolic acids, molecules found on the cell surface of certain *Mycobacteria*, can induce lung macrophages to transform into a phenotype called the "foamy macrophage," an important component of the granuloma characterized by a high lipid content and ablation of bactericidal activity (27). But does induction of this macrophage phenotype only help protect the bacteria from clearance, or does the foamy macrophage contribute to bacterial metabolism? Despite being in a semidormant state, the bacilli within the granuloma associate closely with lipid droplets inside these lipid-rich macrophages (27), and subsequent investigation has confirmed that *M. tuberculosis* is able to accumulate intracellular, host-derived triacylglycerols (28). The use of these host-derived triacylglycerols for bacterial metabolism during the dormant state is strongly supported by the observation that bacterial fatty acid oxidation genes are upregulated during residence within lipid-loaded macrophages (28). As to exactly how the bacteria conduct metabolism *in vivo*, two bacterial homologs of isocitrate lyase (ICL1 and ICL2) are both needed for intracellular replication (29). These proteins are vital for the glyoxylate cycle in *M. tuberculosis*, a pathway needed for replenishment of TCA cycle intermediates during fatty acid metabolism when glycolysis is not being utilized (Fig. 1).

Sugar and fat and, in a pinch, amino acids can be fed into the central metabolism to yield energy. The questions explored in these examples regarding the preferred food sources and metabolic strategies of several bacterial pathogens are relevant for other pathogenic species as well. In the case of the human body, a wide range of tissue types and physiological environments exist where pathogens elicit disease, each one being unique in terms of carbon source content and availability. One might then speculate that pathogens that are able to infect numerous tissue types, such as *Staphylococcus aureus*, display a range of metabolic behavior based on the variable levels of glucose, fatty acids, and other carbon resources at different sites of infection. Also, do bacteria that infect immune-privileged tissues, such as the brain and meninges, have the ability to acquire nutrients that are normally unavailable to other microbes? These and many other questions about energy metabolism during infection will reveal more surprising capabilities of bacterial pathogens.

The Host Is a Crowded and Sometimes Bountiful Place

One of the most exciting developments in microbiology has been the launching of the Human Microbiome Project (30, 31), an undertaking to identify and investigate the myriad microorganisms that reside in and on the human body. This endeavor is now possible due to the availability of new genomic tools that allow researchers to investigate metagenomes, complex microbial communities composed of multiple species. But one of the most important aspects of the Human Microbiome Project is that it has increased appreciation for the ways the nonpathogenic, resident microbiota of the body can contribute to health and disease. In other words, our bodies are complex ecosystems, and when bacterial pathogens cause disease, they are often doing it within an environment where the growth of other microbes may have an influence, for better or worse. In terms of energy metabolism, it is important to appreciate that within a species-rich niche such as the gastrointestinal tract or the oral cavity, a multitude of resident bacterial species are engaging in a wide range of metabolism, consuming different food sources and excreting different waste products, creating a niche that some

bacterial pathogens have found unique ways of exploiting.

One of the most severe pathogens of the gastrointestinal system is the Gram-positive endospore-forming bacterium *Clostridium difficile*. The various classical virulence factors that this microbe, an obligate anaerobe, produces, such as toxins, have been well characterized (32). But how does *C. difficile* make its living, metabolically speaking, within the gut milieu? It is extremely difficult to test this question directly in hosts that harbor a vastly diverse native gut microbiota. To simplify the situation, a model system using gnotobiotic mice (mice harboring a defined and limited microbiota) has helped reveal how *C. difficile* benefits from the fermentation products of one microbe to run its own fermentative metabolism (33). The nonpathogenic, common gut microbe *Bacteroides thetaiotaomicron* produces the metabolite succinate during fermentation of carbohydrates. In *B. thetaiotaomicron*–harboring mice, *C. difficile* is able to grow to higher population densities when the mice are fed a high-carbohydrate diet compared to when they are fed a low-carbohydrate diet. When the global transcriptional profile of *C. difficile* grown in *B. thetaiotaomicron*–harboring mice fed a standard, carbohydrate-rich diet versus a polysaccharide deficient one was compared, the pathogen showed increased expression of multiple carbohydrate metabolism genes under the former condition, in particular, genes involved in the succinate to butyrate fermentation pathway. When mice are colonized with *B. thetaiotaomicron* only, high levels of succinate are detectable in the mouse gut. In mice cocolonized with *B. thetaiotaomicron* and *C. difficile*, higher levels of butyrate are generated than in mice harboring *C. difficile* only. Thus, the *C. difficile* appears to adapt its metabolic strategy to use *B. thetaiotaomicron*–generated succinate when it is present, generating butyrate as an end product. But in the normal gut, succinate levels are generally kept low due to the presence of other resident bacteria that produce other fermentation end products, such as the short-chain fatty acids acetate and butyrate.

However, wild type mice treated with antibiotics have higher levels of succinate in the gut, suggesting that antibiotic treatment changes the microbiota population distribution and thus changes the metabolite content as well. In antibiotic-treated mice, wild type *C. difficile* greatly out-competes an isogenic mutant lacking the succinate transporter (33), supporting the idea that *C. difficile* experiences a growth environment that supports succinate fermentation when members of the microbiota that prevent the accumulation of succinate are absent. This defined experimental approach greatly illuminates our understanding of how a pathogen like *C. difficile* can be present in the gut at nonpathogenic levels under normal conditions but then can expand and cause disease after antibiotic treatment, all due to a simple switch in energy-yielding metabolism.

The benign gut resident *B. thetaiotaomicron* also may assist another enteric pathogen via succinate production. Enterohemorrhagic *E. coli* (EHEC) has a curious way of colonizing the gut by forming what are called "attaching and effacing lesions," causing intestinal epithelial cells to remodel their cytoskeleton to form pedestal-like extensions upon which the EHEC firmly attach themselves. EHEC exhibits lower levels of virulence gene expression in conditions that promote glycolysis (i.e., carbohydrate rich), while virulence expression is increased in sugar-poor conditions where gluconeogenesis is needed by the microbe (34, 35). EHEC grown *in vitro* in the presence of *B. thetaiotaomicron* showed enhanced expression of virulence genes, and attaching and effacing lesion formation was much higher in tissue culture when EHEC was cocultured with *B. thetaiotaomicron* (36). Interestingly, virulence gene expression in the presence of *B. thetaiotaomicron* was decreased in EHEC mutants lacking the protein Cra, which is a regulatory protein that senses sugar concen-

trations (36). Since Cra enhances virulence gene expression in nutritional environments that suppress glycolysis but enhance gluconeogenesis, the authors hypothesized that *in vivo*, EHEC benefits from localized succinate production by the resident microbiota in the sugar-limited region of the gut epithelial surface, as opposed to the carbohydrate-rich gut lumen (34, 36).

A final example of the dynamic metabolic interplay between bacterial pathogens and resident microbiota shows that "cross-feeding" of preferred food sources can alter virulence behavior. The bacterium *Aggregatibacter actinomycetemcomitans* can colonize the human oral cavity and cause aggressive periodontitis. A facultative anaerobe, *A. actinomycetemcomitans* can use several carbon sources but prefers to catabolize L-lactate over glucose, even though growth is slower using L-lactate (37). The microbe does not catabolize L-lactate anaerobically but, rather, oxidizes this food source in an oxygen-dependent manner (38). When grown aerobically with glucose during *in vitro* coculture with the nonpathogenic resident of the oral microbiota, *Streptococcus gordonii*, *A. actinomycetemcomitans* mutants deficient in L-lactate metabolism show diminished growth, though they are able to grow well in high-glucose mono-culture, suggesting that the ability to metabolize L-lactate is important specifically in the presence of *S. gordonii*. Using a mouse thigh abscess model (a common model system for examining oral bacterial pathogenesis), the authors further showed that the ability to metabolize L-lactate is important only for *A. actinomycetemcomitans* infection during coculture with *S. gordonii*, since mutants lacking the ability to catabolize L-lactate establish mono-culture infection as well as wild type but are much less abundant in coculture abscesses (38). These data strongly suggest that L-lactate produced by *S. gordonii*, and also potentially by host lactate dehydrogenase in the subgingival crevice, can enhance the growth of this pathogen in the human oral cavity.

These examples not only further illustrate that the ability to find and utilize preferred food sources during infection is important for bacterial pathogens, but also show that the host resident microbial landscape can have major effects on pathogen energy metabolism by providing specific nutritional environments. More importantly, these studies support the idea that changes to or perturbations in the host microbiota can create environments that can enhance or inhibit a pathogen's ability to engage in its preferred microbial metabolic pathways, thereby supporting or hindering damage to the host.

The Parts that Make It All Go

Yet another way of looking at central metabolism for bacterial pathogens is to ask questions about the enzymatic machinery that is essential for conducting preferred modes of metabolism. Organisms vary widely in their ability to generate essential cellular components from scratch and in their ability to acquire key components from exogenous sources when *de novo* synthesis is not possible. The intracellular pathogen *L. monocytogenes* replicates efficiently within the cytoplasm of host cells, where it is able to acquire a variety of host molecules to support growth, including glucose-6-phosphate as a carbon source (39) and the essential thiol-containing cofactor lipoate (40), which is needed for several enzymes involved in aerobic metabolism (41). The *L. monocytogenes* genome does not contain genes necessary for *de novo* lipoate biosynthesis (42). However, this bacterium does produce two functional lipoate ligase enzymes (LplA1 and LplA2) that are able to catalyze the covalent attachment of lipoate to the enzyme pyruvate dehydrogenase, a critical enzyme for bacterial respiration (40, 43). The LplA1 enzyme is specifically needed for *L. monocytogenes* intracellular growth and virulence in mice (41). More importantly, LplA1 but not LplA2 is needed for utilization of lipoyl-peptides, a specific form of lipoate that is available

within the host cell (40). This example highlights the importance of organic accessory cofactors that bacteria need for running metabolism during infection, and it also shows how pathogens may evolve to have an expanded ability obtain important cofactors that exist in various forms within the host.

The End of the Line: Using a Novel Electron Sink to Outpace the Competitors

The last example illustrating the flexible and opportunistic logic of one bacterial pathogen's approach to metabolism involves *S.* Typhimurium, which is able to make its metabolic living inside the host cell by acquiring intracellular glucose and undergoing standard aerobic respiration (glycolysis + TCA cycle). But this bacterium is also able to replicate within the lumen of the gastrointestinal tract, outside of host cells and among the intestinal microbiota, where oxygen is limiting and where competition for carbon sources is fierce. The key to understanding the significance of these findings is an appreciation of the differences between using fermentation versus respiration for ATP generation. Fermentation can be simple glycolysis run cyclically and is characterized by a low yield of ATP per oxidized carbon source input relative to respiration (Fig. 1). Unlike fermentation, respiration capitalizes on energy released during the process of electron transport to create a proton gradient that drives enzymatic ATP synthesis (oxidative phosphorylation), resulting in a much larger yield of usable energy. But the central difference is that only respiration requires a highly oxidized, terminal electron acceptor to act as a sink at the end of electron transport, whereas fermentation relies on the enzymatic reoxidation of the electron carriers that were reduced along the pathway (NADH to NAD+), generating some waste product in the process, often an acid such as lactate. Although the electron sink that supports the highest theoretical energy yield via respiration is oxygen, many other molecules (such as nitrate or sulfate) can play the role of terminal electron acceptor as well.

And this brings the discussion back to *S*. Typhimurium. Infection of mice with *S*. Typhimurium results in acute intestinal inflammation that is induced by various bacterial virulence factors, including two different bacterial secretion systems (44). The gut inflammation promotes a less hospitable environment for the resident microbiota and allows the *Salmonellae* to out-compete the resident microbiota (45). Part of the mechanism that supports this growth advantage for *S*. Typhimurium in the inflamed gut is its unique ability to use the molecule tetrathionate as a terminal electron acceptor for anaerobic respiration. Bacteria in the mouse colon, a generally anaerobic environment, produce hydrogen sulphide as a fermentation byproduct, which is converted to the less toxic molecule thiosulphate by host mucosal cells. Importantly, thiosulphate can be converted to tetrathionate by a strong oxidant. In a mouse model of colitis, C57BL/6 mice infected with *S*. Typhimurium show acute levels of cecal inflammation, whereas infection with bacteria lacking the ability to use tetrathionate in anaerobic respiration results in inflammation with increased cecal tetrathionate concentration (46). Tetrathionate was not detected in the gut of mice infected with *S*. Typhimurium lacking the virulence factors that cause inflammation, strongly supporting the idea that reactive oxygen species generated by the host during inflammation are responsible for the appearance of tetrathionate that is usable by the bacteria. Bacteria able to use tetrathionate respiration showed a strong growth advantage compared to tetrathionate metabolic mutants in the mouse gut, but not in the spleen, suggesting that this metabolic advantage is site-specific in the host (46). Importantly, generation of reactive oxygen by the host NADPH oxidase during inflammation, and not nitric oxide production by the nitric oxide synthase, seems to be responsible for the generation of tetrathionate in the inflamed gut, since wild type bacteria did not out-compete tetrathionate metabolic mutants in mice lacking the gene encoding the NADPH oxidase. The ability to undergo anaerobic respiration with a terminal electron acceptor generated by the combined activity of both the host (reactive oxygen) and the resident microbiota (hydrogen sulfide) is a remarkably unique strategy to bolster a pathogenic metabolic advantage.

Tetrathionate anaerobic respiration is not the only trick used by *S*. Typhimurium to out-compete the microbiota in the colon. Nitrate is an even more electronegative electron acceptor than tetrathionate, and thus it promotes an even stronger energy yield when used for anaerobic respiration. In a mouse model of colitis, a strain of *S*. Typhimurium lysogenized by a bacteriophage carrying the virulence gene *sopE* was able to switch to nitrate metabolism in the gut to out-compete the native microbiota (47). Like the tetrathionate example, the generation of nitrate in the gut is dependent on host inflammation. However, unlike tetrathionate, luminal nitrate concentration rises due to the host expression of the inducible nitric oxide synthase, which generates nitric oxide that then leads to nitrate. Bacteria with the *sopE*-containing bacteriophage did not have a growth advantage in iNOS-deficient mice. Interestingly, the lysogenized bacteria suppress the genes for tetrathionate metabolism both *in vitro* and *in vivo* when nitrate is available, illustrating a remarkable level of metabolic flexibility and control (47).

The examples outlined thus far clearly show that bacterial pathogens engage in energy-yielding metabolism during infection in ways that take advantage of the specific host environment at the site of infection. The process of bacterial metabolism is extremely dynamic, and pathogens exhibit a wide range of metabolic control and flexibility during infection. A key point to emphasize about energy-yielding metabolic pathways is that, although we consider them mainly in terms of their importance in ATP generation, the reality is that intermediates for both anabolism and catabolism are constantly being fed into and siphoned off these pathways for many other metabolic needs, with constant regulation based on the moment-to-moment needs of the cell. Thus, each of the stories illustrated here represents a "tip of the iceberg" situation, posing new questions about how pathogenic catabolic behavior is connected to the anabolic needs and strategies during infection as well.

ION AND NUTRIENT ACQUISITION BY BACTERIAL PATHOGENS

The human body is a rich reservoir of fundamental nutrients for bacteria that can exploit it, and nutrient acquisition is an essential aspect of host–pathogen interactions. The mechanisms of energy generation described in the previous section require high levels of carbon and other building blocks, and bacteria must extract these nutrients from resources found in the host, including sugars, amino acids, lipids and nitrogen-containing compounds. Moreover, transition metals such as iron, zinc and manganese are essential for survival and proliferation of all living organisms. This section will focus on strategies bacteria use to gain access to these critical nutrients from the complex host environment.

Transition Metal Ions: Precious Metals for Life

Transition metals, including iron, zinc, manganese, and copper, among others, are nutrients required for many biological processes. These metals have unique redox potential because they can undergo change in their oxidation state and serve as essential cofactors for many enzymes (48). In bacteria, it is estimated that 30 to 45% of enzymes require a metal cofactor for function (49). However, at high concentrations, these metals are toxic for the cells because they

perturb cellular redox potential and can drive production of highly reactive hydroxyl radicals. Therefore, all organisms possess biochemical systems to sense and regulate metal levels, and mammals have evolved strategies to sequester free metal ions to limit toxicity and also to restrict availability of these metal ions to invading microorganisms. This concept of growth restriction by limiting access to essential metals is called nutritional immunity (50, 51). As described below, pathogens have evolved numerous mechanisms for metal uptake or efflux to circumvent nutritional immunity (Table 2).

Iron

Iron (Fe) is the most abundant transition metal in the human body, but free iron is almost undetectable. Bacteria need concentrations on the order of 10^{-6}M iron to survive and proliferate, whereas circulation of free iron in human blood is approximately 10^{-18}M. Iron is a cofactor for many enzymes involved in fundamental cellular processes, including DNA replication, transcription, metabolism, and energy generation through respiration.

Iron sequestration by the host

In vertebrates, most iron is stored intracellularly in complex with heme, a tetrapyrrole ring that binds a ferrous iron (Fe^{2+}) atom. Heme is primarily found in the oxygen-transporting protein hemoglobin, contained within circulating erythrocytes. Moreover, free hemoglobin or heme is bound by the serum proteins haptoglobin and hemopexin, respectively (52). At physiological pH, free Fe^{2+} in the extracellular environment is rapidly oxidized to ferric iron (Fe^{3+}) and captured by the serum protein, transferrin, or by lactoferrin, a glycoprotein found in human secretions such as saliva, tears, and breast milk, rendering free ferrous iron unavailable for microorganisms. In cells, Fe^{3+} is captured by the storage protein ferritin. In phagocytic cells of the innate immune system, such as macrophages and neutrophils, the phagosomal membrane protein NRAMP1 (natural

TABLE 2 Summary of bacterial mechanisms for metal ion acquisition

Pathogens	Infection site (model)	Ion	System contributing to virulence	Reference
Salmonella enterica serovar Typhimurium	Systemic infection (mice)	Fe	EntC, EntB, IroN (salmochelin/enterobactin)	62
Streptococcus suis	Systemic infection (mice)	Fe	FeoB, iron transporter	56
Campylobacter jejuni	Gastrointestinal tract (chick)	Fe	FeoB, iron transporter	58
Staphylococcus aureus	Systemic infection (mice)	Fe	Isd heme uptake system	69
Yersinia pestis	Systemic infection/bubonic plague (mice)	Fe	Yef and Feo iron transporter	127
S. aureus	Systemic infection (mice)	Mn	MntABC and MntH Mn transporters	82
Escherichia coli (UPEC)	Bladder and kidney (mice)	Zn	ZnuABC and ZupT Zn transporters	86
S. Typhimurium	Inflamed gut (mice)	Zn	ZnuABC Zn uptake system	84
Acinetobacter baumannii	Lungs (mice)	Zn	ZnuABC Zn uptake system	83
Mycobacterium tuberculosis	Differentiated human macrophages	Zn	CtpC P1-type ATPase, Zn efflux system	85
M. tuberculosis	Lung and lymph nodes (guinea pigs)	Cu	MctB copper transport protein B	95
E. coli	Mouse macrophage-like cells	Cu	CopA ATPase, Cu^+ export system	89
E. coli (UPEC)	Bladder (mice)	Cu	Yersinibactin	96
Pseudomonas aeruginosa	Systemic infection (mice)	Cu	CopA1 P-type ATPase, Cu^+ efflux system	94

resistance-associated macrophage protein 1), pumps Fe^{2+} out of the phagosomal compartment, which physically surrounds bacteria taken up by the host cell, to reduce metal ion availability to intracellular bacteria (53). These mechanisms of iron limitation also exist in plants and invertebrates, which suggests a conserved and universal innate immune response against invading pathogens (54, 55).

Bacterial mechanisms of iron acquisition

The host mechanisms of iron sequestration discussed above efficiently limit the availability of iron, but bacterial pathogens possess their own weapons to counteract host innate defenses and to acquire Fe^{2+} that will be used as a nutrient source. Specific strategies used by a given pathogen mainly depend on the particular sites of infection and the intracellular or extracellular lifestyle. Bacterial mechanisms for iron acquisition can be divided into three major categories: siderophores, heme acquisition systems, and free Fe^{2+} transporters (50). Free Fe^{2+} can enter the periplasm of Gram-negative bacteria through nonspecific porins and gets transported

across the cytoplasmic membrane of Gram-negative and Gram-positive bacteria by the FeoB family of transporters. Members of the FeoB family of metal transporters are important for the virulence of many pathogens, including *Streptococcus suis* and *Campylobacter jejuni* (56–58).

Siderophores are low-molecular-mass iron chelators secreted by bacteria that bind to Fe^{3+} with an affinity higher than mammalian Fe-binding proteins such as lactoferrin and transferrin, allowing them to steal iron from these host proteins. Iron-bound siderophores are recognized at the bacterial surface by specific bacterial receptors and transported into the cytoplasm where bound Fe^{3+} is reduced into Fe^{2+} or released by degradation of the siderophore. Epithelial cells and neutrophils can neutralize some siderophores by secreting the antimicrobial protein lipocalin-2 (also known as neutrophil gelatinase-associated lipocalin), during acute infection (59). Lipocalin-2 expression is controlled by signaling through Toll-like receptors, pattern recognition receptors of the innate immune system responsive to microbial ligands. Lipocalin-2 can sequester the catecholate siderophore enterobactin, which is produced by common pathogenic enterobacteria such as *E. coli* and *S.* Typhimurium, causative agents of gastrointestinal diseases (59). To circumvent this immune defense, some bacteria synthesize a modified siderophore, called salmochelin, which is a glucosylated derivative of enterobactin that is not recognized by lipocalin-2 (60). Production of salmochelin is essential for efficient colonization and growth of *S.* Typhimurium within the inflamed gut (61, 62).

Heme represents one of the most abundant sources of iron, and pathogens have evolved heme uptake systems as well as hemophore systems. To gain access to heme, which is mainly bound to hemoproteins, bacteria secrete exotoxins to degrade hemoglobin (63). Free heme is captured by specific membrane complexes (TonB-dependent heme acquisition systems in Gram-negative bacteria and Isd systems in Gram-positive bacteria) and transported into the cytoplasm, where heme-catabolizing enzymes release Fe^{2+} (50, 64). Heme is the preferred source of iron of *S. aureus*, a member of the skin microbiome that can cause tissue abscesses, as well as more severe diseases including bacteremia and endocarditis (65–67). *S. aureus* can grow *in vitro* with erythrocytes as the sole source of iron. Hemolysins secreted by *S. aureus* lyse erythrocytes, releasing hemoglobin, which is targeted by the IsdB (iron-regulated surface determinant B) cell wall receptor. As alternative routes for iron acquisition, IsdH recognizes the hemogloblin-haptoglobin complex, whereas IsdA captures free heme (68). The Isd system is critical for iron acquisition during systemic *S. aureus* infection and for efficient colonization of spleen, kidneys, and heart (69). In addition to surface heme receptors, some bacteria also secrete hemophores, which are proteins that bind heme and can be reacquired by the bacteria. *Bacillus anthracis*, the causative agent of anthrax, secretes two hemophores, IsdX1 and IsdX2, which bind heme and are re-

quired for growth in iron-depleted environments (70–72).

Zinc and manganese

Sequestration of zinc (Zn) and manganese (Mn) is also an important innate defense strategy used by vertebrates to fight bacterial infection. Zinc is used for its structural and catalytic roles in a large number of proteins. In bacteria, 5 to 6% of the proteome consists of zinc-binding proteins, justifying the need for specific acquisition systems (73). Among them, enzymes involved in central metabolic pathways, DNA repair, response to oxidative stress, and antibiotic resistance require zinc as an essential cofactor (74). Manganese is also an important metal for bacteria, because many Mn-dependent enzymes encoded by pathogens are involved in central carbon metabolism and are necessary for resistance to oxidative stress (75).

Control of Mn^{2+} and Zn^{2+} levels by the host

Vertebrates secrete proteins that belong to the S100 family and inhibit bacterial growth by chelating Mn^{2+} and Zn^{2+}. S100A7 protein (also called psoriasin) is secreted as a homodimer by keratinocytes and inhibits *E. coli* growth on human skin through sequestration and chelation of Zn^{2+} (76). Similarly, calprotectin, which is a heterodimer formed by S100A8 and S100A9 (also known as calgranulin A and B, respectively), represents ~40% of the cytosolic protein pool in neutrophils and exhibits antimicrobial activity against bacterial pathogens through chelation of the nutrients Mn^{2+} and Zn^{2+} (77, 78). Calprotectin is the major neutrophil-derived protein found in abscesses formed by *S. aureus* (77). As is true for iron, immune cells also control Mn^{2+} and Zn^{2+} availability to intracellular bacteria by multiple mechanisms. Manganese is pumped out of the phagosome by the NRAMP1 protein, whereas zinc levels are reduced by the action of members of the ZIP and ZnT zinc transporter family (79–81).

Bacterial acquisition of Mn^{2+} and Zn^{2+}

The fight for metals is a continuous ongoing process between bacteria and the host. As described for iron, bacterial mechanisms exist that minimize the chelation of zinc and manganese by calprotectin. To counteract this antimicrobial response, *S. aureus* expresses specialized manganese transporters, MntABC and MntH, to compete with calprotectin for Mn^{2+} during systemic infection (82). Likewise, *S.* Typhimurium and *Acinetobacter baumannii* express the high-affinity zinc transporter ZnuABC to overcome the antimicrobial effect of calprotectin during infection (83, 84). *S.* Typhimurium, in addition to neutralizing the effect of calprotectin, also exploits the accumulation of this antimicrobial molecule during infection of the inflamed gut to advantageously compete with the resident host microbiota (84).

Use of zinc in host defense

In the constant battle to limit metal access during infection, mammals also exploit the toxicity associated with elevated concentrations of transition metals as an antimicrobial strategy. Macrophages control zinc levels inside the bacteria-containing phagosome during infection by *M. tuberculosis*. This increase in free Zn^{2+} results in accumulation of the metal inside the cytoplasm of *M. tuberculosis*, reducing intracellular growth. *Mycobacterium* resolves this zinc-dependent intoxication by expressing CtpC, a metal efflux P1-type ATPase (85). Similarly, the ZnuABC and ZupT zinc exporters are required for optimal colonization of mice bladders and kidneys during urinary tract infection caused by *E. coli* (86). Thus, it is clear that while bacteria must acquire metal ions for replication and metabolism, levels of these key nutrients within the bacteria themselves are tightly regulated.

Copper

Copper (Cu) is a redox-active metal ion that can exist in a reduced (Cu^+) or an oxidized state (Cu^{2+}) and, as a consequence, is critical for proteins involved in a wide range of cellular processes. Copper is also used by some metalloenzymes involved in electron transfer reactions, such as cytochrome oxidase (87). However, in contrast to Fe, Mn, and Zn, which are required for bacterial growth, copper is mainly recognized for its antimicrobial benefits and its role in innate immune defense against bacteria.

Copper toxicity

In mammals, the innate immune response provoked by secretion of the proinflammatory cytokine, interferon-γ, induces expression of Cu pumps, resulting in an increased Cu concentration at the infection site (88). In activated macrophages, the Cu^+ transport protein 1 (CTR1) takes Cu^+ inside the cell, whereas the P-type ATPase ATP7A pumps Cu^+ inside the phagolysosome, again emphasizing the importance of precise regulation of metal ion levels (89). Multiple mechanisms have been described to explain copper toxicity in bacteria. Macrophages use copper to increase bacterial killing by oxidative damage. In the phagosome, Cu^+ can interact with hydrogen peroxide to produce the highly reactive hydroxyl anion and hydroxyl radical, which in turn causes lethal damage to lipids, proteins, and nucleic acids. Unligated copper also causes disruption of iron-sulfur clusters by replacing the Fe atoms, resulting in the disruption of protein structure. Enzymes that contain an Fe-S cluster, such as dehydratases involved in branch-chain amino acid synthesis in *E. coli*, are targeted by Cu during infection (90). An alternative mechanism has been described during *Neisseria gonorrhoeae* infection, where increased Cu levels result in increased sensitivity to reactive nitrogen species produced by innate immune cells (91).

Copper regulation by bacteria

The recurring theme of measure–countermeasure should be now apparent, because bacteria have evolved strategies to prevent copper toxicity imposed by the host and to tightly regulate the level of cytoplasmic copper (92). In general, bacterial proteomes contain only a few copper-binding proteins (~0.3%), and these proteins are mainly localized in the periplasm or in the cyoplasmic membrane, preventing unligated copper from accessing the cytoplasm. Bacteria can also express Cu-binding proteins to sequester free Cu^+, such as the *Mycobacterium* methallothionein, (MymT), which protects the bacterium from copper toxicity (93). Many pathogenic bacteria encode a P-type ATPase Cu^+ efflux protein that pumps copper outside of the bacterial cytoplasm. For *E. coli*, a mutant lacking the CopA ATPase is hypersensitive to killing by macrophage-like cells (89). Similarly, a CopA1 ATPase mutant of *Pseudomonas aeruginosa* is attenuated in a systemic mouse model of infection (94). *M. tuberculosis* also encodes a membrane copper transporter that is required to ensure resistance to copper toxicity and intracellular survival *in vivo* (95). Lastly, uropathogenic *E. coli* use an unusual method to limit copper toxicity. During bladder infection, uropathogenic *E. coli* secretes the siderophore yersiniabactin, which allows capture of essential iron, but this compound can also bind to copper and prevent its toxicity (96). Consistently, *E. coli* strains that produce yersiniabactin exhibit greater resistance to copper-related toxicity.

Nutrient Acquisition

In the host cell, many nutrients essential for bacterial growth are enclosed within complex molecules such as proteins and higher-order glycolipids and are not readily accessible. Moreover, depending on the particular niche colonized by the pathogen or the local inflammation state, nutrient supply might vary greatly during the course of infection. Therefore, nutritional restriction by the host is an important aspect of the innate immune defense against pathogens (97). The following section will highlight some of the mech-

anisms used by pathogenic bacteria to maximize nutrient acquisition in the complex environment of the host (graphically summarized in Fig. 2).

The arsenal of microbial degradative enzymes

Host macromolecules are a good source of carbon and nitrogen when bacterial enzymes, such as proteases or phospholipases, can degrade these molecules to extract essential nutrients. *Vibrio cholerae*, the causative agent of the severe diarrheal disease cholera, utilizes host sialic acid to generate carbon, nitrogen, and energy (98, 99). Sialic acids are a family of nine-carbon amino sugars found in abundance in the mammalian gut. *V. cholerae* encodes a sialic acid catabolism gene cluster (the *nan-nag* cluster) located in the VPI2 pathogenicity island, which is found only in toxigenic strains that are the primary cause of disease. NanH, a neuraminidase, is required for cleavage of bound sialic acid from higher-order gangliosides found at the cell surface. The free sialic acid (mainly *N*-acetylneuraminic acid or Neu5Ac) is taken up by *V. cholerae* and converted to fructose-6-P that feeds into the glycolytic pathway. This catabolic pathway plays a significant role for *V. cholerae* colonization of infant mice, an important animal model for studying human cholera (98). The *nan* cluster is also found in many other human pathogens that colonize the gut, including *E. coli*, *S.* Typhimurium, *Shigella* spp., and *Clostridium* spp., among others, and a correlation between sialic acid catabolism and bacterial fitness in the gut is now emerging (100). Of note, the use of NanH to hydrolyze host sialic acid as a carbon source is not restricted to gut pathogens but is also required for biofilm formation and lung colonization by *P. aeruginosa* (101).

The γ-glutamyl transpeptidase, GGT, produced by *F. tularensis* is another striking example of a microbial strategy for nutrient acquisition (102). *F. tularensis* is a highly infectious Gram-negative bacterial pathogen

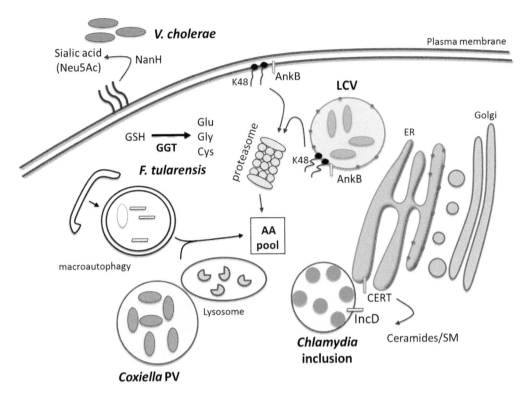

FIGURE 2 Graphical summary of bacterial mechanisms used to release intracellular host nutrients. Pathogenic bacteria perturb host cell functions to provide resources for survival and replication. Abbreviations: GSH, glutathione; GGT, γ-glutamyl transpeptidase; LCV, *Legionella*-containing vacuole; ER, endoplasmic reticulum; AA, amino acids; CERT, ceramide transfer protein; SM, sphingomyelin.

that causes the deadly disease tularemia. After entry into mammalian cells, *F. tularensis* replicates in the cytosol using amino acids as its major source of carbon and energy required for proliferation. *F. tularensis* particularly requires high levels of cysteine to support intracellular proliferation, because cysteine is metabolized into pyruvate, a key substrate of the TCA cycle. Because cysteine is the most limiting amino acid in humans, *F. tularensis* has evolved to use host gluthathione, a tripeptide (L-γ-L-glutamyl-L-cysteinyl-glycine) that is abundant in the cytosol. The GGT enzyme of *F. tularensis* cleaves gluthathione to release cysteine; mutants of *Francisella* that lack this enzyme are severely impaired for growth in mouse macrophages and attenuated for virulence in mice (102).

Raiding the pantry: exploitation of host processes to provide food

Chlamydia species are Gram-negative obligate human intracellular bacteria that manipulate the host cell to enhance nutrient and lipid acquisition. *Chlamydia* resides in a unique *Chlamydia*-containing inclusion in the cytosol of host cells and is one of the few bacterial pathogens that need host-derived lipids such as sphingomyelin (SM) for intracellular proliferation. SM is incorporated into the *Chlamydia* cell wall as well as into the growing inclusion membrane during bacterial replication (103). To acquire host-derived SM, *Chlamydia trachomatis* uses the IncD protein, an effector of the syringe-like bacterial type III secretion system, which is inserted into the inclusion membrane. IncD mediates recruitment of the host ceramide transfer protein, CERT, at the site of contact between the bacterial inclusion and the endoplasmic reticulum membrane (104). CERT is involved in the nonvesicular transfer of ceramides, precursors of SM, from the endoplasmic reticulum to the Golgi apparatus. The recruitment of CERT to the bacterial inclusion is required for *C. trachomatis* intracellular replication (105). Thus, *Chlamydia*, with its reduced genome, illustrates how obligate intracellular pathogens are able to extensively exploit host trafficking pathways to gain essential lipids/nutrients to support replication.

Some bacteria are able to obtain nutrients by manipulating host degradation processes rather than relying on their own degradative mechanisms, including *C. trachomatis* and *Chlamydia pneumoniae*. Lysosomes are cellular degradation compartments within the host cell that contain an array of degradative enzymes that break down proteins, carbohydrates, nucleic acids, and lipids. Depletion of amino acids within the lysosomal compartment results in growth inhibition of *Chlamydia* spp., which suggests that these bacteria rely on degradation of exogenous cargo for nutrient acquisition within the inclusion (106). *Coxiella burnetti*, an obligate intracellular bacterium that causes human Q fever, also uses the degradative properties of the lysosome for nutrient acquisition (107). *C. burnetti* proliferates inside the host cell in a specialized vacuole, termed the parasitophorous vacuole, which is a phagolysosome-like compartment (108). An acidic environment is required for optimal growth of these bacteria, and amino acids and other nutrients required for replication likely reach the parasitophorous vacuole via fusion of protein/peptide-loaded lysosomes.

One of the most well-studied bacterial pathogens that exploits host cell degradation capacity is *Legionella pneumophila*, a bacterium that replicates within alveolar macrophages and causes pneumonia (Legionnaires's disease). Inside macrophages, *L. pneumophila* replicates within the *Legionella*-containing vacuole (LCV), which is remodeled by a series of secreted effectors and resembles the rough endoplasmic reticulum membrane (109). The level of amino acids, the main source of carbon and energy generation for *Legionella*, within the host cytosol is not sufficient to power the robust intracellular replication of this bacterium. To gain access to these key nutrients, *Legionella* boosts the cellular level of amino acids by subverting host proteasomal degradation processes (110). The secreted bacterial effector AnkB is anchored to the cytosolic face of the LCV membrane by a lipid modification and triggers polyubiquitin tagging of proteins at the LCV surface. These ubiquitinated proteins are subsequently targeted to the 26S proteasome and rapidly degraded to generate a localized supply of amino acids (110). AnkB is also injected into the host cell directly after bacterial attachment and is localized to the plasma membrane. This allows rapid polyubiquitination and degradation of host proteins and generates a nutrient-rich environment for the establishment of the LCV (111). Not surprisingly, the *Legionella* AnkB mutant has a severe growth defect for intravacuolar replication in macrophages and has a reduced ability to cause pulmonary disease in mice. *L. pneumophila* also encodes amino acid transporters, such as the PhtA transporter involved in import of threonine, an essential amino acid for *Legionnella*, into the bacteria during infection (112). The PhtA transporter is required for growth, but not survival inside macrophages.

F. tularensis, a bacterium that can replicate up to 1,000-fold in the host cell cytosol, also manipulates host degradation machinery to facilitate nutrient uptake. Acquisition of host amino acids is critical for this intracellular pathogen, because *F. tularensis* is auxotrophic for six amino acids, relying solely on the host to provide them. To promote a permissive growth environment, *F. tularensis* induces macroautophagy, a host recycling pathway normally stimulated by starvation that targets host proteins, organelles, and invading pathogens for degradation (113).

Macroautophagy inhibition results in decreased intracellular replication of *Francisella*, which can be rescued by adding excess amino acids, highlighting the role of this host pathway for bacterial proliferation (113). Autophagy has been studied mainly for its role in innate immune defense, but several bacterial pathogens like *Francisella* have evolved mechanisms to evade killing by autophagic degradation and instead exploit this pathway to increase bacterial proliferation. *Anaplasma phagocytophilum*, an obligate intracellular bacterium that belongs to the *Rickettsiales* order and causes human granulocytic anaplasmosis, is another example of a bacterium that actively induces autophagy to stimulate the richer host nutrient environment essential for proliferation (114).

METABOLIC CONTROL OF HOST–PATHOGEN INTERACTIONS

Pathogenesis is defined by the nature of the interaction between host and pathogen. As described above, bacterial pathogens are adept at exploiting the host as a chemical warehouse of sorts. However, the complex metabolic interactions of the bacteria with its host also signal regulatory processes that expand the bacterial repertoire for successful infection. In this section, we will tie in previous examples of pathogen metabolism with mechanisms used by bacteria to position themselves to take advantage of the host.

Orienteering: Nutrient Sensors Control Metabolism and Niche Adaptations

S. Typhimurium is able to out-compete resident gut microbiota by stimulating intestinal inflammation in a mouse model of colitis and then relying on tetrathionate respiration for robust replication, as described above (46). However, this striking result does not explain how *S.* Typhimurium can position itself at the intestinal interface, where tetrathionate is most abundant. Previous studies had

determined that chemotaxis, the energy-dependent process by which bacteria move up or down chemical gradients, was important for the fitness of *S.* Typhimurium in models of colitis (115). Baumler and colleagues identified tetrathionate as a signal for the Aer methyl-accepting chemotaxis protein (116). Aer regulated chemotaxis toward tetrathionate and only conferred a fitness advantage upon *S.* Typhimurium under conditions of tetrathionate respiration *in vivo*. These findings indicate that *S.* Typhimurium not only has the metabolic capacity to remodel the biochemical environment of the intestine to give itself a competitive edge, but also encodes the machinery to seek areas with the highest concentration of alternative electron acceptors, such as tetrathionate, to enhance the opportunity for rapid replication.

In the previous case, *S.* Typhimurium succeeds by changing the host intestinal environment to a more inflammatory state that favors replication, but other pathogens such as EHEC take advantage of nutrient signals generated by the resident microbiota to control virulence and metabolic gene expression. EHEC encodes a two-component sensing system, FusKR, that consists of a sensor kinase (FusK) and a response regulator (FusR). FusK senses fucose and is required for EHEC colonization of the mammalian intestine (35). Although fucose is present at high levels in the intestine, host cells incorporate most fucose molecules into complex carbohydrate structures such as mucin, which is abundant at the surface of the intestinal epithelium. Fucose can be liberated from mucin by the fucosidase activity of *B. thetaiotaomicron*, a common resident of the microbiota (117). During growth in mucin, *B. thetaiotaomicron* freed fucose for sensing by EHEC FusKR, regulating EHEC virulence and metabolic gene expression and thereby modulating pathogenesis (35). In this case, free fucose enabled EHEC to spatially orient in the mammalian intestine, likely limiting expression of fucose utilization and virulence genes to localized environments where such metabolic capacity provides a competitive advantage.

Evading Immune System Predation

Metabolism can also provide powerful weapons used by bacteria to manipulate host immune responses, promoting pathogen survival. *M. tuberculosis* can be considered one of the most successful human pathogens, having been discovered in human remains thousands of years old. The success of *M. tuberculosis* likely relies in large part on the myriad ways in which the bacterium controls the immune response to its advantage. In a screen for *M. tuberculosis* genes that enhanced fitness in response to immune pressure, Rubin and colleagues identified genes of the tryptophan biosynthesis pathway (118). One established mechanism of nutritional immunity relies on the host enzyme, indoleamine 2,3-dioxygenase (IDO), which degrades the amino acid tryptophan, decreasing its availability to pathogens (119). IDO is induced by the proinflammatory cytokine, interferon-γ, and can be effective in host resistance against pathogens that are tryptophan auxotrophs, such as *Chlamydia* or *Toxoplasma* spp. (120). However, *M. tuberculosis* can upregulate *trp* biosynthesis genes within the infected host to overcome the lack of tryptophan availability. A *trp* mutant strain was hypersusceptible to killing by IFN-γ-treated macrophages compared to wild type *M. tuberculosis*, and that hypersusceptibility was reversed by inhibiting IDO or by addition of exogenous tryptophan (118). Thus, *M. tuberculosis* uses a metabolic strategy to counteract a specific mechanism of host nutritional immunity.

Host immune cell metabolism is increasingly appreciated as a critical determinant of immune function (121). The nucleoside adenosine has powerful immunosuppressive effects on the immune system, promoting T cell tolerance, or anergy (122). Adenosine receptors can play an important role in protecting the host from tissue damage or organ failure

in models of polymicrobial sepsis (123). The Gram-positive pathogen *S. aureus* is a common colonizer of human skin that can also cause abscesses, soft tissue infections, and systemic disease (124). Mutations in the *S. aureus* adenosine synthase *adsA* gene were found to predispose bacteria to killing in human blood (125). AdsA was required for staphylococcal virulence and abscess formation, indicating the importance of this protein during infection *in vivo*. Notably, the AdsA protein is found not in the bacterial cytosol, but rather, outside the bacterial cell, anchored to the cell wall. Incubation of *S. aureus* in blood increased the adenosine concentration in an AdsA-dependent manner, and this enzymatic activity contributed to virulence (125). These results indicate that *S. aureus* is able to synthesize adenosine in human blood, promoting an immunosuppressive environment. *S. aureus adsA* mutants were more susceptible to neutrophil killing, suggesting that at least one mechanism of adenosine-dependent immunosuppression occurs through modulation of innate immune effector functions.

CONCLUSION

The host–pathogen interactions described above indicate that bacterial metabolism is an essential component of the disease process. Acquisition of nutrients to support energy metabolism and biosynthesis drives bacterial replication within the host. The speed and efficiency of bacterial replication likely play a determining role in the outcome of disease. However, it is also apparent that bacterial metabolism can enhance other aspects of pathogenesis, including nutrient sensing and immune evasion. A deeper appreciation for pathogen metabolic capabilities will continue to emerge as we apply more sophisticated methodologies to our understanding of pathogenesis. Defining genomes, transcriptomes, and metabolomes at a global level will paint a more comprehensive picture of how the tremendous metabolic capacity of bacterial pathogens enables them to exploit the human host.

ACKNOWLEDGMENTS

This work was funded by NIH National Institute of Allergy and Infectious Diseases (NIAID) grants RO1 A1109048 and R33 A1102106.

CITATION

Passalacqua KD, Charbonneau M-E, O'Riordan MXD. 2016. Bacterial metabolism shapes the host–pathogen interface. Microbiol Spectrum 4(3):VMBF-0027-2015.

REFERENCES

1. **Rohmer L, Hocquet D, Miller SI.** 2011. Are pathogenic bacteria just looking for food? Metabolism and microbial pathogenesis. *Trends Microbiol* **19:**341–348.

2. **Lipmann F.** 1941. Metabolic generation and utilization of phosphate bond energy. *Adv Enzymol* **1:**99–162.

3. **de Duve C.** 2013. The other revolution in the life sciences. *Science* **339:**1148.

4. **Adler CJ, Dobney K, Weyrich LS, Kaidonis J, Walker AW, Haak W, Bradshaw CJ, Townsend G, Soltysiak A, Alt KW, Parkhill J, Cooper A.** 2013. Sequencing ancient calcified dental plaque shows changes in oral microbiota with dietary shifts of the Neolithic and Industrial Revolutions. *Nat Genet* **45:**450–455.

5. **Moye ZD, Zeng L, Burne RA.** 2014. Fueling the caries process: carbohydrate metabolism and gene regulation by *Streptococcus mutans. J Oral Microbiol* **6**. doi:10.3402/jom.v6.24878.

6. **Abranches J, Nascimento MM, Zeng L, Browngardt CM, Wen ZT, Rivera MF, Burne RA.** 2008. CcpA regulates central metabolism and virulence gene expression in *Streptococcus mutans. J Bacteriol* **190:**2340–2349.

7. **Kietzman CC, Caparon MG.** 2011. Distinct time-resolved roles for two catabolite-sensing pathways during *Streptococcus pyogenes* infection. *Infect Immun* **79:**812–821.

8. **Iyer R, Baliga NS, Camilli A.** 2005. Catabolite control protein A (CcpA) contributes to virulence and regulation of sugar metabolism in *Streptococcus pneumoniae. J Bacteriol* **187:**8340–8349.

9. **Carvalho SM, Kloosterman TG, Kuipers OP, Neves AR.** 2011. CcpA ensures optimal metabolic fitness of *Streptococcus pneumoniae. PLoS One* **6:**e26707. doi:10.1371/journal.pone.0026707.

10. **Bidossi A, Mulas L, Decorosi F, Colomba L, Ricci S, Pozzi G, Deutscher J, Viti C, Oggioni MR.** 2012. A functional genomics approach to establish the complement of carbohydrate transporters in *Streptococcus pneumoniae. PLoS One* **7:**e33320. doi:10.1371/journal.pone.0033320.

11. **King SJ, Hippe KR, Weiser JN.** 2006. Deglycosylation of human glycoconjugates by the sequential activities of exoglycosidases expressed by *Streptococcus pneumoniae. Mol Microbiol* **59:**961–974.

12. **Shelburne SA, Davenport MT, Keith DB, Musser JM.** 2008. The role of complex carbohydrate catabolism in the pathogenesis of invasive streptococci. *Trends Microbiol* **16:**318–325.

13. **Burnaugh AM, Frantz LJ, King SJ.** 2008. Growth of *Streptococcus pneumoniae* on human glycoconjugates is dependent upon the sequential activity of bacterial exoglycosidases. *J Bacteriol* **190:**221–230.

14. **Bowden SD, Rowley G, Hinton JC, Thompson A.** 2009. Glucose and glycolysis are required for the successful infection of macrophages and mice by *Salmonella enterica* serovar Typhimurium. *Infect Immun* **77:**3117–3126.

15. **Tchawa Yimga M, Leatham MP, Allen JH, Laux DC, Conway T, Cohen PS.** 2006. Role of gluconeogenesis and the tricarboxylic acid cycle in the virulence of *Salmonella enterica* serovar Typhimurium in BALB/c mice. *Infect Immun* **74:**1130–1140.

16. **Dougan G, Baker S.** 2014. *Salmonella enterica* serovar Typhi and the pathogenesis of typhoid fever. *Annu Rev Microbiol* **68:**317–336.

17. **Thiennimitr P, Winter SE, Baumler AJ.** 2012. *Salmonella*, the host and its microbiota. *Curr Opin Microbiol* **15:**108–114.

18. **Salcedo SP, Noursadeghi M, Cohen J, Holden DW.** 2001. Intracellular replication of *Salmonella* Typhimurium strains in specific subsets of splenic macrophages *in vivo. Cell Microbiol* **3:**587–597.

19. **Mercado-Lubo R, Leatham MP, Conway T, Cohen PS.** 2009. *Salmonella enterica* serovar Typhimurium mutants unable to convert malate to pyruvate and oxaloacetate are avirulent and immunogenic in BALB/c mice. *Infect Immun* **77:**1397–1405.

20. **Martinez FO, Gordon S.** 2014. The M1 and M2 paradigm of macrophage activation: time for reassessment. *F1000prime Rep* **6:**13.

21. **Xavier MN, Winter MG, Spees AM, den Hartigh AB, Nguyen K, Roux CM, Silva TM, Atluri VL, Kerrinnes T, Keestra AM, Monack DM, Luciw PA, Eigenheer RA, Baumler AJ, Santos RL, Tsolis RM.** 2013. PPARgamma-mediated increase in glucose availability sustains chronic *Brucella abortus* infection in alternatively activated macrophages. *Cell Host Microbe* **14:**159–170.

22. **Kang K, Reilly SM, Karabacak V, Gangl MR, Fitzgerald K, Hatano B, Lee CH.** 2008. Adipocyte-derived Th2 cytokines and myeloid PPARdelta regulate macrophage polarization and insulin sensitivity. *Cell Metab* **7:**485–495.

23. **Eisele NA, Ruby T, Jacobson A, Manzanillo PS, Cox JS, Lam L, Mukundan L, Chawla A, Monack DM.** 2013. *Salmonella* require the fatty acid regulator PPARdelta for the establishment of a metabolic environment essential for long-term persistence. *Cell Host Microbe* **14:**171–182.

24. **Bloch H, Segal W.** 1956. Biochemical differentiation of *Mycobacterium tuberculosis* grown *in vivo* and *in vitro*. *J Bacteriol* **72:**132–141.

25. **Cole ST, Brosch R, Parkhill J, Garnier T, Churcher C, Harris D, Gordon SV, Eiglmeier K, Gas S, Barry CE 3rd, Tekaia F, Badcock K, Basham D, Brown D, Chillingworth T, Connor R, Davies R, Devlin K, Feltwell T, Gentles S, Hamlin N, Holroyd S, Hornsby T, Jagels K, Krogh A, McLean J, Moule S, Murphy L, Oliver K, Osborne J, Quail MA, Rajandream MA, Rogers J, Rutter S, Seeger K, Skelton J, Squares R, Squares S, Sulston JE, Taylor K, Whitehead S, Barrell BG.** 1998. Deciphering the biology of *Mycobacterium tuberculosis* from the complete genome sequence. *Nature* **393:**537–544.

26. **Sassetti CM, Rubin EJ.** 2003. Genetic requirements for mycobacterial survival during infection. *Proc Natl Acad Sci USA* **100:**12989–12994.

27. **Peyron P, Vaubourgeix J, Poquet Y, Levillain F, Botanch C, Bardou F, Daffe M, Emile JF, Marchou B, Cardona PJ, de Chastellier C, Altare F.** 2008. Foamy macrophages from tuberculous patients' granulomas constitute a nutrient-rich reservoir for *M. tuberculosis* persistence. *PLoS Pathog* **4:**e1000204. doi:10.1371/journal.ppat.1000204.

28. **Daniel J, Maamar H, Deb C, Sirakova TD, Kolattukudy PE.** 2011. *Mycobacterium tuberculosis* uses host triacylglycerol to accumulate lipid droplets and acquires a dormancy-like phenotype in lipid-loaded macrophages. *PLoS Pathog* **7:**e1002093. doi:10.1371/journal.ppat.1002093.

29. **Munoz-Elias EJ, McKinney JD.** 2005. *Mycobacterium tuberculosis* isocitrate lyases 1 and 2 are jointly required for *in vivo* growth and virulence. *Nat Med* **11:**638–644.

30. **Gevers D, Knight R, Petrosino JF, Huang K, McGuire AL, Birren BW, Nelson KE, White O, Methe BA, Huttenhower C.** 2012. The Human Microbiome Project: a community resource for the healthy human microbiome. *PLoS Biol* **10:**e1001377. doi:10.1371/journal.pbio.1001377.

31. **Grice EA, Segre JA.** 2012. The human microbiome: our second genome. *Annu Rev Genomics Hum Genet* **13:**151–170.

32. **Vedantam G, Clark A, Chu M, McQuade R, Mallozzi M, Viswanathan VK.** 2012. *Clostridium difficile* infection: toxins and non-toxin virulence factors, and their contributions to disease establishment and host response. *Gut Microbes* **3:**121–134.

33. **Ferreyra JA, Wu KJ, Hryckowian AJ, Bouley DM, Weimer BC, Sonnenburg JL.** 2014. Gut microbiota-produced succinate promotes *C. difficile* infection after antibiotic treatment or motility disturbance. *Cell Host Microbe* **16:**770–777.

34. **Njoroge JW, Gruber C, Sperandio V.** 2013. The interacting Cra and KdpE regulators are involved in the expression of multiple virulence factors in enterohemorrhagic *Escherichia coli*. *J Bacteriol* **195:**2499–2508.

35. **Pacheco AR, Curtis MM, Ritchie JM, Munera D, Waldor MK, Moreira CG, Sperandio V.** 2012. Fucose sensing regulates bacterial intestinal colonization. *Nature* **492:**113–117.

36. **Curtis MM, Hu Z, Klimko C, Narayanan S, Deberardinis R, Sperandio V.** 2014. The Gut commensal *Bacteroides thetaiotaomicron* exacerbates enteric infection through modification of the metabolic landscape. *Cell Host Microbe* **16:**759–769.

37. **Brown SA, Whiteley M.** 2007. A novel exclusion mechanism for carbon resource partitioning in *Aggregatibacter actinomycetemcomitans*. *J Bacteriol* **189:**6407–6414.

38. **Ramsey MM, Rumbaugh KP, Whiteley M.** 2011. Metabolite cross-feeding enhances virulence in a model polymicrobial infection. *PLoS Pathog* **7:**e1002012. doi:10.1371/journal.ppat.1002012.

39. **Chico-Calero I, Suarez M, Gonzalez-Zorn B, Scortti M, Slaghuis J, Goebel W, Vazquez-Boland JA, European Listeria Genome Consortium.** 2002. Hpt, a bacterial homolog of the microsomal glucose-6-phosphate translocase,

mediates rapid intracellular proliferation in *Listeria. Proc Natl Acad Sci USA* **99**:431–436.

40. **Keeney KM, Stuckey JA, O'Riordan MX.** 2007. LplA1-dependent utilization of host lipoyl peptides enables *Listeria* cytosolic growth and virulence. *Mol Microbiol* **66**:758–770.

41. **O'Riordan M, Moors MA, Portnoy DA.** 2003. *Listeria* intracellular growth and virulence require host-derived lipoic acid. *Science* **302**:462–464.

42. **Glaser P, Frangeul L, Buchrieser C, Rusniok C, Amend A, Baquero F, Berche P, Bloecker H, Brandt P, Chakraborty T, Charbit A, Chetouani F, Couve E, de Daruvar A, Dehoux P, Domann E, Dominguez-Bernal G, Duchaud E, Durant L, Dussurget O, Entian KD, Fsihi H, Portillo FG, Garrido P, Gautier L, Goebel W, Gomez-Lopez N, Hain T, Hauf J, Jackson D, Jones LM, Kaerst U, Kreft J, Kuhn M, Kunst F, Kurapkat G, Madueno E, Maitournam A, Vicente JM, Ng E, Nedjari H, Nordsiek G, Novella S, de Pablos B, Perez-Diaz JC, Purcell R, Remmel B, Rose M, Schlueter T, Simoes N, Tierrez A, Vazquez-Boland JA, Voss H, Wehland J, Cossart P.** 2001. Comparative genomics of *Listeria* species. *Science* **294**:849–852.

43. **Zhao X, Miller JR, Jiang Y, Marletta MA, Cronan JE.** 2003. Assembly of the covalent linkage between lipoic acid and its cognate enzymes. *Chem Biol* **10**:1293–1302.

44. **Santos RL, Raffatellu M, Bevins CL, Adams LG, Tukel C, Tsolis RM, Baumler AJ.** 2009. Life in the inflamed intestine, *Salmonella* style. *Trends Microbiol* **17**:498–506.

45. **Stecher B, Robbiani R, Walker AW, Westendorf AM, Barthel M, Kremer M, Chaffron S, Macpherson AJ, Buer J, Parkhill J, Dougan G, von Mering C, Hardt WD.** 2007. *Salmonella enterica* serovar Typhimurium exploits inflammation to compete with the intestinal microbiota. *PLoS Biol* **5**:2177–2189. doi:10.1371/journal.pbio.0050244.

46. **Winter SE, Thiennimitr P, Winter MG, Butler BP, Huseby DL, Crawford RW, Russell JM, Bevins CL, Adams LG, Tsolis RM, Roth JR, Baumler AJ.** 2010. Gut inflammation provides a respiratory electron acceptor for *Salmonella. Nature* **467**:426–429.

47. **Lopez CA, Winter SE, Rivera-Chavez F, Xavier MN, Poon V, Nuccio SP, Tsolis RM, Baumler AJ.** 2012. Phage-mediated acquisition of a type III secreted effector protein boosts growth of *Salmonella* by nitrate respiration. *mBio* **3**:e00143–12. doi:10.1128/mBio.00143-12.

48. **Andreini C, Bertini I, Cavallaro G, Holliday GL, Thornton JM.** 2008. Metal ions in biological catalysis: from enzyme databases to general principles. *J Biol Inorg Chem* **13**:1205–1218.

49. **Klein JS, Lewinson O.** 2011. Bacterial ATP-driven transporters of transition metals: physiological roles, mechanisms of action, and roles in bacterial virulence. *Metallomics* **3**:1098–1108.

50. **Hood MI, Skaar EP.** 2012. Nutritional immunity: transition metals at the pathogen-host interface. *Nat Rev Microbiol* **10**:525–537.

51. **Weinberg ED.** 1975. Nutritional immunity. Host's attempt to withold iron from microbial invaders. *JAMA* **231**:39–41.

52. **Johnson EE, Wessling-Resnick M.** 2012. Iron metabolism and the innate immune response to infection. *Microbes Infect* **14**:207–216.

53. **Cellier MF, Courville P, Campion C.** 2007. Nramp1 phagocyte intracellular metal withdrawal defense. *Microbes Infect* **9**:1662–1670.

54. **Franza T, Expert D.** 2013. Role of iron homeostasis in the virulence of phytopathogenic bacteria: an 'a la carte' menu. *Mol Plant Pathol* **14**:429–438.

55. **Geiser DL, Winzerling JJ.** 2012. Insect transferrins: multifunctional proteins. *Biochim Biophys Acta* **1820**:437–451.

56. **Aranda J, Cortes P, Garrido ME, Fittipaldi N, Llagostera M, Gottschalk M, Barbe J.** 2009. Contribution of the FeoB transporter to *Streptococcus suis* virulence. *Int Microbiol* **12**:137–143.

57. **Cartron ML, Maddocks S, Gillingham P, Craven CJ, Andrews SC.** 2006. Feo-transport of ferrous iron into bacteria. *Biometals* **19**:143–157.

58. **Naikare H, Palyada K, Panciera R, Marlow D, Stintzi A.** 2006. Major role for FeoB in *Campylobacter jejuni* ferrous iron acquisition, gut colonization, and intracellular survival. *Infect Immun* **74**:5433–5444.

59. **Flo TH, Smith KD, Sato S, Rodriguez DJ, Holmes MA, Strong RK, Akira S, Aderem A.** 2004. Lipocalin 2 mediates an innate immune response to bacterial infection by sequestrating iron. *Nature* **432**:917–921.

60. **Hantke K, Nicholson G, Rabsch W, Winkelmann G.** 2003. Salmochelins, siderophores of *Salmonella enterica* and uropathogenic *Escherichia coli* strains, are recognized by the outer membrane receptor IroN. *Proc Natl Acad Sci USA* **100**:3677–3682.

61. **Raffatellu M, George MD, Akiyama Y, Hornsby MJ, Nuccio SP, Paixao TA, Butler BP, Chu H, Santos RL, Berger T, Mak TW, Tsolis RM, Bevins CL, Solnick JV, Dandekar S, Baumler AJ.** 2009. Lipocalin-2 resistance confers an advantage to *Salmonella enterica* serotype Typhimurium for growth and survival in the inflamed intestine. *Cell Host Microbe* **5**:476–486.

62. **Crouch ML, Castor M, Karlinsey JE, Kalhorn T, Fang FC.** 2008. Biosynthesis and IroC-dependent export of the siderophore salmochelin are essential for virulence of *Salmonella enterica* serovar Typhimurium. *Mol Microbiol* **67:**971–983.

63. **Drago-Serrano ME, Parra SG, Manjarrez-Hernandez HA.** 2006. EspC, an autotransporter protein secreted by enteropathogenic *Escherichia coli* (EPEC), displays protease activity on human hemoglobin. *FEMS Microbiol Lett* **265:**35–40.

64. **Porcheron G, Garenaux A, Proulx J, Sabri M, Dozois CM.** 2013. Iron, copper, zinc, and manganese transport and regulation in pathogenic *Enterobacteria*: correlations between strains, site of infection and the relative importance of the different metal transport systems for virulence. *Front Cell Infect Microbiol* **3:**90.

65. **Coates R, Moran J, Horsburgh MJ.** 2014. Staphylococci: colonizers and pathogens of human skin. *Future Microbiol* **9:**75–91.

66. **Lowy FD.** 1998. *Staphylococcus aureus* infections. *N Engl J Med* **339:**520–532.

67. **Skaar EP, Humayun M, Bae T, DeBord KL, Schneewind O.** 2004. Iron-source preference of *Staphylococcus aureus* infections. *Science* **305:**1626–1628.

68. **Hammer ND, Skaar EP.** 2011. Molecular mechanisms of *Staphylococcus aureus* iron acquisition. *Annu Rev Microbiol* **65:**129–147.

69. **Pishchany G, Dickey SE, Skaar EP.** 2009. Subcellular localization of the *Staphylococcus aureus* heme iron transport components IsdA and IsdB. *Infect Immun* **77:**2624–2634.

70. **Fabian M, Solomaha E, Olson JS, Maresso AW.** 2009. Heme transfer to the bacterial cell envelope occurs via a secreted hemophore in the Gram-positive pathogen *Bacillus anthracis*. *J Biol Chem* **284:**32138–32146.

71. **Honsa ES, Fabian M, Cardenas AM, Olson JS, Maresso AW.** 2011. The five near-iron transporter (NEAT) domain anthrax hemophore, IsdX2, scavenges heme from hemoglobin and transfers heme to the surface protein IsdC. *J Biol Chem* **286:**33652–33660.

72. **Maresso AW, Garufi G, Schneewind O.** 2008. *Bacillus anthracis* secretes proteins that mediate heme acquisition from hemoglobin. *PLoS Pathog* **4:**e1000132. doi:10.1371/journal.ppat.1000132.

73. **Andreini C, Banci L, Bertini I, Rosato A.** 2006. Zinc through the three domains of life. *J Proteome Res* **5:**3173–3178.

74. **Cerasi M, Ammendola S, Battistoni A.** 2013. Competition for zinc binding in the host-pathogen interaction. *Front Cell Infect Microbiol* **3:**108.

75. **Kehres DG, Maguire ME.** 2003. Emerging themes in manganese transport, biochemistry and pathogenesis in bacteria. *FEMS Microbiol Rev* **27:**263–290.

76. **Glaser R, Harder J, Lange H, Bartels J, Christophers E, Schroder JM.** 2005. Antimicrobial psoriasin (S100A7) protects human skin from *Escherichia coli* infection. *Nat Immunol* **6:**57–64.

77. **Corbin BD, Seeley EH, Raab A, Feldmann J, Miller MR, Torres VJ, Anderson KL, Dattilo BM, Dunman PM, Gerads R, Caprioli RM, Nacken W, Chazin WJ, Skaar EP.** 2008. Metal chelation and inhibition of bacterial growth in tissue abscesses. *Science* **319:**962–965.

78. **Damo SM, Kehl-Fie TE, Sugitani N, Holt ME, Rathi S, Murphy WJ, Zhang Y, Betz C, Hench L, Fritz G, Skaar EP, Chazin WJ.** 2013. Molecular basis for manganese sequestration by calprotectin and roles in the innate immune response to invading bacterial pathogens. *Proc Natl Acad Sci USA* **110:**3841–3846.

79. **Jabado N, Jankowski A, Dougaparsad S, Picard V, Grinstein S, Gros P.** 2000. Natural resistance to intracellular infections: natural resistance-associated macrophage protein 1 (Nramp1) functions as a pH-dependent manganese transporter at the phagosomal membrane. *J Exp Med* **192:**1237–1248.

80. **Begum NA, Kobayashi M, Moriwaki Y, Matsumoto M, Toyoshima K, Seya T.** 2002. *Mycobacterium bovis* BCG cell wall and lipopolysaccharide induce a novel gene, BIGM103, encoding a 7-TM protein: identification of a new protein family having Zn-transporter and Zn-metalloprotease signatures. *Genomics* **80:**630–645.

81. **Kitamura H, Morikawa H, Kamon H, Iguchi M, Hojyo S, Fukada T, Yamashita S, Kaisho T, Akira S, Murakami M, Hirano T.** 2006. Toll-like receptor-mediated regulation of zinc homeostasis influences dendritic cell function. *Nat Immunol* **7:**971–977.

82. **Kehl-Fie TE, Zhang Y, Moore JL, Farrand AJ, Hood MI, Rathi S, Chazin WJ, Caprioli RM, Skaar EP.** 2013. MntABC and MntH contribute to systemic *Staphylococcus aureus* infection by competing with calprotectin for nutrient manganese. *Infect Immun* **81:**3395–3405.

83. **Hood MI, Mortensen BL, Moore JL, Zhang Y, Kehl-Fie TE, Sugitani N, Chazin WJ, Caprioli RM, Skaar EP.** 2012. Identification of an *Acinetobacter baumannii* zinc acquisition system that facilitates resistance to calprotectin-

mediated zinc sequestration. *PLoS Pathog* **8:** e1003068. doi:10.1371/journal.ppat.1003068.

84. **Liu JZ, Jellbauer S, Poe AJ, Ton V, Pesciaroli M, Kehl-Fie TE, Restrepo NA, Hosking MP, Edwards RA, Battistoni A, Pasquali P, Lane TE, Chazin WJ, Vogl T, Roth J, Skaar EP, Raffatellu M.** 2012. Zinc sequestration by the neutrophil protein calprotectin enhances *Salmonella* growth in the inflamed gut. *Cell Host Microbe* **11:**227–239.

85. **Botella H, Peyron P, Levillain F, Poincloux R, Poquet Y, Brandli I, Wang C, Tailleux L, Tilleul S, Charriere GM, Waddell SJ, Foti M, Lugo-Villarino G, Gao Q, Maridonneau-Parini I, Butcher PD, Castagnoli PR, Gicquel B, de Chastellier C, Neyrolles O.** 2011. Mycobacterial p(1)-type ATPases mediate resistance to zinc poisoning in human macrophages. *Cell Host Microbe* **10:**248–259.

86. **Sabri M, Houle S, Dozois CM.** 2009. Roles of the extraintestinal pathogenic *Escherichia coli* ZnuACB and ZupT zinc transporters during urinary tract infection. *Infect Immun* **77:**1155–1164.

87. **Dupont CL, Grass G, Rensing C.** 2011. Copper toxicity and the origin of bacterial resistance: new insights and applications. *Metallomics* **3:** 1109–1118.

88. **Hodgkinson V, Petris MJ.** 2012. Copper homeostasis at the host-pathogen interface. *J Biol Chem* **287:**13549–13555.

89. **White C, Lee J, Kambe T, Fritsche K, Petris MJ.** 2009. A role for the ATP7A copper-transporting ATPase in macrophage bactericidal activity. *J Biol Chem* **284:**33949–33956.

90. **Macomber L, Imlay JA.** 2009. The iron-sulfur clusters of dehydratases are primary intracellular targets of copper toxicity. *Proc Natl Acad Sci USA* **106:**8344–8349.

91. **Djoko KY, Franiek JA, Edwards JL, Falsetta ML, Kidd SP, Potter AJ, Chen NH, Apicella MA, Jennings MP, McEwan AG.** 2012. Phenotypic characterization of a copA mutant of *Neisseria gonorrhoeae* identifies a link between copper and nitrosative stress. *Infect Immun* **80:**1065–1071.

92. **Samanovic MI, Ding C, Thiele DJ, Darwin KH.** 2012. Copper in microbial pathogenesis: meddling with the metal. *Cell Host Microbe* **11:**106–115.

93. **Gold B, Deng H, Bryk R, Vargas D, Eliezer D, Roberts J, Jiang X, Nathan C.** 2008. Identification of a copper-binding metallothionein in pathogenic mycobacteria. *Nat Chem Biol* **4:**609–616.

94. **Schwan WR, Warrener P, Keunz E, Stover CK, Folger KR.** 2005. Mutations in the cueA

gene encoding a copper homeostasis P-type ATPase reduce the pathogenicity of *Pseudomonas aeruginosa* in mice. *Int J Med Microbiol* **295:**237–242.

95. **Wolschendorf F, Ackart D, Shrestha TB, Hascall-Dove L, Nolan S, Lamichhane G, Wang Y, Bossmann SH, Basaraba RJ, Niederweis M.** 2011. Copper resistance is essential for virulence of *Mycobacterium tuberculosis*. *Proc Natl Acad Sci USA* **108:**1621–1626.

96. **Chaturvedi KS, Hung CS, Crowley JR, Stapleton AE, Henderson JP.** 2012. The siderophore yersiniabactin binds copper to protect pathogens during infection. *Nat Chem Biol* **8:**731–736.

97. **Abu Kwaik Y, Bumann D.** 2013. Microbial quest for food *in vivo*: "nutritional virulence" as an emerging paradigm. *Cell Microbiol* **15:** 882–890.

98. **Almagro-Moreno S, Boyd EF.** 2009. Sialic acid catabolism confers a competitive advantage to pathogenic *Vibrio cholerae* in the mouse intestine. *Infect Immun* **77:**3807–3816.

99. **Jeong HG, Oh MH, Kim BS, Lee MY, Han HJ, Choi SH.** 2009. The capability of catabolic utilization of N-acetylneuraminic acid, a sialic acid, is essential for *Vibrio vulnificus* pathogenesis. *Infect Immun* **77:**3209–3217.

100. **Almagro-Moreno S, Boyd EF.** 2010. Bacterial catabolism of nonulosonic (sialic) acid and fitness in the gut. *Gut Microbes* **1:**45–50.

101. **Soong G, Muir A, Gomez MI, Waks J, Reddy B, Planet P, Singh PK, Kaneko Y, Wolfgang MC, Hsiao YS, Tong L, Prince A.** 2006. Bacterial neuraminidase facilitates mucosal infection by participating in biofilm production. *J Clin Invest* **116:**2297–2305.

102. **Alkhuder K, Meibom KL, Dubail I, Dupuis M, Charbit A.** 2009. Glutathione provides a source of cysteine essential for intracellular multiplication of *Francisella tularensis*. *PLoS Pathog* **5:**e1000284. doi:10.1371/journal.ppat. 1000284.

103. **Scidmore MA.** 2011. Recent advances in *Chlamydia* subversion of host cytoskeletal and membrane trafficking pathways. *Microbes Infect* **13:**527–535.

104. **Derre I, Swiss R, Agaisse H.** 2011. The lipid transfer protein CERT interacts with the *Chlamydia* inclusion protein IncD and participates to ER-*Chlamydia* inclusion membrane contact sites. *PLoS Pathog* **7:**e1002092. doi:10.1371/journal.ppat.1002092.

105. **Elwell CA, Jiang S, Kim JH, Lee A, Wittmann T, Hanada K, Melancon P, Engel JN.** 2011. *Chlamydia trachomatis* co-opts GBF1 and CERT

to acquire host sphingomyelin for distinct roles during intracellular development. *PLoS Pathog* 7: e1002198. doi:10.1371/journal.ppat.1002198.

106. **Ouellette SP, Dorsey FC, Moshiach S, Cleveland JL, Carabeo RA.** 2011. *Chlamydia* species-dependent differences in the growth requirement for lysosomes. *PLoS One* 6:e16783. doi:10.1371/journal.pone.0016783.

107. **Ghigo E, Colombo MI, Heinzen RA.** 2012. The *Coxiella burnetii* parasitophorous vacuole. *Adv Exp Med Biol* 984:141–169.

108. **Heinzen RA, Scidmore MA, Rockey DD, Hackstadt T.** 1996. Differential interaction with endocytic and exocytic pathways distinguish parasitophorous vacuoles of *Coxiella burnetii* and *Chlamydia trachomatis*. *Infect Immun* 64:796–809.

109. **Isberg RR, O'Connor TJ, Heidtman M.** 2009. The *Legionella pneumophila* replication vacuole: making a cosy niche inside host cells. *Nat Rev Microbiol* 7:13–24.

110. **Price CT, Al-Quadan T, Santic M, Rosenshine I, Abu Kwaik Y.** 2011. Host proteasomal degradation generates amino acids essential for intracellular bacterial growth. *Science* 334:1553–1557.

111. **Bruckert WM, Price CT, Abu Kwaik Y.** 2014. Rapid nutritional remodeling of the host cell upon attachment of *Legionella pneumophila*. *Infect Immun* 82:72–82.

112. **Sauer JD, Bachman MA, Swanson MS.** 2005. The phagosomal transporter A couples threonine acquisition to differentiation and replication of *Legionella pneumophila* in macrophages. *Proc Natl Acad Sci USA* 102:9924–9929.

113. **Steele S, Brunton J, Ziehr B, Taft-Benz S, Moorman N, Kawula T.** 2013. *Francisella tularensis* harvests nutrients derived via ATG5-independent autophagy to support intracellular growth. *PLoS Pathog* 9:e1003562. doi:10.1371/journal.ppat.1003562.

114. **Niu H, Xiong Q, Yamamoto A, Hayashi-Nishino M, Rikihisa Y.** 2012. Autophagosomes induced by a bacterial Beclin 1 binding protein facilitate obligatory intracellular infection. *Proc Natl Acad Sci USA* 109:20800–20807.

115. **Stecher B, Hapfelmeier S, Muller C, Kremer M, Stallmach T, Hardt WD.** 2004. Flagella and chemotaxis are required for efficient induction of *Salmonella enterica* serovar Typhimurium colitis in streptomycin-pretreated mice. *Infect Immun* 72:4138–4150.

116. **Rivera-Chavez F, Winter SE, Lopez CA, Xavier MN, Winter MG, Nuccio SP, Russell JM, Laughlin RC, Lawhon SD, Sterzenbach T, Bevins CL, Tsolis RM, Harshey R, Adams LG, Baumler AJ.** 2013. *Salmonella* uses energy taxis to benefit from intestinal inflammation. *PLoS Pathog* 9:e1003267. doi:10.1371/journal.ppat.1003267.

117. **Sonnenburg JL, Xu J, Leip DD, Chen CH, Westover BP, Weatherford J, Buhler JD, Gordon JI.** 2005. Glycan foraging *in vivo* by an intestine-adapted bacterial symbiont. *Science* 307:1955–1959.

118. **Zhang YJ, Reddy MC, Ioerger TR, Rothchild AC, Dartois V, Schuster BM, Trauner A, Wallis D, Galaviz S, Huttenhower C, Sacchettini JC, Behar SM, Rubin EJ.** 2013. Tryptophan biosynthesis protects mycobacteria from CD4 T-cell-mediated killing. *Cell* 155:1296–1308.

119. **Schmidt SV, Schultze JL.** 2014. New insights into IDO biology in bacterial and viral infections. *Front Immunol* 5:384.

120. **MacKenzie CR, Gonzalez RG, Kniep E, Roch S, Daubener W.** 1999. Cytokine mediated regulation of interferon-gamma-induced IDO activation. *Adv Exp Med Biol* 467:533–539.

121. **Pearce EL, Pearce EJ.** 2013. Metabolic pathways in immune cell activation and quiescence. *Immunity* 38:633–643.

122. **Zarek PE, Powell JD.** 2007. Adenosine and anergy. *Autoimmunity* 40:425–432.

123. **Thiel M, Caldwell CC, Sitkovsky MV.** 2003. The critical role of adenosine A2A receptors in downregulation of inflammation and immunity in the pathogenesis of infectious diseases. *Microbes Infect* 5:515–526.

124. **Boucher HW, Corey GR.** 2008. Epidemiology of methicillin-resistant *Staphylococcus aureus*. *Clin Infect Dis* 46(Suppl 5):S344–S349.

125. **Thammavongsa V, Kern JW, Missiakas DM, Schneewind O.** 2009. *Staphylococcus aureus* synthesizes adenosine to escape host immune responses. *J Exp Med* 206:2417–2427.

126. **Chubukov V, Gerosa L, Kochanowski K, Sauer U.** 2014. Coordination of microbial metabolism. *Nat Rev Microbiol* 12:327–340.

127. **Fetherston JD, Mier I Jr, Truszczynska H, Perry RD.** 2012. The Yfe and Feo transporters are involved in microaerobic growth and virulence of *Yersinia pestis* in bubonic plague. *Infect Immun* 80:3880–3891.

Iron Acquisition Strategies of Bacterial Pathogens

3

JESSICA R. SHELDON,[1] HOLLY A. LAAKSO,[1] and DAVID E. HEINRICHS[1]

BIOLOGICAL IMPORTANCE OF IRON

Iron is essential to nearly all life forms on Earth, required for the proper function of enzymes involved in, for example, respiration, photosynthesis, the tricarboxylic acid cycle, nitrogen fixation, electron transport, and amino acid synthesis. The utility of iron in biological processes hinges on its chemical properties as a transition metal, engaging in single electron transfers to interconvert between the ferrous (Fe^{2+}) and ferric (Fe^{3+}) states. While this clearly makes iron advantageous, the same property provides the explanation for why excess, or "free," iron is inherently toxic. Ferrous iron–catalyzed Fenton chemistry results in the generation of the highly toxic hydroxyl radical (OH•) that can compromise cellular integrity through damage to lipids, proteins, and nucleic acids.

Aside from *Borrelia burgdorferi* and *Treponema pallidum*, iron is essential to all microbial pathogens, yet perhaps the most difficult issue facing pathogens is accessing enough iron to support growth. The concentration of iron under physiological conditions (10^{-8} to 10^{-9} M) is orders of magnitude below the $\sim 10^{-6}$ M required for bacterial growth, owing to the formation of insoluble ferric oxyhydroxide precipitates, and host sequestration mechanisms further

[1]Department of Microbiology and Immunology, University of Western Ontario, London, Ontario, Canada N6A 5C1.

Virulence Mechanisms of Bacterial Pathogens, 5th edition
Edited by Indira T. Kudva, Nancy A. Cornick, Paul J. Plummer, Qijing Zhang, Tracy L. Nicholson, John P. Bannantine, and Bryan H. Bellaire
© 2016 American Society for Microbiology, Washington, DC
doi:10.1128/microbiolspec.VMBF-0010-2015

decrease the available concentration to the range of $\sim 10^{-18}$ M. As such, iron plays a fundamental role in host-pathogen interactions, and coevolution has shaped both bacterial and host iron acquisition/sequestration mechanisms.

IRON METABOLISM IN HEALTH AND DISEASE

Host Iron Homeostasis

Perturbations to the balance of iron within the human body can impact both overall health and susceptibility to infectious disease. Sophisticated mechanisms thus exist to control the daily intake of iron that is required for metabolic processes and the synthesis of new erythrocytes. The majority of iron within the body is found intracellularly, in association with heme, a planar tetrapyrrole ring that coordinates a central ferrous iron ion, and is bound within proteins such as hemoglobin or myoglobin. Hemoglobin is typically contained within circulating erythrocytes, but during routine destruction of senescent cells, it is released into the blood. Although the levels of extracellular hemoglobin are usually low, rapid erythrocyte lysis triggered by pathological conditions can increase the concentration of free heme and hemoglobin to harmful levels. Free hemoglobin is thus scavenged by haptoglobin, whereas hemopexin is involved in sequestration of free heme. Through receptor-mediated endocytosis, hemoglobin-haptoglobin and heme-hemopexin complexes are taken up by macrophages or hepatocytes, and the bound iron can either be stored or returned to the iron cycle.

Dietary iron is taken up by enterocytes as either heme-iron or as ferrous iron through apical surface localized heme carrier protein (HCP)-1 or divalent metal transporter (DMT)-1, respectively. Ferric iron is first reduced to ferrous iron prior to uptake, and heme is degraded by heme oxygenase to release ferrous iron. Ferrous iron faces three potential fates inside the enterocyte: (i) utilization in cellular processes, (ii) sequestration in the multimeric, iron-storage protein, ferritin, or (iii) export from the cell into the circulation via ferroportin. Ferroportin is the only known iron exporter in humans, and it functions to mobilize iron primarily from enterocytes and macrophages for transport to sites of demand within the body. Ferrous iron effluxed by ferroportin is oxidized by hephaestin on the surface of enterocytes, and ceruloplasmin on nonintestinal cells and within the plasma, thus permitting iron-loading of transferrin, which has poor affinity for Fe^{2+}.

Iron-Withholding as a Facet of Innate Immunity

Transferrin is an abundant serum glycoprotein capable of reversibly coordinating two molecules of Fe^{3+} with very high affinity ($K_d = 10^{23}$ M^{-1} at neutral pH). Transferrin is invaluable to iron homeostasis in humans, because it delivers iron to various cells but also scavenges free iron in the bloodstream, essentially sequestering it from invading pathogens. The transferrin-like glycoprotein lactoferrin is commonly found extracellularly in secretions and intracellularly in the secondary granules of neutrophils. Lactoferrin functions to sequester iron at mucosal surfaces and is released from neutrophils at infectious foci, thus participating in the host defense against invading microbes.

Many dynamic processes exist within the host to restrict the iron available to pathogens. The withholding of iron, and other essential metals, is referred to as "nutritional immunity" and functions as a key component of innate immunity. Much of this response is orchestrated by the human hormone hepcidin, which is secreted by the liver and directly regulates the internalization and degradation of ferroportin. Hepcidin is released primarily in response to excess levels of extracellular iron, either to combat transferrin saturation or as part of the inflammatory response. With the degradation of ferroportin, iron is stored intracellularly, dietary iron uptake is halted, and iron release from macrophages is stopped. Overall, this process may result in a decrease in serum levels by as much as 30%, and when triggered by invading microbes, is referred to as the "hypoferremia of infection."

To combat infection by intracellular pathogens, the natural resistance macrophage protein 1 functions to export iron and other essential metals from the phagosomal compartment. Natural resistance macrophage protein 1 is also involved in the release of neutrophil gelatinase-associated lipocalin (NGAL; also known as siderocalin, lipocalin 2, and 24p3), an acute-phase protein secreted primarily by neutrophils that scavenges catechol-type siderophores produced by bacteria. NGAL binds enterobactin, a siderophore widely synthesized by the *Enterobacteriaceae*, and NGAL-deficient ($NGAL^{-/-}$) mice are hypersusceptible to Gram-negative bacterial infections (1). Despite lacking an intrinsic ability to bind iron, NGAL appears to function primarily in the maintenance of extracellular and intracellular iron concentrations within the host. The transport of iron by NGAL is purportedly aided by the mammalian siderophore, 2,5-dihydroxybenzoic acid (2,5-DHBA), which is structurally similar to the 2,3-DHBA iron-binding moiety of enterobactin (2, 3). 2,5-DHBA likely scavenges free iron and, when bound to NGAL, may be effectively shuttled across cellular membranes (2). Notably, 2,5-DHBA is capable of promoting growth of *Escherichia coli* in a mammalian model, so it is not surprising that synthesis of 2,5-DHBA is downregulated during infection, freeing NGAL to bind to bacterial siderophores.

Hereditary Diseases Compromising Iron-Withholding Within the Host

Although iron homeostasis is stringently controlled, many hereditary disease states, as well as excess exposure to the element, can result in an imbalance in iron levels, impacting both the overall health of the host and susceptibility to infectious disease. The most common genetic disease influencing host iron metabolism is hereditary hemochromatosis, which is largely caused by defects to the gene encoding human hemochromatosis protein, *HFE* (for high Fe). Although the exact molecular mechanisms governing hereditary hemochromatosis are still unclear, recent insights suggest that HFE is involved in iron-sensing and the regulation of hepcidin production (4). HFE is thought to participate in the formation of an iron-sensing complex, which in the presence of high levels of holo-transferrin activates a signal cascade promoting transcription of the gene encoding hepcidin (*HAMP*) (5). Deactivation of this regulatory complex and/or cascade results in inadequate production of hepcidin, leading to excessive intestinal iron absorption and recycling (6). The net result of the aforementioned dysregulation is abnormally high levels of free iron within the body, broadly referred to as iron overload.

Other less common hereditary iron overload diseases are principally associated with genetic defects in the genes encoding ceruloplasmin (*CP*) and transferrin (*TF*), which result in aceruloplasminemia and atransferrinemia/hypotransferrinemia, respectively (7). The absence of ceruloplasmin impairs the ability of ferroportin to export iron in cells lacking an alternate ferroxidase (e.g., hephaestin), as is the case with astrocytes of the central nervous system, which leads to iron accumulation in the brain and progressive neurodegeneration (8). Reduced or absent serum transferrin similarly impairs the trafficking of iron throughout the body, as well as the production of hepcidin (as discussed above), leading to accretion primarily within the liver and heart. Further, inadequate iron delivery to hematopoietic cells in the bone marrow by transferrin results in decreased hemoglobin availability, leading to anemia (9). The symptoms of hereditary hemo-

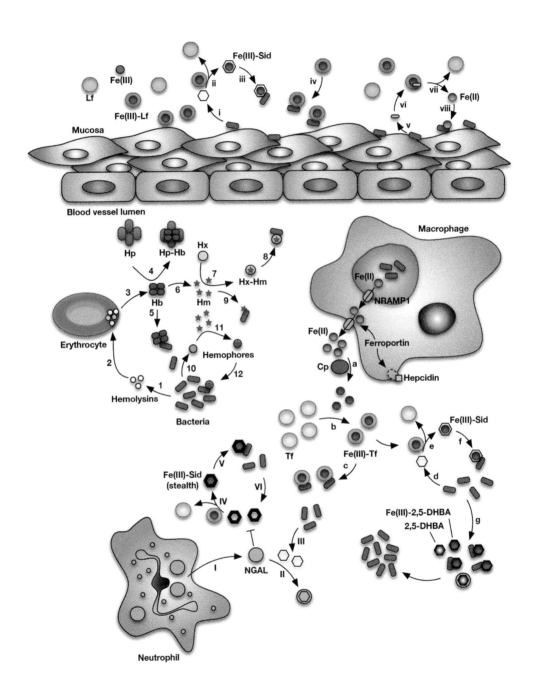

chromatosis and aceruloplasminemia are most effectively delayed or reduced through phlebotomy and/or chelation therapy (5, 10), while atransferrinemia/hypotransferrinemia is managed primarily through transfusion of whole blood or purified apo-transferrin (11). Not only do diseases impacting host iron homeostasis enhance the risk of severe and invasive infections, but often so do their clinical interventions. Indeed, while thalassemia and sickle cell disease (SCD) can result in iron overload, it is often the treatment for these conditions that leads to hyperferremia. Both thalassemia and SCD are characterized by the abnormal formation of adult hemoglobin, a heterotetramer comprised of two α-globin subunits and two β-globin subunits. In thalassemia, genetic defects can impact the synthesis of either of the globin subunits (α-thalassemia and β-thalassemia), resulting in ineffective erythropoiesis and accelerated hemolysis of existing erythrocytes (12). SCD is due specifically to a single amino acid change in the β-globin subunit, which results in the polymerization of hemoglobin tetramers into rigid fibers and gives rise to the sickle-shaped erythrocytes from which the disorder derives its name (13, 14). Sickle cells are inherently fragile, and their instability contributes to the development of hemolytic anemia. As with thalassemia, the symptoms of SCD may be treated with frequent blood transfusions, which enhances not only the risk of iron overload, but also the frequency and severity of bacterial and fungal infections.

To reduce iron content in patients suffering iron overload, treatment can include phlebotomy or chelation therapy. Deferoxamine mesylate, the mesylate salt derivative of the microbial siderophore desferrioxamine B, is frequently used for chelation therapy. Deferoxamine mesylate, however, can promote more severe infection by some bacteria, including *Yersinia* spp., *Klebsiella* spp., and *Staphylococcus aureus* (15–17), which are able to use the siderophore as a source of iron.

OVERVIEW OF BACTERIAL IRON ACQUISITION STRATEGIES

Even within the healthy host, bacterial invaders that scavenge enough iron have the potential to cause infection. Iron has ultimately driven an evolutionary arms race between microbes in pursuit of this essential element and hosts striving to withhold it from them. In effect, for every mechanism

FIGURE 1 The host versus pathogen battle for iron. Cartoon representation of the various strategies used by the host to sequester iron from invading pathogens and the counter strategies used by pathogens to obtain host iron. On mucosal surfaces, lactoferrin sequesters iron, yet bacteria can obtain iron from lactoferrin by secreting siderophores (i to iii), directly binding lactoferrin (iv), or by secreting reductases (pink pill) that reduce iron from FeIII to FeII, releasing it from lactoferrin (v to viii). Bacteria can obtain iron bound to heme by secreting hemolysins which release intracellular hemoglobin and heme into the blood. While the host uses hemoglobin- and heme-scavenging proteins to sequester these iron sources, bacteria have mechanisms to counter these systems (1 to 12). Macrophages move iron from the phagosome and the cell using natural resistance macrophage protein 1 and ferroportin, respectively, to keep iron from intracellular pathogens. In response to binding by the iron homeostasis hormone hepcidin, membrane-bound ferroportin is degraded, thus withholding iron in intracellular compartments. FeII that is secreted is rapidly oxidized by ceruloplasmin (Cp), and the FeIII is quickly picked up by transferrin (a, b). Transferrin-bound iron is scavenged by bacteria using transferrin-binding proteins (c) or through secretion of siderophores (d to f). Bacteria can also obtain iron using the mammalian siderophore 2,5-DHBA (g). Neutrophils secrete NGAL (also known as siderocalin, lipocalin 2, or 24p3) (I) which serves to capture some bacterial siderophores (II, III). Some bacteria synthesize and secrete stealth siderophores which are not bound by NGAL and can remove transferrin-bound iron even in the presence of NGAL (IV to VI). Lf, lactoferrin; Tf, transferrin; sid, siderophore; Hp, haptoglobin; Hx, hemopexin; Hb, hemoglobin; Hm, heme; Cp, ceruloplasmin.

employed by the host to sequester iron, bacterial pathogens have evolved mechanisms to circumvent this withholding strategy (see Fig. 1). Accordingly, a diverse array of iron acquisition strategies exist among bacterial pathogens, some of which are highly conserved and broadly employed, while others are highly specific and intricately linked to the pathophysiology of a given bacterium. Broadly, and as summarized in Fig. 1, the mechanisms for iron uptake by pathogenic bacteria include (i) the extraction and capture of heme-iron from host hemoproteins through the use of secreted proteins or cell surface–associated receptors, (ii) the acquisition of transferrin and lactoferrin-bound iron through specific surface-associated binding proteins or the secretion of siderophores, and (iii) the uptake of free inorganic iron facilitated by ferric iron reductases and associated ferrous iron permeases. Later in the chapter, the mechanisms by which pathogens acquire iron within the host are discussed, with a focus on how these mechanisms are known to impact the virulence of bacterial pathogens.

Coordinated Regulation of Iron Acquisition and Virulence Gene Expression

Iron, or lack thereof, is a fundamental sensory cue in bacterial pathogens, and it triggers the coordinated regulation of genes involved in both iron acquisition and virulence. The response to iron deprivation in prokaryotes is largely controlled by two separate families of highly conserved, iron-responsive regulators that repress transcription of iron acquisition genes when the concentration of intracellular iron is high and alleviate this repression when iron is limiting. In Gram-negative bacteria, and the low–guanine and cytosine (G+C)–content Gram-positive *Firmicutes*, such as *Staphylococcus* spp., *Bacillus* spp., and *Listeria monocytogenes*, iron homeostasis is controlled by members of the ferric uptake regulator (Fur) superfamily

(18). The high-G+C-content Gram-positive *Actinobacteria*, *Corynebacterium diphtheriae*, and *Mycobacterium* spp., utilize an alternative iron-responsive regulator, the d̲iphtheria t̲ox̲in r̲epressor (DtxR; IdeR in the *Mycobacteriaceae*) to mediate both iron uptake and virulence gene expression (19). Notably, while little primary sequence similarity exists between members of these two families, Fur and DtxR-like proteins possess similar domain architecture and function in a comparable manner. In brief, both Fur and DtxR are homodimeric metalloregulators that bear an N-terminal helix-turn-helix DNA-binding domain and a C-terminal metal corepressor binding site that also functions in dimerization of the protein (18, 20). Coordination of Fe^{2+} within each protein subunit induces a conformational change rendering the iron-loaded repressor proficient for DNA binding, which occurs at a consensus sequence located within the promoter/operator region of the targeted gene (18, 21–23). Association of $Fur\text{-}Fe^{2+}$ or $DtxR\text{-}Fe^{2+}$ with the operator of iron-responsive genes effectively bars RNA polymerase from binding the promoter, thereby inhibiting transcription under iron-replete conditions. When intracellular iron concentrations are low, the metal is no longer readily available to interact with the repressor, the complex dissociates from DNA, and transcription proceeds.

The overwhelming majority of iron acquisition strategies employed by bacterial pathogens, and discussed herein, are wholly or at least partially regulated by members of the Fur or DtxR superfamilies. In addition to their role in iron acquisition, Fur and DtxR both play a key role in virulence and have been shown to directly or indirectly (e.g., through small Fur/DtxR-regulated RNAs) control the expression of factors contributing to pathogenicity, including the secretion of toxins, production of adhesins, formation of biofilms, and regulation of quorum sensing (24, 25). Indeed, DtxR was initially identified, as its name implies, as an iron-dependent negative regulator of diphtheria toxin production in *C. diphtheriae* (22, 26). Further, both Fur and DtxR have been demonstrated, through relevant *in vivo* models, to influence the colonization, survival, and/or proliferation of numerous bacterial pathogens within the host including, but not limited to, *S. aureus*, *Helicobacter pylori*, *Haemophilus influenzae*, *L. monocytogenes*, *Campylobacter jejuni*, *Vibrio cholerae*, and *Mycobacterium tuberculosis* (for reviews see 26, 27). The role of these metalloregulatory proteins *in vivo* no doubt is complex and multifactorial, but it appears to reflect a common strategy employed by bacterial pathogens in order to respond appropriately upon sensing their transition into the iron-limited host.

ACCESSING HEME IRON

While bacterial pathogens express a plethora of iron acquisition systems, capable of exploiting a multitude of host iron sources, heme represents a particularly auspicious target because it comprises approximately 75% of the total mammalian iron pool. Indeed, heme is a preferred iron source for pathogens such as *S. aureus* (28) and an obligate requirement for heme auxotrophs including staphylococcal small colony variants (29), *Bartonella* spp., *Bacteroides* spp., *Porphyromonas gingivalis*, and *H. influenzae* (30). Because heme exists primarily in association with hemoglobin within circulating erythrocytes, invading pathogens have evolved sophisticated mechanisms to access heme from intracellular hemoproteins. The secretion of hemolysins is a tactic commonly employed by extracellular and facultative intracellular pathogens to enhance local heme availability. Indeed, the expression of such cytolytic factors is often induced under conditions of iron starvation and during bacteremia and has long been recognized as an important multifactorial determinant of pathogenicity in many bacteria (31).

Upon its release from damaged erythrocytes, hemoglobin, or spontaneously dissociated heme, may be captured by bacteria expressing specific secreted and/or cell surface–associated heme/hemoglobin-binding proteins. Additionally, some pathogens are capable of extracting heme from heme-iron complexes such as heme-hemopexin, hemoglobin-haptoglobin, and serum albumin, thus subverting the efforts of these host iron sequestration proteins in withholding iron from microbial invaders. In this section, archetypical heme acquisition systems will be discussed, as will be less-conserved methods employed by specific pathogens (see also Table 1).

Extracellular Mechanisms of Heme Capture

In a number of bacterial pathogens, the acquisition of extracellular heme as a cofactor or iron source is initiated by the synthesis and secretion of small, soluble, heme-binding proteins referred to as hemophores (32). Hemophores are capable of both capturing free heme and appropriating it from various hemoproteins. Hemophore-bound heme is subsequently transferred to specific heme-binding receptor proteins localized on the outer membrane in Gram-negative bacteria or the cell wall in Gram-positive bacteria, both of which help mediate uptake through the cell envelope. To date, two major types of hemophores have been characterized: the HasA-type hemophores of Gram-negative pathogens and the <u>near</u> iron <u>transporter</u> (NEAT)–domain containing hemophores of Gram-positive pathogens. Additionally, the heme auxotrophic bacteria *H. influenzae* and *P. gingivalis* each produce a distinct hemophore-like protein, HxuA and HmuY (33, 34), respectively, to help fulfill their obligate metabolic requirements for heme. Each hemophore possesses unique mechanisms for export, acquisition of heme, and transfer of heme to the cell surface prior to uptake.

TABLE 1 Examples of heme acquisition systems essential for virulence

Bacterium	Heme system	Model[a]	Reference[b]
Bacillus anthracis	Isd	Mouse (i.t.)	275
Bordetella pertussis	Bhu	Mouse (i.n.)	276
Escherichia coli	Chu	Mouse (t.u.)	277
Haemophilus influenzae	Hbp	Mouse (i.p.)	278
Listeria monocytogenes	Hup	Mouse (i.v.)	279
Neisseria meningitidis	HmbR	Rat (i.p.)	280
Staphylococcus aureus	Isd	Mouse (i.v.)	128
Streptococcus pyogenes	Shr	Zebrafish (i.m.)	281
Vibrio vulnificus	Hup	Mouse (i.p.)	282

[a]i.t., intratracheal; i.n., intranasal; t.u., transurethral; i.p., intraperitoneal; i.v., intravenous; i.m., intramuscular.
[b]Due to space limitations, we cite only one reference even though there are multiple studies published in many cases.

HasA-type hemophores of Gram-negative pathogens

HasA (for h̲eme a̲cquisition s̲ystem) of *Serratia marcescens* was the first extracellular heme-binding protein to be isolated and characterized within the bacterial domain (35). HasA-homologous hemophores have since been identified in a number of pathogenic or opportunistically pathogenic bacteria including *Pseudomonas aeruginosa, Pseudomonas fluorescens, Yersinia pestis, Yersinia pseudotuberculosis, Yersinia enterocolitica,* and the soft rot-causing plant pathogens *Pectobacterium carotovorum* and *Pectobacterium atrosepticum* (32). HasA-type proteins lack significant sequence homology to other known proteins, and indeed to other types of hemophores, but display a high degree of structural conservation within the family. HasA of *S. marcescens* (HasA$_{SM}$) and *P. aeruginosa* (HasA$_{PA}$) have been structurally characterized and are nearly identical globular monomeric proteins with a unique α/β fold, capable of coordinating a single molecule of ferric heme with very high affinity (HasA$_{SM}$; K_d = 1.8 × 10^{-11} M) (36). Common to substrates of type I secretion systems, these hemophores possess a C-terminal export motif and are transported to the external milieu by a dedicated ATP-binding cassette (ABC) exporter (37). Upon secretion, HasA-type hemophores are capable of acquiring heme from a broad range of host hemoproteins including hemoglobin, hemopexin, and myoglobin (38), but the means by which HasA facilitates heme acquisition is currently a matter of debate. The broad substrate range of HasA, and its ability to nondiscriminately acquire heme from hemoglobin of unrelated organisms (e.g., human and bovine, leghemoglobin from leguminous plants) (32, 38), supports the notion that HasA acquires heme without direct interaction with these hemoproteins (38).

Upon binding at the cell surface, holo-HasA is not internalized but, rather, transfers heme to an iron-regulated, outer membrane receptor protein for import (HasR) (Fig. 2) (39, 40). The hemophore is known to complex tightly with HasR, although the mechanism of heme transfer between the two is not yet fully understood (41, 42). HasR binds heme with lower affinity than HasA (39), and the binding of holo-HasA to the receptor is thought to induce conformational changes that successively weaken the binding of heme to HasA (43). Heme binding by HasR is mediated by two highly conserved histidine residues (44), found in numerous other outer membrane heme receptor proteins including HemR of *Y. enterocolitica* (45), ShuA of *Shigella dysenteriae* (46), and HmuR of *P. gingivalis* (47). Notably, HasR can independently mediate the uptake of free and hemoglobin-bound heme, but HasR and HasA function synergistically to enhance

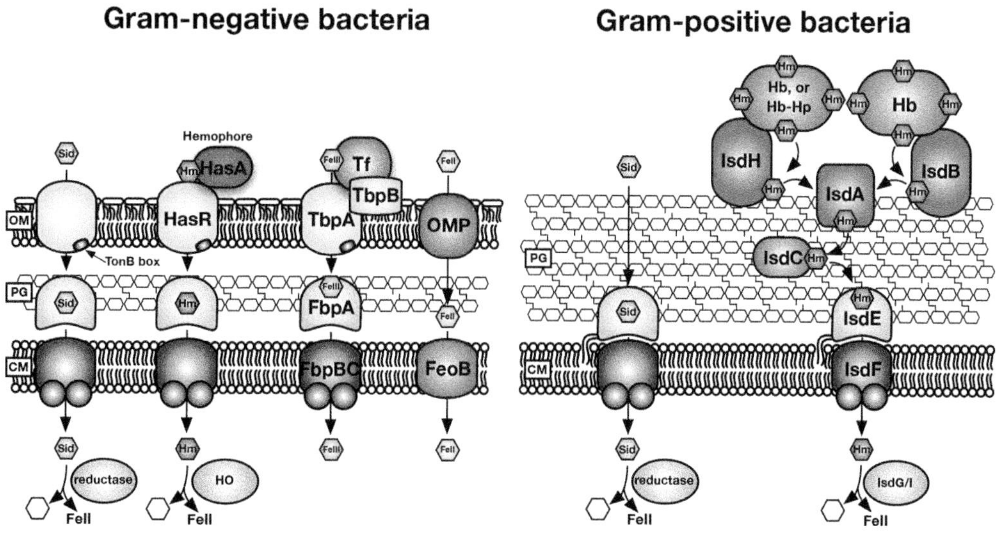

FIGURE 2 **Model of iron uptake mechanisms in Gram-negative and Gram-positive bacteria. Diagrams depicting the envelope proteins required for the uptake of iron, or iron scavenged from siderophores, heme, or transferrin. This is a composite diagram and represents mechanisms used by many pathogenic bacteria, as described in the text. OM, outer membrane; PG, peptidoglycan; CM, cytoplasmic membrane; sid, FeIII-siderophore; Hm, heme; Tf, transferrin; OMP, outer membrane porin; HO, heme oxygenase; Hb, hemoglobin; Hp, haptoglobin. Adapted by permission from Macmillan Publishers Ltd: Nature Reviews Microbiology (274), copyright 2012.**

heme uptake by approximately 100-fold over the outer membrane receptor alone (48).

HasR is a member of the TonB-dependent transporter (TBDT) family (Fig. 3). The uptake of heme by TBDTs is an energetic process driven by TonB and the proton motive force or, in the case of the *has* system of *S. marcescens*, the HasR-specific TonB ortholog, HasB (49, 50). In addition to the expected negative regulation by iron and Fur, expression of the *has* operon is further modulated by heme and extracytoplasmic function sigma (σ) and anti-σ factors (HasI and HasS, respectively), through a signal cascade induced by the binding of heme-loaded HasA to HasR (51–53). Despite the known regulation of *has* by heme, it is not known how expression of this hemophore-based heme acquisition system influences the *in vivo* survival and virulence of pathogens in which it is employed. Indeed, to date, the role of *has* has been assessed solely in a murine model of bubonic plague, where it was

shown that neither *has* nor the hemin uptake system, *hmu* (discussed below), are required for the pathogenicity of *Y. pestis* under the conditions assessed (54).

HxuA, a Gram-negative pseudohemophore
Restricted to members of the *Pasteurellaceae* and characterized only in *H. influenzae* type b (Hib) and unencapsulated nontypeable *H. influenzae* (NTHi) isolates, the heme-hemopexin utilization protein, HxuA, contrasts with HasA-type hemophores in its extremely limited range of substrate specificity and its means of facilitating heme acquisition (33, 55, 56). HxuA bears an N-terminal signal peptide and belongs to a two-partner secretion system, where export of the "pseudohemophore" is mediated by the outer membrane partner protein, HxuB (57, 58). Depending upon the strain, Hxu A is either anchored to the outer membrane or at least partially released into the supernatant, whereupon it facilitates the release

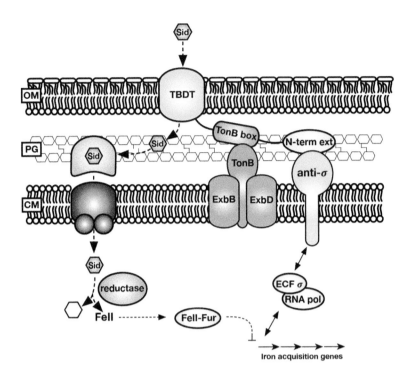

FIGURE 3 Model of TonB-dependent transport in Gram-negative bacteria. An iron-siderophore complex (blue hexagon) entering through a TonB-dependent transporter (TBDT) in the outer membrane (OM). Although the transport of an iron siderophore complex is shown here, iron, or other iron complexes, use similar uptake mechanisms (e.g., FeIII, heme) (see Fig. 1). Movement through the TBDT requires an interaction of the TonB box (located near the N-terminus of the TBDT sequence) with the TonB protein, with the energy for conformational changes provided by the proton motive force captured by the ExbB and ExbD proteins. Once in the periplasm, the iron-loaded siderophore complex is recognized by a substrate-binding protein which delivers the complex to an ABC transporter in the cytoplasmic membrane (CM). Depending on the particular system, iron is released from the siderophore in the cytoplasm by either destruction of the siderophore or reduction on the metal (as shown). Intracellular iron, via Fur, negatively regulates transcription of genes encoding high-affinity iron acquisition systems. In some TBDTs, an N-terminal extension is present to provide an extra layer of control of gene expression, in addition to Fur. This involves an anti-σ factor and extracytoplasmic function σ-factor, allowing for gene expression in response to the uptake of particular iron chelates. Modified with permission from Annual Review of Microbiology, volume 64 © by Annual Reviews, http://www.annualreviews.org. See Noinaj et al. (91).

of heme solely from heme-hemopexin complexes (59). Although the exact mechanism by which HxuA liberates heme from heme-hemopexin is unknown, it differs from HasA in that direct protein-protein interactions are required (56, 60). Further, by strict definition, HxuA is not a hemophore, because it lacks a specific heme-binding domain. Instead, HxuA appears to release heme from heme-hemopexin for capture by HxuC, a TBDT (60). Similar to HasR, HxuC is capa-

ble of mediating heme uptake independently of HxuA and is additionally capable of acquiring heme from serum albumin and hemoglobin (61, 62). The role of *hxuA* and *hxuB* in *H. influenzae* heme-iron acquisition should not be overlooked, however, because both are essential to the utilization of heme-hemopexin by this heme auxotroph (57). Further, the Hxu-encoding locus, *hxuCBA*, has been implicated in *H. influenzae* pathogenicity, because strains lacking this operon are less virulent in an infant rat model of hematogenous meningitis (61). Interestingly, the expression of HxuA, as well as transferrin-binding proteins A and B (TbpA and TbpB, respectively), has been detected in middle ear aspirates of children afflicted with otitis media (63), although further investigation is required to fully elucidate the role of *hxuCBA* in the utilization of heme-hemopexin by *H. influenzae* during infection.

NEAT domains and NEAT-containing Gram-positive hemophores

The hemophores of *Bacillus anthracis*, IsdX1 and IsdX2, are components of an iron-regulated surface determinant (Isd) pathway (64, 65) that includes cell surface–associated proteins involved in the acquisition and transfer of heme-iron through the Gram-positive cell wall. Heme coordination by IsdX1 and IsdX2 is mediated by NEAT domains, of which IsdX1 has one and IsdX2 has five (64, 65). NEAT domains were first identified in genetic loci encoding for putative ferric iron transporters (66), although it has since been revealed that these diverse ~120-amino-acid-residue sequences actually encode for discrete modules involved in heme and/or hemoprotein binding, heme extraction, and NEAT:NEAT-mediated heme transfer (67–69). NEAT domains are found in both pathogenic and nonpathogenic members of the phylum *Firmicutes* and, while lacking conformity in their amino acid sequences, are highly conserved at a structural level. A prototypical NEAT domain is comprised of eight β-strands and a small α-helix, which together fold to form a hydrophobic pocket in which heme may be bound (67). Heme coordination by a NEAT domain is mediated by a conserved YXXXY motif, where preservation of the first tyrosine residue reliably predicts heme-binding functionality (70). The mechanisms of hemoprotein-binding and heme extraction by NEAT domains appear to differ between organisms but have been most extensively explored for the Isd system of *S. aureus* (see below).

Each NEAT domain of IsdX1 and IsdX2 of *B. anthracis* has been functionally characterized, and together, both hemophores are capable of liberating heme from hemoglobin, binding heme through NEAT domains possessing the aforementioned YXXXY motif, and transferring extracted heme to the cell wall–associated heme-binding protein, IsdC, for eventual uptake (64, 65, 71, 72). Unlike the heme-extracting Isd proteins of *S. aureus* (IsdB and IsdH), where NEAT domains function synergistically in extracting heme from hemoglobin, the sole NEAT domain of IsdX1 appears to independently fulfill this task (65). Further, IsdX1 is capable of transferring heme to IsdX2 and, while heme transfer between two hemophores may seem counter-intuitive, it has been suggested that the multiple heme-binding domains of IsdX2 may serve to sequester heme when present in excess and thus limit the rate of uptake (71, 72). Alternatively, given that IsdX2 is partially cell wall–associated, it is possible that this hemophore doubles as a surface receptor for heme.

Encoded from an otherwise uncharacterized Isd-like locus, *L. monocytogenes* expresses two NEAT domain–containing, heme-extracting proteins: hemin-binding proteins 1 and 2 (Hbp1 and Hbp2), respectively (12, 73). Apart from the hemophores of *B. anthracis*, Hbp2 is the only other hemophore conclusively identified in the Gram-positive pathogens. While Hbp1 is thought to be cell wall–associated, Hbp2 is both secreted as a true hemophore and, to a lesser extent, anchored to the cell surface (12, 73). In the current model, heme is extracted from hemoglobin or captured from the external milieu by Hbp2, using a unique coordination method not involving the YXXXY motif, and is subsequently transferred to surface-associated Hbp2 or Hbp1 for uptake (73). Hbp1 and Hbp2 both have a high affinity for heme and hemoglobin, suggesting that, as with other Isd-like systems, they are advantageous at physiological concentrations (nM range) (12, 73). The means by which heme delivered by Hbp2 is transported through the listerial cell envelope is not known, but likely it occurs in a manner analogous to other Isd-containing bacteria and/or may involve the uncharacterized heme/hemoglobin-uptake ABC transporter, HupDGC (73).

HmuY and the gingipain proteases: a collaborative system for heme acquisition in *P. gingivalis*

Iron acquisition by the Gram-negative, oral anaerobe *P. gingivalis* is a fascinating and complex example of how pathogens have evolved unique iron uptake mechanisms central to their distinct pathophysiology. *P. gingivalis* is a key etiological agent of periodontitis, a disease characterized by inflammation, bleeding, and degradation of the tissues supporting teeth. The destructive process initiated by *P. gingivalis* leads to the formation of periodontal pockets suffused with an inflammatory exudate containing iron complexes including transferrin, serum albumin, hemoglobin, haptoglobin, and heme-hemopexin (74). *P. gingivalis*, despite lacking endogenous siderophores, grows robustly within these pockets due to a versatile means of accessing heme (75). Indeed, heme is essential to the virulence of *P. gingivalis*, not only because it is incapable of synthesizing protoporphyrin IX (PPIX), but also because heme is a fundamental component of the black pigment employed by the bacterium, purportedly to protect against peroxide stress (76). Heme acquisition in *P. gingivalis* is distinctively aided by the secretion of arginine- and lysine-specific cysteine proteases (RgpA and RgpB, and Kgp, respectively), collectively referred to as "gingipains." Additionally, these gingipains contribute to the inflammation and tissue destruction characteristic of periodontitis, promote adherence to epithelial cells, and assist in multispecies biofilm development and thus, are multifactorial virulence determinants of *P. gingivalis* (77). Both RgpA and Kgp are multidomain proteins consisting of an N-terminal proteolytic domain and C-terminal hemagglutinin domain.

In a cooperative fashion, gingipains act first to oxidize heme within hemoglobin through RgpA, which functions both to reduce the affinity of hemoglobin for bound heme and to render the resulting methemoglobin more susceptible to proteolysis by Kgp (78, 79). Heme released through this sequential proteolytic degradation is then rapidly sequestered by the lipoprotein hemophore, HmuY (for heme utilization), and is transported into the periplasm by the cognate TBDT, HmuR (80). HmuY is found both attached to the outer membrane and released to the external milieu as a classical hemophore, where it is proposed that Kgp is responsible for cleaving the protein from the surface of the cell (34). HmuY is additionally capable of independently capturing free heme and removing heme directly from methemoglobin and methemalbumin (81), thus highlighting its utility in accessing heme sources commonly encountered by the pathogen. Further, the gingipains nonspecifically degrade other host iron-containing proteins, including haptoglobin, hemopexin, transferrin, and albumin, as a source of both iron and peptides (82), suggesting that together with the HmuY hemophore, these proteases play a crucial role in the survival and virulence of *P. gingivalis* within its discrete host niche. The mechanism for translocation of heme into the cytosol of *P. gingivalis* is not known, but it is proposed that genes within the *hmuYRSTUV* locus encode for a heme-specific ABC-type transporter (83).

Other secreted proteases as putative liberators of heme

As demonstrated for the gingipain proteases of *P. gingivalis*, the secretion of proteolytic enzymes capable of degrading host heme-iron complexes would be a valuable asset to pathogens, particularly those lacking dedicated systems for the acquisition of iron or heme from these substrates. The prevalence of secreted hemoprotein proteases may perhaps be underappreciated and, outside of *P. gingivalis*, have only been marginally characterized in pathogenic strains of *E. coli.* As members of the diverse serine protease autotransporter of *Enterobacteriaceae* (SPATE) family, these enzymes possess an N-terminal leader peptide that targets them to the periplasm via type V secretion, a functional passenger domain carrying a serine protease motif, and a C-terminal translocator domain, which forms a β-barrel in the outer membrane and allows for external release of the passenger domain through proteolytic cleavage (84). The passenger domain of hemoglobin protease and enteropathogenic *E. coli* secreted protein C (EspC) is thought to facilitate both hemoglobin degradation and heme-binding in enteropathogenic *E. coli* (85, 86), suggesting that they function like hemophores. The observed *in vitro* activity of hemoglobin protease and EspC in heme-iron extraction, however, has not been confirmed, nor has a TBDT that interacts with hemoglobin protease or EspC been identified. The expression of hemoglobin protease by *E. coli* has been implicated, however, in the development of cospecies intra-abdominal abscesses with *Bacteroides fragilis,* a heme auxotroph, through what is thought to be pathogenic synergy; *B. fragilis* provides fibrin deposition that facilitates abscess development and immune evasion, whereas *E. coli* liberates heme from hemoglobin via hemoglobin protease for utilization by both bacteria (87). The exploitation of heme liberated from host complexes by heterologous microorganisms is a potentially important facet of polymicrobial infections.

Heme Capture at the Cell Surface

A universal mechanism for iron transport through the Gram-negative cell envelope

The outer membrane in Gram-negative bacteria serves as a coarse selective barrier, restricting potentially toxic compounds, such as antibiotics, from unfettered access to the periplasmic space. Porins allow for the non-specific diffusion of small (<600 kDa), hydrophilic molecules and ions, including Fe^{2+} (Fig. 2), through the outer membrane, while the uptake of some nutrients, including disaccharides, nucleosides, and phosphates, occurs through facilitated diffusion (88). In contrast, the uptake of larger molecules and/or those present at exceedingly low concentrations in the extracellular milieu requires dedicated high-affinity, energy-dependent transporters to traverse the outer membrane (88, 89). Iron complexes, such as heme, transferrin, and most siderophores, exceed the size exclusion criteria for unimpeded diffusion across the outer membrane, and thus, the uptake of iron from these substrates is invariably facilitated by iron-regulated, TonB-dependent outer membrane receptors (Fig. 2 and Fig. 3).

Structure, function, and regulation of TonB-dependent transporters

As discussed above for hemophores, specific outer membrane receptors in Gram-negative bacteria serve as the recipients of heme, either through transfer from hemophores or directly from the external environment, whereupon they facilitate the transport of heme, intact, into the periplasm. Acquisition of iron from transferrin and lactoferrin is similarly mediated by TBDTs that directly bind these host glycoproteins or bind siderophores that have stripped iron from them. While the vast majority of TBDTs are involved in the acquisition of iron, other substrates such as vitamin B_{12}, nickel complexes, colicins, phages, and carbohydrates may also gain entry to the periplasmic space through these transporters (90). To date, approximately 50 TBDT structures have been solved, alone and in complex with various ligands, and each consists of a transmembrane-spanning β-barrel encircling an independently folded N-terminal plug domain (see Fig. 4). Substrate-binding residues are located on the exofacial side of the plug, lining the interior of the pore, and on extracellular loops of the β-barrel and are customized to accommodate binding of the preferred substrate (91). The N-terminus of the pore domain also contains a weakly

SIDE VIEW

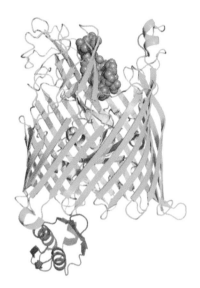

TOP VIEW

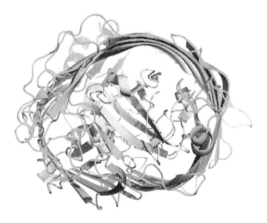

FIGURE 4 **Structure of a representative TBDT. A ribbon diagram of the *Pseudomonas aeruginosa* ferric pyoverdine (FpvA) receptor, bound to pyoverdine. The structure (PDB 2W16) illustrates the 22-stranded β-barrel (green) surrounding the N-terminal "plug" domain (yellow), which is attached to the N-terminal extension signaling domain (red). Pyoverdine bound to the receptor is shown using orange space filling. The side and top views of the structure are illustrated. In the latter view, the pyoverdine has been removed.**

conserved motif of approximately seven amino acid residues, referred to as the TonB-box, which are responsible for interacting with the TonB protein that is part of the TonB-ExbB-ExbD complex, as described below.

In addition to the plug and barrel domains of canonical TBDTs, a subset of these proteins, including HasR of *S. marcescens* (53), the ferric citrate receptor, FecA, of *E. coli* (92), and the ferric pyoverdine receptor, FpvA, of *P. aeruginosa* (93), possess a third domain, localized within the periplasm and designated the "N-terminal extension" or "signaling domain" (Fig. 3) (94–96). TBDTs bearing such a domain not only are subject to regulation by Fur, but are also capable of fine-tuning their own expression through a α-/anti-α-factor signaling cascade induced upon binding of the iron-loaded substrate to the transporter. Briefly, and in general, an anti-α factor localized to the inner membrane sequesters an associated and often cotranscribed extracytoplasmic function α-factor under nonactivating conditions (i.e., in the absence of substrate). In the presence of a substrate, the N-terminal extension of the TBDT interacts with the associated anti-α-factor, promoting release of the once-bound α-factor into the cytosol. The extracytoplasmic function α-factor in turn directs RNA polymerase to transcribe the operon encoding the transporter and any accompanying genes involved in substrate acquisition (e.g., hemophore or siderophore biosynthesis genes). In this manner, a signal can be relayed from the cell surface to the cytoplasm indicating the availability of substrates for acquisition, and the bacterium can respond with commensurate expression of the cognate TBDT for uptake.

The outer membrane of Gram-negative bacteria lacks an energy source, and thus the proton motive force of the cytoplasmic membrane is required to fuel the active transport of iron complexes into the periplasm. Transduction of energy to the outer membrane is mediated by the inner membrane complex

TonB-ExbB-ExbD (97), through a mechanism which is not yet fully understood and the details of which are outside the scope of this chapter, although several comprehensive reviews on the subject are available (89, 91, 98, 99). In brief, TonB bears three functional domains: an N-terminal signal sequence that targets the protein for translocation to the cytoplasmic membrane, a proline-rich periplasmic spacer region thought to confer flexibility to TonB and allowing it to span the periplasmic space, and a C-terminal domain which interacts with TonB-boxes of TBDTs. Binding of an iron complex to its respective TBDT promotes unfolding of the TonB box, which signals to TonB-ExbB-ExbD that a substrate is bound and ready for transport. Although the exact nature of the signaling between the TonB-box and TonB-ExbB-ExbD is unknown, it induces the TonB-box to physically engage TonB (Fig. 3) (100, 101), energizing the transporter for uptake of the bound iron complex. While it is commonly acknowledged that the plug domain, which otherwise occludes the β-barrel pore, must then undergo a conformational change to allow for passage of the substrate into the periplasm and likely involves at least partial expulsion of the plug from the pore (102), the nature of this domain rearrangement has yet to be fully characterized and indeed remains a point of contention (91, 103).

ABC transporters for heme transport across the inner membrane

Once in the periplasm, heme must subsequently be transported across the Gram-negative inner membrane and into the cytosol, a process mediated by ABC-type transporters. Notably, while this discussion specifically pertains to heme transport in Gram-negative bacteria, transport occurs analogously in Gram-positive bacteria across the cytoplasmic membrane and is similarly applicable to the uptake of other iron substrates, including siderophores and Fe^{3+} (Fig. 2). As depicted in Fig. 5, canonical prokaryotic ABC-type transporters consist of three central components: (i) a dedicated high-affinity substrate-binding protein (SBP), which captures and shuttles the substrate through the periplasmic space in Gram-negative bacteria or is lipid-anchored to the cytoplasmic membrane and captures heme from the external milieu in Gram-positive bacteria, (ii) an associated permease, usually comprised of two integral transmembrane protein subunits, and (iii) two peripheral ATPases, which power substrate translocation via ATP hydrolysis (104). In Gram-negative bacteria, the periplasm is a dynamic and congested space, and thus SBPs

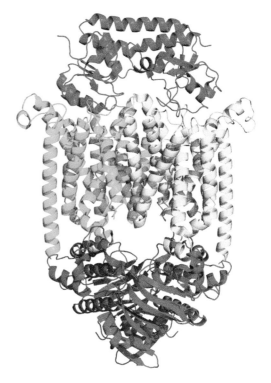

FIGURE 5 Structure of *E. coli* BtuCDF. A ribbon diagram of the *E. coli* BtuCDF complex (PDB 2QI9), representative of the iron-siderophore/cobalamin family of cytoplasmic membrane transporters. The two lobes of the substrate-binding protein BtuF (magenta) are docked on top of the two permease domains (BtuC, monomers colored yellow and green) which are associated with ATP-binding proteins (BtuD, monomers colored red and blue).

play an essential role in the trafficking of scantily available substrates, such as heme, to the inner membrane. Further, the specificity of an ABC-type transporter is usually governed by the ligand(s) bound by its cognate SBP. To date, over 50 heme-specific SBPs have been putatively identified (105), although few have been structurally and functionally characterized.

The vast majority of SBPs involved in the coordination of inorganic iron and organic iron complexes, such as heme, siderophores, and cobalamin, are categorized as cluster A, class III SBPs (106). These proteins are found exclusively in association with ABC transporters and possess two independently folded domains, each comprised of a central β-sheet surrounded by α-helices, that are joined by an α-helical linker of approximately 20 amino acid residues (Fig. 5). The substrate (e.g., heme) is coordinated in an interdomain cleft and, in class III SBPs, binding involves minimal conformational changes to the protein, owing to inflexibility of the α-helical spine. Docking of an SBP with its cognate ABC transporter is facilitated by salt bridges formed between highly conserved glutamic acid residues located at the apex of each SBP lobe and positively charged patches of arginine and/or lysine residues on the periplasmic face of the permease subunits. The formation of this stable SBP:ABC transporter complex, as illustrated in the paradigmatic example of the *E. coli* vitamin B_{12}-specific SBP, BtuF, and its associated transporter, BtuCD (Fig. 5) (107), is necessary to induce translocation of the substrate.

The first functionally characterized prokaryotic heme ABC transport system, encoded by the hemin uptake locus, *hemRSTUV*, of *Y. enterocolitica* is comprised of the heme-specific periplasmic SBP HemT, the integral transmembrane protein HemU, and the ATP-binding protein HemV (108). In total, this locus encodes for a complete heme uptake system in *Y. enterocolitica*, including a TBDT capable of independently binding and extracting heme from host hemoproteins at the cell surface (HemR) (109), and a cytosolic heme-carrier protein which sequesters free heme upon transport into the cell (HemS) (110). HemTUV-homologous heme ABC transporters have been functionally interrogated in a number of Gram-negative pathogens, including HmuTUV of *Y. pestis* (111, 112), ShuTUV of *Shigella dysenteriae* (113), HutBCD of *V. cholerae* (114), and PhuTUV of *P. aeruginosa* (115), and in each case, the transporter is required for efficient heme transport into the cytosol. Structural elucidation of both the apo- and holo- forms of the heme-binding SBPs ShuT and PhuT confirmed that both proteins exhibit classical class III SBP architecture, where heme is coordinated in a deep but narrow groove between the globular N- and C-terminal domains with little domain rearrangement upon binding. Although the binding pockets of the two proteins differ substantially, in both ShuT and PhuT heme is pentacoordinate, with a conserved tyrosine residue located within the N-terminal domain of the SBP serving as the heme axial ligand (116). Indeed, despite poor overall primary sequence homology, nearly every putative periplasmic heme-specific SBP identified to date appears to possess such a tyrosine residue, suggesting a common mechanism for heme binding in these proteins (105). Obviously, exceptions exist, and HmuT of *Y. pestis* appears to represent a unique subset of heme-specific SBPs, where two stacked heme molecules are coordinated in a single, comparatively large, binding cleft by a tyrosine and a histidine residue. The presence of these two residues may predict dual heme binding in other SBPs, and it has been proposed that in these systems, the two heme molecules are transported simultaneously (117).

Structural and functional characterization of the representative ABC transporters BtuCDF of *E. coli* and HmuTUV of *Y. pestis* suggests that the mechanism of substrate translocation (vitamin B_{12} and heme, respectively) is conserved (118, 119). In brief, it appears that in the absence of a loaded SBP and

ATP, the transporter is closed to the cytoplasm but open to the periplasm, forming an outward-facing cavity large enough to accommodate most of the substrate. The binding of the holo-SBP together with ATP permits release of the substrate into the lumen of the transporter, which undergoes a conformational change, trapping the substrate within a centrally located cavity. Upon ATP hydrolysis, the substrate is effectively expelled from the lumen into the cytosol, and the transporter collapses, likely to avoid leakage of cytoplasmic contents. The mechanism by which the apo-SBP is released back into the periplasm and the transporter is reset is currently unknown but likely involves ATP hydrolysis (For a comprehensive review of ABC transporters see reference 120). The potential toxicity of heme necessitates that it be rapidly sequestered or degraded upon transport into the cytosol and, notably, many loci encoding heme ABC transporters also include genes expressing cytosolic heme-binding proteins. Such heme carrier proteins have been characterized in *S. dysenteriae* (ShuS), *P. aeruginosa* (PhuS), and *Y. enterocolitica* (HemS), where heme is received directly from the associated ABC transporter at the cytoplasmic membrane (110, 121, 122) and ostensibly is shuttled safely to either heme storage or degradation pathways within the cell.

The iron-regulated surface determinant pathway: a Gram-positive heme acquisition mechanism

While not possessing an outer membrane through which heme must be actively transported, the thick peptidoglycan layer (~20 to 40 nm) of Gram-positive bacteria impedes the accessibility of heme to cell membrane–associated receptor proteins. This impediment necessitates a means by which heme can be conveyed through the cell wall, particularly when the concentration of available extracellular heme is low (<50 nM range) (12, 123, 124). Indeed, mechanisms that shuttle heme from the cell surface to the

cytoplasmic membrane have been described in a number of Gram-positive pathogens including *S. aureus*, *Staphylococcus lugdunensis*, *B. anthracis*, *L. monocytogenes*, *Streptococcus pyogenes*, and *C. diphtheriae* (for a recent comprehensive review see reference 125). As introduced above, the Isd pathway is the best characterized of these mechanisms, has been most extensively investigated in *S. aureus* (see Fig. 2), and herein is discussed as a paradigmatic example of such heme transfer systems in the Gram-positive pathogens.

Unlike *B. anthracis* and *L. monocytogenes*, *S. aureus* is not known to elaborate hemophores, and thus heme extraction, binding, and transfer are all performed by cell surface–associated proteins. In its entirety, the Isd pathway of *S. aureus* consists of nine iron-regulated proteins, IsdA through IsdI, and a genetically linked sortase B enzyme (SrtB) (126, 127). Three of these proteins (IsdA, IsdB, and IsdH) are anchored to the cell wall by sortase A (127), where the latter two proteins bind and extract heme from hemoproteins at the cell surface (124, 128, 129). IsdB and IsdH transfer freed heme to IsdA or directly to a fourth cell wall–associated heme-binding protein, IsdC (130, 131). IsdC is positioned deep within the cell wall by SrtB (126), and this localization is purportedly ideal for funneling heme from IsdA, IsdB, and/or IsdH to the membrane-associated protein, IsdE (130–134). Heme transfer through the cell wall is a passive process that is driven, in part, by the successive increase in affinity that each Isd protein has for heme, relative to the preceding protein (IsdB/IsdH < IsdA < IsdC < IsdE) (132–135). Transient, ultraweak (≥ micromolar affinity), "hand-clasp"-type interactions facilitate the movement of heme specifically between the NEAT domains of interacting Isd proteins (130, 136–138). IsdE does not contain a NEAT domain, and instead is a type III SBP, which along with its cognate membrane permease, IsdF, is a member of the ABC transporter superfamily (133, 134). The requisite ATPase for energizing the transfer of heme across the cytoplasmic membrane by IsdEF in *S. aureus* has yet to be identified.

The Isd pathway in *S. aureus* is required for uptake of iron from physiological concentrations of heme or hemoglobin (124), and indeed IsdA, IsdB, IsdC, IsdH, and the heme-degrading enzymes IsdG and IsdI are all required for maximal virulence of *S. aureus* in murine models of infection (124, 128, 139–141). As with the hemophores of Gram-positive pathogens, NEAT domains, ranging from one in each IsdA and IsdC, to two in IsdB, and three in IsdH, are the functional units involved in heme-iron acquisition in *S. aureus* (70, 136, 142–145). Each of the staphylococcal NEAT domains bears distinct specificities, where the N-terminal NEAT domains of IsdB ($IsdB_{N1}$) and IsdH ($IsdH_{N1}$ and $IsdH_{N2}$) bind hemoglobin (or hemoglobin-haptoglobin) (129, 146–150), and the C-terminal NEAT domains of these proteins ($IsdB_{N2}$ and $IsdH_{N3}$), as well as those of IsdA and IsdC, bind heme (70, 136, 143, 151). Unlike the sole NEAT domain of IsdX1, which is independently capable of mediating heme extraction from hemoglobin, the individual NEAT domains of IsdB and IsdH appear to function cooperatively as a conserved unit to fulfill this purpose. In brief, this extraction module is comprised of an N-terminal hemoglobin-binding domain ($IsdB_{N1}$ or $IsdH_{N2}$), an intervening and inflexible α-helical linker region, and a contiguous C-terminal heme-binding domain ($IsdB_{N2}$ or $IsdH_{N3}$) (148, 150, 152–154). Working in concert with the hemoglobin-binding domain, the indispensable linker region is proposed to induce steric strain on hemoglobin, thereby facilitating the dissociation of heme (148, 150, 153), while at the same time positioning the associated heme-binding domain in close proximity to the globin heme-binding pocket (148). Upon release from hemoglobin, heme is rapidly seized by the C-terminal heme-binding domain of IsdB or IsdH for subsequent transfer to IsdA or IsdC, prior to transport into the cytoplasm for use by the bacterium (130, 131).

The Isd pathway has been sparsely characterized outside of *S. aureus*. Aside from atypically pathogenic *S. lugdunensis* (155–157), coagulase-negative staphylococci do not encode for an Isd system. *L. monocytogenes* appears to encode an *isd*-like locus for uptake of heme from Hbp1 and Hbp2, but the functionality of this system has not yet been explored (12, 73). In *B. anthracis*, IsdC performs a central role in receiving heme from IsdX1 and IsdX2, but homologs of other cell surface–associated Isd proteins are missing in this organism (65, 158). Uptake of heme by *B. anthracis* hemophores may be aided by an alternative NEAT-domain-containing protein, BslK (for <u>B</u>. anthracis <u>S</u>-layer homology protein K), which has been proposed to facilitate heme transfer through the S-layer crystalline array of this pathogen to IsdC (70, 159). Notably, mutation of none of the Isd systems characterized to date fully abrogates growth on heme/hemoglobin as an iron source, except at low nM heme/hemoglobin concentrations, suggesting that alternative mechanisms for heme-iron acquisition likely exist in the Gram-positive pathogens.

Alternative Mechanisms for Heme Acquisition in Gram-Positive Pathogens

An extensive review of all heme-iron acquisition systems in bacterial pathogens is outside the scope of this chapter, but some of the known mechanisms are summarized in Table 1 (for an in-depth discussion, see reference 125). Two notable non-Isd heme shuttle pathways have been identified in the Gram-positive pathogens: the streptococcal iron acquisition system of *S. pyogenes* and the <u>hem</u>in-<u>u</u>ptake and <u>h</u>eme <u>t</u>ransport-<u>a</u>ssociated locus (Hmu-Hta) of *C. diphtheriae* (160, 161). The streptococcal iron acquisition system functions analogously to the Isd system of *S. aureus* and appears to include divergent members of the NEAT family of proteins, including the <u>s</u>treptococcal <u>h</u>emoprotein <u>r</u>eceptor (Shr; an IsdB/IsdH analog), and the <u>s</u>treptococcal <u>h</u>eme-associated cell surface protein (Shp; an IsdC analog) (160, 162). Hemoprotein binding by Shr, however, does not occur by way of the NEAT domain, but rather by a unique N-terminal domain (162). Heme extracted from host hemoproteins by Shr, using the composite N-terminal–NEAT domain, is transferred via Shp to a heme ABC transporter (HtsABC; an IsdEF homolog) for uptake (160, 162, 163). Notably, Shr is both highly immunogenic and promotes the survival of *S. pyogenes* in whole human blood and thus has been investigated as a vaccine target (164).

In contrast, the Hmu-Hta system of *C. diphtheriae* is distinct from heme acquisition systems in other Gram-positive pathogens. Hmu-Hta is comprised of six DtxR-regulated genes: three that encode an ABC transporter bearing homology to *hmuTUV* of *Y. pestis* (161), two that encode heme-binding cell surface-associated proteins (HtaA and HtaB), and one protein of unknown function (HtaC) (165). Similar to Shr, HtaA and HtaB are not anchored to the cell wall by sortases but, rather, possess a C-terminal transmembrane domain for attachment (165, 166). Further, these two proteins lack NEAT domains and instead mediate heme extraction and binding using a unique conserved region of ~150 amino acid residues. HtaA appears to facilitate heme uptake from host hemoproteins, whereas HtaB is proposed to function as an intermediary in transferring heme to HmuTUV (165–167). Heme uptake by *C. diphtheriae* may additionally be aided by the corynebacterial heme transport-associated proteins (ChtA, ChtB, and ChtC), but further efforts are required to elucidate the means by which these systems cooperatively promote heme-iron acquisition in this pathogen (168).

The Fate of Intracellular Heme

Heme that is not incorporated as a prosthetic group into bacterial enzymes must be sequestered, degraded, or effluxed to guard against toxicity. As previously discussed, the import of heme in some bacteria is coupled with its rapid seizure by heme-carrier molecules such as ShuS, PhuS, and HemS (of *S. dysenteriae*, *P. aeruginosa*, and *Y. enterocolitica*, respectively), and homologs of these proteins are found widely dispersed among the *Proteobacteria*. Heme-degrading enzymes are required by eukaryotes and prokaryotes alike to liberate iron from the porphyrin ring.

Until recently, heme degradation in bacteria was thought to occur solely through the action of heme oxygenases (HOs) that function analogously to eukaryotic HOs and catalyze the conversion of heme to biliverdin with the release of iron and CO (169). Indeed, such canonical HOs have been identified in both Gram-positive and Gram-negative pathogens including HmuO of *C. diphtheriae* (170, 171) and HemO of *Neisseria* spp. (172) and *P. aeruginosa* (173). A novel class of heme-degrading enzymes was recently identified in Gram-positive pathogens including *S. aureus*, *S. lugdunensis*, *Bacillus* spp., and *M. tuberculosis* (174). For a detailed discussion on heme degradation by both canonical and noncanonical HOs, readers are referred to recent comprehensive reviews by Wilks and colleagues (175, 176).

Several mechanisms exist for guarding microbes against the toxicity associated with excess intracellular heme and include inhibiting uptake or endogenous synthesis through Fur or DtxR-mediated repression, sequestration in heme-binding proteins, degradation by canonical and noncanonical HOs, and efflux. Heme is generally more toxic to Gram-positive pathogens than to Gram-negative pathogens, and although the reasons for this are unclear, mechanisms for heme efflux have almost exclusively been identified in Gram-positive organisms. Heme toxicity and efflux will not be discussed in detail here, and we refer the reader to an excellent review on the subject (177).

ACCESSING TRANSFERRIN-IRON

An important facet of innate immunity, and indeed one of the first lines of defense against invading bacterial pathogens, is the low availability of iron at host mucosal surfaces and within the serum and lymph, owing to sequestration by lactoferrin and transferrin, respectively. As with the utilization of heme-iron complexes, many successful pathogens are capable of circumventing iron withholding by transferrin and lactoferrin, by usurping iron sequestered by these host glycoproteins. Three main mechanisms exist for the utilization of transferrin and/or lactoferrin by bacteria: the elaboration of cell surface–associated transferrin- or lactoferrin-specific binding proteins (Tbps and Lbps, respectively), the secretion of small iron-chelating molecules, referred to as siderophores, and the extracellular release of broad substrate range reductases, which reduce ferric iron to ferrous iron for subsequent uptake by inorganic iron permeases. All three mechanisms ultimately function to liberate iron from transferrin and/or lactoferrin prior to its transport into the cell (see Tables 2 and 3).

Transferrin- and Lactoferrin-Binding Proteins: the TbpA/TbpB Paradigm

The establishment of infection by pathogenic *Neisseriaceae*, *Pasteurellaceae*, and *Moraxellaceae* species unequivocally begins with colonization of a specific mucosal surface such as the urogenital tract (*Neisseria gonorrhoeae*) or the upper respiratory tract (*Neisseria meningitidis*, *Moraxella catarrhalis*, and *H. influenzae*). Iron available to mucosal pathogens exists predominantly in the extracellular state and, as such, survival and proliferation of the aforementioned bacteria are undoubtedly aided by their capacity to exploit host transferrin and/or lactoferrin directly as iron sources. Unlike most Gram-negative pathogens, the ability of these microbes to utilize iron-containing host glycoproteins is not facilitated by the production of siderophores (as discussed below) but instead is mediated by highly specific, cell surface–associated transferrin- or lactoferrin-binding proteins (178–180).

TABLE 2 Examples of siderophore and transferrin-binding protein-dependent iron acquisition systems essential for virulence

Bacterium	Siderophore	Model[a]	Reference
Acinetobacter baumannii	Acinetobactin	Mouse (i.p.)	283
Bacillus anthracis	Petrobactin	Mouse (s.c.)	211
Campylobacter jejuni	Enterobactin	Chick	284
Dickeya dadantii	Chrysobactin	African violet	285
Klebsiella pneumoniae	Aerobactin	Mouse (s.c. and i.p.)	286
	Yersiniabactin	Mouse (i.n.)	287
Legionella pneumophila	Legiobactin	Mouse (i.t.)	288
Mycobacterium tuberculosis	Mycobactin	Mouse (aerosol)	289
Pantoea stewartii	Aerobactin	Sweet Corn	290
Proteus mirabilis	Yersiniabactin	Mouse (t.u.)	291
Pseudomonas aeruginosa	Pyochelin	Mouse (i.n. and i.m.)	292
	Pyoverdine	Mouse (i.n. and i.m.)	292
Pseudomonas syringae	Pyoverdine	Tobacco plant	293
Salmonella enterica	Enterobactin	Mouse (i.p.)	294
	Salmochelin	Mouse (o.g.)	219
Shigella flexneri	Aerobactin	Chicken embryo	295
Staphylococcus aureus	Staphyloferrin A	Mouse (s.c.)	125
	Staphyloferrin B	Mouse (i.v.)	213
Yersinia pestis	Yersiniabactin	Mouse (i.v.)	296
Actinobacillus pleuropneumoniae	Tbp	Pigs (aerosol)	297
Neisseria meningitidis	Tbp	Mouse (i.p.)	298
Neisseria gonorrhoeae	Tbp	Human male (urethritis)	299

[a]i.n., intranasal; i.m., intramuscular; i.p., intraperitoneal; i.t., intratracheal; i.v., intravenous; o.g., orogastric; s.c., subcutaneous.

TABLE 3 **Examples of inorganic iron uptake systems essential for virulence**

Bacterium	Uptake system	Model[a]	Reference
Campylobacter jejuni	Feo	Piglet	300
Escherichia coli	Feo	Mouse (o.g.)	301
Francisella tularensis	Feo	Mouse (i.d.)	302
Helicobacter pylori	Feo	Mouse (oral)	221
Legionella pneumophila	Feo	Mouse (i.t.)	303
Porphyromonas gingivalis	Feo	Mouse (s.c.)	304
Salmonella enterica	Sit	Mouse (i.p. and oral)	305
Xanthomonas oryzae	Feo	Rice plants	306

[a]i.d., intradermal; i.p., intraperitoneal; i.t., intratracheal; o.g., orogastric; s.c., subcutaneous.

The paradigmatic transferrin-receptor in Gram-negative bacteria is a Fur-regulated bipartite system consisting of an outer membrane receptor protein, TbpA (181), and a surface-associated lipoprotein, TbpB (182) (Fig. 2). Both TbpA and TbpB bind transferrin, but TbpA nondiscriminantly binds both apo- and holo-transferrin, whereas TbpB selectively binds holo-transferrin (183). TbpB purportedly functions as bait to capture iron-loaded transferrin from the extracellular milieu and deliver it to TbpA for TonB-dependent uptake. Similar to the mechanism of heme uptake by HasA/HasR, TbpA is capable of independently mediating transferrin-iron acquisition (182, 184), and the presence of TbpB substantially enhances the efficiency of transferrin-iron acquisition by the bacterium.

In contrast to heme and siderophores, which are transported intact through the outer membrane, iron must first be liberated from transferrin prior to uptake by TbpA. Both TbpA and TbpB of the human pathogen *N. meningitidis* exclusively bind the C-lobe of human transferrin (hTf) (185, 186), through nonoverlapping binding sites (186, 187). As depicted in Fig. 6, TbpB is a bilobate protein, where each lobe is comprised of an eight-stranded β-barrel and an adjacent four-stranded "handle" domain (187). The C-lobe of holo-hTf effectively docks onto the "cap" of the N-lobe of TbpB with minimal conformational change to either protein, and the two are held together by extensive interactions along a large binding interface (for details see reference 187). The structural

characterization of TbpB in complex with hTf has provided insight into both the specificity of TbpB for transferrin solely of its host species and its role in iron acquisition from transferrin. First, TbpB interacts with a region of hTf (loop $L_{496-515}$) that is highly variable in sequence and length between mammalian transferrin homologs, where variations within the TbpB recognition site

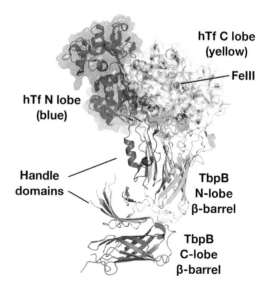

FIGURE 6 **Structure of *Neisseria meningitidis* TbpB bound to iron-loaded human transferrin. Depicted is a ribbon diagram of PDB 3VE1 illustrating the binding of human transferrin (also illustrated with transparent surface; N lobe colored blue, C lobe colored yellow, iron depicted with red sphere) by *N. meningitidis* TbpB colored from the N terminus (in blue) to the C terminus (in red). Some relevant domains are indicated. More detail on this structure can be found in Calmettes et al. (187).**

sterically hinder binding of the protein and help to explain the lack of cross-species transferrin-iron acquisition by TbpB (187). Second, instead of helping to liberate ferric iron from hTf, the interaction between hTf and TbpB stabilizes iron binding, where the formation of the holo-hTf-TbpB complex is proposed to block protonation of a critical residue (H349) in hTf which acts as a pH-dependent trigger for iron release (187, 188); in this manner, iron is maintained within holo-hTf-TbpB until delivery to TbpA.

TbpA is similar to other TonB-dependent outer membrane receptors, as described previously. TbpA, however, is substantially larger (~20%) than other TBDTs, owing to extensive extracellular loop regions extending from both the β-barrel and plug domains, the latter of which has been proposed to function as a sensor for ligand binding (186). In contrast to TbpB, TbpA induces a large conformational change in hTf upon binding, where an α-helical extension of TbpA inserts itself into the iron-binding cleft of the hTf C-lobe, effectively prying the iron coordination site partially open and thus facilitating iron release. Transfer of ferric iron from TbpB to TbpA for subsequent uptake is mediated by the formation of a TbpB-holo-hTf-TbpA complex, which forms a bounded compartment that directs ferric iron toward the TbpA plug domain, although the mechanism by which this occurs has not yet been fully elucidated (186). Transport of insoluble ferric iron through TbpA is thought to be mediated by transient binding of iron to a conserved motif (EIEYE) in the plug domain (189).

As with TbpB, TbpA of *N. meningitidis* binds several human-specific residues on hTf (186), further explicating the specificity of these Tbps for hTf. The human-specific tropism of *N. meningitidis* and *N. gonorrhoeae* is due in part to the specificity of TbpA/TbpB for hTf and has largely precluded the use of animal models for meningococcal and gonococcal infections. The recent development of transgenic mice expressing hTf represents a major breakthrough for studying the pathogenicity of *Neisseria* spp. (190, 191). Interestingly, TbpA binds several distinct transferrin residues that have evolved rapidly within primate lineages, suggesting that coevolution of pathogenic *Neisseriaceae*, *Pasteurellaceae*, and *Moraxellaceae* with their primate host has driven adaptive changes within transferrin to evade this particular aspect of bacterial iron piracy (192). In contrast, the binding site of TbpB on hTf partially overlaps that of the mammalian transferrin receptor, TfR (187), thus protecting the TbpB binding site from rapid evolution that would otherwise mitigate binding of TbpB to hTf.

In addition to transferrin use, many pathogenic *Neisseriaceae* and *Moraxellaceae* are capable of exploiting lactoferrin as an iron source (193). Comprised of a TonB-dependent outer membrane lactoferrin-binding protein (LbpA) (194) and an accessory lactoferrin-binding lipoprotein (LbpB) (195), the lactoferrin acquisition system functions analogously to the TbpA/TbpB system described above, with notable differences. LbpB purportedly binds the N-lobe of holo-lactoferrin, in contrast to the binding of TbpB to the C-lobe of holo-transferrin (196). Further, LbpB appears to stabilize the iron-loaded form of lactoferrin not through manipulating a pH-dependent switch, but rather, by barring conformational changes that allow for iron release from holo-lactoferrin (196). Last, LbpB fulfills the unique function of conferring protection against the antimicrobial cationic peptide, lactoferricin, a degradation product of lactoferrin (197), by sequestering the peptide at negatively charged residues predominantly within the C-lobe of the lipoprotein and by potentially sheltering bound lactoferrin from proteolysis (196, 198, 199).

Despite these differences, it is thought that key structural and functional features of TbpA/TbpB and LbpA/LbpB are maintained. Notably, the α-helical extension of TbpA that was proposed to help extract iron from holo-transferrin is structurally conserved in LbpA, and thus the mechanism of iron release between these two proteins is believed to be comparable (196). Further, both TbpA and LbpA possess a periplasmic loop region that may mediate docking of the ferric-iron-binding protein A (FbpA) (200). Interestingly, FbpA, which is structurally similar to a single lobe of eukaryotic transferrin, effectively serves as a bacterial transferrin, shuttling insoluble and potentially toxic Fe^{3+} and small Fe^{3+}-complexes between biological membranes (201). FbpA delivers Fe^{3+} to its associated permease, FbpBC, which together comprise an ABC transporter that represents a "nodal point" for ferric iron utilization in a number of Gram-negative pathogens (201–204). Indeed, FbpABC is required for iron uptake from transferrin, lactoferrin, and ferric iron chelates, such as ferric citrate and iron pyrophosphate in pathogenic *Neisseria* spp. (203–205). Together, TbpA/TbpB and LbpA/LbpB, coupled with FbpABC, form a distinct mechanism by which mucosal pathogens lacking endogenous siderophore production can exploit predominant iron sources within their host environment.

Siderophores

In contrast to the relatively limited prevalence of transferrin- and lactoferrin-binding proteins among bacterial pathogens, siderophores are ubiquitously employed as a tool to pirate iron from host glycoproteins and to scavenge residual free iron from the external milieu. Synthesized and secreted in response to iron deprivation, siderophores are low molecular weight (generally less than 1 kDa), soluble molecules with high specificity and affinity for Fe^{3+} (206). Enterobactin, a siderophore produced by Gram-negative enterics, is one of the strongest iron chelators known, with an estimated affinity of 10^{-52} M (207). Not only are siderophores widely expressed by both pathogenic and nonpathogenic bacteria, but they are often produced by fungi and graminaceous plants to promote growth under iron-limited conditions (208), and 2,5-DHBA was most recently identified as a

mammalian siderophore (2, 3). To date, several hundred siderophores have been identified, over 270 of which have been structurally characterized. This has revealed a diverse array of structures yet a limited number of iron-coordinating functional groups (for a comprehensive list see Appendix 1 in reference 208). Broadly, siderophores can be categorized based on the functional groups involved in iron coordination and include catecholate, hydroxamate, and α-hydroxycarboxylate types. A fourth, nondescript category is comprised of siderophores employing more than one of the aforementioned classes of coordinating moieties and is thus referred to as "mixed type" (206). Regardless of type, siderophores tend to stably coordinate a single Fe^{3+} ion in a hexadentate fashion, with oxygen atoms serving as the most common ligand (208).

The biosynthesis of siderophores typically follows one of two modes of assembly, delineated by the requirement, or lack thereof, for large multimodular enzymatic scaffolds referred to as <u>n</u>on<u>r</u>ibosomal <u>p</u>eptide <u>s</u>ynthetases (NRPSs). NRPS-based siderophore synthesis involves the activation and incorporation of nonproteinogenic amino acids into an elongating chain, the sequence of which is dictated by the order of the NRPS domains, in lieu of an RNA template (for a detailed discussion of NRPS siderophore synthesis, see reference 209). In addition to the synthesis of numerous macrocyclic, or "aryl capped," peptidic siderophores (206), including enterobactin, bacillibactin of *Bacillus* spp. (Fig. 7), mycobactin of *M. tuberculosis*, yersiniabactin of *Yersinia* spp., and vibriobactin of *V. cholerae*, NRPS enzymes also give rise to antimicrobial peptides and peptide-based antibiotics such as penicillin, daptomycin, and vancomycin (209). In contrast, <u>N</u>RPS-<u>i</u>ndependent <u>s</u>iderophore (NIS) synthesis employs an alternative family of synthetases, which catalyze the condensation of alternating amino alcohols, alcohols, dicarboxylic acids, and diamines via amine or ester bond formation, giving rise to

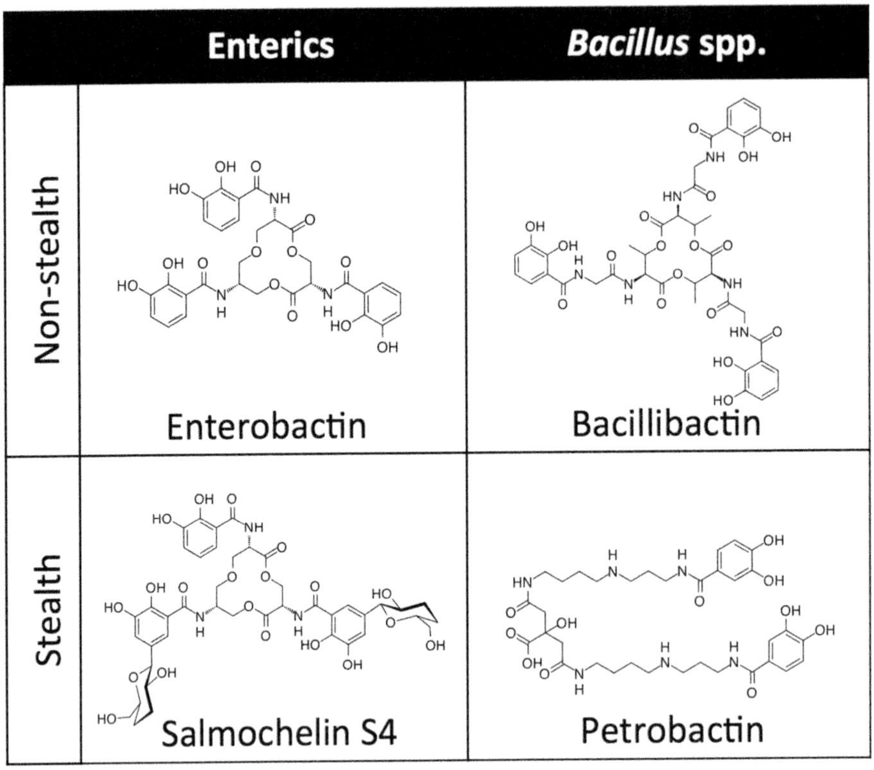

FIGURE 7 Structures of representative catechol-containing stealth and nonstealth siderophores. Stealth siderophores are not bound by mammalian siderocalin.

nonpeptidic siderophores (for a detailed discussion of NIS siderophore synthesis, see reference 210). The majority of carboxylate and α-hydroxycarboxylate type siderophores are synthesized using NIS-type pathways, including staphyloferrins A and B of *S. aureus*, alcaligin of *Bordetella pertussis* and *Bordetella bronchiseptica*, and aerobactin of the *Enterobacteriaceae* (208). Interestingly, petrobactin (Fig. 7), which is produced by pathogenic *Bacillus* spp., is synthesized using a unique NIS/NRPS hybrid system (211).

To mediate iron uptake from the external milieu, newly synthesized siderophores must first be exported from the cytoplasm. Siderophore export is, to date, poorly characterized, but in both Gram-negative and Gram-positive bacteria, transport across the cytoplasmic membrane appears to be mediated by exporters of the major facilitator superfamily (212). Subsequent transport across the outer membrane in Gram-negative bacteria is performed by multidomain efflux pumps of the resistance-nodulation cell division or ABC transporter-type families, and most often these export proteins are encoded from the biosynthetic locus of the associated siderophore. As discussed above, the transport of iron-loaded siderophores back across the Gram-negative outer membrane is mediated by specific TBDTs, and in both Gram-negative and Gram-positive pathogens, ABC transporters facilitate passage of the siderophore, intact, across the cytoplasmic membrane (Fig. 2). While some SBPs and ABC transporters are highly specific for a given siderophore, others possess broad substrate specificity for catecholate, carboxylate, or α-hydroxycarboxylate-type siderophores and, as such, may allow for the appropriation of siderophores from heterologous microorganisms.

Bacteria capable of exploiting these "xenosiderophores" may be afforded a competitive advantage in polymicrobial communities, where they are potentially able to pilfer multiple iron-chelating molecules without the energetic demands of synthesizing siderophores *de novo*. Indeed, some bacteria including *S. lugdunensis* (157), *L. monocytogenes* (12), and *S. pyogenes*, are wholly dependent on the uptake of xenosiderophores to access the transferrin-iron pool within the host, and the general trend is for the expression of several more siderophore importers than exporters overall. The conserved ferric hydroxamate uptake (Fhu) system is but one example of a broad substrate range Fe^{3+}-siderophore importer, homologs of which are found in each of the aforementioned organisms, along with many other Gram-negative and Gram-positive pathogens. *Staphylococcus* spp. and *Bacillus* spp. are additionally capable of utilizing catecholate-type siderophores, as well as ferrated catecholamine stress hormones, such as epinephrine, norepinephrine, and/or dopamine as "pseudosiderophores" using the staphylococcal siderophore transporter, SstABCD (213), and FeuABCD (214), respectively. Notably, catecholamine stress hormones do not directly strip iron from transferrin but, rather, promote its reduction from Fe^{3+} to Fe^{2+}, thus facilitating iron release from transferrin and allowing for uptake by the hormone (215).

Upon delivery of the iron-loaded siderophore to the cytoplasm, two possible mechanisms exist for the release of iron for cellular processes: (i) reductive iron release from the siderophore using a ferrisiderophore reductase, leaving the molecule intact for possible recycling, and (ii) reduction of iron concurrent with hydrolysis of the siderophore backbone, as has been shown for *tris*-catecholate siderophores such as enterobactin and bacillibactin (206). The dissociation of iron from the intact siderophore is considered to be the more prevalent method, because specialized enzymes are not required and reutilization of the siderophore would ostensibly be more energetically favorable.

Stealth siderophores

In defense against siderophore-mediated iron piracy, neutrophils of the mammalian host secrete NGAL, an acute-phase protein capable of sequestering bacterial siderophores; unsurprisingly, bacterial invaders have responded by evolving tactics to counter this affront to their acquisition of iron. NGAL coordinates ferric-siderophores within a cup-shaped ligand-binding pocket (calyx) that is large, broad, and shallow and is uniquely lined with polar and positively charged residues (216, 217). As such, the NGAL calyx is ideally suited to the sequestration of negatively charged ferric siderophores, such as the catecholates. To circumvent the effects of NGAL, some pathogenic bacteria elaborate more than one siderophore, often including an NGAL-sensitive (e.g., catecholate) and an NGAL-immune siderophore (e.g., a structurally modified aromatic or one that simply lacks aromatic-binding motifs). Siderophores that evade the effects of NGAL are aptly referred to as "stealth siderophores" and are often associated with virulence potential. The production of a stealth siderophore is exemplified by uropathogenic *E. coli* and *Salmonella enterica* serovars, where iron acquisition by NGAL-sensitive enterobactin is complemented by production of glucosylated enterobactin derivatives, such as salmochelin S4 (Fig. 7) (218); the addition of bulky glucose residues to the catechol moieties of the siderophore renders it sterically discordant for NGAL-binding. Indeed, despite the extremely high affinity of enterobactin for Fe^{3+}, salmochelin appears to be required for the virulence of *S. enterica* (219). Similarly, pathogenic *Bacillus* spp. secrete both bacillibactin and petrobactin, the latter of which bears 3,4-DHBA moieties in lieu of the common 2,3-DHBA moieties, where the position of the carboxylates also renders the siderophore incompatible for binding by

NGAL. Petrobactin is uniquely required for the virulence of *B. anthracis* (211).

Extracellular Ferric Iron Reductases

In theory, bacterial pathogens could utilize cell surface–associated or –secreted ferric iron reductases, which reduce Fe^{3+} to Fe^{2+}, not only to access insoluble Fe^{3+}-precipitates, but also to nonspecifically liberate iron from host iron complexes such as transferrin, lactoferrin, and ferritin (Fig. 1). The uptake of solubilized Fe^{2+} through the cell envelope occurs by way of inorganic iron permeases (Fig. 2), obviating the need for dedicated uptake mechanisms for each individual iron chelate. Indeed, extracellular and/or cell surface–associated reductase activity has been reported for *H. pylori* (220, 221) and the facultatively intracellular, ruminant pathogen *Mycobacterium avium* subsp. *paratuberculosis* (222), although the molecular determinants and substrate specificities of these enzymes are not well defined. Similarly, *L. monocytogenes* is capable of mobilizing iron from a wide range of complexes, including transferrin, lactoferrin, hemoglobin, catecholamine stress hormones, and exogenous siderophores, through what is thought to be a potent broad-substrate-specificity ferric iron reductase (223–226). A ferric reductase (FepB) recently described in *L. monocytogenes* functions as part of the ferric iron permease system, FepABC (for <u>Fe</u>-dependent <u>p</u>eroxidase), but it is unclear if the aforementioned activity can fully be ascribed to this enzyme (227). Interestingly, homogentisic acid of *Legionella pneumophila* and the associated pyomelanin pigment, HGA-melanin, were both shown reduce Fe^{3+} complexes such as transferrin and ferritin, where mobilized Fe^{2+} was subsequently transported by the <u>fe</u>rrous <u>iro</u>n permease, FeoB (228, 229). Notably, siderophore production by *L. pneumophila* was found to be inversely correlated to homogentisic acid–melanin secretion, suggesting that the two mechanisms are likely differentially regulated and may fulfill distinct roles in iron acquisition by this bacterium (228).

The interplay between well-defined iron acquisition strategies and ferric iron reductases has not yet been investigated, nor is it known if these enzymes contribute to the *in vivo* survival or pathogenicity of these organisms. It is interesting to speculate that ferric iron reductases may provide a means of accessing host intracellular iron stores, such as ferritin, but this notion has only been preliminarily investigated in *M. avium* subsp. *paratuberculosis*, where ferric reductase expression was observed in an association with intracellular mycobacteria of naturally infected bovine intestinal tissue (222). Clearly, while reductive iron release seems to be a viable means for pathogens to access a multitude of host iron complexes, to which they may not have specific receptors or acquisition pathways, it is a currently underappreciated and underexplored facet of bacterial iron acquisition.

INORGANIC IRON TRANSPORT

While Fe^{2+} uptake is important, particularly in anoxic and/or acidic environments, such systems are sparsely characterized in most microorganisms, owing to the obscuring influence of siderophore and heme-iron uptake systems. In Gram-negative bacteria, it is believed that ferrous iron ions are capable of diffusing across the outer membrane in a TonB-independent fashion and that elemental iron is actively transported across the cytoplasmic membrane. Two inorganic iron acquisition systems are widely conserved in both Gram-positive and Gram-negative pathogens: the <u>fe</u>rrous <u>iro</u>n transport system, Feo (see Table 3), and functional analogs of Fet3p-Ftrp1, a high-affinity, reductive iron permease in *Saccharomyces cerevisiae* (230).

FeoAB(C): a Dedicated Ferrous Iron Transporter

The *Enterobacteriaceae*, including key human pathogens such as pathogenic *E. coli*, *Shigella* spp., *Salmonella* spp., and *Y. pestis*, acquire inorganic iron in part through the highly conserved and dedicated ferrous iron transporter, Feo. In most γ-proteobacteria, Feo is encoded from the three-gene operon *feoABC* (231) and is regulated by Fur and anaerobic transcriptional activators, Fnr and/or AcrA, in response to iron and oxygen deprivation, respectively (232, 233). Surprisingly, despite the initial identification of Feo in *E. coli* K-12 nearly 30 years ago (234), the functions of the individual components of transporters are still somewhat unclear. FeoB is an integral membrane protein and likely functions as the main Fe^{2+}-permease, although it lacks homology to other known Fe^{2+}-transporters (231, 235). The activity of FeoB requires binding of GTP to a G protein domain located within its N-terminal cytoplasmic region, and while mutation of this binding site abolishes Fe^{2+} transport (236), it is not known whether GTP hydrolysis energizes iron uptake by FeoB. FeoA is a small, hydrophilic, cytoplasmic protein of unknown function, bearing homology to eukaryotic Src homology-3 domains, which often facilitate protein-protein interactions. While conflicting evidence exists concerning whether FeoA interacts directly with FeoB, it is nevertheless required for FeoB-mediated Fe^{2+} acquisition in *S. enterica*, *V. cholerae*, and *E. coli* (232, 237, 238).

FeoC is another small, hydrophilic, cytoplasmic protein that is only readily apparent in the γ-proteobacteria, although genes encoding other small proteins of undefined function are present in proximity to *feo* in other organisms (235). FeoC contains an Fe-S cluster and a putative winged-helix DNA-binding motif (232, 234, 239) and, accordingly, was once thought to serve as a transcriptional regulator of *feoABC* (235). Instead, it appears, at least in the case of *S. enterica*, that FeoC binds and protects FeoB from proteolytic degradation in iron-deplete, anoxic environments (240). FeoC itself is subject to oxygen-sensitive proteolysis, where the Fe-S cluster is thought to serve as an oxygen sensor, promoting degradation of the protein during aerobiosis (241). Thus, FeoC may provide assurance that FeoB is stably expressed when oxygen and iron are limiting and that it is rapidly degraded when they are not, thus levying further control over Fe^{2+} acquisition by the bacterium. Together, FeoABC represents a key means by which enteric pathogens, in particular, acquire iron in microaerophilic or anaerobic niches of the gastrointestinal tract. Indeed, *feoABC* has been implicated in the virulence of many of these pathogens, as summarized in Table 3. While considerable gaps exist in our understanding of how FeoABC functions in Fe^{2+} uptake in the γ-proteobacteria, even less is known about the transporter in Gram-positive pathogens. Homologs of *feoAB* have been identified in a number of Gram-positive pathogens, including *B. anthracis*, *S. aureus*, and *L. monocytogenes*, and although the operon is upregulated during iron-restricted growth in the latter two (235, 242, 243), Feo has yet to be functionally characterized in any of these organisms.

EfeUOB/FepABC: a Conserved but Enigmatic Pathway for Inorganic Iron Uptake

The Fur-regulated, acid-induced elemental ferrous iron uptake system of *E. coli*, EfeUOB, is a tripartite inorganic iron transporter that bears homology to the Fe^{2+} acquisition system Fet3p-Ftrp1 of baker's yeast (244, 245). Homologs of *efeUOB* are widely distributed among many bacterial phyla, although for nearly every characterized system, the preferred substrate remains a matter of debate. In *E. coli*, EfeUOB has been implicated not only in the acquisition of Fe^{2+} and Fe^{3+}, but also in the extraction and subsequent uptake of iron from heme (246), as has similarly been postulated for the staphylococcal EfeUOB ortholog, FepABC (247, 248). In *B. subtilis*, EfeUOB is involved in the acquisition of both Fe^{2+} and Fe^{3+} (249), whereas a similar four-component system in pathogenic *Bordetella* spp. and *Brucella* spp. appears to be a dedicated ferrous iron transporter

(FtrABCD) (250, 251). As discussed above, FepABC of *L. monocytogenes* may facilitate access to a plethora of host Fe^{3+}-complexes through robust ferric reductase activity, but a substrate of this transporter has not yet been defined (227).

EfeU and FepC are integral transmembrane proteins bearing homology to the yeast ferric iron permease, Ftrp1. While *efeUOB* is required for Fe^{2+} acquisition in *E. coli* under acidic conditions (244, 245), it is likely that the EfeU (FepC) serves as a transporter of Fe^{3+}, where Fe^{2+} captured from the external milieu is oxidized to Fe^{3+} by the uncharacterized substrate-binding protein, EfeO (FepA), prior to uptake. In most organisms, EfeO (FepA) possesses a putative divalent metal cation-binding motif (GxHxxE) and an N-terminal cupredoxin (Cup) domain, the latter of which is thought to confer the aforementioned ferroxidase activity, similar to the yeast multicopper oxidase, Fet3p (252). Contention regarding the substrate specificity of EfeUOB/FepABC largely hinges on the function of EfeB (FepB), an extracytoplasmic protein of the dye-decolorizing heme peroxidase (DyP) superfamily. Members of the DyP family possess highly varied functions, and in *E. coli* and *S. aureus*, EfeB (and a paralog YfeX) and FepB, respectively, have been credited with a novel heme deferrochelatase activity. Deferrochelation is a process wherein iron is removed from heme through a reductive process that, remarkably, conserves the porphyrin ring, thus yielding free iron and PPIX (247, 253, 254). Given that PPIX is not readily metabolized by bacteria and is potentially toxic, questions have been raised about the biological utility of generating PPIX as a byproduct of heme-iron extraction. As such, other research suggests that EfeB, YfeX, and FepB may instead function as typical DyP peroxidases to oxidize porphyrinogens to porphyrins (255). In *B. subtilis*, EfeB does appear to function as a DyP peroxidase but uniquely functions as a switch between Fe^{2+} and Fe^{3+} acquisition in this organism. Notably, EfeO in *B. subtilis*

lacks a Cup domain (and thus ferroxidase activity) and instead is capable of receiving Fe^{3+} directly from the external milieu in the absence of EfeB. Under microaerobic conditions, when Fe^{2+} predominates, EfeB oxidizes Fe^{2+} to Fe^{3+} prior to transfer to EfeO and subsequent uptake into the cytosol by EfeU (249). Although inconsistencies remain, it appears that EfeUOB/FepABC has distinctively evolved in specific microorganisms to facilitate access to the iron sources most frequently encountered and/or to which no other means of uptake exist. While investigations into the *in vivo* role of EfeUOB/FepABC are limited, orthologous transporters in both *S. aureus* (*fepABC*) and *Brucella abortus* (*ftrABCD*) have been implicated in the survival and virulence of these pathogens within murine models of infection (248, 251). Thus, inorganic iron acquisition via *efeUOB/fepABC* and similar ferric iron permeases should not be disregarded as an inconsequential means of iron uptake.

IRON ACQUISITION SYSTEMS AS THERAPEUTIC TARGETS

Given the essentiality of iron to bacterial pathogens and the known expression of iron acquisition systems within the host, these systems have evoked much interest in developing antibacterial strategies, for either the development of vaccines, the design of iron acquisition inhibitors, or the utility of iron acquisition systems to deliver toxic substances into the cell in a "Trojan horse" type of approach. Below, we present a very brief summary of a few examples of how iron acquisition systems are being used as therapeutic targets.

Iron-Acquisition Proteins as Vaccine Targets

For many pathogenic species of bacteria, there is no approved vaccine. Many proteins involved in iron acquisition satisfy several key requirements for vaccine candidates in that they are exposed at the cell surface, expressed *in vivo*, frequently essential to virulence, and are conserved within species. Space limitations dictate that we limit our discussion here to only two examples.

Several components of the Isd system in *S. aureus* have generated interest in vaccine development. IsdB, IsdA, and IsdH are immunogenic in laboratory animals and can provide a protective response in mice (256–259), and IsdB also elicited a strong immune response in rhesus macaques (260). The IsdB vaccine, V710, showed immunogenic properties in humans in phase I trials (261) and moved to phase II/III trials in adults, at which point, unfortunately, the trials on V710 were halted due to an inability of the vaccine to protect against postoperative *S. aureus* infection (262). Research continues to examine the utility of other Isd components as part of an effective *S. aureus* vaccine, and multivalent approaches appear to provide much promise. In one example, immunization of mice with a combination of IsdA and IsdB, along with two other surface-expressed proteins, SdrD and SdrE, substantially increased survival of *S. aureus*–challenged mice compared to unimmunized controls (259).

TbpA and TbpB have been examined as vaccine candidates for over two decades for *N. meningitidis* and *N. gonorrhoeae* (263). Denatured TbpA and/or TbpB from *N. meningitidis* elicited an immune response in animals and provided protection from *N. meningitidis* infection (264, 265), and humans generate an antibody response to these proteins (263, 266, 267). In contrast, *N. gonorrhoeae* TbpA and TbpB do not evoke a strong immune response in humans, because IgG, IgA, and IgM antibody levels in the serum of individuals with a previous gonococcal infection were low and comparable to the control group (268). However, a TbpB-cholera toxin B (Ctb) conjugate administered to mice had significantly higher antibody levels in serum than TbpB alone (269). Although there is currently a vaccine for *N. meningitidis*, it is not effective against serogroup B or *N. gonorrhoeae*. Because TbpB is conserved in all isolates of *N. meningitidis* and *N. gonorrhoeae*, it remains a promising vaccine candidate.

Exploiting Iron Acquisition Systems for Antibiotic/Inhibitor Design

Among the diverse array of siderophore structures are those that possess antibiotic properties, termed sideromycins. Naturally occurring sideromycins include albomycin and the salmycins that contain the antibiotic moieties thioribosyl pyrimidine or aminoglycosides, respectively. The molecules gain access to the cell via the normal route of entry for the siderophore component. Sideromycins have not seen extensive use as therapeutics because of the development of rapid resistance, owing to mutations in the siderophore transport system or to the protein required for intracellular antibiotic activation. However, significant research has been performed to generate synthetic siderophore-antibiotic conjugates, exploiting the versatility of synthetic iron chelators to improve efficacy as therapeutic agents. The reader is referred to a comprehensive review on the topic (270).

For bacteria for which siderophore synthesis is an important virulence determinant, siderophore biosynthesis inhibitors offer promise as a novel class of antibacterial. The biosynthetic pathway for catechol-type siderophores, such as mycobactin, yersiniabactin, enterobactin, and pyochelin, for example, proceeds from chorismate using chorismate-utilizing enzymes such as salicylate synthase and isochorismate synthase. That these enzymes are not present in mammalian cells makes them ideal targets for bacterial inhibition. For a more detailed discussion on the development of inhibitors to chorismate-utilizing enzymes, we refer the reader to a recent review (271).

An alternative strategy to target iron metabolism in bacteria is through intoxication by alternative transition metals. Noniron metalloporphyrins, such as gallium-PPIX, have potent antibacterial activity against both Gram-negative and Gram-positive bacteria (272). These compounds exploit heme uptake systems as a means to enter cells, and since heme acquisition is important to many pathogens, these compounds offer exciting possibilities to treat problematic human pathogens. Alternatively, conjugating gallium to siderophores, such as deferoxamine mesylate, has been shown to be effective in killing *P. aeruginosa*, blocking biofilm for mation, and decreasing corneal infection in rabbits when combined with gentamicin, as opposed to gentamicin treatment alone (273). These data provide the incentive to initiate research into the testing of this and other siderophore gallium conjugates for efficacy in other bacterial pathogens.

CONCLUSIONS

The past decade of study of iron acquisition strategies employed by human, animal, and plant pathogens has brought rapid progress and led to breakthroughs in our understanding of how pathogens have evolved to deal with iron limitation imposed by the host. Although this field has been one of the most intensely studied for decades, new and fascinating information continues to be uncovered with regard to the role of iron on bacterial physiology, metabolism, adaptation, and virulence. Important new insights into mechanisms of iron scavenging continue to be derived from a continuum of work from many laboratories in the disciplines of microbiology, cellular microbiology, pathogenesis, biochemistry, and structural biology. We are now closer than ever to seeing the translation of knowledge on iron acquisition systems into valuable inhibitors, antibiotics, and vaccines aimed at decreasing the burden of infectious disease by ever-evolving drug-resistant bacterial pathogens.

ACKNOWLEDGMENTS

This work was supported by operating grants from the Canadian Institutes of Health Research (CIHR) and the Natural Sciences and Engineering Research Council. JRS was supported by a CIHR Frederick Banting and Charles Best Doctoral Research Award, and an Ontario Graduate Scholarship.

CITATION

Sheldon JR, Laakso HA, Heinrichs DE. 2016. Iron acquisition strategies of bacterial pathogens. Microbiol Spectrum 4(2):VMBF-0010-2015.

REFERENCES

1. **Flo TH, Smith KD, Sato S, Rodriguez DJ, Holmes MA, Strong RK, Akira S, Aderem A.** 2004. Lipocalin 2 mediates an innate immune response to bacterial infection by sequestrating iron. *Nature* **432:**917–921.
2. **Liu Z, Reba S, Chen W-D, Porwal SK, Boom WH, Petersen RB, Rojas R, Viswanathan R, Devireddy L.** 2014. Regulation of mammalian siderophore 2,5-DHBA in the innate immune response to infection. *J Exp Med* **211:**1197–1213.
3. **Devireddy LR, Hart DO, Goetz DH, Green MR.** 2010. A mammalian siderophore synthesized by an enzyme with a bacterial homolog involved in enterobactin production. *Cell* **141:**1006–1017.
4. **Vujić M.** 2014. Molecular basis of HFE-hemochromatosis. *Front Pharmacol* **5:**42.
5. **Pietrangelo A.** 2015. Genetics, genetic testing and management of hemochromatosis: 15 years since hepcidin. *Gastroenterology* **149:** 1240–1251.
6. **Babitt JL, Lin HY.** 2011. The molecular pathogenesis of hereditary hemochromatosis. *Semin Liver Dis* **31:**280–292.
7. **Anderson GJ.** 2001. Ironing out disease: inherited disorders of iron homeostasis. *IUBMB Life* **51:**11–17.
8. **Levi S, Finazzi D.** 2014. Neurodegeneration with brain iron accumulation: update on pathogenic mechanisms. *Drug Metab Transp* **5:**99.
9. **Bartnikas TB.** 2012. Known and potential roles of transferrin in iron biology. *Biometals* **25:**677–686.

10. **Miyajima H.** 2015. Investigated and available therapeutic options for treating aceruloplasminemia. *Expert Opin Orphan Drugs* **3**:1011–1020.

11. **Shamsian BS, Rezaei N, Arzanian MT, Alavi S, Khojasteh O, Eghbali A.** 2009. Severe hypochromic microcytic anemia in a patient with congenital atransferrinemia. *Pediatr Hematol Oncol* **26**:356–362.

12. **Xiao Q, Jiang X, Moore KJ, Shao Y, Pi H, Dubail I, Charbit A, Newton SM, Klebba PE.** 2011. Sortase independent and dependent systems for acquisition of haem and haemoglobin in *Listeria monocytogenes*. *Mol Microbiol* **80**:1581–1597.

13. **Sankaran VG, Weiss MJ.** 2015. Anemia: progress in molecular mechanisms and therapies. *Nat Med* **21**:221–230.

14. **Edelstein SJ, Telford JN, Crepeau RH.** 1973. Structure of fibers of sickle cell hemoglobin. *Proc Natl Acad Sci USA* **70**:1104–1107.

15. **Chan GC-F, Chan S, Ho P-L, Ha S-Y.** 2009. Effects of chelators (deferoxamine, deferiprone and deferasirox) on the growth of *Klebsiella pneumoniae* and *Aeromonas hydrophila* isolated from transfusion-dependent thalassemia patients. *Hemoglobin* **33**:352–360.

16. **Schubert S, Autenrieth IB.** 2000. Conjugation of hydroxyethyl starch to desferrioxamine (DFO) modulates the dual role of DFO in *Yersinia enterocolitica* infection. *Clin Diagn Lab Immunol* **7**:457–462.

17. **Arifin AJ, Hannauer M, Welch I, Heinrichs DE.** 2014. Deferoxamine mesylate enhances virulence of community-associated methicillin resistant *Staphylococcus aureus*. *Microbes Infect* **16**:967–972.

18. **Escolar L, Pérez-Martin J, de Lorenzo V.** 1999. Opening the iron box: transcriptional metalloregulation by the Fur protein. *J Bacteriol* **181**:6223–6229.

19. **Hantke K.** 2001. Iron and metal regulation in bacteria. *Curr Opin Microbiol* **4**:172–177.

20. **White A, Ding X, vanderSpek JC, Murphy JR, Ringe D.** 1998. Structure of the metal-ion-activated diphtheria toxin repressor/tox operator complex. *Nature* **394**:502–506.

21. **De Lorenzo V, Wee S, Herrero M, Neilands JB.** 1987. Operator sequences of the aerobactin operon of plasmid ColV-K30 binding the ferric uptake regulation (*fur*) repressor. *J Bacteriol* **169**:2624–2630.

22. **Boyd J, Oza MN, Murphy JR.** 1990. Molecular cloning and DNA sequence analysis of a diphtheria *tox* iron-dependent regulatory element (*dtxR*) from *Corynebacterium diphtheriae*. *Proc Natl Acad Sci USA* **87**:5968–5972.

23. **Baichoo N, Helmann JD.** 2002. Recognition of DNA by Fur: a reinterpretation of the *fur* box consensus sequence. *J Bacteriol* **184**:5826–5832.

24. **Carpenter BM, Whitmire JM, Merrell DS.** 2009. This is not your mother's repressor: the complex role of fur in pathogenesis. *Infect Immun* **77**:2590–2601.

25. **Fillat MF.** 2014. The FUR (ferric uptake regulator) superfamily: diversity and versatility of key transcriptional regulators. *Arch Biochem Biophys* **546**:41–52.

26. **Schmitt MP, Holmes RK.** 1991. Iron-dependent regulation of diphtheria toxin and siderophore expression by the cloned *Corynebacterium diphtheriae* repressor gene *dtxR* in *C. diphtheriae* C7 strains. *Infect Immun* **59**:1899–1904.

27. **Troxell B, Hassan HM.** 2013. Transcriptional regulation by ferric uptake regulator (Fur) in pathogenic bacteria. *Front Cell Infect Microbiol* **3**:59.

28. **Skaar EP, Humayun M, Bae T, DeBord KL, Schneewind O.** 2004. Iron-source preference of *Staphylococcus aureus* infections. *Science* **305**:1626–1628.

29. **Proctor RA, von Eiff C, Kahl BC, Becker K, McNamara P, Herrmann M, Peters G.** 2006. Small colony variants: a pathogenic form of bacteria that facilitates persistent and recurrent infections. *Nat Rev Microbiol* **4**:295–305.

30. **Gruss A, Borezée-Durant E, Lechardeur D.** 2012. Environmental heme utilization by heme-auxotrophic bacteria. *Adv Microb Physiol* **61**:69–124.

31. **Los FCO, Randis TM, Aroian RV, Ratner AJ.** 2013. Role of pore-forming toxins in bacterial infectious diseases. *Microbiol Mol Biol Rev* **77**:173–207.

32. **Cescau S, Cwerman H, Létoffé S, Delepelaire P, Wandersman C, Biville F.** 2007. Heme acquisition by hemophores. *Biometals* **20**:603–613.

33. **Hanson MS, Pelzel SE, Latimer J, Müller-Eberhard U, Hansen EJ.** 1992. Identification of a genetic locus of *Haemophilus influenzae* type b necessary for the binding and utilization of heme bound to human hemopexin. *Proc Natl Acad Sci USA* **89**:1973–1977.

34. **Wójtowicz H, Guevara T, Tallant C, Olczak M, Sroka A, Potempa J, Solà M, Olczak T, Gomis-Rüth FX.** 2009. Unique structure and stability of HmuY, a novel heme-binding protein of *Porphyromonas gingivalis*. *PLoS Pathog* **5**:e1000419. doi:10.1371/journal.ppat.1000419.

35. **Létoffé S, Ghigo JM, Wandersman C.** 1994. Iron acquisition from heme and hemoglobin by a *Serratia marcescens* extracellular protein. *Proc Natl Acad Sci USA* **91**:9876–9880.

36. **Arnoux P, Haser R, Izadi N, Lecroisey A, Delepierre M, Wandersman C, Czjzek M.** 1999. The crystal structure of HasA, a hemophore secreted by *Serratia marcescens*. *Nat Struct Biol* **6:**516–520.

37. **Létoffé S, Ghigo JM, Wandersman C.** 1994. Secretion of the *Serratia marcescens* HasA protein by an ABC transporter. *J Bacteriol* **176:**5372–5377.

38. **Wandersman C, Delepelaire P.** 2012. Haemophore functions revisited. *Mol Microbiol* **85:**618–631.

39. **Izadi-Pruneyre N, Huche F, Lukat-Rodgers GS, Lecroisey A, Gilli R, Rodgers KR, Wandersman C, Delepelaire P.** 2006. The heme transfer from the soluble HasA hemophore to its membrane-bound receptor HasR is driven by protein-protein interaction from a high to a lower affinity binding site. *J Biol Chem* **281:**25541–25550.

40. **Krieg S, Huche F, Diederichs K, Izadi-Pruneyre N, Lecroisey A, Wandersman C, Delepelaire P, Welte W.** 2009. Heme uptake across the outer membrane as revealed by crystal structures of the receptor-hemophore complex. *Proc Natl Acad Sci USA* **106:**1045–1050.

41. **Létoffé S, Deniau C, Wolff N, Dassa E, Delepelaire P, Lecroisey A, Wandersman C.** 2001. Haemophore-mediated bacterial haem transport: evidence for a common or overlapping site for haem-free and haem-loaded haemophore on its specific outer membrane receptor. *Mol Microbiol* **41:**439–450.

42. **Létoffé S, Debarbieux L, Izadi N, Delepelaire P, Wandersman C.** 2003. Ligand delivery by haem carrier proteins: the binding of *Serratia marcescens* haemophore to its outer membrane receptor is mediated by two distinct peptide regions. *Mol Microbiol* **50:**77–88.

43. **Wolff N, Izadi-Pruneyre N, Couprie J, Habeck M, Linge J, Rieping W, Wandersman C, Nilges M, Delepierre M, Lecroisey A.** 2008. Comparative analysis of structural and dynamic properties of the loaded and unloaded hemophore HasA: functional implications. *J Mol Biol* **376:**517–525.

44. **Létoffé S, Wecker K, Delepierre M, Delepelaire P, Wandersman C.** 2005. Activities of the *Serratia marcescens* heme receptor HasR and isolated plug and beta-barrel domains: the beta-barrel forms a heme-specific channel. *J Bacteriol* **187:**4637–4645.

45. **Bracken CS, Baer MT, Abdur-Rashid A, Helms W, Stojiljkovic I.** 1999. Use of hemeprotein complexes by the *Yersinia enterocolitica* HemR receptor: histidine residues are essential for receptor function. *J Bacteriol* **181:**6063–6072.

46. **Burkhard KA, Wilks A.** 2007. Characterization of the outer membrane receptor ShuA from the heme uptake system of *Shigella dysenteriae*: substrate specificity and identification of the heme protein ligands. *J Biol Chem* **282:**15126–15136.

47. **Simpson W, Olczak T, Genco CA.** 2000. Characterization and expression of HmuR, a TonB-dependent hemoglobin receptor of *Porphyromonas gingivalis*. *J Bacteriol* **182:**5737–5748.

48. **Ghigo JM, Létoffé S, Wandersman C.** 1997. A new type of hemophore-dependent heme acquisition system of *Serratia marcescens* reconstituted in *Escherichia coli*. *J Bacteriol* **179:**3572–3579.

49. **Paquelin A, Ghigo JM, Bertin S, Wandersman C.** 2001. Characterization of HasB, a *Serratia marcescens* TonB-like protein specifically involved in the haemophore-dependent haem acquisition system. *Mol Microbiol* **42:**995–1005.

50. **Benevides-Matos N, Wandersman C, Biville F.** 2008. HasB, the *Serratia marcescens* TonB paralog, is specific to HasR. *J Bacteriol* **190:**21–27.

51. **Cwerman H, Wandersman C, Biville F.** 2006. Heme and a five-amino-acid hemophore region form the bipartite stimulus triggering the has signaling cascade. *J Bacteriol* **188:**3357–3364.

52. **Rossi MS, Paquelin A, Ghigo JM, Wandersman C.** 2003. Haemophore-mediated signal transduction across the bacterial cell envelope in *Serratia marcescens*: the inducer and the transported substrate are different molecules. *Mol Microbiol* **48:**1467–1480.

53. **Biville F, Cwerman H, Létoffé S, Rossi M-S, Drouet V, Ghigo JM, Wandersman C.** 2004. Haemophore-mediated signalling in *Serratia marcescens*: a new mode of regulation for an extra cytoplasmic function (ECF) sigma factor involved in haem acquisition. *Mol Microbiol* **53:**1267–1277.

54. **Rossi MS, Fetherston JD, Létoffé S, Carniel E, Perry RD, Ghigo JM.** 2001. Identification and characterization of the hemophore-dependent heme acquisition system of *Yersinia pestis*. *Infect Immun* **69:**6707–6717.

55. **Cope LD, Thomas SE, Latimer JL, Slaughter CA, Müller-Eberhard U, Hansen EJ.** 1994. The 100 kDa haem:haemopexin-binding protein of *Haemophilus influenzae*: structure and localization. *Mol Microbiol* **13:**863–873.

56. **Cope LD, Thomas SE, Hrkal Z, Hansen EJ.** 1998. Binding of heme-hemopexin complexes by soluble HxuA protein allows utilization of this complexed heme by *Haemophilus influenzae*. *Infect Immun* **66:**4511–4516.

57. **Cope LD, Yogev R, Müller-Eberhard U, Hansen EJ.** 1995. A gene cluster involved in the utilization of both free heme and heme: hemopexin by *Haemophilus influenzae* type b. *J. Bacteriol* 177:2644–2653.

58. **Baelen S, Dewitte F, Clantin B, Villeret V.** 2013. Structure of the secretion domain of HxuA from *Haemophilus influenzae. Acta Crystallograph Sect F Struct Biol Cryst Commun* 69:1322–1327.

59. **Wong JC, Patel R, Kendall D, Whitby PW, Smith A, Holland J, Williams P.** 1995. Affinity, conservation, and surface exposure of hemopexin-binding proteins in *Haemophilus influenzae. Infect Immun* 63:2327–2333.

60. **Fournier C, Smith A, Delepelaire P.** 2011. Haem release from haemopexin by HxuA allows *Haemophilus influenzae* to escape host nutritional immunity. *Mol Microbiol* 80:133–148.

61. **Morton DJ, Seale TW, Madore LL, VanWagoner TM, Whitby PW, Stull TL.** 2007. The haem-haemopexin utilization gene cluster (*hxuCBA*) as a virulence factor of *Haemophilus influenzae. Microbiology* 153:215–224.

62. **Cope LD, Love RP, Guinn SE, Gilep A, Usanov S, Estabrook RW, Hrkal Z, Hansen EJ.** 2001. Involvement of HxuC outer membrane protein in utilization of hemoglobin by *Haemophilus influenzae. Infect Immun* 69:2353–2363.

63. **Whitby PW, Sim KE, Morton DJ, Patel JA, Stull TL.** 1997. Transcription of genes encoding iron and heme acquisition proteins of *Haemophilus influenzae* during acute otitis media. *Infect Immun* 65:4696–4700.

64. **Gat O, Zaide G, Inbar I, Grosfeld H, Chitlaru T, Levy H, Shafferman A.** 2008. Characterization of *Bacillus anthracis* iron-regulated surface determinant (Isd) proteins containing NEAT domains. *Mol Microbiol* 70:983–999.

65. **Maresso AW, Garufi G, Schneewind O.** 2008. *Bacillus anthracis* secretes proteins that mediate heme acquisition from hemoglobin. *PLoS Pathog* 4:e1000132. doi:10.1371/journal.ppat.1000132.

66. **Andrade MA, Ciccarelli FD, Perez-Iratxeta C, Bork P.** 2002. NEAT: a domain duplicated in genes near the components of a putative Fe3+ siderophore transporter from Gram-positive pathogenic bacteria. *Genome Biol* 3:research00471–research00475.

67. **Honsa ES, Maresso AW, Highlander SK.** 2014. Molecular and evolutionary analysis of NEAr-iron Transporter (NEAT) domains. *PloS One* 9:e104794. doi:10.1371/journal.pone.0104794.

68. **Grigg JC, Ukpabi G, Gaudin CF, Murphy ME.** 2010. Structural biology of heme binding in the *Staphylococcus aureus* Isd system. *J Inorg Biochem* 104:341–348.

69. **Honsa ES, Maresso AW.** 2011. Mechanisms of iron import in anthrax. *Biometals* 24:533–545.

70. **Grigg JC, Vermeiren CL, Heinrichs DE, Murphy ME.** 2007. Haem recognition by a *Staphylococcus aureus* NEAT domain. *Mol Microbiol* 63:139–149.

71. **Fabian M, Solomaha E, Olson JS, Maresso AW.** 2009. Heme transfer to the bacterial cell envelope occurs via a secreted hemophore in the Gram-positive pathogen *Bacillus anthracis. J Biol Chem* 284:32138–32146.

72. **Honsa ES, Fabian M, Cardenas AM, Olson JS, Maresso AW.** 2011. The five near-iron transporter (NEAT) domain anthrax hemophore, IsdX2, scavenges heme from hemoglobin and transfers heme to the surface protein IsdC. *J Biol Chem* 286:33652–33660.

73. **Malmirchegini GR, Sjodt M, Shnitkind S, Sawaya MR, Rosinski J, Newton SM, Klebba PE, Clubb RT.** 2014. Novel mechanism of hemin capture by Hbp2, the hemoglobin-binding hemophore from *Listeria monocytogenes. J Biol Chem* 289:34886–34899.

74. **Mukherjee S.** 1985. The role of crevicular fluid iron in periodontal disease. *J Periodontol* 56:22–27.

75. **Shizukuishi S, Tazaki K, Inoshita E, Kataoka K, Hanioka T, Amano A.** 1995. Effect of concentration of compounds containing iron on the growth of *Porphyromonas gingivalis. FEMS Microbiol Lett* 131:313–317.

76. **Smalley JW, Silver J, Marsh PJ, Birss AJ.** 1998. The periodontopathogen *Porphyromonas gingivalis* binds iron protoporphyrin IX in the mu-oxo dimeric form: an oxidative buffer and possible pathogenic mechanism. *Biochem J* 331:681–685.

77. **Li N, Collyer CA.** 2011. Gingipains from *Porphyromonas gingivalis*: complex domain structures confer diverse functions. *Eur J Microbiol Immunol* 1:41–58.

78. **Smalley JW, Birss AJ, Szmigielski B, Potempa J.** 2007. Sequential action of R- and K-specific gingipains of *Porphyromonas gingivalis* in the generation of the heam-containing pigment from oxyhaemoglobin. *Arch Biochem Biophys* 465:44–49.

79. **Smalley JW, Birss AJ, Szmigielski B, Potempa J.** 2008. Mechanism of methaemoglobin breakdown by the lysine-specific gingipain of the periodontal pathogen *Porphyromonas gingivalis. Biol Chem* 389:1235–1238.

80. **Olczak T, Sroka A, Potempa J, Olczak M.** 2008. *Porphyromonas gingivalis* HmuY and HmuR: further characterization of a novel mechanism of heme utilization. *Arch Microbiol* 189:197–210.

81. Smalley JW, Byrne DP, Birss AJ, Wójtowicz H, Sroka A, Potempa J, Olczak T. 2011. HmuY haemophore and gingipain proteases constitute a unique syntrophic system of haem acquisition by *Porphyromonas gingivalis*. *PLoS One* **6**:e17182. doi:10.1371/journal.pone.0017182.

82. Sroka A, Sztukowska M, Potempa J, Travis J, Genco CA. 2001. Degradation of host heme proteins by lysine- and arginine-specific cysteine proteinases (gingipains) of *Porphyromonas gingivalis*. *J Bacteriol* **183**:5609–5616.

83. Lewis JP, Plata K, Yu F, Rosato A, Anaya C. 2006. Transcriptional organization, regulation and role of the *Porphyromonas gingivalis* W83 hmu haemin-uptake locus. *Microbiology* **152**:3367–3382.

84. Dautin N. 2010. Serine protease autotransporters of *Enterobacteriaceae* (SPATEs): biogenesis and function. *Toxins* **2**:1179–1206.

85. Drago-Serrano ME, Parra SG, Manjarrez-Hernández HA. 2006. EspC, an autotransporter protein secreted by enteropathogenic *Escherichia coli* (EPEC), displays protease activity on human hemoglobin. *FEMS Microbiol Lett* **265**:35–40.

86. Otto BR, van Dooren SJ, Nuijens JH, Luirink J, Oudega B. 1998. Characterization of a hemoglobin protease secreted by the pathogenic *Escherichia coli* strain EB1. *J Exp Med* **188**: 1091–1103.

87. Otto BR, van Dooren SJM, Dozois CM, Luirink J, Oudega B. 2002. *Escherichia coli* hemoglobin protease autotransporter contributes to synergistic abscess formation and heme-dependent growth of *Bacteroides fragilis*. *Infect Immun* **70**:5–10.

88. Nikaido H. 1992. Porins and specific channels of bacterial outer membranes. *Mol Microbiol* **6**:435–442.

89. Braun V, Günter K, Hantke K. 1991. Transport of iron across the outer membrane. *Biol Met* **4**:14–22.

90. Schauer K, Rodionov DA, de Reuse H. 2008. New substrates for TonB-dependent transport: do we only see the "tip of the iceberg"? *Trends Biochem Sci* **33**:330–338.

91. Noinaj N, Guillier M, Barnard TJ, Buchanan SK. 2010. TonB-dependent transporters: regulation, structure, and function. *Annu Rev Microbiol* **64**:43–60.

92. Härle C, Kim I, Angerer A, Braun V. 1995. Signal transfer through three compartments: transcription initiation of the *Escherichia coli* ferric citrate transport system from the cell surface. *EMBO J* **14**:1430–1438.

93. Lamont IL, Beare PA, Ochsner U, Vasil AI, Vasil ML. 2002. Siderophore-mediated signaling regulates virulence factor production in *Pseudomonas aeruginosa*. *Proc Natl Acad Sci USA* **99**:7072–7077.

94. Kim I, Stiefel A, Plantör S, Angerer A, Braun V. 1997. Transcription induction of the ferric citrate transport genes via the N-terminus of the FecA outer membrane protein, the Ton system and the electrochemical potential of the cytoplasmic membrane. *Mol Microbiol* **23**:333–344.

95. Braun V, Mahren S, Ogierman M. 2003. Regulation of the FecI-type ECF sigma factor by transmembrane signalling. *Curr Opin Microbiol* **6**:173–180.

96. Welz D, Braun V. 1998. Ferric citrate transport of *Escherichia coli*: functional regions of the FecR transmembrane regulatory protein. *J Bacteriol* **180**:2387–2394.

97. Bradbeer C. 1993. The proton motive force drives the outer membrane transport of cobalamin in *Escherichia coli*. *J Bacteriol* **175**: 3146–3150.

98. Krewulak KD, Vogel HJ. 2011. TonB or not TonB: is that the question? *Biochem Cell Biol Biochim Biol Cell* **89**:87–97.

99. Braun V. 1995. Energy-coupled transport and signal transduction through the Gram-negative outer membrane via TonB-ExbB-ExbD-dependent receptor proteins. *FEMS Microbiol Rev* **16**:295–307.

100. Pawelek PD, Croteau N, Ng-Thow-Hing C, Khursigara CM, Moiseeva N, Allaire M, Coulton JW. 2006. Structure of TonB in complex with FhuA, *E. coli* outer membrane receptor. *Science* **312**:1399–1402.

101. Shultis DD, Purdy MD, Banchs CN, Wiener MC. 2006. Outer membrane active transport: structure of the BtuB:TonB complex. *Science* **312**:1396–1399.

102. Udho E, Jakes KS, Finkelstein A. 2012. TonB-dependent transporter FhuA in planar lipid bilayers: partial exit of its plug from the barrel. *Biochemistry* **51**:6753–6759.

103. Schalk IJ, Mislin GLA, Brillet K. 2012. Structure, function and binding selectivity and stereoselectivity of siderophore-iron outer membrane transporters. *Curr Top Membr* **69**:37–66.

104. Davidson AL, Dassa E, Orelle C, Chen J. 2008. Structure, function, and evolution of bacterial ATP-binding cassette systems. *Microbiol Mol Biol Rev* **72**:317–364.

105. Tong Y, Guo M. 2009. Bacterial heme-transport proteins and their heme-coordination modes. *Arch Biochem Biophys* **481**:1–15.

106. Berntsson RPA, Smits SHJ, Schmitt L, Slotboom D-J, Poolman B. 2010. A structural

classification of substrate-binding proteins. *FEBS Lett* **584:**2606–2617.

107. **Borths EL, Locher KP, Lee AT, Rees DC.** 2002. The structure of *Escherichia coli* BtuF and binding to its cognate ATP binding cassette transporter. *Proc Natl Acad Sci USA* **99:** 16642–16647.

108. **Stojiljkovic I, Hantke K.** 1994. Transport of haemin across the cytoplasmic membrane through a haemin-specific periplasmic binding-protein-dependent transport system in *Yersinia enterocolitica. Mol Microbiol* **13:**719–732.

109. **Stojiljkovic I, Hantke K.** 1992. Hemin uptake system of *Yersinia enterocolitica*: similarities with other TonB-dependent systems in Gram-negative bacteria. *EMBO J* **11:**4359–4367.

110. **Schneider S, Paoli M.** 2005. Crystallization and preliminary X-ray diffraction analysis of the haem-binding protein HemS from *Yersinia enterocolitica. Acta Crystallograph Sect F Struct Biol Cryst Commun* **61:**802–805.

111. **Hornung JM, Jones HA, Perry RD.** 1996. The *hmu* locus of *Yersinia pestis* is essential for utilization of free haemin and haem-protein complexes as iron sources. *Mol Microbiol* **20:** 725–739.

112. **Thompson JM, Jones HA, Perry RD.** 1999. Molecular characterization of the hemin uptake locus (*hmu*) from *Yersinia pestis* and analysis of *hmu* mutants for hemin and hemoprotein utilization. *Infect Immun* **67:**3879–3892.

113. **Wyckoff EE, Duncan D, Torres AG, Mills M, Maase K, Payne SM.** 1998. Structure of the *Shigella dysenteriae* haem transport locus and its phylogenetic distribution in enteric bacteria. *Mol Microbiol* **28:**1139–1152.

114. **Occhino DA, Wyckoff EE, Henderson DP, Wrona TJ, Payne SM.** 1998. *Vibrio cholerae* iron transport: haem transport genes are linked to one of two sets of *tonB, exbB, exbD* genes. *Mol Microbiol* **29:**1493–1507.

115. **Ochsner UA, Johnson Z, Vasil ML.** 2000. Genetics and regulation of two distinct haem-uptake systems, *phu* and *has*, in *Pseudomonas aeruginosa. Microbiology* **146:**185–198.

116. **Ho WW, Li H, Eakanunkul S, Tong Y, Wilks A, Guo M, Poulos TL.** 2007. Holo- and apo-bound structures of bacterial periplasmic heme-binding proteins. *J Biol Chem* **282:**35796–35802.

117. **Mattle D, Zeltina A, Woo J-S, Goetz BA, Locher KP.** 2010. Two stacked heme molecules in the binding pocket of the periplasmic heme-binding protein HmuT from *Yersinia pestis. J Mol Biol* **404:**220–231.

118. **Woo J-S, Zeltina A, Goetz BA, Locher KP.** 2012. X-ray structure of the *Yersinia pestis* heme transporter HmuUV. *Nat Struct Mol Biol* **19:**1310–1315.

119. **Lewinson O, Lee AT, Locher KP, Rees DC.** 2010. A distinct mechanism for the ABC transporter BtuCD-BtuF revealed by the dynamics of complex formation. *Nat Struct Mol Biol* **17:**332–338.

120. **ter Beek J, Guskov A, Slotboom DJ.** 2014. Structural diversity of ABC transporters. *J Gen Physiol* **143:**419–435.

121. **Wyckoff EE, Lopreato GF, Tipton KA, Payne SM.** 2005. *Shigella dysenteriae* ShuS promotes utilization of heme as an iron source and protects against heme toxicity. *J Bacteriol* **187:** 5658–5664.

122. **Tripathi S, O'Neill MJ, Wilks A, Poulos TL.** 2013. Crystal structure of the *Pseudomonas aeruginosa* cytoplasmic heme binding protein, Apo-PhuS. *J Inorg Biochem* **128:**131–136.

123. **Beveridge TJ, Matias VRF.** 2006. Ultrastructure of Gram-positive cell walls, p 3–11. *In* Fischetti V, Novick R, Ferretti J, Portnoy D, Rood J (ed), *Gram-Positive Pathogens*, 2nd ed. ASM Press, Washington, DC.

124. **Pishchany G, Sheldon JR, Dickson CF, Alam MT, Read TD, Gell DA, Heinrichs DE, Skaar EP.** 2014. IsdB-dependent hemoglobin binding is required for acquisition of heme by *Staphylococcus aureus. J Infect Dis* **209:**1764–1772.

125. **Sheldon JR, Heinrichs DE.** 2015. Recent developments in understanding the iron acquisition strategies of Gram positive pathogens. *FEMS Microbiol Rev* **39:**592–630.

126. **Mazmanian SK, Ton-That H, Su K, Schneewind O.** 2002. An iron-regulated sortase anchors a class of surface protein during *Staphylococcus aureus* pathogenesis. *Proc Natl Acad Sci USA* **99:** 2293–2298.

127. **Mazmanian SK, Skaar EP, Gaspar AH, Humayun M, Gornicki P, Jelenska J, Joachmiak A, Missiakas DM, Schneewind O.** 2003. Passage of heme-iron across the envelope of *Staphylococcus aureus. Science* **299:**906–909.

128. **Torres VJ, Pishchany G, Humayun M, Schneewind O, Skaar EP.** 2006. *Staphylococcus aureus* IsdB is a hemoglobin receptor required for heme iron utilization. *J Bacteriol* **188:**8421–8429.

129. **Dryla A, Hoffmann B, Gelbmann D, Giefing C, Hanner M, Meinke A, Anderson AS, Koppensteiner W, Konrat R, von Gabain A, Nagy E.** 2007. High-affinity binding of the staphylococcal HarA protein to haptoglobin and hemoglobin involves a domain with an antiparallel eight-stranded beta-barrel fold. *J Bacteriol* **189:**254–264.

130. **Muryoi N, Tiedemann MT, Pluym M, Cheung J, Heinrichs DE, Stillman MJ.** 2008. Demonstration of the iron-regulated surface determinant (Isd) heme transfer pathway in *Staphylococcus aureus*. *J Biol Chem* **283:**28125–28136.

131. **Liu M, Tanaka WN, Zhu H, Xie G, Dooley DM, Lei B.** 2008. Direct hemin transfer from IsdA to IsdC in the iron-regulated surface determinant (Isd) heme acquisition system of *Staphylococcus aureus*. *J Biol Chem* **283:**6668–6676.

132. **Tiedemann MT, Heinrichs DE, Stillman MJ.** 2012. Multiprotein heme shuttle pathway in *Staphylococcus aureus*: iron-regulated surface determinant cog-wheel kinetics. *J Am Chem Soc* **134:**16578–16585.

133. **Grigg JC, Vermeiren CL, Heinrichs DE, Murphy ME.** 2007. Heme coordination by *Staphylococcus aureus* IsdE. *J Biol Chem* **282:**28815–28822.

134. **Pluym M, Vermeiren CL, Mack J, Heinrichs DE, Stillman MJ.** 2007. Heme binding properties of *Staphylococcus aureus* IsdE. *Biochemistry* **46:**12777–12877.

135. **Moriwaki Y, Terada T, Caaveiro JMM, Takaoka Y, Hamachi I, Tsumoto K, Shimizu K.** 2013. Heme binding mechanism of structurally similar iron-regulated surface determinant near transporter domains of *Staphylococcus aureus* exhibiting different affinities for heme. *Biochemistry* **52:**8866–8877.

136. **Villareal VA, Pilpa RM, Robson SA, Fadeev EA, Clubb RT.** 2008. The IsdC protein from *Staphylococcus aureus* uses a flexible binding pocket to capture heme. *J Biol Chem* **283:**31591–31600.

137. **Abe R, Caaveiro JMM, Kozuka-Hata H, Oyama M, Tsumoto K.** 2012. Mapping ultraweak protein-protein interactions between heme transporters of *Staphylococcus aureus*. *J Biol Chem* **287:**16477–16487.

138. **Grigg JC, Mao CX, Murphy MEP.** 2011. Iron-coordinating tyrosine is a key determinant of NEAT domain heme transfer. *J Mol Biol* **413:**684–698.

139. **Reniere ML, Skaar EP.** 2008. *Staphylococcus aureus* haem oxygenases are differentially regulated by iron and haem. *Mol Microbiol* **69:**1304–1315.

140. **Cheng AG, Kim HK, Burts ML, Krausz T, Schneewind O, Missiakas DM.** 2009. Genetic requirements for *Staphylococcus aureus* abscess formation and persistence in host tissues. *FASEB J* **23:**3393–3404.

141. **Visai L, Yanagisawa N, Josefsson E, Tarkowski A, Pezzali I, Rooijakkers SH, Foster TJ, Speziale P.** 2009. Immune evasion by *Staphylococcus aureus* conferred by iron-regulated surface determinant protein IsdH. *Microbiology* **155:**667–679.

142. **Pilpa RM, Fadeev EA, Villareal VA, Wong ML, Phillips M, Clubb RT.** 2006. Solution structure of the NEAT (NEAr Transporter) domain from IsdH/HarA: the human hemoglobin receptor in *Staphylococcus aureus*. *J Mol Biol* **360:**435–447.

143. **Sharp KH, Schneider S, Cockayne A, Paoli M.** 2007. Crystal structure of the heme-IsdC complex, the central conduit of the Isd iron/heme uptake system in *Staphylococcus aureus*. *J Biol Chem* **282:**10625–10631.

144. **Watanabe M, Tanaka Y, Suenaga A, Kuroda M, Yao M, Watanabe N, Arisaka F, Ohta T, Tanaka I, Tsumoto K.** 2008. Structural basis for multimeric heme complexation through a specific protein-heme interaction: the case of the third neat domain of IsdH from *Staphylococcus aureus*. *J Biol Chem* **283:**28649–28659.

145. **Gaudin CFM, Grigg JC, Arrieta AL, Murphy MEP.** 2011. Unique heme-iron coordination by the hemoglobin receptor IsdB of *Staphylococcus aureus*. *Biochemistry* **50:**5443–5452.

146. **Dryla A, Gelbmann D, von Gabain A, Nagy E.** 2003. Identification of a novel iron regulated staphylococcal surface protein with haptoglobin-haemoglobin binding activity. *Mol Microbiol* **49:**37–53.

147. **Pilpa RM, Robson SA, Villareal VA, Wong ML, Phillips M, Clubb RT.** 2009. Functionally distinct NEAT (NEAr Transporter) domains within the *Staphylococcus aureus* IsdH/HarA protein extract heme from methemoglobin. *J Biol Chem* **284:**1166–1176.

148. **Dickson CF, Krishna Kumar K, Jacques DA, Malmirchegini GR, Spirig T, Mackay JP, Clubb RT, Guss JM, Gell DA.** 2014. Structure of the hemoglobin-IsdH complex reveals the molecular basis of iron capture by *Staphylococcus aureus*. *J Biol Chem* **289:**6728–6738.

149. **Krishna Kumar K, Jacques DA, Pishchany G, Caradoc-Davies T, Spirig T, Malmirchegini GR, Langley DB, Dickson CF, Mackay JP, Clubb RT, Skaar EP, Guss JM, Gell DA.** 2011. Structural basis for hemoglobin capture by *Staphylococcus aureus* cell-surface protein, IsdH. *J Biol Chem* **286:**38439–38447.

150. **Bowden CFM, Verstraete MM, Eltis LD, Murphy MEP.** 2014. Hemoglobin binding and catalytic heme extraction by IsdB near iron transporter domains. *Biochemistry* **53:**2286–2294.

151. **Pluym M.** 2008. Heme binding in the NEAT domains of IsdA and IsdC of *Staphylococcus aureus*. *J Inorg Biochem* **102:**480–488.

152. Fonner BA, Tripet BP, Eilers B, Stanisich J, Sullivan-Springhetti RK, Moore R, Liu M, Lei B, Copie V. 2014. Solution structure and molecular determinants of hemoglobin binding of the first NEAT domain of IsdB in *Staphylococcus aureus*. *Biochemistry* **53:**3922–3933.

153. Spirig T, Malmirchegini GR, Zhang J, Robson SA, Sjodt M, Liu M, Krishna Kumar K, Dickson CF, Gell DA, Lei B, Loo JA, Clubb RT. 2013. *Staphylococcus aureus* uses a novel multidomain receptor to break apart human hemoglobin and steal its heme. *J Biol Chem* **288:**1065–1078.

154. Zhu H, Li D, Liu M, Copié V, Lei B. 2014. Non-heme-binding domains and segments of the *Staphylococcus aureus* IsdB protein critically contribute to the kinetics and equilibrium of heme acquisition from methemoglobin. *PLoS One* **9:**e100744. doi:10.1371/journal.pone.0100744.

155. Haley KP, Janson EM, Heilbronner S, Foster TJ, Skaar EP. 2011. *Staphylococcus lugdunensis* IsdG liberates iron from host heme. *J Bacteriol* **193:**4749–4757.

156. Zapotoczna M, Heilbronner S, Speziale P, Foster TJ. 2012. Iron-regulated surface determinant (Isd) proteins of *Staphylococcus lugdunensis*. *J Bacteriol* **194:**6453–6467.

157. Brozyna JR, Sheldon JR, Heinrichs DE. 2014. Growth promotion of the opportunistic human pathogen, *Staphylococcus lugdunensis*, by heme, hemoglobin, and coculture with *Staphylococcus aureus*. *MicrobiologyOpen* **3:**182–195.

158. Maresso AW, Chapa TJ, Schneewind O. 2006. Surface protein IsdC and Sortase B are required for heme-iron scavenging of *Bacillus anthracis*. *J Bacteriol* **188:**8145–8152.

159. Tarlovsky Y, Fabian M, Solomaha E, Honsa E, Olson JS, Maresso AW. 2010. A *Bacillus anthracis* S-layer homology protein that binds heme and mediates heme delivery to IsdC. *J Bacteriol* **192:**3503–3511.

160. Bates CS, Montañez GE, Woods CR, Vincent RM, Eichenbaum Z. 2003. Identification and characterization of a *Streptococcus pyogenes* operon involved in binding of hemoproteins and acquisition of iron. *Infect Immun* **71:**1042–1055.

161. Drazek ES, Hammack CA, Schmitt MP. 2000. *Corynebacterium diphtheriae* genes required for acquisition of iron from haemin and haemoglobin are homologous to ABC haemin transporters. *Mol Microbiol* **36:**68–84.

162. Ouattara M, Cunha EB, Li X, Huang Y-S, Dixon D, Eichenbaum Z. 2010. Shr of group A *Streptococcus* is a new type of composite NEAT protein involved in sequestering haem from methaemoglobin. *Mol Microbiol* **78:**739–756.

163. Lei B, Liu M, Voyich JM, Prater CI, Kala SV, DeLeo FR, Musser JM. 2003. Identification and characterization of HtsA, a second heme-binding protein made by *Streptococcus pyogenes*. *Infect Immun* **71:**5962–5969.

164. Dahesh S, Nizet V, Cole JN. 2012. Study of streptococcal hemoprotein receptor (Shr) in iron acquisition and virulence of M1T1 group A streptococcus. *Virulence* **3:**566–575.

165. Allen CE, Schmitt MP. 2009. HtaA is an iron-regulated hemin binding protein involved in the utilization of heme iron in *Corynebacterium diphtheriae*. *J Bacteriol* **191:**2638–2648.

166. Allen CE, Schmitt MP. 2011. Novel hemin binding domains in the *Corynebacterium diphtheriae* HtaA protein interact with hemoglobin and are critical for heme iron utilization by HtaA. *J Bacteriol* **193:**5374–5385.

167. Allen CE, Schmitt MP. 2014. Utilization of host iron sources by *Corynebacterium diphtheriae*: multiple hemoglobin-binding proteins are essential for the use of iron from the hemoglobin/haptoglobin complex. *J Bacteriol* **197:**553–562.

168. Allen CE, Burgos JM, Schmitt MP. 2013. Analysis of novel iron-regulated, surface-anchored hemin-binding proteins in *Corynebacterium diphtheriae*. *J Bacteriol* **195:**2852–2863.

169. Wilks A. 2002. Heme oxygenase: evolution, structure, and mechanism. *Antioxid Redox Signal* **4:**603–614.

170. Schmitt MP. 1997. Utilization of host iron sources by *Corynebacterium diphtheriae*: identification of a gene whose product is homologous to eukaryotic heme oxygenases and is required for acquisition of iron from heme and hemoglobin. *J Bacteriol* **179:**838–845.

171. Wilks A, Schmitt MP. 1998. Expression and characterization of a heme oxygenase (HmuO) from *Corynebacterium diphtheriae*. Iron acquisition requires oxidative cleavage of the heme macrocycle. *J Biol Chem* **273:**837–841.

172. Zhu W, Wilks A, Stojiljkovic I. 2000. Degradation of heme in Gram-negative bacteria: the product of the *hemO* gene of *Neisseriae* is a heme oxygenase. *J Bacteriol* **182:**6783–6790.

173. Ratliff M, Zhu W, Deshmukh R, Wilks A, Stojiljkovic I. 2001. Homologues of neisserial heme oxygenase in Gram-negative bacteria: degradation of heme by the product of the *pigA* gene of *Pseudomonas aeruginosa*. *J Bacteriol* **183:**6394–6403.

174. Nambu S, Matsui T, Goulding CW, Takahashi S, Ikeda-Saito M. 2013. A new way to degrade

heme: the *Mycobacterium tuberculosis* enzyme MhuD catalyzes heme degradation without generating CO. *J Biol Chem* **288:**10101–10109.

175. **Wilks A, Heinzl G.** 2014. Heme oxygenation and the widening paradigm of heme degradation. *Arch Biochem Biophys* **544:**87–95.

176. **Wilks A, Ikeda-Saito M.** 2014. Heme utilization by pathogenic bacteria: not all pathways lead to biliverdin. *Acc Chem Res* **47:**2291–2298.

177. **Anzaldi LL, Skaar EP.** 2010. Overcoming the heme paradox: heme toxicity and tolerance in bacterial pathogens. *Infect Immun* **78:**4977–4989.

178. **West SE, Sparling PF.** 1985. Response of *Neisseria gonorrhoeae* to iron limitation: alterations in expression of membrane proteins without apparent siderophore production. *Infect Immun* **47:**388–394.

179. **Campagnari AA, Shanks KL, Dyer DW.** 1994. Growth of *Moraxella catarrhalis* with human transferrin and lactoferrin: expression of iron-repressible proteins without siderophore production. *Infect Immun* **62:**4909–4914.

180. **Schryvers AB, Gray-Owen S.** 1992. Iron acquisition in *Haemophilus influenzae*: receptors for human transferrin. *J Infect Dis* **165:**S103–S104.

181. **Cornelissen CN, Biswas GD, Tsai J, Paruchuri DK, Thompson SA, Sparling PF.** 1992. Gonococcal transferrin-binding protein 1 is required for transferrin utilization and is homologous to TonB-dependent outer membrane receptors. *J Bacteriol* **174:**5788–5797.

182. **Anderson JE, Sparling PF, Cornelissen CN.** 1994. Gonococcal transferrin-binding protein 2 facilitates but is not essential for transferrin utilization. *J Bacteriol* **176:**3162–3170.

183. **Boulton IC, Gorringe AR, Allison N, Robinson A, Gorinsky B, Joannou CL, Evans RW.** 1998. Transferrin-binding protein B isolated from *Neisseria meningitidis* discriminates between apo and diferric human transferrin. *Biochem J* **334:**269–273.

184. **Irwin SW, Averil N, Cheng CY, Schryvers AB.** 1993. Preparation and analysis of isogenic mutants in the transferrin receptor protein genes, *tbpA* and *tbpB*, from *Neisseria meningitidis*. *Mol Microbiol* **8:**1125–1133.

185. **Alcantara J, Yu RH, Schryvers AB.** 1993. The region of human transferrin involved in binding to bacterial transferrin receptors is localized in the C-lobe. *Mol Microbiol* **8:**1135–1143.

186. **Noinaj N, Easley NC, Oke M, Mizuno N, Gumbart J, Boura E, Steere AN, Zak O, Aisen P, Tajkhorshid E, Evans RW, Gorringe AR, Mason AB, Steven AC, Buchanan SK.** 2012. Structural basis for iron piracy by pathogenic *Neisseria*. *Nature* **483:**53–58.

187. **Calmettes C, Alcantara J, Yu R-H, Schryvers AB, Moraes TF.** 2012. The structural basis of transferrin sequestration by transferrin-binding protein B. *Nat Struct Mol Biol* **19:**358–360.

188. **Steere AN, Byrne SL, Chasteen ND, Smith VC, MacGillivray RTA, Mason AB.** 2010. Evidence that His349 acts as a pH-inducible switch to accelerate receptor-mediated iron release from the C-lobe of human transferrin. *J Biol Inorg Chem* **15:**1341–1352.

189. **Noto JM, Cornelissen CN.** 2008. Identification of TbpA residues required for transferrin-iron utilization by *Neisseria gonorrhoeae*. *Infect Immun* **76:**1960–1969.

190. **Zarantonelli M-L, Szatanik M, Giorgini D, Hong E, Huerre M, Guillou F, Alonso J-M, Taha M-K.** 2007. Transgenic mice expressing human transferrin as a model for meningococcal infection. *Infect Immun* **75:**5609–5614.

191. **Szatanik M, Hong E, Ruckly C, Ledroit M, Giorgini D, Jopek K, Nicola M-A, Deghmane A-E, Taha M-K.** 2011. Experimental meningococcal sepsis in congenic transgenic mice expressing human transferrin. *PLoS One* **6:**e22210. doi:10.1371/journal.pone.0022210.

192. **Barber MF, Elde NC.** 2014. Escape from bacterial iron piracy through rapid evolution of transferrin. *Science* **346:**1362–1366.

193. **Beddek AJ, Schryvers AB.** 2010. The lactoferrin receptor complex in Gram negative bacteria. *Biometals* **23:**377–386.

194. **Schryvers AB, Morris LJ.** 1988. Identification and characterization of the human lactoferrin-binding protein from *Neisseria meningitidis*. *Infect Immun* **56:**1144–1149.

195. **Bonnah RA, Yu R, Schryvers AB.** 1995. Biochemical analysis of lactoferrin receptors in the *Neisseriaceae*: identification of a second bacterial lactoferrin receptor protein. *Microb Pathog* **19:**285–297.

196. **Brooks CL, Arutyunova E, Lemieux MJ.** 2014. The structure of lactoferrin-binding protein B from *Neisseria meningitidis* suggests roles in iron acquisition and neutralization of host defences. *Acta Crystallogr Sect F Struct Biol Commun* **70:**1312–1317.

197. **Bellamy W, Takase M, Wakabayashi H, Kawase K, Tomita M.** 1992. Antibacterial spectrum of lactoferricin B, a potent bactericidal peptide derived from the N-terminal region of bovine lactoferrin. *J Appl Bacteriol* **73:**472–479.

198. **Morgenthau A, Livingstone M, Adamiak P, Schryvers AB.** 2012. The role of lactoferrin binding protein B in mediating protection against human lactoferricin. *Biochem Cell Biol* **90:**417–423.

199. **Morgenthau A, Partha SK, Adamiak P, Schryvers AB.** 2014. The specificity of protection against cationic antimicrobial peptides by lactoferrin binding protein B. *Biometals* **27**:923–933.

200. **Noinaj N, Cornelissen CN, Buchanan SK.** 2013. Structural insight into the lactoferrin receptors from pathogenic *Neisseria. J Struct Biol* **184**:83–92.

201. **Parker Siburt CJ, Mietzner TA, Crumbliss AL.** 2012. FbpA: a bacterial transferrin with more to offer. *Biochim Biophys Acta* **1820**:379–392.

202. **Anderson DS, Adhikari P, Nowalk AJ, Chen CY, Mietzner TA.** 2004. The hFbpABC transporter from *Haemophilus influenzae* functions as a binding-protein-dependent ABC transporter with high specificity and affinity for ferric iron. *J Bacteriol* **186**:6220–6229.

203. **Khun HH, Kirby SD, Lee BC.** 1998. A *Neisseria meningitidis fbpABC* mutant is incapable of using nonheme iron for growth. *Infect Immun* **66**:2330–2336.

204. **Adhikari P, Berish SA, Nowalk AJ, Veraldi KL, Morse SA, Mietzner TA.** 1996. The *fbpABC* locus of *Neisseria gonorrhoeae* functions in the periplasm-to-cytosol transport of iron. *J Bacteriol* **178**:2145–2149.

205. **Biville F, Brézillon C, Giorgini D, Taha M-K.** 2014. Pyrophosphate-mediated iron acquisition from transferrin in *Neisseria meningitidis* does not require TonB activity. *PLoS One* **9**: e107612. doi:10.1371/journal.pone.0107612.

206. **Miethke M, Marahiel MA.** 2007. Siderophore-based iron acquisition and pathogen control. *Microbiol Mol Biol Rev* **71**:413–451.

207. **Carrano CJ, Raymond KN.** 1979. Ferric ion sequestering agents. 2. Kinetics and mechanism of iron removal from transferrin by enterobactin and synthetic tricatechols. *J Am Chem Soc* **101**:5401–5404.

208. **Hider RC, Kong X.** 2010. Chemistry and biology of siderophores. *Nat Prod Rep* **27**:637–657.

209. **Crosa JH, Walsh CT.** 2002. Genetics and assembly line enzymology of siderophore biosynthesis in bacteria. *Microbiol Mol Biol Rev* **66**:223–249.

210. **Challis GL.** 2005. A widely distributed bacterial pathway for siderophore biosynthesis independent of nonribosomal peptide synthetases. *Chembiochem* **6**:601–11.

211. **Cendrowski S, MacArthur W, Hanna P.** 2004. *Bacillus anthracis* requires siderophore biosynthesis for growth in macrophages and mouse virulence. *Mol Microbiol* **51**:407–417.

212. **Hannauer M, Sheldon JR, Heinrichs DE.** 2015. Involvement of major facilitator superfamily proteins SfaA and SbnD in staphyloferrin secretion in *Staphylococcus aureus. FEBS Lett* **589**:730–737.

213. **Beasley FC, Marolda CL, Cheung J, Buac S, Heinrichs DE.** 2011. *Staphylococcus aureus* transporters Hts, Sir, and Sst capture iron liberated from human transferrin by staphyloferrin A, staphyloferrin B, and catecholamine stress hormones, respectively, and contribute to virulence. *Infect Immun* **79**:2345–2355.

214. **Zawadzka AM, Abergel RJ, Nichiporuk R, Andersen UN, Raymond KN.** 2009. Siderophore-mediated iron acquisition systems in *Bacillus cereus*: identification of receptors for anthrax virulence-associated petrobactin. *Biochemistry* **48**:3645–3657.

215. **Sandrini SM, Shergill R, Woodward J, Muralikuttan R, Haigh RD, Lyte M, Freestone PP.** 2010. Elucidation of the mechanism by which catecholamine stress hormones liberate iron from the innate immune defense proteins transferrin and lactoferrin. *J Bacteriol* **192**:587–594.

216. **Goetz DH, Holmes MA, Borregaard N, Blumh ME, Raymond KN, Strong RK.** 2002. The neutrophil lipocalin NGAL is a bacteriostatic agent that interferes with siderophore-mediated iron acquisition. *Mol Cell* **10**:1033–1043.

217. **Goetz DH, Willie ST, Armen RS, Bratt T, Borregaard N, Strong RK.** 2000. Ligand preference inferred from the structure of neutrophil gelatinase associated lipocalin. *Biochemistry* **39**:1935–1941.

218. **Hantke K, Nicholson G, Rabsch W, Winkelmann G.** 2003. Salmochelins, siderophores of *Salmonella enterica* and uropathogenic *Escherichia coli* strains, are recognized by the outer membrane receptor IroN. *Proc Natl Acad Sci USA* **100**:3677–3682.

219. **Crouch M-LV, Castor M, Karlinsey JE, Kalhorn T, Fang FC.** 2008. Biosynthesis and IroC-dependent export of the siderophore salmochelin are essential for virulence of *Salmonella enterica* serovar Typhimurium. *Mol Microbiol* **67**:971–983.

220. **Worst DJ, M. Gerrits M, Vandenbroucke-Grauls CMJE, Kusters JG.** 1998. *Helicobacter pylori ribBA*-mediated riboflavin production is involved in iron acquisition. *J Bacteriol* **180**:1473–1479.

221. **Velayudhan J, Hughes NJ, McColm AA, Bagshaw J, Clayton CL, Andrews SC, Kelly DJ.** 2000. Iron acquisition and virulence in *Helicobacter pylori*: a major role for FeoB, a high-affinity ferrous iron transporter. *Mol Microbiol* **37**:274–286.

222. **Homuth M, Valentin-Weigand P, Rohde M, Gerlach G-F.** 1998. Identification and characterization of a novel extracellular ferric reductase from *Mycobacterium paratuberculosis*. *Infect Immun* **66:**710–716.

223. **Coulanges V, Andre P, Ziegler O, Buchheit L, Vidon DJ.** 1997. Utilization of iron-catecholamine complexes involving ferric reductase activity in *Listeria monocytogenes*. *Infect Immun* **65:**2778–2785.

224. **Deneer HG, Healey V, Boychuk I.** 1995. Reduction of exogenous ferric iron by a surface-associated ferric reductase of *Listeria* spp. *Microbiology* **141:**1985–1892.

225. **Coulanges V, Andre P, Vidon DJ.** 1998. Effect of siderophores, catecholamines, and catechol compounds on *Listeria* spp.: growth in iron-complexed medium. *Biochem Biophys Res Commun* **249:**526–530.

226. **Cowart RE.** 2002. Reduction of iron by extracellular iron reductases: implications for microbial iron acquisition. *Arch Biochem Biophys* **400:**273–281.

227. **Tiwari KB, Birlingmair J, Wilkinson BJ, Jayaswal RK.** 2014. The role of the twin-arginine translocase (*tat*) system in iron uptake in *Listeria monocytogenes*. *Microbiology* **161:**264–271.

228. **Zheng H, Chatfield CH, Liles MR, Cianciotto NP.** 2013. Secreted pyomelanin of *Legionella pneumophila* promotes bacterial iron uptake and growth under iron-limiting conditions. *Infect Immun* **81:**4182–4191.

229. **Chatfield CH, Cianciotto NP.** 2007. The secreted pyomelanin pigment of *Legionella pneumophila* confers ferric reductase activity. *Infect Immun* **75:**4062–4070.

230. **Kwok EY, Severance S, Kosman DJ.** 2006. Evidence for iron channeling in the Fet3p-Ftr1p high-affinity iron uptake complex in the yeast plasma membrane. *Biochemistry* **45:**6317–6327.

231. **Hantke K.** 2003. Is the bacterial ferrous iron transporter FeoB a living fossil? *Trends Microbiol* **11:**192–195.

232. **Kammler M, Schön C, Hantke K.** 1993. Characterization of the ferrous iron uptake system of *Escherichia coli*. *J Bacteriol* **175:**6212–6219.

233. **Carpenter C, Payne SM.** 2014. Regulation of iron transport systems in *Enterobacteriaceae* in response to oxygen and iron availability. *J Inorg Biochem* **133:**110–117.

234. **Hantke K.** 1987. Ferrous iron transport mutants in *Escherichia coli* K12. *FEMS Microbiol Lett* **44:**53–57.

235. **Cartron ML, Maddocks S, Gillingham P, Craven CJ, Andrews SC.** 2006. Feo: transport of ferrous iron into bacteria. *Biometals* **19:**143–157.

236. **Marlovits TC, Haase W, Herrmann C, Aller SG, Unger VM.** 2002. The membrane protein FeoB contains an intramolecular G protein essential for Fe(II) uptake in bacteria. *Proc Natl Acad Sci USA* **99:**16243–16248.

237. **Kim H, Lee H, Shin D.** 2012. The FeoA protein is necessary for the FeoB transporter to import ferrous iron. *Biochem Biophys Res Commun* **423:**733–738.

238. **Weaver EA, Wyckoff EE, Mey AR, Morrison R, Payne SM.** 2013. FeoA and FeoC are essential components of the *Vibrio cholerae* ferrous iron uptake system, and FeoC interacts with FeoB. *J Bacteriol* **195:**4826–4835.

239. **Hung K-W, Juan T-H, Hsu Y-L, Huang TH.** 2012. NMR structure note: the ferrous iron transport protein C (FeoC) from *Klebsiella pneumoniae*. *J Biomol NMR* **53:**161–165.

240. **Kim H, Lee H, Shin D.** 2013. The FeoC protein leads to high cellular levels of the Fe(II) transporter FeoB by preventing FtsH protease regulation of FeoB in *Salmonella enterica*. *J Bacteriol* **195:**3364–3370.

241. **Kim H, Lee H, Shin D.** 2015. Lon-mediated proteolysis of the FeoC protein prevents *Salmonella enterica* from accumulating the Fc(II) transporter FeoB under high-oxygen conditions. *J Bacteriol* **197:**92–98.

242. **Ledala N, Sengupta M, Muthaiyan A, Wilkinson BJ, Jayaswal RK.** 2010. Transcriptomic response of *Listeria monocytogenes* to iron limitation and Fur mutation. *Appl Environ Microbiol* **76:**406–416.

243. **Ledala N, Zhang B, Seravalli J, Powers R, Somerville GA.** 2014. Influence of iron and aeration on *Staphylococcus aureus* growth, metabolism, and transcription. *J Bacteriol* **196:**2178–2189.

244. **Grosse C, Scherer J, Koch D, Otto M, Taudte N, Grass G.** 2006. A new ferrous iron-uptake transporter, EfeU (YcdN), from *Escherichia coli*. *Mol Microbiol* **62:**120–131.

245. **Cao J, Woodhall MR, Alvarez J, Cartron ML, Andrews SC.** 2007. EfeUOB (YcdNOB) is a tripartite, acid-induced and CpxAR-regulated, low-pH Fe2+ transporter that is cryptic in *Escherichia coli* K-12 but functional in *E. coli* O157:H7. *Mol Microbiol* **65:**857–875.

246. **Létoffé S, Delepelaire P, Wandersman C.** 2006. The housekeeping dipeptide permease is the *Escherichia coli* heme transporter and functions with two optional peptide binding proteins. *Proc Natl Acad Sci USA* **103:**12891–12896.

247. **Turlin E, Débarbouillé M, Augustyniak K, Gilles A-M, Wandersman C.** 2013. *Staphylo-*

coccus aureus FepA and FepB proteins drive heme iron utilization in *Escherichia coli*. *PloS One* **8**:e56529. doi:10.1371/journal.pone.0056529.

248. **Biswas L, Biswas R, Nerz C, Ohlsen K, Schlag M, Schäfer T, Lamkemeyer T, Ziebandt AK, Hantke K, Rosenstein R, Götz F.** 2009. Role of the twin-arginine translocation pathway in *Staphylococcus*. *J Bacteriol* **191**:5921–5929.

249. **Miethke M, Monteferrante CG, Marahiel MA, van Dijl JM.** 2013. The *Bacillus subtilis* EfeUOB transporter is essential for high-affinity acquisition of ferrous and ferric iron. *Biochim Biophys Acta* **1833**:2267–2278.

250. **Brickman TJ, Armstrong SK.** 2012. Iron and pH-responsive FtrABCD ferrous iron utilization system of *Bordetella* species: *Bordetella* ferrous iron transport system. *Mol Microbiol* **86**:580–593.

251. **Elhassanny AEM, Anderson ES, Menscher EA, Roop RM.** 2013. The ferrous iron transporter FtrABCD is required for the virulence of *Brucella abortus* 2308 in mice. *Mol Microbiol* **88**:1070–1082.

252. **Rajasekaran MB, Nilapwar S, Andrews SC, Watson KA.** 2010. EfeO-cupredoxins: major new members of the cupredoxin superfamily with roles in bacterial iron transport. *Biometals* **23**:1–17.

253. **Létoffé S, Heuck G, Delepelaire P, Lange N, Wandersman C.** 2009. Bacteria capture iron from heme by keeping tetrapyrrol skeleton intact. *Proc Natl Acad Sci USA* **106**:11719–11724.

254. **Liu X, Du Q, Wang Z, Zhu D, Huang Y, Li N, Wei T, Xu S, Gu L.** 2011. Crystal structure and biochemical features of EfeB/YcdB from *Escherichia coli* O157: ASP235 plays divergent roles in different enzyme-catalyzed processes. *J Biol Chem* **286**:14922–14931.

255. **Dailey HA, Septer AN, Daugherty L, Thames D, Gerdes S, Stabb EV, Dunn AK, Dailey TA, Phillips JD.** 2011. The *Escherichia coli* protein YfeX functions as a porphyrinogen oxidase, not a heme dechelatase. *mBio* **2**:e00248-11. doi:10.1128/mBio.00248-11.

256. **Clarke SR, Brummell KJ, Horsburgh MJ, McDowell PW, Mohamad SA, Stapleton MR, Acevedo J, Read RC, Day NP, Peacock SJ, Mond JJ, Kokai-Kun JF, Foster SJ.** 2006. Identification of *in vivo*-expressed antigens of *Staphylococcus aureus* and their use in vaccinations for protection against nasal carriage. *J Infect Dis* **193**:1098–1108.

257. **Kim HK, DeDent A, Cheng AG, McAdow M, Bagnoli F, Missiakas DM, Schneewind O.** 2010. IsdA and IsdB antibodies protect mice against *Staphylococcus aureus* abscess forma-tion and lethal challenge. *Vaccine* **28**:6382–6392.

258. **Ster C, Beaudoin F, Diarra MS, Jacques M, Malouin F, Lacasse P.** 2010. Evaluation of some *Staphylococcus aureus* iron-regulated proteins as vaccine targets. *Vet Immunol Immunopathol* **136**:311–318.

259. **Stranger-Jones YK, Bae T, Schneewind O.** 2006. Vaccine assembly from surface proteins of *Staphylococcus aureus*. *Proc Natl Acad Sci USA* **103**:16942–16947.

260. **Kuklin NA, Clark DJ, Secore S, Cook J, Cope LD, McNeely T, Noble L, Brown MJ, Zorman JK, Wang XM, Pancari G, Fan H, Isett K, Burgess B, Bryan J, Brownlow M, George H, Meinz M, Liddell ME, Kelly R, Schultz L, Montgomery D, Onishi J, Losada M, Martin M, Ebert T, Tan CY, Schofield TL, Nagy E, Meineke A, Joyce JG, Kurtz MB, Caulfield MJ, Jansen KU, McClements W, Anderson AS.** 2006. A novel *Staphylococcus aureus* vaccine: iron surface determinant B induces rapid antibody responses in rhesus macaques and specific increased survival in a murine *S. aureus* sepsis model. *Infect Immun* **74**:2215–2223.

261. **Harro CD, Betts RF, Hartzel JS, Onorato MT, Lipka J, Smugar SS, Kartsonis NA.** 2011. The immunogenicity and safety of different formulations of a novel *Staphylococcus aureus* vaccine (V710): results of two phase I studies. *Vaccine* **30**:1729–1736.

262. **Fowler VG, Allen KB, Moreira ED, Moustafa M, Isgro F, Boucher HW, Corey GR, Carmeli Y, Betts R, Hartzel JS, Chan ISF, McNeely TB, Kartsonis NA, Guris D, Onorato MT, Smugar SS, DiNubile MJ, Sobanjo-ter Meulen A.** 2013. Effect of an investigational vaccine for preventing *Staphylococcus aureus* infections after cardiothoracic surgery: a randomized trial. *JAMA* **309**:1368–1378.

263. **Gorringe AR, Borrow R, Fox AJ, Robinson A.** 1995. Human antibody response to meningo-coccal transferrin binding proteins: evidence for vaccine potential. *Vaccine* **13**:1207–1212.

264. **West D, Reddin K, Matheson M, Heath R, Funnell S, Hudson M, Robinson A, Gorringe A.** 2001. Recombinant *Neisseria meningitidis* transferrin binding protein A protects against experimental meningococcal infection. *Infect Immun* **69**:1561–1567.

265. **Lissolo L, Maitre-Wilmotte G, Dumas P, Mignon M, Danve B, Quentin-Millet MJ.** 1995. Evaluation of transferrin-binding protein 2 within the transferrin-binding protein complex as a potential antigen for future meningococcal vaccines. *Infect Immun* **63**:884–890.

266. **Ferreirós CM, Ferrón L, Criado MT.** 1994. *In vivo* human immune response to transferrin-binding protein 2 and other iron-regulated proteins of *Neisseria meningitidis*. *FEMS Immunol Med Microbiol* **8:**63–68.

267. **Johnson AS, Gorringe AR, Fox AJ, Borrow R, Robinson A.** 1997. Analysis of the human Ig isotype response to individual transferrin binding proteins A and B from *Neisseria meningitidis*. *FEMS Immunol Med Microbiol* **19:**159–167.

268. **Price GA, Hobbs MM, Cornelissen CN.** 2004. Immunogenicity of gonococcal transferrin binding proteins during natural infections. *Infect Immun* **72:**277–283.

269. **Price GA, Russell MW, Cornelissen CN.** 2005. Intranasal administration of recombinant *Neisseria gonorrhoeae* transferrin binding proteins A and B conjugated to the cholera toxin B subunit induces systemic and vaginal antibodies in mice. *Infect Immun* **73:**3945–3953.

270. **Ji C, Juárez-Hernández RE, Miller MJ.** 2012. Exploiting bacterial iron acquisition: siderophore conjugates. *Future Med Chem* **4:**297–313.

271. **Švarcová M, Krátký M, Vinšová J.** 2015. Investigation of potential inhibitors of chorismate-utilizing enzymes. *Curr Med Chem* **22:**1383–1399.

272. **Stojiljkovic I, Kumar V, Srinivasan N.** 1999. Non-iron metalloporphyrins: potent antibacterial compounds that exploit haem/Hb uptake systems of pathogenic bacteria. *Mol Microbiol* **31:**429–442.

273. **Banin E, Lozinski A, Brady KM, Berenshtein E, Butterfield PW, Moshe M, Chevion M, Greenberg EP, Banin E.** 2008. The potential of desferrioxamine-gallium as an anti-*Pseudomonas* therapeutic agent. *Proc Natl Acad Sci USA* **105:**16761–16766.

274. **Hood MI, Skaar EP.** 2012. Nutritional immunity: transition metals at the pathogen-host interface. *Nat Rev Microbiol* **10:**525–537.

275. **Carlson PE, Carr KA, Janes BK, Anderson EC, Hanna PC.** 2009. Transcriptional profiling of *Bacillus anthracis* Sterne (34F2) during iron starvation. *PloS One* **4:**e6988. doi:10.1371/journal.pone.0006988.

276. **Brickman TJ, Vanderpool CK, Armstrong SK.** 2006. Heme transport contributes to *in vivo* fitness of *Bordetella pertussis* during primary infection in mice. *Infect Immun* **74:**1741–1744.

277. **Torres AG, Redford P, Welch RA, Payne SM.** 2001. TonB-dependent systems of uropathogenic *Escherichia coli*: aerobactin and heme transport and TonB are required for virulence in the mouse. *Infect Immun* **69:**6179–6185.

278. **Rosadini CV, Wong SMS, Akerley BJ.** 2008. The periplasmic disulfide oxidoreductase DsbA contributes to *Haemophilus influenzae* pathogenesis. *Infect Immun* **76:**1498–1508.

279. **Jin B, Newton SM, Shao Y, Jiang X, Charbit A, Klebba PE.** 2006. Iron acquisition systems for ferric hydroxamates, haemin and haemoglobin in *Listeria monocytogenes*. *Mol Microbiol* **59:**1185–1198.

280. **Stojiljkovic I, Hwa V, de Saint Martin L, O'Gaora P, Nassif X, Heffron F, So M.** 1995. The *Neisseria meningitidis* haemoglobin receptor: its role in iron utilization and virulence. *Mol Microbiol* **15:**531–541.

281. **Fisher M, Huang Y-S, Li X, McIver KS, Toukoki C, Eichenbaum Z.** 2008. Shr is a broad-spectrum surface receptor that contributes to adherence and virulence in group A streptococcus. *Infect Immun* **76:**5006–5015.

282. **Oh MH, Lee SM, Lee DH, Choi SH.** 2009. Regulation of the *Vibrio vulnificus* hupA gene by temperature alteration and cyclic AMP receptor protein and evaluation of its role in virulence. *Infect Immun* **77:**1208–1215.

283. **Gaddy JA, Arivett BA, McConnell MJ, López-Rojas R, Pachón J, Actis LA.** 2012. Role of acinetobactin-mediated iron acquisition functions in the interaction of *Acinetobacter baumannii* strain ATCC 19606T with human lung epithelial cells, *Galleria mellonella* caterpillars, and mice. *Infect Immun* **80:**1015–1024.

284. **Palyada K, Threadgill D, Stintzi A.** 2004. Iron acquisition and regulation in *Campylobacter jejuni*. *J Bacteriol* **186:**4714–4729.

285. **Enard C, Diolez A, Expert D.** 1988. Systemic virulence of *Erwinia chrysanthemi* 3937 requires a functional iron assimilation system. *J Bacteriol* **170:**2419–2426.

286. **Russo TA, Olson R, Macdonald U, Metzger D, Maltese LM, Drake EJ, Gulick AM.** 2014. Aerobactin mediates virulence and accounts for increased siderophore production under iron-limiting conditions by hypervirulent (hypermucoviscous) *Klebsiella pneumoniae*. *Infect Immun* **82:**2356–2367.

287. **Lawlor MS, O'connor C, Miller VL.** 2007. Yersiniabactin is a virulence factor for *Klebsiella pneumoniae* during pulmonary infection. *Infect Immun* **75:**1463–1472.

288. **Allard KA, Dao J, Sanjeevaiah P, McCoy-Simandle K, Chatfield CH, Crumrine DS, Castignetti D, Cianciotto NP.** 2009. Purification of legiobactin and importance of this siderophore in lung infection by *Legionella pneumophila*. *Infect Immun* **77:**2887–2895.

289. **Rodriguez GM, Smith I.** 2006. Identification of an ABC transporter required for iron acquisition and virulence in *Mycobacterium tuberculosis*. *J Bacteriol* **188:**424–430.

290. **Burbank L, Mohammadi M, Roper MC.** 2015. Siderophore-mediated iron acquisition influences motility and is required for full virulence of the xylem-dwelling bacterial phytopathogen *Pantoea stewartii* subsp. stewartii. *Appl Environ Microbiol* **81**:139–148.

291. **Himpsl SD, Pearson MM, Arewång CJ, Nusca TD, Sherman DH, Mobley HLT.** 2010. Proteobactin and a yersiniabactin-related siderophore mediate iron acquisition in *Proteus mirabilis. Mol Microbiol* **78**:138–157.

292. **Takase H, Nitanai H, Hoshino K, Otani T.** 2000. Impact of siderophore production on *Pseudomonas aeruginosa* infections in immunosuppressed mice. *Infect Immun* **68**:1834–1839.

293. **Taguchi F, Suzuki T, Inagaki Y, Toyoda K, Shiraishi T, Ichinose Y.** 2010. The siderophore pyoverdine of *Pseudomonas syringae* pv. tabaci 6605 is an intrinsic virulence factor in host tobacco infection. *J Bacteriol* **192**:117–126.

294. **Yancey RJ, Breeding SA, Lankford CE.** 1979. Enterochelin (enterobactin): virulence factor for *Salmonella typhimurium. Infect Immun* **24**:174–180.

295. **Lawlor KM, Daskaleros PA, Robinson RE, Payne SM.** 1987. Virulence of iron transport mutants of *Shigella flexneri* and utilization of host iron compounds. *Infect Immun* **55**:594–599.

296. **Bobrov AG, Kirillina O, Fetherston JD, Miller MC, Burlison JA, Perry RD.** 2014. The *Yersinia pestis* siderophore, yersiniabactin, and the ZnuABC system both contribute to zinc acquisition and the development of lethal septicaemic plague in mice. *Mol Microbiol* **93**:759–775.

297. **Baltes N, Hennig-Pauka I, Gerlach G-F.** 2002. Both transferrin binding proteins are virulence factors in *Actinobacillus pleuropneumoniae* serotype 7 infection. *FEMS Microbiol Lett* **209**:283–287.

298. **Renauld-Mongénie G, Poncet D, Mignon M, Fraysse S, Chabanel C, Danve B, Krell T, Quentin-Millet M-J.** 2004. Role of transferrin receptor from a *Neisseria meningitidis tbpB* isotype II strain in human transferrin binding and virulence. *Infect Immun* **72**:3461–3470.

299. **Cornelissen CN, Kelley M, Hobbs MM, Anderson JE, Cannon JG, Cohen MS, Sparling PF.** 1998. The transferrin receptor expressed by gonococcal strain FA1090 is required for the experimental infection of human male volunteers. *Mol Microbiol* **27**:611–616.

300. **Naikare H, Palyada K, Panciera R, Marlow D, Stintzi A.** 2006. Major role for FeoB in *Campylobacter jejuni* ferrous iron acquisition, gut colonization, and intracellular survival. *Infect Immun* **74**:5433–5444.

301. **Stojiljkovic I, Cobeljic M, Hantke K.** 1993. *Escherichia coli* K-12 ferrous iron uptake mutants are impaired in their ability to colonize the mouse intestine. *FEMS Microbiol Lett* **108**:111–115.

302. **Thomas-Charles CA, Zheng H, Palmer LE, Mena P, Thanassi DG, Furie MB.** 2013. FeoB-mediated uptake of iron by *Francisella tularensis. Infect Immun* **81**:2828–2837.

303. **Robey M, Cianciotto NP.** 2002. *Legionella pneumophila feoAB* promotes ferrous iron uptake and intracellular infection. *Infect Immun* **70**:5659–5669.

304. **Dashper SG, Butler CA, Lissel JP, Paolini RA, Hoffmann B, Veith PD, O'Brien-Simpson NM, Snelgrove SL, Tsiros JT, Reynolds EC.** 2005. A novel *Porphyromonas gingivalis* FeoB plays a role in manganese accumulation. *J Biol Chem* **280**:28095–28102.

305. **Janakiraman A, Slauch JM.** 2000. The putative iron transport system SitABCD encoded on SPI1 is required for full virulence of *Salmonella typhimurium. Mol Microbiol* **35**:1146–1155.

306. **Pandey A, Sonti RV.** 2010. Role of the FeoB protein and siderophore in promoting virulence of *Xanthomonas oryzae* pv. oryzae on rice. *J Bacteriol* **192**:3187–3203.

BACTERIAL COMMUNICATION
AND VIRULENCE

Sociomicrobiology and Pathogenic Bacteria

4

JOAO B. XAVIER[1]

INTRODUCTION

Microbiology has gathered much attention in recent years in part thanks to major scientific advancements in the microbiome field. Large-scale projects such as the NIH-funded Human Microbiome Project (1–3) provide extensive catalogues of the microbes that live in and on the human body. Statements like "the human body is home to bacteria that outnumber human cells by more than 10:1" or "the genetic content of these bacteria can be 100x that of the human genome" are often used by mainstream media and are known to the general public. Vast explorations of the human and nonhuman microbiomes are to a large extent boosted by recent breakthroughs in DNA sequencing and community metagenomics (4–6), and the many studies that have emerged reveal an expanding role of multispecies host-associated microbial communities in several host functions (7, 8). Arguably, one of the most notable functions of commensal microbiota, i.e., nonpathogenic microbes, is protecting the host from colonization by other microbes (9). This is an exciting area of research that aims to address open questions in pathogenesis such as why individuals exposed to the same pathogen can differ in their levels of infection. It can also explain why patients can have increased risk of infections after antibiotic

[1]Program for Computational Biology, Memorial Sloan Kettering Cancer Center, New York, NY 10065.
Virulence Mechanisms of Bacterial Pathogens, 5th edition
Edited by Indira T. Kudva, Nancy A. Cornick, Paul J. Plummer, Qijing Zhang, Tracy L. Nicholson, John P. Bannantine, and Bryan H. Bellaire
© 2016 American Society for Microbiology, Washington, DC
doi:10.1128/microbiolspec.VMBF-0019-2015

therapy destroys the commensal microbiota that would naturally protect against pathogen invasion.

Understanding the ability of microbiomes to protect against colonization by pathogens and other related aspects of microbial pathogenesis requires a new set of experimental and theoretical tools. The focus must broaden beyond the single pathogen as the cause of disease and start to include the host-resident microbiota. Understanding how microbial communities function, how they are assembled, and how they change in time after perturbations such as antibiotics or diet changes, is a complex problem that is best suited to an integrative approach. Fortunately, there is an extensive body of knowledge on the functioning of complex biological consortia in the fields of ecology and evolution from which we can learn.

I start by reviewing the findings of sociomicrobiology, a discipline that aims to address how bacteria function in communities (10). I then analyze how seemingly cooperative microbes may actually be driven by selfish motives even within communities where every microbe is of the same species. I move on to multispecies communities, a more complex scenario where both conflict and cooperation occur and may both be essential components of the robust behaviors that microecosystems often have. I end with an ecologist's view of the human microbiome and a discussion of how resistance against pathogen colonization can be interpreted as a problem in theoretical ecology.

BIOFILMS, QUORUM SENSING, AND THE DAWN OF SOCIOMICROBIOLOGY

Most species of bacteria are social. Biofilms, dense communities of bacteria, are a common cause of persistent infections, and the list of biofilm-forming pathogens includes common threats such as *Pseudomonas aeruginosa* (11), *Escherichia coli* (12), *Salmonella enterica* (13), *Klebsiella pneumoniae* (14), *Vibrio cholerae*

(15, 16), and *Clostridium difficile* (17). Clinical microbiologists came to realize the importance of biofilm formation in pathogenesis in part because bacteria in biofilms have much higher tolerance to antibiotics, and the mechanism of this tolerance appears to be distinct from conventional antibiotic resistance (18, 19).

Biofilms saw a surge in interest among microbiologists in the late 1990s. Even though it was well known that microbes form dense surface-attached films and that these films have medical implications, the topic of how bacteria form biofilms seemed to get more interest from engineers who were interested their detrimental roles in industrial biofouling but also beneficial applications such as biofilm reactors for wastewater treatment (20, 21). When experimentalists first showed that quorum sensing played a role in regulating biofilm formation (22, 23), the search for genetic mechanisms of biofilm formation became a very hot topic. The excitement in the field quickly grew as new molecular mechanisms of biofilm formation came to light (24, 25). The growing field generated a new model (Fig. 1), primarily inspired by experiments in *P. aeruginosa* but later supported by other species, in which biofilm formation follows a developmental program with different stages and phases, each one potentially driving expression of a distinct set of genes, much a like the developmental programs of multicellular eukaryotic organisms (26).

The excitement experienced at the time was understandable. If a genetic program similar to developmental pathways in multicellular organisms controls biofilm formation, then this would open the way to new therapies. Antibiofilm drugs such as quorum sensing inhibitors (27) would be a huge new opportunity for medicine when resistance to traditional antibiotics is a growing problem at the global scale and pharmaceutical companies invest less in new antibiotic discovery (28). Could we find ways to fight bacteria by jamming their cell-to-cell communication

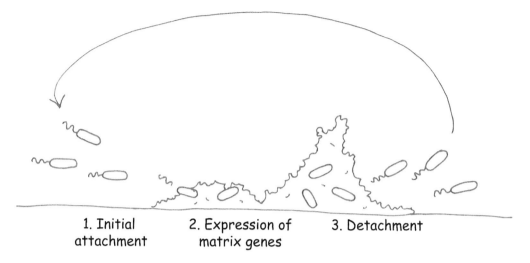

1. Initial
attachment

2. Expression of
matrix genes

3. Detachment

FIGURE 1 A model of biofilm development and life cycle proposed in reference 18. Planktonic bacteria attach to surfaces, initiate expression of biofilm genes such as synthesis of extracellular polymeric matrices, and grow a biofilm. A cell can detach from a mature biofilm and go back to the planktonic state, closing the biofilm life cycle.

channels and preventing them from organizing themselves in communities that make them harder to treat?

The years that followed the onset of sociomicrobiology were a boom for biofilm research, leading to important findings. A notable example is the role of the secondary messenger cyclic-di-GMP in regulating the bacterial transition from motile to biofilm modes (29). This small molecule, which can regulate many other functions in multiple species of bacteria, plays a key role in biofilm formation by informing when the cell should downregulate genes for motility and upregulate biofilm genes. In *P. aeruginosa*, there is an emerging picture in which the bacterium mechanically senses a surface using the transmembrane Wsp system (30). This system is a multiprotein complex composed of WspA, WspB, WspC, WspD, WspE, and WspF. The transmembrane WspA protein possibly changes conformation when cells contact an attachment surface. This triggers phosphorylation of a response regulator called WspR that then leads to cyclic-diGMP production. Downstream of the Wsp complex, the transcriptional activator FleQ

regulates expression of flagella genes when cyclic-diGMP levels are low but switches to expression of biofilm matrix genes (the *pel* operon) when cyclic-diGMP levels are high. The ability of FleQ to bind to c-diGMP and regulate the motility-to-biofilm transition depends on a protein-protein interaction between FleQ and the antiactivator FleN (31, 32). Knocking out FleN produces *P. aeruginosa* cells that are multiflagellated but immotile (33), whereas point mutations in that protein can produce multiflagellated mutants that are hypermotile, the so-called hyperswarmers (34). Hyperswarmers are locked in a perpetual motility mode and cannot make proper biofilms. Similarly, a number of mutants in c-diGMP-related genes have been found to be locked in either motility or biofilm modes (35). c-diGMP is therefore key to the molecular decision making process that dictates how cells transition from the planktonic mode to the surface-attached mode of bacterial living (Fig. 1). Work in this area may reveal new molecular mechanisms that can become targets to prevent pathogens from forming biofilms (36).

Molecular biology often seems to take for granted the view of biofilms as highly organized communities. It is not uncommon to find descriptions of a "city of microbes" (37) where bacteria live together in synergy, communicate via cell-cell signaling, and share secreted resources. But how realistic is that view? Natural selection is a selfish process whereby the fittest survive and leave more offspring. Could we expect biofilms with millions of individual bacteria to be immune to the evolution of exploitative mutants that benefit from the cooperation of others? In the next section I discuss the arrival of social evolutionary theory to the field of microbiology and how the view of natural selection acting primarily at the level of the gene can help clarify some of these issues and shed light on microbial pathogenesis.

BACTERIAL SOCIAL BEHAVIOR: COOPERATION OR CONFLICT?

Social evolution theory is a field that aims to dissect the evolutionary mechanisms of social behavior. The evolution of cooperative

behavior, in particular, is an old problem that puzzled Darwin, yet even 10 years ago this problem was recognized as one of the top "125 unknowns" by the journal *Science* (38). Around that time, the field of social evolutionary theory started its foray into bacterial pathogenesis (39, 40).

A landmark paper at the time looked at the production of iron-scavenging siderophores under the lens of social evolution (39). Siderophores are compounds secreted by bacteria that have high affinity to iron. Once in the extracellular space, siderophores scavenge iron that would otherwise be inaccessible to the bacteria and free it up to be taken up by bacterial cells (Fig. 2). Siderophore scavenging allows bacteria such as *P. aeruginosa* to grow in iron-limited environments such as host tissues, where extracellular iron is normally maintained at very low concentrations exactly to prevent the growth of pathogens. The problem from an evolutionary perspective is that siderophores are what is called a "public good" in a bacterial society. A public good is a concept taken from economics that means a resource that is available to all individuals within a population, irrespective

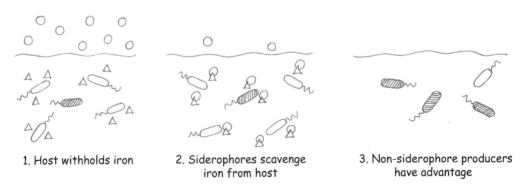

1. Host withholds iron   2. Siderophores scavenge iron from host   3. Non-siderophore producers have advantage

Legend: ◯ Iron   △ Siderophore   〰️🝙 Cheater

FIGURE 2 Siderophore production as a cooperative trait (74). Some bacterial pathogens like *Pseudomonas aeruginosa* secrete siderophores to scavenge iron the in iron-limited environments of host tissues (panel 1). Siderophores have high affinity to iron and can be taken up by bacteria including non-siderophore producers that still have the siderophore receptors (panel 2). Non-siderophore producers exploit wild-type producers by not paying the cost of siderophore production, but this cheating behavior can lead to the extinction of siderophore production in the population (panel 3).

of who's producing it. When the production of a public good is costly, there is a strong incentive for cheating, meaning that individuals would not produce the public good but just exploit the public goods produced by others. In these situations, what prevents cheaters from taking over and causing the collapse of the population?

The study by Griffin and colleagues (39) first showed experimentally that siderophores of *P. aeruginosa* are costly public goods. They compared the growth of a siderophore-producing strain and a nonproducing strain in iron-limited conditions where siderophores are key to bacterial growth. As expected, they saw that the siderophore-producing strain grows much better than the nonproducing strain when the two are compared in monocultures. However, when mixed together in a coculture, the non-siderophore-producing strain grew better than the producing strain because it could use the siderophores without paying a metabolic cost of their production.

Importantly, the final numbers in the population were lower for the coculture than for the monoculture of siderophore producers. The nonproducing strain benefited from being mixed with the producer, but the whole population suffered as a consequence (Fig. 3A).

This dramatic outcome is a hallmark of cheating and captures the essence of the problem of the evolution of cooperation (41). Cheaters gain a selfish benefit from being in a mixed population with cooperators, but the whole population suffers from cheating compared to a population that is composed 100% of cooperators. So how can we observe so many cooperative traits in nature, where organisms seem to altruistically sacrifice their own fitness for the benefit of others? This question has been on the minds of evolutionary biologists for a long time. One answer is kin selection. J. B. S. Haldane, one of the architects of modern synthesis, reportedly joked that he would altruistically give

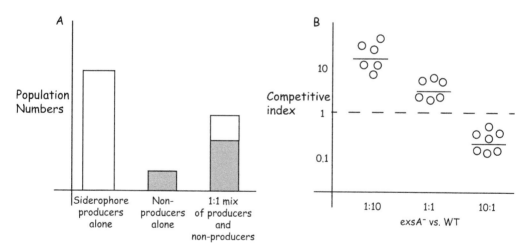

FIGURE 3 Laboratory experiments reveal the hallmarks of cheating. (A) Siderophore-producing *Pseudomonas aeruginosa* grow reasonably well in iron-depleted media by increasing iron uptake thanks to siderophore scavenging (Fig. 2). Non–siderophore producers (cheaters) grow poorly in the same environment when alone but do better when mixed with producers by not paying the cost of siderophore production. The advantage of nonproducers comes at the expense of the whole population (74). **(B)** The competitive advantage of cheaters decreases as their frequency increases because there are fewer cooperators to exploit in the population. This example is taken from a study of type III secretion systems in *P. aeruginosa* where *exsA⁻* mutants lacking the type III system could cheat over wild-type bacteria (WT), but their measured competitive index decreased as cheater numbers increased in the population (53).

his life for two brothers or eight cousins, reflecting the Mendelian inheritance probability of one-third of sharing a gene with a brother and one-eighth of sharing a gene with a first-degree cousin. Kin selection explains that a cooperative strategy can evolve if the fitness costs that the cooperative behavior has to the actor are less than the fitness benefit to the recipient multiplied by a relatedness coefficient between actor and recipient. This relationship, $r \times b > c$, is known as Hamilton's rule, in honor of William Hamilton, who's seminal work laid the foundations for investigating the genetic basis of social behavior (42, 43). The insight behind this elegant rule is that selection acts at the level of the genes, and a gene encoding for a cooperative behavior will increase in frequency within a population if its function is to make the organism that carries it help other carriers of that gene. Since fitness concerns the increase of gene frequency in a population, a gene may be fit if it increases other copies of itself, and social evolutionary biologists often use the term "inclusive fitness" to account for social effects. The concepts of social evolution theory were popularized in large part thanks to the book *The Selfish Gene* by Richard Dawkins (44).

Why is this relevant to microbial pathogens? Spontaneous mutants that lose function in a gene occur commonly in bacterial populations. If a mutant has a loss of function in a cooperative gene, for example, in the gene *pvdA* that catalyzes a key step in the synthesis of the siderophore pyoverdin (45), then this mutant could become a cheater. A way for cooperation to be maintained in the face of cheaters is if the remaining cooperators cooperate only with individuals that still carry a functional copy, but not with mutants that lack the gene. This would be the case where *r* would have a high value.

Griffin and colleagues (39) tested this prediction by mixing bacteria in different ways to manipulate relatedness experimentally. Their experiments revealed that conditions of high relatedness favored siderophore producers (cooperators), whereas conditions of low relatedness, where strains mixed more frequently with other clones, favored nonproducing strains (cheaters), which is in accordance with social evolution theory.

Mechanisms Stabilizing Cooperation in Bacterial Pathogens

Mixing reduces the likelihood that cooperative benefits will be received by related individuals. In nature and in the clinic we expect that bacterial strains and species will often be in mixed communities. Are there other mechanisms stabilizing cooperation in communities where relatedness is low?

The extracellular polymeric substances of biofilms could naïvely be viewed as a public good. These substances, which make up the gooey matrix that sticks bacteria to each other and to the solid substratum in a biofilm (Fig. 1), require significant metabolic resources to be produced. Mutants that do not produce matrix could still benefit from the matrix produced by others. However, a series of studies, first with computer simulations (46) and later with experiments with *V. cholerae* (47) and *Pseudomonas fluorescens* (48) showed this not to be the case and provided a new mechanism to explain the evolutionary stability of biofilm communities. The reason is that bacterial biofilms have very steep gradients of nutrients and other solute substances. For example, in biofilms of aerobic bacteria and in colonies growing on agar plates, diffusional gradients are often so steep that bacteria on the inside of the biofilm cannot grow because all oxygen is consumed before it reaches the interior. In a mixed biofilm of polymer producers and non–polymer producers the producers gain an advantage because the polymers allow them to be pushed to the top and reach higher concentrations of nutrients. By secreting polymers, a polymer-producing bacterium benefits itself and its lineage and literally suffocates non–polymer producers in the inner layers of the biofilm. This mechanism of "competitive smothering" proposes that polymer production is a competitive strategy, not a cooperative behavior. What could at first glance be perceived as a cooperation reveals a selfish motive.

Bacteria have alternative ways to tilt Hamilton's equation in their favor, even when a trait is clearly cooperative. *P. aeruginosa* colonies are capable of a remarkable collective motility behavior called swarming behavior (49, 50). Swarming allows the colony to spread across large surfaces in a way that single cells cannot, and this benefits the population. However, swarming requires that cells produce and secrete large amounts of biosurfactants, called rhamnolipids, that lubricate the surface and allow the bacteria to slide on top of it (50). Rhamnolipids are a public good, like siderophores. Strains that do not produce surfactants, such as an $rhlA^-$ mutant, cannot swarm on their own but will do so when mixed with surfactant producers (51). However, unlike with siderophores, there is no public good dilemma. With a 1:1 mixture of wild-type bacteria, $rhlA^-$ remains roughly at 1:1 even though the wild type is producing copious amounts of surfactants and the $rhlA^-$ strain is benefiting from them. How do we explain this conundrum?

The *rhlA* gene is an operon (*rhlAB*) that is tightly regulated by a combination of quorum sensing and metabolic sensing. The regulatory circuit ensures that *P. aeruginosa* wild-type cells express rhamnolipids not only when they have reached a quorum but also when they have a carbon source in excess of that needed to grow. This regulation, called metabolic prudence, ensures that *P. aeruginosa* delays expression of cooperation to times when it becomes affordable because it has an abundance of carbon. By doing this, *P. aeruginosa* uses transcriptional regulation to decrease the cost of cooperation, the c in Hamilton's equation (51). Metabolic prudence allows cooperation even in situations of low relatedness where constitutive cooperation is not possible (52).

Cheating Can Explain Clonal Diversity in Infections

In the absence of a mechanism to reduce costs or increase relatedness, a social trait that provides a benefit to others may be doomed. This is the case in opportunistic infections by *P. aeruginosa* where virulence mediated by a type III secretion system can be seen as an altruistic trait. Type III systems are important factors in pathogenesis that consist of huge needle-like transmembrane protein complexes that inject toxins into host cells. The system is essential for pathogenesis, but the protein complex is costly. Experiments using a mouse model of lung infection by *P. aeruginosa* showed that cheating by mutants lacking type III secretion can happen in vivo (53). Although these mutants fail to infect mice on their own, they do well when coinfected with type III–positive isogenic strains at a 1:1 ratio. When coinfected at different ratios, the type III advantage was high when they were the minority in the mix, but this advantage decreased when they were in the majority. This is called frequency-dependent selection in evolutionary theory (54), and the finding that fitness decreases with increasing frequency is a hallmark of cheating (Fig. 3B). The public goods in this case are likely the metabolic products released by the killing of eukaryotic host cells, which should benefit all individuals in a bacterial population irrespective of which ones have a type III system. Type III secretion mutants are often found in patients with *P. aeruginosa*, and their rise may be due to cheating (53). In the absence of a mechanism to protect against cheating, cheaters are fated to dominate, and cooperation is doomed to extinction. Perhaps this type of phenomenon could be exploited in the development of "Trojan horse" approaches (55), where engineered cheaters exploit wild-type pathogens.

MULTISPECIES COMMUNITIES AND THE MICROBIOME

In the previous section I gave several examples of cooperation and conflict between bacteria of the same species. However, many bacterial communities are multispecies, and the number and richness of social behaviors can grow exponentially, making them harder to dissect experimentally. Computer models of multispecies biofilms suggest that the presence of competing strains can have a strong influence on within-species cooperation and that both within-species and between-species interactions are highly influenced by environmental conditions (56). In spite of this complexity, understanding how bacteria interact within multispecies communities can be an essential step toward a mechanistic basis of host-associated microbiomes relevant for many aspects of host health (57–60) and even host behavior (61).

Low biodiversity in the gut microbiota seems to increase the risk of enteric infection (9). We can learn a lot from extreme examples, and here the infectious diseases of bone marrow transplantation patients is providing an insightful model. Patients receiving bone marrow transplants typically have a blood or bone marrow cancer such as leukemia or lymphoma, and they are hospitalized during the procedure. During this time the patients become immunocompromised and may have to receive large doses of antibiotics in different combinations to prevent opportunistic infections. In many cases the patients are diagnosed with infection by pathogens such as *C. difficile* and vancomycin-resistant *Enterococcus* (VRE) following administration of antibiotics.

Resistance Against Pathogen Colonization

A recent large-scale study analyzed the gut microbiota of a cohort of 94 allogeneic hematopoietic stem cell transplantation patients at Memorial Sloan Kettering (62).

Metagenomics from fecal samples taken at several time points relative to the day of the transplant showed many cases in which the biodiversity of the microbiota fell sharply during antibiotic treatment. This drop in biodiversity is typically due to the expansion of a single member of the gut microbiota. When a single member dominates the microbiome this boosts the risk of infection.

The observation that intestinal domination in bone marrow transplants increases the risk of infection suggests an ecological interpretation in which the commensal gut microbiota is a biodiverse ecosystem that naturally resists invasion by a foreign species. When the host takes antibiotics, the composition of the gut microbiota is perturbed which can cause a cascading loss of species that interact with each other and lead to a drop in biodiversity that opens the way to invasions (Fig. 4). This ecological interpretation is supported by mathematical models that take into account the dynamic social interactions between species. Computer simulations show that sudden shifts in microbiota composition can lead the system to a state of dysbiosis that is difficult to recover from (63). The same effect was replicated in mouse models in which antibiotics were given to mice to perturb their gut microbiota before they received a dose of pathogens. The procedure has been tested in a range of antibiotics and at least two pathogens, *C. difficile* and vancomycin-resistant *Enterococcus* (64, 65). In these mouse models pretreatment with antibiotics increases infection rates dramatically.

Understanding resistance to invasion in the gut microbiota is a problem in ecology, and it makes sense to apply the tools of mathematical ecology to dissect its mechanisms. A recent approach used the classical model of predator-prey dynamics, called the generalized Lotka-Volterra equation, to describe the interactions between microbes in the gut (66–68). In its most detailed form, the model includes three terms to describe (i) the specific growth rate of each microbe,

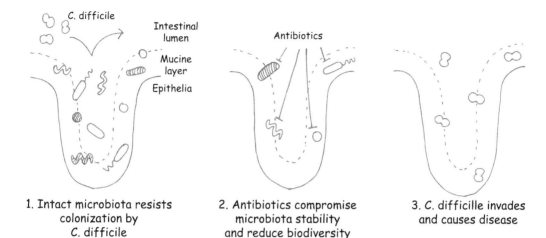

1. Intact microbiota resists colonization by C. difficile

2. Antibiotics compromise microbiota stability and reduce biodiversity

3. C. difficille invades and causes disease

FIGURE 4 **Colonization resistance by the gut microbiota can be harmed by antibiotic therapy. (Panel 1) The gut microbiota can resist colonization by pathogens such as** *Clostridium difficile*. **(Panel 2) Antibiotics disrupt the ecology of the commensal microbiota. (Panel 3) Antibiotic-challenged microbiota open the way to colonization.**

(ii) the pairwise interactions between all microbial species, and (iii) the effects of external factors such as antibiotics on each species. These models have a large lumber of parameters, and determining their values can be challenging. It is nonetheless possible by using large enough data sets and computational techniques to avoid overfitting. Once a model is correctly parameterized it reveals the network of interactions occurring between members of the microbiota, which is valuable information for the investigation of mechanisms of resilience to antibiotic perturbations but also to identify microbes that protect against pathogen invasion (67).

The Lotka-Volterra approach was applied recently to model the microbiota of human patients and mouse models following antibiotic treatment and *C. difficile* infection. The model revealed that a single commensal microbe, *Clostridium scindens*, explained a significant part of the protection in both mice and humans. However, a community was always better than a single microbe. Experimental follow-up studies unveiled the mechanism by showing that the capability of *C. scindens* to metabolize secondary bile

acids is key to hindering *C. difficile* colonization (69).

CONCLUSION

Microbes have rich and diverse social lives (70), and pathogenic bacteria are not an exception. In many cases, pathogens invading a human host encounter a commensal community that may be viewed as the first line of defense against pathogen invasion. Understanding how these communities function requires an investigation of its social behaviors, both cooperative and competitive, and how they produce a biodiverse and robust microbiota.

These are exciting times for the field of the human microbiome. Although the millions of bacteria that live in and on our bodies have been long recognized to play important roles in health and disease, their study has traditionally been hampered because most microbes are difficult to cultivate in laboratory conditions. Recent advancements in DNA sequencing, metagenomic analysis, and culturing of microbial communities (71, 72) enable a direct mechanistic analysis of microbiome biology. The booming field of metagenomics-based analysis of the microbiota is opening a new perspective that presents new challenges and many opportunities. We can anticipate that microbiome analysis of patients may become routine in the future, enabling the use of computer models based on ecological theory to assist medicine, for example, in the rational design of antibiotic therapies (73).

Before this is possible we must gain a better understanding of the ecology and evolution of social interaction in microbial communities. As we discussed here, even monospecies communities have conflict and cooperation. Analyzing the features of microbial communities requires new frameworks that expand the field of sociomicrobiology to include concepts from evolution. There is a tremendous potential for the field of microbial pathogenesis, because the social behaviors of microbes may reveal new therapeutic targets.

ACKNOWLEDGMENTS

I thank Joana S. Torres for making the figures.

This work was supported by the Office of the Director, National Institutes of Health under award number DP2OD008440 to J.B. X. and a seed grant from the Lucille Castori Center for Microbes, Inflammation, and Cancer.

CITATION

Xavier JB. 2016. Sociomicrobiology and pathogenic bacteria. Microbiol Spectrum 4 (3):VMBF-0019-2015.

REFERENCES

1. **Peterson J, Garges S, Giovanni M, McInnes P, Wang L, Schloss JA, Bonazzi V, McEwen JE, Wetterstrand KA, Deal C.** 2009. The NIH human microbiome project. *Genome Res* **19:**2317–2323.

2. **Turnbaugh PJ, Ley RE, Hamady M, Fraser-Liggett CM, Knight R, Gordon JI.** 2007. The human microbiome project. *Nature* **449:**804–810.

3. **The Human Microbiome Project Consortium.** 2012. A framework for human microbiome research. *Nature* **486:**215–221.

4. **Eckburg PB, Bik EM, Bernstein CN, Purdom E, Dethlefsen L, Sargent M, Gill SR, Nelson KE, Relman DA.** 2005. Diversity of the human intestinal microbial flora. *Science* **308:**1635–1638.

5. **Turnbaugh PJ, Hamady M, Yatsunenko T, Cantarel BL, Duncan A, Ley RE, Sogin ML, Jones WJ, Roe BA, Affourtit JP.** 2009. A core gut microbiome in obese and lean twins. *Nature* **457:**480–484.

6. **Ley RE, Bäckhed F, Turnbaugh P, Lozupone CA, Knight RD, Gordon JI.** 2005. Obesity alters gut microbial ecology. *Proc Natl Acad Sci USA* **102:**11070–11075.

7. **Cho I, Blaser MJ.** 2012. The human microbiome: at the interface of health and disease. *Nat Rev Genet* **13:**260–270.

8. **Morgan XC, Tickle TL, Sokol H, Gevers D, Devaney KL, Ward DV, Reyes JA, Shah SA, LeLeiko N, Snapper SB.** 2012. Dysfunction of the intestinal microbiome in inflammatory bowel disease and treatment. *Genome Biol* **13:**R79.

9. **Taur Y, Pamer EG.** 2013. The intestinal microbiota and susceptibility to infection in immunocompromised patients. *Curr Opin Infect Dis* **26:**332–337.

10. **Parsek MR, Greenberg EP.** 2005. Sociomicrobiology: the connections between quorum sensing and biofilms. *Trends Microbiol* **13:**27–33.

11. **Costerton J, Stewart PS, Greenberg E.** 1999. Bacterial biofilms: a common cause of persistent infections. *Science* **284:**1318–1322.

12. **Ashby M, Neale J, Knott S, Critchley I.** 1994. Effect of antibiotics on non-growing planktonic cells and biofilms of *Escherichia coli*. *J Antimicrob Chemother* **33:**443–452.

13. **Ledeboer NA, Jones BD.** 2005. Exopolysaccharide sugars contribute to biofilm formation by *Salmonella enterica* serovar Typhimurium on HEp-2 cells and chicken intestinal epithelium. *J Bacteriol* **187:**3214–3226.

14. **Anderl JN, Franklin MJ, Stewart PS.** 2000. Role of antibiotic penetration limitation in *Klebsiella pneumoniae* biofilm resistance to ampicillin and ciprofloxacin. *Antimicrob Agents Chemother* **44:**1818–1824.

15. **Drescher K, Nadell CD, Stone HA, Wingreen NS, Bassler BL.** 2014. Solutions to the public goods dilemma in bacterial biofilms. *Curr Biol* **24:**50–55.

16. **Nadell CD, Drescher, Wingreen NS, Bassler BL.** 2015. Extracellular matrix structure governs invasion resistance in bacterial biofilms. *ISME J* **9:**1700–1709.

17. **Dapa T, Unnikrishnan M.** 2013. Biofilm formation by *Clostridium difficile. Gut Microbes* **4:**397–402.

18. **O'Toole G, Kaplan HB, Kolter R.** 2000. Biofilm formation as microbial development. *Annu Rev Microbiol* **54:**49–79.

19. **Stewart PS, Costerton JW.** 2001. Antibiotic resistance of bacteria in biofilms. *Lancet* **358:** 135–138.

20. **Characklis W, Cooksey K.** 1983. Biofilms and microbial fouling. *Adv Appl Microbiol* **29:**93–138.

21. **Henze M, Harremoës P.** 1983. Anaerobic treatment of wastewater in fixed film reactors: a literature review. *Water Sci Technol* **15:**1–101.

22. **Davies DG, Parsek MR, Pearson JP, Iglewski BH, Costerton J, Greenberg E.** 1998. The involvement of cell-to-cell signals in the development of a bacterial biofilm. *Science* **280:**295–298.

23. **Parsek MR, Greenberg E.** 2005. Sociomicrobiology: the connections between quorum sensing and biofilms. *Trends Microbiol* **13:**27–33.

24. **O'Toole GA, Kolter R.** 1998. Flagellar and twitching motility are necessary for *Pseudomonas aeruginosa* biofilm development. *Mol Microbiol* **30:**295–304.

25. **O'Toole GA, Pratt LA, Watnick PI, Newman DK, Weaver VB, Kolter R.** 1999. Genetic approaches to study of biofilms. *Methods Enzymol* **310:**91–109.

26. **O'Toole G, Kaplan HB, Kolter R.** 2000. Biofilm formation as microbial development. *Annu Rev Microbiol* **54:**49–79.

27. **Hentzer M, Riedel K, Rasmussen TB, Heydorn A, Andersen JB, Parsek MR, Rice SA, Eberl L, Molin S, Høiby N, Kjelleberg S, Givskov M.** 2002. Inhibition of quorum sensing in *Pseudomonas aeruginosa* biofilm bacteria by a halogenated furanone compound. *Microbiology* **148:**87–102.

28. **Boyle KE, Heilmann S, van Ditmarsch D, Xavier JB.** 2013. Exploiting social evolution in biofilms. *Curr Opin Microbiol* **16:**207–212.

29. **Jenal U, Malone J.** 2006. Mechanisms of cyclic-di-GMP signaling in bacteria. *Annu Rev Genet* **40:**385–407.

30. **Güvener ZT, Harwood CS.** 2007. Subcellular location characteristics of the *Pseudomonas aeruginosa* GGDEF protein, WspR, indicate that it produces cyclic-di-GMP in response to growth on surfaces. *Mol Microbiol* **66:**1459–1473.

31. **Hickman JW, Harwood CS.** 2008. Identification of FleQ from *Pseudomonas aeruginosa* as a c-di-GMP-responsive transcription factor. *Mol Microbiol* **69:**376–389.

32. **Baraquet C, Murakami K, Parsek MR, Harwood CS.** 2012. The FleQ protein from *Pseudomonas aeruginosa* functions as both a repressor and an activator to control gene expression from the pel operon promoter in response to c-di-GMP. *Nucleic Acids Res* **40:** 7207–7218.

33. **Dasgupta N, Arora SK, Ramphal R.** 2000. *fleN*, a gene that regulates flagellar number in *Pseudomonas aeruginosa. J Bacteriol* **182:**357–364.

34. **van Ditmarsch D, Boyle KE, Sakhtah H, Oyler JE, Nadell CD, Deziel E, Dietrich LE, Xavier JB.** 2013. Convergent evolution of hyperswarming leads to impaired biofilm formation in pathogenic bacteria. *Cell Rep* **4:**697–708.

35. **Kuchma SL, Brothers KM, Merritt JH, Liberati NT, Ausubel FM, O'Toole GA.** 2007. BifA, a cyclic-di-GMP phosphodiesterase, inversely regulates biofilm formation and swarming motility by *Pseudomonas aeruginosa* PA14. *J Bacteriol* **189:**8165–8178.

36. **Kearns DB.** 2013. You get what you select for: better swarming through more flagella. *Trends Microbiol* **21:**508–509.

37. **Watnick P, Kolter R.** 2000. Biofilm, city of microbes. *J Bacteriol* **182:**2675–2679.

38. **Pennisi E.** 2005. How did cooperative behavior evolve? *Science* **309:**93.

39. **Griffin AS, West SA, Buckling A.** 2004. Cooperation and competition in pathogenic bacteria. *Nature* **430:**1024–1027.

40. **Keller L, Surette MG.** 2006. Communication in bacteria: an ecological and evolutionary perspective. *Nat Rev Microbiol* **4:**249–258.

41. **West SA, Griffin AS, Gardner A, Diggle SP.** 2006. Social evolution theory for microorganisms. *Nat Rev Microbiol* **4:**597–607.

42. **Hamilton WD.** 1964. Genetical evolution of social behaviour. I. *J Theor Biol* **7:**1–16.

43. **Hamilton WD.** 1964. The genetical evolution of social behaviour. II. *J Theor Biol* **7:**17–52.

44. **Dawkins R.** 2006. *The Selfish Gene.* Oxford University Press, Oxford, UK.

45. **Visca P, Ciervo A, Orsi N.** 1994. Cloning and nucleotide sequence of the *pvdA* gene encoding the pyoverdin biosynthetic enzyme L-ornithine N5-oxygenase in *Pseudomonas aeruginosa. J Bacteriol* **176:**1128–1140.

46. **Xavier JB, Foster KR.** 2007. Cooperation and conflict in microbial biofilms. *Proc Natl Acad Sci USA* **104:**876–881.

47. **Nadell CD, Bassler BL.** 2011. A fitness trade-off between local competition and dispersal in *Vibrio cholerae* biofilms. *Proc Natl Acad Sci USA* **108:**14181–14185.

48. **Kim W, Racimo F, Schluter J, Levy SB, Foster KR.** 2014. Importance of positioning for microbial evolution. *Proc Natl Acad Sci USA* **111:**E1639–E1647.

49. **Köhler T, Curty LK, Barja F, Van Delden C, Pechère JC.** 2000. Swarming of *Pseudomonas aeruginosa* is dependent on cell-to-cell signaling and requires flagella and pili. *J Bacteriol* **182:**5990–5996.

50. **Rashid MH, Kornberg A.** 2000. Inorganic polyphosphate is needed for swimming, swarming, and twitching motilities of *Pseudomonas aeruginosa*. *Proc Natl Acad Sci USA* **97:** 4885–4890.

51. **Xavier JB, Kim W, Foster KR.** 2011. A molecular mechanism that stabilizes cooperative secretions in *Pseudomonas aeruginosa*. *Mol Microbiol* **79:**166–179.

52. **de Vargas Roditi L, Boyle KE, Xavier JB.** 2013. Multilevel selection analysis of a microbial social trait. *Mol Syst Biol* **9:**684.

53. **Czechowska K, McKeithen-Mead S, Al Moussawi K, Kazmierczak BI.** 2014. Cheating by type 3 secretion system-negative *Pseudomonas aeruginosa* during pulmonary infection. *Proc Natl Acad Sci USA* **111:**7801–7806.

54. **van Ditmarsch D, Xavier JB.** 2014. Seeing is believing: what experiments with microbes reveal about evolution. *Trends Microbiol* **22:**2–4.

55. **Brown SP, West SA, Diggle SP, Griffin AS.** 2009. Social evolution in micro-organisms and a Trojan horse approach to medical intervention strategies. *Philos Trans R Soc Lond B Biol Sci* **364:**3157–3168.

56. **Mitri S, Xavier JB, Foster KR.** 2011. Social evolution in multispecies biofilms. *Proc Natl Acad Sci USA* **108**(Suppl 2):10839–10846.

57. **Grice EA, Kong HH, Conlan S, Deming CB, Davis J, Young AC, Bouffard GG, Blakesley RW, Murray PR, Green ED, Turner ML, Segre JA, Progra NCS.** 2009. Topographical and temporal diversity of the human skin microbiome. *Science* **324:**1190–1192.

58. **Dewhirst FE, Chen T, Izard J, Paster BJ, Tanner ACR, Yu W-H, Lakshmanan A, Wade WG.** 2010. The human oral microbiome. *J Bacteriol* **192:**5002–5017.

59. **Kau AL, Ahern PP, Griffin NW, Goodman AL, Gordon JI.** 2011. Human nutrition, the gut microbiome and the immune system. *Nature* **474:**327–336.

60. **Wu GD, Chen J, Hoffmann C, Bittinger K, Chen Y-Y, Keilbaugh SA, Bewtra M, Knights D, Walters WA, Knight R, Sinha R, Gilroy E, Gupta K, Baldassano R, Nessel L, Li H, Bushman FD, Lewis JD.** 2011. Linking long-term dietary patterns with gut microbial enterotypes. *Science* **334:**105–108.

61. **Ezenwa VO, Gerardo NM, Inouye DW, Medina M, Xavier JB.** 2012. Microbiology. Animal behavior and the microbiome. *Science* **338:**198–199.

62. **Taur Y, Xavier JB, Lipuma L, Ubeda C, Goldberg J, Gobourne A, Lee YJ, Dubin KA, Socci ND, Viale A, Perales MA, Jenq RR, van den Brink MR, Pamer EG.** 2012. Intestinal domination and the risk of bacteremia in patients undergoing allogeneic hematopoietic stem cell transplantation. *Clin Infect Dis* **55:**905–914.

63. **Bucci V, Bradde S, Biroli G, Xavier JB.** 2012. Social interaction, noise and antibiotic-mediated switches in the intestinal microbiota. *PLoS Comput Biol* **8:**e1002497. doi:10.1371/journal.pcbi.1002497.

64. **Ubeda C, Taur Y, Jenq RR, Equinda MJ, Son T, Samstein M, Viale A, Socci ND, van den Brink MR, Kamboj M, Pamer EG.** 2010. Vancomycin-resistant *Enterococcus* domination of intestinal microbiota is enabled by antibiotic treatment in mice and precedes bloodstream invasion in humans. *J Clin Invest* **120:**4332–4341.

65. **Buffie CG, Jarchum I, Equinda M, Lipuma L, Gobourne A, Viale A, Ubeda C, Xavier J, Pamer EG.** 2012. Profound alterations of intestinal microbiota following a single dose of clindamycin results in sustained susceptibility to *Clostridium difficile*-induced colitis. *Infect Immun* **80:**62–73.

66. **Marino S, Baxter NT, Huffnagle GB, Petrosino JF, Schloss PD.** 2014. Mathematical modeling of primary succession of murine intestinal microbiota. *Proc Natl Acad Sci USA* **111:**439–444.

67. **Stein RR, Bucci V, Toussaint NC, Buffie CG, Ratsch G, Pamer EG, Sander C, Xavier JB.** 2013. Ecological modeling from time-series inference: insight into dynamics and stability of intestinal microbiota. *PLoS Comput Biol* **9:** e1003388. doi:10.1371/journal.pcbi.1003388.

68. **Fisher CK, Mehta P.** 2014. Identifying keystone species in the human gut microbiome from metagenomic timeseries using sparse linear regression. *PloS One* **9:**e102451. doi:10.1371/journal.pone.0102451.

69. **Buffie CG, Bucci V, Stein RR, McKenney PT, Ling L, Gobourne A, No D, Liu H, Kinnebrew M, Viale A, Littmann E, van den Brink MR, Jenq RR, Taur Y, Sander C, Cross J,**

Toussaint NC, Xavier JB, Pamer EG. 2014. Precision microbiome reconstitution restores bile acid mediated resistance to *Clostridium difficile. Nature.* [Epub ahead of print.]

70. Nadell CD, Xavier JB, Foster KR. 2009. The sociobiology of biofilms. *FEMS Microbiol Rev* **33:**206–224.

71. Goodman AL, Kallstrom G, Faith JJ, Reyes A, Moore A, Dantas G, Gordon JI. 2011. Extensive personal human gut microbiota culture collections characterized and manipulated in gnotobiotic mice. *Proc Natl Acad Sci USA* **108:**6252–6257.

72. Cullen TW, Schofield WB, Barry NA, Putnam EE, Rundell EA, Trent MS, Degnan PH, Booth CJ, Yu H, Goodman AL. 2015. Gut microbiota. Antimicrobial peptide resistance mediates resilience of prominent gut commensals during inflammation. *Science* **347:**170–175.

73. Bucci V, Xavier JB. 2014. Towards predictive models of the human gut microbiome. *J Mol Biol.* [Epub ahead of print.]

74. Griffin AS, West SA, Buckling A. 2004. Cooperation and competition in pathogenic bacteria. *Nature* **430:**1024–1027.

Candida–Bacteria Interactions: Their Impact on Human Disease

5

DEVON L. ALLISON,[1,2] HUBERTINE M. E. WILLEMS,[3] J.A.M.S. JAYATILAKE,[4] VINCENT M. BRUNO,[5,6] BRIAN M. PETERS,[3] and MARK E. SHIRTLIFF[2,5]

INTRODUCTION

Candida species are the most common commensal fungus that coexists with hundreds of species of bacteria in the human body. Between 24 and 70% of humans harbor *Candida* species in various body niches, including the oral and vaginal mucosa and the skin (1). Out of over 150 *Candida* species, *Candida albicans* is the principal pathogenic species that causes infections, especially in patient populations with immune dysfunction due to HIV infection, malignancy, immunosuppressive therapy, and organ transplantation. Therefore, these opportunistic infections of *Candida* in topical or systemic forms have become widespread and account for 8 to 10% of bloodstream infections in hospitals (2). Nearly 70% of denture wearers experience denture stomatitis, or inflammation of oral mucosa covered by denture prostheses, with *C. albicans* being a primary etiological factor (3, 4). Almost 75% of the female population

[1]Graduate Program in Life Sciences, Molecular Microbiology and Immunology Program, University of Maryland-Baltimore, Baltimore, MD 21201; [2]Department of Microbial Pathogenesis, University of Maryland-Baltimore, Dental School, Baltimore, MD 21201; [3]Department of Clinical Pharmacy, University of Tennessee Health Science Center, Memphis, TN 38163; [4]Department of Oral Medicine and Periodontology, Faculty of Dental Sciences, University of Peradeniya, Sri Lanka; [5]The Institute for Genomic Sciences; [6]Department of Microbiology and Immunology, School of Medicine, University of Maryland-Baltimore, Baltimore, MD 21201.

Virulence Mechanisms of Bacterial Pathogens, 5th edition
Edited by Indira T. Kudva, Nancy A. Cornick, Paul J. Plummer, Qijing Zhang, Tracy L. Nicholson, John P. Bannantine, and Bryan H. Bellaire
© 2016 American Society for Microbiology, Washington, DC
doi:10.1128/microbiolspec.VMBF-0030-2016

has experienced an episode of vulvovaginal candidiasis at least once in their lifetime, and many have recurring episodes (5). In many of these conditions, there is a phenotypic change for *Candida* from harmless commensal to invasive pathogen. Adhesion to various surfaces, morphogenesis, phenotypic and genotypic switching, and production of lytic enzymes are major virulence mechanisms facilitating this conversion (6). However, properties of the host are also complicit in enabling *Candida* to act as an invasive pathogen since compromise in the interleukin-17 (IL-17)/Th17 arm of the host immune response (e.g., AIDS, Job's syndrome, etc.) or an imbalance in the host microbiome (7) both can contribute to candidiasis (7). During this shift, commensal or transient organisms living with *Candida* species in various locations may play diverse roles in the process of pathogenesis; environmental bacteria may also be introduced via catheters, cannulae, and prosthetic appliances and interact with the already present *Candida*. Such interactions may be detrimental to the health of the human host, leading to mortality.

Currently, fungal-bacterial relations have gained attention due to their impact on human health, the environment, and the health care economy (8). However, polymicrobial infections associated with *Candida* have been reported in the past at variable levels and in a variety of locations. A previous study that analyzed both veteran's affair and university hospital patients concluded that 27% of candidemic infections had a polymicrobial composition (9). *Candida* species have been found to coexist frequently with *Staphylococcus aureus* and *Streptococcus mutans* on denture surfaces and oral mucosa of denture users (10). Polymicrobial infective endocarditis cases among intravenous drug abusers have increased in frequency, with mixtures of *Candida* species and bacteria becoming common etiologies (11). Alarmingly, *Candida*-associated polymicrobial infections have often resulted in high mortality and morbidity in both adults and children because of their increased

dissemination behavior and the current lack of diagnostic sensitivity (9, 12). The interplay between resident microbes, the host, and the compartment environment contributes toward virulence seen in the host and must be taken into account when discussing *Candida*, especially in a biofilm mode of growth (see Fig. 1). Here we review some of the important interactions between *Candida* species, with a focus on *C. albicans*, and clinically relevant bacteria with reference to their regulation of virulence and pathogenicity as well as the current diagnostic and management strategies for these polymicrobial infections.

CANDIDA BIOFILMS

Biofilms are comprised of heterogeneous communities of microorganisms that attach to biotic or abiotic surfaces and/or to one another and are embedded within a host- and/or microbe derived hydrated extracellular matrix, with a complex three-dimensional architecture (13–15) (see Fig. 2). Biofilm-associated infections have unique clinical significance because of the tendency of embedded microbes to harbor resistance against antimicrobials and host defenses. Biofilms are known to utilize multiple strategies to withstand antimicrobial agents, such as physical barriers, dramatically downregulated metabolic rates, and persister phenotypes (16). These complex communities develop both on mucosa and on the surfaces of indwelling medical devices, incorporating endogenous and exogenous microorganisms, thereby creating polymicrobial environments. Many common infections such as dental caries, periodontitis, otitis media, and diabetic foot wound infections are associated with polymicrobial biofilms (17). With the help of advanced culture-independent molecular techniques (e.g., next-generation sequencing), interspecies interactions have been demonstrated to play a significant role in colonization, survival, infection dynamics, and resistance to antimicrobials and host

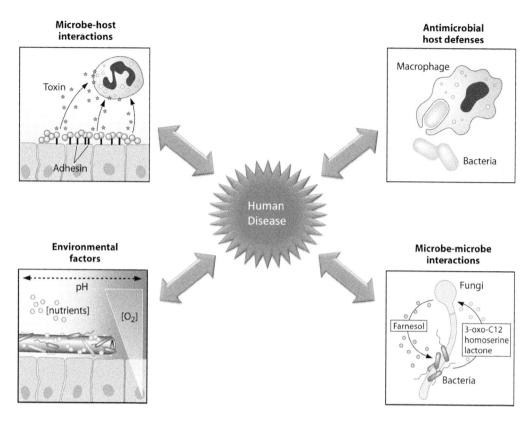

FIGURE 1 Schematic showing the interdependent relationships required for development of human disease. Infection is influenced by microbe–microbe interactions, microbe–host interactions, antimicrobial host defenses, and environmental factors. Significant changes in any of these factors can lead to the development of or predisposition to infection. For example, microbes lacking virulence factors may become apathogenic. Similarly, host immunodeficiencies will encourage infectious processes. It is now becoming increasingly appreciated that intermicrobial interactions and environmental cues also determine infection outcomes such that specific microbial populations under certain conditions may enhance or predict disease progression (184).

defenses (18, 19). Recently, dual-species transcriptomics has been utilized to examine gene expression of *C. albicans* in the presence of other organisms. Dutton and colleagues used RNA-sequencing to analyze the transcriptomes of *Streptococcus gordonii* and *C. albicans* during coculture and found that *C. albicans* genes contributing to hyphal development and arginine biosynthesis were highly upregulated in the presence of *S. gordonii* (20). The presence of multiple and differing organisms within the biofilm community may also provide growth advantages to pathogens and increase the ability to share

genetic information encoding antimicrobial resistance (17). In particular, *Staphylococcus epidermidis* and *C. albicans* form thicker biofilms in the presence of extracellular DNA (eDNA) (21).

C. albicans is the leading pathogenic biofilm former among *Candida* species, and its ability to form biofilms is dependent on the morphogenetic switch from yeast to filamentous hyphae (22). Through multiple knockouts and genetic manipulation, genes governing the transition between yeast and hyphae as well as those factors affected downstream have been determined to create

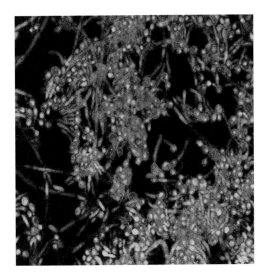

FIGURE 2 *Candida albicans* **strain DAY185 stained with a combination of calcofluor white (blue)/ Syto9 (green) and imaged by confocal laser scanning microscopy (195).**

"yeast-locked" and "hyphae-locked" mutants (23, 24). In particular, *EFG1* and *CPH1* have been implicated in the phenotypic change of yeast to hyphae; *EFG1* is considered the master transcription regulator for hyphal transition and is required in most conditions found in a human host, including neutral pH, carbon dioxide, and sera presence (25); while many transcriptional factors affect hyphal formation, EFG1 has been shown repeatedly to be important and is commonly used in genetic knock-outs to force *C. albicans* to stay in the yeast form in most environmental situations. *In vivo* infection studies with *C. albicans* strains harboring homozygous deletions of *EFG1* and *CPH1* have demonstrated that hyphal morphogenesis is required for the development of oropharyngeal, vulvovaginal, and hematogenously disseminated candidiasis (26–28). Hyphae facilitate intermicrobial interactions and adhesion to surfaces, knitting the complex biofilm architecture together. One of the earliest *in vitro* studies demonstrated that certain piliated strains of bacteria enhanced *C. albicans* attachment to epithelial cells, showing how bacteria could

assist fungi (29). Several subsequent studies have focused on these bacterial interactions with *C. albicans* biofilms in the context of disease. *Pseudomonas aeruginosa*, another potent former of biofilms and a pathogen in immunocompromised cystic fibrosis patients, has been shown to create a thick biofilm on *C. albicans* hyphae which results in killing of the fungus (30). *S. aureus* also favors binding to *C. albicans* hyphae; however, both bacteria and fungus coexist in a live, mature biofilm on biomedical surfaces and oral epithelium (31, 32).

Several species of bacteria have been shown to alter the expression of hyphae-associated genes in *C. albicans*, such as *CDR4*, when grown in coculture (33). *S. mutans*, a major bacterial player in the formation of dental caries, possesses specific glycosyltransferase enzymes that allow it to tightly bind to *C. albicans*, providing a possible explanation for both species being frequently isolated together from caries in children (34). The large scope of unique interactions observed in *Candida*–bacteria biofilms has created a need to better understand how these interactions occur and are maintained.

CANDIDA AND COAGGREGATION

Adhesion to various microbial cells, or coaggregation, is the initial step in intermicrobial interactions, making the adhesion between *Candida* and bacteria a key factor in colonization and pathogenesis (35). Deletion of *C. albicans ALS3*, which encodes a surface glycoprotein, results in the loss of *C. albicans* attachment to saliva-coated surfaces as the biofilm matures, promoting the importance of the ALS proteins in maintaining adhesion throughout the biofilm lifecycle (36). Coaggregation has been known for many years to be a vital component in cross-kingdom interactions. Utilizing a simple agglutination assay, Bagg and Silverwood demonstrated that *C. albicans* yeast cells coaggregated well with oral bacteria including *Streptococcus sanguinis*,

Streptococcus salivarius, S. mutans, Streptococcus mitis, Fusobacterium nucleatum, and *Actinomyces viscosus* but not with *Bacteroides melaninogenicus* (*Prevotella melaninogenica*) (see Fig. 3). Their study provided evidence that bacterial surface lectins and yeast cell surface carbohydrates may interact to allow coagulation with specific bacteria species, such as *Fusobacterium*, but could not explain all adherence mechanisms, including those of oral streptococci (37). Jenkinson and colleagues followed up on the mechanisms of aggregation in regard to oral streptococci and *C. albicans* by starving yeast cells of glucose and testing their adherence with *S. gordonii* and *S. sanguis.* They determined that starvation promoted adherence of oral streptococci to *C. albicans* yeast and that since the conditions may have triggered expression of new surface molecules, the biofilm environment must also be taken into account when thinking about adhesion mechanisms (38).

Holmes and others further evaluated the interaction of *C. albicans* and *S. gordonii,* concluding that cell wall polysaccharides from *S. gordonii* participate in binding to *C. albicans* and that treatment with antipolysaccharide antibodies can abolish the adherence between the organisms (39). Advances in *in vitro* biofilm growth have recently provided better insights into biofilm formation and its core components. Diaz and colleagues utilized a novel flow cell apparatus that incorporated mucosal tissue from the oral cavity and esophagus to better characterize the interaction between *C. albicans* and oral *Streptococcus* species. They saw that there was a cooperative interaction, as the presence of *C. albicans* increased the amount of *Streptococcus oralis* on oral mucosal tissue, and that invasion of *C. albicans* into the tissue increased when in coculture (40). Recently, Arzmi and others examined aggregation of polymicrobial biofilms using artificial saliva media and cocultured combinations of *S. mutans* and *Actinomyces naeslundii* with different strains of *C. albicans.* They discovered that the aggregation of bacteria and fungus was variable, depending on the specific strain of *C. albicans* present (41). These studies suggest that different surface receptors, each of which contributes to aggregation, may be expressed at different times during dual-species biofilm development, particularly in the oral cavity.

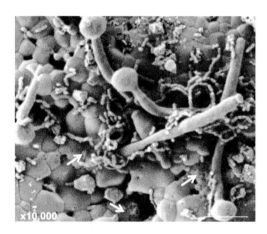

FIGURE 3 Scanning electron micrographs of a polymicrobial biofilm formed on discs of hydroxyapatite. This shows the affinity of *Streptococcus mutans* to the *Candida albicans* hyphal elements as the streptococcal chains wrap around the hyphae. Small perforations are evident on the surfaces of the hydroxyapatite due to the highly acidic local microenvironment induced by the acidogenic bacterial species, *S. mutans* (196). Bar = 10 mm.

CANDIDA–BACTERIA INTERACTIONS IN THE HUMAN HOST

C. albicans often exists in a milieu of other microbial species. These relations are likely to affect how *C. albicans* interacts with the host. This section will discuss the various interspecies interactions that are dependent upon not only the environment of the host compartment, but also the resident microbial species in these compartments. While certain intermicrobial interactions can occur in multiple host compartments, we have grouped *C. albicans* with the historically recognized bacterial partner(s) in each compartment.

Interactions on the Skin and into Systemic Disease: *Candida–Staphylococcus* Species

Clinical Coisolation

Staphylococcus aureus, a Gram-positive bacterium, is a common colonizer of the skin and mucosa, such as the nasal cavity. Clearance of *S. aureus* from this particular body niche is dependent on a functioning Th17 axis of the immune system and neutrophil access (42). This requirement becomes problematic in immunocompromised patients, predominantly HIV-positive patients with low T-cell counts, in whom *S. aureus* may have an increased opportunity to interact with *C. albicans*. Such an interaction may be lethal to the host, with *S. aureus* frequently isolated from the blood of patients with candidemia, suggesting that patients with candidemia may have higher rates of bacteremia (9, 11). This coisolation in bloodstream infections is present even in the neonatal population, where *S. aureus* and *Candida* species were coisolated in about 9% of polymicrobial bloodstream infections (12). Infective endocarditis, a major health concern due to the significant 16% in-hospital mortality, has occasionally been associated with polymicrobial infection with both staphylococcal and fungal species (43, 44).

Infectious Synergy

Multiple animal models have shown a significant increase in the virulence of both *Candida* and *Staphylococcus* species when coinfection exists. When mice were given intraperitoneal injections of *C. albicans* and *S. aureus*, mortality resulted within 2 days but was not seen when each organism was injected alone. In these mice, both fungus and bacteria were found together in the spleen, pancreas, and esophagus, indicating dissemination from the intraperitoneal site. *S. aureus* was always accompanied by *C. albicans* in these disseminated pockets of infection, suggesting a synergistic role between organisms (45–47). A neonatal colonization model has demonstrated that coinfection of

C. albicans and *S. epidermidis*, another skin colonizer, caused delays in weight gain as the rat pups aged and an increase in morbidity at sublethal doses delivered subcutaneously. When young rat pups were given fluconazole prophylaxis prior to coinfection, there was a substantial increase in survival and weight gain, providing evidence of the importance of *C. albicans* in this infection process (48). A mouse model mimicking polymicrobial peritonitis, a complication that has increased with the usage of peritoneal dialysis methods, further supported previous studies that mono-infection of *C. albicans* or *S. aureus* are nonlethal, but dual-species infections raise mortality significantly. Larger bacterial and fungal burden was detected in kidneys and spleens of dual-infected mice compared to mono-infected mice, and increases in proinflammatory cytokines, such as IL-6 and G-CSF, were seen within 1 day in these organs. Increased neutrophil presence was also detected in the dual-species infection, and when mice were treated with nonsteroidal anti-inflammatory drugs (NSAIDs), all mice survived with lower bacterial and fungal burdens in kidneys and spleens. This protective effect was countered by application of PGE_2 (prostaglandin E_2), an oxylipin known to increase proinflammatory cytokines, and it suggests that polymicrobial infection control may involve modulating the host innate immune response (49).

With indwelling medical devices serving as excellent substrates to form biofilms, a polymicrobial infection model was developed using subcutaneous implanted titanium discs in mice and proximately injecting *S. aureus* and *C. albicans* nearby. These discs, coated with antimicrobial agents, were able to decrease some of the microbial burden on the implant but could not decrease the burden in nearby tissue. Such results exemplify how polymicrobial infections can be tenacious and difficult to treat, as well as the need for new and functional treatment methods (50). Taken together, these animal models have thoroughly demonstrated the potent power of *C. albicans–Staphylococcus* species infections in causing morbidity and mortality in multiple body niches.

In testing the impact of hyphae-formation in polymicrobial biofilm development, *S. aureus* adherence to mutants in the regulators of morphogenesis *CPH* and *EFG* was evaluated. It was found that *S. aureus* bound in high numbers to *C. albicans* hyphae produced by *cph1/cph1* and *efg1/efg1* single mutants. In contrast, when staphylococcal adherence to the *cph1/cph1, efg1/efg1* double mutant was evaluated, binding was nearly abolished. This is probably because of the tendency for *S. aureus* to preferentially bind hyphae since the double mutant produced a majority of yeast cells compared to the complete or partial hyphal production in the *cph1/cph1* and *efg1/efg1* single mutants, respectively. While this hyphae dependence on staphylococcal binding is very important, it should be noted that increased concentrations of serum strongly promote even nonspecific polymicrobial adherence within these biofilms. This alternative effector of adherence serves as a reminder that the proximal environment around the biofilm can play a potent role in its development (51, 52). When grown in dual-species biofilm models with *C. albicans* and *S. aureus*, the bacterial cells preferably bound and associated with the hyphae within the biofilm mass (see Figs. 4 and 5) (32, 45–48, 51).

Harriot and Noverr elucidated part of this interaction by using different killing methods on *C. albicans* biofilms to see if this changed the polymicrobial biofilm dynamic with *S. aureus*. They saw that formalin- and heat-killed, but not antifungal-treated (51), *C. albicans* hyphae were unable to sustain a thick and closely associated biofilm with *S. aureus*, suggesting that a fungal protein was the major player in this dual-species interaction (51). With yeast and hyphae being

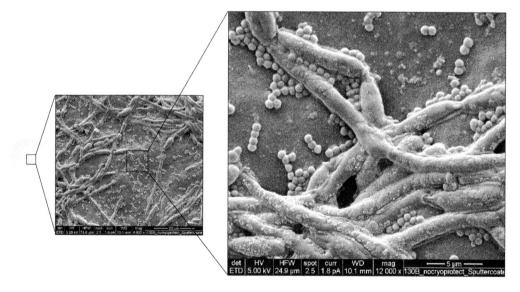

FIGURE 4 We and others have previously reported the association of *Staphylococcus aureus* with *Candida albicans* hyphae during polymicrobial biofilm growth. High-resolution scanning electron microscopy confirmed these findings and demonstrated a three-dimensionally distributed pattern of *S. aureus* hyphal attachment. Not only can *S. aureus* be found bordering the basal layer of the hyphae-substratum interface, but bacterial cells are also seen attached to the upper portion of the hyphal surface. The precise architectural details and spatial arrangement cannot be fully appreciated like those in the cryo-SEM image of a *C. albicans–S. aureus* dual species biofilm on PVC catheter disks.

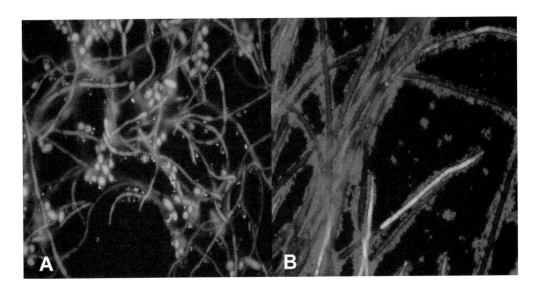

FIGURE 5 **Images of biofilm probed with (A) TAMRA-labeled universal yeast probe and FITC-labeled** *Staphylococcus aureus* **probe and (B) TAMRA-labeled** *S. aureus* **probe and FITC-labeled** *Candida albicans* **probe (31).**

distinct forms in *C. albicans*, the protein composition as well as the secretome of both stages differs, opening the chance for new interactions that could explain the specificity of *C. albicans* hyphae and *S. aureus* association. Utilizing two-dimensional gel electrophoresis on protein extracts from dual-species biofilms, Peters and colleagues demonstrated that specific proteins for yeast and hyphae stages were upregulated when *C. albicans* was grown with *S. aureus* (31, 53). The yeast–*S. aureus* biofilm had the most changes in protein expression for both species; this may be because yeast-form *C. albicans* produces a unique quorum sensing molecule called farnesol, which causes a loss in *S. aureus* membrane integrity and decreased bacterial viability. Such a harsh environment may further explain the upregulation of *S. aureus* stress proteins in this interaction (31, 53).

Candida Adhesins that Bind *S. aureus*

The determination of fungal and bacterial adhesion mechanisms has been a central focus in the study of *C. albicans* and *S. aureus* interaction. These studies have concentrated on previously noted *Candida* surface adhesins, such as ALS (agglutinin-like sequence) proteins and Hwp1p (hyphal wall proteins), as well as hyphal transcription factors *Bcr1p* and *Tec1p* (54). Initially, Harriot and Noverr took their cues from studies looking at *S. epidermidis* and *C. albicans* and decided to use mutants in multiple ALS proteins and *HWP1*. They found no significant effect of deleting any of these proteins when *C. albicans* and *S. aureus* were grown in dual-species biofilms with large concentrations of serum. However, these large concentrations of serum may have compensated for some of the mutations. The authors suspected that the *Candida* biofilm matrix was a key to polymicrobial development (51). This work was followed by Peters and colleagues, who used ALS mutants in serum-free media and noted a significant defect in *S. aureus* binding to *C. albicans* lacking *Als3p* (52) (see Fig. 6). These results suggest that environmental conditions can alter polymicrobial biofilm development and that there may be some nonspecific *S. aureus*–*C. albicans* interactions that involve sera components such as fibro-

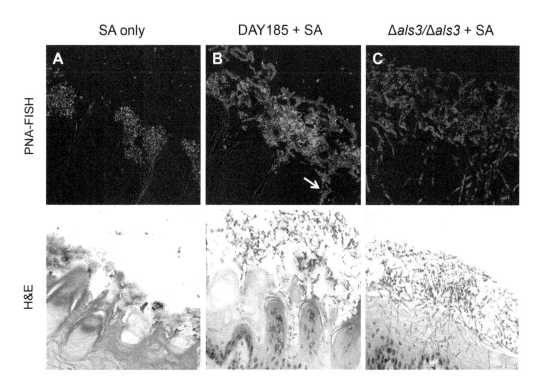

FIGURE 6 **Infection of CD-1 mouse tongue tissue b** *Staphylococcus aureus* **alone,** *Candida albicans* **DAY185 + *S. aureus* (DAY185+SA), or *C. albicans* als3 mutant + *S. aureus* (Δals3/Δals3 + SA) and subsequently stained by PNA-FISH or hematoxylin and eosin (H&E). (A) Monomicrobial *S. aureus* (green) infections were confined to the epithelial surface but were noninvasive as confirmed by a lack of inflammatory infiltrate by H&E staining. (B) Coinfection with DAY185+SA showed staphylococci attached to the hyphal surface of *C. albicans* (red) and in some instances where hyphae had pierced the epithelial layer, *S. aureus* (green) could be seen coembedded within the epithelium (white arrow). (C) However, coinfection with Δals3/Δals3 +SA demonstrated a fully invasive *C. albicans* infection with relatively few staphylococci seen attached to the hyphae and an absence of epithelial coinvasion (195).**

nectin and albumin. Beaussart and others used single force spectroscopy to examine the molecular interactions of *S. epidermidis* with *C. albicans* Als1/Als3 proteins, noticing that there was a reduced amount of binding in yeast cells compared to germ tube, the previous lacking Als proteins. They performed single force spectroscopy with *Als1/Als3* double knockouts as well as mannosyltransferase mutants and concluded that *Candida*–staphylococci adherence required ALS proteins with correct o-mannosylations (55).

The importance of *Als3p* was verified in a recent study by Schlecht and colleagues using a dual-species oral infection model in an immunocompromised murine host, simulating the environment of a patient with oral candidiasis. In infected tongue tissues, *S. aureus* was shown to invade only with wild-type and *Als3*-complemented *C. albicans* strains. Such specificity was shown to impact systemic disease, with no *S. aureus* dissemination found in kidney tissues when coinfected on the tongue with the *als3Δ* mutant strain. Since the *als3Δ* mutant can still form hyphae and actively penetrate tissue, the authors concluded that this defect was attributed to specific *S. aureus–C. albicans* binding and that it prevented *S. aureus* from attaching with these invasive hyphae (32). However, other factors such as complicity of the host immune response or augmented microbial virulence may also come into play in this interaction. These results support one of the first studies examining polymicrobial intra-abdominal infections, which was completed in 1983. Similar to the kidney dissemination witnessed by Schlecht and colleagues with dual infections of bacteria and fungus, Carlson observed that even at sublethal doses, *S. aureus* could be recovered from the bloodstream of mice coinfected with *C. albicans*. These findings were also shown during dual-species infection of *Serratia marcescens* and *Enterococcus faecalis* (46). The translation of the binding mechanism of *S. aureus* to Als3p protein in *C. albicans* from *in vitro* to *in vivo* is an important finding and suggests the need for biofilm treatments that address both organisms.

Staphylococcus Adhesins that Bind C. albicans

While the *C. albicans* binding protein in the *C. albicans–S. aureus* interaction has been elucidated, the *S. aureus* binding partner remains unknown, as does the impact of *S. aureus*–produced factors on the polymicrobial biofilm. Fehrmann and colleagues used biopanning to see which peptides produced by *S. aureus* would have strong binding to *C. albicans* biofilms in the presence of fibronectin and noted consistent binding with staphylococcal coagulase and extracellular fibrinogen binding protein (Efb). Since these staphylococcal components can block complement pathways used by the innate immune system, Fehrmann and others examined how these might play into the host-pathogen response with *C. albicans* present. Phagocytosis of *C. albicans* was inhibited in the presence of staphylococcal Efb and coagulase. Confocal images demonstrated that a fibrin shield coated *C. albicans* and protected the fungus, formed as the coagulase broke down the fibronectin in the media (56). These findings show that *C. albicans* could derive benefit from secreted staphylococcal factors, particularly against the innate immune system, which is the front line of defense in a dual-species infection. Meanwhile, low levels of farnesol produced by *C. albicans* biofilms, but not tryosol (a *C. albicans* quorum sensing molecule produced during early biofilm development), have shown a modest increase in *S. aureus* biofilm production (57). This same study also noted that the small amounts of PGE_2 produced by *C. albicans* stimulated biofilm growth in *S. aureus*, with this being attenuated by the addition of indomethacin, a cyclooxygenase inhibitor. These results also support the findings of Peter and Noverr and suggest that prostaglandins produced during the host inflammatory response may feed into polymicrobial biofilm development (49). It is evident that fungal and bacterial aspects can work together to potentiate virulence while circumventing host immune systems in *Candida*–staphylococci interactions.

Antimicrobial Resistance with Staphylococcus Species Induced by C. albicans

Staphylococcus species are known for developing antimicrobial resistance in multiple clinical situations. The CDC's most current report on invasive methicillin-resistant *S. aureus* (MRSA) infections has shown that health care–associated MRSA infections remain the deadliest in the United States even though overall rates of MRSA infection are decreasing in portions of the nation (58). Development of antimicrobial resistance by the biofilm organisms has traditionally been attributed to the complex matrix of the biofilm, rendering weak diffusion of the drug throughout the structure. Some *in vitro* studies have noted that *S. aureus* and *S. epidermidis* gain antimicrobial resistance in the presence of *C. albicans* (59, 60). Utilizing an *in vitro* catheter disk model system, Adam and colleagues demonstrated that some *S. epidermidis* strains released extracellular polymer slime that hindered fluconazole activity against *C. albicans* in a mixed-species biofilm. The authors also tested the effects of coculture with vancomycin treatment, a last resort drug for highly resistant staphylococcal infections, and discovered that even in slime-negative *S. epidermidis* strains, coculture could protect against clinical levels of vancomycin (59). These findings show that *C. albicans* and *S. epidermidis* share mutual benefits to counteract the action of antimicrobials in polymicrobial biofilm development. Similarly, Al-Fattani and Douglas examined the biofilm matrices of *C. albicans* and *Candida tropicalis*, noting stark differences in their major constituents, with *C. albicans* matrix comprised of glucose and *C. tropicalis* matrix comprised of hexosamine. These differences made significant contributions to drug resistance in *Candida* biofilms, with *C. tropicalis* biofilms being almost completely resistant to both fungicidal and fungistatic agents (61).

Harriot and Noverr followed up on these observations by looking at *S. aureus*–*C. albicans* biofilms in the presence of antimicrobials and reported increased vancomycin resistance in *S. aureus* during coculture. They postulated that the resistance was conferred by secretion of extracellular matrix components of *C. albicans* into the biofilm. Through immunofluorescence microscopy, the authors showed that *S. aureus* could become coated in *C. albicans* matrix and that this could help block vancomycin from reaching its target of peptidoglycan (60). However, it should be noted that addition of *C. albicans* matrix alone did not restore vancomycin resistance in *S. aureus* to levels similar to that seen in polymicrobial biofilm culture, suggesting that several components mediate this interaction. Importantly, *C. albicans* mutant *Bcr1p* was unable to adhere to plastic, formed a weak biofilm matrix, and was incapable of conferring vancomycin resistance when grown with *S. aureus*, supporting the concept that adhesion and biofilm matrix can be vital factors in antimicrobial resistance. However, dual-species biofilms grown with als3Δ and *hwp1Δ* *C. albicans* mutants were capable of conferring the vancomycin resistance as closely as to the wild-type strain. It is important to remember that Als proteins and Hwp1p are surface-expressed adhesins, some

of which can be rendered unnecessary in the presence of large amounts of sera (utilized in these experiments) and that these mutants can still form biofilms (51). Such conditions with large concentrations of sera could possibly simulate growth on bloodstream catheters but would not be as applicable in deep tissue infections, further suggesting that staphylococcal factors may be important in this induced resistance.

Interactions in the Lungs

Candida–P. aeruginosa

P. aeruginosa is a Gram-negative bacterium that is ubiquitous in the environment but can become an opportunistic pathogen in the immunocompromised population. In the CDC's 2013 report on antibiotic resistance, multidrug-resistant *P. aeruginosa* was listed as a serious threat, alongside pathogens such as MRSA and multidrug-resistant tuberculosis (62). Strikingly, *P. aeruginosa* engages in an antagonistic relationship when grown with *C. albicans* in *in vitro* biofilms, with a noticeable killing of hyphal filaments (30). However, these organisms have the opportunity to engage within an immunocompromised patient in multiple locations. Early studies utilized mouse burn models to examine if *P. aeruginosa* infection could influence or amplify a concurrent *C. albicans* infection. These studies demonstrated that a low-virulence *P. aeruginosa* strain could prime a mouse for lethal candidiasis; it should be noted that as *C. albicans* CFUs increased in these studies, *P. aeruginosa* CFUs decreased. The authors speculate that the large amount of elastase produced by this *P. aeruginosa* strain may have further damaged tissues and facilitated *C. albicans* dissemination from the skin into the kidneys, because purified elastase injected with *C. albicans* produced similar deaths (63). Yu and colleagues noted the similarities in structure of the *P. aeruginosa* pilus adhesin and the *C. albicans* fimbrial adhesin and investigated if the two structures could share a common epitope for immune recognition. Through agglutination assays, they detailed how monoclonal antibodies raised against bacteria could bind to fungus and vice versa (64). Since both pilus adhesin and fimbrial adhesin recognize glycosphingolipids on cell surfaces, a common antibody against each could be utilized in the prevention of *P. aeruginosa* or *C. albicans* biofilms through the action of neutralizing antibodies.

On the contrary, the fungicidal effects of *P. aeruginosa* on *C. albicans* in multiple *in vitro* coculture settings have been reported by several investigators (65–67). Hogan and Kolter provided a foundation in this work by showing that *P. aeruginosa* can attach to *C. albicans* hyphae and kill them. They also examined mutations in *P. aeruginosa* pili, structures responsible for adhesion to a variety of surfaces, and noted an overall decrease in attachment to hyphae with these pili mutants (30). This correlates with the data of Yu and others and suggests that pili are important to *Pseudomonas* in this relationship (64). Corroborating this antagonism, live/dead imaging revealed that *P. aeruginosa* bound to *C. albicans* hyphae and remained stationed on these particular hyphae as they caused cell lysis in the immediate area. Brand and colleagues further tested if direct contact was needed for *P. aeruginosa* to kill using spent media on fungal cultures and determined that secreted products in the media did have a modest inhibitory effect on *C. albicans* (68). Overall, most evidence suggests that direct interaction between *P. aeruginosa* and *C. albicans* is detrimental to *C. albicans*.

Like many bacteria, *P. aeruginosa* can use quorum sensing to signal between cells within biofilm structures; Gram-negative bacteria use homoserine lactones to accomplish these tasks. *P. aeruginosa* secretes *N*-3-oxo-C12 homoserine lactone (3OC12HSL) at large micromolar amounts in biofilms; when smaller amounts were introduced into *C. albicans* cultures, complete repression of filamentation was witnessed. This effect could also be seen when *C. albicans* was treated with similar 12-carbon backbone molecules, suggesting that *C. albicans* may be able to sense its environment and respond through detection of these small molecules (69). McAlester and colleagues followed these observations by examining multiple strains of *P. aeruginosa* and noticed that production of HSL varied between strains; when supernatant from these strains was placed on yeast-form *C. albicans*, only high HSL producers could inhibit the yeast-hyphae switch, while low HSL producers did not have any effects on fungal transition. Since *C. albicans* can also produce its own quorum sensing molecule, farnesol, the authors decided to see if this could alter growth or other aspects of *P. aeruginosa* and determined that micromolar concentrations of farnesol could stop swarming activity, an important method of dispersal for *P. aeruginosa* (70). At the molecular level concerning *P. aeruginosa*, Cugini and colleagues utilized qualitative PCR to show that while transcripts of genes in the *Pseudomonas* quinolone signal operon, another quorum sensing mechanism in *P. aeruginosa*, are decreased in the presence of farnesol, the modulating transcription factor for the operon was unaffected. Through electrophoretic mobility shift assays, the authors were able to show that farnesol interfered with the transcription factor and directed it toward an alternative site, ultimately reducing production of the bacterial virulence factor pyocyanin (71). Such findings strongly support the idea of an antagonistic relationship in the immunocompromised patient, with bacteria and fungus each producing their own molecules to silence the opponent.

In an early report, Kerr and colleagues demonstrated that pyocyanin produced by *P. aeruginosa* could be an antifungal agent, though not at the same levels as current antifungal treatments such as fluconazole (66). Since *P. aeruginosa* is known to produce phenazine compounds that can act as antimicrobial agents and because pyocyanin is a phenazine derivative through the shikimate pathway, Gibson and others examined if phenazines were important in these dual-species interactions. The authors documented a red pigment on *C. albicans* lawns inoculated with single points of *P. aeruginosa*; knocking out the *Pseudomonas* quinolone signal operon abolished this pigmentation, suggesting an association with pyocyanin. Through further genetic knockouts, the component responsible for the red pigment was determined to be a pyocyanin precursor, 5-methyl-phenazinium-1-carboxylate (5MPCA), and it appeared only in areas of fungal cell death, supporting the concept that pyocyanin components may act as antifungal agents (72). Further studies on 5MPCA by Morales and colleagues demonstrated that the phenazine compound was taken up by *C. albicans* cells and interacted with oxygen, generating reactive oxygen species (ROS) that could be detected by probes. When testing catalase-deficient *C. albicans* mutants to confirm the role of reactive oxygen species damage in this interaction, the authors saw that these *C. albicans* mutants, which could not handle oxidative stress, had increased death when treated with 5MPCA (73). All of these current studies show that quorum sensing molecules may play an important role in the cross-talks between *Candida* and *Pseudomonas* in coculture, and as such, purified molecules may be exploited in controlling biofilm-associated infections in the face of rapidly developing antimicrobial and antifungal resistance.

To further dissect the genetic effects of *P. aeruginosa* secreted factors on *C. albicans* biofilms, Holcombe and others performed a transcriptomic screen on the fungus and discovered that the expression of genes related to drug or toxin efflux increased, while biofilm and adhesion genes decreased (74). This inhibitory effect of *P. aeruginosa* on *Candida* biofilms has been shown for multiple *Candida* species. Biofilms of *C. tropicalis* and *Candida dubliniensis* grown with *P. aeruginosa* had decreased fungal viability and were thinner compared to mono-species fungal biofilms alone (75). Further studies by Bandara and colleagues on *P. aeruginosa* interactions

with different *Candida* species have revealed that *P. aeruginosa* lipopolysaccharide (LPS) inhibited *Candida glabrata*, *Candida krusei*, and *C. dubliniensis* biofilm formation and maturation, suggesting that bacterial LPS can have an effect throughout biofilm development (76).

However, *Candida* species are not without their own defenses; Chen and colleagues pointed out that ethanol produced by the fungus can halt swarming behavior and promote biofilm development. Using a transposon screen, the authors determined that levels of cyclic-di-GMP, an important secondary messenger molecule, were decreased through WspR, a factor that stimulates exopolysaccharide production for biofilms (77). Lopez-Medina and others further examined *C. albicans* defense mechanisms against *P. aeruginosa* using a neutropenic murine mouse model and inoculated the gut with both pathogens. Their results demonstrated that *P. aeruginosa* virulence was attenuated in the presence of *C. albicans* and that when the transcriptome of *P. aeruginosa* was analyzed via RNAseq, genes encoding pyochelin and pyoverdine, siderophores used to sequester iron for bacteria, were highly downregulated. Utilizing spent media, the authors concluded that *C. albicans* secreted proteins that inhibited the pyochelin and pyoverdine produced by *P. aeruginosa* and that virulence of the bacteria could be rescued by the addition of iron in the murine model (78). While *P. aeruginosa* and *Candida* species maintain an antagonistic relationship, these studies elucidating defense mechanisms of each opportunistic pathogen might be applied to other polymicrobial biofilm situations and provide unique therapeutic targets.

Candida–Burkholderia cenocepacia

Burkholderia cepacia complex is comprised of 17 distinct species of Gram-negative bacteria that survive in a wide range of environments, including some antiseptic solutions, and can cause serious infection in immunocompromised patients (79). These bacteria possess important virulence factors such as quorum sensing mechanisms, the ability to form biofilms on plastics and epithelial cells, and intrinsic resistance to several antibiotics (80). *B. cenocepacia*, one of the members of this complex, is responsible for causing an invasive respiratory disease called cepacia syndrome in individuals with cystic fibrosis, which can lead to death (81). The reports on interactions between *B. cenocepacia* and *Candida* are rare; however, they have the potential for interaction by overlap of niche in the cystic fibrosis lung environment. Boon and colleagues noted a molecule produced in most of the *B. cepacia* complex species, cis-2-dodecenoic acid (BDSF), was important to produce biofilms and extracellular polysaccharides in *B. cenocepacia*. In both coculture and with the addition of BDSF, *C. albicans* hyphal formation was stunted, and this was further supported by rescue of hyphal health through knocking out the genes controlling BDSF production (82). How this suppression of fungal growth is accomplished is currently unknown, as is any effect on *C. albicans* quorum sensing molecules on *B. cepacia* complex members. Such molecules may serve as a mechanism to establish dominance in the cystic fibrosis lung, and further analysis on the therapeutic potential of the purified BDSF molecule is needed.

Candida–Mycobacterium tuberculosis

While tuberculosis is not a major health concern in the Western world, throughout sub-Saharan Africa and portions of Asia, the disease is endemic. Patients with latent tuberculosis can serve as reservoirs and may progress to active disease once their immune system falters (83). With an increase in multidrug-resistant strains as well as patients immunocompromised from HIV infection, this provides a suitable environment for interaction of the acid-fast bacteria with *Candida* species. Examining a hospital in South India, Kali and colleagues noted that 40% of their surveyed population infected with *M. tuberculosis* also had *C. albicans*

coinfection. The authors recovered several species of *Candida*, particularly in patients displaying pulmonary disease symptoms. This suggests that it may be clinically beneficial to screen patients with tuberculosis infection for fungal pathogens, especially female patients, who were determined to have a significantly higher chance of harboring dual infection (84). An earlier study in five hospitals across northern Kenya examined HIV-positive patients with positive tuberculosis tests, and of the 11 patients determined to harbor both virus and mycobacterium, 4 were coinfected with *Candida* species (85). Because there are such limited reports regarding the coisolation of *Candida* and *M. tuberculosis* in patients, little research has been conducted on the interaction between these pathogens of the immunocompromised.

Both *M. tuberculosis* and *Candida* infection have immunocompromise as a common point, though traditionally *M. tuberculosis* is associated with Th1 cytotoxic killing through interferon-γ, while *Candida* is associated with neutrophils, IL-17, and Th17 lineage. Genetic errors in IL-17A/F result in mucocutaneous candidiasis, while errors in interferon-γ genes lead to increased mycobacterial diseases, even from weak strains such as the tuberculosis vaccine strain, *Mycobacterium bovis*. A recent study noted that some pediatric patients have been infected with both pathogens, suggesting a common genetic mutation. Okada and others used genomic sequencing of seven pediatric patients over many ethnic backgrounds and found a common loss-of-function mutation in both copies of RAR-related orphan receptor C (RORC). This alteration led to a nonfunctioning RORγ, the vital transcription factor for the Th17 linage, and the production of T-cells that could no longer produce IL-17A/F. Further examination of this genetic defect through analysis of the T-cell receptor repertoire demonstrated a decrease in rearrangement of 5′ portions of the V regions in the T-cell receptor, resulting in the absence of type 1 NK T-cells, which are important in recognizing the unique glycolipids of mycobacterium species (86). While no current literature has examined the phenotypic or genetic effects of mycobacterium and *Candida* coinfection on the respective organisms, it may prove important to further an understanding of different T-cell subsets, primarily invariant T-cells, of which little is currently known.

Interactions in the Oral Cavity

S. aureus and C. albicans

The discussion above of the interaction of *S. aureus* and *C. albicans* is also relevant to the oral cavity. *S. aureus* is often carried within the nares and on the skin of colonized hosts. Although *S. aureus* is generally thought to be a noncommensal, increasing numbers of culture and molecular-based studies have shown that this pathogenic species is more common on mucosal surfaces from healthy subjects than originally hypothesized (87–97). While this pathogen may not directly contribute to localized mucosal virulence in the oral cavity, the transient or persistent carriage of *S. aureus* on various mucosal surfaces can provide an infectious source for systemic disease, particularly when *C. albicans* is present (9, 32, 98–101).

Candida–Streptococcus species

The oral microbiome is comprised of many *Streptococcus* species, providing multiple locations for contact with *Candida* species, including dental appliances and the periodontal pocket. Some of the earliest work on cross-kingdom interactions reported on coaggregation between *Candida* and various oral bacteria species, including *S. mutans* and *S. salivarius* (37, 102). These studies suggested that binding of *C. albicans* with viridans streptococci (oral streptococcus that are α-hemolytic and optochin-resistant) was important for yeast colonization on the oral surfaces. Holmes and colleagues determined that *S. gordonii*, a streptococcus species that rapidly adheres to tooth surfaces, was able to bind to *C. albicans* through streptococcal

surface proteins A and B (SspA and SspB) in addition to surface-associated proteins cshA and B. By expressing SspB on the surface of *E. faecalis*, the authors enabled *Candida–Enterococcus* binding, supporting their hypothesis (102). These original studies implied that a complex environment exists within the oral cavity, with salivary factors such as mucus interacting with *Candida* species and oral bacteria to provide multiple ligand–receptor interactions.

Recently, with a better understanding of the role of the oral microbiome in human health, studies have focused on determining how *Candida–Streptococcus* interactions occur in biofilms. Bamford and others showed that *S. gordonii* enhanced hyphal development and biofilm formation in *C. albicans* when in the presence of human saliva but that streptococcal contact with *C. albicans* through SspA and SspB was not the only factor for polymicrobial biofilm development. They investigated quorum sensing within *S. gordonii* through knockouts of the *luxS* system, which produces universal quorum sensing molecule autoinducer-2 (AI-2), and discovered that these mutants could no longer form dense biofilms with *C. albicans* (103). These results suggest that cross-talk between *Candida* and *S. gordonii* could be vital for promoting biofilm formation in the oral cavity and on oral appliances and that *Candida* species may be a bridge from a healthy microbiome to a pathogenic microbiome.

Candida adhesins ALS proteins have also been found to mediate interactions with streptococci during many steps in polymicrobial biofilm formation. Silverman and colleagues demonstrated that Als3 in *C. albicans* was required to form and sustain biofilms on a salivary pellicle (initial stage of attachment to tooth surfaces) when *S. gordonii* was present. To further support their conclusions, the authors used genetic alterations of *Saccharomyces cerevisiae*, yeast that cannot attach to *S. gordonii*, to express Als3p on the surface of *S. cerevisiae* and established yeast–bacteria adherence (36). However, several

ALS proteins have similarities in structure, and it is not illogical for multiple ALS proteins to take part in these interactions. Hoyer and others reported that Als1 was also bound with *S. gordonii* during interkingdom interactions using NT-Als crystal structures to visualize the adhesion of Als1p to SspB on *S. gordonii* (104). Meanwhile, Dutton and colleagues have demonstrated that *O*-mannosylation of the *C. albicans* cell wall is required for hyphae to bind with *S. gordonii* (105). However, Hoyer and others noticed that even though the ALS protein of *C. albicans* bound open C-termini of respective ligands, in the case of *S. gordonii* SspB, the C-terminus is bound to peptidoglycans and obscured, suggesting that there must be some type of editing to free the SspB ligand (104).

S. mutans, the principle bacteria found in human caries, is another member of the viridans streptococci group that can interact directly with *C. albicans* and may exchange secretory products with the fungus. Jarosz and others examined the effects of spent media from *S. mutans* and a mutated strain of *S. mutans* that lacked the comC gene, encoding for both competence and a quorum sensing molecule, CSP. When these media were placed on *C. albicans*, only the wild-type *S. mutans*–derived media could inhibit hyphae formation; this was further supported by the use of synthetic CSP in a dose-dependent fashion also preventing hyphal formation and forcing reversion to yeast forms (106). Vilchez and colleagues continued exploration into components secreted by *S. mutans* and observed that one small molecule could inhibit the AI-2 quorum sensing. They pursued this further with nuclear magnetic resonance spectrometry to determine that the molecule was trans-2-decenoic acid and that when placed on *C. albicans*, it prevented hyphal formation but did not stunt growth overall. A possible mechanism of action for trans-2-decenoic acid is altering surface protein expression, because Hwp1 expression on *C. albicans* was terminated in the presence of the compound. This secreted molecule has a similar structure to molecules of the diffusible signal factor family, previously seen in *Burkholderia* species, and was also determined to be secreted from other cariogenic bacteria, such as *S. sanguinis* (107). These findings demonstrate that oral streptococcus species and *C. albicans* can interact with each other but may limit each other, perhaps in the attempt to secure nutrients or other materials in the oral cavity.

Examination of young children with dental caries has shown that *Candida* species are found at a higher prevalence in caries-positive children than in caries-free children, with most children carrying *C. albicans* (108). Dental plaque collected from children with early childhood caries (where caries can be seen in those as young as six months) was found to have a positive association with *C. albicans* and *S. mutans*, whereas plaque from an older group of children with caries only had a positive association with *S. mutans* (109). These clinical findings promote the concept that *C. albicans* and *S. mutans* together may facilitate survival in the cariogenic environment; *in vitro* examination of these dual-species biofilms showed that even though extrapolysaccharide matrix (EPS) production was reduced in *S. mutans*, induction of quorum sensing systems in the bacteria increased production of mutacin, a broad-spectrum bacteriocin (110). Since the *S. mutans* quorum sensing system also controls competence, induction by *C. albicans* may enable the bacteria to acquire new genetic information quickly, which may alter cariogenicity and the landscape of the oral microbiome.

Previously, Gregoire and colleagues demonstrated that *S. mutans* preferred to bind to *C. albicans* cells that had glucans on their surfaces and that these reactions involved glucosyltransferases produced by *S. mutans*. Utilizing a micropipette technique to visualize individual adhesion events, the authors saw that beads coated with saliva adhered better to glucan-coated *C. albicans*. When *S. mutans* was added to the mixture, there was a significant increase in bacteria bound to saliva-coated structures with glucan-positive *C. albicans* (111). This study suggested that the glucosyltransferases from *S. mutans* can help to increase a glucan and fructan matrix on the tooth surface, promoting caries. While this appears to be contradicted by Sztajer and others, who reported a decrease of EPS production by *S. mutans*, it may be that in the earlier stages (as noted by Gregoire and others) a more intense matrix is produced, which decreases over time as *C. albicans* takes up more sucrose, and forces *S. mutans* to induce its quorum sensing machinery (110, 111). When these findings are taken together, it is obvious that the interaction between *Candida* and streptococci is more complex than just synergistic, but with their interaction positively associated with early childhood caries, it can be concluded that treatments for this disease must include a multikingdom approach to be successful.

Candida–Porphyromonas gingivalis

Candida species have been isolated from periodontal lesions; however, the association of *Candida* species with periodontal disease has not been solidified—only speculated. Periodontal disease affects the gingival tissue and tooth attachment/anchoring in the alveolar bone of the mouth. These diseases can range from mild gingival inflammation (gingivitis) to chronic gingival inflammation and alveolar bone loss (periodontitis) (112). It was shown that subgingival colonization of *C. albicans* was associated with the severity of chronic periodontitis and was the only yeast species to be present in all yeast-positive cases (113).

P. gingivalis is well known for its role in chronic periodontitis, with a variety of virulence factors such as LPS, gingipains, and fimbriae along with the ability to form biofilms (114). Unfortunately, interactions between *Candida* species and *P. gingivalis* have not been thoroughly assessed. Pretreatment of human gingival epithelial cells and human gingival fibroblasts with heat-killed *C. albicans* or mannoprotein-b-glucan complex (a major cell wall and biofilm matrix component of the fungus) derived from *C. albicans*

enhanced *P. gingivalis* invasion of the cells. However, this enhancement was not through adhesion or upregulation of typical adhesive molecules, such as ICAM-1. These results suggest that *C. albicans* exacerbates periodontal disease by providing assistance to *P. gingivalis* invasion of epithelial cells, possibly by serving as a scaffold to allow the bacterium time to invade (115). In the presence of some evidence of symbiotic interactions between *Candida* and *P. gingivalis*, it is important to further explore the molecular mechanisms involved to determine better treatment methods for periodontal disease.

Candida–Aggregatibacter actinomycetemcomitans

Localized juvenile/aggressive periodontitis is an acute form of periodontal disease associated with anaerobic bacteria in the oral cavity, resulting in bone loss and periodontal ligament destruction around specific clusters of teeth. *A. actinomycetemcomitans* has been identified as a causative agent of localized juvenile/aggressive periodontitis (116). This organism produces a variety of virulence factors such as leukotoxin, cytolethal distending toxin, Fc-binding factors, and proteases (117). It was shown that in dual-species biofilms, *A. actinomycetemcomitans* adhered to *C. albicans* and inhibited biofilm formation via the general quorum sensing molecule AI-2, synthesized by the *luxS* gene (118). This molecule can be used to communicate between both Gram-positive and Gram-negative bacteria, and Bachtiar and colleagues demonstrated that synthetic AI-2 could also inhibit *C. albicans* biofilm formation, providing a possible treatment option by modulating the oral flora through quorum sensing. Periodontitis is linked with several systemic conditions, particularly diabetes mellitus, and patients with both diseases have been shown to harbor various *Candida* species, strikingly *C. albicans* (119). Determining how periodontal bacteria and *Candida* species interact within the gingival pocket will be vital to developing more effective oral health biomaterials.

Candida–Acinetobacter baumannii

A. baumannii, a Gram-negative bacterium, has emerged as one of the most troublesome pathogens for health care institutions globally. The ability of *A. baumannii* to adhere to and persist on surfaces in a biofilm, particularly on medical devices, has made the bacterium a concern in hospitals and war zones. *A. baumannii* is emerging as a pertinent opportunistic human pathogen and is part of the ESKAPE pathogens due to its development of multidrug resistance along with the biofilm-forming capability, earning it the term "superbug" (120). Given that *C. albicans* and *A. baumannii* are common etiological agents of nosocomial infections in the immunocompromised and that they overlap niches in the oral cavity, it is vital to understand any interactions between these organisms. It was demonstrated that outer membrane protein A (OmpA) of *A. baumannii*19606, a standard lab strain, was essential for bacterial attachment to *C. albicans* filaments through knockout and complement experiments (121). OmpA was also shown to be important for attachment and invasion of epithelial cells; since *C. albicans* binds to N-cadherins on epithelial cells through its protein Als3, it is possible that OmpA may bind to Als3 on *C. albicans* (122). This interaction between bacteria and fungus resulted in fungal death, visualized with fluorescent microscopy and only when *A. baumannii* was in direct contact with *C. albicans* filaments through a functional OmpA protein (121). These findings show antagonism between these two opportunists; determination of the mechanism of fungal killing by *A. baumannii* deserves further exploration to minimize serious infections in the immunocompromised population.

Interactions in the Gastrointestinal Tract

Candida–E. faecalis

The Gram-positive bacterium *E. faecalis* and *C. albicans* often coinhabit the human large intestine and the oral cavity, with *E. faecalis*

consistently isolated after failing endodontic (root canal) treatments (123, 124). Unfortunately, to date, the interactions between *C. albicans* and enterococci have not been thoroughly examined. Several studies showed that the relationship between *E. faecalis* and *C. albicans* in polymicrobial biofilms is antagonistic. In a *Caenorhabditis elegans* model of a coinfection with *E. faecalis* and *C. albicans*, *E. faecalis* inhibited *C. albicans* hyphal formation and protected *C. elegans* from being killed by *C. albicans*. Interestingly, the presence of *C. albicans* reduced *E. faecalis* cell death. These results correspond with findings *in vitro*, where *E. faecalis* inhibits *Candida* hyphal formation in a dual-species biofilm. The inhibition of *Candida* hyphal morphogenesis by *E. faecalis* was caused by a secreted heat-stable protein of approximately 10 kDa and was partially dependent on the Fsr quorum-sensing system, which regulates virulence in *E. faecalis* (125). Shekh and Roy identified an *E. faecalis* strain that produces an anti-Candida protein (APC), an anti-mycotic protein that was nonhemolytic and different from the one Cruz and colleagues discovered (126). Heat-killed *E. faecalis* prevented *C. albicans* from adhering to plastic substrates, and in a murine oral infection model, heat-killed *E. faecalis* protected against oral candidiasis, showing that direct cell contact between the two species plays an important role in cross-kingdom interactions (127). These findings indicate a role for quorum sensing molecules and other proteins produced by both *C. albicans* and *E. faecalis* in the interaction between these two organisms. These molecules may be promising in the quest to find new therapeutic strategies in the battle against antimicrobial drug resistance, and additional research may further elucidate the role of these molecules and their mechanism of action.

Candida–Escherichia coli

E. coli remains one of the most important organisms found in the gastrointestinal tract, and different virotypes of *E. coli* are responsible for causing a variety of infections, including diarrhea, respiratory tract infections, wound infections, and septicemia. *E. coli* and *C. albicans* are often found together in human tissues and body fluids (128). Polymicrobial intra-abdominal infections involving fungi result in higher mortality rates (up to 75%) compared to bacterial polymicrobial infections (up to 30%), and *Candida* species are the most commonly found fungi in these infections (129–132). In an experimental murine model of peritonitis, *C. albicans* showed synergism with *E coli*. In this model, co-infection with both *C. albicans* and *E. coli* resulted in higher mortality in mice compared to a single-species infection (133). This *Candida*-associated mortality of experimental animals was augmented by *E. coli* and its LPS (134). Bandara and colleagues evaluated the effect of *E. coli* LPS on different *Candida* species biofilms *in vitro* and found that *E. coli* LPS caused a significant reduction in the growth of *C. tropicalis*, *Candida parapsilosis*, *C. krusei*, and *C. dubliniensis* (135). In addition, *E. coli* secretory elements significantly impair *Candida* biofilm development, possibly by modulating hyphal-specific genes and their transcriptional regulation (136). Interestingly, when *Candida–E. coli* biofilms were treated with the fluoroquinolone antibiotic ofloxacin, the β-1, 3-glucan produced by *C. albicans* increased *E. coli* tolerance of ofloxacin (137).

These findings suggest that the interaction between *Candida* and *E. coli* is synergistic. Since they are commonly isolated from infection sites and seem to increase mortality and tolerance to antibacterial agents, they can cause serious problems in immunocompromised individuals. More research on the interaction between these two species is needed, and targeting β-1, 3-glucan production by *C. albicans* is currently used in the clinic through the echinocandin class of antifungals. These drugs may be useful in combination therapy with other antimicrobial agents, because there is still little fungal resistance to echinocandins (138).

Candida–Salmonella species

Salmonella species can survive intracellularly within epithelial cells, dendritic cells, and macrophages, causing chronic inflammation. The bacterium is well known for its ability to cause gastrointestinal pathology, ranging from asymptomatic carriage to gastroenteritis and typhoid fever (139). Since *Candida* appears as a commensal in the gastrointestinal tract, the overlap of niches provides an excellent point for interaction between species. In a *C. elegans* polymicrobial infection model, *Salmonella enterica* serovar Typhimurium inhibited *C. albicans* filamentation, stunting fungal virulence. Moreover, an *in vitro* co-culture model showed that *S.* Typhimurium inhibits *C. albicans* viability and its ability to form a biofilm (140). The type III secretion systems are important virulence factors for *Salmonella* pathogenesis and are encoded by *Salmonella* pathogenicity island 1 (SPI-1) and SPI-2 on the bacterial chromosome (141). The type III secretion system allows the bacterium to inject effector proteins directly into the host cell (141, 142). There are more than 30 known SPI-1- and SPI-2-regulated effectors in *Salmonella* species that utilize these systems (143). One of these effectors, sopB, plays a critical role in interaction and competition with *C. albicans* by killing filaments. Deletion of *sopB* significantly increased the survival of *C. albicans in vitro*. The sopB effector translocates into filaments via SipB, killing *C. albicans* hyphae. In *C. elegans*, *S.* Typhimurium sopB decreased the viability of *C. albicans* filaments and repressed elongation of filaments, germ tubes, and biofilm formation during infection. Remarkably, researchers found that the sopB effector is associated with the transcriptional repression of CDC42 in *C. albicans* (which encodes a Rho-type GTPase related to viability) and suggested that the sopB effector of *S.* Typhimurium is important for competing against fungi (144).

Considering these findings, it is reasonable to conclude that interaction between *S.* Typhimurium and *C. albicans* is multifactorial and that the viability of *C. albicans* is associated with the *S.* Typhimurium sopB and sipB type III secretion system translocation machinery. However, only limited research has been done on the interaction of *C. albicans* with intestinal bacterial pathogens. The human intestinal tract has a remarkable microbial community, including *Candida*. Understanding the interactions between the diverse organisms within the complex milieu of the intestinal tract may expose important pathogenic and therapeutic insights.

Candida–Helicobacter pylori

H. pylori has been found to colonize the human gastrointestinal tract and is responsible for many conditions, ranging from gastritis and peptic ulcers to adenocarcinoma (145). In terms of association to *Candida*, *Helicobacter* has shown unique interactions with the fungus as illustrated by a handful of reports. *H. pylori* DNA was found within *Candida* yeasts isolated from cheek swabs of dyspeptic Iranian patients, a location that has an endemic *H. pylori* presence (146). This is an important finding in the cohabitation of these two pathogens, with reference to treatment, prevention, and the control of cross-transmission.

Analysis of the relationship between *H. pylori* and *Candida* using specimens obtained from patients with specific upper gastrointestinal tract disorders suggested a positive relationship of *Helicobacter* with *Candida*, which may help maintain the persistence of *H. pylori* in the oral cavity, possibly favoring reinoculation of the stomach with the bacterium and allowing the bacterium to exist in these endemic regions. Analysis of samples taken from patients with severe gastric ulcerations confirmed coinhabitation of *Candida* and *Helicobacter* in human disease conditions (147).

The intracellular existence of *Helicobacter* within *Candida* yeast cells was investigated by several groups in an attempt to explore the underlying mechanisms of this interaction. Fluorescent microscopy showed that labeled *H. pylori* survives as viable, fast-moving bodies inside the vacuoles of *Candida* yeast cells obtained from multiple niches (148–150). It has been suggested that the yeast vacuoles serve as a niche that protects *H. pylori* against environmental stresses while nourishing the bacteria and providing it with sterols such as ergosterol (150). *H. pylori* seems to be vertically transmitted to the daughter cells of *C. albicans* and continues to express its own proteins to survive safely within the yeast cells (148, 149). The bacteria inside yeast cells produce peroxiredoxin and thiol peroxidase, substances which can counteract the respiratory bursts of most phagocytic immune cells. In addition, urease and VacA, two virulence factors of *H. pylori*, are produced when *H. pylori* is taken into *C. albicans* and are capable of modulating the host innate immune response to promote bacterial survival (150). These virulence mechanisms may thus play a crucial role in intracellular survival of *H. pylori* in both epithelial cells and yeast cells. Human gastric epithelial cells and human immune cells have been recognized as the only eukaryotic cells that host *H. pylori*. *H. pylori* might use this intracellular establishment within the yeast cells as a "Trojan horse" mechanism to invade and persist inside human epithelial and immune cells. This could be a crucial step in the colonization of the human gastrointestinal tract, as well as persistence in a variety of environmental conditions, being masked from the host immune defenses.

Interactions in the Vulvovagina

Candida–Lactobacillus species

Lactobacillus species are known for their probiotic effects and are widely known to negate the colonization of pathogens in the gastrointestinal tract and the female genitourinary tract (151). In the female genital tract, lactobacilli function as a barrier against infection with other pathogens by competing for adherence and producing several antimicrobial compounds, such as H_2O_2 and lactic acid. These compounds lower the vaginal pH to an inhospitable level for many microbial species

(152–156). Lactobacilli isolated from the oral cavity were shown to inhibit the growth of *C. albicans* through the production of H_2O_2 (157). Lactobacilli vaginal isolates also inhibited the growth of *C. albicans*, but this effect was only partially attributed to the production of peroxides (158). It was shown that supernatants obtained from cultures of four *Lactobacillus* species (*Lactobacillus rhamnosus*, *Lactobacillus acidophilus*, *Lactobacillus plantarum*, and *Lactobacillus reuteri*) impaired hyphal and biofilm formation of *Candida* (159). Taken together, these data show an inhibiting effect of lactobacilli on *Candida* growth, hyphal formation, and biofilm production.

Kohler and others showed that the growth of *Candida* was suppressed by lactic acid (produced by lactobacilli), and using fluorescent microscopy, they showed a loss in metabolic activity and cell viability. Moreover, when kept under coculture conditions, *C. albicans* showed an increase in expression of stress-related genes (e.g., SIS1, TPS3, HSP78, TPO3, SEO1), indicating that the cells were in hostile environments, most likely through the lower pH created by lactobacilli acid production (160). Interestingly, Wagner and Johnson showed that *Candida* activated the NF-κB pathway–associated genes Iκκα and ELK1 upon infection of VK2/E6E7 vaginal epithelial cells. Lactobacilli suppressed this expression of NF-κB-related inflammatory genes and induced IL-1α and IL-1β expression via alternative signal transduction pathways, such as mitogen-activated protein kinase/AP-1. Activation of such alternative signaling mechanisms by lactobacilli may provide a mechanism to decrease the inflammatory damage caused by vulvovaginal candidiasis and demonstrates the importance of IL-1β to stimulate anti-*Candida* defenses in the innate immune system (161). *Lactobacillus crispatus*, a common species found in the female genital tract, inhibited growth and adhesion of *C. albicans* to HeLa cells. Toll-like receptors (TLR)-2 and -4 expressed by HeLa cells are modulated by both *L. crispatus*

and *C. albicans*, and the production of IL-8 and human beta defensin (HBD)2/3 by both species is modulated via the TLR2/4 pathway. Given that *L. crispatus* inhibited *C. albicans* growth and adhesion to epithelial cells, this pathway could be a promising target in antifungal treatment (162).

Two other lactobacilli strains found in healthy vaginal microflora, *L. reuteri* RC-14 and *L. rhamnosus* GR-1, were found to inhibit *C. albicans* growth and attenuated virulence in vaginal cell cultures (163). In addition, Martinez and colleagues demonstrated that use of probiotic lactobacilli and antifungal drug combinations were more effective in controlling the *C. albicans* growth in vaginal candidiasis than antifungal agents alone (164). Chew and others expanded these findings, showing that inhibition of *C. glabrata* growth by *L. rhamnosus* GR-1 and *L. reuteri* RC-1 strains leads to cell death, an important observation due to an increase in non–*C. albicans* infections in some populations (165). Romani and colleagues described that some bacteria can support host-fungal symbiosis (166). Commensal lactobacilli and mammals together increase immune tolerance in response to *C. albicans* through the tryptophan catabolic pathway production of indoleamine 2,3-dioxygenase 1, which drives resources away from inflammatory T-cell lineages and promotes a T-regulatory state. Given the commensal cohabitation by these microorganisms in humans and the frequency of vulvovaginal candidiasis among women worldwide, it is important to ascertain the inhibitory mechanisms of *Lactobacillus* on *Candida* so that its probiotic nature can be fine-tuned to work with the host and prevent recurring infections.

DIAGNOSTICS FOR *CANDIDA*-ASSOCIATED POLYMICROBIAL INFECTIONS

History and examination are the cornerstones of the diagnosis of infections, irrespective of their mono- or polymicrobial etiology. Evidence of contamination, presence of a foreign body, use of a prosthetic or iatrogenic instrument often can be ruled out by the clinical history that can be easily gathered from the patient. Further, the signs of inflammation and infection may be elucidated by a systematic clinical examination. In addition, the general assessment of the patient for hygiene and health is also important in the assessment of the degree of contamination and the level of the host's immune competence, respectively. In case of the patient using prosthetic appliance therapy, the nature and quality of the prosthesis and its use should also be assessed and monitored.

Following the history and examination, various investigations including microbiological methods play a role in the diagnostic process. Conventional microbiological cultures using Sabourauds dextrose agar have been useful in isolating *Candida* from clinical samples. However, investigations using bacteria–fungi coculture both in blood cultures and animal models showed that usual microbiological techniques, including Gram stain and culture on solid media, were inadequate to detect fungemia when concomitant bacteremia was present (167). These investigators have suggested that the likely mechanisms for this fungal growth suppression included nutritional depletion and elaboration of a toxic substance by the bacteria. Consequently, the reported incidence of blood cultures with synchronous bacteremia and candidemia may underestimate the definite incidence. One possible alternative is to perform an additional and simultaneous culture using chrome-agar *Candida* medium that prevents bacterial growth and is an excellent growth platform for identification of most commonly encountered *Candida* species (168). In addition, the advances in molecular microbiology technology using PCR improved the rate of detection of *Candida* in blood cultures and has demonstrated *Candida* in the blood of patients with culture-

negative results, confirming the lack of sensitivity of blood culture in disseminated candidiasis (169). Several other factors have been suggested to avert the synchronous isolation of *Candida* and bacteria in blood cultures. One of the reasons for difficulty in isolating *Candida* in blood culture is rapid bacterial proliferation that often inhibits the fungal proliferation (167). This phenomenon, if occurring in actual patient specimens, would lead to a reduction in numbers of blood cultures isolating *Candida* species. On the other hand, early commencement of antibacterial drugs immediately upon detection of fever in patients would lead to a reduced incidence of synchronous bacteremia and candidemia because of the presence of bactericidal antibiotics in the blood.

In the context of polymicrobial infections often related to biofilms, novel methods with the potential to identify and quantify each individual member of the polymicrobial community have the utmost importance. In particular, molecular biological methods have demonstrated the ability to precisely define the identity and the quantity of each species of a polymicrobial biofilm infection. For example, advanced techniques including metagenomic analyses are helpful to describe polymicrobial ecosystems (170). Flow cells are used to study microbial interactions in biofilms (171). Recently, microbiome-level analyses involving either conserved, phylogenetically informative genes such as bacterial 16S rRNA gene or whole shotgun metagenomic sequencing have provided promising results. Comprehensive, quantitative molecular diagnostic methods are the most efficient and effective ways to appropriately identify and characterize the complex bacterial and fungal components of such polymicrobial infections (172). Although various high-tech diagnostic methods have been suggested such as metagenomics analyses and flow cells, they have yet to reach clinical diagnostic laboratories in many parts of the world.

MANAGING *CANDIDA*–BACTERIA POLYMICROBIAL INFECTIONS

Importance of Recognizing the Potential for Polymicrobial Infection

In cases of bacterial or fungal infection, it is important to recognize that the infection may not be only bacterial or only fungal since standard diagnostic modalities (see above) for polymicrobial infections can often miss major players in the infectious milieu. Considering a polymicrobial infection in the differential diagnosis is important for three reasons: (i) designing appropriate chemotherapy, (ii) taking into account systemic bacterial infections due to *Candida* infections, and (iii) recognizing the importance of infectious synergy on patient morbidity and mortality.

Designing appropriate chemotherapy

When *Candida* is missed during diagnosis, and a polymicrobial infection is treated as a bacterial infection, treatment and cure will not be obtained. A clinical assumption of a mono-species or mono-kingdom infection ignores the potential for a polymicrobial infection that necessarily impacts the disease management (i.e., antibiotic +/- antifungal administration). Therefore, patients often undergo an unnecessary infection cycle during which antibiotics are first used, followed by a fungal infection. Antibiotic therapy is halted and replaced by antifungal therapy, allowing the pathogenic bacterial species that was not eliminated by the abbreviated antibiotic regimen to become a fulminant infection again. Chasing this moving target of antimicrobially based infection resolution only increases the risk of patient morbidity and mortality as well as the development of antimicrobial-resistant strains. Therefore, once a *Candida* or fungal infection is found following an initial bacterial infection diagnosis and initiation of antibiotic therapy, the initial broad-spectrum or antibiotic sensitivity-directed antibiotic therapy should be continued to avoid the return and exacerbation of the original

bacterial infection as well as the acquisition of multidrug-resistant bacteria such as vancomycin-resistant enterococci (173).

Since a contribution of *Candida* is often missed during diagnosis by standard culture, advanced techniques (e.g., PCR, IBIS, or differential/selective media) should be used, or if not present, can be considered during the differential diagnosis by noting particular risk factors for invasive candidiasis. Invasive candidiasis that can predispose patients to the potential for polymicrobial infection can be considered when patients demonstrate certain risk factors. Besides maintaining a good diet and avoiding social risk factors (obesity, smoking, alcohol/drug abuse), there are a number of other risk factors associated with developing invasive candidiasis. Some of these include broad-spectrum antibiotic usage, immunosuppression due to disease (e.g., Job's disease, AIDS following uncontrolled HIV infection, etc.), administration of immunosuppressive agents (e.g., chemotherapy, steroids, or antirejection agents following organ transplant), some indwelling medical devices (e.g., endotracheal tubes, urinary catheters, intravenous catheters, and parenteral nutrition), diabetes and diabetic foot wounds, and extremes of age. These risk factors can result in failure of the host to keep *Candida* in check, an imbalance between commensal bacteria and fungi, or invasion of particular host niches by opportunistic bacterial and fungal pathogens (8).

Taking into account systemic bacterial infections due to *Candida* infections

Systemic bacterial infections and complications may result from localized invasive candidiasis or even superficial infections by this fungal pathogen (32, 101). Patient morbidity and mortality may increase due to systemic infections that result from the ability of *Candida* to deliver other microbial species into deep tissue layers or the circulatory system of the host. Therefore, systemic complications such as bacterial infections due to candidiasis should be considered and may require more empirical antibacterial coverage (174). As such, when selecting antibiotics it is important to consider the sensitivity, bioavailability, toxicity, degree of resistance formation, and stability (175). It has been demonstrated that *Candida* facilitated the invasion of bacteria into host tissues. The findings in the above studies demonstrate that superficial candidiasis may constitute a risk factor for disseminated bacterial disease, warranting awareness of therapeutic management of immunocompromised individuals. The identification of superficial candidiasis as a risk factor for disseminated bacterial disease has serious clinical implications. For instance, it is very important to improve awareness in terms of therapeutic management, particularly in immunocompromised individuals, who often experience recurrent episodes of superficial candidiasis affecting oral and vaginal mucosae, to avoid disseminated bacterial infections.

Impact of microbial infectious synergy on patient morbidity and mortality

Coinfection by *C. albicans* and microbial species may produce a synergistic infection due to the interaction of the host, *Candida*, and the bacterial species, thereby dramatically increasing the severity and unpredictability of the infection (9, 45, 174, 176). Therefore, coinfections should be taken extremely seriously. Characterizing the nature of the complex interaction between *Candida* and bacteria may be the first step in understanding the nature of their coexistence in the host. Unraveling the mechanisms that *Candida* and bacteria use in a competitive, polymicrobial environment would not only deepen our understanding of their coinhabitation but may also provide important insights into novel pathways that help the development of new antimicrobial drugs.

Control of Biofilm Formation

Since the interaction between *Candida* species and bacteria often occurs in a biofilm mode of growth, it is important to describe biofilm resolution strategies. Microbes can produce biofilms on synthetic materials or devitalized tissue that results in the failure of antimicrobial agents and the host immune response to resolve these infections. Management of biofilm-related polymicrobial infections, particularly those involving *Candida*, can be challenging. Removal of the infected device is generally needed to establish cure of *Candida* infections of medical devices. The mainstay for the resolution of biofilm-associated infections continues to be the removal of the nidus of infection (e.g., indwelling medical device, devitalized tissue, periodontal scaling, and/or debridement) (14, 177–188). There are a number of other biofilm resolution strategies: small molecules that interfere with either bacterial and fungal quorum sensing systems, signaling pathways that control biofilm formation and maintenance, or unique nutrient requirements by biofilm microorganisms to maintain localized pH and redox conditions. Also, macromolecular approaches to biofilm eradication have been proposed that include matrix-digesting enzymes and the development of biofilm-specific antibodies. Some examples that that have been proposed include promoting programmed detachment, mechanical disruption, dispersal agents, DNAse, nanoparticles (modified silver and gold), lyase, lactonase, alpha-amylases, lysostaphin (for staphylococcal strains), photodynamic therapy (see references 189 and 190 for a review of some of these strategies), and antibody-directed photoacoustic killing (191).

Probiotics and prebiotics may have a role in preventing or even treating polymicrobial infections. Live microorganisms when administered in proper concentrations that have health benefits are known as probiotics. There are sets of particular bacterial species that are found in different body niches and are able to control *Candida* through their probiotic action (192). Probiotics are able to control various infections by exploiting the microbial interference as a mechanism for novel prophylactic or therapeutic management of polymicrobial diseases. Prebiotics, defined as an oligosaccharide indigestible by humans but able to be fermented by beneficial gut bacteria such as *Lactobacillus* and *Bifidobacterium* species, may also play a role. By combining a probiotic and a prebiotic (called a synbiotic [193]), microbial mucosal health can be dramatically improved. It is evident that bacteria such as *Lactobacillus* species have the potential to control yeast colonization in various body niches and therefore could be used in the management of *Candida* infections.

Phage therapy could also be used to control these polymicrobial infections. Phages are viruses that act against bacteria and that demonstrate a particular tropism for specific species. These phages infect and lyse bacterial populations by undergoing rounds of phage replication, thereby reducing bacterial populations. While bactericidal activity was once thought to primarily be a consequence of lytic events, it has been shown that phage particles encode depolymerases that exhibit enzymatic activity against bacterial matrices, including exopolymeric compounds. However, phage therapy has not entered phase III clinical trials or showed effective biofilm infection therapy *in vivo* against multiple microbial strains, even with decades of research attempts.

Polymicrobial vaccines may also play a role in the future control of polymicrobial infections. Now that we are aware that chronic and polymicrobial infections involve *Candida* and bacterial biofilms, investigators can develop appropriate vaccines that prevent these coinfections. When *Candida* or bacteria invade the host they can either be removed by the host innate immune response or get attached to the host extracellular matrix proteins to develop a localized biofilm community. The resulting proteome of the microorganisms becomes distinct once the population transforms into a biofilm phenotype and deviates remarkably from the characteristics of the planktonic proteome.

According to Harro et al. (194), two components of the biofilm, i.e., bacterial cells within the biofilm and the biofilm matrix, although they vary between bacterial genera, species, and strains, could be considered as targets for vaccine development if common antigens are found. Moreover, to prevent polymicrobial infection, a vaccine composed of a multivalent cocktail of antigenic proteins from all microorganisms involved in disease pathology may have to be considered.

Once combined with conventional antibiotics to battle the microbial cells existing in the planktonic state, nonsurgical biofilm eradication may finally be realized. However, many of these antibiofilm strategies are in early *in vitro*, animal, or topical development and are not approved for use for invasive disease. Therefore, infections caused by *Candida*–bacteria interactions have significant complexity and are still in the infancy stages in vaccine development. Vaccine design for *Candida*–bacteria polymicrobial infections should consider the unique virulence attributes of the yeast and the bacteria in question to achieve success.

SUMMARY, CONCLUSIONS, AND FUTURE DIRECTIONS

Candida can exist in a polymicrobial biofilm mode of growth attached to biotic and abiotic surfaces. Some microbes have evolved mutualistic or even synergistic relationships to facilitate cohabitation on epithelial surfaces and deep wounds, while others have developed competitive antagonistic approaches during cocolonization. Biofilm formation occurs within a complex milieu of host factors and other members of the human microbiota. Thus, bacteria can attenuate or enhance fungal invasion and virulence in *C. albicans* mucosal biofilms, not to mention the candidal effect of augmentation or abrogation of virulence on bacteria.

Complex *Candida*–bacteria interactions are not a rare occurrence; they do exist, interact, and coaggregate with common bacteria (both commensals and frank pathogens), and this interaction has great clinical significance. The effects of such interactions are relevant to the host, the microbe, and the environment. Elucidating the nature of these interactions at the proteomic, genetic, transcriptomic, metabolomics, and systems levels is imperative in the understanding, prevention, and management of polymicrobial infections. It is likely that interaction between host, *Candida*, and commensal microbiota dictates the types of host–fungus relationship, and the microbial dysbiosis may predispose to a variety of chronic fungal infections and diseases at local and distant sites. The elucidation of these complex interactions is important not only for a better understanding of the pathobiology of infections and microbial interactions but also for the identification of novel targets for future antimicrobial strategies as the age of antibiotics begins to wane.

ACKNOWLEDGMENTS

This work was funded by National Institutes of Health, NIDCR grant DE025679.

CITATION

Allison DL, Willems HM, Jayatilake JAMS, Bruno VM, Peters BM, Shirtliff ME. 2016. Candida–bacteria interactions: their impact on human disease. Microbiol Spectrum 4(3): VMBF-0030-2016.

REFERENCES

1. **Abu-Elteen K, Hamad M.** 2012. Changing epidemiology of classical and emerging human fungal infections: a review. *Jordan J Biol Sci* **5:**215–230.
2. **Pfaller MA, Diekema DJ.** 2007. Epidemiology of invasive candidiasis: a persistent public health problem. *Clin Microbiol Rev* **20:**133–163.
3. **Budtz-Jorgensen E.** 2000. Ecology of *Candida*-associated denture stomatitis. *Microb Ecol Health Dis* **12:**170–185.
4. **Gendreau L, Loewy ZG.** 2011. Epidemiology and etiology of denture stomatitis. *J Prosthodont* **20:**251–260.
5. **Achkar JM, Fries BC.** 2010. *Candida* infections of the genitourinary tract. *Clin Microbiol Rev* **23:**253–273.
6. **Calderone RA, Fonzi WA.** 2001. Virulence factors of *Candida albicans*. *Trends Microbiol* **9:**327–335.
7. **Conti HR, Shen F, Nayyar N, Stocum E, Sun JN, Lindemann MJ, Ho AW, Hai JH, Yu JJ, Jung JW, Filler SG, Masso-Welch P, Edgerton M, Gaffen SL.** 2009. Th17 cells and IL-17 receptor signaling are essential for mucosal host defense against oral candidiasis. *J Exp Med* **206:**299–311.
8. **Peleg AY, Hogan DA, Mylonakis E.** 2010. Medically important bacterial-fungal interactions. *Nat Rev Microbiol* **8:**340–349.
9. **Klotz SA, Chasin BS, Powell B, Gaur NK, Lipke PN.** 2007. Polymicrobial bloodstream infections involving *Candida* species: analysis of patients and review of the literature. *Diagn Microbiol Infect Dis* **59:**401–406.
10. **Baena-Monroy T, Moreno-Maldonado V, Franco-Martinez F, Aldape-Barrios B, Quindos G, Sanchez-Vargas LO.** 2005. *Candida albicans*, *Staphylococcus aureus* and *Streptococcus mutans* colonization in patients wearing dental prosthesis. *Med Oral Patol Oral Cir Bucal* **10**(Suppl 1): E27–E39.
11. **Sousa C, Botelho C, Rodrigues D, Azeredo J, Oliveira R.** 2012. Infective endocarditis in intravenous drug abusers: an update. *Eur J Clin Microbiol Infect Dis* **31:**2905–2910.
12. **Pammi M, Zhong D, Johnson Y, Revell P, Versalovic J.** 2014. Polymicrobial bloodstream infections in the neonatal intensive care unit are associated with increased mortality: a case-control study. *BMC Infect Dis* **14:**390.
13. **Douglas LJ.** 2003. *Candida* biofilms and their role in infection. *Trends Microbiol* **11:**30–36.
14. **Shirtliff ME, Mader JT, Camper AK.** 2002. Molecular interactions in biofilms. *Chem Biol* **9:**859–871.
15. **Donlan RM, Costerton JW.** 2002/4. Biofilms: survival mechanisms of clinically relevant microorganisms. *Clin Microbiol Rev* **15:**167–193.
16. **Mah TF, O'Toole GA.** 2001. Mechanisms of biofilm resistance to antimicrobial agents. *Trends Microbiol* **9:**34–39.
17. **Peters BM, Jabra-Rizk MA, O'May GA, Costerton JW, Shirtliff ME.** 2012. Polymicrobial interactions: impact on pathogenesis and human disease. *Clin Microbiol Rev* **25:**193–213.

18. **Wolcott R, Costerton JW, Raoult D, Cutler SJ.** 2013. The polymicrobial nature of biofilm infection. *Clin Microbiol Infect* **19:**107–112.

19. **Diaz PI, Strausbaugh LD, Dongari-Bagtzoglou A.** 2014. Fungal-bacterial interactions and their relevance to oral health: linking the clinic and the bench. *Front Cell Infect Microbiol* **4:**101.

20. **Dutton LC, Paszkiewicz KH, Silverman RJ, Splatt PR, Shaw S, Nobbs AH, Lamont RJ, Jenkinson HF, Ramsdale M.** 2016. Transcriptional landscape of trans-kingdom communication between *Candida albicans* and *Streptococcus gordonii*. *Mol Oral Microbiol* **31:**136–161.

21. **Pammi M, Liang R, Hicks J, Mistretta TA, Versalovic J.** 2013. Biofilm extracellular DNA enhances mixed species biofilms of *Staphylococcus epidermidis* and *Candida albicans*. *BMC Microbiol* **13:**257.

22. **Garcia-Sanchez S, Aubert S, Iraqui I, Janbon G, Ghigo JM, d'Enfert C.** 2004. *Candida albicans* biofilms: a developmental state associated with specific and stable gene expression patterns. *Eukaryot Cell* **3:**536–545.

23. **Fonzi WA, Irwin MY.** 1993. Isogenic strain construction and gene mapping in *Candida albicans*. *Genetics* **134:**717–728.

24. **Nakayama H, Mio T, Nagahashi S, Kokado M, Arisawa M, Aoki Y.** 2000. Tetracycline-regulatable system to tightly control gene expression in the pathogenic fungus *Candida albicans*. *Infect Immun* **68:**6712–6719.

25. **Stoldt VR, Sonneborn A, Leuker CE, Ernst JF.** 1997. Efg1p, an essential regulator of morphogenesis of the human pathogen *Candida albicans*, is a member of a conserved class of bHLH proteins regulating morphogenetic processes in fungi. *EMBO J* **16:**1982–1991.

26. **Park H, Myers CL, Sheppard DC, Phan QT, Sanchez AA, Edwards JE, Filler SG.** 2005. Role of the fungal Ras-protein kinase A pathway in governing epithelial cell interactions during oropharyngeal candidiasis. *Cell Microbiol* **7:**499–510.

27. **Peters BM, Palmer GE, Nash AK, Lilly EA, Fidel PL Jr, Noverr MC.** 2014. Fungal morphogenetic pathways are required for the hallmark inflammatory response during *Candida albicans* vaginitis. *Infect Immun* **82:**532–543.

28. **Lo HJ, Kohler JR, DiDomenico B, Loebenberg D, Cacciapuoti A, Fink GR.** 1997. Nonfilamentous *C. albicans* mutants are avirulent. *Cell* **90:**939–949.

29. **Centeno A, Davis CP, Cohen MS, Warren MM.** 1983. Modulation of *Candida albicans* attachment to human epithelial cells by bacteria and carbohydrates. *Infect Immun* **39:**1354–1360.

30. **Hogan DA, Kolter R.** 2002. *Pseudomonas-Candida* interactions: an ecological role for virulence factors. *Science* **296:**2229–2232.

31. **Peters BM, Jabra-Rizk MA, Scheper MA, Leid JG, Costerton JW, Shirtliff ME.** 2010. Microbial interactions and differential protein expression in *Staphylococcus aureus-Candida albicans* dual-species biofilms. *FEMS Immunol Med Microbiol* **59:**493–503.

32. **Schlecht LM, Peters BM, Krom BP, Freiberg JA, Hansch GM, Filler SG, Jabra-Rizk MA, Shirtliff ME.** 2015. Systemic *Staphylococcus aureus* infection mediated by *Candida albicans* hyphal invasion of mucosal tissue. *Microbiology* **161:**168–181.

33. **Fox SJ, Shelton BT, Kruppa MD.** 2013. Characterization of genetic determinants that modulate *Candida albicans* filamentation in the presence of bacteria. *PLoS One* **8:**e71939. doi:10.1371/journal.pone.0071939.

34. **Hwang G, Marsh G, Gao L, Waugh R, Koo H.** 2015. Binding force dynamics of *Streptococcus mutans*-glucosyltransferase B to *Candida albicans*. *J Dent Res* **94:**1310–1317.

35. **Katharios-Lanwermeyer S, Xi C, Jakubovics NS, Rickard AH.** 2014. Mini-review: microbial coaggregation: ubiquity and implications for biofilm development. *Biofouling* **30:**1235–1251.

36. **Silverman RJ, Nobbs AH, Vickerman MM, Barbour ME, Jenkinson HF.** 2010. Interaction of *Candida albicans* cell wall Als3 protein with *Streptococcus gordonii* SspB adhesin promotes development of mixed-species communities. *Infect Immun* **78:**4644–4652.

37. **Bagg J, Silverwood RW.** 1986. Coagglutination reactions between *Candida albicans* and oral bacteria. *J Med Microbiol* **22:**165–169.

38. **Jenkinson HF, Lala HC, Shepherd MG.** 1990. Coaggregation of *Streptococcus sanguis* and other streptococci with *Candida albicans*. *Infect Immun* **58:**1429–1436.

39. **Holmes AR, Gopal PK, Jenkinson HF.** 1995. Adherence of *Candida albicans* to a cell surface polysaccharide receptor on *Streptococcus gordonii*. *Infect Immun* **63:**1827–1834.

40. **Diaz PI, Xie Z, Sobue T, Thompson A, Biyikoglu B, Ricker A, Ikonomou L, Dongari-Bagtzoglou A.** 2012. Synergistic interaction between *Candida albicans* and commensal oral streptococci in a novel *in vitro* mucosal model. *Infect Immun* **80:**620–632.

41. **Arzmi MH, Dashper S, Catmull D, Cirillo N, Reynolds EC, McCullough M.** 2015. Coaggregation of *Candida albicans*, *Actinomyces naeslundii* and *Streptococcus mutans* is *Candida albicans* strain dependent. *FEMS Yeast Res* **15:**fov038.

42. **Archer NK, Harro JM, Shirtliff ME.** 2013. Clearance of *Staphylococcus aureus* nasal carriage is T cell dependent and mediated through interleukin-17A expression and neutrophil influx. *Infect Immun* **81**:2070–2075.

43. **Marks DJ, Hyams C, Koo CY, Pavlou M, Robbins J, Koo CS, Rodger G, Huggett JF, Yap J, Macrae MB, Swanton RH, Zumla AI, Miller RF.** 2015. Clinical features, microbiology and surgical outcomes of infective endocarditis: a 13-year study from a UK tertiary cardiothoracic referral centre. *QJM* **108**:219–229.

44. **Thuny F, Grisoli D, Collart F, Habib G, Raoult D.** 2012. Management of infective endocarditis: challenges and perspectives. *Lancet* **379**:965–975.

45. **Carlson E.** 1982. Synergistic effect of *Candida albicans* and *Staphylococcus aureus* on mouse mortality. *Infect Immun* **38**:921–924.

46. **Carlson E.** 1983. Enhancement by *Candida albicans* of *Staphylococcus aureus, Serratia marcescens*, and *Streptococcus faecalis* in the establishment of infection in mice. *Infect Immun* **39**:193–197.

47. **Carlson E, Johnson G.** 1985. Protection by *Candida albicans* of *Staphylococcus aureus* in the establishment of dual infection in mice. *Infect Immun* **50**:655–659.

48. **Venkatesh MP, Pham D, Fein M, Kong L, Weisman LE.** 2007. Neonatal coinfection model of coagulase-negative *Staphylococcus* (*Staphylococcus epidermidis*) and *Candida albicans*: fluconazole prophylaxis enhances survival and growth. *Antimicrob Agents Chemother* **51**:1240–1245.

49. **Peters BM, Noverr MC.** 2013. *Candida albicans-Staphylococcus aureus* polymicrobial peritonitis modulates host innate immunity. *Infect Immun* **81**:2178–2189.

50. **Kucharikova S, Gerits E, De Brucker K, Braem A, Ceh K, Majdic G, Spanic T, Pogorevc E, Verstraeten N, Tournu H, Delattin N, Impellizzeri F, Erdtmann M, Krona A, Lovenklev M, Knezevic M, Frohlich M, Vleugels J, Fauvart M, de Silva WJ, Vandamme K, Garcia-Forgas J, Cammue BP, Michiels J, Van Dijck P, Thevissen K.** 2016. Covalent immobilization of antimicrobial agents on titanium prevents *Staphylococcus aureus* and *Candida albicans* colonization and biofilm formation. *J Antimicrob Chemother* **71**:936–945.

51. **Harriott MM, Noverr MC.** 2010. Ability of *Candida albicans* mutants to induce *Staphylococcus aureus* vancomycin resistance during polymicrobial biofilm formation. *Antimicrob Agents Chemother* **54**:3746–3755.

52. **Peters BM, Ovchinnikova ES, Krom BP, Schlecht LM, Zhou H, Hoyer LL, Busscher HJ, van der Mei HC, Jabra-Rizk MA, Shirtliff ME.** 2012. *Staphylococcus aureus* adherence to *Candida albicans* hyphae is mediated by the hyphal adhesin Als3p. *Microbiology* **158**:2975–2986.

53. **Jabra-Rizk MA, Falkler WA Jr, Merz WG, Kelley JI, Baqui AA, Meiller TF.** 1999. Coaggregation of *Candida dubliniensis* with *Fusobacterium nucleatum. J Clin Microbiol* **37**:1464–1468.

54. **Nobile CJ, Mitchell AP.** 2005. Regulation of cell-surface genes and biofilm formation by the *C. albicans* transcription factor Bcr1p. *Curr Biol* **15**:1150–1155.

55. **Beaussart A, Herman P, El-Kirat-Chatel S, Lipke PN, Kucharikova S, Van Dijck P, Dufrene YF.** 2013. Single-cell force spectroscopy of the medically important *Staphylococcus epidermidis-Candida albicans* interaction. *Nanoscale* **5**:10894–10900.

56. **Fehrmann C, Jurk K, Bertling A, Seidel G, Fegeler W, Kehrel BE, Peters G, Becker K, Heilmann C.** 2013. Role for the fibrinogen-binding proteins coagulase and Efb in the *Staphylococcus aureus-Candida* interaction. *Int J Med Microbiol* **303**:230–238.

57. **Krause J, Geginat G, Tammer I.** 2015. Prostaglandin E2 from *Candida albicans* stimulates the growth of *Staphylococcus aureus* in mixed biofilms. *PLoS One* **10**:e0135404. doi:10.1371/journal.pone.0135404.

58. **Centers for Disease Control and Prevention.** 2012. Active Bacterial Core Surveillance Report, Emerging Infections Program Network, Methicillin-Resistant *Staphylococcus aureus*, 2011. http://www.cdc.gov/abcs/reports-findings/surveyreports/mrsa11.pdf.

59. **Adam B, Baillie GS, Douglas LJ.** 2002. Mixed species biofilms of *Candida albicans* and *Staphylococcus epidermidis. J Med Microbiol* **51**:344–349.

60. **Harriott MM, Noverr MC.** 2009. *Candida albicans* and *Staphylococcus aureus* form polymicrobial biofilms: effects on antimicrobial resistance. *Antimicrob Agents Chemother* **53**:3914–3922.

61. **Al-Fattani MA, Douglas LJ.** 2004. Penetration of *Candida* biofilms by antifungal agents. *Antimicrob Agents Chemother* **48**:3291–3297.

62. **Centers for Disease Control and Prevention.** 2013. Antibiotic Resistance Threats in the United States, 2013. http://www.cdc.gov/drugresistance/threat-report-2013/pdf/ar-threats-2013-508.pdf.

63. **Neely AN, Law EJ, Holder IA.** 1986. Increased susceptibility to lethal *Candida* infections in burned mice preinfected with *Pseudomonas*

aeruginosa or pretreated with proteolytic enzymes. *Infect Immun* **52**:200–204.

64. **Yu L, Lee KK, Hodges RS, Paranchych W, Irvin RT.** 1994. Adherence of *Pseudomonas aeruginosa* and *Candida albicans* to glycosphingolipid (Asialo-GM1) receptors is achieved by a conserved receptor-binding domain present on their adhesins. *Infect Immun* **62**:5213–5219.

65. **Kerr JR.** 1994. Suppression of fungal growth exhibited by *Pseudomonas aeruginosa*. *J Clin Microbiol* **32**:525–527.

66. **Kerr JR, Taylor GW, Rutman A, Hoiby N, Cole PJ, Wilson R.** 1999. *Pseudomonas aeruginosa* pyocyanin and 1-hydroxyphenazine inhibit fungal growth. *J Clin Pathol* **52**:385–387.

67. **Kaleli I, Cevahir N, Demir M, Yildirim U, Sahin R.** 2007. Anticandidal activity of *Pseudomonas aeruginosa* strains isolated from clinical specimens. *Mycoses* **50**:74–78.

68. **Brand A, Barnes JD, Mackenzie KS, Odds FC, Gow NA.** 2008. Cell wall glycans and soluble factors determine the interactions between the hyphae of *Candida albicans* and *Pseudomonas aeruginosa*. *FEMS Microbiol Lett* **287**:48–55.

69. **Hogan DA, Vik A, Kolter R.** 2004. A *Pseudomonas aeruginosa* quorum-sensing molecule influences *Candida albicans* morphology. *Mol Microbiol* **54**:1212–1223.

70. **McAlester G, O'Gara F, Morrissey JP.** 2008. Signal-mediated interactions between *Pseudomonas aeruginosa* and *Candida albicans*. *J Med Microbiol* **57**:563–569.

71. **Cugini C, Calfee MW, Farrow JM 3rd, Morales DK, Pesci EC, Hogan DA.** 2007. Farnesol, a common sesquiterpene, inhibits PQS production in *Pseudomonas aeruginosa*. *Mol Microbiol* **65**:896–906.

72. **Gibson J, Sood A, Hogan DA.** 2009. *Pseudomonas aeruginosa-Candida albicans* interactions: localization and fungal toxicity of a phenazine derivative. *Appl Environ Microbiol* **75**:504–513.

73. **Morales DK, Jacobs NJ, Rajamani S, Krishnamurthy M, Cubillos-Ruiz JR, Hogan DA.** 2010. Antifungal mechanisms by which a novel *Pseudomonas aeruginosa* phenazine toxin kills *Candida albicans* in biofilms. *Mol Microbiol* **78**:1379–1392.

74. **Holcombe LJ, McAlester G, Munro CA, Enjalbert B, Brown AJ, Gow NA, Ding C, Butler G, O'Gara F, Morrissey JP.** 2010. *Pseudomonas aeruginosa* secreted factors impair biofilm development in *Candida albicans*. *Microbiology* **156**:1476–1486.

75. **Bandara HM, Yau JY, Watt RM, Jin LJ, Samaranayake LP.** 2010. *Pseudomonas aeruginosa* inhibits *in-vitro Candida* biofilm development. *BMC Microbiol* **10**:125.

76. **Bandara HM, Lam OL, Watt RM, Jin LJ, Samaranayake LP.** 2010. Bacterial lipopolysaccharides variably modulate *in vitro* biofilm formation of *Candida* species. *J Med Microbiol* **59**:1225–1234.

77. **Chen AI, Dolben EF, Okegbe C, Harty CE, Golub Y, Thao S, Ha DG, Willger SD, O'Toole GA, Harwood CS, Dietrich LE, Hogan DA.** 2014. *Candida albicans* ethanol stimulates *Pseudomonas aeruginosa* WspR-controlled biofilm formation as part of a cyclic relationship involving phenazines. *PLoS Pathog* **10**:e1004480. doi:10.1371/journal.ppat.1004480.

78. **Lopez-Medina E, Fan D, Coughlin LA, Ho EX, Lamont IL, Reimmann C, Hooper LV, Koh AY.** 2015. *Candida albicans* inhibits *Pseudomonas aeruginosa* virulence through suppression of pyochelin and pyoverdine biosynthesis. *PLoS Pathog* **11**:e1005129. doi:10.1371/journal. ppat.1005129.

79. **Suppiger A, Schmid N, Aguilar C, Pessi G, Eberl L.** 2013. Two quorum sensing systems control biofilm formation and virulence in members of the *Burkholderia cepacia* complex. *Virulence* **4**:400–409.

80. **Coenye T.** 2010. Social interactions in the *Burkholderia cepacia* complex: biofilms and quorum sensing. *Future Microbiol* **5**:1087–1099.

81. **Drevinek P, Holden MT, Ge Z, Jones AM, Ketchell I, Gill RT, Mahenthiralingam E.** 2008. Gene expression changes linked to antimicrobial resistance, oxidative stress, iron depletion and retained motility are observed when *Burkholderia cenocepacia* grows in cystic fibrosis sputum. *BMC Infect Dis* **8**:121.

82. **Boon C, Deng Y, Wang LH, He Y, Xu JL, Fan Y, Pan SQ, Zhang LH.** 2008. A novel DSF-like signal from *Burkholderia cenocepacia* interferes with *Candida albicans* morphological transition. *ISME J* **2**:27–36.

83. **Rangaka MX, Cavalcante SC, Marais BJ, Thim S, Martinson NA, Swaminathan S, Chaisson RE.** 2015. Controlling the seedbeds of tuberculosis: diagnosis and treatment of tuberculosis infection. *Lancet* **386**:2344–2353.

84. **Kali A, Charles MP, Noyal MJ, Sivaraman U, Kumar S, Easow JM.** 2013. Prevalence of *Candida* co-infection in patients with pulmonary tuberculosis. *Australas Med J* **6**:387–391.

85. **Ochieng W, Wanzala P, Bii C, Oishi I, Ichimura H, Lihana R, Mpoke S, Mwaniki D, Okoth FA.** 2005. Tuberculosis and oral *Candida* species surveillance in HIV infected individuals in northern Kenya, and the implications on tuberculin skin

test screening for DOPT-P. *East Afr Med J* **82**:609–613.

86. **Okada S, Markle JG, Deenick EK, Mele F, Averbuch D, Lagos M, Alzahrani M, Al-Muhsen S, Halwani R, Ma CS, Wong N, Soudais C, Henderson LA, Marzouqa H, Shamma J, Gonzalez M, Martinez-Barricarte R, Okada C, Avery DT, Latorre D, Deswarte C, Jabot-Hanin F, Torrado E, Fountain J, Belkadi A, Itan Y, Boisson B, Migaud M, Arlehamn CS, Sette A, Breton S, McCluskey J, Rossjohn J, de Villartay JP, Moshous D, Hambleton S, Latour S, Arkwright PD, Picard C, Lantz O, Engelhard D, Kobayashi M, Abel L, Cooper AM, Notarangelo LD, Boisson-Dupuis S, Puel A, Sallusto F, Bustamante J, Tangye SG, Casanova JL.** 2015. IMMUNODEFICIENCIES. Impairment of immunity to *Candida* and *Mycobacterium* in humans with bi-allelic RORC mutations. *Science* **349**:606–613.

87. **Kukita K, Kawada-Matsuo M, Oho T, Nagatomo M, Oogai Y, Hashimoto M, Suda Y, Tanaka T, Komatsuzawa H.** 2013. *Staphylococcus aureus* SasA is responsible for binding to the salivary agglutinin gp340, derived from human saliva. *Infect Immun* **81**:1870–1879.

88. **Nelson-Filho P, Borba IG, Mesquita KS, Silva RA, Queiroz AM, Silva LA.** 2013. Dynamics of microbial colonization of the oral cavity in newborns. *Braz Dent J* **24**:415–419.

89. **Merghni A, Ben Nejma M, Hentati H, Mahjoub A, Mastouri M.** 2014. Adhesive properties and extracellular enzymatic activity of *Staphylococcus aureus* strains isolated from oral cavity. *Microb Pathog* **73**:7–12.

90. **Kim GY, Lee CH.** 2015. Antimicrobial susceptibility and pathogenic genes of *Staphylococcus aureus* isolated from the oral cavity of patients with periodontitis. *J Periodontal Implant Sci* **45**:223–228.

91. **Koukos G, Sakellari D, Arsenakis M, Tsalikis L, Slini T, Konstantinidis A.** 2015. Prevalence of *Staphylococcus aureus* and methicillin resistant *Staphylococcus aureus* (MRSA) in the oral cavity. *Arch Oral Biol* **60**:1410–1415.

92. **McCormack MG, Smith AJ, Akram AN, Jackson M, Robertson D, Edwards G.** 2015. *Staphylococcus aureus* and the oral cavity: an overlooked source of carriage and infection? *Am J Infect Control* **43**:35–37.

93. **O'Donnell LE, Smith K, Williams C, Nile CJ, Lappin DF, Bradshaw D, Lambert M, Robertson DP, Bagg J, Hannah V, Ramage G.** 2016. Dentures are a reservoir for respiratory pathogens. *J Periodontal Implant Sci* **25**:99–104.

94. **Sanford BA, Thomas VL, Ramsay MA, Jones TO.** 1986. Characterization of clinical strains of *Staphylococcus aureus* associated with pneumonia. *J Clin Microbiol* **24**:131–136.

95. **Ohara-Nemoto Y, Haraga H, Kimura S, Nemoto TK.** 2008. Occurrence of staphylococci in the oral cavities of healthy adults and nasal oral trafficking of the bacteria. *J Med Microbiol* **57**:95–99.

96. **Smith AJ, Robertson D, Tang MK, Jackson MS, MacKenzie D, Bagg J.** 2003. *Staphylococcus aureus* in the oral cavity: a three-year retrospective analysis of clinical laboratory data. *Br Dent J* **195**:701–703; discussion 694.

97. **Miyake Y, Iwai T, Sugai M, Miura K, Suginaka H, Nagasaka N.** 1991. Incidence and characterization of *Staphylococcus aureus* from the tongues of children. *J Dent Res* **70**:1045–1047.

98. **Pulimood S, Ganesan L, Alangaden G, Chandrasekar P.** 2002. Polymicrobial candidemia. *Diagn Microbiol Infect Dis* **44**:353–357.

99. **Carlson E.** 1983. Enhancement by *Candida albicans* of *Staphylococcus aureus*, *Serratia marcescens*, and *Streptococcus faecalis* in the establishment of infection in mice. *Infect Immun* **39**:193–197.

100. **Carlson E.** 1983. Effect of strain of *Staphylococcus aureus* on synergism with *Candida albicans* resulting in mouse mortality and morbidity. *Infect Immun* **42**:285–292.

101. **Kong EF, Kucharikova S, Van Dijck P, Peters BM, Shirtliff ME, Jabra-Rizk MA.** 2015. Clinical implications of oral candidiasis: host tissue damage and disseminated bacterial disease. *Infect Immun* **83**:604–613.

102. **Holmes AR, McNab R, Jenkinson HF.** 1996. *Candida albicans* binding to the oral bacterium *Streptococcus gordonii* involves multiple adhesin-receptor interactions. *Infect Immun* **64**:4680–4685.

103. **Bamford CV, d'Mello A, Nobbs AH, Dutton LC, Vickerman MM, Jenkinson HF.** 2009. *Streptococcus gordonii* modulates *Candida albicans* biofilm formation through intergeneric communication. *Infect Immun* **77**:3696–3704.

104. **Hoyer LL, Oh SH, Jones R, Cota E.** 2014. A proposed mechanism for the interaction between the *Candida albicans* Als3 adhesin and streptococcal cell wall proteins. *Front Microbiol* **5**:564.

105. **Dutton LC, Nobbs AH, Jepson K, Jepson MA, Vickerman MM, Aqeel Alawfi S, Munro CA, Lamont RJ, Jenkinson HF.** 2014. O-mannosylation in *Candida albicans* enables development of interkingdom biofilm communities. *MBio* **5**:e00911–14. doi:10.1128/mBio.00911-14.

106. Jarosz LM, Deng DM, van der Mei HC, Crielaard W, Krom BP. 2009. *Streptococcus mutans* competence-stimulating peptide inhibits *Candida albicans* hypha formation. *Eukaryot Cell* **8:**1658–1664.

107. Vilchez R, Lemme A, Ballhausen B, Thiel V, Schulz S, Jansen R, Sztajer H, Wagner-Dobler I. 2010. *Streptococcus mutans* inhibits *Candida albicans* hyphal formation by the fatty acid signaling molecule trans-2-decenoic acid (SDSF). *Chembiochem* **11:**1552–1562.

108. Raja M, Hannan A, Ali K. 2010. Association of oral candidal carriage with dental caries in children. *Caries Res* **44:**272–276.

109. de Carvalho FG, Silva DS, Hebling J, Spolidorio LC, Spolidorio DM. 2006. Presence of mutans streptococci and *Candida* spp. in dental plaque/dentine of carious teeth and early childhood caries. *Arch Oral Biol* **51:**1024–1028.

110. Sztajer H, Szafranski SP, Tomasch J, Reck M, Nimtz M, Rohde M, Wagner-Dobler I. 2014. Cross-feeding and interkingdom communication in dual-species biofilms of *Streptococcus mutans* and *Candida albicans*. *ISME J* **8:**2256–2271.

111. Gregoire S, Xiao J, Silva BB, Gonzalez I, Agidi PS, Klein MI, Ambatipudi KS, Rosalen PL, Bauserman R, Waugh RE, Koo H. 2011. Role of glucosyltransferase B in interactions of *Candida albicans* with *Streptococcus mutans* and with an experimental pellicle on hydroxyapatite surfaces. *Appl Environ Microbiol* **77:**6357–6367.

112. Savage A, Eaton KA, Moles DR, Needleman I. 2009. A systematic review of definitions of periodontitis and methods that have been used to identify this disease. *J Clin Periodontol* **36:**458–467.

113. Canabarro A, Valle C, Farias MR, Santos FB, Lazera M, Wanke B. 2013. Association of subgingival colonization of *Candida albicans* and other yeasts with severity of chronic periodontitis. *J Periodontal Res* **48:**428–432.

114. Bostanci N, Belibasakis GN. 2012. *Porphyromonas gingivalis*: an invasive and evasive opportunistic oral pathogen. *FEMS Microbiol Lett* **333:**1–9.

115. Tamai R, Sugamata M, Kiyoura Y. 2011. *Candida albicans* enhances invasion of human gingival epithelial cells and gingival fibroblasts by *Porphyromonas gingivalis*. *Microb Pathog* **51:**250–254.

116. Herbert BA, Novince CM, Kirkwood KL. 2015. *Aggregatibacter actinomycetemcomitans*, a potent immunoregulator of the periodontal host defense system and alveolar bone homeostasis. *Mol Oral Microbiol* [Epub ahead of print.] doi:10.1111/omi.12119.

117. Raja M, Ummer F, Dhivakar CP. 2014. *Aggregatibacter actinomycetemcomitans*: a tooth killer? *J Clin Diagn Res* **8:**ZE13–ZE16.

118. Bachtiar EW, Bachtiar BM, Jarosz LM, Amir LR, Sunarto H, Ganin H, Meijler MM, Krom BP. 2014. AI-2 of *Aggregatibacter actinomycetemcomitans* inhibits *Candida albicans* biofilm formation. *Front Cell Infect Microbiol* **4:**94.

119. Al Mubarak S, Robert AA, Baskaradoss JK, Al-Zoman K, Al Sohail A, Alsuwyed A, Ciancio S. 2013. The prevalence of oral *Candida* infections in periodontitis patients with type 2 diabetes mellitus. *J Infect Public Health* **6:**296–301.

120. Richards AM, Abu Kwaik Y, Lamont RJ. 2015. Code blue: *Acinetobacter baumannii*, a nosocomial pathogen with a role in the oral cavity. *Mol Oral Microbiol* **30:**2–15.

121. Gaddy JA, Tomaras AP, Actis LA. 2009. The *Acinetobacter baumannii* 19606 OmpA protein plays a role in biofilm formation on abiotic surfaces and in the interaction of this pathogen with eukaryotic cells. *Infect Immun* **77:**3150–3160.

122. Phan QT, Myers CL, Fu Y, Sheppard DC, Yeaman MR, Welch WH, Ibrahim AS, Edwards JE Jr, Filler SG. 2007. Als3 is a *Candida albicans* invasin that binds to cadherins and induces endocytosis by host cells. *PLoS Biol* **5:**e64.

123. Donskey CJ. 2004. The role of the intestinal tract as a reservoir and source for transmission of nosocomial pathogens. *Clin Infect Dis* **39:**219–226.

124. Stuart CH, Schwartz SA, Beeson TJ, Owatz CB. 2006. *Enterococcus faecalis*: its role in root canal treatment failure and current concepts in retreatment. *J Endod* **32:**93–98.

125. Cruz MR, Graham CE, Gagliano BC, Lorenz MC, Garsin DA. 2013. *Enterococcus faecalis* inhibits hyphal morphogenesis and virulence of *Candida albicans*. *Infect Immun* **81:**189–200.

126. Shekh RM, Roy U. 2012. Biochemical characterization of an anti-*Candida* factor produced by *Enterococcus faecalis*. *BMC Microbiol* **12:**132.

127. Ishijima SA, Hayama K, Ninomiya K, Iwasa M, Yamazaki M, Abe S. 2014. Protection of mice from oral *Candidiasis* by heat-killed *Enterococcus faecalis*, possibly through its direct binding to *Candida albicans*. *Med Mycol J* **55:**E9–E19.

128. Hermann C, Hermann J, Munzel U, Ruchel R. 1999. Bacterial flora accompanying *Candida* yeasts in clinical specimens. *Mycoses* **42:**619–627.

129. **Goldstein EJ.** 2002. Intra-abdominal anaerobic infections: bacteriology and therapeutic potential of newer antimicrobial carbapenem, fluoroquinolone, and desfluoroquinolone therapeutic agents. *Clin Infect Dis* **35:**S106–S111.

130. **Edey M, Hawley CM, McDonald SP, Brown FG, Rosman JB, Wiggins KJ, Bannister KM, Johnson DW.** 2010. Enterococcal peritonitis in Australian peritoneal dialysis patients: predictors, treatment and outcomes in 116 cases. *Nephrol Dial Transplant* **25:**1272–1278.

131. **Barraclough K, Hawley CM, McDonald SP, Brown FG, Rosman JB, Wiggins KJ, Bannister KM, Johnson DW.** 2010. Polymicrobial peritonitis in peritoneal dialysis patients in Australia: predictors, treatment, and outcomes. *Am J Kidney Dis* **55:**121–131.

132. **Dupont H, Paugam-Burtz C, Muller-Serieys C, Fierobe L, Chosidow D, Marmuse JP, Mantz J, Desmonts JM.** 2002. Predictive factors of mortality due to polymicrobial peritonitis with *Candida* isolation in peritoneal fluid in critically ill patients. *Arch Surg* **137:**1341–1346; discussion 1347.

133. **Klaerner HG, Uknis ME, Acton RD, Dahlberg PS, Carlone-Jambor C, Dunn DL.** 1997. *Candida albicans* and *Escherichia coli* are synergistic pathogens during experimental microbial peritonitis. *J Surg Res* **70:**161–165.

134. **Henry-Stanley MJ, Hess DJ, Erickson EA, Garni RM, Wells CL.** 2003. Effect of lipopolysaccharide on virulence of intestinal *Candida albicans*. *J Surg Res* **113:**42–49.

135. **Bandara HM, Yau JY, Watt RM, Jin LJ, Samaranayake LP.** 2009. *Escherichia coli* and its lipopolysaccharide modulate *in vitro Candida* biofilm formation. *J Med Microbiol* **58:**1623–1631.

136. **Bandara HM, Cheung BP, Watt RM, Jin LJ, Samaranayake LP.** 2013. Secretory products of *Escherichia coli* biofilm modulate *Candida* biofilm formation and hyphal development. *J Investig Clin Dent* **4:**186–199.

137. **De Brucker K, Tan Y, Vints K, De Cremer K, Braem A, Verstraeten N, Michiels J, Vleugels J, Cammue BP, Thevissen K.** 2015. Fungal beta-1,3-glucan increases ofloxacin tolerance of *Escherichia coli* in a polymicrobial *E. coli/Candida albicans* biofilm. *Antimicrob Agents Chemother* **59:**3052–3058.

138. **Baixench MT, Aoun N, Desnos-Ollivier M, Garcia-Hermoso D, Bretagne S, Ramires S, Piketty C, Dannaoui E.** 2007. Acquired resistance to echinocandins in *Candida albicans*: case report and review. *J Antimicrob Chemother* **59:**1076–1083.

139. **Hurley D, McCusker MP, Fanning S, Martins M.** 2014. *Salmonella*-host interactions: modulation of the host innate immune system. *Front Immunol* **5:**481.

140. **Tampakakis E, Peleg AY, Mylonakis E.** 2009. Interaction of *Candida albicans* with an intestinal pathogen, *Salmonella enterica* serovar Typhimurium. *Eukaryot Cell* **8:**732–737.

141. **Zhou D, Galan J.** 2001. *Salmonella* entry into host cells: the work in concert of type III secreted effector proteins. *Microbes Infect* **3:**1293–1298.

142. **Ly KT, Casanova JE.** 2007. Mechanisms of *Salmonella* entry into host cells. *Cell Microbiol* **9:**2103–2111.

143. **McGhie EJ, Brawn LC, Hume PJ, Humphreys D, Koronakis V.** 2009. *Salmonella* takes control: effector-driven manipulation of the host. *Curr Opin Microbiol* **12:**117–124.

144. **Kim Y, Mylonakis E.** 2011. Killing of *Candida albicans* filaments by *Salmonella enterica* serovar Typhimurium is mediated by sopB effectors, parts of a type III secretion system. *Eukaryot Cell* **10:**782–790.

145. **Haley KP, Gaddy JA.** 2015. *Helicobacter pylori*: genomic insight into the host-pathogen interaction. *Int J Genomics* **2015:**386905.

146. **Salmanian AH, Siavoshi F, Akbari F, Afshari A, Malekzadeh R.** 2008. Yeast of the oral cavity is the reservoir of *Heliobacter pylori*. *J Oral Pathol Med* **37:**324–328.

147. **Ince AT, Kocaman O, Ismailova M, Tozlu M, Gucin Z, Iraz M.** 2014. A rare co-existence of *Helicobacter pylori*, *Candida albicans* and *Candida keyfr* in a giant gastric ulcer. *Turk J Gastroenterol* **25:**435–436.

148. **Saniee P, Siavoshi F, Nikbakht Broujeni G, Khormali M, Sarrafnejad A, Malekzadeh R.** 2013. Localization of *H. pylori* within the vacuole of *Candida* yeast by direct immunofluorescence technique. *Arch Iran Med* **16:**705–710.

149. **Saniee P, Siavoshi F, Nikbakht Broujeni G, Khormali M, Sarrafnejad A, Malekzadeh R.** 2013. Immunodetection of *Helicobacter pylori*-specific proteins in oral and gastric *Candida* yeasts. *Arch Iran Med* **16:**624–630.

150. **Siavoshi F, Saniee P.** 2014. Vacuoles of *Candida* yeast as a specialized niche for *Helicobacter pylori*. *World J Gastroenterol* **20:**5263–5273.

151. **Di Cerbo A, Palmieri B, Aponte M, Morales-Medina JC, Iannitti T.** 2016. Mechanisms and therapeutic effectiveness of lactobacilli. *J Clin Pathol* **69:**187–203.

152. **Kunz J.** 1995. Causes and consequences of an unbalanced vaginal ecosystem. *Praxis* (Bern 1994) **84:**1405–1415. [In German.]

153. Martinez RC, Franceschini SA, Patta MC, Quintana SM, Nunes AC, Moreira JL, Anukam KC, Reid G, De Martinis EC. 2008. Analysis of vaginal lactobacilli from healthy and infected Brazilian women. *Appl Environ Microbiol* **74:**4539–4542.

154. McLean NW, Rosenstein IJ. 2000. Characterisation and selection of a *Lactobacillus* species to re-colonise the vagina of women with recurrent bacterial vaginosis. *J Med Microbiol* **49:**543–552.

155. Kaewsrichan J, Peeyananjarassri K, Kongprasertkit J. 2006. Selection and identification of anaerobic lactobacilli producing inhibitory compounds against vaginal pathogens. *FEMS Immunol Med Microbiol* **48:**75–83.

156. Mijac VD, Dukic SV, Opavski NZ, Dukic MK, Ranin LT. 2006. Hydrogen peroxide producing lactobacilli in women with vaginal infections. *Eur J Obstet Gynecol Reprod Biol* **129:**69–76.

157. Fitzsimmons N, Berry DR. 1994. Inhibition of *Candida albicans* by *Lactobacillus acidophilus*: evidence for the involvement of a peroxidase system. *Microbios* **80:**125–133.

158. Strus M, Kucharska A, Kukla G, Brzychczy-Wloch M, Maresz K, Heczko PB. 2005. The *in vitro* activity of vaginal *Lactobacillus* with probiotic properties against *Candida*. *Infect Dis Obstet Gynecol* **13:**69–75.

159. Orsi CF, Sabia C, Ardizzoni A, Colombari B, Neglia RG, Peppoloni S, Morace G, Blasi E. 2014. Inhibitory effects of different lactobacilli on *Candida albicans* hyphal formation and biofilm development. *J Biol Regul Homeost Agents* **28:**743–752.

160. Kohler GA, Assefa S, Reid G. 2012. Probiotic interference of *Lactobacillus rhamnosus* GR-1 and *Lactobacillus reuteri* RC-14 with the opportunistic fungal pathogen *Candida albicans*. *Infect Dis Obstet Gynecol* **2012:**636474.

161. Wagner RD, Johnson SJ. 2012. Probiotic *Lactobacillus* and estrogen effects on vaginal epithelial gene expression responses to *Candida albicans*. *J Biomed Sci* **19:**58.

162. Rizzo A, Losacco A, Carratelli CR. 2013. *Lactobacillus crispatus* modulates epithelial cell defense against *Candida albicans* through Toll-like receptors 2 and 4, interleukin 8 and human beta-defensins 2 and 3. *Immunol Lett* **156:**102–109.

163. Martinez RC, Seney SL, Summers KL, Nomizo A, De Martinis EC, Reid G. 2009. Effect of *Lactobacillus rhamnosus* GR-1 and *Lactobacillus reuteri* RC-14 on the ability of *Candida albicans* to infect cells and induce inflammation. *Microbiol Immunol* **53:**487–495.

164. Martinez RC, Franceschini SA, Patta MC, Quintana SM, Candido RC, Ferreira JC, De Martinis EC, Reid G. 2009. Improved treatment of vulvovaginal candidiasis with fluconazole plus probiotic *Lactobacillus rhamnosus* GR-1 and *Lactobacillus reuteri* RC-14. *Lett Appl Microbiol* **48:**269–274.

165. Chew SY, Cheah YK, Seow HF, Sandai D, Than LT. 2015. Probiotic *Lactobacillus rhamnosus* GR-1 and *Lactobacillus reuteri* RC-14 exhibit strong antifungal effects against vulvovaginal candidiasis-causing *Candida glabrata* isolates. *J Appl Microbiol* **118:**1180–1190.

166. Romani L, Zelante T, Palmieri M, Napolioni V, Picciolini M, Velardi A, Aversa F, Puccetti P. 2015. The cross-talk between opportunistic fungi and the mammalian host via microbiota's metabolism. *Semin Immunopathol* **37:**163–171.

167. Hockey LJ, Fujita NK, Gibson TR, Rotrosen D, Montgomerie JZ, Edwards JE Jr. 1982. Detection of fungemia obscured by concomitant bacteremia: *in vitro* and *in vivo* studies. *J Clin Microbiol* **16:**1080–1085.

168. Daef E, Moharram A, Eldin SS, Elsherbiny N, Mohammed M. 2014. Evaluation of chromogenic media and seminested PCR in the identification of *Candida* species. *Braz J Microbiol* **45:**255–262.

169. Ahmad S, Khan Z, Mustafa AS, Khan ZU. 2002. Seminested PCR for diagnosis of candidemia: comparison with culture, antigen detection, and biochemical methods for species identification. *J Clin Microbiol* **40:**2483–2489.

170. Fredricks DN, Relman DA. 1996. Sequence-based identification of microbial pathogens: a reconsideration of Koch's postulates. *Clin Microbiol Rev* **9:**18–33.

171. Foster JS, Kolenbrander PE. 2004. Development of a multispecies oral bacterial community in a saliva-conditioned flow cell. *Appl Environ Microbiol* **70:**4340–4348.

172. Dowd SE, Delton Hanson J, Rees E, Wolcott RD, Zischau AM, Sun Y, White J, Smith DM, Kennedy J, Jones CE. 2011. Survey of fungi and yeast in polymicrobial infections in chronic wounds. *J Wound Care* **20:**40–47.

173. Webb D, Thadepalli H. 1979. Skin and soft tissue polymicrobial infections from intravenous abuse of drugs. *West J Med* **130:**200–204.

174. Klotz SA, Gaur NK, De Armond R, Sheppard D, Khardori N, Edwards JE Jr, Lipke PN, El-Azizi M. 2007. *Candida albicans* Als proteins mediate aggregation with bacteria and yeasts. *Med Mycol* **45:**363–370.

175. Brook I. 2002. Microbiology of polymicrobial abscesses and implications for therapy. *J Antimicrob Chemother* **50:**805–810.

176. **Carlson E.** 1983. Enhancement by *Candida albicans* of *Staphylococcus aureus*, *Serratia marcescens*, and *Streptococcus faecalis* in the establishment of infection in mice. *Infect Immun* **39**:193–197.

177. **Bertesteanu S, Triaridis S, Stankovic M, Lazar V, Chifiriuc MC, Vlad M, Grigore R.** 2014. Polymicrobial wound infections: pathophysiology and current therapeutic approaches. *Int J Pharm* **463**:119–126.

178. **Archer NK, Mazaitis MJ, Costerton JW, Leid JG, Powers ME, Shirtliff ME.** 2011. *Staphylococcus aureus* biofilms: properties, regulation, and roles in human disease. *Virulence* **2**:445–459.

179. **Brady RA, Leid JG, Calhoun JH, Costerton JW, Shirtliff ME.** 2008. Osteomyelitis and the role of biofilms in chronic infection. *FEMS Immunol Med Microbiol* **52**:13–22.

180. **Mader JT, Shirtliff M, Calhoun JH.** 1999. The host and the skeletal infection: classification and pathogenesis of acute bacterial bone and joint sepsis. *Baillieres Best Pract Res Clin Rheumatol* **13**:1–20.

181. **Mader JT, Shirtliff ME, Bergquist SC, Calhoun J.** 1999. Antimicrobial treatment of chronic osteomyelitis. *Clin Orthop Relat Res* **(360)**:47–65.

182. **Miclau T, Schmidt AH, Wenke JC, Webb LX, Harro JM, Prabhakara R, Shirtliff ME.** 2010. Infection. *J Orthop Trauma* **24**:583–586.

183. **Parvizi J, Alijanipour P, Barberi EF, Hickok NJ, Phillips KS, Shapiro IM, Schwarz EM, Stevens MH, Wang Y, Shirtliff ME.** 2015. Novel developments in the prevention, diagnosis, and treatment of periprosthetic joint infections. *J Am Acad Orthop Surg* **23**(Suppl): S32–S43.

184. **Peters BM, Jabra-Rizk MA, O'May GA, Costerton JW, Shirtliff ME.** 2012. Polymicrobial interactions: impact on pathogenesis and human disease. *Clin Microbiol Rev* **25**:193–213.

185. **Shirtliff ME, Leid JG, Costerton JW.** 2002. Basic science of musculoskeletal infections, p 1–62. *In* Mader JT, Calhoun JH (ed), *Musculoskeletal Infections*. Marcel Dekker, Inc., New York, New York.

186. **Shirtliff ME, Mader JT.** 2000. Osteomyelitis: clinical features and molecular aspects of persistence, p 375–395. *In* Nataro JP, Blaser MJ, Cunningham-Rundles S (ed), *Persistent Bacterial Infections*. ASM Press, Washington, DC.

187. **Shirtliff ME, Peters BM, Jabra-Rizk MA.** 2009. Cross-kingdom interactions: *Candida albicans* and bacteria. *FEMS Microbiol Lett* **299**:1–8.

188. **Xu Z, Li L, Shirtliff ME, Peters BM, Li B, Peng Y, Alam MJ, Yamasaki S, Shi L.** 2011. Resistance class 1 integron in clinical methicillin-resistant *Staphylococcus aureus* strains in southern China, 2001-2006. *Clin Microbiol Infect* **17**:714–718.

189. **Melander RJ, Melander C.** 2015. Innovative strategies for combating biofilm-based infections. *Adv Exp Med Biol* **831**:69–91.

190. **Taraszkiewicz A, Fila G, Grinholc M, Nakonieczna J.** 2013. Innovative strategies to overcome biofilm resistance. *Biomed Res Int* **2013**:150653.

191. **Galanzha EI, Shashkov E, Sarimollaoglu M, Beenken KE, Basnakian AG, Shirtliff ME, Kim JW, Smeltzer MS, Zharov VP.** 2012. *In vivo* magnetic enrichment, photoacoustic diagnosis, and photothermal purging of infected blood using multifunctional gold and magnetic nanoparticles. *PLoS One* **7**:e45557. doi:10.1371/journal.pone.0045557.

192. **Ishikawa KH, Mayer MP, Miyazima TY, Matsubara VH, Silva EG, Paula CR, Campos TT, Nakamae AE.** 2015. A multispecies probiotic reduces oral Candida colonization in denture wearers. *J Prosthodont* **24**:194–199.

193. **Roberfroid MB.** 2000. Prebiotics and probiotics: are they functional foods? *Am J Clin Nutr* **71**:1682S–1687S; discussion 1688S–1690S.

194. **Harro JM, Peters BM, O'May GA, Archer N, Kerns P, Prabhakara R, Shirtliff ME.** 2010. Vaccine development in *Staphylococcus aureus*: taking the biofilm phenotype into consideration. *FEMS Immunol Med Microbiol* **59**:306–323.

195. **Peters BM, Ovchinnikova ES, Krom BP, Schlecht LM, Zhou H, Hoyer LL, Busscher HJ, van der Mei HC, Jabra-Rizk MA, Shirtliff ME.** 2012. *Staphylococcus aureus* adherence to *Candida albicans* hyphae is mediated by the hyphal adhesin Als3p. *Microbiology* **158**:2975–2986.

196. **Metwalli KH, Khan SA, Krom BP, Jabra-Rizk MA.** 2013. *Streptococcus mutans*, *Candida albicans*, and the human mouth: a sticky situation. *PLoS Pathog* **9**:e1003616. doi:10.1371/journal.ppat.1003616.

Microbial Endocrinology in the Pathogenesis of Infectious Disease

6

MARK LYTE[1]

MICROBIAL ENDOCRINOLOGY: CONCEPTUAL FRAMEWORK

Microbial endocrinology represents the intersection of two seemingly disparate fields: microbiology and neurobiology (Fig 1). The field of microbial endocrinology was founded in 1993 when the term was first coined by Lyte (1, 2) based on experimental data obtained the prior year (3, 4). Although the concept of microbial endocrinology was founded just over 2 decades ago (1, 3–5), there has been published evidence by numerous investigators over the preceding 6 decades going back to 1930 (6), that demonstrate the validity of uniting the fields of microbiology and neurobiology as a conceptual framework with which to understand interactions between the microbiota and the host in the pathogenesis of infectious disease. It should be appreciated, however, that approaching microbiology through an interdisciplinary "lens" such as microbial endocrinology has relevance outside of the field of infectious disease. As will be discussed in this article, the ability of microorganisms to not only respond to, but also produce the very same neurochemicals that are more typically thought in the context of mammalian systems, means that host interactions with microorganisms are much more interactive than previously envisioned. This is the basis of microbial endocrinology (1, 2, 7–9). As such,

[1]Department of Veterinary Microbiology and Preventive Medicine, College of Veterinary Medicine, Iowa State University, Ames, IA 50011.
Virulence Mechanisms of Bacterial Pathogens, 5th edition
Edited by Indira T. Kudva, Nancy A. Cornick, Paul J. Plummer, Qijing Zhang, Tracy L. Nicholson, John P. Bannantine, and Bryan H. Bellaire
© 2016 American Society for Microbiology, Washington, DC
doi:10.1128/microbiolspec.VMBF-0021-2015

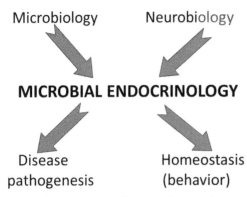

FIGURE 1 The conceptual basis of microbial endocrinology represents the intersection of microbiology and neurobiology and is based on the commonly shared neurochemicals that form the evolutionary basis of cell-to-cell communication in vertebrates (see text for in-depth discussion).

microbial endocrinology has found applications outside of infectious disease (where it has its developmental roots) including other aspects of host health such as the ability of the gut microbiota to influence the brain and behavior through the microbiota-gut-brain axis (10–12). This review will address how and why the fields of microbiology and neurobiology should intersect and what the relevance of this interaction is for infectious disease.

Note Regarding Definitions

When attempting to unite certain aspects of two seemingly disparate fields, the use of terms which originated in one field need to be addressed if they carry the same meaning in the other. The use of the terms "neurotransmitter," "neuromodulator," and "neurohormone" are designations that are associated with neurobiology and not microbiology. In neurobiology, a neurotransmitter is any chemical messenger that can act locally between two different neurons. In doing so, it is released from one neuron and diffuses across a small gap separating the two neurons, referred to as a synaptic cleft, where it binds to a receptor on the second neuron,

thus communicating and possibly propagating a signal. A neuromodulator is similar to a neurotransmitter but does not need to be released at a synaptic site and can act across longer distances and possibly act through a second messenger. The term neurohormone is used to identify those substances secreted by neuroendocrine cells into the systemic circulation that can exert effects on distant sites. To further complicate matters, any one chemical can have multiple roles; a neurochemical such as norepinephrine can be both a neurotransmitter and a neurohormone.

Given that microorganisms can form communities, a case can be made that the local release by cells within one community adjacent to another in a section of the gut fulfills the requirement of a neurotransmitter. Or release by one community in the cecum can have downstream effects on another microbial community in the colon, thus fulfilling a neurohormone-type definition. How one should apply these neurobiological terms to microbiology has yet to reach any consensus within the scientific community. Thus, for the purposes of consistency and ease of presentation, any chemical produced by a microorganism that is also recognized within neurobiology as either a neurotransmitter, neuromodulator, or neurohormone in a mammalian system will be referred to in this article as simply a "neurochemical." For the neurochemicals discussed in this article, the reader is referred to any standard neuroendocrinology reference book such as reference 13 for the current definitions and spectrum of biological activities in animals, encompassing their role in homeostasis and various disease pathologies.

HISTORICAL EVIDENCE FOR MICROBIAL ENDOCRINOLOGY IN INFECTIOUS DISEASE

In 1983 a clinical report appeared which described the development of gas gangrene in a 13-year-old girl following the intramuscular injection of epinephrine (14). That the administration of a neurochemical more commonly associated with a stress response should result in the appearance of a life-threatening infection should not have come as a surprise to the authors. Even as late as 1968, Harvey and Purnell, commenting on a fatal case of gas gangrene in a 22-year-old man who had received an intramuscular injection of epinephrine, wrote that the practice of epinephrine administration in the buttocks must be discontinued due to the probability of the injection site harboring clostridial spores (15). However, knowledge of such associations between an injectable neurochemical that has varied uses from treatment of urticaria to suppression of local inflammatory reactions and the development of a life-threatening infectious disease had been known since the 1930s (6).

The curious history of a dreaded infectious disease, gas gangrene, and an injectable catecholamine (epinephrine is a member of the catecholamine family; Fig. 2) that is used to treat a wide spectrum of medical conditions ranging from anaphylaxis to urticaria is illustrative of the intersection of neurobiology and microbiology in the pathogenesis of infectious disease. The latter part of the 19th century and early 20th century was a time that saw both the rise of modern endocrinology as personified by the first synthesis and application of a purified endocrine compound, epinephrine (16), and at the same time the continued development of modern bacteriology. Individually, each field continued its upward trajectory of increased understanding of the mechanisms by which they had respective roles to play in disease and homeostasis. Little research was done into how the fields might interact with one another. Undoubtedly, much of this was due to the prevailing view that the microbe could not be equated on the same level as multicellular organisms. However, a more interactive role of the microbiota with the host beyond the more fundamental aspects of pathogenesis was envisioned by some at the

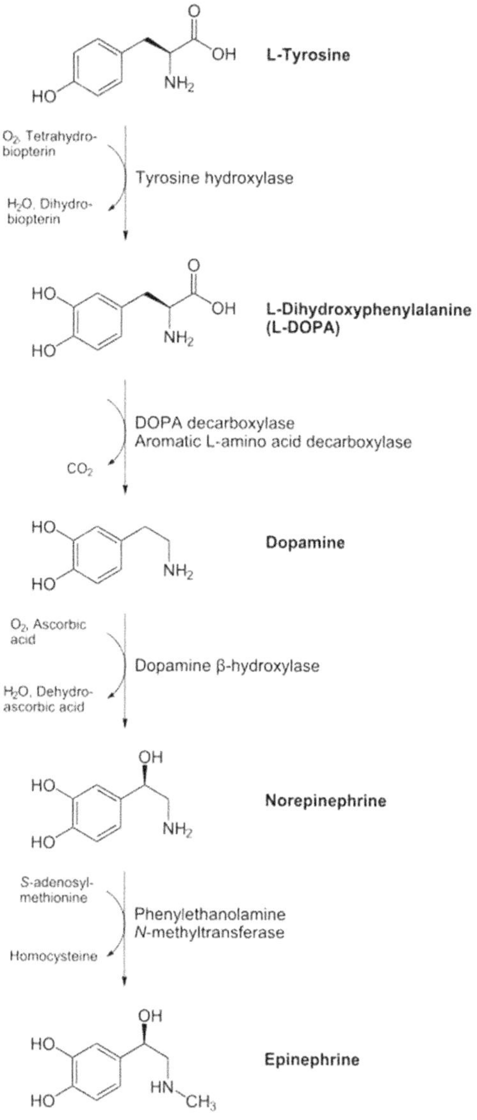

FIGURE 2 The chemical biosynthetic pathway for catecholamines utilizes the same pathway (substrates and cofactors) in microorganisms as it does in animals (47). Courtesy of NEUROtiker, licensed under CC-BY-SA 3.0 (https://creativecommons.org/licenses/by/3.0/us/).

time. Concepts that were in many ways the forerunner of modern thinking in the ability of the microbiota-gut-brain axis to influence behavior (discussed later in this article) were advanced by a number of individuals at the time (17).

From the early to mid-20th century, both clinicians and microbiologists were aware of the association of endocrinology and microbiology thanks in large measure to the cases of epinephrine and gas gangrene reported in the literature. In fact, these researchers early on identified the mechanism by which the association of epinephrine with *Clostridium perfringens*, the causative agent of gas gangrene, often proved to be a fatal one for the patient. Prior to the advent of disposable syringes, metal needles and glass syringes were reused constantly between patients, with only a cursory cleaning in alcohol. Patient to patient transmission of infectious disease was frequently encountered due to the inadequate alcohol treatment of syringe needles, which could only marginally kill actively growing (vegetative) bacterial cells, but not bacterial spores. As is well understood today, certain vegetative bacteria such as *C. perfringens*, can undergo sporulation. Such spores, which are formed from the vegetative cells under conditions of nutritional deprivation, are totally resistant to alcohol treatment and can only be killed by autoclaving. From those early reports (6) it was determined that a previously used syringe needle that had been employed to treat a gas gangrene patient was then used to administer epinephrine to a patient for urticaria. Within 6 hours a fatal fulminating gas gangrene infection developed. These reports noting the rapidity of infectious spread in patients receiving epinephrine injections with contaminated needles led A. A. Miles and colleagues in 1948 to begin a series of experiments examining the role of catecholamines in bacterial pathogenesis (18). In these experiments, the ability of epinephrine to modulate the *in vivo* growth of both Gram-positive and Gram-negative bacteria in a guinea pig model was conclusively demonstrated in tissue slices with enhancement of growth of bacteria coinjected with epinephrine that was log orders greater than that for control slices coinjected with saline (18). It should be noted that norepinephrine was not investigated. The authors concluded that the ability of epinephrine to dramatically enhance bacterial growth was due to some protective coating of the bacteria by epinephrine or an epinephrine-induced inhibition of immune cell function. The testing of each of these possible mechanisms, however, met with failure (18).

Significantly, at no time did these authors or others suggest that the action of epinephrine on bacterial growth was due to a direct, nonimmune effect as is discussed in this article. Interestingly, one technique that has been used by microbiologists to enable gas gangrene infections to "take" in mice has been the coinjection of epinephrine along with *C. perfringens* (19). As *C. perfringens* infections are difficult to establish in a mouse model, the finding that coinjection with epinephrine could enhance infectivity proved to be a valuable tool for medicinal chemists to use in the design of new chemotherapeutic drugs against infection. Interestingly, Traub (19) described that only fresh, and not oxidized, epinephrine solutions were successful in enhancing *C. perfringens* infectivity in mice. With a new generation of microbiologists and the advent of molecular techniques to evaluate potential antimicrobials *in vitro*, the use of animal models decreased, and this technique was no longer utilized. In a larger scope, this and the history that preceded it did not make its presence felt in mainstream microbiological thought. However, as detailed in the following section, a flurry of activity by a number of investigators highlighted the evolutionary relationship of host neurochemicals in microorganisms and what this meant for health and the pathogenesis of infectious disease.

WIDESPREAD PRESENCE OF NEUROCHEMICALS IN MICROORGANISMS

It is perhaps somewhat surprising to learn that neurochemicals which are more commonly associated with mammalian nervous systems are in fact widely dispersed through-out nature. For example, the biogenic amines, particularly the catecholamine family, have been identified in plants (20) as well as in-sects (21) and fish (22), in addition to most vertebrates. Although textbooks which deal with neurobiology, endocrinology, and neu-rophysiology certainly do not mention the presence of the very same neurochemicals in microorganisms, it should be recognized that their presence in microorganisms (both pro-karyotic and eukaryotic) had been the sub-ject of intensive research and debate in the 1970s and 1980s. But more importantly, these groups of investigators were among the first to ascribe an evolutionary basis to the shared presence of hormonal peptides in vertebrates and unicellular microorganisms (23, 24). Others, such as Mayer and Baldi (25), were among the first to propose that the evolu-tionary basis for these shared regulatory peptides represented a "universal structured code for biological communication" between individual systems. In discussing these earlier studies, the terms "hormonal peptide" and "regulatory peptide" are used as in the orig-inal text instead of "neurochemicals," as discussed in the note at the beginning of this article. The reason is that these early papers were chiefly concerned with shared peptides and not neurochemicals such as the catecholamines (23, 24).

What is perhaps most surprising to micro-biologists and neurobiologists is that micro-organisms themselves possess the very same neurochemicals that are found in vertebrates. The range of neurochemicals and the vari-ety of microorganisms in which they have been identified is very large (26). These in-clude, but are not limited to, acetylcholine (27, 28), histamine (29–31), serotonin (32–34), catecholamines (33–36), and agmatine (37, 38). All of the preceding neurochemicals are important components of an animal's nervous system. The presence of insulin-like material in microorganisms has also been ex-tensively documented, with its biological ac-tivity demonstrated in every microorganism

examined to date (26, 39). Other neurochemi-cals isolated from microorganisms which have been shown to have biological activity in mammalian cells include corticotropin from *Tetrahymena pyriformis* (40), somato-statin from *Bacillus subtilis* (41), and proges-terone from *Trichophyton mentagrophytes* (42). Numerous other neurochemicals iden-tified by radioimmunoassay and chromato-graphic behavior, as well as the presence of the corresponding putative receptor, have also been demonstrated in various microor-ganisms (for reviews see references 23, 26, 43).

Investigators have debated the signifi-cance of such neurochemicals in microorga-nisms for decades. The most widely accepted theory concerns the use of such neurochemi-cals as a form of intercellular communication (24, 44). Indeed, studies have shown that the growth of colonies of *Escherichia coli* involves a high degree of specialization of function by individual bacteria (45, 46) and, presum-ably, the need for some form of intercellu-lar communication to accomplish this goal. It should not, therefore, be surprising that the development of intercellular signaling systems in animals has been proposed to be due to horizontal gene transfer from bac-teria (47). For example, the complete bio-synthetic pathway for the catecholamines is found in bacteria. This includes all the same substrates and cofactors that are used in ani-mals (47).

While the ubiquitous distribution of neuro-chemicals and receptors throughout nature is not fully appreciated in the fields of micro-biology and neurobiology, it should be borne in mind that this widespread distribution implies that microorganisms have had ample opportunity to interact with multicellular systems along a very long evolutionary time frame. For example, there is an extensive literature documenting the presence of neu-rochemicals in normal plant physiology extending from pollen germination to stimulation of flowering and catecholamines in particular (48). From an evolutionary

viewpoint, since the upregulation of neurochemicals in nonvertebrates is also temporally associated with times of increased rate
of infection susceptibility, bacteria have
probably evolved to exploit neurochemicals
as biomarkers of stress and thus host weak-
ness. It then follows during this evolutionary
process that organisms, such as plants that
have to combat bacterial challenges during
periods of stress, have developed means based
on interruption of the microorganisms-
neurochemical interface to combat stress-
induced infection.

Critically, evidence has been published that
supports this line of reasoning. In response to
the challenge with the plant pathogen *Pseudomonas syringae*, which causes bacterial
speck on the leaves of tomato plants, especially
during cold periods, tomato plants produce
the metabolite *p*-coumaroylnorepinephrine
(Fig. 3). As can be seen in Fig. 3, *p*-coumaroyl-
norepinephrine is a conjugate of hydroxycinnamic acid with norepinephrine. Although
the purported mechanism of action of *p*-
coumaroylnorepinephrine is in maintaining
plant cell wall integrity (49), no data was actually presented to demonstrate this facet of
activity. Instead a role for antimicrobial activity role was demonstrated by Zacares et al.
(50), who reported not only direct antimicrobial activity of *p*-coumaroyldopamine against
P. syringae, but also that tomato plants can also
synthesize the hydroxycinnamic acid amides
of dopamine to yield *p*-coumaroyldopamine
(50). Interestingly, the production of these
hydroxycinnamic acid amides of biogenic
amines has also been reported in as diverse
plant species as pepper (51–53), potato (54, 55),
and wheat (56), thereby indicating evolutionary conservation of an important metabolite
that is only produced in times of plant stress
to protect against bacterial pathogens. This
phenomenon highlights that microorganisms
can interact with potential hosts, be they other
bacteria, plants, insects, fish, or vertebrates,
through the microbial endocrinology-based
mechanism of shared neurochemicals. The
most thoroughly researched interactions be-

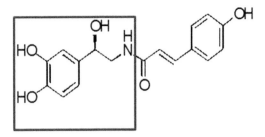

**FIGURE 3 The plant metabolite *p*-coumaroylnor-
epinephrine is synthesized in response to stress
and infection. This compound as well as *p*-
coumaroyldopamine are hydroxycinnamic acid
amides of norepinephrine (box designates norepinephrine part of the structure) and dopamine,
respectively, and have been shown to have direct
antimicrobial activity against the plant pathogen
Pseudomonas syringae (50).**

tween host (regardless whether the host is
plant, fish, or animal) and infectious microorganism have been concerned in some fashion
with stress, as will be discussed in the following sections.

Note Regarding Bidirectionality of Microbial Endocrinology

As discussed previously, there is a common
evolutionary pathway in which stress-related
neurochemicals first evolved in bacteria and,
through lateral gene transfer, were acquired
by mammals (47). This means that a "mechanistic bidirectional" signaling pathway for
these neurochemicals exists between microbiota and the host in which neurochemicals
produced by the host can influence the microorganism (Fig. 4A), and neurochemicals
produced by the microorganism, in turn,
can affect the host (Fig. 4B) (5, 57, 58).
Although the direction shown in Fig. 4A is
more thoroughly addressed in this article
than the one shown in Fig. 4B, the latter is
of no less significance in the ability of microorganisms to influence host health. For
example, the ability of probiotics to produce
neurochemicals has been known for decades
(28). Recently, this ability has been proposed
as a means to influence the microbiota-

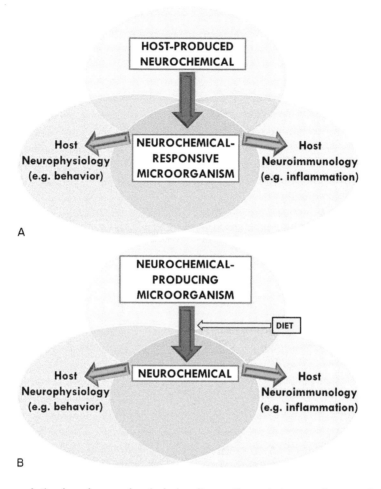

FIGURE 4 **The evolution-based neurochemical signaling pathway between microorganism and host means that a neurochemical(s) produced by the host can influence the microorganism (A), and at the same time a neurochemical(s) produced by the microorganism can, in turn, influence the host (B). As shown in part B, diet plays a crucial part in the latter because it provides the substrates and cofactors necessary for the microorganism to produce a specific neurochemical according to a biosynthetic pathway that is the same as that found in the host.**

gut-brain axis and thereby influence host brain and behavior as well as potentially influence disease processes that have a neuroimmune component and can thus be regulated by compounds that interact with neurochemical receptors on immune cells (59, 60). It should be noted that in Fig. 4B, diet is included as it can provide the substrates and cofactors needed by the microorganisms to produce the neurochemical as part of the biosynthetic pathway (61–63).

NEUROPHYSIOLOGICAL CONSIDERATIONS AND THEIR RELEVANCE TO MICROBIAL ENDOCRINOLOGY

In considering the microorganism-host interface as regards infectious disease, the neurophysiological environment that is present becomes a pivotal factor influencing whether a productive infection may develop. It must be stated at the outset of this section that the dynamic and multifactorial nature of both host and microbial factors underlying any infectious disease episode are highly complex. As such, it should be recognized that a microbial endocrinology-based mechanism represents only that which may be present at a specific time point during the infective process. Thus, it is expressly not the objective of this chapter to obviate or diminish in any way the multitude of other factors, whether host or microbial, that are involved in the pathogenesis of infectious disease.

At the same time, from a conceptual point of view, any consideration of the neurophysiological environment must take into account both the host and the microbe itself. This is because both are equally capable of producing and responding to neurochemical signals produced by one another. Further contributing complexity into this already complex equation is the recent demonstration that neurochemicals produced by one bacterial genera in the gut can affect another. A recent example of this can be found in the work by Strandwitz et al. (64), who showed that production of gamma-amino butyric acid (GABA) by one gut bacterial species is required for the growth of another. In this preliminary work, growth and subsequent isolation of the gut microbe *Flavonifractor* spp. from fecal matter was dependent upon a neighboring GABA-producing bacterium, such as *Bacteroides fragilis*. This preliminary report suggests that production of any neurochemical by a microbe may also affect neighboring microbial communities. Whether the consequences are beneficial or harmful in creating an environment which may favor or hinder any potential pathogen has yet to be investigated. Much will depend on a number of factors such as where in the gut the neurochemical-producing and neurochemical-responsive microbial communities are regionally located as well as whether the communities are luminal or mucosal associated. While an in-depth discussion of neurophysiology and the production of neurochemicals is beyond the scope of this

article (the reader is directed to standard neuroendocrinological texts such as reference 13), a discussion of the neurochemical environment of the two main avenues in which pathogenic microorganisms can enter a host is warranted.

Lung Environment

The lungs are extensively innervated by nerves belonging to the autonomic nervous system. For example, adrenergic and cholinergic components of the autonomic nervous system have been demonstrated to extensively innervate pulmonary tissue in the pig (65). Such extensive innervation serves a number of functions in the regulation of normal pulmonary homeostasis such as control of smooth muscle tone, secretion of mucus from submucosal glands, and blood flow within the lungs themselves (66). While there is understandably a large body of literature on autonomic nervous system–related receptors in the human regarding treatment option for a number of pulmonary–related disease states, there is little knowledge of the neural innervation of the bovine lung and correspondingly little, if in fact any, reports of the neuroendocrine environment within the nonhuman lung following a stress-related event. It can reasonably be assumed that given the extensive blood flow in the lung, as well as the abundant noradrenergic nerve innervation which is also present throughout the organ, that a stress-related event would result in substantial amounts of catecholamines being present within the lung space. These stress-released catecholamines would be then available to interact with any bacterial pathogens that might also be present in the lung. One study which indicated that this would indeed be the case was performed in sheep where endotoxin-mediated injury to the lung resulted in elevated plasma levels of both norepinephrine and epinephrine within the lung space (67).

If concentrations of catecholamines such as norepinephrine are indeed elevated within the stressed lung, it is likely that it would contribute to the infective process by directly interacting with bacterial pathogens. Anderson and Armstrong (68) have shown that the *in vitro* growth of the respiratory pathogen *Bordetella bronchiseptica* is greatly increased in the presence of norepinephrine and that this ability is, in part, mediated by the ability of norepinephrine to increase acquisition of transferrin-bound iron by *B. bronchiseptica.* That the interaction of stress-related neurochemicals with the lung may be an area worth investigating can also be seen in a study which examined the interaction of the *Mycoplasma hyopneumoniae* with norepinephrine. Global transcriptional analysis of *M. hyopneumoniae* following exposure to norepinephrine revealed numerous changes within the overall pattern of upregulation of protein expression and downregulation of general metabolism (69).

Gastrointestinal Environment

A cursory examination of the papers dealing with gastrointestinal infections and the host environment will find a predominance of investigations dealing with immune responses. Fewer numbers of reports have dealt with the host nervous system that innervates the gut, specifically the division of the nervous system known as the enteric nervous system (ENS) (70, 71). The ENS is composed of over 500 million neurons and is in constant communication with the central nervous system through nerves such as the vagus nerve, which directly connects portions of the gut to the brain. It is through this ENS-vagus connection that information derived from elements of the ENS that innervate the gut is transmitted to the brain (70). Further contributing to the amount of information obtained in the gut are the luminal epithelial chemosensors, which can respond to and transmit information regarding bacterial metabolites such as neuroactive compounds that are contained within the luminal space (72). This gut-to-brain communication has

been the subject of intensive study for many years and is now recognized to play an important role in the ability of gut-related pathologies to also result in mental health–related issues such as depression (73). The inclusion and recognition that microorganisms interact with elements of the ENS and thereby contribute to the information that is received by the brain concerning the physiological state of the gut has led to the relatively new field of study known as the microbiota-gut-brain axis (11).

To give an idea how extensive is the neuronal innervation of the gut and that such innervation can contribute to neurochemicals being present at the mucosal interface as well as in the mesenteric organs that are available to interact with microorganisms, the stomach provides an instructive example since it is essentially a dopaminergic organ producing the highest amount of dopamine in the body (74, 75). In fact, the entire length of the gut contains extensive arrays of neuronal innervation extending to the tips of the gut villi that produce biogenic amines which can be detected in the luminal space and are accessible to the microbiota (76, 77). Recent data has also shown that even epithelial cells are capable of producing neurochemicals such as the catecholamines dopamine and norepinephrine, albeit in the vaginal tract (78). Brosnahan et al. (78) reported that in response to infection with *Staphylococcus aureus*, the production of norepinephrine and dopamine by vaginal epithelial cells contributed to an enhanced state of inflammation as reflected by increased levels of the cytokines IL-6 and IL-8 and the chemokine MIP-3α. This recently reported ability of a vaginal epithelial cell to produce neurochemicals further highlights that bacterial-neurochemical interactions can occur at a number of host-bacterial interfaces and that the possible anatomical sites that can serve as an infectious entry point where microbial endocrinology can play a part in the infective process should not be thought to be restricted only to the gastrointestinal tract (79). Indeed, corneal epithelial cells have been reported to contain detectable intracellular concentrations of epinephrine that would be available to an infectious agent to utilize as it seeks to establish a productive infection (80). Thus, the examination of gut epithelial cells for the production of neurochemicals would seem warranted.

While host contributions of neurochemicals into the lumen of the gut, as well as presumably interstitial spaces in the lung, are easily understood due to extensive neuronal innervation in surrounding tissue, contributions by the microbiota itself have recently been recognized. Asano et al. (35) reported that while the catecholamines norepinephrine and dopamine were produced in appreciable physiological amounts in the luminal contents of specific pathogen-free mice, in germ-free animals substantially lower amounts were detected. Critically, whereas the majority of catecholamines in pathogen-free animals were structurally determined to be free and biologically active, those found in germ-free animals were present in a biologically inactive, conjugated form. Inoculation of germ-free animals with the flora from specific pathogen-free mice resulted in the production of free, biologically active catecholamines within the gut lumen. As such, this report clearly established that *in vivo* the microbiota is capable of producing neurochemicals that are commonly only associated with host production (35).

Other neurochemicals for which host levels were solely thought to be only due to host-derived production have also been found to have a portion contributed by the microbiota. Production of serotonin had been noted in the intestinal tract of the parasitic nematode *Ascaris suum* nearly three decades ago (81, 82). Comparison of the plasma level of serotonin in conventionally colonized mice with that in germ-free animals revealed that plasma serotonin levels were nearly 3-fold higher in the conventionally colonized mice as compared to the germ-free animals due to the presence of the microbiota in the conventionally colonized animals (83). More recently, Sridharan and colleagues demonstrated that gut microbiota in specific pathogen-free mice are able to produce serotonin (84).

STRESS AND INFECTIOUS DISEASE AS A MODEL OF THE RELEVANCE OF MICROBIAL ENDOCRINOLOGY FOR UNDERSTANDING MECHANISMS GOVERNING THE PATHOGENESIS OF INFECTIOUS DISEASE

The study of stress and how it relates to infectious disease has been the most intensely studied facet of microbial endocrinology to date. It provides the best example of how the study of the intersection of microbiology and neurobiology, otherwise referred to as microbial endocrinology, can lead to new insights regarding the ability of microorganisms to cause disease. The majority of our understanding of the neurochemical outflow from stress has been through the examination of blood-borne catecholamine levels (85), reflective of an extensive catecholaminergic system in the gut (86). A handful of studies have found high concentrations of neurochemicals being produced within the gut for which little explanation exists (75, 87). As already mentioned, the stomach is a dopaminergic organ producing the highest amount of dopamine in the body (74). The entire length of the gut contains extensive arrays of neuronal innervation extending to the tips of the gut villi that produce biogenic amines which can be detected in the luminal space and are accessible to the microbiota (76, 77, 79). Throughout the body, most of the neurochemical degradation that is associated with stress is due to enzymes contained within the gut, not by extragastrointestinal systems as was once commonly believed (85). The gut is, therefore, the site where stress and microbiota can interact with consequences for the pathogenesis of infectious disease.

Both physical and psychosocial stress, as well as alteration of circadian rhythm, have been shown to alter microbiota community structure within the gut (88–92). These studies have relied on the analysis of *ex vivo* biological samples, primarily fecal matter. Given that the gut is not homogenously innervated by the ENS, it is likely that the elaboration of stress-related neurochemicals is primarily located in areas of high innervation. Recent work performed in murine (89, 93) and porcine (94) models has shown that the ability of stress to alter community structure within the gut strongly depends on the anatomical region of the gut in which the community is located (presumably correlated with high enteric innervation as these studies did not also examine neuroanatomical innervation in the microbiota sample regions). This highlights the inability of simple examination of fecal material to gain an understanding of the degree to which stress can influence host microbiota. Because of these limitations in methods, regional differences in microbiota community structure throughout the different gut regions are only now beginning to be elucidated (89, 93, 94).

A pivotal study which demonstrated the rapidity with which the microbiota community structure within the gut can rapidly change due to the influx of host stress-related neurochemicals into the lumen was shown in a neurotoxin-induced model of trauma (95). One of the consequences of severe trauma is the massive release of stress-related neurochemicals, primarily the catecholamines (96, 97). At the same time, gut-related infections primarily due to the emergence of commensal microorganisms, such as *E. coli*, are a well-recognized surgical issue (98–100). The use of a neurotoxin-induced model of injury was able to demonstrate that these two events were not just correlated, but the sudden and massive release of stress-related neurochemicals was actually the cause of the altered microbial community structure in the gut and the emergence of potential Gram-negative pathogens (95). Within 24

hours following the administration of the neurotoxin 6-hydroxydopamine, the release of catecholamines from neurotoxin-injured enteric neurons into the lumen resulted in the rapid alteration of microbiota community from one that was dominated by Gram-positive taxa to one dominated by a single Gram-negative bacterial species, namely *E. coli* (95). Further evidence of the association of neuronal activity to microbiota composition was observed as injured nerves rehealed over a 2-week period; the microbiota community structure returned to normal (95). Examination of a number of commensal *E. coli* strains obtained from the feces of healthy donors demonstrated their ability to rapidly increase their rate of growth in response to physiological levels of norepinephrine, thereby suggesting that the release of catecholamines within the gut may be a contributory factor in trauma-related sepsis (101).

Note Regarding Experimental Design Used in the Examination of Microbial Endocrinology–Based Mechanisms in Infectious Disease

As the spectrum of neurochemicals that have been identified in microorganisms is quite extensive, there is not one mechanism that can be identified that applies to all. Although it could quite correctly be proposed that another reason for the lack of common mechanisms being identified to date is the sheer number and diversity of microorganisms, the principal reason can, in part, be found in the art of microbial culture itself. The use of the word "art" is not taken lightly since many of the media which are used today, especially the rich media, had their origins in clinical diagnosis and surgical treatment where the rapid growth and quantitation of bacterial numbers determined when to amputate an infected limb or to simply debride (102). These media were, and still remain, largely of animal origin and contain highly undefined source materials such as brains and hearts as can be found in a prototypical example of brain-heart infusion broth. The end result is that each microbiological medium will contain variable amounts of substrates and cofactors that can be used by the microorganism in the production of any one specific neurochemical. Further, the origin of the source material can change, especially if it is of animal origin. For example, media producers will obtain meat from the lowest-cost providers, leading to use of cattle from different regions and countries. In this common case, cattle will be of different genetic origins and undoubtedly will have been raised on different feed sources. The end result is that the concentration of neurochemical precursors and cofactors that are needed as part of the biochemical synthesis pathway for a particular neurochemical will vary greatly, leading to incorrect conclusions concerning the ability of a microorganism to produce or respond to a specific neurochemical.

An example of this can be seen in a report which concluded that the addition of epinephrine to trypticase soy broth did not result in any change in growth (103). The authors did not even consider that the medium employed already allowed optimal growth of their test bacterial species, which in this case was *S. aureus*. Further increases in growth were therefore highly unlikely. The principal difference between this report from Magee et al. (103) and the large numbers of other reports discussed in this article which have demonstrated the ability of a wide range of microbial species to respond to catecholamines is that the former used a rich microbiological medium while the latter studies used more *in vivo*–relevant media. That an incorrect interpretation of *in vivo* results can arise from results based on a less than ideal *in vitro* experimental design can be seen in a report which demonstrated the ability of epinephrine at a wound site to increase the rate of *S. aureus* growth by log orders over the nonepinephrine control (104). In explaining this *in vivo* result, Tran et al. (104)

dismissed any consideration of a direct effect of the epinephrine on the microorganism itself based on the *in vitro* results obtained by Magee et al. (103) and instead ascribed the result due to inhibition of immune responses, although prior reports, such as those by Miles and colleagues (18, 105), found no evidence of immune suppression as a mechanism by which epinephrine potentiated intradermal infections. It should be noted that subsequent studies have shown that epinephrine actually potentiates the ability of neutrophils to accumulate at the site of infection (106), which would lead to less bacterial growth, not more.

Other considerations in experimental design have been covered in detail elsewhere (for review see reference 107). Among the specific points that need to be emphasized in addition to those already discussed regarding medium selection is that of inoculum density. O'Donnell et al. (108) reported that the lower the inoculum density in *in vitro* culture, the greater the response to exogenously added catecholamines. This is not an unexpected result if considered from an infectious disease standpoint where the host most often encounters not high infectious loads, but instead, low doses that then result in disease. Inoculum densities in the millions or even hundreds of thousands of colony forming units in tissue culture are not reflective of the *in vivo* situation, where as little as 10 colony forming units of an infectious bacterium such as *E. coli* O157:H7 can result in infection (109). Utilization of doses of microorganisms that reflect the amount that actually results in the development of a productive infection in the host is critical to elucidating the mechanism(s) by which host and microbial factors interact in the pathogenesis of infection. As such, the overall consideration that must govern any examination of the microbial endocrinology–based mechanisms underlying the pathogenesis of infectious disease is the design of an experimental system which more closely mimics the *in vivo* milieu that the microorganism finds itself in at the time of initiation of the pathogenic process.

Throughout this article, stress has served as a unifying theme to illustrate the extent to which microbial endocrinology plays a role in infectious disease. This is not as much owing to any specific editorial design but instead due to the majority of publications which have utilized stress-related neurochemicals in experimental design. As such, the mechanisms underlying the ability of the main family of stress-related neurochemicals, the catecholamines (Fig. 2), to influence the pathogenesis of infectious disease will be the primary focus of this section. Other neurochemicals not related to the stress response will also be discussed following the catecholamines.

Catecholamine biochemistry

Principal among the catecholamines that are released during stress events are epinephrine from the adrenal medulla and norepinephrine from sympathetic nerve terminals. Interest in the role that catecholamines may play in bacterial pathogenesis has been heightened by the demonstration that catecholamines can directly stimulate bacterial growth and elaboration of virulence-associated properties as well as production of autoinducer-like substances (4, 9, 77, 108, 110–117). The biochemical pathway for the synthesis of catecholamines is L-dopa (most commonly derived from food sources) → dopamine → norepinephrine → epinephrine (Fig. 2). Given the close structural similarity between the 2,3-dihydroxybenzoylserine ring of catecholamines to the catecholate siderophores, it is not surprising to find the involvement of iron as a mechanism (113).

The question may be asked whether most of the results seen are simply due to the catecholamine-facilitated provision of iron. Results from a number of studies in which iron was *not* a limiting factor demonstrate

that this is not the case. These include, but are not limited to, studies such as that of Peterson et al. (118), who showed that exposure to norepinephrine increased the ratio of horizontal gene transfer of antibiotic-resistant genes between enteric pathogens. They further demonstrated that the ability of norepinephrine to increase horizontal gene transfer between bacteria was blocked by α but not β-adrenergic receptor antagonists and that, critically, these results were observed in iron-replete medium.

Other studies have also demonstrated that the effects of stress-related neurochemicals are not simply due to the facilitated provision of iron; some of these include studies in which exclusively enteric pathogens such as *Yersinia enterocolitica* increase growth in the presence of norepinephrine and dopamine, but not when exposed to epinephrine (4), despite having been shown in other studies to increase provision of iron (113). This specificity in the utilization of specific catecholamines may have an evolutionary explanation in that bacteria may have developed the ability to recognize host neurochemicals based on the evolutionary association with specific anatomical regions of the host. In the case of epinephrine in the gut, enteric microorganisms would not encounter this neurochemical since the neurons contained within the ENS that innervates the entire length of the gut do not possess the enzyme phenylethanolamine-N-methyltransferase, which is needed for conversion of norepinephrine to epinephrine in the catecholamine biosynthetic pathway (Fig. 2) (119). As such, intestinal pathogens which are not commonly associated with extraintestinal infection, such as *Y. enterocolitica*, have not developed the ability to respond to the stress neurochemical epinephrine despite its ability to facilitate the provision of iron.

Work performed in the 1970s further points out that iron is simply not the only mechanism. Okamura et al. (120) demonstrated that while dopamine and norepinephrine can be oxidized by membrane-bound tyramine oxidase at relative rates of 99% and 77%, respectively, epinephrine cannot be utilized at all. Again, specificity in the utilization of individual members of the catecholamine family of stress-related neurochemicals by unique microorganisms provides key insights into mechanisms and demonstrates that we need to look beyond simple, albeit critical, mechanisms such as the provision of iron. That iron provision may be happening at the same time as part of an infectious microorganism's response to any neurochemical should not obscure the search for other mechanisms. More recently, Xu et al. in 2015 (121) demonstrated that analysis of the transcriptomic profiles of the foodborne pathogen *Campylobacter jejuni* NCTC 11168 grown in iron-restricted medium in the presence or absence of norepinephrine or epinephrine revealed that each catecholamine elicited the expression of unique numbers of genes. For example, of the 183 and 156 genes that were differentially expressed by *C. jejuni* as a result of growth in epinephrine- or norepinephrine-containing medium, respectively, only 102 genes were common to both catecholamine conditions. Those genes that were differentially expressed encompassed a wide variety of cellular functions beyond simply iron uptake extending from DNA repair and metabolism to oxidative stress response and ribosomal protein biosynthesis as well as virulence and motility (121). In a similar fashion, earlier work by Li et al. (122) demonstrated that culture of the respiratory pathogen *Actinobacillus pleuropneumoniae* with epinephrine or norepinephrine resulted in the differential expression of 158 and 105 genes, respectively, as compared to controls. Critically, among the catecholamine-induced differentially regulated genes, only 18 genes were common to both epinephrine and norepinephrine, which suggested that bacterial pathogens such as *A. pleuropneumoniae* may possess multiple responsive systems for individual members of the catecholamine family that impact bacterial physiology.

One of these possible neurochemical-related mechanisms may be the induction of growth factors produced by microorganisms as part of their response to neurochemicals. The first description of a neurochemical-induced growth factor produced by a bacterium was reported in 1996 when *E. coli* O157:H7 cocultured with norepinephrine resulted in a supernatant that contained a growth factor that when applied to naïve *E. coli* O157:H7 increased the growth rate over 5 logs as compared to controls (110). Remarkably, only amounts as low as 0.391% of conditioned supernatant from norepinephrine-stimulated bacteria were needed to induce rapid growth in naïve cells. Subsequent work demonstrated that a number of bacterial strains were capable of production of neurochemical conditioned medium that could stimulate the growth of naïve cells (123). Use of this neurochemical-produced conditioned media has been successfully employed in the resuscitation of *Salmonella enterica* serovar Typhimurium and enterohemorrhagic *E. coli* from the viable but nonculturable state (124) as well as used in the design of a new selective chromogenic plating medium for the identification of *Bacillus cereus* (125). To date, concerted attempts at elucidating the chemical structure of this neurochemical-induced growth factor have been unsuccessful (M. Lyte, unpublished work), although prior work has shown it not to be a siderophore (110). However, a report by Burton et al. (126) disputed the nonsiderophore nature of the norepinephrine-conditioned medium and argued that it was in fact enterobactin and its breakdown product 2,3-dihydroxybenzoylserine.

Catecholamine receptor pharmacology

Catecholamines bind to specific receptors: norepinephrine to adrenergic receptors (divided into α and β types) and dopamine and related synthetic compounds based on catecholamine structure such as dobutamine to dopaminergic receptors (divided into D1 to D5 subtypes). Dobutamine is a synthetic derivative of dopamine and is widely used in the treatment of congestive heart failure. Although the vast majority of catecholamine receptor pharmacology has been done in mammalian systems, the characterization of adrenergic receptors in nonmammalian systems utilizing pharmacological reagents developed for mammalian systems has enabled the identification of adrenergic receptors in *T. pyriformis* (127) and *Trypanosoma cruzi* (128). The small numbers of studies that have attempted to examine adrenergic receptor pharmacology in bacteria have produced conflicting results. The first reported study which examined the ability of adrenergic receptor antagonists to block the ability of norepinephrine to induce growth of *E. coli* suggested the presence of a novel non-α, non-β adrenergic receptor in a variety of Gram-negative bacteria (129). Work by Sperandio and colleagues (130, 131) has shown that α-adrenergic antagonists could block the ability of catecholamines to induce the production of autoinducer-3 in *E. coli* O157:H7, suggesting cross-communication between host endocrine signals and bacterial quorum sensing system(s). Additionally, Freestone et al. (132) demonstrated the ability of involvement of dopaminergic antagonists to block catecholamine-induced growth in *E. coli* O157:H7, *S. enterica*, and *Y. enterocolitica*.

Catecholamines in the hospital setting and relevance to infectious disease susceptibility

A majority of infections that are life-threatening occur in the hospital setting (133). Among these nosocomial pathogens, two specific genera stand out: *Staphylococcus* spp. (134) and *Clostridium* spp. (135). In the case of the former, coagulase-negative staphylococci, specifically *Staphylococcus epidermidis*, and for the latter *Clostridium difficile*, are the primary species contributing to high rates of infection (135–137).

In the hospital setting patients are exposed to high levels of stress either through clinical protocols involved in treatment or through the administration of drugs that dramatically elevate the level of systemic catecholamines. Treatments that contribute to high levels of circulating stress-related neurochemicals include mechanical ventilation and parenteral feeding. Mechanical ventilation is a method of assisted breathing in which positive pressure is applied via an endotracheal or tracheostomy tube to force air into the patient's lungs. Parenteral nutrition refers to feeding nutritional formula to a patient via an intravenous tube thereby bypassing the normal oral route of digestion. Human studies have shown that both mechanical ventilation and parenteral nutrition result in a sustained elevation of circulating levels of catecholamines (138, 139). As will be described in the following sections, these procedures ultimately play an iatrogenic role in the development of nosocomial infections.

Coagulase-negative staphylococci as nosocomial pathogens

Of the 5 million intravascular catheters employed each year, approximately 250,000 catheter-related bloodstream infections are reported, with an attributable mortality of 12 to 25% (140, 141). The organisms most commonly isolated from indwelling medical devices belong to the coagulase-negative staphylococci (C-NS). The C-NS constitute a major component of the skin microflora and were for many years regarded as saprophytes, or at least as organisms with no or low virulence. However, the C-NS, in particular *S. epidermidis*, have become recognized as serious nosocomial pathogens associated with indwelling medical devices such as catheters (142–145) and prosthetic joints (146). The increasing incidence of infections caused by these bacteria can be attributed to their particular affinity for the biomaterials of the invasive technologies integral to much of modern medicine. In association with appropriate biomaterial surfaces, such as those ranging from polysilicone in catheters to steel in hip replacements, *S. epidermidis* adheres and proliferates to form biofilms, highly complex structures that represent functional communities of microbes (147, 148). Under-standing the environmental factors that can contribute to the ability of C-NS to act as nosocomial pathogens would be of obvious benefit to high-risk patients.

Evidence to support a role for catecholamines in the formation of *S. epidermidis* biofilms

S. epidermidis biofilms are multilayered mi-crobial cell clusters embedded within a diffuse extracellular polysaccharide (EPS) matrix often referred to as slime (149). Although the mechanics of biofilm formation are not yet fully understood (150), it is generally agreed that the process takes place in two stages: rapid attachment to the surface followed by a prolonged phase that involves cellular pro-liferation and intercellular adhesion (151). Adherence depends on cell-surface character-istics of the bacteria, in particular, hydropho-bicity (152, 153), the presence of adhesive surface-associated proteins (154, 155), EPS production (156), the nature of the biomaterial (157, 158), and the presence on the indwelling device of deposited host proteins, such as fibrinogen, fibronectin, and vitronectin (151). Characterization of transposon mutants of *S. epidermidis* deficient in biofilm formation (159, 160) has shown that initial attachment is mediated in part by the *atlE* gene product, a surface-associated autolysin which also possesses vitronectin-binding activity (161). Intercellular adhesion and the formation of multicellular layers requires EPS synthesis, which is composed of the polysaccharide intercellular adhesin (PIA), a linear 1,6-linked glucosaminoglycan (149). Production of PIA is dependent on the *icaABC* operon (162). While relatively little is known about control of *atlE* expression in *S. epidermidis*, synthesis of PIA has recently been shown to be phase-variable (163).

Initial studies had shown that among the Gram-positive bacteria that could re-spond to micromolar concentrations of neu-rochemicals were members belonging to *Staphylococcus* genera (164). In particular,

norepinephrine increased the planktonic growth of *S. epidermidis* by log orders (164). As the vast majority of infections occur not as planktonic growth, but instead as biofilms, Lyte et al. (114) examined the ability of the catecholamines, and synthetic drugs based on catecholamines such as dobutamine that are most often employed in the clinical setting, to influence the formation of *S. epidermidis* biofilms. The exposure of *S. epidermidis* to pharmacologically relevant concentrations of the widely used inotropic drugs, do-butamine and norepinephrine, resulted in increased biofilm growth and production of EPS as shown by both scanning electron microscopy and immunofluorescence, re-spectively (114). In demonstrating catechol-amine and catecholamine-based synthetic drug-induced induction of *S. epidermidis* biofilm, two methodological aspects were employed that differed from previous stud-ies of biofilm formation and emphasize the importance of experimental design in the examination of possible microbial endocri-nology–based mechanisms in an infective pro-cess as already discussed.

First, only 10 to 100 colony forming units of *S. epidermidis* were used to seed the bio-materials (114). This small amount of bacteria was chosen to reflect physiologically relevant infecting doses that were likely to be encoun-tered in the clinical setting. This is in con-trast to the majority of prior biofilm studies which have used log-orders higher amounts of bacteria to establish biofilms (165–167). Second was the use of the culture conditions which employed a plasma-supplemented minimal media. This also differs from other studies which have used rich microbiological media to study biofilm formation, but which may be argued do not reflect *in vivo* condi-tions in which host factors present in plasma which are recognized to play a role in initial bacterial adhesion are not present. This observation is of particular consequence since a number of previous publications had noted that plasma actually prevented *S. epi-dermidis* biofilm formation (167–169). Thus, this work was the first demonstration that catecholamines and synthetic drugs based on the catecholamine structure may serve as an etiological factor in the bacterial colonization of indwelling medical devices due to their ability to stimulate *S. epidermidis* growth and biofilm formation (114, 164).

Possible mechanisms by which stress-related neurochemicals and catecholamine-based synthetic drugs influence infection in the clinical setting

Due to their catechol moieties (as previously discussed), catecholamines have been shown to facilitate the provision of iron from host iron-sequestering transferrin enabling *S. epidermidis* biofilm formation (114, 164). The recognized inability of *S. epidermidis* to grow in normal human plasma without extra iron supplementation has been ascribed to the presence of transferrin (170, 171). The ability of transferrin to sequester iron, coupled with the lack of a demonstrable mechanism by which *S. epidermidis* could acquire such bound iron except in the presence of therapeutic administration of catecholamines and synthetic catecholamine-based drugs, suggests that the use of catecholamine antagonists may provide a means by which to prevent biofilm formation (172).

Another report which has expanded the relevance of understanding microbial endocrinology–based mechanisms in the clinical setting concerns the ability of catecholamines to facilitate physiological recovery of antimicrobial-damaged bacteria (173). In an effort to decrease the incidence of catheter-related bloodstream infections, the use of antimicrobial-impregnated catheters has taken on increasing usage (174, 175). However, the utilization of these catheters, which are usually impregnated on their surface with the antimicrobials rifampin and minocycline, has not decreased the incidence of catheter-related bloodstream infections. Freestone et al. (173) demonstrated that while exposure of C-NS to concentrations of rifampin and minocycline that

exceeded the minimum inhibitory concentration resulted in nonviable bacteria as confirmed by failure to grow in culture, the addition of norepinephrine and dopamine at clinically relevant concentrations resulted in the physiological and growth recovery of antimicrobial-damaged C-NS.

More recent examinations of the role of catecholamines in the formation of biofilms and their relevance to the clinical setting have been published. Lanter et al. (176) have reported that addition of physiologically relevant amounts of norepinephrine induced the ability of individual clusters of bacteria under conditions of low iron availability to break off from established *Pseudomonas aeruginosa* biofilms. The authors proposed that this may be a mechanism by which bacteria such as *P. aeruginosa* that can colonize atherosclerotic plaques can break off due to the hormonal state of the patient, thereby causing disruption of the plaque integrity ultimately increasing the chance of heart attack and stroke (176). An earlier report by Freestone et al. (177) had demonstrated that catecholamines and catecholamine-based synthetic drugs may also be a causative factor contributing to the ability of *P. aeruginosa* to colonize the airways of critically ill patients, leading to ventilator-associated pneumonia. Another clinically important bacterium that forms biofilms as part of its infectious etiology, *Streptococcus pneumoniae*, has also been shown to be responsive to neurochemicals. Sandrini et al. (178) demonstrated that *S. pneumoniae*, which is responsible for community-acquired and nosocomial pneumonia, is responsive to clinically relevant concentrations of norepinephrine such that exposure not only increased the expression of genes that are functionally relevant in metabolism and subsequent host colonization, but also resulted in increased growth and biofilm formation.

It must be emphasized, however, that (as already discussed previously) the ability to provide iron may not be the sole mechanism by which catecholamines and catecholamine-based synthetic drugs may interact with microorganisms in the clinical setting to promote growth and alter virulence-related properties. Data from other laboratories have shown that catecholamines may modulate bacterial physiology and virulence in non-growth-, noniron-related contexts. Vlisidou et al. (179) used a ligated ileal loop model of virulence to show that norepinephrine significantly enhanced attachment of *E. coli* 0157:H7 to calf intestinal tissue, while it has been reported that epinephrine stimulates expression of a type III protein secretion apparatus and motility in *E. coli* 0157 in a *LuxS* mutant as well as production of an autoinducer-3 molecule (180). Interestingly, both the autoinducer-3 and epinephrine-dependent motility responses could be blocked by the adrenergic receptor blockers propranolol and phentolamine, suggesting the presence of a receptor-mediated, non-iron-related, process.

More recently, Pasupuleti et al. (181) has shown that the ability of norepinephrine to function as a chemoattractant for enterohemorrhagic *E. coli* is dependent on the conversion of norepinephrine to 3,4-dihydroxymandelic acid following the norepinephrine-dependent induction of genes encoding tyramine oxidase. The continued production of a chemoattractant by enterohemorrhagic *E. coli* already colonizing the intestinal mucosa due to exposure to host norepinephrine has been proposed by the authors to serve as a recruitment vehicle by which additional *E. coli*, and potentially other bacteria, may be attracted to the infection site, thereby contributing to the pathogenic process (181). And as regards the role of catecholamines in the ability of bacteria to attach onto surfaces as a first step in biofilm formation, recent data has further shown the involvement of non-iron-dependent mechanisms. For example, Park et al. (182) has demonstrated that exposure of engineered *E. coli* which displays a catecholamine-based surface moiety results in increased adhesion onto a variety of surface materials.

SPECTRUM OF INFECTIOUS DISEASE–ASSOCIATED MICROORGANISMS IS EXTENSIVE AND GROWING

As can be expected, the more one digs into the literature to find instances of where neurochemicals and bacteria have been examined, the more one finds papers which provide tantalizing clues that these two systems, one the neurophysiological and the other microbial, could interact in totally unexpected ways. For example, *C. jejuni* is a highly prevalent food-borne pathogen that requires a microaerophilic environment in the laboratory for its propagation. However, the addition of norepinephrine to the microbiological growth medium was shown by Bowdre et al. to result in tolerance to and growth of *C. jejuni* in an aerobic environment (183). At the time, the wider implications of this important finding as to the role of neurochemicals in general in the pathogenesis of infectious disease had not yet been fully envisioned.

Examination of the literature often reveals interesting reports of the association of neurochemicals and infectious disease in the same manner as in the case of the early reports on the role of catecholamines in the development of gas gangrene. These reports can stimulate insightful ideas that inform the design of microbial endocrinology–based experimental design. For example, it has been well recognized that certain strains of bacteria that are associated with food spoilage can produce histamine (184–186). Based on these reports, an examination of microorganisms that can colonize the respiratory tract revealed that infectious bacteria can produce histamine by decarboxylation of histidine (29). The possible role of bacteria-produced histamine as an inflammatory mediator contributing to respiratory illness was subsequently proposed (187). Subsequent to these studies, Voropaeva (188) examined a large cohort of microbial strains isolated from children with bronchial asthma for antimicrobial resistance and the ability to produce histamine (188). It was demonstrated that a positive correlation existed between the ability of a particular infectious strain to produce histamine and antimicrobial resistance. Whether this could causally account for the ability of the infectious microorganisms to colonize the airways of children with bronchial asthma has yet to be shown.

As already noted, a number of groups have shown the ability of neurochemicals to influence virulence-related properties of infectious microorganisms in an increasing number of studies (4, 9, 77, 108, 110–117). In terms of known virulence factors that contribute to invasion of host cells, exposure of enterotoxigenic *E. coli* to norepinephrine was shown to increase the expression of the K99 pilus adhesion that facilitates attachment to the gastrointestinal mucosa by over 235-fold (111). Stress-related neurochemicals have been shown to increase conjugative transfer of antibiotic-resistant genes between enteric bacteria, thereby contributing to the increased prevalence of antibiotic-resistant food-borne bacterial pathogens in the food supply (118). Additionally, the ability of monoamines such as norepinephrine and dopamine to alter gene expression has now been shown for a number of pathogenic microorganisms including *M. hyopneumoniae* (69), *S. enterica* serovar Typhimurium (189), and *Vibrio parahaemolyticus* (190).

More recently, the motility and biofilm formation of the aquatic Gram-negative bacterium *Vibrio harveyi* has been shown to be responsive to norepinephrine and dopamine (191). Since *V. harveyi* is an opportunistic pathogen for a wide variety of marine animals including shrimp and oysters, it has been suggested that stress in these marine animals (such as cold stress) and the subsequent elaboration of stress-related neurochemicals represent a microbial endocrinology–based mechanism facilitating infection (192). Similar results have also now been reported by others for other pathogenic *Vibrio* spp. such as *Vibrio anguillarum* and *Vibrio campbellii* (193).

It should be noted that although this article has dealt mainly with prokaryotic microorganisms, the role of neurochemicals in infectious disease involving eukaryotic microorganisms such as yeasts and parasites has also been well documented. In the case of yeasts, the production and response of yeasts to neurochemicals such as the stress-related biogenic amines has been demonstrated (194). An excellent review of the role of endocrinology in the pathogenesis of fungal infections has been published (195). Interestingly, reports dealing with the interaction of parasites with neurochemicals have also consistently appeared in the literature. For example, *Plasmodium falciparum* was shown to produce a somatostatin-like peptide similar in structure to that of mammalian somatostatin (196). The ability of intracellular forms of the parasite *T. cruzi* to differentiate from the amastigote for the trypomastigote form was shown to be able to be triggered when exposed to adrenergic ligands present in host cells (197). Coppi et al. (198) have reported that catecholamines could induce the ability of the enteric parasites *Entamoeba invadens* and *Entamoeba histolytica* to differentiate into the infectious cyst stage. Remarkably, only mucin had previously been shown to be able to induce cyst stage formation (199). As such, the authors have proposed that *Entamoeba* spp. possess an autocrine catecholamine system to stimulate encystation and thereby increase subsequent infectivity for other animals (198).

Another protozoal parasite, *Cryptosporidium parvum*, has also been shown to be responsive to a neurochemical. Pretreatment of infant mice with agmatine inhibited infection with *C. parvum* by altering the cellular metabolism to such a degree that colonization of the intestine was reduced (200). Agmatine, which is a polyamine synthesized within the gastrointestinal tract, has a number of functions including that as a novel neurotransmitter whose spectrum of host targets within the nervous system is still poorly understood (201, 202). This incomplete understanding of the cellular targets for agmatine only further highlights the relevance of the intersection of microbiology and neurobiology that forms the theoretical basis of microbial endocrinology. Since agmatine is also synthesized by bacteria (37), the possibility that a bacteria-produced neurochemical affecting host neurophysiology must be considered. Such bacteria-host interactions which are governed by a neurochemical produced by both points out the bidirectionality of microbe-host interactions inherent in a microbial endocrinology–based approach.

MICROBIAL ENDOCRINOLOGY AND THE MICROBIOTA-GUT-BRAIN AXIS: WHY IT MATTERS IN INFECTIOUS DISEASE

The concept that bacteria in the gut can communicate with the brain, thereby influencing behavior, and that the host nervous system can, in turn, influence the composition of the gut microbiota, has given rise to the concept of a microbiota-gut-brain axis (11). An ever-growing number of studies have demonstrated the ability of bacteria to influence brain function, for which a number of possible mechanistic routes have been proposed (10, 12, 59, 60, 203–207). Due to shared neurochemicals between host and microbe, microbial endocrinology has been proposed as one of the mechanisms by which such reciprocal communication between brain (nervous system) and microorganisms in the gut can occur (208, 209).

A number of anatomical similarities can be found between the ENS and the central nervous system (210). Multiple pathways underlie communication from the gastrointestinal tract to the brain, with sensory neurons in the gastrointestinal tract providing a route, via the vagus nerve, to provide early signaling to the brain regarding the presence of potential pathogens within the gut (211, 212). These studies clearly demonstrate that host-derived central nervous system–based mechanisms are capable of

detecting changes in the microbial flora contained within the gastrointestinal system. From an evolutionary viewpoint, this should make elegant sense that over the long evolutionary period in which host and microorganisms have coexisted, that this evolutionary symbiosis should, in addition to the well-recognized functions of nutrition etc., also contain an element in which monitoring of the microbiota is in the best interests of the host. The bidirectional nature of microbial endocrinology implies that the microbiota also responds to the host with the microbiota-gut-brain axis (7, 208, 209).

While the role of microbial endocrinology in the microbiota-gut-brain axis as regards behavior is straightforward and immediately apparent, its role in infectious disease may be less so but of no less consequence. Microbial endocrinology, as previously discussed, is an evolutionary-based concept (2, 5). And as highlighted already, a number of past investigators have also utilized evolution as a theoretical basis for examining the possible health implications of shared messenger molecules between host and microbe, albeit not in the context of infectious disease (23–25, 213). Such consideration of clinical-related disease which has an infectious disease etiology, as will be discussed in the following section, holds the potential for the development of new clinical-based therapies in which the consideration of the recognition of the infectious agent as a neurochemical-responsive organism plays a central role.

SIRS: A Possible Model for the Use of Microbial Endocrinology in Treatment of Disease with Infectious Etiology

As the prototypical example of how microbial endocrinology can lead to potential new therapies in which the microbiota-gut-brain is involved, the clinical condition of systemic inflammatory response syndrome (SIRS) will be employed. SIRS is one of the leading causes of mortality and morbidity in the surgical intensive care unit (214). The development of SIRS is characterized by the production of multiple cytokines as part of an inflammatory cascade due to an insult that may be of infectious origin (215). The incidence of mortality and morbidity increases dramatically if SIRS progress on to multiple organ dysfunction syndrome or multiple organ failure (216). While a number of theories, most prominently the gut as a motor organ of failure (217–219), have offered some insight into the pathophysiology, treatment still remains problematic (220). Ongoing research into the microbial-based mechanisms responsible for injury-induced alterations in gut bacterial diversity has continued in an effort to identify mechanisms that can lead to effective therapies (221–223). For example, enteral nutrition contributes favorably to changes in bacterial populations, but also to maintenance of mucosal integrity including the nerves within the villi that serve as sensory reporters of gut status, and its use has contributed to a reduction in mortality (224). Intestinal villi are innervated by catecholaminergic nerves within the ENS. Although these adrenergic nerves terminate near the basolateral membranes of the mucosal epithelial cells within the gut, they are nonetheless responsive to general sympathetic activity since enteric adrenergic neurons are located in the prevertebral ganglia outside the gut wall (extrinsic to the gut) and hence are susceptible to modulation by central nervous system activity.

The continued development of new theories emphasizing the interplay of the intestinal mucosa with the altered gut microbiota emphasizes the critical role of the gut microbiota in the development of inflammation. Indeed, use of a probiotic/synbiotic combinatory therapy has resulted in improvement in mortality and morbidity in critically ill patients to reduce complications such as the development of SIRS and multiple organ failure following trauma (225). However, none of the current treatments specifically address the contributory role of altered bidirectional gut-brain neural communication resulting from damaged intestinal mucosal integrity to the development of inflammation.

Acknowledging that infectious agents are only infrequently isolated from patients who have already undergone multiple rounds of antibiotics during hospitalization, the proposed microbial endocrinology–based hypothesis proposes that the central nervous system promotes an inflammatory response directed against an iatrogenically transformed enteric microbiota. During hospitalization, the immediate and sustained induced changes in microbial ecology coupled with the widespread damage to intestinal villi, and the enteric nerves which innervate them, along with the overall high levels of circulating catecholamines, all synergistically exacerbate the altered neurophysiology of the individual. Critically, these profound gut-related changes cannot go unnoticed by the brain in the overall regulation of homeostasis and may, therefore, represent the perceived threat that is responsible for the ever-escalating inflammatory response.

Why Current Treatment Regimens Promote Microbial Endocrinology–Based Interactions

As viewed from an evolutionary perspective, two distinct, but interrelated, phases evolve in the development of SIRS. In the immediate phase following the initial inciting traumatic event, the pronounced release of large amounts of stress-related catecholamines coupled with the loss of enteral nutrition leads to alteration of the gut microbiome, the so-called undrained abscess of multiple organ failure (226). Following trauma, altered bacterial diversity within the gut is well recognized to occur in the intensive care setting to the extent that the gut has long been viewed as a reservoir of occult infection (227). Animal models have revealed an association between the release of catecholamines and a dramatic shift from largely Gram-positive anaerobic bacteria to Gram-negative bacteria, with *E. coli* as the overwhelmingly predominant Gram-negative species increasing by log orders in absolute numbers (95, 228). Further, Alverdy et al. (229) demonstrated that increases in luminal levels of norepinephrine following surgical stress resulted in increased expression of the PA-I lectin/adhesin of *P. aeruginosa*, leading to greater attachment and colonization of the gut and increasing the eventual likelihood of lethal gut-derived sepsis. The gut has therefore long served as a focal point of inquiry (230).

Within the intensive care unit, interventional strategies may enhance the unwanted consequence of ramping up the inflammatory cycle. Interventional support, notably the use of total parenteral nutrition, exacerbated by the administration of synthetic catecholamine-based drugs, and mechanical ventilation, all contribute to increased sympathetic activation (138, 139). The resultant highly increased systemic level of catecholamines contributes to the maintenance of a Gram-negative bacterial population in the gut through direct neuroendocrine-bacterial interactions as defined by microbial endocrinology (231). The overall effect of current interventional care thus perpetuates the altered gut environment and most importantly provides continuous signaling to the central nervous system that the initial inflammatory response has been inadequate to deal with the altered gut microbiota. Indeed, as the patient progresses along a path leading to SIRS, heroic interventional support measures further increase the components of the "fight or flight response," thereby ensuring a continuing high level of circulating stress-related neurochemicals derived from both endogenous and exogenous sources. Thus, from an evolutionary perspective, the response of an organism to a threat (altered Gram-negative predominant gut microbiota perceived as an infectious threat) which has not been contained by an initial response (inflammatory response) is to continually increase that response until it proves effective. The end result of this interventional-driven evolutionary response is the continual ramping up of the inflammatory response and the eventual development of SIRS (231).

How a Microbial Endocrinology–Based Understanding Can Lead to New Treatment Modalities

Since one of the principal drivers of an altered, largely Gram-negative, microbiota in the gut is the continual provision of high levels of catecholamine-based synthetic drugs as previously discussed (as well, of course, as the patient's own trauma-induced host production), more judicious administration of such drugs, the currently accepted conversion from total parenteral nutrition to enteral nutrition, and the use of selective beta blockers should each diminish the overall stress response and allow the microbiota to return to a more normal composition. Beta blockers have already been used successfully in the management of severe pediatric burns to reverse burn injury–induced muscle-protein catabolism (232). Other points of entry exist that may serve as potential targets for therapeutic intervention. A dual motor system based on the microbial endocrinology and the evolutionary symbiosis between the gut and the brain has been proposed as the basis for the design of new treatment modalities for SIRS (231).

CONCLUDING THOUGHTS

In the nearly quarter of a century since the introduction of the proposal that microbial endocrinology has a role to play in the pathogenesis of infectious disease, increasing numbers of reports (as discussed in this article) have begun to examine the ability of a wide panoply of neurochemicals to influence the infectivity of microorganisms. There is a rich historical context dating back to the early 1930s which has shown that neurochemicals have a decisive role to play in infection. As already discussed, the use of an experimental design that seeks to more closely mimic the *in vivo* milieu will continue to play a critical role in furthering continued examination of the mechanisms by which microbial endocrinology can influence the pathogenesis of infectious disease. This is not an easy undertaking, as experiments cannot be conducted in the same manner that is widespread in current microbiological research, namely the use of rich medium that does not reflect the host environment that the microorganism must deal with during the infective process. And the continued development of the microbiota-gut-brain axis and its relevance regarding infection will continue to be an area of high interest. The intersection of microbiology and neurobiology as embodied in microbial endocrinology represents a translational-oriented research direction that may yield new insights into the mechanisms responsible for the development of infectious disease but also point the way to interrupt such interactions and in this aspect provide a new generation of anti-infective strategies.

CITATION

Lyte M. 2016. Microbial endocrinology in the pathogenesis of infectious disease. Microbiol Spectrum 4(2):VMBF-0021-2015.

REFERENCES

1. **Lyte M.** 1993. The role of microbial endocrinology in infectious disease. *J Endocrinol* **137:**343–345.
2. **Lyte M.** 2010. Microbial endocrinology: a personal journey, p 1–16. *In* Lyte M, Freestone PPE (ed), *Microbial Endocrinology: Interkingdom Signaling in Infectious Disease and Health.* Springer, New York.
3. **Lyte M.** 1992. The role of catecholamines in Gram-negative sepsis. *Med Hypotheses* **37:**255–258.
4. **Lyte M, Ernst S.** 1992. Catecholamine induced growth of Gram negative bacteria. *Life Sci* **50:**203–212.
5. **Lyte M.** 2004. Microbial endocrinology and infectious disease in the 21st century. *Trends Microbiol* **12:**14–20.
6. **Renaud M, Miget A.** 1930. Role favorisant des perturbations locales causees par l'adrenaline sur le developpement des infections microbiennes. *C R Seances Soc Biol Fil* **103:**1052–1054.
7. **Lyte M.** 2010. The microbial organ in the gut as a driver of homeostasis and disease. *Med Hypotheses* **74:**634–638.
8. **Sandrini S, Aldriwesh M, Alruways M, Freestone P.** 2015. Microbial endocrinology: host-bacteria communication within the gut microbiome. *J Endocrinol* **225:**R21–R34.
9. **Karavolos MH, Williams P, Khan CM.** 2011. Interkingdom crosstalk: host neuroendocrine stress hormones drive the hemolytic behavior of *Salmonella typhi. Virulence* **2:**371–374.
10. **Lyte M.** 2013. Microbial endocrinology in the microbiome-gut-brain axis: how bacterial production and utilization of neurochemicals influence behavior. *PLoS Pathog* **9:**e1003726. doi:10.1371/journal.ppat.1003726.
11. **Lyte M, Cryan JF.** 2014. *Microbial Endocrinology: the Microbiota-Gut-Brain Axis in Health and Disease.* Springer, New York, NY.
12. **Wall R, Cryan JF, Ross RP, Fitzgerald GF, Dinan TG, Stanton C.** 2014. Bacterial neuroactive compounds produced by psychobiotics. *Adv Exp Med Biol* **817:**221–239.
13. **Fink G, Pfaff DW, Levine JE.** 2012. *Handbook of Neuroendocrinology*, 1st ed. Academic Press, Boston, MA.
14. **Teo WS, Balasubramaniam P.** 1983. Gas gangrene after intramuscular injection of adrenaline. *Clin Orthop Relat Res* **174:**206–207.
15. **Harvey PW, Purnell GV.** 1968. Fatal case of gas gangrene associated with intramuscular injections. *Br Med J* **1:**744–746.
16. **Yamashima T.** 2003. Jokichi Takamine (1854–1922), the samurai chemist, and his work on adrenalin. *J Med Biogr* **11:**95–102.
17. **Bested AC, Logan AC, Selhub EM.** 2013. Intestinal microbiota, probiotics and mental health: from Metchnikoff to modern advances. Part I. Autointoxication revisited. *Gut Pathog* **5:**5.
18. **Evans DG, Miles AA, Niven JS.** 1948. The enhancement of bacterial infections by adrenaline. *Br J Exp Pathol* **29:**20–39.
19. **Traub WH, Bauer D, Wolf U.** 1991. Virulence of clinical and fecal isolates of *Clostridium perfringens* type A for outbred NMRI mice. *Chemotherapy* **37:**426–435.
20. **Kulma A, Szopa J.** 2007. Catecholamines are active compounds in plants. *Plant Sci* **172:**433–440.
21. **Pitman RM.** 1971. Transmitter substances in insects: a review. *Comp Gen Pharmacol* **2:**347–371.
22. **Guerrero HY, Caceres G, Paiva CL, Marcano D.** 1990. Hypothalamic and telencephalic catecholamine content in the brain of the teleost

fish, *Pygocentrus notatus*, during the annual reproductive cycle. *Gen Comp Endocrinol* **80**:257–263.

23. **Roth J, LeRoith D, Shiloach J, Rosenzweig JL, Lesniak MA, Havrankova J.** 1982. The evolutionary origins of hormones, neurotransmitters, and other extracellular chemical messengers: implications for mammalian biology. *N Engl J Med* **306**:523–527.

24. **Dohler KD.** 1986. Development of hormone receptors: conclusion. *Experientia* **42**:788–794.

25. **Mayer EA, Baldi JP.** 1991. Can regulatory peptides be regarded as words of a biological language. *Am J Physiol* **261**:G171–G184.

26. **Lenard J.** 1992. Mammalian hormones in microbial cells. *Trends Biochem Sci* **17**:147–150.

27. **Kawashima K, Misawa H, Moriwaki Y, Fujii YX, Fujii T, Horiuchi Y, Yamada T, Imanaka T, Kamekura M.** 2007. Ubiquitous expression of acetylcholine and its biological functions in life forms without nervous systems. *Life Sci* **80**:2206–2209.

28. **Stephenson M, Rowatt E.** 1947. The production of acetylcholine by a strain of *Lactobacillus plantarum*. *J Gen Microbiol* **1**:279–298.

29. **Devalia JL, Harmanyeri Y, Cundell DR, Davies RJ, Grady D, Tabaqchali S.** 1988. Variation in histamine synthesis by Gram-negative and Gram-positive respiratory tract bacteria and the effect of cefaclor. *Royal Society of Medicine Services Ltd International Congress and Symposium Series* **128**:49–55.

30. **Masson F, Talon R, Montel MC.** 1996. Histamine and tyramine production by bacteria from meat products. *Int J Food Microbiol* **32**:199–207.

31. **Thomas CM, Hong T, van Pijkeren JP, Hemarajata P, Trinh DV, Hu W, Britton RA, Kalkum M, Versalovic J.** 2012. Histamine derived from probiotic *Lactobacillus reuteri* suppresses TNF via modulation of PKA and ERK signaling. *PLoS One* **7**:e31951. doi:10.1371/journal.pone.0031951.

32. **Hurley R, Leask BG, Ruthven CR, Sandler M, Southgate J.** 1971. Investigation of 5-hydroxytryptamine production by *Candida albicans in vitro* and *in vivo*. *Microbios* **4**:133–143.

33. **Ozogul F.** 2011. Effects of specific lactic acid bacteria species on biogenic amine production by foodborne pathogens. *Int J Food Sci Technol* **46**:478–484.

34. **Shishov VA, Kirovskaia TA, Kudrin VS, Oleskin AV.** 2009. Amine neuromediators, their precursors, and oxidation products in the culture of *Escherichia coli* K-12. *Prikl Biokhim Mikrobiol* **45**:550–554. [In Russion.]

35. **Asano Y, Hiramoto T, Nishino R, Aiba Y, Kimura T, Yoshihara K, Koga Y, Sudo N.** 2012. Critical role of gut microbiota in the production of biologically active, free catecholamines in the gut lumen of mice. *Am J Physiol Gastrointest Liver Physiol* **303**:G1288–G1295.

36. **Tsavkelova EA, Botvinko IV, Kudrin VS, Oleskin AV.** 2000. Detection of neurotransmitter amines in microorganisms with the use of high-performance liquid chromatography. *Dokl Biochem* **372**:115–117.

37. **Raasch W, Regunathan S, Li G, Reis DJ.** 1995. Agmatine, the bacterial amine, is widely distributed in mammalian tissues. *Life Sci* **56**:2319–2330.

38. **Arena ME, Manca de Nadra MC.** 2001. Biogenic amine production by *Lactobacillus*. *J Appl Microbiol* **90**:158–162.

39. **LeRoith D, Shiloach J, Heffron R, Rubinovitz C, Tanenbaum R, Roth J.** 1985. Insulin-related material in microbes: similarities and differences from mammalian insulins. *Can J Biochem Cell Biol* **63**:839–849.

40. **Leroith D, Liotta AS, Roth J, Shiloach J, Lewis ME, Pert CB, Krieger DT.** 1982. Corticotropin and beta-endorphin-like materials are native to unicellular organisms. *Proc Natl Acad Sci USA* **79**:2086–2090.

41. **LeRoith D, Pickens W, Vinik AI, Shiloach J.** 1985. *Bacillus subtilis* contains multiple forms of somatostatin-like material. *Biochem Biophys Res Commun* **127**:713–719.

42. **Schar G, Stover EP, Clemons KV, Feldman D, Stevens DA.** 1986. Progesterone binding and inhibition of growth in *Trichophyton mentagrophytes*. *Infect Immun* **52**:763–767.

43. **Roshchina VV.** 2010. Evolutionary considerations of neurotransmitters in microbial, plant and animal cells, p 17–52. *In* Lyte M, Freestone PP (ed), *Microbial Endocrinology: Interkingdom Signaling in Infectious Disease and Health*. Springer, New York, NY.

44. **LeRoith D, Roberts CJ, Lesniak MA, Roth J.** 1986. Receptors for intercellular messenger molecules in microbes: similarities to vertebrate receptors and possible implications for diseases in man. *Experientia* **42**:782–788.

45. **Shapiro JA, Hsu C.** 1989. *Escherichia coli* K-12 cell-cell interactions seen by time-lapse video. *J Bacteriol* **171**:5963–5974.

46. **Budrene EO, Berg HC.** 1995. Dynamics of formation of symmetrical patterns by chemotactic bacteria. *Nature* **376**:49–53.

47. **Iyer LM, Aravind L, Coon SL, Klein DC, Koonin EV.** 2004. Evolution of cell-cell signaling in animals: did late horizontal gene transfer from bacteria have a role? *Trends Genet* **20**:292–299.

48. **Roshchina VV.** 2001. *Neurotransmitters in Plant Life.* Science Publishers, Enfield, NH.

49. **Von Roepenack-Lahaye E, Newman MA, Schornack S, Hammond-Kosack KE, Lahaye T, Jones JD, Daniels MJ, Dow JM.** 2003. p-Coumaroylnoradrenaline, a novel plant metabolite implicated in tomato defense against pathogens. *J Biol Chem* **278:**43373–43383.

50. **Zacares L, Lopez-Gresa MP, Fayos J, Primo J, Belles JM, Conejero V.** 2007. Induction of p-coumaroyldopamine and feruloyldopamine, two novel metabolites, in tomato by the bacterial pathogen *Pseudomonas syringae. Mol Plant Microbe Interact* **20:**1439–1448.

51. **Kang S, Back K.** 2006. Enriched production of N-hydroxycinnamic acid amides and biogenic amines in pepper (*Capsicum annuum*) flowers. *Scientia Horticulturae* **108:**337–341.

52. **Newman MA, von Roepenack-Lahaye E, Parr A, Daniels MJ, Dow JM.** 2001. Induction of hydroxycinnamoyl-tyramine conjugates in pepper by *Xanthomonas campestris,* a plant defense response activated by hrp gene-dependent and hrp gene-independent mechanisms. *Mol Plant Microbe Interact* **14:**785–792.

53. **Newman MA, von Roepenack-Lahaye E, Parr A, Daniels MJ, Dow JM.** 2002. Prior exposure to lipopolysaccharide potentiates expression of plant defenses in response to bacteria. *Plant J* **29:**487–495.

54. **King RR, Calhoun LA.** 2005. Characterization of cross-linked hydroxycinnamic acid amides isolated from potato common scab lesions. *Phytochemistry* **66:**2468–2473.

55. **Mittelstrass K, Treutter D, Plessl M, Heller W, Elstner EF, Heiser I.** 2006. Modification of primary and secondary metabolism of potato plants by nitrogen application differentially affects resistance to *Phytophthora infestans* and *Alternaria solani. Plant Biol (Stuttg)* **8:**653–661.

56. **Morant M, Schoch GA, Ullmann P, Ertunc T, Little D, Olsen CE, Petersen M, Negrel J, Werck-Reichhart D.** 2007. Catalytic activity, duplication and evolution of the CYP98 cytochrome P450 family in wheat. *Plant Mol Biol* **63:**1–19.

57. **Lyte M, Freestone PPE.** 2010. *Microbial Endocrinology: Interkingdom Signaling in Infectious Disease and Health.* Springer, New York, NY.

58. **Everest P.** 2007. Stress and bacteria: microbial endocrinology. *Gut* **56:**1037–1038.

59. **Lyte M.** 2011. Probiotics function mechanistically as delivery vehicles for neuroactive compounds: microbial endocrinology in the design and use of probiotics. *Bioessays* **33:**574–581.

60. **Cryan JF, Dinan TG.** 2012. Mind-altering microorganisms: the impact of the gut microbiota on brain and behaviour. *Nat Rev Neurosci* **13:**701–712.

61. **Lyte M.** 2013. Microbial endocrinology and nutrition: a perspective on new mechanisms by which diet can influence gut-to-brain communication. *PharmaNutrition* **1:**35–39.

62. **Norris V, Molina F, Gewirtz AT.** 2013. Hypothesis: bacteria control host appetites. *J Bacteriol* **195:**411–416.

63. **Alcock J, Maley CC, Aktipis CA.** 2014. Is eating behavior manipulated by the gastrointestinal microbiota? Evolutionary pressures and potential mechanisms. *Bioessays* **36:**940–949.

64. **Strandwitz P, Kim K-H, Stewart E, Clardy J, Lewis K.** 2014. GABA modulating bacteria in the human gut microbiome, abstr 417, RISE:2014: Research, Innovation, and Scholarship Expo, Northeastern University, Boston, MA.

65. **Wojtarowicz A, Podlasz P, Czaja K.** 2003. Adrenergic and cholinergic innervation of pulmonary tissue in the pig. *Folia Morphol (Warsz)* **62:**215–218.

66. **Belvisi MG.** 2002. Overview of the innervation of the lung. *Curr Opin Pharmacol* **2:**211–215.

67. **Hofford JM, Milakofsky L, Pell S, Vogel W.** 1996. A profile of amino acid and catecholamine levels during endotoxin-induced acute lung injury in sheep: searching for potential markers of the acute respiratory distress syndrome. *J Lab Clin Med* **128:**545–551.

68. **Anderson MT, Armstrong SK.** 2008. Norepinephrine mediates acquisition of transferrin-iron in *Bordetella bronchiseptica. J Bacteriol* **190:**3940–3947.

69. **Oneal MJ, Schafer ER, Madsen ML, Minion FC.** 2008. Global transcriptional analysis of *Mycoplasma hyopneumoniae* following exposure to norepinephrine. *Microbiology* **154:**2581–2588.

70. **Furness JB, Callaghan BP, Rivera LR, Cho HJ.** 2014. The enteric nervous system and gastrointestinal innervation: integrated local and central control. *Adv Exp Med Biol* **817:**39–71.

71. **Lomax AE, Sharkey KA, Furness JB.** 2010. The participation of the sympathetic innervation of the gastrointestinal tract in disease states. *Neurogastroenterol Motil* **22:**7–18.

72. **Breer H, Eberle J, Frick C, Haid D, Widmayer P.** 2012. Gastrointestinal chemosensation: chemosensory cells in the alimentary tract. *Histochem Cell Biol* **138:**13–24.

73. **Foster JA, McVey Neufeld KA.** 2013. Gut-brain axis: how the microbiome influences anxiety and depression. *Trends Neurosci* **36:**305–312.

74. **Eisenhofer G, Aneman A, Friberg P, Hooper D, Fandriks L, Lonroth H, Hunyady B, Mezey E.** 1997. Substantial production of dopamine in the human gastrointestinal tract. *J Clin Endocrinol Metab* **82:**3864–3871.

75. **Eisenhofer G, Aneman A, Hooper D, Holmes C, Goldstein DS, Friberg P.** 1995. Production and metabolism of dopamine and norepinephrine in mesenteric organs and liver of swine. *Am J Physiol* **268:**G641–G649.

76. **Chen C, Lyte M, Stevens MP, Vulchanova L, Brown DR.** 2006. Mucosally-directed adrenergic nerves and sympathomimetic drugs enhance non-intimate adherence of *Escherichia coli* O157:H7 to porcine cecum and colon. *Eur J Pharmacol* **539:**116–124.

77. **Green BT, Lyte M, Chen C, Xie Y, Casey MA, Kulkarni-Narla A, Vulchanova L, Brown DR.** 2004. Adrenergic modulation of *Escherichia coli* O157:H7 adherence to the colonic mucosa. *Am J Physiol Gastrointest Liver Physiol* **287:** G1238–G1246.

78. **Brosnahan AJ, Vulchanova L, Witta SR, Dai Y, Jones BJ, Brown DR.** 2013. Norepinephrine potentiates proinflammatory responses of human vaginal epithelial cells. *J Neuroimmunol* **259:**8–16.

79. **Lyte M, Vulchanova L, Brown DR.** 2011. Stress at the intestinal surface: catecholamines and mucosa-bacteria interactions. *Cell Tissue Res* **343:**23–32.

80. **Pullar CE, Zhao M, Song B, Pu J, Reid B, Ghoghawala S, McCaig C, Isseroff RR.** 2007. Beta-adrenergic receptor agonists delay while antagonists accelerate epithelial wound healing: evidence of an endogenous adrenergic network within the corneal epithelium. *J Cell Physiol* **211:**261–272.

81. **Hsu SC, Johansson KR, Donahue MJ.** 1986. The bacterial flora of the intestine of *Ascaris suum* and 5-hydroxytryptamine production. *J Parasitol* **72:**545–549.

82. **Shahkolahi AM, Donahue MJ.** 1993. Bacterial flora, a possible source of serotonin in the intestine of adult female *Ascaris suum. J Parasitol* **79:**17–22.

83. **Wikoff WR, Anfora AT, Liu J, Schultz PG, Lesley SA, Peters EC, Siuzdak G.** 2009. Metabolomics analysis reveals large effects of gut microflora on mammalian blood metabolites. *Proc Natl Acad Sci USA* **106:**3698–3703.

84. **Sridharan GV, Choi K, Klemashevich C, Wu C, Prabakaran D, Pan LB, Steinmeyer S, Mueller C, Yousofshahi M, Alaniz RC, Lee K, Jayaraman A.** 2014. Prediction and quantification of bioactive microbiota metabolites in the mouse gut. *Nat Commun* **5:**5492.

85. **Goldstein DS.** 2010. Catecholamines 101. *Clin Auton Res* **20:**331–352.

86. **Furness JB.** 2012. The enteric nervous system and neurogastroenterology. *Nat Rev Gastroenterol Hepatol* **9:**286–294.

87. **Bertrand PP, Bertrand RL.** 2010. Serotonin release and uptake in the gastrointestinal tract. *Auton Neurosci* **153:**47–57.

88. **Bailey MT, Dowd SE, Galley JD, Hufnagle AR, Allen RG, Lyte M.** 2011. Exposure to a social stressor alters the structure of the intestinal microbiota: implications for stressor-induced immunomodulation. *Brain Behav Immun* **25:**397–407.

89. **Galley JD, Yu Z, Kumar P, Dowd SE, Lyte M, Bailey MT.** 2014. The structures of the colonic mucosa-associated and luminal microbial communities are distinct and differentially affected by a prolonged murine stressor. *Gut Microbes* **5:**748–760.

90. **Bangsgaard Bendtsen KM, Krych L, Sorensen DB, Pang W, Nielsen DS, Josefsen K, Hansen LH, Sorensen SJ, Hansen AK.** 2012. Gut microbiota composition is correlated to grid floor induced stress and behavior in the BALB/c mouse. *PLoS One* **7:**e46231. doi:10.1371/journal.pone.0046231.

91. **Aguilera M, Vergara P, Martinez V.** 2013. Stress and antibiotics alter luminal and wall-adhered microbiota and enhance the local expression of visceral sensory-related systems in mice. *Neurogastroenterol Motil* **25:**e515–e529.

92. **Thaiss CA, Zeevi D, Levy M, Zilberman-Schapira G, Suez J, Tengeler AC, Abramson L, Katz MN, Korem T, Zmora N, Kuperman Y, Biton I, Gilad S, Harmelin A, Shapiro H, Halpern Z, Segal E, Elinav E.** 2014. Transkingdom control of microbiota diurnal oscillations promotes metabolic homeostasis. *Cell* **159:**514–529.

93. **Galley JD, Nelson MC, Yu Z, Dowd SE, Walter J, Kumar PS, Lyte M, Bailey MT.** 2014. Exposure to a social stressor disrupts the community structure of the colonic mucosa-associated microbiota. *BMC Microbiol* **14:**189.

94. **Looft T, Allen HK, Cantarel BL, Levine UY, Bayles DO, Alt DP, Henrissat B, Stanton TB.** 2014. Bacteria, phages and pigs: the effects of in-feed antibiotics on the microbiome at different gut locations. *ISME J* **8:**1566–1576.

95. **Lyte M, Bailey MT.** 1997. Neuroendocrine-bacterial interactions in a neurotoxin-induced model of trauma. *J Surg Res* **70:**195–201.

96. **Woolf PD, McDonald JV, Feliciano DV, Kelly MM, Nichols D, Cox C.** 1992. The catecholamine response to multisystem trauma. *Arch Surg* **127:**899–903.

97. **Zetterström BEM, Palmerio C, Fine J.** 1964. Changes in tissue content of catechol amines in traumatic shock. *Acta Chir Scand* **128:**13–11.

98. **Alverdy JC, Aoys E, Moss GS.** 1988. Total parenteral nutrition promotes bacterial translocation from the gut. *Surgery* **104:**185–190.

99. **Hendrickson BA, Guo J, Laughlin R, Chen Y, Alverdy JC.** 1999. Increased type 1 fimbrial expression among commensal *Escherichia coli* isolates in the murine cecum following catabolic stress. *Infect Immun* **67:**745–753.

100. **Deitch EA.** 1990. Bacterial translocation of gut flora. *J Trauma* **30:**S184–S189.

101. **Freestone PP, Williams PH, Haigh RD, Maggs AF, Neal CP, Lyte M.** 2002. Growth stimulation of intestinal commensal *Escherichia coli* by catecholamines: a possible contributory factor in trauma-induced sepsis. *Shock* **18:**465–470.

102. **Heggers JP, Robson MC.** 1991. *Quantitative Bacteriology: Its Role in the Armamentarium of the Surgeon.* CRC Press, Boca Raton, FL.

103. **Magee C, Rodeheaver GT, Edgerton MT, Golden GT, Haury B, Edlich RF.** 1977. Studies of the mechanisms by which epinephrine damages tissue defenses. *J Surg Res* **23:**126–131.

104. **Tran DT, Miller SH, Buck D, Imatani J, Demuth RJ, Miller MA.** 1985. Potentiation of infection by epinephrine. *Plast Reconstr Surg* **76:**933–934.

105. **Miles AA, Miles EM, Burke J.** 1957. The value and duration of defence reactions of the skin to the primary lodgement of bacteria. *Br J Exp Pathol* **38:**79–96.

106. **Morken JJ, Warren KU, Xie Y, Rodriguez JL, Lyte M.** 2002. Epinephrine as a mediator of pulmonary neutrophil sequestration. *Shock* **18:**46–50.

107. **Haigh RD.** 2010. Experimental design considerations for *in vitro* microbial endocrinology investigations, p 291–308. *In* Lyte M, Freestone PE (ed), *Microbial Endocrinology: Interkingdom Signaling in Infectious Disease and Health.* Springer, New York, NY.

108. **O'Donnell PM, Aviles H, Lyte M, Sonnenfeld G.** 2006. Enhancement of *in vitro* growth of pathogenic bacteria by norepinephrine: importance of inoculum density and role of transferrin. *Appl Environ Microbiol* **72:**5097–5099.

109. **Tarr PI, Neill MA.** 2001. *Escherichia coli* O157: H7. *Gastroenterol Clin North Am* **30:**735–751.

110. **Lyte M, Frank CD, Green BT.** 1996. Production of an autoinducer of growth by norepinephrine cultured *Escherichia coli* O157:H7. *FEMS Microbiol Lett* **139:**155–159.

111. **Lyte M, Erickson AK, Arulanandam BP, Frank CD, Crawford MA, Francis DH.** 1997. Norepinephrine-induced expression of the K99 pilus adhesin of enterotoxigenic *Escherichia coli. Biochem Biophys Res Commun* **232:**682–686.

112. **Lyte M, Nguyen KT.** 1997. Alteration of *Escherichia coli* O157:H7 growth and molecular fingerprint by the neuroendocrine hormone noradrenaline. *Microbios* **89:**197–213.

113. **Freestone PP, Lyte M, Neal CP, Maggs AF, Haigh RD, Williams PH.** 2000. The mammalian neuroendocrine hormone norepinephrine supplies iron for bacterial growth in the presence of transferrin or lactoferrin. *J Bacteriol* **182:**6091–6098.

114. **Lyte M, Freestone PP, Neal CP, Olson BA, Haigh RD, Bayston R, Williams PH.** 2003. Stimulation of *Staphylococcus epidermidis* growth and biofilm formation by catecholamine inotropes. *Lancet* **361:**130–135.

115. **Rasko D, Moreira C, Li de R, Reading N, Ritchie J, Waldor M, Williams N, Taussig R, Wei S, Roth M, Hughes D, Huntley J, Fina M, Falck J, Sperandio V.** 2008. Targeting QseC signaling and virulence for antibiotic development. *Science* **321:**1078–1080.

116. **Karavolos M, Spencer H, Bulmer D, Thompson A, Winzer K, Williams P, Hinton J, Khan C.** 2008. Adrenaline modulates the global transcriptional profile of *Salmonella* revealing a role in the antimicrobial peptide and oxidative stress resistance responses. *BMC Genomics* **9:**458.

117. **Kinney KS, Austin CE, Morton DS, Sonnenfeld G.** 1999. Catecholamine enhancement of *Aeromonas hydrophila* growth. *Microb Pathog* **26:**85–91.

118. **Peterson G, Kumar A, Gart E, Narayanan S.** 2011. Catecholamines increase conjugative gene transfer between enteric bacteria. *Microb Pathog* **51:**1–8.

119. **Furness JB.** 2006. *The Enteric Nervous System*, 2nd ed. Blackwell, Malden, MA.

120. **Okamura H, Murooka Y, Harada T.** 1976. Regulation of tyramine oxidase synthesis in *Klebsiella aerogenes. J Bacteriol* **127:**24–31.

121. **Xu F, Wu C, Guo F, Cui G, Zeng X, Yang B, Lin J.** 2015. Transcriptomic analysis of *Campylobacter jejuni* NCTC 11168 in response to epinephrine and norepinephrine. *Front Microbiol* **6:**452.

122. **Li L, Xu Z, Zhou Y, Sun L, Liu Z, Chen H, Zhou R.** 2012. Global effects of catecholamines on *Actinobacillus pleuropneumoniae* gene expression. *PLoS One* **7:**e31121. doi:10.1371/journal.pone.0031121.

123. **Freestone PP, Haigh RD, Williams PH, Lyte M.** 1999. Stimulation of bacterial growth by heat-stable, norepinephrine-induced autoinducers. *FEMS Microbiol Lett* **172:**53–60.

124. **Reissbrodt R, Rienaecker I, Romanova JM, Freestone PP, Haigh RD, Lyte M, Tschape H, Williams PH.** 2002. Resuscitation of *Salmonella enterica* serovar typhimurium and enterohemorrhagic *Escherichia coli* from the viable but nonculturable state by heat-stable enterobacterial autoinducer. *Appl Environ Microbiol* **68:**4788–4794.

125. **Reissbrodt R, Rassbach A, Burghardt B, Rienacker I, Mietke H, Schleif J, Tschape H, Lyte M, Williams PH.** 2004. Assessment of a new selective chromogenic *Bacillus cereus* group plating medium and use of enterobacterial autoinducer of growth for cultural identification of *Bacillus* species. *J Clin Microbiol* **42:**3795–3798.

126. **Burton CL, Chhabra SR, Swift S, Baldwin TJ, Withers H, Hill SJ, Williams P.** 2002. The growth response of *Escherichia coli* to neurotransmitters and related catecholamine drugs requires a functional enterobactin biosynthesis and uptake system. *Infect Immun* **70:**5913–5923.

127. **Iwata H, Kariya K, Fujimoto S.** 1969. Effect of compounds affecting the adrenergic mechanism on cell growth and division of *Tetrahymena pyriformis* W. *Jpn J Pharmacol* **19:**275–281.

128. **de Castro SL, Oliveira MM.** 1987. Radioligand binding characterization of beta-adrenergic receptors in the protozoa *Trypanosoma cruzi*. *Comp Biochem Physiol C* **87:**5–8.

129. **Lyte M, Ernst S.** 1993. Alpha and beta adrenergic receptor involvement in catecholamine-induced growth of Gram-negative bacteria. *Biochem Biophys Res Commun* **190:**447–452.

130. **Reading NC, Rasko DA, Torres AG, Sperandio V.** 2009. The two-component system QseEF and the membrane protein QseG link adrenergic and stress sensing to bacterial pathogenesis. *Proc Natl Acad Sci USA* **106:**5889–5894.

131. **Clarke MB, Hughes DT, Zhu C, Boedeker EC, Sperandio V.** 2006. The QseC sensor kinase: a bacterial adrenergic receptor. *Proc Natl Acad Sci USA* **103:**10420–10425.

132. **Freestone PP, Haigh RD, Lyte M.** 2007. Blockade of catecholamine-induced growth by adrenergic and dopaminergic receptor antagonists in *Escherichia coli* O157:H7, *Salmonella enterica* and *Yersinia enterocolitica*. *BMC Microbiol* **7:**8.

133. **Rello J, Ricart M, Mirelis B, Quintana E, Gurgui M, Net A, Prats G.** 1994. Nosocomial bacteremia in a medical-surgical intensive care unit: epidemiologic characteristics and factors influencing mortality in 111 episodes. *Intensive Care Med* **20:**94–98.

134. **Rupp ME, Archer GL.** 1994. Coagulase-negative staphylococci: pathogens associated with medical progress. *Clin Infect Dis* **19:**231–243.

135. **Gabriel L, Beriot-Mathiot A.** 2014. Hospitalization stay and costs attributable to *Clostridium difficile* infection: a critical review. *J Hosp Infect* **88:**12–21.

136. **Drekonja DM.** 2014. *Clostridium difficile* infection: current, forgotten and emerging treatment options. *J Comp Eff Res* **3:**547–557.

137. **Becker K, Heilmann C, Peters G.** 2014. Coagulase-negative staphylococci. *Clin Microbiol Rev* **27:**870–926.

138. **Helton WS, Rockwell M, Garcia RM, Maier RV, Heitkemper M.** 1995. TPN-induced sympathetic activation is related to diet, bacterial translocation, and an intravenous line. *Arch Surg* **130:**209–214.

139. **Mutlu GM, Mutlu EA, Factor P.** 2001. GI complications in patients receiving mechanical ventilation. *Chest* **119:**1222–1241.

140. **Crump JA, Collignon PJ.** 2000. Intravascular catheter-associated infections. *Eur J Clin Microbiol Infect Dis* **19:**1–8.

141. **Pittet D, Tarara D, Wenzel RP.** 1994. Nosocomial bloodstream infection in critically ill patients. Excess length of stay, extra costs, and attributable mortality. *JAMA* **271:**1598–1601.

142. **Cho SH, Naber K, Hacker J, Ziebuhr W.** 2002. Detection of the icaADBC gene cluster and biofilm formation in *Staphylococcus epidermidis* isolates from catheter-related urinary tract infections. *Int J Antimicrob Agents* **19:**570–575.

143. **Ganderton L, Chawla J, Winters C, Wimpenny J, Stickler D.** 1992. Scanning electron microscopy of bacterial biofilms on indwelling bladder catheters. *Eur J Clin Microbiol Infect Dis* **11:**789–796.

144. **Mermel LA, Farr BM, Sherertz RJ, Raad II, O'Grady N, Harris JS, Craven DE.** 2001. Guidelines for the management of intravascular catheter-related infections. *Clin Infect Dis* **32:**1249–1272.

145. **Molina J, Penuela I, Lepe JA, Gutierrez-Pizarraya A, Gomez MJ, Garcia-Cabrera E, Cordero E, Aznar J, Pachon J.** 2013. Mortality and hospital stay related to coagulase-negative *Staphylococci bacteremia* in non-critical patients. *J Infect* **66:**155–162.

146. **Inman RD, Gallegos KV, Brause BD, Redecha PB, Christian CL.** 1984. Clinical and microbial features of prosthetic joint infection. *Am J Med* **77:**47–53.

147. **Costerton JW, Stewart PS, Greenberg EP.** 1999. Bacterial biofilms: a common cause of persistent infections. *Science* **284:**1318–1322.

148. **Stoodley P, Sauer K, Davies DG, Costerton JW.** 2002. Biofilms as complex differentiated communities. *Annu Rev Microbiol* **56:**187–209.

149. **Mack D, Fischer W, Krokotsch A, Leopold K, Hartmann R, Egge H, Laufs R.** 1996. The intercellular adhesin involved in biofilm accumulation of *Staphylococcus epidermidis* is a linear beta-1,6-linked glucosaminoglycan: purification and structural analysis. *J Bacteriol* **178:**175–183.

150. **Gotz F.** 2002. *Staphylococcus* and biofilms. *Mol Microbiol* **43:**1367–1378.

151. **Dunne WM Jr.** 2002. Bacterial adhesion: seen any good biofilms lately? *Clin Microbiol Rev* **15:**155–166.

152. **Molnar C, Hevessy Z, Rozgonyi F, Gemmell CG.** 1994. Pathogenicity and virulence of coagulase negative staphylococci in relation to adherence, hydrophobicity, and toxin production *in vitro. J Clin Pathol* **47:**743–748.

153. **Steer JA, Hill GB, Srinivasan S, Southern J, Wilson AP.** 1997. Slime production, adherence and hydrophobicity in coagulase-negative staphylococci causing peritonitis in peritoneal dialysis. *J Hosp Infect* **37:**305–316.

154. **Rupp ME, Archer GL.** 1992. Hemagglutination and adherence to plastic by *Staphylococcus epidermidis. Infect Immun* **60:**4322–4327.

155. **Fey PD, Ulphani JS, Gotz F, Heilmann C, Mack D, Rupp ME.** 1999. Characterization of the relationship between polysaccharide intercellular adhesin and hemagglutination in *Staphylococcus epidermidis. J Infect Dis* **179:** 1561–1564.

156. **Rohde H, Knobloch JK, Horstkotte MA, Mack D.** 2001. Correlation of biofilm expression types of *Staphylococcus epidermidis* with polysaccharide intercellular adhesin synthesis: evidence for involvement of icaADBC genotype-independent factors. *Med Microbiol Immunol (Berl)* **190:**105–112.

157. **Koerner RJ, Butterworth LA, Mayer IV, Dasbach R, Busscher HJ.** 2002. Bacterial adhesion to titanium-oxy-nitride (TiNOX) coatings with different resistivities: a novel approach for the development of biomaterials. *Biomaterials* **23:**2835–2840.

158. **Arciola CR, Campoccia D, Montanaro L.** 2002. Effects on antibiotic resistance of *Staphylococcus epidermidis* following adhesion to polymethylmethacrylate and to silicone surfaces. *Biomaterials* **23:**1495–1502.

159. **Heilmann C, Gerke C, Perdreau-Remington F, Gotz F.** 1996. Characterization of Tn917 insertion mutants of *Staphylococcus epidermidis* affected in biofilm formation. *Infect Immun* **64:** 277–282.

160. **Heilmann C, Schweitzer O, Gerke C, Vanittanakom N, Mack D, Gotz F.** 1996. Molecular basis of intercellular adhesion in the biofilm-forming *Staphylococcus epidermidis. Mol Microbiol* **20:**1083–1091.

161. **Heilmann C, Hussain M, Peters G, Gotz F.** 1997. Evidence for autolysin-mediated primary attachment of *Staphylococcus epidermidis* to a polystyrene surface. *Mol Microbiol* **24:**1013–1024.

162. **McKenney D, Hubner J, Muller E, Wang Y, Goldmann DA, Pier GB.** 1998. The ica locus of *Staphylococcus epidermidis* encodes production of the capsular polysaccharide/adhesin. *Infect Immun* **66:**4711–4720.

163. **Ziebuhr W, Lossner I, Rachid S, Dietrich K, Gotz F, Hacker J.** 2000. Modulation of the polysaccharide intercellular adhesin (PIA) expression in biofilm forming *Staphylococcus epidermidis*. Analysis of genetic mechanisms. *Adv Exp Med Biol* **485:**151–157.

164. **Neal CP, Freestone PP, Maggs AF, Haigh RD, Williams PH, Lyte M.** 2001. Catecholamine inotropes as growth factors for *Staphylococcus epidermidis* and other coagulase-negative staphylococci. *FEMS Microbiol Lett* **194:**163–169.

165. **Christensen GD, Simpson WA, Younger JJ, Baddour LM, Barrett FF, Melton DM, Beachey EH.** 1985. Adherence of coagulase-negative staphylococci to plastic tissue culture plates: a quantitative model for the adherence of staphylococci to medical devices. *J Clin Microbiol* **22:**996–1006.

166. **Deighton MA, Balkau B.** 1990. Adherence measured by microtiter assay as a virulence marker for *Staphylococcus epidermidis* infections. *J Clin Microbiol* **28:**2442–2447.

167. **Linton CJ, Sherriff A, Millar MR.** 1999. Use of a modified Robbins device to directly compare the adhesion of *Staphylococcus epidermidis* RP62A to surfaces. *J Appl Microbiol* **86:**194–202.

168. **Vacheethasanee K, Temenoff JS, Higashi JM, Gary A, Anderson JM, Bayston R, Marchant RE.** 1998. Bacterial surface properties of clinically isolated *Staphylococcus epidermidis* strains determine adhesion on polyethylene. *J Biomed Mater Res* **42:**425–432.

169. **Galliani S, Viot M, Cremieux A, Van der Auwera P.** 1994. Early adhesion of bacteremic strains of *Staphylococcus epidermidis* to polystyrene: influence of hydrophobicity, slime production, plasma, albumin, fibrinogen, and fibronectin. *J Lab Clin Med* **123:**685–692.

170. **Matinaho S, von Bonsdorff L, Rouhiainen A, Lonnroth M, Parkkinen J.** 2001. Dependence of *Staphylococcus epidermidis* on non-transferrin-bound iron for growth. *FEMS Microbiol Lett* **196:**177–182.

171. **Lindsay JA, Riley TV, Mee BJ.** 1995. *Staphylococcus aureus* but not *Staphylococcus epidermidis* can acquire iron from transferrin. *Microbiology* **141**(Pt 1):197–203.

172. **Stewart PS.** 2003. New ways to stop biofilm infections. *Lancet* **361**:97.

173. **Freestone PP, Haigh RD, Lyte M.** 2008. Catecholamine inotrope resuscitation of antibiotic-damaged staphylococci and its blockade by specific receptor antagonists. *J Infect Dis* **197**:1044–1052.

174. **Crnich CJ, Maki DG.** 2004. Are antimicrobial-impregnated catheters effective? Don't throw out the baby with the bathwater. *Clin Infect Dis* **38**:1287–1292.

175. **Marciante KD, Veenstra DL, Lipsky BA, Saint S.** 2003. Which antimicrobial impregnated central venous catheter should we use? Modeling the costs and outcomes of antimicrobial catheter use. *Am J Infect Control* **31**:1–8.

176. **Lanter BB, Sauer K, Davies DG.** 2014. Bacteria present in carotid arterial plaques are found as biofilm deposits which may contribute to enhanced risk of plaque rupture. *MBio* **5**:e01206-14. doi:10.1128/mBio.01206-14.

177. **Freestone PP, Hirst RA, Sandrini SM, Sharaff F, Fry H, Hyman S, O'Callaghan C.** 2012. *Pseudomonas aeruginosa*-catecholamine inotrope interactions: a contributory factor in the development of ventilator-associated pneumonia? *Chest* **142**:1200–1210.

178. **Sandrini S, Alghofaili F, Freestone P, Yesilkaya H.** 2014. Host stress hormone norepinephrine stimulates pneumococcal growth, biofilm formation and virulence gene expression. *BMC Microbiol* **14**:180.

179. **Vlisidou I, Lyte M, van Diemen PM, Hawes P, Monaghan P, Wallis TS, Stevens MP.** 2004. The neuroendocrine stress hormone norepinephrine augments *Escherichia coli* O157:H7-induced enteritis and adherence in a bovine ligated ileal loop model of infection. *Infect Immun* **72**:5446–5451.

180. **Kendall MM, Sperandio V.** 2007. Quorum sensing by enteric pathogens. *Curr Opin Gastroenterol* **23**:10–15.

181. **Pasupuleti S, Sule N, Cohn WB, MacKenzie DS, Jayaraman A, Manson MD.** 2014. Chemotaxis of *Escherichia coli* to norepinephrine (NE) requires conversion of NE to 3,4-dihydroxymandelic acid. *J Bacteriol* **196**:3992–4000.

182. **Park JP, Choi MJ, Kim SH, Lee SH, Lee H.** 2014. Preparation of sticky *Escherichia coli* through surface display of an adhesive catecholamine moiety. *Appl Environ Microbiol* **80**:43–53.

183. **Bowdre JH, Krieg NR, Hoffman PS, Smibert RM.** 1976. Stimulatory effect of dihydroxyphenyl compounds on the aerotolerance of *Spirillum volutans* and *Campylobacter fetus* subspecies *jejuni*. *Appl Environ Microbiol* **31**:127–133.

184. **Ienistea C.** 1971. Bacterial production and destruction of histamine in foods, and food poisoning caused by histamine. *Nahrung* **15**:109–113.

185. **Tarjan V, Janossy G.** 1978. The role of biogenic amines in foods. *Nahrung* **22**:285–289.

186. **Stratton JE.** 1990. Biogenic amines in cheese and other fermented foods: a review. *J Food Prot* **54**:460–470.

187. **Devalia JL, Grady D, Harmanyeri Y, Tabaqchali S, Davies RJ.** 1989. Histamine synthesis by respiratory tract micro-organisms: possible role in pathogenicity. *J Clin Pathol* **42**:516–522.

188. **Voropaeva EA.** 2002. Resistance to antibiotics and histamine production at the bacteria, isolated from the stomatopharynx of the children with bronchial asthma. *Antibiot Khimioter* **47**:8–13. [In Russian.]

189. **Bearson BL, Bearson SM, Uthe JJ, Dowd SE, Houghton JO, Lee I, Toscano MJ, Lay DC Jr.** 2008. Iron regulated genes of *Salmonella enterica* serovar Typhimurium in response to norepinephrine and the requirement of fepDGC for norepinephrine-enhanced growth. *Microbes Infect* **10**:807–816.

190. **Nakano M, Takahashi A, Sakai Y, Nakaya Y.** 2007. Modulation of pathogenicity with norepinephrine related to the type III secretion system of *Vibrio parahaemolyticus*. *J Infect Dis* **195**:1353–1360.

191. **Yang Q, Anh ND, Bossier P, Defoirdt T.** 2014. Norepinephrine and dopamine increase motility, biofilm formation, and virulence of *Vibrio harveyi*. *Front Microbiol* **5**:584.

192. **Lacoste A, Jalabert F, Malham SK, Cueff A, Poulet SA.** 2001. Stress and stress-induced neuroendocrine changes increase the susceptibility of juvenile oysters (*Crassostrea gigas*) to *Vibrio splendidus*. *Appl Environ Microbiol* **67**:2304–2309.

193. **Pande GS, Suong NT, Bossier P, Defoirdt T.** 2014. The catecholamine stress hormones norepinephrine and dopamine increase the virulence of pathogenic *Vibrio anguillarum* and *Vibrio campbellii*. *FEMS Microbiol Ecol* **90**:761–769.

194. **Malikina KD, Shishov VA, Chuvelev DI, Kudrin VS, Oleskin AV.** 2010. Regulatory role of monoamine neurotransmitters in *Saccharomyces cerevisiae* cells. *Prikl Biokhim Mikrobiol* **46**:672–677. [In Russian.]

195. **Clemons KV, Shankar J, Stevens DA.** 2010. Mycologic endocrinology, p 269–290. *In* Lyte

M, Freestone PPE (ed), *Microbial Endocrinology Interkingdom Signaling in Infectious Disease and Health.* Springer, New York, NY.

196. **Pan JX, Mikkelsen RB, Wallach DF, Asher CR.** 1987. Synthesis of a somatostatin-like peptide by *Plasmodium falciparum. Mol Biochem Parasitol* **25:**107–111.

197. **Zavala-Castro JE, Guzman-Marin E, Zavala-Velazquez J.** 1995. Adrenergic ligands trigger intracellular differentiation of *Trypanosoma cruzi. Arch Med Res* **26:**449–450.

198. **Coppi A, Merali S, Eichinger D.** 2002. The enteric parasite *Entamoeba* uses an autocrine catecholamine system during differentiation into the infectious cyst stage. *J Biol Chem* **277:** 8083–8090.

199. **Coppi A, Eichinger D.** 1999. Regulation of *Entamoeba invadens* encystation and gene expression with galactose and N-acetylglucosamine. *Mol Biochem Parasitol* **102:**67–77.

200. **Moore D, Waters WR, Wannemuehler MJ, Harp JA.** 2001. Treatment with agmatine inhibits *Cryptosporidium parvum* infection in infant mice. *J Parasitol* **87:**211–213.

201. **Molderings GJ, Haenisch B.** 2012. Agmatine (decarboxylated L-arginine): physiological role and therapeutic potential. *Pharmacol Ther* **133:**351–365.

202. **Haenisch B, von Kugelgen I, Bonisch H, Gothert M, Sauerbruch T, Schepke M, Marklein G, Hofling K, Schroder D, Molderings GJ.** 2008. Regulatory mechanisms underlying agmatine homeostasis in humans. *Am J Physiol Gastrointest Liver Physiol* **295:**G1104–G1110.

203. **Reid G.** 2011. Neuroactive probiotics. *Bioessays* **33:**562.

204. **Collins SM, Kassam Z, Bercik P.** 2013. The adoptive transfer of behavioral phenotype via the intestinal microbiota: experimental evidence and clinical implications. *Curr Opin Microbiol* **16:**240–245.

205. **Neufeld KA, Kang N, Bienenstock J, Foster JA.** 2011. Effects of intestinal microbiota on anxiety-like behavior. *Commun Integr Biol* **4:**492–494.

206. **Bravo JA, Forsythe P, Chew MV, Escaravage E, Savignac HM, Dinan TG, Bienenstock J, Cryan JF.** 2011. Ingestion of *Lactobacillus* strain regulates emotional behavior and central GABA receptor expression in a mouse via the vagus nerve. *Proc Natl Acad Sci USA* **108:**16050–16055.

207. **Desbonnet L, Clarke G, Shanahan F, Dinan TG, Cryan JF.** 2013. Microbiota is essential for social development in the mouse. *Mol Psychiatry* [Epub ahead of print.] doi:10.1038/mp.2013.65.

208. **Lyte M.** 2014. Microbial endocrinology: host-microbiota neuroendocrine interactions influencing brain and behavior. *Gut Microbes* **5:**381–389.

209. **Lyte M.** 2014. Microbial endocrinology and the microbiota-gut-brain axis. *Adv Exp Med Biol* **817:**3–24.

210. **Jessen KR, Mirsky R.** 1983. Astrocyte-like glia in the peripheral nervous system: an immunohistochemical study of enteric glia. *J Neurosci* **3:**2206–2218.

211. **Goehler LE, Gaykema RP, Opitz N, Reddaway R, Badr N, Lyte M.** 2005. Activation in vagal afferents and central autonomic pathways: early responses to intestinal infection with *Campylobacter jejuni. Brain Behav Immun* **19:**334–344.

212. **Lyte M, Gaykema R, Goehler L.** 2009. Behavior modification of host by microbes, p 121–127. *In* Schaechter M (ed), *Encyclopedia of Microbiology*, 3rd ed. Elsevier, Oxford, UK.

213. **Le Roith D, Shiloach J, Berelowitz M, Frohman LA, Liotta AS, Krieger DT, Roth J.** 1983. Are messenger molecules in microbes the ancestors of the vertebrate hormones and tissue factors? *Fed Proc* **42:**2602–2607.

214. **Frohlich M, Lefering R, Probst C, Paffrath T, Schneider MM, Maegele M, Sakka SG, Bouillon B, Wafaisade A, Committee on Emergency Medicine, Intensive Care and Trauma Management of the German Trauma Society (Sektion NIS).** 2014. Epidemiology and risk factors of multiple-organ failure after multiple trauma: an analysis of 31,154 patients from the TraumaRegister DGU. *J Trauma Acute Care Surg* **76:**921–927; discussion 927–928.

215. **Tsukamoto T, Chanthaphavong RS, Pape HC.** 2010. Current theories on the pathophysiology of multiple organ failure after trauma. *Injury* **41:**21–26.

216. **Baue AE, Durham R, Faist E.** 1998. Systemic inflammatory response syndrome (SIRS), multiple organ dysfunction syndrome (MODS), multiple organ failure (MOF): are we winning the battle? *Shock* **10:**79–89.

217. **Swank GM, Deitch EA.** 1996. Role of the gut in multiple organ failure: bacterial translocation and permeability changes. *World J Surg* **20:**411–417.

218. **Wang P, Ba ZF, Cioffi WG, Bland KI, Chaudry IH.** 1998. Is gut the "motor" for producing hepatocellular dysfunction after trauma and hemorrhagic shock? *J Surg Res* **74:**141–148.

219. **Mittal R, Coopersmith CM.** 2014. Redefining the gut as the motor of critical illness. *Trends Mol Med* **20:**214–223.

220. **Balk RA.** 2014. Systemic inflammatory response syndrome (SIRS): where did it come from and is it still relevant today? *Virulence* **5:**20–26.

221. **Bengmark S.** 2012. Pro- and synbiotics to prevent sepsis in major surgery and severe emergencies. *Nutrients* **4:**91–111.

222. **Boyd JH, Russell JA, Fjell CD.** 2014. The meta-genome of sepsis: host genetics, pathogens and the acute immune response. *J Innate Immun* **6:**272–283.

223. **Madan JC, Salari RC, Saxena D, Davidson L, O'Toole GA, Moore JH, Sogin ML, Foster JA, Edwards WH, Palumbo P, Hibberd PL.** 2012. Gut microbial colonisation in premature neonates predicts neonatal sepsis. *Arch Dis Child Fetal Neonatal Ed* **97:**F456–F462.

224. **Sultan S, Forsmark CE.** 2010. Therapeutics. Review: enteral nutrition reduces mortality, multiple organ failure, and systemic infection more than TPN in acute pancreatitis. *Ann Intern Med* **153:**JC1–6.

225. **Shimizu K, Ogura H, Asahara T, Nomoto K, Morotomi M, Tasaki O, Matsushima A, Kuwagata Y, Shimazu T, Sugimoto H.** 2013. Probiotic/synbiotic therapy for treating critically ill patients from a gut microbiota perspective. *Dig Dis Sci* **58:**23–32.

226. **Marshall JC, Christou NV, Meakins JL.** 1993. The gastrointestinal tract. The "undrained abscess" of multiple organ failure. *Ann Surg* **218:**111–119.

227. **Marshall JC, Christou NV, Horn R, Meakins JL.** 1988. The microbiology of multiple organ failure. The proximal gastrointestinal tract as an occult reservoir of pathogens. *Arch Surg* **123:**309–315.

228. **Rocha F, Laughlin R, Musch MW, Hendrickson BA, Chang EB, Alverdy J.** 2001. Surgical stress shifts the intestinal *Escherichia coli* population to that of a more adherent phenotype: role in barrier regulation. *Surgery* **130:**65–73.

229. **Alverdy J, Holbrook C, Rocha F, Seiden L, Wu RL, Musch M, Chang E, Ohman D, Suh S.** 2000. Gut-derived sepsis occurs when the right pathogen with the right virulence genes meets the right host: evidence for *in vivo* virulence expression in *Pseudomonas aeruginosa*. *Ann Surg* **232:**480–489.

230. **Alverdy JC, Chang EB.** 2008. The re-emerging role of the intestinal microflora in critical illness and inflammation: why the gut hypothesis of sepsis syndrome will not go away. *J Leukoc Biol* **83:**461–466.

231. **Lyte M.** 2009. Reciprocal gut-brain evolutionary symbiosis provokes and amplifies the postinjury systemic inflammatory response syndrome. *Surgery* **146:**950–954.

232. **Herndon DN, Hart DW, Wolf SE, Chinkes DL, Wolfe RR.** 2001. Reversal of catabolism by beta-blockade after severe burns. *N Engl J Med* **345:**1223–1229.

Small RNAs in Bacterial Virulence and Communication

7

SARAH L. SVENSSON[1] and CYNTHIA M. SHARMA[1]

INTRODUCTION

Many pathogenic bacteria transit between free-living lifestyles and the markedly different environments presented by their hosts. This requires detection, integration, and response to different external and intracellular conditions and subsequent realignment of physiology and metabolism, as well as virulence factor expression via coordinated gene expression changes. Signals detected by pathogens include not only changes in temperature, pH, or nutrient availability, but also cues from the host and neighboring bacteria. How virulence genes are regulated at the transcriptional level has been studied extensively, and the regulons of several master regulators of virulence and survival gene transcription have been described in detail (1, 2). This has provided insight into both general regulatory mechanisms used by bacteria, and the lifestyles of pathogenic species.

Besides transcriptional control, gene expression can also be regulated at the posttranscriptional level. The importance of diverse posttranscriptional mechanisms (i.e., regulation of mRNA translation, stability, and processing) in bacterial virulence gene expression is becoming increasingly apparent (3–5). The central players in posttranscriptional control in bacteria are

[1]Research Center for Infectious Diseases (ZINF), University of Würzburg, Josef-Schneider-Straße 2 / Bau D15, 97080 Würzburg, Germany.
Virulence Mechanisms of Bacterial Pathogens, 5th edition
Edited by Indira T. Kudva, Nancy A. Cornick, Paul J. Plummer, Qijing Zhang, Tracy L. Nicholson, John P. Bannantine, and Bryan H. Bellaire
© 2016 American Society for Microbiology, Washington, DC
doi:10.1128/microbiolspec.VMBF-0028-2015

small noncoding (sRNAs), which mainly use their base-pairing capacity to directly interact with mRNAs, ultimately leading to repression or activation of protein expression (3). Recently, there has been an explosion in identification of candidate sRNAs in bacterial pathogens by global transcriptome studies using deep sequencing, revealing a previously unappreciated capacity for RNA-based regulation (6–9). In addition, an ever-increasing diversity of mechanisms of action, beyond the canonical translational repression via base-pairing interactions, has been described for riboregulators. These include activation of target gene expression, direct modulation of protein activity, and effects on transcription (3). Relatively limited conservation of sRNA repertoires between even closely related bacteria (10) suggests that this class of regulators is diverse. Many of the known mechanisms and functions of sRNAs are based on work in *Gammaproteobacteria* spp. and especially model organisms such as *Escherichia coli* and *Salmonella*. Insights from ongoing functional characterization of sRNA candidates outside the enterobacteria, including in a variety of important pathogens, is identifying additional mechanisms of gene regulation by sRNAs. This work is deepening the understanding of how virulence programs are regulated in bacterial pathogens. Also, in addition to sRNAs, endogenous highly conserved and structured regions within mRNAs themselves, such as riboswitches, are now known to factor centrally in posttranscriptional regulation. An emerging class of dual-function mRNAs that act both as templates for protein synthesis and as *trans*-acting regulators themselves, or act by sequestering proteins or sRNAs, has been reported (11, 12). These mechanisms also utilize various protein accomplices, such as RNA-binding proteins or ribonucleases (RNases). For example, the RNA chaperone Hfq is required for sRNA stability and function in enterobacteria and has also been linked to virulence regulation in pathogens (13, 14).

While the first sRNAs characterized had relatively restricted functions in bacterial reg-

ulatory networks, it is now also clear that sRNAs can regulate multiple genes in the same pathway or phenotypic response (15). Similar to the protein master-regulators of transcription, they can be global regulators of metabolic processes or pathways that are central to pathogenesis, including outer membrane integrity, quorum sensing, iron homeostasis, biofilm formation, or host–pathogen interactions (4). Several sRNAs are also either induced in response to antibiotic treatment or are required for antibiotic tolerance (16, 17). Many transcription factor master-regulators of virulence and survival are themselves regulated by sRNAs or include sRNAs as part of their regulons. sRNAs encoded on pathogenicity islands (PAIs) or virulence plasmids are prime candidates for regulators with a central role in virulence (18–20). Nevertheless, PAI-encoded sRNAs can also regulate genes of the core genome (21, 22).

While once thought to be rare novelties of bacterial gene regulation, sRNAs are now taking center stage in bacterial virulence control. Many recent reviews discuss the emerging roles and mechanisms of sRNAs in human pathogens such as *Salmonella enterica* (23, 24), one of the main model organisms for riboregulation, but also, for example, in diverse pathogens such as *Listeria* (25, 26), *Vibrio* spp. (27, 28), *Yersinia* spp. (29, 30), *Staphylococcus aureus* (31, 32), *Mycobacterium tuberculosis* (33), *Helicobacter pylori* (34), *Pseudomonas aeruginosa* (35), and streptococci (36).

In this article, we provide an overview of the diversity of regulatory mechanisms used by sRNAs, especially in pathogens, as well as their various protein "accomplices." We apologize for any studies or sRNA examples that cannot be mentioned here due to space restrictions. We provide a general overview of how deep sequencing methods have revolutionized prokaryotic transcriptome analysis and sRNA identification and how they have provided novel means to study their functions and regulons on a genome-wide scale

(37). We refer the reader to more in-depth reviews for more detailed descriptions of methods to identify and verify sRNAs (38–40) and to study their functions (41, 42). Finally, pathways central to virulence and bacterial communication, such as quorum sensing, that employ sRNAs in the pathogens *S. aureus* and *Vibrio cholerae*, will be discussed in more detail to illustrate how riboregulation is integrated into gene regulatory circuits.

IDENTIFICATION OF A WEALTH OF sRNAs IN BACTERIAL GENOMES

The first sRNAs known were serendipitously discovered as curious noncoding transcripts in biochemical or functional genetic screens, aided by their relative abundance in the bacterial cell (38). Many of the first sRNAs to be functionally characterized were identified on mobile genetic elements such as plasmids, phages, and transposons, where they were shown to control replication, maintenance, or transposition (43). The abundant OmpR-dependent sRNA MicF was identified as the first chromosomally encoded sRNA that represses translation of an mRNA (encoding the OmpF porin) (44), making it a prototype for environmental posttranscriptional regulation by sRNAs. The first sRNA shown to directly affect virulence, RNAIII of *S. aureus* (see section on RNAIII, below), was then revealed to regulate multiple virulence factor-encoding transcripts (45).

Genome-Wide Approaches to Identify sRNAs

Approximately 15 years ago, numerous global studies were initiated to gauge the potential for sRNA-mediated regulation in bacteria, mainly in *E. coli* but also in pathogens (reviewed in 38, 40). These genome-wide searches used comparative genomics, secondary structure predictions, and/or computational searches for promoters and terminators in "intergenic" regions to identify potential

sRNA candidates (46–49). Confirmation of transcriptional activity with high-density or tiling microarrays increased the confidence of predictions (50–52) and also revealed many sRNAs that are expressed under pathogenesis-related conditions or involved in virulence of bacterial pathogens (53). RNomics approaches (either shotgun cloning or microarray analysis of cDNA) in multiple species, including *E. coli* and the pathogens *P. aeruginosa* and *S. aureus*, added to the pool of putative sRNAs (18, 54, 55). Identification of RNAs that copurify with the RNA chaperone Hfq by either microarrays (56) or direct enzymatic sequencing (57) was also utilized.

Going Deeper: Global Sequencing Approaches Identify Numerous sRNA Candidates and Place Riboregulators Centrally into Posttranscriptional Regulatory Networks

The development of a variety of next-generation sequencing technologies (so-called deep sequencing) to sequence cDNA ("RNA-sequencing" or "RNA-seq") has revolutionized transcriptome annotation and identification of novel noncoding transcripts in many pro- and eukaryotes and vastly increased the number of potential riboregulators (37). Furthermore, an increasing number of novel deep sequencing applications have been developed, such as global mapping of transposon insertion sites (transposon-sequencing) (58), surveying and measuring translatomes using ribosome profiling (59), and analysis of RNA-protein complexes (60). These approaches greatly facilitate the identification, verification, and functional characterization of sRNAs and are summarized below.

RNA-seq-based transcriptome analysis

Global transcriptome analyses at single-nucleotide resolution using RNA-seq technology have identified a wealth of sRNA candidates in prokaryotic genomes in recent years (6–8, 37, 39). While initial approaches in *V. cholerae* and *Listeria* employed deep sequencing of size-selected RNA that had been depleted of tRNA and 5S rRNA ("sRNA-seq") (2, 61, 62), a variety of RNA-seq methodologies to cover full transcriptomes have also been developed (8). These include approaches that specifically analyze primary transcriptomes and annotate transcriptional start sites, such as differential RNA-seq (dRNA-seq; reviewed in reference 9). RNA-seq studies have revealed a wealth of novel sRNAs and regulatory elements in diverse prokaryotes including numerous human pathogens such as *Burkholderia cenocepacia* (63), *H. pylori* (64), *Salmonella* (65–67), *Campylobacter jejuni* (68–71), *Neisseria gonorrhoeae* (72), *V. cholerae* (73, 74), *Chlamydia* spp. (75, 76), *Listeria* spp. (77, 78), *P. aeruginosa* (79), *M. tuberculosis* (80), *Streptococcus pneumoniae* (81), staphylococci (82, 83), and *Legionella* (84). Comparative transcriptome analysis in different pathogenic species or strains has revealed both conserved sRNAs and strain-specific sRNAs that might contribute to differences in pathovar gene regulation and colonization of different niches or hosts (68, 77). Strikingly, a large reservoir of potential noncoding regulatory RNAs have also been identified transcribed antisense to open reading frames (ORFs) (85–87). It remains unclear how many of these "pervasive" transcripts are due to spurious transcription and how many have real functions.

Besides genome-wide transcriptome analysis, global RNA-seq analysis of RNA copurifying with RNA-binding proteins (so-called RIP-seq: RNA-immunoprecipitation-sequencing) has also played an important part in the recent large-scale identification of sRNA candidates. RIP-seq of the RNA chaperone Hfq has revealed a surprising number of sRNA candidates arising not only from intergenic regions, but also in untranslated regions (UTRs) of mRNAs, such as 3′UTRs (88–90). As a result, mRNAs/coding regions are now accepted as an important source of sRNAs. Sequencing of cross-linked Hfq-binding RNAs in enterohemorrhagic *E. coli* has identified numerous candidate sRNAs,

including some that are encoded by PAIs (22). Likewise, RIP-seq of *S. aureus* RNase III revealed global regulatory functions for this enzyme, as well as novel mechanisms of gene coregulation (91).

These approaches have together greatly expanded the number of candidate sRNAs in bacteria. In *Salmonella*, for example, there are 280 strong sRNA candidates (66). However, functional characterization of sRNAs and identification of their mRNA targets can be laborious. For most of the candidate sRNAs their functions and targets still need to be identified. The limited number of currently characterized sRNAs available for comparative analyses, together with their short overall length (50 to 400 nucleotides [nt]) and short region of complementarity to target mRNAs (sometimes as few as 7 nt) has made *in silico* predictions of regulons challenging (42). A variety of methods have been developed to identify and study sRNA regulons using global approaches (39). Quantitative RNA-seq now serves as the gold standard for studying and comparing bacterial transcriptomes (92), replacing hybridization-based technologies such as microarrays and providing both single-nucleotide resolution and a higher dynamic range. Comparative transcriptomics of sRNA deletion and over-expression strains, as well as following pulse-expression of sRNAs, has both identified direct sRNA targets and revealed the global physiological functions of sRNAs and bacterial RNases (93).

Transposon-sequencing

The power of deep sequencing has also been harnessed for unbiased, global genetic screens for sRNAs. The location of transposon insertions in high-density mutant libraries can be identified by "transposon-sequencing" (Tn-seq) based on deep sequencing of transposon-chromosome junctions (58, 94). Due to the use of deep sequencing, a high insertion density (so far, as high as one insertion for every 8 bp) can be screened. This provides the resolution necessary to identify short genomic regions that might encode sRNAs or regulatory regions, which might have been missed in traditional transposon screens. Furthermore, combination of Tn-seq with whole-transcriptome RNA-seq data allows for the identification of transcriptionally active regions. As proof-of-principle, Tn-seq of two serovars of pathogenic *Salmonella* (Typhimurium and Typhi) with different host ranges and tissue tropisms identified an essential core genome conserved with nonpathogenic *E. coli* K12, as well as differences in sRNA repertoires that may underlie variations in pathogenicity (95). Tn-seq has been used to define the essential gene content and/or candidate virulence-associated sRNAs of numerous other pathogens, including *N. gonorrhoeae* (72), *S. pneumoniae* (81, 96), *M. tuberculosis* (97), *Salmonella* (95, 98, 99), enterohemorrhagic *E. coli* (100), *C. jejuni* (101), and *Haemophilus influenzae* (102).

HOW REGULATORY RNAs POSTTRANSCRIPTIONALLY REGULATE GENE EXPRESSION IN BACTERIA

While many sRNAs directly interact with mRNAs via base-pairing, other mechanisms of riboregulation have also been described. These include sRNAs that directly modulate protein activity, *cis*-acting elements of mRNAs themselves, and even dual-function sRNAs, which act as both riboregulators and code for small proteins (11). In this section, we provide an overview of the steadily expanding diversity of mechanisms employed by regulatory RNA (3, 103). We focus, where possible, on examples identified in pathogenic species that control virulence- and survival-associated phenotypes or regulate virulence genes (Table 1).

Regulation by *cis*-Encoded Antisense RNAs

Most of the functionally characterized sRNAs regulate their target mRNAs by an antisense

mechanism using direct base-pairing interactions. Base-pairing sRNAs are generally divided into two categories based on their genomic relationship with their mRNA targets: (i) *Cis*-encoded sRNAs are transcribed from the opposite DNA strand and therefore show perfect, often extensive (>75 nt), complementarity with their target mRNAs (Fig. 1A), and (ii) *Trans*-encoded sRNAs are transcribed from different genomic locations than their targets and interact, often with multiple mRNAs, via imperfect base-pairing (Fig. 1B).

The first identified *cis*-encoded antisense RNAs (asRNAs) were found opposite to replication genes of plasmids or to transposase genes. They control maintenance and stability of mobile genetic elements through, for example, inhibition of primer maturation, transcriptional attenuation, translational repression, or induction of RNA degradation or cleavage (43). Many *cis*-encoded asRNAs are components of so-called type I toxin–antitoxin (TA) systems (104). These are two-gene elements consisting of a stable protein toxin and an unstable *cis*-encoded RNA antitoxin that base-pairs with the toxin mRNA, thereby inhibiting its translation and leading to degradation (105). While type I TA systems were initially found to be involved in plasmid stability and addiction, an increasing number of TA loci have since been identified in the chromosomes of many bacteria, including pathogens (106). The function of these chromosomally encoded TA systems remains enigmatic, but they may mediate adaptation of metabolism under stress, persister cell formation, or antibiotic resistance (107, 108). For example, TisB is an SOS-induced membrane-interacting toxic peptide that has been implicated in persister cell formation, which may increase intrinsic antibiotic resistance of bacterial populations (reviewed in 109). Its asRNA antitoxin, IstR, acts by sequestering a ribosome standby site on the *tisB* mRNA, thereby preventing its translation (110). TisB-dependent persister cells are tolerant to multiple antibiotics, and deletion of *Salmonella*

TABLE 1 Examples of PAI-encoded sRNAs and of riboregulators of bacterial virulence/colonization factors

Type	RNA	Pathogen	Target(s)	Related phenotypes/comment	Reference(s)
cis-acting sRNAs	5'ureB	Helicobacter pylori	ureB	Urease expression/acid adaptation	116
	AmgR	Salmonella enterica	mgtC	Survival in macrophages	114
	IesR-1	S. enterica serovar Typhimurium	Unknown	Expressed from pSLT virulence plasmid, required for replication in fibroblasts	115
trans-acting sRNAs	AbcR-1, AbcR-2	Brucella abortus	Unknown	Infection of macrophages and chronic infection of mice	152
	DapZ	S. Typhimurium	oppA, dppA	3'UTR-encoded sRNA that regulates amino acid/oligopeptide metabolism	88
	DsrA	Borrelia burgdorferi	rpoS	Expression of virulence-associated surface proteins	163
	FasX	Group A streptococci	ska, cpa	Streptokinase and pilus expression	173
	IhtA	Chlamydia trachomatis	hctA	Differentiation between the RB and EB developmental stages	150
	InvR	S. Typhimurium	ompD	PAI-encoded, activated by SPI-1 regulator HilD, represses a porin of the core genome	21
	IsrJ	S. Typhimurium	Unknown	Affects translocation of SptP and invasion into nonphagocytic cells	19
	IsrM	S. Typhimurium	sopA, hilE	Invasion, intracellular replication, virulence, and colonization of mice	155
	IstR	Escherichia coli	tisB	Persister cell formation	340
	IstR	Salmonella	tisB	Type I TA system, colonization	111
	LhrC	Listeria monocytogenes	lapB	Represses a virulence-associated adhesin	57, 133
	PapR	Uropathogenic E. coli	papI	Population-level type I fimbriae expression	149
	RepG	H. pylori	tlpB	Chemotaxis receptor levels	137
	Rli27	L. monocytogenes	Lmo0514	Activation of expression of a cell wall protein inside cells	164
	RyhB	Shigella dysenteriae	virB	Affects T3SS/effectors and virulence	148
	RprA	S. enterica	rpoS, ricI	Control of conjugation of the pSLT virulence plasmid in response to membrane conditions	171
	SgrS	S. Typhimurium	sopD	Core genome sRNA that regulates a SPI-1 effector	132
	SprD	Staphylococcus aureus	sbi	Immune evasion	316
	SprX	S. aureus	spoVG	Glycopeptide resistance	135
	SroA	S. Typhimurium	Unknown	Riboswitch-derived sRNA required for infection of mice	111
	sX13	Xanthomonas campestris	hrpX	Affects levels of T3SS regulator	138
	TarB	Vibrio cholerae	tcpF	Regulates a virulence factor and affects colonization	2
	VqmR	V. cholerae	vpsT, rtx	Biofilm formation and toxin expression	73
	VR-RNA	Clostridium perfringens	colA	Toxin expression	168
Dual-function (sRNA with ORF,	fim 5'UTR	S. Typhimurium	CsrA	Hierarchical fimbriae expression	279
	RNAIII	S. aureus	spa, hla, coa, rot, sbi	δ-haemolysin-encoding; quorum sensing control of toxin and surface protein expression	45, 315

Category	Name	Organism	Target	Function	Reference
mRNA with regulatory function	SprA1-SprA1$_{AS}$	S. aureus	SprA1-encoded cytolysin	Cytolysin-encoding, cis-encoded trans-sRNA	318
Riboswitches (ligand/signal)	PhrS	Pseudomonas aeruginosa	pqsR	Quorum sensing	170
	mgtA 5'UTR (Mg^{2+})	Salmonella	mgtA	Intracellular magnesium uptake	239
	pilA1 5'UTR (c-di-GMP)	Clostridium difficile	pilA1	Expression of type IV pili and aggregation	250
	Vc2 (c-di-GMP)	V. cholerae	VC1722	Present in the mRNA encoding a TfoX competence regulator homologue	248
	alx 5'UTR (pH)	Salmonella	alx	Controls expression of the Alx transporter by forming a translationally active structure at low pH	246
Thermosensors	css 5'UTR	Neisseria meningitidis	css	Controls capsule biosynthesis and immune evasion	264
	lasI 5'UTR	P. aeruginosa	lasI	Quorum sensing	266
	prfA 5'UTR	L. monocytogenes	prfA	Virulence factor expression	263
	rhlAB 5'UTR	P. aeruginosa	rhlR	Quorum sensing	266
	toxT 5'UTR	V. cholerae	toxT	Virulence factor expression	289
Protein-modulating	6S	L. pneumophila	RNAP	Required for optimal replication in amoeba and mammalian host cells	231
	6S	S. Typhimurium	RNAP	Repressed during intracellular replication	341
	CsrB/C	V. cholerae	CsrA	Quorum sensing	306
	CsrB/C	S. Typhimurium	CsrA	Motility and pathogenesis	220
	Ms1	Mycobacterium smegmatis	RNAP	Implicated in stationary phase adaptation	232
	Rli55	L. monocytogenes	EutV	Ethanolamine utilization	259
	RsmX/Y/Z	P. aeruginosa	RsmA	T3SS, T6SS, virulence, exopolysaccharide	222, 223
	RsmX/Y/Z	L. pneumophila	CsrA	Motility and replication in macrophages, expression of T4SS effectors	84, 225, 226
IasRNA/excludon	CsrB/C	Yersinia pseudotuberculosis	CsrA	Virulence regulator RovA	216
	Anti0677	L. monocytogenes	Flagellar operon	Motility/flagellum biosynthesis	53, 289
CRISPR/Cas	Cas2	L. pneumophila	Unknown	Cas2 is required for infection of amoeba	331
	CRISPR/Cas	Streptococcus pyogenes	Foreign DNA	DNA uptake and capsule genotype	327
	CRISPR/Cas	Enterococcus spp.	Foreign DNA	Mobile DNA/antibiotic resistance uptake	326
	RliB	L. monocytogenes	Unknown	Deletion of rliB affects virulence in mice	53, 342
	scal/tracr/Cas9	Francisella novicida	FTN_1103	Regulates a lipoprotein and affects immune evasion, antibiotic resistance	328, 329
Other	pilE upstream	N. gonorrhoeae	pilE upstream G-quadruplex	Recombination of expressed pilin locus/antigenic variation	343

^{a}Abbreviations: ORF, open reading frame; RB, reticulate body; EB, elementary body; PAI, pathogenicity island; TA, toxin–antitoxin; T3/4/6SS, type III/IV/VI secretion system RNAP, RNA polymerase; UTR, untranslated region

A

cis-encoded sRNAs

complementary to 5'/3'UTR

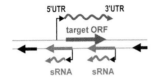

complementary to ORF

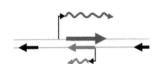

B

trans-encoded sRNAs

stand-alone (intergenic)

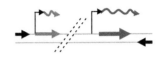

mRNA (3'UTR)-derived

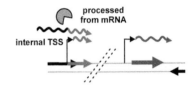

C

excludon / overlapping UTRs

lasRNA / excludon

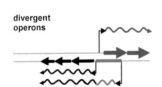

extended 3'UTR

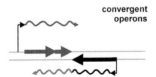

D

cis-acting mRNA elements

riboswitch

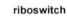
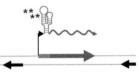

thermosensor

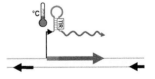

istR also reduces fitness in pooled deletion mutant infections in mice, supporting a role in pathogenesis (111).

Besides the asRNAs of ORFs encoding small toxic proteins, an increasing number of transcripts have been reported that are expressed antisense to other mRNAs, including examples that are antisense to UTRs or coding regions (Fig. 1A) or even to sRNAs (85, 86). Some asRNAs have, in fact, been shown to regulate virulence-associated genes. The *Salmonella* PhoPQ two-component regulatory system (TCRS) responds to the acidified environment of the phagolysosome, among other signals, to activate expression of factors that allow for intracellular replication. These include MgtC, an inner membrane protein required for survival in macrophages and virulence in mice (112, 113), as well as the MgtB Mg^{2+} transporter. PhoP also activates expression of the 1.2-kb AmgR transcript, which is encoded antisense to *mgtCBR*. AmgR promotes decay of *mgtC* mRNA via an RNase E–dependent mechanism (114). Absence of the AmgR asRNA both increases MgtC and MgtB levels and enhances bacterial virulence. A second asRNA, lesR-1, has also been identified on the pSLT virulence plasmid of *S.* Typhimurium (115). Expression of lesR-1 is 300-fold higher during infection of fibroblasts compared to its expression in broth culture, and it is required for replication in this cell type. In the gastric pathogen

H. pylori, the urease enzyme, encoded in part by the *ureAB* operon, is required for adaptation to the acidic environment of the stomach. An sRNA (named 5′*ureB*-sRNA) on the opposite strand to *ureAB* is expressed dependent on the ArsRS TCRS and binds to the 5′-end of the *ureB* message (116, 117). This promotes premature transcription termination of the *ureAB* transcript and thereby represses urease levels at neutral pH, where the enzyme is presumably dispensable.

Recent work has identified asRNAs in *Neisseria* that may act at the DNA level, rather than by base-pairing with mRNA. Adherence to the epithelium of the urogenital tract by *N. gonorrhoeae* is mediated by type IV pili. Pilin genes are a prime target of antigenic variation, which provides population-level fitness and mediates immune evasion and persistent infection. A G-quadruplex (G4) structure upstream of the promoter of *pilE* has been shown to be required for recombination between the "expressed" *pilE* locus and one of the 19 remaining "silent" *pilS* pilin loci (118). Transcription of a short, C-rich RNA antisense to this G4 structure is also required for switching (119). It has been suggested that transcription of the asRNA may aid in formation of the G4 structure via a DNA:RNA hybrid between the asRNA and the complementary C-rich strand of the *pilE* G4. However, it is not yet clear whether it is solely the act of transcription (rather than

---

FIGURE 1 Genomic location and regulatory relationships between bacterial riboregulators and their mRNA targets. Riboregulators are depicted in red; target mRNAs are shown in blue. Flanking open reading frames (ORFs) are shown in black. Arrows indicate transcriptional start sites. (A) *Cis*-encoded antisense RNAs are transcribed from the opposite strand to their target mRNAs and can overlap with target 5′/3′ untranslated regions (UTRs) (top panel) and/or the mRNA ORF (bottom panel). (B)*Trans*-encoded sRNAs can be expressed from distinct regions of the chromosome from their target genes: either from stand-alone genes encoded intergenically (top panel) or from ORFs/3′UTRs via either processing or internal transcriptional start sites (bottom panel). (C) Extended UTR elements of adjacent operons can allow for coregulation of related genes at the posttranscriptional level. The long-antisense RNA (lasRNA) of the excludon paradigm arises from transcription of an extended 5′UTR that has complementarity to a divergently transcribed operon (top panel). Also, extended 3′UTR elements can potentially base-pair with transcripts expressed from convergently transcribed operons (bottom panel). (D)*Cis*-elements within mRNAs themselves can regulate expression of their associated transcripts. These include ligand-binding riboswitches (top panel) and temperature-responsive RNA thermosensors (bottom panel).

the sRNA itself) that mediates G4 formation. Recombination also contributes to pilin antigenic variation in *N. meningitidis*. However, in meningococci, an asRNA conditionally expressed from a region downstream of *pilE*, complementary to the entire *pilE* coding sequence and 5′UTR, may instead influence the rate of variation (120).

A large reservoir of potential *cis*-encoded sRNAs is the pervasive antisense transcription that has been noted in recent global bacterial transcriptome studies (121). For example, dRNA-seq analysis of *H. pylori* found that approximately half of all ORFs had at least one antisense TSS (64). Likewise, it has been proposed that 75% of *S. aureus* coding genes could be subject to regulation by asRNAs resulting from widespread transcription antisense to coding mRNAs, which provides double-stranded substrates for processing and/or degradation by RNase III (87). Extensive asRNA expression has also been noted from the Ti plasmid of the plant pathogen *Agrobacterium*, many of which are antisense to known virulence genes (122). Presumably, these transcripts are well suited to interfere with transcription or translation of mRNAs on the opposite strand or to stimulate their degradation by RNase III. However, whether these asRNAs are simply transcriptional noise or play a general regulatory role is still unclear, as many are neither significantly conserved nor very abundant.

Transcriptome maps of *Listeria* spp. identified a new class of asRNA species, the long antisense RNAs (lasRNAs), and a new concept in riboregulation, the "excludon" (53, 77) (reviewed in 123) (Fig. 1C). Often, lasRNAs arise in divergently transcribed ORFs/operons with mutually exclusive or related functions and can overlap multiple ORFs. Expression from a conditional promoter upstream of one operon provides an asRNA, likely part of an extended leader, which can base-pair with the mRNA of the operon on the opposite strand (Fig. 1C, top panel). One such "excludon" in the *Listeria* flagellum biosynthesis locus has been identified and characterized (53). The *mogR* mRNA, encoding the MogR repressor of flagellum biosynthesis, can be expressed from a promoter immediately upstream of the start codon. However, expression of *mogR* from a second σ^B-dependent promoter further upstream leads to a transcript with a longer 5′UTR. This extra leader (lasRNA Anti0677) extends into the adjacent divergently transcribed operon, which encodes three genes required for flagellum export. Overexpression of the longer *mogR* transcript leads to decreased motility and flagellin transcript levels, possibly due to antisense interactions with this adjacent motility-associated operon. Likewise, transcription of extended 3′UTRs in convergently transcribed operons could potentially interfere with transcripts on the opposite strand, also leading to coregulation (Fig. 1C, bottom panel). Numerous examples of such situations were identified in tiling-array analysis of the *Listeria monocytogenes* transcriptome (53) but still await functional characterization.

Regulation by *trans*-Encoded sRNAs

Trans-encoded sRNAs (Fig. 1B) are a diverse family of short (50 to 300 nt), usually untranslated, transcripts. While *trans*-sRNAs (also referred to as simply "sRNAs") are often encoded intergenically, they can also be derived from UTRs (5′ or 3′UTRs) or even from coding regions themselves (89) (Fig. 1B, bottom). Many sRNAs are global regulators of gene expression and are often induced in response to stress or inside host cells (3, 4, 15, 124). They can control extensive regulons that include mRNAs in similar physiological pathways such as outer membrane biogenesis (125, 126), iron or carbon metabolism (127, 128), or amino acid transport/biosynthesis and peptide uptake (129).

Comparison of sRNAs that require the RNA chaperone Hfq for their stability or function (see below) has led to the proposal of a modular sRNA structure: a short single-stranded "seed region" required to interact with target mRNAs, an AU-rich Hfq-binding region, and a structured terminal loop, which facilitates Rho-independent transcription termination and protects the sRNA from degradation by 3′-exonucleases (3). The seed region, which base-pairs with target mRNAs, often has only a surprisingly short region of complementarity—sometimes only 6 to 7 nt (130, 131). Extended interactions between sRNAs and their target mRNAs can also be imperfect, with multiple nonpairing bases. The consequence of imperfect base-pairing is two-fold: first, an sRNA can be a global regulator, interacting with numerous target mRNAs in related pathways, and second, one mRNA may be targeted by multiple sRNAs and can thus be regulated posttranscriptionally in response to numerous signals. Yet, still, the seed-pairing strategy maintains regulatory specificity. Only a single base pair difference in the targeting region of the mRNAs encoding two paralog effector proteins of *S.* Typhimurium, *sopD* and *sopD2*, is sufficient for the sRNA SgrS to discriminate between them (132). While expression of *sopD* is repressed by SgrS, *sopD2* is not regulated by this sRNA.

Functional characterization of sRNAs outside the enterobacteria and in those lacking Hfq has uncovered other common themes of sRNA structure and function. Many sRNAs use unpaired sequences in apical hairpin loops to interact with target mRNAs. An increasing number of sRNAs with C- or C/U-rich loops have been reported that are well suited for base-pairing with G-rich sequences of mRNAs, such as the consensus ribosome binding site (RBS). Examples of these C-rich sRNAs are widespread in bacterial pathogens, such as *L. monocytogenes* (133), *S. aureus* (134, 135), *V. cholerae* (73), *Salmonella* (136), *H. pylori* (137), and *Xanthomonas campestris* (138). Thus, like the seed-pairing sRNAs of enterobacteria, such C-rich sRNAs may represent another common family of riboregulators.

While some sRNAs share structural themes, the diversity of mechanisms and regulatory consequences of *trans*-acting sRNAs is ever-increasing. Base-pairing by sRNAs can lead to repression or activation of target gene expression (3, 139) (Fig. 2A). Here, we will discuss a selection of *trans*-acting sRNAs that control genes associated with virulence or survival in bacterial pathogens (see also Table 1).

trans-encoded sRNAs that repress virulence gene expression

The prototypical sRNA represses protein levels by interfering with translation initiation and/or elongation through base-pairing with the translation initiation region (TIR), often at or near the RBS and start codon (Fig. 2A, left). However, RNAs can also interact with other mRNA regions (Fig. 2B), such as far upstream of the TIR in the 5′UTR. For example, ribosome standby sites or translational enhancers can be targeted (110, 140). Targeting can also occur within coding sequences (141). As the ribosome protects mRNAs from the RNA turnover machinery of the cell (142), translation inhibition often results in degradation of a message since it can be more directly targeted for degradation by RNases. In addition, interaction of some sRNAs with their target can expose RNase cleavage sites, recruit ribonucleases such as RNase E, and/or stimulate the cleavage activity of RNase E by providing a 5′ monophosphate (141, 143, 144), thereby affecting mRNA stability. sRNAs can be catalytic (recycled to repress other mRNA molecules) or noncatalytic (codegraded with their targets) (145, 146). Single sRNAs can show amazing versatility, using different mechanisms depending on the target mRNA and nature of base-paring interaction (145).

Several sRNAs that repress virulence genes, such as the above-mentioned *Salmonella* SgrS sRNA that represses expression of the SopD effector protein (132), or genes crucial for replication within the host have been reported (4) (see Table 1). The virulence plasmid of the gastrointestinal pathogen *Shigella dysenteriae* encodes genes required for invasion of host cells and disease, including a type III secretion system (T3SS) and its

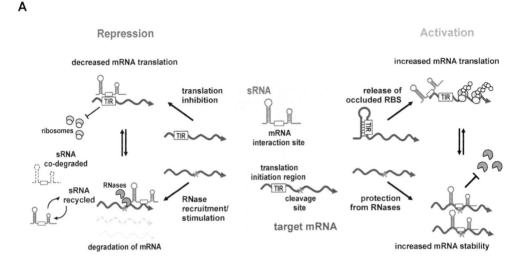

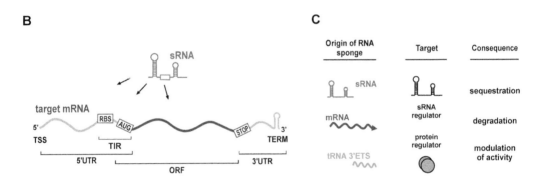

FIGURE 2 Mechanisms of posttranscriptional control by regulatory RNAs. (A) Gene repression (left) and activation (right) mechanisms used by base-pairing sRNAs (depicted in red) for direct regulation of target mRNAs (shown in blue) at the level of translation or stability. Base-pairing interaction sites in mRNAs and sRNAs are shown with blue- and red-lined boxes, respectively. Potential RNase cleavage sites are indicated with an orange asterisk. Also participating are ribosomes and RNases. TIR, translation initiation region including RBS and start codon. (B) Potential sRNA interaction sites in regulated target mRNAs, starting from the TSS (transcriptional start site) to the transcriptional terminator (TERM). (C) Targeting/titration of other regulatory molecules by riboregulators acting as so-called sponges to affect gene expression. RNA sponges can be stand-alone sRNAs, regions of mRNAs themselves (either intact or processed), or those derived from housekeeping RNAs such as the 3′ external transcribed spacer (3′ ETS) of tRNAs. They can target either sRNA or protein regulators and have been shown to sequester them away from their targets, trigger their degradation, and/or modulate their regulatory activity.

effectors. These genes are coordinately regulated in response to environmental signals by two transcriptional regulators, VirF and VirB (147). The iron-responsive sRNA RyhB represses levels of VirB, thereby indirectly repressing its entire regulon (148). Overexpression of RyhB decreases VirB levels,

reduces effector secretion, and causes defects compared to the wild-type strain for invasion *in vitro*. In uropathogenic *E. coli*, comparative deep-sequencing of Hfq-bound RNAs during infection identified PapR, an sRNA that represses a protein involved in phase variation and appears to affect expression of P-fimbriae, an important epithelial adhesion factor at the population level (149).

The obligate intracellular pathogen *Chlamydia trachomatis* cycles between two physiological states during infection: elementary bodies and reticulate bodies. The infectious, extracellular elementary bodies are transcriptionally and translationally silent due to chromatin condensation, which is mediated in part by the histone-like protein HctA (also called Hc1). During differentiation into metabolically active reticulate bodies, HctA levels are reduced, and this correlates with expression of the IhtA sRNA (150). IhtA interacts with the *hctA* mRNA *in vitro* and appears to repress its translation (151).

Two apparently redundant sRNAs, AbcR-1 and AbcR-2, are conserved in *Alphaproteobacteria* such as *Brucella abortus* and *Agrobacterium tumefaciens* (152, 153). In *B. abortus*, these sRNAs regulate genes involved in amino acid transport and are required for infection of macrophages, as well as chronic infection of mice.

Several *Salmonella* sRNAs are induced under virulence-associated stress conditions or inside eukaryotic cells, including PAI-encoded sRNAs (19, 66, 154). One such sRNA of *S.* Typhimurium, IsrM, regulates virulence factors essential for invasion of host cells (155). IsrM targets the 5′UTR of *sopA* mRNA, encoding a SPI-1 effector, as well as the leader of *hilE*, a global regulator of the expression of SPI-1 proteins. Deletion of *isrM* results in defects in epithelial cell invasion and replication inside macrophages, as well as reduced virulence and extraintestinal growth in mice. A second PAI-encoded sRNA, InvR, is activated by the SPI-1 regulator HilD and represses the *ompD* porin mRNA encoded in the core genome (21). A third PAI-encoded sRNA, IsrJ, is required for invasion into host cells and secretion of the SPI-1 T3SS effector SptP (19). However, the mRNA targets and mode of regulation for IsrJ have not yet been determined. The conserved enterobacterial sRNA OxyS is induced under oxidative stress by OxyR and acts as

both a repressor and activator of gene expression in *E. coli*. OxyS represses levels of the FhlA regulator and the RpoS sigma factor (156–158), and interestingly, an *oxyS* deletion mutant in *Salmonella* shows increased fitness in mice during infections with pooled deletion mutants (111).

Small RNAs that repress important virulence and colonization factors have also been identified in Gram-positive pathogens. Profiling of *L. monocytogenes* sRNA expression in macrophages has detected 71 noncoding transcripts not previously identified under routine laboratory conditions (62). *L. monocytogenes* requires the surface protein LapB for adhesion and entry into host cells. The multicopy LhrC sRNA, induced by the stress-associated LisRK TCRS, uses three UCCC sequences to interact with G-rich sequences near the start codon of the *lapB* message to inhibit its translation (133). ChIP-seq of the *M. tuberculosis* PhoP regulon identified the sRNA Mcr7, which was predicted to interact with *tatC* mRNA, encoding a component of the twin-arginine translocation system (159). Deletion of *phoP*, which is required for Mcr7 expression, increases twin-arginine translocation–dependent substrates in the *M. tuberculosis* secretome, some of which contribute to infection of the host.

trans-encoded sRNAs that activate virulence gene expression

sRNAs can activate gene expression by mechanisms that increase mRNA translation or transcript stability (139, 160) (Fig. 2A, right). Increased translation can result from base-pairing interactions that disrupt inhibitory secondary structures sequestering the RBS, as observed for activation of the alpha toxin–encoding *hla* mRNA by RNAIII in *S. aureus* (161). In the Lyme disease spirochete *Borrelia burgdorferi*, the alternative sigma factor RpoS reciprocally regulates expression of two virulence-associated surface proteins, OspC and OspA (162). *B. burgdorferi* RpoS expression is activated at higher temperatures, and this requires the sRNA DsrA, which may allow unfolding of a structured region in the 5'UTR of the *rpoS* mRNA that sequesters its RBS (163). Inside host cells, *L. monocytogenes* upregulates cell wall–associated proteins, including Lmo0514, which is encoded by an mRNA with two different 5'UTR lengths of 28 and 234 nucleotides (164). The longer message is induced inside cells, and the extended leader of this transcript can base-pair with Rli27 sRNA, which is also upregulated inside cells. This interaction activates translation of the mRNA.

Like decreased mRNA stability due to translational repression, increased translation can also protect transcripts from the RNA turnover machinery of the cell (Fig. 2A). Pathogen sRNAs have also been reported to activate mRNAs by selective stabilization of decay intermediates or longer isoforms (165, 166) or by mediating processing into more stable transcripts (167). For example, VR-RNA of *Clostridium perfringens* activates expression of collagenase by mediating processing of the leader of the *colA* transcript to increase its stability (168).

Activation by sRNAs can occur by mechanistic twists on the above themes that combine different regulatory modules. *P. aeruginosa* uses multiple quorum sensing systems to coordinately control expression of group-associated phenotypes, including virulence. The *Pseudomonas* quinolone system (PQS) generates and detects the signal 2-heptyl-3-hydroxy-4-quinolone and controls expression of virulence genes, including elastase, phospholipase, and phenazine via the activator PqsR (169). Levels of PqsR are regulated indirectly by an sRNA via translational activation of a short upstream ORF (uORF) in the *pqsR* leader (170). Translation of *pqsR* is coupled to translation of the uORF; i.e., increased translation of the uORF releases a structure that occludes the RBS of *pqsR*. The RBS of the uORF is also occluded by the inhibitory secondary structure. Upon induction under low oxygen conditions, the PhrS sRNA base-pairs with a region upstream of the uORF and releases

sequestration of its RBS. The resulting translation of the uORF thereby allows expression of the translationally coupled *pqsR* gene.

sRNAs can also activate multiple targets posttranscriptionally, and this can integrate different signals into regulatory logic modules, such as those commonly seen in transcription factor networks (124). In feed-forward loops, one regulator is controlled by a second regulator, and both act upon a third target. In *Salmonella*, the RicI protein inhibits conjugation of the virulence plasmid pSLT and is the target of such a feed-forward loop, modulated by an sRNA (171). Full expression of RicI requires translational activation of both its transcriptional regulator (RpoS) and its own mRNA by a single sRNA, RprA. RprA has two separate targeting seed sequences (one for *rpoS* and one for *ricI*). While the full-length RprA, which has both seed sequences, is induced under conditions such as envelope stress, the sRNA is processed by RNase E to a more stable 3' form with only the *ricI* seed. This lower stability of full-length RprA allows another level of control: while activating conditions lead to immediate upregulation of both RpoS and RicI seed pairing regions, differential decay allows for resetting of the signal or even activation by only the second (*ricI*-targeting) seed when input from other conditions that activate RpoS are present. This module ensures that expression of the RicI conjugation inhibitor occurs only under conditions of significant membrane damage.

trans-acting sRNAs that both activate and repress virulence genes

The versatility of sRNAs as gene regulators also lies in their potential to either repress or activate different targets. One of the best-characterized sRNA that can both activate and repress targets is RNAIII of *S. aureus* (see section on RNAIII, below). However, RNAIII is far from the exception. The Qrr3 sRNA involved in *Vibrio* quorum sensing uses four distinct mechanisms to either repress or activate different target mRNAs depending on a particular pairing strategy that dictates the regulatory mechanism (145). FasX, conserved in group A streptococci (i.e., *Streptococcus pyogenes*), activates expression of the secreted virulence factor streptokinase via base-pairing interactions that stabilize the *ska* transcript (172). The same sRNA can also bind to the 5′-end of a pilus operon mRNA, thereby reducing mRNA stability and repressing translation of the first gene of this mRNA, *cpa*, encoding a minor pilin component (173).

The gastric pathogen *H. pylori* expresses at least 60 candidate sRNAs (64). The abundant, conserved sRNA RepG regulates expression of the TlpB chemotaxis receptor, involved in pH, autoinducer, and urea chemotaxis (174–176), at the level of *tlpB* mRNA stability and translation. Interaction between a C-rich terminator loop of RepG with a variable homopolymeric G-repeat in the *tlpB* mRNA leader differentially represses or activates expression of TlpB depending on the G-repeat length (137). Therefore, RepG has the potential to act as either an activator or repressor based on phase variation in its targeting sequence.

The RNA chaperone Hfq and auxiliary protein factors that cooperate with *trans*-acting sRNAs

The Hfq RNA chaperone is present in about 50% of bacteria with sequenced genomes (14). Hfq is a homo-hexameric, doughnut-shaped protein, with each subunit containing two domains similar to the Sm proteins of eukaryotes (177). It binds sRNAs on one of two binding faces, with a preference for single-stranded A-, U-, or A/U-rich sequences near structured regions (178–180). Through these interactions, Hfq mediates numerous aspects of sRNA metabolism and activity (reviewed in 13). Hfq aids the interaction between many *trans*-acting sRNAs and their targets and can either facilitate presentation of seed regions for base-pairing to targets, open target structures, or increase the local concentration of sRNAs, thereby lowering the effective dissociation constant between sRNA and mRNA targets. It is also required for the stability of some sRNAs by protecting A/U-rich sites from degradation by RNase E (181). Together with sRNAs, Hfq can also recruit RNase E to degrade the target (182). The chaperone itself can also bind and affect translation of some mRNAs (183, 184), even being recruited to target mRNAs by an sRNA, such as has been reported for the Spot42 sRNA and *sdhC* mRNA (185). Competition for Hfq by sRNAs may be yet another layer of global regulation, with sRNAs actively cycling on Hfq in a concentration-dependent manner (186–188). In fact, in *S.* Typhimurium, the Hfq-bound sRNA profile changes with bacterial growth phase (14), and in uropathogenic *E. coli*, the Hfq-bound sRNA profile differs between intracellular and extracellular environments (149).

Not surprisingly, deletion of *hfq* has pleiotropic effects in numerous bacteria, including virulence (14). However, not all bacteria encode Hfq, and not all sRNAs in Hfq-containing bacteria require this protein for their activity or stability (189). In fact, sRNAs are often divided into Hfq-dependent and Hfq-independent, based on whether stability and/or interaction with target mRNAs by the sRNA is dependent on the RNA chaperone. Numerous sRNAs of Gram-positive bacteria show Hfq-independence in stability and/or target interactions, despite being identified in Hfq-binding screens. LhrC of *L. monocytogenes* was first identified in an Hfq-RNA coIP study (57), although it regulates at least one target, *lapB* mRNA, in the absence of *hfq* (133). This raises the question as to whether unidentified RNA chaperones exist that replace or complement the functions of Hfq.

Several ribonucleases also factor centrally into multiple levels of riboregulation, including the biogenesis/maturation and activity of *trans*-encoded sRNAs (190). Many RNases are essential for viability in diverse species and/or have pleiotropic effects on bacterial physiology or virulence of pathogens, including RNase III, RNase E, RNase R, PNPase (polynucleotide phosphorylase), and RNase Y (191–198). Some RNases, such as RNase E, cooperate with sRNAs to degrade target mRNAs, after either exposure of specific cleavage sites or release from the protection of the translational machinery (199, 200). RNase III can cleave double-stranded regions formed by loop–loop interactions between sRNAs and mRNAs, such as those between *S. aureus* RNAIII and several virulence factor–encoding mRNAs (201–204) (see section on RNAIII, below). RNases themselves also have direct effects on gene expression independent of an sRNA accomplice via cleavage of specific coding transcripts implicated in virulence. This has been especially apparent for RNases III and Y in Gram-positive bacteria (reviewed in 205, 206). For example, RNase Y of *S. aureus* is required for processing and stabilization of the transcript encoding the SaePQRS TCRS, a global regulator of virulence, thereby contributing to activation of expression of virulence genes (192). RIP-seq of a catalytically inactive mutant has likewise identified substrates of RNase III in *S. aureus* (91). RNase III was revealed to process mRNAs, such as the *cspA* major cold shock protein mRNA, to increase their stability, as well as to cleave overlapping transcripts from divergently transcribed genes to generate leaderless mRNAs. Therefore, widely conserved RNases in bacterial pathogens, such as RNase III, RNase Y, and RNase E, have key roles in virulence-associated posttranscriptional control, despite their central housekeeping roles. The diverse repertoire of RNases in different pathogens suggests there may be yet unidentified examples of RNases that act either alone or in concert with sRNAs on virulence-associated transcripts.

RNAs that Regulate or Antagonize Protein Activity

While the above-described *cis-* and *trans-*acting sRNAs function through base-pairing interactions with their target RNAs, some sRNAs instead interact with proteins and modulate their activity (3, 207) (Fig. 2C). A hallmark of these RNAs is substrate mimicry, and activity modulation is thus often directed toward RNA-binding proteins. Some abundant sRNAs, such as ChiX and CrcZ, can even titrate the RNA chaperone Hfq away from target mRNAs (208, 209).

Csr/Rsm regulatory networks

Perhaps the most widespread and well-studied posttranscriptional regulatory system in bacteria is the Csr (carbon storage regulator)/Rsm (repressor of secondary metabolites) network (210). Csr/Rsm has been linked to virulence control in several pathogens (29, 211). The central protein regulator of the system, CsrA (RsmA in some species) is a global posttranscriptional regulator conserved in many Gram-positive and Gram-negative bacteria. Generally, CsrA binds GGA-containing stem-loops near the TIR of target mRNAs, inhibiting translation and/or affecting their stability. CsrA can also stabilize or activate transcripts, such as the *flhDC* mRNA of *E. coli*, encoding the master regulator of the flagellar biosynthesis cascade (212). PGA (poly-*N*-acetylglucosamine) is a major component of the *E. coli* and *Salmonella* biofilm matrix, exported by the PGA export protein (213). In *Salmonella*, CsrA binds the 5′UTR of *pga* mRNA (214). However, this binding unexpectedly releases a secondary structure that sequesters a Rho entry site, which stimulates transcription termination. A hallmark of the Csr/Rsm system of *Gammaproteobacteria* is the presence of multiple environmentally regulated sRNAs (CsrB/C or RsmX/Y/Z), which bind and antagonize CsrA (RsmA) function. These sRNAs contain multiple CsrA-binding sites and sequester the regulator from target mRNAs, thereby interfering with their repression or activation.

In many bacteria, effects of *csrA* deletion are pleiotropic, and CsrA directly controls translation of mRNAs related to carbon metabolism (reviewed in 211). Csr networks also reciprocally control motility and biofilm formation, two phenotypes central to pathogen survival and colonization. In several pathogens, the CsrA regulon also includes important virulence factors (5, 29). In *Yersinia pseudotuberculosis*, CsrA has global effects on the transcriptome (215). In particular, CsrA has been shown to indirectly repress RovA, a global regulator of virulence that is required to activate expression of virulence factors such as the primary invasin and pili (216). Transcription of the antagonizing sRNAs CsrB/C in *Y. pseudotuberculosis* is controlled by at least three regulators, including Crp (the cAMP regulatory protein, involved in catabolite repression), the Mg^{2+}-dependent PhoPQ TCRS, and the BarA/UvrY TCRS, indicating that the *Yersinia* Csr system links multiple environmental cues to virulence gene expression (29, 217, 218).

In *Salmonella*, CsrA specifically represses translation of *hilD*, which activates the positive regulators of the SPI-1 and SPI-2 PAIs, HilA and SsrAB, respectively, as well as multiple proteins involved in c-di-GMP metabolism (219, 220). Gram-negative phytopathogens, such as various xanthomonads, use a T3SS to deliver effectors that modify the plant host. Biogenesis of the *Xanthomonas* T3SS machinery, encoded by the *hrp/hrc* loci, is controlled transcriptionally by the master regulator HrpG, and in *Xanthomonas citri*, RsmA binds and stabilizes the 5′UTR of the *hrpG* mRNA (221). In *P. aeruginosa*, RsmA represses translation of factors associated with chronic colonization including a type VI secretion system (T6SS) and biofilm matrix exopolysaccharide (222, 223). A second RsmA homologue, RsmF, has also been identified in *P. aeruginosa*, which has in part overlapping but also unique regulatory roles (224). In *Legionella*, the RsmX and RsmY sRNAs are induced in stationary phase and relieve CsrA-mediated repression of Dot/Icm effectors (225). Deletion of both sRNAs attenuates growth in the protozoan host

Acanthamoeba castellanii and macrophages (225, 226). Overall, CsrA is the most highly conserved posttranscriptional regulator of virulence (5, 211).

6S RNA

Another widespread sRNA that modulates protein activity and can also affect pathogen survival is the highly conserved and abundant housekeeping 6S RNA, which accumulates during stationary phase and controls activity of RNA polymerase (RNAP) (227). 6S RNA forms an extended hairpin with a single-stranded bulge, which mimics the DNA structure of an open transcription complex. Binding of 6S to the σ^{70}-containing holoenzyme reduces transcription from housekeeping promoters and reprograms RNAP (228). 6S RNA also acts as a template for transcription of short pRNAs ("product RNAs") that might facilitate unwinding of 6S from RNAP and thus recycling of the polymerase during outgrowth of bacteria (229). The 6S homologue of *Coxiella burnetii*, an obligate intracellular pathogen, is induced in Vero cells, suggesting a role during infection (230). *L. pneumophila* 6S is also required for its replication inside cells (231). A novel RNAP-interacting sRNA has also been identified in *Mycobacterium smegmatis* (232). Like 6S RNA, Ms1 sRNA is most highly expressed in stationary phase. However, Ms1 interacts with core RNAP, rather than the housekeeping holoenzyme bound to σ^A. Whether homologues of Ms1, or other novel sRNA regulators of RNAP, exist in pathogens is not yet clear. Overall, this class of RNAP-interacting sRNAs has the potential to globally effect transcription during stationary phase and persistent infection.

cis-Regulation by Endogenous mRNA Elements: Riboswitches, Thermosensors, and 3′UTR Elements

Riboswitches

Global TSS mapping in multiple species suggests that 5′UTRs of bacterial mRNAs are relatively short (20 to 40 nt). However, some transcripts have longer, structured leaders that can mediate their own regulation post-transcriptionally (Fig. 1D, upper panel). Metabolite-sensing "riboswitches" are structured 5'UTR elements that provide allosteric feedback control for many biosynthetic pathways (reviewed in 233, 234). Riboswitches often detect pathway intermediates and end products related to the protein encoded by the mRNA. As such, conserved riboswitch elements have been identified that detect metabolites such as thiamine pyrophosphate, Mg^{2+}, purines, amino acids, charged tRNAs, and phosphosugars. In Gram-positive bacteria, up to 2 to 4% of genes may be regulated by these structures (235, 236). Riboswitches are generally composed of two independently structured domains that determine signal sensitivity (the "aptamer") and regulatory output (the "expression platform"), respectively. Binding of a specific small-molecule ligand to the aptamer domain causes structural changes that affect the conformation of the adjacent expression platform. Conformational changes of the output domain can affect RBS accessibility, exposure of RNase E cleavage sites, or transcription termination/antitermination of the associated mRNA.

Salmonella senses numerous metabolic cues inside host cells. Magnesium levels, detected by the PhoPQ TCRS, represent an important signal for expression of virulence factors, including MgtC and the high-affinity Mg^{2+} transporter MgtA (237, 238). The promoter of *mgtA* is induced by PhoPQ under low Mg^{2+}. However, the leader of the *mgtA* transcript also contains a magnesium-sensing riboswitch element which maintains a Rho termination factor binding site under low Mg^{2+}, thereby promoting premature termination of transcription (239, 240). High magnesium also allows for translation of a short proline-rich leader peptide, MgtL (241, 242). Under proline limitation, ribosome stalling on the leader favors formation of a structure that promotes transcript elonga-

tion. Therefore, the *mgtA* leader integrates two disparate intracellular signals to affect elongation of the *mgtA* transcript. In addition to Mg^{2+}, riboswitches can also sense other metal ions such as Mn^{2+}, Co^{2+}, and Ni^{2+} (243–245). Also in *Salmonella*, a pH-responsive riboswitch has been reported upstream of the *alx* gene encoding a transporter (246). This element increases expression of the transporter in response to high pH through formation of a translationally active structure depending on transcriptional pausing.

Cyclic diguanylate (c-di-GMP) is a nucleotide second messenger that regulates biofilm formation and virulence in many bacteria (247). Protein receptors for c-di-GMP have been identified; however, bacteria have also evolved two riboswitch types to respond to this second messenger. Many genes that are part of c-di-GMP metabolism themselves contain such riboswitches (248), suggesting a role in feedback control or signal adaptation. Some are present in leaders of ORFs encoding factors known to be under control of c-di-GMP. For example, a riboswitch in the leader of a *Clostridium difficile* mRNA binds c-di-GMP to stimulate alternative RNA processing by an allosteric group I ribozyme (249). Alternative splicing produces an mRNA with an unmasked start codon and canonical ribosome-binding site, supporting translation of the putative virulence factor encoded by the mRNA. A second *C. difficile* c-di-GMP riboswitch has been identified upstream of *pilA1* of the pilin locus which allows transcription elongation under high second messenger levels (250) and thus may influence cell aggregation. In *V. cholerae*, a c-di-GMP responsive GEMM (Genes for the Environment, Membranes and Motility) motif is found in the leader of *gbpA* (248). The *gbpA* gene encodes an *N*-acetylglucosamine-binding protein that mediates adhesion to GlcNAc oligosaccharides and is required for both environmental survival and colonization (251, 252). A second GEMM element is present upstream of VC1722, which is similar to the TfoX regulator of competence (248).

Recently, a riboswitch specific for another emerging second messenger, cyclic diadenylate (c-di-AMP) has also been reported (253, 254).

Riboswitches can also either be a source for *trans*-acting sRNAs or regulate expression of sRNAs. The *Salmonella* sroA sRNA appears to arise from terminated transcription of the *thiB* riboswitch element (54). A mutant carrying a deletion in *sroA* shows reduced fitness during pooled mutant infections in mice (111). Two terminated SAM (*S*-adenosyl methionine) riboswitches of *L. monocytogenes*, SreA and SreB, bind the 5′UTR of the mRNA encoding the PrfA virulence regulator and repress its expression, thereby linking metabolism and virulence (255). Riboswitches not only control mRNAs, but can also control expression of antisense RNAs in response to cellular conditions. For example, in *Clostridium acetobutylicum*, a sulfur metabolic operon is controlled by T-box and S-box riboswitch-controlled antisense RNAs (256). In *Listeria*, a vitamin B12 riboswitch is transcribed as part of a noncoding antisense RNA (257). The riboswitch controls the length of the asRNA depending on B12 levels by a transcription termination mechanism. In the absence of the cofactor, the asRNA is transcribed and can repress the *cis*-encoded *pocR* transcript, encoding an activator of the Pdu propanediol catabolism pathway, which requires B12. When ligand levels are sufficient, the riboswitch prevents expression of the asRNA and allows activation of the pathway. The ANTAR (AmiR and NasR transcriptional antiterminator regulator) domain family of response regulators is characterized by an output domain that binds target mRNAs to affect transcription antitermination. (258). A B12 riboswitch-controlled sRNA was recently found to sequester an ANTAR-family response regulator EutV in *L. monocytogenes* and *Enterococcus faecalis* to control ethanol utilization genes (259, 260). This exemplifies the potential for high complexity through integration of multiple RNA-based regulatory mechanisms.

Thermosensors

Structured regions of 5′UTRs can also regulate gene expression in response to temperature changes (Fig. 1D, lower panel). These thermosensor modules, or "RNA thermometers," generally fold in a temperature-dependent manner into alternative structures that occlude or expose the RBS to affect translation (261). Hallmarks of these elements, such as the FourU or ROSE thermosensors, are structured regions that base-pair with and sequester the TIR at low temperatures (262). Elevated temperature unfolds this region and allows ribosome access. Thermosensor modules have, not surprisingly, been identified in many heat shock genes, playing a role in sensing and adaptation to heat stress. Temperature is also a key signal for bacterial pathogens, because changes in temperature are experienced upon transition between environment and host or during inflammation. RNA thermosensors have been identified in virulence genes of many bacterial pathogens, including master regulators of virulence gene expression (reviewed in 262).

L. monocytogenes relies on a master regulator, PrfA, for induction of virulence gene transcription. PrfA regulates virulence factors such as listeriolysin O, the InlA and InlB invasions, and the phospholipases PlcA and PlcB (1). Expression of these factors is almost undetectable at lower temperatures (i.e., 30°C). The 5′UTR of *prfA* contains a structured region that sequesters the RBS at low temperature but allows its translation at 37°C (263) and thereby activation of virulence genes once *Listeria* is within the host. *N. meningitidis* is primarily a commensal of the human nasopharynx but can cause serious diseases such as sepsis and meningitis upon entry into other body sites. Expression of the capsule, sialylated lipopolysaccharide, as well as recruitment of complement regulator factor H, contribute to complement resistance and immune evasion of *N. meningitidis*. In response to elevated temperature, i.e., upon inflammation in the nasopharynx, expression of immune-evasion factors and complement resistance increases as a result of thermosensor-based control of three genes required for expression of these phenotypes (264). This also has implications for meningococcal success upon coinfection with inflammation-inducing pathogens such as influenza.

P. aeruginosa is ubiquitous in environmental niches such as soil and water. Many *P. aeruginosa* virulence phenotypes, such as rhamnolipid biosynthesis and type III secretion, are under control of RhlR, the regulator of the Rhl C_4-HSL (butanoyl-homoserine lactone)–sensing quorum sensing system (265). Many RhlR-dependent phenotypes are more highly expressed at 37°C, and a thermosensitive ROSE-like element has been identified in the 5′UTR of *rhlA*, upstream of *rhlR* (266). The thermosensor is structured at lower temperatures, having a polar negative effect on transcription of downstream *rhlB* and *rhlR*. However, thermosensor melting at the permissive temperature (37°C) allows transcription of *rhlR*. A second thermosensor has also been identified in the 5′UTR of *lasI* mRNA (266). In this context, melting of the ROSE-like element at 37°C allows translation of LasI, which is responsible for production of 3O-C_{12}-HSL (3-oxo-dodecanoyl-homoserine lactone). A global screen for RNA thermometers in *P. aeruginosa* revealed four additional thermosensor candidates, including one that regulates *ptxS*, which is involved in exotoxin A production (267).

Expression of many virulence genes on the *Yersinia* virulence plasmid, such as those encoding the T3SS and Yop effectors, is minimal outside the host but strongly induced at the 37°C host body temperature. Temperature-dependent expression of these genes is controlled by the transcriptional regulator LcrF. While transcription of *lcrF* is controlled by the thermo-labile transcription factor YmoA, a second, posttranscriptional, layer of temperature control of LcrF has been shown (268). A novel, structured element in the intergenic region of the *yscW-lcrF* polycistron sequesters the *lcrF* RBS at 25°C. Melting of the element at 37°C allows LcrF translation and induction of downstream virulence genes. *Y. pseudotuberculosis* strains with stabilized or destabilized versions of the thermosensor are attenuated for dissemination following oral infection in mice, suggesting that the *lcrF* thermosensor is critical for virulence factor expression.

3′UTR elements

While eukaryotic 3′UTRs are thought to actively participate in gene regulation, for example, by acting as microRNA sponges (269, 270), the role of bacterial 3′UTRs in posttranscriptional control is only now being revealed. In *S. aureus*, up to one third of mRNAs were found to have long 3′UTRs (greater than 100 nt) which could have regulatory function (271). The long 3′UTR of *icaR*, encoding a repressor of the major exopolysaccharide, was revealed to use a C-rich sequence to interact with its own RBS, thereby interfering with translation initiation and providing a substrate for RNase III cleavage (271). Whether this interaction is inter- or intramolecular is not yet clear. Likewise, the *Salmonella hilD* mRNA, encoding an activator of pathogenicity island 1 (SPI-1), carries a 310-nt long 3′UTR which is important for turnover of its own mRNA (272). However, the underlying molecular mechanism remains unclear.

Dual-Function mRNAs with *trans*-Regulatory Functions and RNA Sponges

The function of mRNAs has traditionally been viewed as a template for protein synthesis. The identification of UTR elements with endogenous regulatory activity, such as riboswitches and thermosensors, demonstrated that mRNAs themselves can have regulatory functions. An increasing number of coding transcripts have been reported in bacteria that also regulate other targets, i.e., in *trans* (Fig. 2C). First, coding or UTR regions can be sources of *trans*-acting sRNAs, such as the terminated transcripts resulting from riboswitch repression, as mentioned above (see "cis-Regulation by Endogenous mRNA Elements"). Also, bacterial 3′UTRs are a source of base-pairing sRNAs (see "Regulation by trans-Encoded sRNAs"), via processing from coding transcripts or via transcription from internal promoters (89). Salmonella SroC sRNA is derived from the 3′ UTR of the gltI gene, which is part of the gltIJKL mRNA, a target of repression by the sRNA GcvB (140, 273). The mRNA-derived SroC sRNA acts as a sponge to sequester and trigger degradation of GcvB, thereby regulating the expression of its own parent mRNA (273).

Full-length messenger RNAs themselves can also regulate other genes by base-pairing or modulating activity of regulatory proteins. The 5′UTR of S. pyogenes irvA mRNA interacts with the gbpC transcript, protecting it from RNase J-mediated degradation (274). The role of mRNAs as sRNA sponges and/or decoys has also become apparent. In Salmonella, carbohydrate utilization pathways are hierarchically regulated. ChiP is a porin required for transport of chitin-derived oligosaccharides across the outer membrane, while the ChbBCA transporter mediates uptake of chitosugars across the inner membrane. Expression of ChiP is repressed by the ChiX sRNA, which base-pairs with the 5′-end of chiPQ mRNA and causes premature transcription termination (275–277). In this interaction, ChiX activity toward chiPQ is catalytic; i.e., ChiX is not codegradated with its target, which preserves the pool of the inhibitory sRNA. Induction of ChiP expression in the presence of chitosugars requires silencing of ChiX by a third player, the chbBC mRNA. The intercistronic region of chbBC acts as a so-called trap-mRNA that acts as a decoy via base-pairing with ChiX (276, 278). Because this interaction opens the ChiX terminator, which in turn increases its susceptibility to degradation, repression of chiPQ mRNA is relieved. This ensures that translation of the porin component occurs

when transcription of the inner membrane transporter is induced.

Cross-talk by mRNA leaders is not limited to base-pairing interactions with other RNAs, and mRNA interactions can also affect activity of protein regulators such as CsrA (see "RNAs that Regulate or Antagonize Protein Activity," above). For example, in Salmonella, in addition to the CsrB/C sRNAs mentioned above, a fimbrial mRNA (fimAICDHF) modulates CsrA activity to mediate hierarchical expression of chromosome-encoded (fim) or plasmid-encoded (pef) fimbriae (279). In C. jejuni, which lacks homologues of the CsrA antagonizing sRNAs, the mRNA of the major flagellin FlaA is not only translationally repressed by CsrA but also acts as an RNA antagonist of CsrA. The abundant flaA mRNA controls, together with the main CsrA antagonist the protein FliW, CsrA-mediated regulation of other flagellar genes (G. Dugar, S. Svensson, C. Sharma, unpublished). Finally, other cellular RNAs that were previously thought to be metabolic byproducts, which have sRNA sponge activity, have been identified using deep sequencing–based approaches. RNA-seq of potential RNA binding partners that copurified with aptamer-tagged sRNAs revealed that the 3′ external transcribed spacers (ETSs) of tRNA genes can also act as sRNA sponges to absorb transcriptional noise from repressed sRNAs (280) (Fig. 2C). Together, the increasing number of newly identified regulatory functions for bacterial mRNAs as well as RNAs not previously thought to have regulatory function demonstrates the complexity of bacterial posttranscriptional networks and shows that riboregulators are not restricted to noncoding transcripts.

RIBOREGULATORS IN QUORUM SENSING AND VIRULENCE REGULATORY NETWORKS OF BACTERIAL PATHOGENS

Quorum sensing allows pathogenic bacteria to sense cell density and coordinate group behaviors such as virulence factor expression or biofilm formation that would be of little benefit in solitary cells and are also important for survival and colonization (281). Quorum sensing involves the release of signaling molecules (autoinducers [AIs]) by producer cells and detection of the signal above a certain threshold by neighbors expressing the appropriate receptors. Signal detection elicits broad changes in gene expression and, subsequently, physiology. Quorum sensing networks are highly regulated at both the transcriptional and posttranscriptional levels. In this section we discuss examples of bacterial pathogens where riboregulation has been shown to factor centrally in quorum sensing and virulence.

Multiple Riboregulators Control *V. cholerae* Quorum Sensing and Virulence

The Gram-negative gammaproteobacterium *V. cholerae* causes epidemics of waterborne diarrheal illness that sweep the globe (282). Its pathogenesis and life cycle are well studied, and it serves as a model for understanding quorum sensing and regulation of virulence gene expression during transmission or colonization. *V. cholerae* is primarily a marine bacterium and lives in brackish waters, either free-living or associated with biofilms. Following ingestion by a human host, expression of two primary virulence factors mediate colonization of the intestine and induce diarrheal disease (reviewed in 283). The TCP (toxin-coregulated pilus), encoded by the *tcpA-F* genes of the phage-encoded *Vibrio* PAI (VPIΦ), mediates adhesion to the intestinal epithelium. The TCP also serves as a receptor for the CTXΦ prophage, which carries the *ctxAB* genes, encoding the cholera toxin (CT). CT is an AB-type toxin which stimulates cyclic-AMP production in host enterocytes, leading to a massive efflux of chloride and water into the intestinal lumen to cause diarrheal disease. In addition to these two virulence factors, competence, the T6SS,

and biofilms are also central to *V. cholerae* fitness (284–286).

Virulence phenotypes of *V. cholerae* are regulated in response to numerous environmental signals. In the intestine, expression of TCP and CT is activated by the AraC-type transcriptional activator ToxT (287), considered a master regulator of virulence. ToxT activates transcription of numerous operons encoding factors required for colonization and disease (Fig. 3A). Expression of *toxT* itself is regulated at multiple levels, including direct induction of transcription from the *toxT* promoter by the cooperative action of the inner membrane-localized regulators TcpPH and ToxR (288) and transcriptional autoregulation. However, ToxT protein levels are also activated posttranscriptionally in response to temperature using an RNA thermometer (289). At environmental temperatures (20°C), a FourU element in the *toxT* mRNA leader, containing an anti-Shine-Dalgarno sequence, sequesters the TIR (Fig. 3A, left). At the host temperature of 37°C, destabilization of this inhibitory structure allows for translation of *toxT* and, in turn, expression of downstream virulence factors such as CT, Acf (accessory colonization factor), and TCP, as well as its own autoregulation (Fig. 3A). A strain carrying a more stable thermosensor variant, which remains folded at 37°C *in vitro*, was found to be defective for mouse colonization, providing evidence that "RNA-melting" *in vivo* is required for regulation of virulence factors.

sRNAs also contribute to *V. cholerae* virulence regulation. ToxT induces transcription of two *trans*-acting sRNAs expressed from the VPIΦ: TarA and TarB (ToxT activated RNAs) (Fig. 3A, right). TarA represses translation of *ptsG*, encoding a glucose transporter, and deletion of *tarA* negatively affects colonization in an infant mouse model in the classical biotype of *V. cholerae* (290). TarA was also reidentified in a global sRNA-seq screen for virulence-regulating sRNAs induced by overexpression of ToxT, together with pull-down and sequencing of ToxT-bound promoters (2). The same study also identified a second ToxT-dependent sRNA, TarB. TarB interacts with *tcpF* of the *tcpA-F* transcript, encoding the secreted TcpF colonization factor. Loss of TarB has a mild effect on colonization, depending on infection conditions (2). Thus, TarB may be required to fine-tune or temporally control expression of TcpF. The RpoE-regulated VrrA sRNA posttranscriptionally regulates multiple genes, including those encoding the outer membrane protein OmpA and TcpA of the TCP. VrrA also represses the mRNA encoding the OmpT porin, which is important during infection (291), as well as the stationary phase survival factor Vrp (292). VrrA may negatively control virulence since a *vrrA* deletion mutant out-competes the wild type during infant mice colonization (293).

Many *V. cholerae* virulence and survival factors, including those activated by ToxT, are under quorum sensing control. It is thought that *V. cholerae* enters the host intestine at low density, where it expresses virulence factors such as CT. At high cell density, virulence factors are repressed. The *Vibrio* quorum sensing network relies on a set of sRNAs that posttranscriptionally control expression of the reciprocally acting master transcription regulators of quorum sensing, AphA and HapR (294, 295) (Fig. 3B). AphA is the regulator of low-density gene expression (Fig. 3B, left) and activates the ToxT virulence regulon as well as genes required for biofilm formation by activation of the VpsT biofilm transcriptional activator (296). In contrast, high-density phenotypes are regulated by the master regulator HapR (Fig. 3B, right). HapR activates genes involved in dispersal (e.g., the *hapA* hemagglutinin/protease gene) and competence (*com*) and also reduces virulence gene expression and biofilm formation through repression of *aphA* and *vpsT*, respectively.

There is a reciprocal gradient of the two transcription factors, depending on bacterial cell density, which is largely mediated via riboregulation (295). *Vibrio* quorum sensing

pathways converge on a set of four nearly homologous, Hfq-dependent base-pairing sRNAs called Qrrs (quorum-regulated RNAs) (reviewed in 27) (Fig. 3B). *Vibrio* secretes and detects two AI signals to sense population density. The two AIs, CAI-1 (cholera autoinducer-1, produced by CqsA) and AI-2 (synthesized by LuxS), are detected via the CqsS and LuxPQ TCRS proteins, respectively. Both CqsS and LuxPQ converge on the LuxU-LuxO phosphorelay system. At low density, when autoinducer concentrations are low and phosphotransfer to the LuxO response regulator is active, transcription of the Qrr sRNAs is activated by phosphorylated LuxO~P and the alternative sigma factor σ^{54} (297) (Fig. 3B, left). In contrast, at high density and high extracellular AI concentrations (Fig. 3B, right), reverse phosphorelay is favored, and phosphorylated LuxO is not available to activate the *qrr* genes.

The "sibling" Qrr sRNAs (*Vibrio* species variably harbor one to five Qrrs) show apparent regulatory redundancy (297), a recurring theme in bacterial sRNA biology (298). They also have regulatory flexibility and interact with different target mRNAs, including both quorum sensing master regulator mRNAs (*aphA* and *hapR* mRNA), using diverse regulatory mechanisms with distinct outcomes (145, 299). The molecular details of Qrr-mediated posttranscriptional quorum sensing regulation have been studied in detail in *V. cholerae* as well as its cousin *V. harveyi*. The Qrrs each have four conserved stem-loops with different functions (300). The first mediates base-pairing with a subset of targets and protects the sRNAs from RNase E–mediated degradation. The second stem-loop contains conserved sequences required for base-pairing with many of the target mRNAs, while the third plays an accessory role in base-pairing and stability. The fourth and final stem-loop, like for many sRNAs, functions as a Rho-independent terminator. Each Qrr conserves a 32-nt core region that allows each to interact with many of the confirmed target mRNAs (27). However,

A

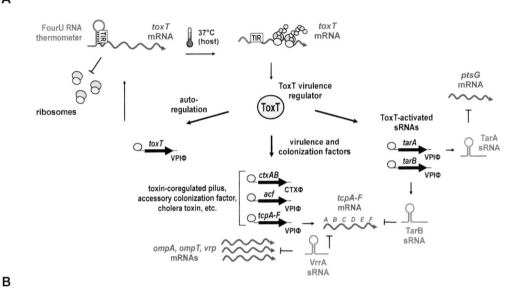

B

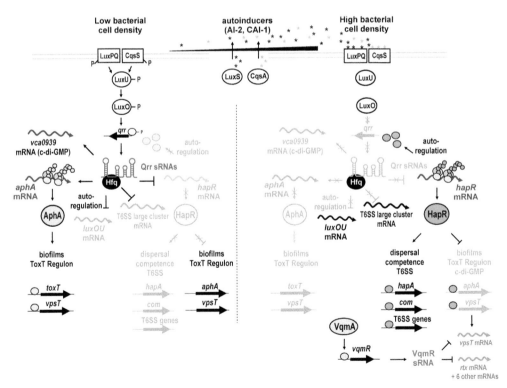

some differences in Qrr sequence and mRNA targeting do exist. For example, Qrr1 of *V. harveyi* lacks nine nucleotides near its 5′-end, which precludes its interaction with some targets, such as *aphA* (300).

In *V. cholerae*, at low density, the Qrrs, aided by Hfq, interact with the *aphA* and *hapR* mRNAs with reciprocal consequences to determine phenotypic output (Fig. 3B, left). Interactions with *aphA* are activating, whereas base-pairing with the *hapR* transcript is destabilizing. At low AI concentrations, Qrr activation of *aphA* translation allows downstream activation of regulons controlled by AphA, such as the ToxT virulence regulon and the VpsT biofilm regulon. However, the Qrrs also activate other mRNAs. For example, they promote translation of a diguanylate cyclase domain protein (Vca0939), thereby raising c-di-GMP levels to, like VpsT activation, promote biofilm formation (301). In addition to activating low-density genes, the Qrrs also repress high-density gene expression by destabilizing the transcript of the high-density regulator HapR (Fig. 3B, left). Therefore, high-density HapR-dependent phenotypes, such

as dispersal, competence, and the T6SS are not expressed. The Qrrs also directly repress the mRNA encoding the large T6SS gene cluster (VCA0107-0123) (302). In contrast, low-density genes that are repressed by HapR (but activated by AphA) such as those of the ToxT regulon and biofilm genes, are de-repressed in the absence of Qrr repression of HapR translation. This ensures that when few bacteria are present, AphA-dependent, low-density genes are expressed/de-repressed, whereas HapR-dependent high-density phenotypes are repressed.

At high cell density, accumulation of AI promotes dephosphorylation of LuxO, and the LuxO~P-dependent Qrr sRNAs are not expressed. Absence of the Qrrs allows expression of high-density phenotypes (Fig. 3B, right panel), largely due to de-repression of *hapR* translation. HapR promotes expression of genes mediating dispersal (*hapA*) and competence (*com*), as well as encoding the T6SS, while also inhibiting expression of virulence factors by repressing *aphA* transcription. The *vpsT* gene, activated by AphA, is also the target of HapR repression

---

FIGURE 3 **Numerous riboregulators participate in quorum sensing and virulence regulation of *Vibrio cholerae*. (A) Riboregulation of the *V. cholerae* ToxT virulence regulon in response to temperature. The central transcriptional regulator ToxT (blue circles, center) activates virulence and colonization factor genes, such as *tcp* (toxin-coregulated pilus), *ctxAB* (cholera toxin), and *acf* (accessory colonization factor). ToxT also autoregulates its own transcription. Levels of ToxT are also modulated in response to temperature by a FourU RNA thermometer, with increased translation at the 37°C host temperature. ToxT also activates the sRNAs TarB, which represses translation of the *tcpF* ORF of *tcpA-F* mRNA, and TarA, which represses *ptsG* mRNA (glucose uptake). The VrrA sRNA also represses *tcpA*. (B) The Qrr sRNAs mediate the switch between *Vibrio* low and high cell-density physiologies via reciprocal posttranscriptional regulation of the master regulators AphA and HapR. *Vibrio* autoinducers (AI-2 and CAI-1) are made by LuxS and CqsA, respectively, and accumulate extracellularly. Phosphorelay systems headed by LuxPQ or CqsS (AI-2 and CAI-1, respectively) detect autoinducers. Left panel: Low bacterial density. Continued phosphorylation of LuxO at low autoinducer conditions leads to transcription of the Qrr sRNAs, which act along with the RNA chaperone Hfq to activate translation of *aphA* mRNA. In turn, AphA expression induces the ToxT virulence regulon (see panel A), as well as genes required for biofilm formation (*vpsT*). The Qrrs also repress the *hapR* mRNA, which encodes the high-density master regulator (see right panel). Right panel: High bacterial density. High autoinducer concentration reduces levels of phosphorylated LuxO and, thus, Qrr expression. The *hapR* mRNA is no longer destabilized, allowing translation of the HapR regulator. HapR activates genes that mediate biofilm dispersal and competence. In addition, genes activated by AphA at low density, such as *vpsT*, as well as *aphA* itself and its regulated genes, are repressed by HapR. Genes encoding the type VI secretion system are also induced. Finally, feedback regulation occurs via HapR activation of Qrr expression and Qrr repression of the *luxO* mRNA. The sRNA VqmR is activated by the transcriptional regulator VqmA and posttranscriptionally represses *vpsT* mRNA and *rtx* mRNA, encoding the RTX toxin, as well as six other mRNAs.**

(303). HapR also controls transcription of 14 c-di-GMP-metabolizing genes, with the net effect of decreasing c-di-GMP levels, which further represses biofilm formation (303). The sRNA VqmR, which is activated by the transcriptional regulator VqmA, represses multiple mRNAs including those of the RTX toxin as well as of VpsT, thereby also inhibiting biofilm formation (73). Overall, absence of Qrr sRNA-mediated posttranscriptional repression and activation of multiple targets, including the master-regulator mRNAs, at high density suppresses virulence and biofilm formation and promotes phenotypes such as dispersal and competence.

Vibrio quorum sensing also incorporates feedback control of the sRNAs. The HapR protein, itself repressed by the Qrrs, has also been shown to activate their transcription (304). This feedback is most significant under high density, which allows efficient switching to low-density expression. The Qrr sRNAs can also repress the mRNA encoding their activator, LuxO (305), providing additional feedback. The *V. cholerae* CsrA system also feeds into quorum sensing upstream of LuxO (306). The Qrrs are some of the best-characterized bacterial sRNAs. Their functional characterization has been central to understanding not only *V. cholerae* quorum sensing and pathogenesis, but also to revealing mechanisms of Hfq-dependent sRNAs, the integration of posttranscriptional control with transcription factors, and the regulatory logic of bacterial gene regulation circuits.

RNAIII: A Dual-Function sRNA Mediates Quorum Sensing Control of *S. aureus* Virulence

S. aureus is a model for understanding sRNA-mediated posttranscriptional control in Gram-positive pathogens, including sRNA-mediated cell density control of virulence factor expression (31, 307). *S. aureus* is an opportunistic human pathogen that resides on the skin and the respiratory tract. Secretion of toxins, exoenzymes, superant-

igens, and capsule modulate and/or subvert the host immune system and underlie serious manifestations of *S. aureus* infection. Biofilm formation and antibiotic resistance also contribute to recalcitrant nosocomial infections.

S. aureus biofilm formation and virulence factor expression are controlled by products of the *agr* (accessory gene regulator) quorum sensing locus, which employs a cyclic octapeptide autoinducer to reciprocally control expression of surface-associated proteins and secreted virulence factors based on bacterial cell density (308). The *agr* locus is transcribed as two transcripts, RNAII and RNAIII (Fig. 4A). The RNAII transcript encodes the AgrB and AgrD enzymes required for synthesis of the Agr octapeptide pheromone. It accumulates upon high cell density to signal when a quorum of the pathogen—suitable for phenotypic switch—has been reached. RNAII also encodes the components of the AgrAC TCRS that detects and responds to the accumulating autoinducer and subsequently activates expression of high-density phenotypes. The primary effector of high-density phenotypes that is activated by the AgrA response regulator is the transcript RNAIII (Fig. 4B), the first sRNA shown to have a central role in bacterial virulence (45). Expression of RNAIII is induced by the AgrA response regulator in late exponential phase upon accumulation of autoinducers (309). RNAIII is a 514-nt transcript with 14 stem-loops, 3 of which have C-rich sequences (Fig. 4B). It was initially identified as the message encoding δ-haemolysin (310), a small protein toxin that targets host cell membranes to cause lysis (311). Later work showed that the 3′-end of RNAIII is a base-pairing regulator of numerous mRNAs encoding virulence factors with the overall effect of increased toxin secretion and decreased expression of surface-associated proteins (reviewed in 31, 312).

RNAIII mediates global antisense repression of *S. aureus* surface proteins upon activation of the Agr quorum sensing system

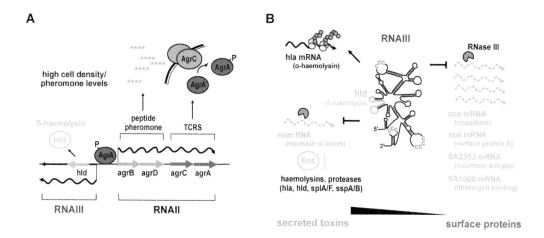

FIGURE 4 The dual-function sRNA RNAIII of *Staphylococcus aureus* reciprocally regulates expression of secreted virulence factors and surface proteins in response to cell density. **(A)** Genomic context and transcriptional regulation of the *S. aureus agr* quorum sensing locus, including the dual-function RNAIII. The RNAII mRNA (black) encodes proteins required for synthesis and detection of the peptide pheromone (*agrBDCA*, green and red open reading frames [ORFs]). Under high cell density and high autoinducer concentration, phosphorylated AgrA (red) activates transcription of the RNAIII sRNA (blue). RNAIII encodes δ-haemolysin (*hld* ORF) and is the major mediator of Agr regulation. **(B)** Overall integration of RNAIII posttranscriptional activities promotes toxin expression and represses expression of secreted proteins. Center: General structure of RNAIII with the *hld* coding region (light blue) and C-rich loops (red). The RNAIII molecule directly activates the mRNA encoding α-haemolysin (*hla*). Also, together with the double-strand-specific RNase III, the sRNA directly represses numerous genes encoding surface-associated proteins (*coa*, *spa*, SA2353, SA1000). RNAIII also represses translation of Rot, a repressor of toxin gene expression.

(202). It directly represses surface protein A, as well as a fibrinogen-binding protein, via base-pairing with the *spa* mRNA and SA1000 mRNAs, respectively. In both cases, translation is inhibited and RNase III-mediated degradation of the message is promoted (202, 203). A similar mechanism also represses SA2353, encoding a secretory antigen, and *coa*, encoding coagulase (201). RNAIII also exerts positive regulatory effects both directly and indirectly. Indirect effects on toxin gene expression are a consequence of direct repression of the mRNA encoding the transcription factor Rot (repressor of toxins) by RNAIII. Rot represses numerous genes encoding toxins that contribute to tissue invasion, including α-haemolysin, staphylococcal protease, and lipase (313). Rot also activates *spa* expression. RNAIII represses translation of *rot* mRNA through base-pairing

interactions that promote RNase III–mediated cleavage of the transcript (202, 314), resulting in downstream release of Rot repression of toxin expression. However, RNAIII can also directly activate toxin expression. Direct activation of *hla* occurs via base-pairing interactions that interfere with mRNA structures that inhibit translation (161). In summary, RNAIII is a dual-function transcript: it both acts as an mRNA, encoding the δ-haemolysin toxin and acts as an sRNA that posttranscriptionally regulates expression of surface proteins and additional secreted toxins in response to cell density cues. The *S. aureus* Agr system thus demonstrates not only the importance of bacterial communication in control of virulence factors, but also the importance of sRNAs as versatile posttranscriptional regulators, allowing the reciprocal and/or coordinate regulation of virulence genes.

Besides RNAIII, several other *S. aureus* sRNAs have been identified that affect virulence and antibiotic resistance. *S. aureus* Sbi is an immunoglobulin-binding protein that interferes with host complement and mediates immune evasion. Transient expression of *sbi* during infection is controlled by the cooperative activities of the sRNA SprD, expressed from the *Staphylococcus* PAI, and RNAIII (315, 316). RNAIII interacts directly with multiple sites on the *sbi* transcript, including its translation initiation region, to suppress translation (315). However, the SprD sRNA also interacts with the 5′-region of the *sbi* mRNA (316). Emergence of *S. aureus* strains resistant to last-line antibiotics is also central to prevalence of the species as a cause of untreatable infections. Resistance to vancomycin is affected by changes in expression of the SprX sRNA, which represses translation of SpoVG, a regulator known to affect glycopeptide resistance (135). The σ^B-dependent RsaA sRNA promotes bacterial persistence through suppression of acute infections (317). RsaA represses translation of the global transcriptional regulator MgrA via two interactions with *mgrA* mRNA: a duplex with the RBS and a loop–loop interaction within the coding region. MgrR repression leads to increased biofilm formation and decreased capsule synthesis, which in turn increases opsonophagocytic killing of *S. aureus* by polymorphonuclear leukocytes. Mice infections showed that RsaA contributes to reduced severity of systemic infections and enhanced chronic infections.

The gene encoding the *S. aureus* SprA sRNA is present in varying copy numbers, depending on the strain, and is encoded on both the core genome and PAIs (18). One copy, SprA1, is encoded in the SaPIn3-PAI of strain Newman. Messenger RNA targets of SprA1 are so far unknown. However, the *sprA1* locus encodes a second sRNA, antisense to SprA1 (SprA1$_{AS}$), and the locus was originally proposed to be a TA system, due to the presence of a short ORF in SprA1 (318).

Intriguingly, the *cis*-encoded asRNA interacts with SprA1 with imperfect *trans*-sRNA-like interactions. These involve the 5′-end of SprA1$_{AS}$ and the RBS/start codon of SprA1, rather than the perfectly complementary 3′-ends. SprA1$_{AS}$ binding prevents translation of the SprA1 ORF, and possibly even more interesting for virulence, the protein encoded by SprA1 is cytotoxic to human cells.

OUTLOOK: RIBOREGULATORS AS CENTRAL PLAYERS IN VIRULENCE NETWORKS

sRNAs are now accepted as central global regulators of bacterial gene expression that facilitate stress adaptation or control virulence traits. Study of sRNA regulons has added to our understanding of how pathogens sense and adapt to different environments, has identified new virulence strategies, and has provided many previously missing links in the complex regulatory networks that control virulence and group-associated behaviors, such as quorum sensing. Identification of structured mRNA leaders with regulatory function, such as thermosensors, has expanded our understanding of how bacteria sense the host environment. Many master regulators of virulence gene transcription are also direct targets of posttranscriptional regulation by sRNAs or UTR elements, such as *Listeria* PrfA, *V. cholerae* ToxT, and *S. aureus* Rot, adding a layer of posttranscriptional control to that contributed by transcription factors. sRNAs have also provided insight into the evolution of bacterial regulatory networks, including regulatory cross-talk between horizontally acquired, virulence-associated genomic elements and the core genome (10).

Functional characterization of pathogen sRNAs has identified novel mechanisms of RNA-mediated regulation. This includes the ability of RNAs to play both regulator and target of regulation, such as mRNA sponges that regulate proteins or mRNAs, or the sRNAs that are subject to antisense regulation themselves (279, 319). RNA-seq has uncovered widespread antisense transcription that may also serve a broad regulatory role, and the functional role of these potential asRNAs remains a major area to be clarified. The "excludon" concept also increases the potential for cross-talk between mRNAs in pathways of related and/or opposing function. One must also wonder if RNA molecules, like effector proteins from pathogens, may have roles outside the bacterial cell. Fungal pathogens have been revealed to secrete RNAs into host cells to modulate the host RNAi immunity system (320). In *S. aureus*, a conserved region of 23S rRNA is recognized by mouse TLR13 and triggers an immune response (321). Moreover, *L. monocytogenes* was found to secrete nucleic acids, including RNAs, into host cells, and this triggers host innate immunity, including the RIG-I-dependent inflammasome (322). Whether this is an active process that benefits that pathogen is still unknown.

Study of RNA-binding proteins such as the RNA chaperone Hfq and RNases has also identified many new modes of posttranscriptional gene regulation. More recently characterized RNA-protein complexes, such as components of the bacterial RNA-based CRISPR/Cas immune system, are revealing additional mechanisms of regulation. CRISPR/Cas systems provide an adaptive immunity by sequence-specific restriction of exogenous nucleic acids such as bacteriophage DNA (reviewed in 323). However, new "moonlighting" roles, outside of phage immunity, for CRISPR/Cas have been identified in bacterial pathogens. For example, they have been shown also to mediate endogenous gene regulation or have even been implicated in pathogenicity (324, 325), and there is an inverse correlation between antibiotic resistance genes on mobile DNA elements with the presence of intact CRISPR loci in enterococci (326). *S. pneumoniae* CRISPR/Cas, when primed with specific sequences, can prevent acquisition of genes encoding virulence-associated traits, such as capsule, by horizontal gene transfer (327). Together, these observations suggest that the presence or absence of CRISPR/Cas could contribute significantly to the fitness of bacterial populations. CRISPR/Cas can also play a direct role in gene regulation. *Francisella* CRISPR/Cas represses an mRNA encoding a lipoprotein, which is a stimulator of innate immune receptors, and the Cas9 nuclease and RNA components are required for evasion of TLR2 signaling and inflammasome evasion, as well as polymyxin resistance (328, 329). The Cas2 nuclease of *L. pneumophila*, which shows significant RNase activity, is also required for replication in amoeba (330, 331). A novel CRISPR locus of *L. monocytogenes*, which interestingly lacks associated *cas* genes, expresses an sRNA RliB and has been associated with virulence (53). Certainly, additional roles in gene regulation in bacterial pathogens will be uncovered as the strong interest in CRISPR/Cas continues.

A dramatic increase in our understanding of RNA biology due to technical advances provided by deep sequencing has revealed a central role for posttranscriptional regulation and sRNAs in bacterial virulence. New approaches based on deep sequencing promise to provide even more insight into posttranscriptional control by RNA, as well as the regulatory events (in both pathogen and host) that underlie infection and immunity. Because posttranscriptional regulation is sometimes most apparent at the level of translation initiation or the proteome, new approaches based on RNA-seq to monitor "translatomes," such as ribosome profiling ("Ribo-seq," deep-sequencing of ribosome-protected mRNA fragments), hold much promise for the identification of sRNA targets, which are sometimes only regulated on the translational level (332). Ribo-seq has already demonstrated repression of the *E. coli* major outer lipoprotein Lpp by a σ^E-dependent 3′UTR-derived sRNA, MicL (333). Also, Dual RNA-seq (simultaneous sequencing of both bacterial and host transcriptomes during infection, either in batch or at the single-cell level) (334–336, 344) promises to be especially relevant for identifying ribo-regulators and transcriptome changes, of both pathogen and host, that are important during infection. This has the potential to identify novel RNA biomarkers, such as microRNAs or long-noncoding RNAs, that indicate infection or predict disease susceptibility/outcomes and can be readily detected with high sensitivity in biological fluids (337). Finally, as the catalogue of functionally characterized sRNA-mRNA target pairs has increased, comparative genomics studies of bacterial pathogens have shed light on the evolution of bacterial regulatory circuits and how horizontally acquired sequences can regulate genes of the core genome (21, 22). Bioinformatics tools arising from these catalogues are also aiding the process of functional characterization (338).

In addition to classical virulence factors, stress response pathways and basic physiology are central to the virulence and survival of bacterial pathogens. Many of these pathways are regulated by RNA and can also impact antibiotic resistance. RNAs are a family of bacterial molecules relatively unexploited by antimicrobial design, and those that control essential processes may serve as candidate drug targets. Many RNA modules, such as SAM and B12 riboswitches, are widely conserved in bacteria but absent in humans, interact with small-molecule ligands, and are well-suited for structure-based drug design. The central role of c-di-GMP sensors in biofilm formation, a significant contributor to antibiotic resistance in the clinic, also makes them promising targets. Recently, a phenotypic screen revealed a small molecule as a synthetic mimic of the flavin mononucleotide natural ligand of the riboflavin riboswitch (339). This structurally distinct mimic (ribocil) inhibits bacterial cell growth via repressing riboswitch-regulated biosynthesis of the essential cofactor riboflavin. Therefore, RNA regulators or RNA-controlled pathways are attractive targets for novel antimicrobials.

ACKNOWLEDGMENTS

We thank Sandy R. Pernitzsch, Kathrin Fröhlich, Mona Alzheimer, and Kai Papenfort for critical comments on this book chapter.

Work in the Sharma lab is supported by Young Investigator program of the Research Center for Infectious Diseases in Würzburg (ZINF), the Young Academy program of the Bavarian Academy of Sciences and Humanities (BAdW), the Bavarian Research Network for Molecular Biosystems (BioSysNet), and DFG project Sh580/1-1. SLS is supported by the PostDocPlus program of the Graduate School for Life Sciences in Würzburg, Germany.

CITATION

Svensson SL, Sharma CM. 2016. Small RNAs in bacterial virulence and communication. Microbiol Spectrum 4(3):VMBF-0028-2015.

REFERENCES

1. **de las Heras A, Cain RJ, Bielecka MK, Vazquez-Boland JA.** 2011. Regulation of *Listeria* virulence: PrfA master and commander. *Curr Opin Microbiol* **14:**118–127.
2. **Bradley ES, Bodi K, Ismail AM, Camilli A.** 2011. A genome-wide approach to discovery of small RNAs involved in regulation of virulence in *Vibrio cholerae*. *PLoS Pathog* **7:**e1002126. doi:10.1371/journal.ppat.1002126.
3. **Storz G, Vogel J, Wassarman KM.** 2011. Regulation by small RNAs in bacteria: expanding frontiers. *Mol Cell* **43:**880–891.
4. **Caldelari I, Chao Y, Romby P, Vogel J.** 2013. RNA-mediated regulation in pathogenic bacteria. *Cold Spring Harbor Perspect Med* **3:**a010298.
5. **Papenfort K, Vogel J.** 2010. Regulatory RNA in bacterial pathogens. *Cell Host Microbe* **8:** 116–127.
6. **Croucher NJ, Thomson NR.** 2010. Studying bacterial transcriptomes using RNA-seq. *Curr Opin Microbiol* **13:**619–624.
7. **van Vliet AH.** 2010. Next generation sequencing of microbial transcriptomes: challenges and opportunities. *FEMS Microbiol Lett* **302:** 1–7.
8. **Sorek R, Cossart P.** 2010. Prokaryotic transcriptomics: a new view on regulation, physiology and pathogenicity. *Nat Rev Genet* **11:**9–16.

9. **Sharma CM, Vogel J.** 2014. Differential RNA-seq: the approach behind and the biological insight gained. *Curr Opin Microbiol* **19C:**97–105.

10. **Updegrove TB, Shabalina SA, Storz G.** 2015. How do base-pairing small RNAs evolve? *FEMS Microbiol Rev* **39:**379–391.

11. **Vanderpool CK, Balasubramanian D, Lloyd CR.** 2011. Dual-function RNA regulators in bacteria. *Biochimie* **93:**1943–1949.

12. **Mellin JR, Cossart P.** 2015. Unexpected versatility in bacterial riboswitches. *Trends Genet* **31:**150–156.

13. **Vogel J, Luisi BF.** 2011. Hfq and its constellation of RNA. *Nat Rev Microbiol* **9:**578–589.

14. **Chao Y, Vogel J.** 2010. The role of Hfq in bacterial pathogens. *Curr Opin Microbiol* **13:**24–33.

15. **Papenfort K, Vogel J.** 2009. Multiple target regulation by small noncoding RNAs rewires gene expression at the post-transcriptional level. *Res Microbiol* **160:**278–287.

16. **Lalaouna D, Eyraud A, Chabelskaya S, Felden B, Masse E.** 2014. Regulatory RNAs involved in bacterial antibiotic resistance. *PLoS Pathog* **10:**e1004299. doi:10.1371/journal.ppat.1004299.

17. **Kim T, Bak G, Lee J, Kim KS.** 2015. Systematic analysis of the role of bacterial Hfq-interacting sRNAs in the response to antibiotics. *J Antimicrob Chemother* **70:**1659–1668.

18. **Pichon C, Felden B.** 2005. Small RNA genes expressed from *Staphylococcus aureus* genomic and pathogenicity islands with specific expression among pathogenic strains. *Proc Natl Acad Sci USA* **102:**14249–14254.

19. **Padalon-Brauch G, Hershberg R, Elgrably-Weiss M, Baruch K, Rosenshine I, Margalit H, Altuvia S.** 2008. Small RNAs encoded within genetic islands of *Salmonella typhimurium* show host-induced expression and role in virulence. *Nucleic Acids Res* **36:**1913–1927.

20. **Wilms I, Overloper A, Nowrousian M, Sharma CM, Narberhaus F.** 2012. Deep sequencing uncovers numerous small RNAs on all four replicons of the plant pathogen *Agrobacterium tumefaciens*. *RNA Biol* **9:**446–457.

21. **Pfeiffer V, Sittka A, Tomer R, Tedin K, Brinkmann V, Vogel J.** 2007. A small noncoding RNA of the invasion gene island (SPI-1) represses outer membrane protein synthesis from the *Salmonella* core genome. *Mol Microbiol* **66:**1174–1191.

22. **Tree JJ, Granneman S, McAteer SP, Tollervey D, Gally DL.** 2014. Identification of bacteriophage-encoded anti-sRNAs in pathogenic *Escherichia coli*. *Mol Cell* **55:**199–213.

23. **Vogel J.** 2009. A rough guide to the noncoding RNA world of *Salmonella*. *Mol Microbiol* **71:**1–11.

24. **Hebrard M, Kroger C, Srikumar S, Colgan A, Handler K, Hinton JC.** 2012. sRNAs and the virulence of *Salmonella enterica* serovar Typhimurium. *RNA Biol* **9:**437–445.

25. **Mellin JR, Cossart P.** 2012. The non-coding RNA world of the bacterial pathogen *Listeria monocytogenes*. *RNA Biol* **9:**372–378.

26. **Izar B, Mraheil MA, Hain T.** 2011. Identification and role of regulatory non-coding RNAs in *Listeria monocytogenes*. *Int J Mol Sci* **12:**5070–5079.

27. **Bardill JP, Hammer BK.** 2012. Non-coding sRNAs regulate virulence in the bacterial pathogen *Vibrio cholerae*. *RNA Biol* **9:**392–401.

28. **Nguyen AN, Jacq A.** 2014. Small RNAs in the *Vibrionaceae*: an ocean still to be explored. *Wiley Interdiscip Rev RNA* **5:**381–392.

29. **Heroven AK, Bohme K, Dersch P.** 2012. The Csr/Rsm system of *Yersinia* and related pathogens: a post-transcriptional strategy for managing virulence. *RNA Biol* **9:**379–391.

30. **Schiano CA, Lathem WW.** 2012. Post-transcriptional regulation of gene expression in *Yersinia* species. *Front Cell Infect Microbiol* **2:**129.

31. **Fechter P, Caldelari I, Lioliou E, Romby P.** 2014. Novel aspects of RNA regulation in *Staphylococcus aureus*. *FEBS Lett* **588:**2523–2529.

32. **Guillet J, Hallier M, Felden B.** 2013. Emerging functions for the *Staphylococcus aureus* RNome. *PLoS Pathog* **9:**e1003767. doi:10.1371/journal.ppat.1003767.

33. **Arnvig K, Young D.** 2012. Non-coding RNA and its potential role in *Mycobacterium tuberculosis* pathogenesis. *RNA Biol* **9:**427–436.

34. **Pernitzsch SR, Sharma CM.** 2012. Transcriptome complexity and riboregulation in the human pathogen *Helicobacter pylori*. *Front Cell Infect Microbiol* **2:**14.

35. **Sonnleitner E, Romeo A, Blasi U.** 2012. Small regulatory RNAs in *Pseudomonas aeruginosa*. *RNA Biol* **9:**364–371.

36. **Le Rhun A, Charpentier E.** 2012. Small RNAs in streptococci. *RNA Biol* **9:**414–426.

37. **Barquist L, Vogel J.** 2015. Accelerating discovery and functional analysis of small RNAs with new technologies. *Annu Rev Genet* **49:**367–394.

38. **Vogel J, Sharma CM.** 2005. How to find small non-coding RNAs in bacteria. *Biol Chem* **386:**1219–1238.

39. **Sharma CM, Vogel J.** 2009. Experimental approaches for the discovery and characterization of regulatory small RNA. *Curr Opin Microbiol* **12:**536–546.

40. **Altuvia S.** 2007. Identification of bacterial small non-coding RNAs: experimental approaches. *Curr Opin Microbiol* **10**:257–261.

41. **Vogel J, Wagner EG.** 2007. Target identification of small noncoding RNAs in bacteria. *Curr Opin Microbiol* **10**:262–270.

42. **Backofen R, Hess WR.** 2010. Computational prediction of sRNAs and their targets in bacteria. *RNA Biol* **7**:32–42.

43. **Brantl S.** 2007. Regulatory mechanisms employed by *cis*-encoded antisense RNAs. *Curr Opin Microbiol* **10**:102–109.

44. **Mizuno T, Chou MY, Inouye M.** 1984. A unique mechanism regulating gene expression: translational inhibition by a complementary RNA transcript (micRNA). *Proc Natl Acad Sci USA* **81**:1966–1970.

45. **Novick RP, Ross HF, Projan SJ, Kornblum J, Kreiswirth B, Moghazeh S.** 1993. Synthesis of staphylococcal virulence factors is controlled by a regulatory RNA molecule. *EMBO J* **12**:3967–3975.

46. **Argaman L, Hershberg R, Vogel J, Bejerano G, Wagner EG, Margalit H, Altuvia S.** 2001. Novel small RNA-encoding genes in the intergenic regions of *Escherichia coli*. *Curr Biol* **11**:941–950.

47. **Rivas E, Eddy SR.** 2000. Secondary structure alone is generally not statistically significant for the detection of noncoding RNAs. *Bioinformatics* **16**:583–605.

48. **Rivas E, Eddy SR.** 2001. Noncoding RNA gene detection using comparative sequence analysis. *BMC Bioinformatics* **2**:8.

49. **Rivas E, Klein RJ, Jones TA, Eddy SR.** 2001. Computational identification of noncoding RNAs in *E. coli* by comparative genomics. *Curr Biol* **11**:1369–1373.

50. **Wassarman KM, Repoila F, Rosenow C, Storz G, Gottesman S.** 2001. Identification of novel small RNAs using comparative genomics and microarrays. *Genes Dev* **15**:1637–1651.

51. **Tjaden B, Saxena RM, Stolyar S, Haynor DR, Kolker E, Rosenow C.** 2002. Transcriptome analysis of *Escherichia coli* using high-density oligonucleotide probe arrays. *Nucleic Acids Res* **30**:3732–3738.

52. **Tjaden B, Haynor DR, Stolyar S, Rosenow C, Kolker E.** 2002. Identifying operons and untranslated regions of transcripts using *Escherichia coli* RNA expression analysis. *Bioinformatics* **18**(Suppl 1):S337–344.

53. **Toledo-Arana A, Dussurget O, Nikitas G, Sesto N, Guet-Revillet H, Balestrino D, Loh E, Gripenland J, Tiensuu T, Vaitkevicius K, Barthelemy M, Vergassola M, Nahori MA, Soubigou G, Regnault B, Coppee JY, Lecuit M, Johansson J, Cossart P.** 2009. The *Listeria* transcriptional landscape from saprophytism to virulence. *Nature* **459**:950–956.

54. **Vogel J, Bartels V, Tang TH, Churakov G, Slagter-Jager JG, Huttenhofer A, Wagner EG.** 2003. RNomics in *Escherichia coli* detects new sRNA species and indicates parallel transcriptional output in bacteria. *Nucleic Acids Res* **31**:6435–6443.

55. **Sonnleitner E, Sorger-Domenigg T, Madej MJ, Findeiss S, Hackermuller J, Huttenhofer A, Stadler PF, Blasi U, Moll I.** 2008. Detection of small RNAs in *Pseudomonas aeruginosa* by RNomics and structure-based bioinformatic tools. *Microbiology* **154**:3175–3187.

56. **Zhang A, Wassarman KM, Rosenow C, Tjaden BC, Storz G, Gottesman S.** 2003. Global analysis of small RNA and mRNA targets of Hfq. *Mol Microbiol* **50**:1111–1124.

57. **Christiansen JK, Nielsen JS, Ebersbach T, Valentin-Hansen P, Sogaard-Andersen L, Kallipolitis BH.** 2006. Identification of small Hfq-binding RNAs in *Listeria monocytogenes*. *RNA* **12**:1383–1396.

58. **Barquist L, Boinett CJ, Cain AK.** 2013. Approaches to querying bacterial genomes with transposon-insertion sequencing. *RNA Biol* **10**:1161–1169.

59. **Ingolia NT.** 2014. Ribosome profiling: new views of translation, from single codons to genome scale. *Nat Rev Genet* **15**:205–213.

60. **Konig J, Zarnack K, Luscombe NM, Ule J.** 2012. Protein-RNA interactions: new genomic technologies and perspectives. *Nat Rev Genet* **13**:77–83.

61. **Liu JM, Livny J, Lawrence MS, Kimball MD, Waldor MK, Camilli A.** 2009. Experimental discovery of sRNAs in *Vibrio cholerae* by direct cloning, 5S/tRNA depletion and parallel sequencing. *Nucleic Acids Res* **37**:e46.

62. **Mraheil MA, Billion A, Mohamed W, Mukherjee K, Kuenne C, Pischimarov J, Krawitz C, Retey J, Hartsch T, Chakraborty T, Hain T.** 2011. The intracellular sRNA transcriptome of *Listeria monocytogenes* during growth in macrophages. *Nucleic Acids Res* **39**:4235–4248.

63. **Yoder-Himes DR, Chain PS, Zhu Y, Wurtzel O, Rubin EM, Tiedje JM, Sorek R.** 2009. Mapping the *Burkholderia cenocepacia* niche response via high-throughput sequencing. *Proc Natl Acad Sci USA* **106**:3976–3981.

64. **Sharma CM, Hoffmann S, Darfeuille F, Reignier J, Findeiss S, Sittka A, Chabas S, Reiche K, Hackermuller J, Reinhardt R, Stadler PF, Vogel J.** 2010. The primary transcriptome of the major human pathogen *Helicobacter pylori*. *Nature* **464**:250–255.

65. Kroger C, Dillon SC, Cameron AD, Papenfort K, Sivasankaran SK, Hokamp K, Chao Y, Sittka A, Hebrard M, Handler K, Colgan A, Leekitcharoenphon P, Langridge GC, Lohan AJ, Loftus B, Lucchini S, Ussery DW, Dorman CJ, Thomson NR, Vogel J, Hinton JC. 2012. The transcriptional landscape and small RNAs of *Salmonella enterica* serovar Typhimurium. *Proc Natl Acad Sci USA* **109**:E1277–E1286.

66. Kroger C, Colgan A, Srikumar S, Handler K, Sivasankaran SK, Hammarlof DL, Canals R, Grissom JE, Conway T, Hokamp K, Hinton JC. 2013. An Infection-relevant transcriptomic compendium for *Salmonella enterica* serovar Typhimurium. *Cell Host Microbe* **14**:683–695.

67. Perkins TT, Kingsley RA, Fookes MC, Gardner PP, James KD, Yu L, Assefa SA, He M, Croucher NJ, Pickard DJ, Maskell DJ, Parkhill J, Choudhary J, Thomson NR, Dougan G. 2009. A strand-specific RNA-Seq analysis of the transcriptome of the typhoid bacillus *Salmonella typhi. PLoS Genet* **5**: e1000569. doi:10.1371/journal.pgen.1000569.

68. Dugar G, Herbig A, Forstner KU, Heidrich N, Reinhardt R, Nieselt K, Sharma CM. 2013. High-resolution transcriptome maps reveal strain-specific regulatory features of multiple *Campylobacter jejuni* isolates. *PLoS Genet* **9**: e1003495. doi:10.1371/journal.pgen.1003495.

69. Porcelli I, Reuter M, Pearson BM, Wilhelm T, van Vliet AH. 2013. Parallel evolution of genome structure and transcriptional landscape in the *Epsilonproteobacteria. BMC Genomics* **14**:616.

70. Taveirne ME, Theriot CM, Livny J, DiRita VJ. 2013. The complete *Campylobacter jejuni* transcriptome during colonization of a natural host determined by RNAseq. *PLoS One* **8**: e73586. doi:10.1371/journal.pone.0073586.

71. Butcher J, Stintzi A. 2013. The transcriptional landscape of *Campylobacter jejuni* under iron replete and iron limited growth conditions. *PLoS One* **8**:e79475. doi:10.1371/journal. pone.0079475.

72. Remmele CW, Xian Y, Albrecht M, Faulstich M, Fraunholz M, Heinrichs E, Dittrich MT, Muller T, Reinhardt R, Rudel T. 2014. Transcriptional landscape and essential genes of *Neisseria gonorrhoeae. Nucleic Acids Res* **42**:10579–10595.

73. Papenfort K, Forstner KU, Cong JP, Sharma CM, Bassler BL. 2015. Differential RNA-seq of *Vibrio cholerae* identifies the VqmR small RNA as a regulator of biofilm formation. *Proc Natl Acad Sci USA* **112**:E766–E775.

74. Mandlik A, Livny J, Robins WP, Ritchie JM, Mekalanos JJ, Waldor MK. 2011. RNA-Seq-based monitoring of infection-linked changes in *Vibrio cholerae* gene expression. *Cell Host Microbe* **10**:165–174.

75. Albrecht M, Sharma CM, Reinhardt R, Vogel J, Rudel T. 2010. Deep sequencing-based discovery of the *Chlamydia trachomatis* transcriptome. *Nucleic Acids Res* **38**:868–877.

76. Albrecht M, Sharma CM, Dittrich MT, Muller T, Reinhardt R, Vogel J, Rudel T. 2011. The transcriptional landscape of *Chlamydia pneumoniae. Genome Biol* **12**:R98.

77. Wurtzel O, Sesto N, Mellin JR, Karunker I, Edelheit S, Becavin C, Archambaud C, Cossart P, Sorek R. 2012. Comparative transcriptomics of pathogenic and non-pathogenic *Listeria* species. *Mol Syst Biol* **8**:583.

78. Oliver HF, Orsi RH, Ponnala L, Keich U, Wang W, Sun Q, Cartinhour SW, Filiatrault MJ, Wiedmann M, Boor KJ. 2009. Deep RNA sequencing of *L. monocytogenes* reveals overlapping and extensive stationary phase and sigma B-dependent transcriptomes, including multiple highly transcribed noncoding RNAs. *BMC Genomics* **10**:641.

79. Wurtzel O, Yoder-Himes DR, Han K, Dandekar AA, Edelheit S, Greenberg EP, Sorek R, Lory S. 2012. The single-nucleotide resolution transcriptome of *Pseudomonas aeruginosa* grown in body temperature. *PLoS Pathog* **8**:e1002945. doi:10.1371/journal.ppat.1002945.

80. Cortes T, Schubert OT, Rose G, Arnvig KB, Comas I, Aebersold R, Young DB. 2013. Genome-wide mapping of transcriptional start sites defines an extensive leaderless transcriptome in *Mycobacterium tuberculosis. Cell Rep* **5**:1121–1131.

81. Mann B, van Opijnen T, Wang J, Obert C, Wang YD, Carter R, McGoldrick DJ, Ridout G, Camilli A, Tuomanen EI, Rosch JW. 2012. Control of virulence by small RNAs in *Streptococcus pneumoniae. PLoS Pathog* **8**:e1002788. doi:10.1371/journal.ppat.1002788.

82. Bohn C, Rigoulay C, Chabelskaya S, Sharma CM, Marchais A, Skorski P, Borezee-Durant E, Barbet R, Jacquet E, Jacq A, Gautheret D, Felden B, Vogel J, Bouloc P. 2010. Experimental discovery of small RNAs in *Staphylococcus aureus* reveals a riboregulator of central metabolism. *Nucleic Acids Res* **38**:6620–6636.

83. Beaume M, Hernandez D, Farinelli L, Deluen C, Linder P, Gaspin C, Romby P, Schrenzel J, Francois P. 2010. Cartography of methicillin-resistant *S. aureus* transcripts: detection, orientation and temporal expression during growth phase and stress conditions. *PLoS One* **5**:e10725. doi:10.1371/journal.pone.0010725.

84. Sahr T, Rusniok C, Dervins-Ravault D, Sismeiro O, Coppee JY, Buchrieser C. 2012.

Deep sequencing defines the transcriptional map of *L. pneumophila* and identifies growth phase-dependent regulated ncRNAs implicated in virulence. *RNA Biol* **9**:503–519.

85. **Georg J, Hess WR.** 2011. *cis*-antisense RNA, another level of gene regulation in bacteria. *Microbiol Mol Biol Rev* **75**:286–300.

86. **Thomason MK, Storz G.** 2010. Bacterial antisense RNAs: how many are there, and what are they doing? *Annu Rev Genet* **44**:167–188.

87. **Lasa I, Toledo-Arana A, Dobin A, Villanueva M, de los Mozos IR, Vergara-Irigaray M, Segura V, Fagegaltier D, Penades JR, Valle J, Solano C, Gingeras TR.** 2011. Genome-wide antisense transcription drives mRNA processing in bacteria. *Proc Natl Acad Sci USA* **108**:20172–20177.

88. **Chao Y, Papenfort K, Reinhardt R, Sharma CM, Vogel J.** 2012. An atlas of Hfq-bound transcripts reveals 3′UTRs as a genomic reservoir of regulatory small RNAs. *EMBO J* **31**:4005–4019.

89. **Miyakoshi M, Chao Y, Vogel J.** 2015. Regulatory small RNAs from the 3′ regions of bacterial mRNAs. *Curr Opin Microbiol* **24**:132–139.

90. **Sittka A, Lucchini S, Papenfort K, Sharma CM, Rolle K, Binnewies TT, Hinton JC, Vogel J.** 2008. Deep sequencing analysis of small noncoding RNA and mRNA targets of the global post-transcriptional regulator, Hfq. *PLoS Genet* **4**:e1000163. doi:10.1371/journal.pgen.1000163.

91. **Lioliou E, Sharma CM, Caldelari I, Helfer AC, Fechter P, Vandenesch F, Vogel J, Romby P.** 2012. Global regulatory functions of the *Staphylococcus aureus* endoribonuclease III in gene expression. *PLoS Genet* **8**:e1002782. doi:10.1371/journal.pgen.1002782.

92. **Creecy JP, Conway T.** 2015. Quantitative bacterial transcriptomics with RNA-seq. *Curr Opin Microbiol* **23C**:133–140.

93. **Clarke JE, Kime L, Romero AD, McDowall KJ.** 2014. Direct entry by RNase E is a major pathway for the degradation and processing of RNA in *Escherichia coli*. *Nucleic Acids Res* **42**:11733–11751.

94. **van Opijnen T, Camilli A.** 2013. Transposon insertion sequencing: a new tool for systems-level analysis of microorganisms. *Nat Rev Microbiol* **11**:435–442.

95. **Barquist L, Langridge GC, Turner DJ, Phan MD, Turner AK, Bateman A, Parkhill J, Wain J, Gardner PP.** 2013. A comparison of dense transposon insertion libraries in the *Salmonella* serovars Typhi and Typhimurium. *Nucleic Acids Res* **41**:4549–4564.

96. **van Opijnen T, Camilli A.** 2010. Genome-wide fitness and genetic interactions determined by Tn-seq, a high-throughput massively parallel sequencing method for microorganisms. *Curr Protoc Microbiol* **Chapter 1**:Unit1E 3.

97. **Zhang YJ, Ioerger TR, Huttenhower C, Long JE, Sassetti CM, Sacchettini JC, Rubin EJ.** 2012. Global assessment of genomic regions required for growth in *Mycobacterium tuberculosis*. *PLoS Pathog* **8**:e1002946. doi:10.1371/journal.ppat.1002946.

98. **Khatiwara A, Jiang T, Sung SS, Dawoud T, Kim JN, Bhattacharya D, Kim HB, Ricke SC, Kwon YM.** 2012. Genome scanning for conditionally essential genes in *Salmonella enterica* serotype Typhimurium. *Appl Environ Microbiol* **78**:3098–3107.

99. **Langridge GC, Phan MD, Turner DJ, Perkins TT, Parts L, Haase J, Charles I, Maskell DJ, Peters SE, Dougan G, Wain J, Parkhill J, Turner AK.** 2009. Simultaneous assay of every *Salmonella* Typhi gene using one million transposon mutants. *Genome Res* **19**:2308–2316.

100. **Eckert SE, Dziva F, Chaudhuri RR, Langridge GC, Turner DJ, Pickard DJ, Maskell DJ, Thomson NR, Stevens MP.** 2011. Retrospective application of transposon-directed insertion site sequencing to a library of signature-tagged mini-Tn5Km2 mutants of *Escherichia coli* O157:H7 screened in cattle. *J Bacteriol* **193**:1771–1776.

101. **Gao B, Lara-Tejero M, Lefebre M, Goodman AL, Galan JE.** 2014. Novel components of the flagellar system in epsilonproteobacteria. *MBio* **5**:e01349-14. doi:10.1128/mBio.01349-14.

102. **Gawronski JD, Wong SM, Giannoukos G, Ward DV, Akerley BJ.** 2009. Tracking insertion mutants within libraries by deep sequencing and a genome-wide screen for *Haemophilus* genes required in the lung. *Proc Natl Acad Sci USA* **106**:16422–16427.

103. **Waters LS, Storz G.** 2009. Regulatory RNAs in bacteria. *Cell* **136**:615–628.

104. **Brantl S, Jahn N.** 2015. sRNAs in bacterial type I and type III toxin-antitoxin systems. *FEMS Microbiol Rev* **39**:413–427.

105. **Jahn N, Brantl S.** 2013. One antitoxin—two functions: SR4 controls toxin mRNA decay and translation. *Nucleic Acids Res* **41**:9870–9880.

106. **Fozo EM, Makarova KS, Shabalina SA, Yutin N, Koonin EV, Storz G.** 2010. Abundance of type I toxin-antitoxin systems in bacteria: searches for new candidates and discovery of novel families. *Nucleic Acids Res* **38**:3743–3759.

107. **Koyanagi S, Levesque CM.** 2013. Characterization of a *Streptococcus mutans* intergenic region containing a small toxic peptide and its *cis*-encoded antisense small RNA antitoxin. *PloS One* **8**:e54291. doi:10.1371/journal.pone.0054291.

108. **Guo Y, Quiroga C, Chen Q, McAnulty MJ, Benedik MJ, Wood TK, Wang X.** 2014. RalR (a DNase) and RalA (a small RNA) form a type I toxin-antitoxin system in *Escherichia coli*. *Nucleic Acids Res* **42**:6448–6462.

109. **Wagner EG, Unoson C.** 2012. The toxin-antitoxin system *tisB-istR1*: expression, regulation, and biological role in persister phenotypes. *RNA Biol* **9**:1513–1519.

110. **Darfeuille F, Unoson C, Vogel J, Wagner EG.** 2007. An antisense RNA inhibits translation by competing with standby ribosomes. *Mol Cell* **26**:381–392.

111. **Santiviago CA, Reynolds MM, Porwollik S, Choi SH, Long F, Andrews-Polymenis HL, McClelland M.** 2009. Analysis of pools of targeted *Salmonella* deletion mutants identifies novel genes affecting fitness during competitive infection in mice. *PLoS Pathog* **5**: e1000477. doi:10.1371/journal.ppat.1000477.

112. **Alix E, Blanc-Potard AB.** 2007. MgtC: a key player in intramacrophage survival. *Trends Microbiol* **15**:252–256.

113. **Lee EJ, Pontes MH, Groisman EA.** 2013. A bacterial virulence protein promotes pathogenicity by inhibiting the bacterium's own F_1F_o ATP synthase. *Cell* **154**:146–156.

114. **Lee EJ, Groisman EA.** 2010. An antisense RNA that governs the expression kinetics of a multifunctional virulence gene. *Mol Microbiol* **76**:1020–1033.

115. **Gonzalo-Asensio J, Ortega AD, Rico-Perez G, Pucciarelli MG, Garcia-Del Portillo F.** 2013. A novel antisense RNA from the *Salmonella* virulence plasmid pSLT expressed by non-growing bacteria inside eukaryotic cells. *PLoS One* **8**:e77939. doi:10.1371/journal. pone.0077939.

116. **Wen Y, Feng J, Sachs G.** 2013. *Helicobacter pylori* 5′*ureB*-sRNA, a *cis*-encoded antisense small RNA, negatively regulates *ureAB* expression by transcription termination. *J Bacteriol* **195**:444–452.

117. **Wen Y, Feng J, Scott DR, Marcus EA, Sachs G.** 2011. A cis-encoded antisense small RNA regulated by the HP0165-HP0166 two-component system controls expression of *ureB* in *Helicobacter pylori*. *J Bacteriol* **193**:40–51.

118. **Cahoon LA, Seifert HS.** 2009. An alternative DNA structure is necessary for pilin antigenic variation in *Neisseria gonorrhoeae*. *Science* **325**:764–767.

119. **Cahoon LA, Seifert HS.** 2013. Transcription of a *cis*-acting, noncoding, small RNA is required for pilin antigenic variation in *Neisseria gonorrhoeae*. *PLoS Pathog* **9**:e1003074. doi:10.1371/journal.ppat.1003074.

120. **Tan FY, Wormann ME, Loh E, Tang CM, Exley RM.** 2015. Characterization of a novel antisense RNA in the major pilin locus of *Neisseria meningitidis* influencing antigenic variation. *J Bacteriol* **197**:1757–1768.

121. **Wade JT, Grainger DC.** 2014. Pervasive transcription: illuminating the dark matter of bacterial transcriptomes. *Nat Rev Microbiol* **12**:647–653.

122. **Dequivre M, Diel B, Villard C, Sismeiro O, Durot M, Coppee JY, Nesme X, Vial L, Hommais F.** 2015. Small RNA deep-sequencing analyses reveal a new regulator of virulence in *Agrobacterium fabrum* C58. *Mol Plant Microbe Interact* **28**:580–589.

123. **Sesto N, Wurtzel O, Archambaud C, Sorek R, Cossart P.** 2013. The excludon: a new concept in bacterial antisense RNA-mediated gene regulation. *Nat Rev Microbiol* **11**:75–82.

124. **Beisel CL, Storz G.** 2010. Base pairing small RNAs and their roles in global regulatory networks. *FEMS Microbiol Rev* **34**:866–882.

125. **Guillier M, Gottesman S, Storz G.** 2006. Modulating the outer membrane with small RNAs. *Genes Dev* **20**:2338–2348.

126. **Vogel J, Papenfort K.** 2006. Small non-coding RNAs and the bacterial outer membrane. *Curr Opin Microbiol* **9**:605–611.

127. **Salvail H, Masse E.** 2012. Regulating iron storage and metabolism with RNA: an overview of posttranscriptional controls of intracellular iron homeostasis. *Wiley Interdiscip Rev RNA* **3**:26–36.

128. **Papenfort K, Vogel J.** 2014. Small RNA functions in carbon metabolism and virulence of enteric pathogens. *Front Cell Infect Microbiol* **4**:91.

129. **Sharma CM, Papenfort K, Pernitzsch SR, Mollenkopf HJ, Hinton JC, Vogel J.** 2011. Pervasive post-transcriptional control of genes involved in amino acid metabolism by the Hfq-dependent GcvB small RNA. *Mol Microbiol* **81**:1144–1165.

130. **Papenfort K, Bouvier M, Mika F, Sharma CM, Vogel J.** Evidence for an autonomous 5′ target recognition domain in an Hfq-associated small RNA. *Proc Natl Acad Sci USA* **107**:20435–20440.

131. **Guillier M, Gottesman S.** 2008. The 5′ end of two redundant sRNAs is involved in the regulation of multiple targets, including their own regulator. *Nucleic Acids Res* **36**:6781–6794.

132. **Papenfort K, Podkaminski D, Hinton JC, Vogel J.** 2012. The ancestral SgrS RNA discriminates horizontally acquired *Salmonella* mRNAs through a single G-U wobble pair. *Proc Natl Acad Sci USA* **109**:E757–E764.

133. **Sievers S, Sternkopf Lillebaek EM, Jacobsen K, Lund A, Mollerup MS, Nielsen PK, Kallipolitis BH.** 2014. A multicopy sRNA of *Listeria monocytogenes* regulates expression of the virulence adhesin LapB. *Nucleic Acids Res* **42:**9383–9398.

134. **Geissmann T, Chevalier C, Cros MJ, Boisset S, Fechter P, Noirot C, Schrenzel J, Francois P, Vandenesch F, Gaspin C, Romby P.** 2009. A search for small noncoding RNAs in *Staphylococcus aureus* reveals a conserved sequence motif for regulation. *Nucleic Acids Res* **37:**7239–7257.

135. **Eyraud A, Tattevin P, Chabelskaya S, Felden B.** 2014. A small RNA controls a protein regulator involved in antibiotic resistance in *Staphylococcus aureus*. *Nucleic Acids Res* **42:**4892–4905.

136. **Papenfort K, Pfeiffer V, Lucchini S, Sonawane A, Hinton JC, Vogel J.** 2008. Systematic deletion of *Salmonella* small RNA genes identifies CyaR, a conserved CRP-dependent riboregulator of OmpX synthesis. *Mol Microbiol* **68:**890–906.

137. **Pernitzsch SR, Tirier SM, Beier D, Sharma CM.** 2014. A variable homopolymeric G-repeat defines small RNA-mediated posttranscriptional regulation of a chemotaxis receptor in *Helicobacter pylori*. *Proc Natl Acad Sci USA* **111:**E501–E510.

138. **Schmidtke C, Abendroth U, Brock J, Serrania J, Becker A, Bonas U.** 2013. Small RNA sX13: a multifaceted regulator of virulence in the plant pathogen *Xanthomonas*. *PLoS Pathog* **9:**e1003626. doi:10.1371/journal.ppat.1003626.

139. **Papenfort K, Vanderpool CK.** 2015. Target activation by regulatory RNAs in bacteria. *FEMS Microbiol Rev* **39:**362–378.

140. **Sharma CM, Darfeuille F, Plantinga TH, Vogel J.** 2007. A small RNA regulates multiple ABC transporter mRNAs by targeting C/A-rich elements inside and upstream of ribosome-binding sites. *Genes Dev* **21:**2804–2817.

141. **Pfeiffer V, Papenfort K, Lucchini S, Hinton JC, Vogel J.** 2009. Coding sequence targeting by MicC RNA reveals bacterial mRNA silencing downstream of translational initiation. *Nat Struct Mol Biol* **16:**840–846.

142. **Deana A, Belasco JG.** 2005. Lost in translation: the influence of ribosomes on bacterial mRNA decay. *Genes Dev* **19:**2526–2533.

143. **Bandyra KJ, Said N, Pfeiffer V, Gorna MW, Vogel J, Luisi BF.** 2012. The seed region of a small RNA drives the controlled destruction of the target mRNA by the endoribonuclease RNase E. *Mol Cell* **47:**943–953.

144. **Morita T, Maki K, Aiba H.** 2005. RNase E-based ribonucleoprotein complexes: mechanical basis of mRNA destabilization mediated by bacterial noncoding RNAs. *Genes Dev* **19:**2176–2186.

145. **Feng L, Rutherford ST, Papenfort K, Bagert JD, van Kessel JC, Tirrell DA, Wingreen NS, Bassler BL.** 2015. A qrr noncoding RNA deploys four different regulatory mechanisms to optimize quorum-sensing dynamics. *Cell* **160:**228–240.

146. **Masse E, Escorcia FE, Gottesman S.** 2003. Coupled degradation of a small regulatory RNA and its mRNA targets in *Escherichia coli*. *Genes Dev* **17:**2374–2383.

147. **Adler B, Sasakawa C, Tobe T, Makino S, Komatsu K, Yoshikawa M.** 1989. A dual transcriptional activation system for the 230 kb plasmid genes coding for virulence-associated antigens of *Shigella flexneri*. *Mol Microbiol* **3:**627–635.

148. **Murphy ER, Payne SM.** 2007. RyhB, an iron-responsive small RNA molecule, regulates *Shigella dysenteriae* virulence. *Infect Immun* **75:**3470–3477.

149. **Khandige S, Kronborg T, Uhlin BE, Moller-Jensen J.** 2015. sRNA-mediated regulation of P-fimbriae phase variation in uropathogenic *Escherichia coli*. *PLoS Pathog* **11:**e1005109. doi:10.1371/journal.ppat.1005109.

150. **Grieshaber NA, Grieshaber SS, Fischer ER, Hackstadt T.** 2006. A small RNA inhibits translation of the histone-like protein Hc1 in *Chlamydia trachomatis*. *Mol Microbiol* **59:**541–550.

151. **Tattersall J, Rao GV, Runac J, Hackstadt T, Grieshaber SS, Grieshaber NA.** 2012. Translation inhibition of the developmental cycle protein HctA by the small RNA IhtA is conserved across *Chlamydia*. *PLoS One* **7:**e47439. doi:10.1371/journal.pone.0047439.

152. **Caswell CC, Gaines JM, Ciborowski P, Smith D, Borchers CH, Roux CM, Sayood K, Dunman PM, Roop Ii RM.** 2012. Identification of two small regulatory RNAs linked to virulence in *Brucella abortus* 2308. *Mol Microbiol* **85:**345–360.

153. **Wilms I, Voss B, Hess WR, Leichert L, Narberhaus F.** 2011. Small RNA-meodiated control of *Agrobacterium tumefaciens* GABA binding protein. *Mol Microbiol* **80:**492–506.

154. **Ortega AD, Quereda JJ, Pucciarelli MG, Garcia-del Portillo F.** 2014. Non-coding RNA regulation in pathogenic bacteria located inside eukaryotic cells. *Front Cell Infect Microbiol* **4:**162.

155. **Gong H, Vu GP, Bai Y, Chan E, Wu R, Yang E, Liu F, Lu S.** 2011. A *Salmonella* small noncoding RNA facilitates bacterial invasion and

intracellular replication by modulating the expression of virulence factors. *PLoS Pathog* 7:e1002120. doi:10.1371/journal.ppat.1002120.

156. **Altuvia S, Zhang A, Argaman L, Tiwari A, Storz G.** 1998. The *Escherichia coli* OxyS regulatory RNA represses *fhlA* translation by blocking ribosome binding. *EMBO J* 17:6069–6075.

157. **Altuvia S, Weinstein-Fischer D, Zhang A, Postow L, Storz G.** 1997. A small, stable RNA induced by oxidative stress: role as a pleiotropic regulator and antimutator. *Cell* 90:43–53.

158. **Zhang A, Altuvia S, Tiwari A, Argaman L, Hengge-Aronis R, Storz G.** 1998. The OxyS regulatory RNA represses *rpoS* translation and binds the Hfq (HF-I) protein. *EMBO J* 17:6061–6068.

159. **Solans L, Gonzalo-Asensio J, Sala C, Benjak A, Uplekar S, Rougemont J, Guilhot C, Malaga W, Martin C, Cole ST.** 2014. The PhoP-dependent ncRNA Mcr7 modulates the TAT secretion system in *Mycobacterium tuberculosis*. *PLoS Pathog* 10:e1004183. doi:10.1371/journal.ppat.1004183.

160. **Fröhlich KS, Papenfort K, Berger AA, Vogel J.** 2012. A conserved RpoS-dependent small RNA controls the synthesis of major porin OmpD. *Nucleic Acids Res* 40:3623–3640.

161. **Morfeldt E, Taylor D, Vongabain A, Arvidson S.** 1995. Activation of alpha-toxin translation in *Staphylococcus aureus* by the *trans*-encoded antisense RNA, RNAIII. *EMBO J* 14:4569–4577.

162. **Hubner A, Yang X, Nolen DM, Popova TG, Cabello FC, Norgard MV.** 2001. Expression of *Borrelia burgdorferi* OspC and DbpA is controlled by a RpoN-RpoS regulatory pathway. *Proc Natl Acad Sci USA* 98:12724–12729.

163. **Lybecker MC, Samuels DS.** 2007. Temperature-induced regulation of RpoS by a small RNA in *Borrelia burgdorferi*. *Mol Microbiol* 64:1075–1089.

164. **Quereda JJ, Ortega AD, Pucciarelli MG, Garcia-Del Portillo F.** 2014. The *Listeria* small RNA Rli27 regulates a cell wall protein inside eukaryotic cells by targeting a long 5′-UTR variant. *PLoS Genet* 10:e1004765. doi:10.1371/journal.pgen.1004765.

165. **Papenfort K, Sun Y, Miyakoshi M, Vanderpool CK, Vogel J.** 2013. Small RNA-mediated activation of sugar phosphatase mRNA regulates glucose homeostasis. *Cell* 153:426–437.

166. **Frohlich KS, Papenfort K, Fekete A, Vogel J.** 2013. A small RNA activates CFA synthase by isoform-specific mRNA stabilization. *EMBO J* 32:2963–2979.

167. **Opdyke JA, Kang JG, Storz G.** 2004. GadY, a small-RNA regulator of acid response genes in *Escherichia coli*. *J Bacteriol* 186:6698–6705.

168. **Obana N, Shirahama Y, Abe K, Nakamura K.** 2010. Stabilization of *Clostridium perfringens* collagenase mRNA by VR-RNA-dependent cleavage in 5′ leader sequence. *Mol Microbiol* 77:1416–1428.

169. **Cao H, Krishnan G, Goumnerov B, Tsongalis J, Tompkins R, Rahme LG.** 2001. A quorum-sensing-associated virulence gene of *Pseudomonas aeruginosa* encodes a LysR-like transcription regulator with a unique self-regulatory mechanism. *Proc Natl Acad Sci USA* 98:14613–14618.

170. **Sonnleitner E, Gonzalez N, Sorger-Domenigg T, Heeb S, Richter AS, Backofen R, Williams P, Huttenhofer A, Haas D, Blasi U.** 2011. The small RNA PhrS stimulates synthesis of the *Pseudomonas aeruginosa* quinolone signal. *Mol Microbiol* 80:868–885.

171. **Papenfort K, Espinosa E, Casadesus J, Vogel J.** 2015. Small RNA-based feedforward loop with AND-gate logic regulates extrachromosomal DNA transfer in *Salmonella*. *Proc Natl Acad Sci USA* 112:E4772–E4781.

172. **Ramirez-Pena E, Trevino J, Liu Z, Perez N, Sumby P.** 2010. The group A *Streptococcus* small regulatory RNA FasX enhances streptokinase activity by increasing the stability of the *ska* mRNA transcript. *Mol Microbiol* 78:1332–1347.

173. **Liu Z, Trevino J, Ramirez-Pena E, Sumby P.** 2012. The small regulatory RNA FasX controls pilus expression and adherence in the human bacterial pathogen group A *Streptococcus*. *Mol Microbiol* 86:140–154.

174. **Huang JY, Sweeney EG, Sigal M, Zhang HC, Remington SJ, Cantrell MA, Kuo CJ, Guillemin K, Amieva MR.** 2015. Chemodetection and destruction of host urea allows *Helicobacter pylori* to locate the epithelium. *Cell Host Microbe* 18:147–156.

175. **Croxen MA, Sisson G, Melano R, Hoffman PS.** 2006. The *Helicobacter pylori* chemotaxis receptor TlpB (HP0103) is required for pH taxis and for colonization of the gastric mucosa. *J Bacteriol* 188:2656–2665.

176. **Rader BA, Wreden C, Hicks KG, Sweeney EG, Ottemann KM, Guillemin K.** 2011. *Helicobacter pylori* perceives the quorum-sensing molecule AI-2 as a chemorepellent via the chemoreceptor TlpB. *Microbiology* 157:2445–2455.

177. **Sauer E.** 2013. Structure and RNA-binding properties of the bacterial LSm protein Hfq. *RNA Biol* 10:610–618.

178. **Folichon M, Arluison V, Pellegrini O, Huntzinger E, Regnier P, Hajnsdorf E.** 2003. The poly(A) binding protein Hfq protects RNA from RNase E and exoribonucleolytic degradation. *Nucleic Acids Res* 31:7302–7310.

179. **Ishikawa H, Otaka H, Maki K, Morita T, Aiba H.** 2012. The functional Hfq-binding module of bacterial sRNAs consists of a double or single hairpin preceded by a U-rich sequence and followed by a 3' poly(U) tail. *RNA* **18**:1062–1074.

180. **Zhang A, Schu DJ, Tjaden BC, Storz G, Gottesman S.** 2013. Mutations in interaction surfaces differentially impact *E. coli* Hfq association with small RNAs and their mRNA targets. *J Mol Biol* **425**:3678–3697.

181. **Moll I, Afonyushkin T, Vytvytska O, Kaberdin VR, Blasi U.** 2003. Coincident Hfq binding and RNase E cleavage sites on mRNA and small regulatory RNAs. *RNA* **9**:1308–1314.

182. **Prevost K, Desnoyers G, Jacques JF, Lavoie F, Masse E.** 2011. Small RNA-induced mRNA degradation achieved through both translation block and activated cleavage. *Genes Dev* **25**:385–396.

183. **Ellis MJ, Trussler RS, Haniford DB.** 2015. Hfq binds directly to the ribosome binding site of IS*10* transposase mRNA to inhibit translation. *Mol Microbiol* **96**:633–650.

184. **Moll I, Leitsch D, Steinhauser T, Blasi U.** 2003. RNA chaperone activity of the Sm-like Hfq protein. *EMBO Rep* **4**:284–289.

185. **Desnoyers G, Masse E.** 2012. Noncanonical repression of translation initiation through small RNA recruitment of the RNA chaperone Hfq. *Genes Dev* **26**:726–739.

186. **Moon K, Gottesman S.** 2011. Competition among Hfq-binding small RNAs in *Escherichia coli*. *Mol Microbiol* **82**:1545–1562.

187. **Wagner EG.** 2013. Cycling of RNAs on Hfq. *RNA Biol* **10**:619–626.

188. **Fender A, Elf J, Hampel K, Zimmermann B, Wagner EG.** 2010. RNAs actively cycle on the Sm-like protein Hfq. *Genes Dev* **24**:2621–2626.

189. **Jousselin A, Metzinger L, Felden B.** 2009. On the facultative requirement of the bacterial RNA chaperone, Hfq. *Trends Microbiol* **17**:399–405.

190. **Viegas SC, Pfeiffer V, Sittka A, Silva IJ, Vogel J, Arraiano CM.** 2007. Characterization of the role of ribonucleases in *Salmonella* small RNA decay. *Nucleic Acids Res* **35**:7651–7664.

191. **Vercruysse M, Kohrer C, Davies BW, Arnold MF, Mekalanos JJ, RajBhandary UL, Walker GC.** 2014. The highly conserved bacterial RNase YbeY is essential in *Vibrio cholerae*, playing a critical role in virulence, stress regulation, and RNA processing. *PLoS Pathog* **10**: e1004175. doi:10.1371/journal.ppat.1004175.

192. **Marincola G, Schafer T, Behler J, Bernhardt J, Ohlsen K, Goerke C, Wolz C.** 2012. RNase Y of *Staphylococcus aureus* and its role in the activation of virulence genes. *Mol Microbiol* **85**:817–832.

193. **Haddad N, Matos RG, Pinto T, Rannou P, Cappelier JM, Prevost H, Arraiano CM.** 2014. The RNase R from *Campylobacter jejuni* has unique features and is involved in the first steps of infection. *J Biol Chem* **289**:27814–27824.

194. **Viegas SC, Mil-Homens D, Fialho AM, Arraiano CM.** 2013. The virulence of *Salmonella enterica* serovar Typhimurium in the insect model *Galleria mellonella* is impaired by mutations in RNase E and RNase III. *Appl Environ Microbiol* **79**:6124–6133.

195. **Haddad N, Tresse O, Rivoal K, Chevret D, Nonglaton Q, Burns CM, Prevost H, Cappelier JM.** 2012. Polynucleotide phosphorylase has an impact on cell biology of *Campylobacter jejuni*. *Front Cell Infect Microbiol* **2**:30.

196. **Chen Z, Itzek A, Malke H, Ferretti JJ, Kreth J.** 2013. Multiple roles of RNase Y in *Streptococcus pyogenes* mRNA processing and degradation. *J Bacteriol* **195**:2585–2594.

197. **Durand S, Gilet L, Condon C.** 2012. The essential function of *B. subtilis* RNase III is to silence foreign toxin genes. *PLoS Genet* **8**: e1003181. doi:10.1371/journal.pgen.1003181.

198. **Durand S, Gilet L, Bessieres P, Nicolas P, Condon C.** 2012. Three essential ribonucleases—RNase Y, J1, and III—control the abundance of a majority of *Bacillus subtilis* mRNAs. *PLoS Genet* **8**:e1002520. doi:10.1371/journal. pgen.1002520.

199. **Caron MP, Lafontaine DA, Masse E.** 2010. Small RNA-mediated regulation at the level of transcript stability. *RNA Biol* **7**:140–144.

200. **Lalaouna D, Simoneau-Roy M, Lafontaine D, Masse E.** 2013. Regulatory RNAs and target mRNA decay in prokaryotes. *Biochim Biophys Acta* **1829**:742–747.

201. **Chevalier C, Boisset S, Romilly C, Masquida B, Fechter P, Geissmann T, Vandenesch F, Romby P.** 2010. *Staphylococcus aureus* RNAIII binds to two distant regions of *coa* mRNA to arrest translation and promote mRNA degradation. *PLoS Pathog* **6**:e1000809. doi:10.1371/journal.ppat.1000809.

202. **Boisset S, Geissmann T, Huntzinger E, Fechter P, Bendridi N, Possedko M, Chevalier C, Helfer AC, Benito Y, Jacquier A, Gaspin C, Vandenesch F, Romby P.** 2007. *Staphylococcus aureus* RNAIII coordinately represses the synthesis of virulence factors and the transcription regulator Rot by an antisense mechanism. *Genes Dev* **21**:1353–1366.

203. **Huntzinger E, Boisset S, Saveanu C, Benito Y, Geissmann T, Namane A, Lina G, Etienne J, Ehresmann B, Ehresmann C, Jacquier A,**

Vandenesch F, Romby P. 2005. *Staphylococcus aureus* RNAIII and the endoribonuclease III coordinately regulate *spa* gene expression. *EMBO J* **24:**824–835.

204. Romilly C, Chevalier C, Marzi S, Masquida B, Geissmann T, Vandenesch F, Westhof E, Romby P. 2012. Loop-loop interactions involved in antisense regulation are processed by the endoribonuclease III in *Staphylococcus aureus. RNA Biol* **9:**1461–1472.

205. Durand S, Tomasini A, Braun F, Condon C, Romby P. 2015. sRNA and mRNA turnover in Gram-positive bacteria. *FEMS Microbiol Rev* **39:**316–330.

206. Jester BC, Romby P, Lioliou E. 2012. When ribonucleases come into play in pathogens: a survey of Gram-positive bacteria. *Int J Microbiol* **2012:**592196.

207. Pichon C, Felden B. 2007. Proteins that interact with bacterial small RNA regulators. *FEMS Microbiol Rev* **31:**614–625.

208. Ellis MJ, Trussler RS, Haniford DB. 2015. Hfq binds directly to the ribosome-binding site of IS*10* transposase mRNA to inhibit translation. *Mol Microbiol* **96:**633–650.

209. Sonnleitner E, Blasi U. 2014. Regulation of Hfq by the RNA CrcZ in *Pseudomonas aeruginosa* carbon catabolite repression. *PLoS Genet* **10:**e1004440. doi:10.1371/journal.pgen.1004440.

210. Romeo T, Vakulskas CA, Babitzke P. 2013. Post-transcriptional regulation on a global scale: form and function of Csr/Rsm systems. *Environ Microbiol* **15:**313–324.

211. Vakulskas CA, Potts AH, Babitzke P, Ahmer BM, Romeo T. 2015. Regulation of bacterial virulence by Csr (Rsm) systems. *Microbiol Mol Biol Rev* **79:**193–224.

212. Wei BL, Brun-Zinkernagel AM, Simecka JW, Pruss BM, Babitzke P, Romeo T. 2001. Positive regulation of motility and *flhDC* expression by the RNA-binding protein CsrA of *Escherichia coli. Mol Microbiol* **40:**245–256.

213. Mika F, Hengge R. 2013. Small regulatory RNAs in the control of motility and biofilm formation in *E. coli* and *Salmonella. Int J Mol Sci* **14:**4560–4579.

214. Figueroa-Bossi N, Schwartz A, Guillemardet B, D'Heygere F, Bossi L, Boudvillain M. 2014. RNA remodeling by bacterial global regulator CsrA promotes Rho-dependent transcription termination. *Genes Dev* **28:**1239–1251.

215. Heroven AK, Dersch P. 2014. Coregulation of host-adapted metabolism and virulence by pathogenic yersiniae. *Front Cell Infect Microbiol* **4:**146.

216. Heroven AK, Bohme K, Rohde M, Dersch P. 2008. A Csr-type regulatory system, including small non-coding RNAs, regulates the global virulence regulator RovA of *Yersinia pseudotuberculosis* through RovM. *Mol Microbiol* **68:**1179–1195.

217. Heroven AK, Sest M, Pisano F, Scheb-Wetzel M, Steinmann R, Bohme K, Klein J, Munch R, Schomburg D, Dersch P. 2012. Crp induces switching of the CsrB and CsrC RNAs in *Yersinia pseudotuberculosis* and links nutritional status to virulence. *Front Cell Infect Microbiol* **2:**158.

218. Nuss AM, Schuster F, Kathrin Heroven A, Heine W, Pisano F, Dersch P. 2014. A direct link between the global regulator PhoP and the Csr regulon in *Y. pseudotuberculosis* through the small regulatory RNA CsrC. *RNA Biol* **11:**580–593.

219. Martinez LC, Yakhnin H, Camacho MI, Georgellis D, Babitzke P, Puente JL, Bustamante VH. 2011. Integration of a complex regulatory cascade involving the SirA/BarA and Csr global regulatory systems that controls expression of the *Salmonella* SPI-1 and SPI-2 virulence regulons through HilD. *Mol Microbiol* **80:**1637–1656.

220. Jonas K, Edwards AN, Ahmad I, Romeo T, Romling U, Melefors O. 2010. Complex regulatory network encompassing the Csr, c-di-GMP and motility systems of *Salmonella* Typhimurium. *Environ Microbiol* **12:**524–540.

221. Andrade MO, Farah CS, Wang N. 2014. The post-transcriptional regulator *rsmA/csrA* activates T3SS by stabilizing the 5′ UTR of *hrpG*, the master regulator of *hrp/hrc* genes, in *Xanthomonas. PLoS Pathog* **10:**e1003945. doi:10.1371/journal.ppat.1003945.

222. Brencic A, Lory S. 2009. Determination of the regulon and identification of novel mRNA targets of *Pseudomonas aeruginosa* RsmA. *Mol Microbiol* **72:**612–632.

223. Goodman AL, Kulasekara B, Rietsch A, Boyd D, Smith RS, Lory S. 2004. A signaling network reciprocally regulates genes associated with acute infection and chronic persistence in *Pseudomonas aeruginosa. Dev Cell* **7:**745–754.

224. Marden JN, Diaz MR, Walton WG, Gode CJ, Betts L, Urbanowski ML, Redinbo MR, Yahr TL, Wolfgang MC. 2013. An unusual CsrA family member operates in series with RsmA to amplify posttranscriptional responses in *Pseudomonas aeruginosa. Proc Natl Acad Sci USA* **110:**15055–15060.

225. Rasis M, Segal G. 2009. The LetA-RsmYZ-CsrA regulatory cascade, together with RpoS and PmrA, post-transcriptionally regulates stationary phase activation of *Legionella pneumophila* Icm/Dot effectors. *Mol Microbiol* **72:**995–1010.

226. Sahr T, Bruggemann H, Jules M, Lomma M, Albert-Weissenberger C, Cazalet C, Buchrieser C. 2009. Two small ncRNAs jointly govern virulence and transmission in *Legionella pneumophila*. *Mol Microbiol* **72**:741–762.

227. Cavanagh AT, Wassarman KM. 2014. 6S RNA, a global regulator of transcription in *Escherichia coli, Bacillus subtilis*, and beyond. *Annu Rev Microbiol* **68**:45–60.

228. Wassarman KM, Storz G. 2000. 6S RNA regulates *E. coli* RNA polymerase activity. *Cell* **101**:613–623.

229. Wassarman KM, Saecker RM. 2006. Synthesis-mediated release of a small RNA inhibitor of RNA polymerase. *Science* **314**:1601–1603.

230. Warrier I, Hicks LD, Battisti JM, Raghavan R, Minnick MF. 2014. Identification of novel small RNAs and characterization of the 6S RNA of *Coxiella burnetii*. *PloS One* **9**:e100147. doi:10.1371/journal.pone.0100147.

231. Faucher SP, Friedlander G, Livny J, Margalit H, Shuman HA. 2010. *Legionella pneumophila* 6S RNA optimizes intracellular multiplication. *Proc Natl Acad Sci USA* **107**:7533–7538.

232. Hnilicova J, Jirat Matejckova J, Sikova M, Pospisil J, Halada P, Panek J, Krasny L. 2014. Ms1, a novel sRNA interacting with the RNA polymerase core in mycobacteria. *Nucleic Acids Res* **42**:11763–11776.

233. Roth A, Breaker RR. 2009. The structural and functional diversity of metabolite-binding riboswitches. *Annu Rev Biochem* **78**:305–334.

234. Dambach MD, Winkler WC. 2009. Expanding roles for metabolite-sensing regulatory RNAs. *Curr Opin Microbiol* **12**:161–169.

235. Mandal M, Boese B, Barrick JE, Winkler WC, Breaker RR. 2003. Riboswitches control fundamental biochemical pathways in *Bacillus subtilis* and other bacteria. *Cell* **113**: 577–586.

236. Irnov, Kertsburg A, Winkler WC. 2006. Genetic control by *cis*-acting regulatory RNAs in *Bacillus subtilis*: general principles and prospects for discovery. *Cold Spring Harbor Symp Quant Biol* **71**:239–249.

237. Blanc-Potard AB, Groisman EA. 1997. The *Salmonella selC* locus contains a pathogenicity island mediating intramacrophage survival. *EMBO J* **16**:5376–5385.

238. Soncini FC, Garcia Vescovi E, Solomon F, Groisman EA. 1996. Molecular basis of the magnesium deprivation response in *Salmonella typhimurium*: identification of PhoP-regulated genes. *J Bacteriol* **178**:5092–5099.

239. Cromie MJ, Shi Y, Latifi T, Groisman EA. 2006. An RNA sensor for intracellular Mg(2+). *Cell* **125**:71–84.

240. Hollands K, Proshkin S, Sklyarova S, Epshtein V, Mironov A, Nudler E, Groisman EA. 2012. Riboswitch control of Rho-dependent transcription termination. *Proc Natl Acad Sci USA* **109**:5376–5381.

241. Zhao G, Kong W, Weatherspoon-Griffin N, Clark-Curtiss J, Shi Y. 2011. Mg^{2+} facilitates leader peptide translation to induce riboswitch-mediated transcription termination. *EMBO J* **30**:1485–1496.

242. Park SY, Cromie MJ, Lee EJ, Groisman EA. 2010. A bacterial mRNA leader that employs different mechanisms to sense disparate intracellular signals. *Cell* **142**:737–748.

243. Price IR, Gaballa A, Ding F, Helmann JD, Ke A. 2015. Mn(2+)-sensing mechanisms of *yybP-ykoY* orphan riboswitches. *Mol Cell* **57**:1110–1123.

244. Furukawa K, Ramesh A, Zhou Z, Weinberg Z, Vallery T, Winkler WC, Breaker RR. 2015. Bacterial riboswitches cooperatively bind Ni(2+) or Co(2+) ions and control expression of heavy metal transporters. *Mol Cell* **57**:1088–1098.

245. Dambach M, Sandoval M, Updegrove TB, Anantharaman V, Aravind L, Waters LS, Storz G. 2015. The ubiquitous *yybP-ykoY* riboswitch is a manganese-responsive regulatory element. *Mol Cell* **57**:1099–1109.

246. Nechooshtan G, Elgrably-Weiss M, Sheaffer A, Westhof E, Altuvia S. 2009. A pH-responsive riboregulator. *Genes Dev* **23**:2650–2662.

247. Romling U, Galperin MY, Gomelsky M. 2013. Cyclic di-GMP: the first 25 years of a universal bacterial second messenger. *Microbiol Mol Biol Rev* **77**:1–52.

248. Sudarsan N, Lee ER, Weinberg Z, Moy RH, Kim JN, Link KH, Breaker RR. 2008. Riboswitches in eubacteria sense the second messenger cyclic di-GMP. *Science* **321**:411–413.

249. Lee ER, Baker JL, Weinberg Z, Sudarsan N, Breaker RR. 2010. An allosteric self-splicing ribozyme triggered by a bacterial second messenger. *Science* **329**:845–848.

250. Bordeleau E, Purcell EB, Lafontaine DA, Fortier LC, Tamayo R, Burrus V. 2015. Cyclic di-GMP riboswitch-regulated type IV pili contribute to aggregation of *Clostridium difficile*. *J Bacteriol* **197**:819–832.

251. Kirn TJ, Jude BA, Taylor RK. 2005. A colonization factor links *Vibrio cholerae* environmental survival and human infection. *Nature* **438**:863–866.

252. Wong E, Vaaje-Kolstad G, Ghosh A, Hurtado-Guerrero R, Konarev PV, Ibrahim AF, Svergun DI, Eijsink VG, Chatterjee NS, van Aalten DM. 2012. The *Vibrio cholerae* colonization factor

GbpA possesses a modular structure that governs binding to different host surfaces. *PLoS Pathog* **8:**e1002373. doi:10.1371/journal.pone.0100147.

253. Ren A, Patel DJ. 2014. c-di-AMP binds the *ydaO* riboswitch in two pseudo-symmetry-related pockets. *Nat Chem Biol* **10:**780–786.

254. Gao A, Serganov A. 2014. Structural insights into recognition of c-di-AMP by the *ydaO* riboswitch. *Nat Chem Biol* **10:**787–792.

255. Loh E, Dussurget O, Gripenland J, Vaitkevicius K, Tiensuu T, Mandin P, Repoila F, Buchrieser C, Cossart P, Johansson J. 2009. A trans-acting riboswitch controls expression of the virulence regulator PrfA in *Listeria monocytogenes*. *Cell* **139:**770–779.

256. Andre G, Even S, Putzer H, Burguiere P, Croux C, Danchin A, Martin-Verstraete I, Soutourina O. 2008. S-box and T-box riboswitches and antisense RNA control a sulfur metabolic operon of *Clostridium acetobutylicum*. *Nucleic Acids Res* **36:**5955–5969.

257. Mellin JR, Tiensuu T, Becavin C, Gouin E, Johansson J, Cossart P. 2013. A riboswitch-regulated antisense RNA in *Listeria monocytogenes*. *Proc Natl Acad Sci USA* **110:**13132–13137.

258. Ramesh A, DebRoy S, Goodson JR, Fox KA, Faz H, Garsin DA, Winkler WC. 2012. The mechanism for RNA recognition by ANTAR regulators of gene expression. *PLoS Genet* **8:**e1002666. doi:10.1371/journal.pgen.1002666.

259. Mellin JR, Koutero M, Dar D, Nahori MA, Sorek R, Cossart P. 2014. Riboswitches. Sequestration of a two-component response regulator by a riboswitch-regulated noncoding RNA. *Science* **345:**940–943.

260. DebRoy S, Gebbie M, Ramesh A, Goodson JR, Cruz MR, van Hoof A, Winkler WC, Garsin DA. 2014. Riboswitches. A riboswitch-containing sRNA controls gene expression by sequestration of a response regulator. *Science* **345:**937–940.

261. Kortmann J, Narberhaus F. 2012. Bacterial RNA thermometers: molecular zippers and switches. *Nat Rev Microbiol* **10:**255–265.

262. Krajewski SS, Narberhaus F. 2014. Temperature-driven differential gene expression by RNA thermosensors. *Biochim Biophys Acta* **1839:**978–988.

263. Johansson J, Mandin P, Renzoni A, Chiaruttini C, Springer M, Cossart P. 2002. An RNA thermosensor controls expression of virulence genes in *Listeria monocytogenes*. *Cell* **110:**551–561.

264. Loh E, Kugelberg E, Tracy A, Zhang Q, Gollan B, Ewles H, Chalmers R, Pelicic V, Tang CM. 2013. Temperature triggers immune evasion by *Neisseria meningitidis*. *Nature* **502:**237–240.

265. Jimenez PN, Koch G, Thompson JA, Xavier KB, Cool RH, Quax WJ. 2012. The multiple signaling systems regulating virulence in *Pseudomonas aeruginosa*. *Microbiol Mol Biol Rev* **76:**46–65.

266. Grosso-Becerra MV, Croda-Garcia G, Merino E, Servin-Gonzalez L, Mojica-Espinosa R, Soberon-Chavez G. 2014. Regulation of *Pseudomonas aeruginosa* virulence factors by two novel RNA thermometers. *Proc Natl Acad Sci USA* **111:**15562–15567.

267. Delvillani F, Sciandrone B, Peano C, Petiti L, Berens C, Georgi C, Ferrara S, Bertoni G, Pasini ME, Deho G, Briani F. 2014. Tet-Trap, a genetic approach to the identification of bacterial RNA thermometers: application to *Pseudomonas aeruginosa*. *RNA* **20:**1963–1976.

268. Bohme K, Steinmann R, Kortmann J, Seekircher S, Heroven AK, Berger E, Pisano F, Thiermann T, Wolf-Watz H, Narberhaus F, Dersch P. 2012. Concerted actions of a thermo-labile regulator and a unique intergenic RNA thermosensor control *Yersinia* virulence. *PLoS Pathog* **8:**e1002518. doi:10.1371/journal.ppat.1002518.

269. Kartha RV, Subramanian S. 2014. Competing endogenous RNAs (ceRNAs): new entrants to the intricacies of gene regulation. *Front Genet* **5:**8.

270. Seitz H. 2009. Redefining microRNA targets. *Curr Biol* **19:**870–873.

271. Ruiz de los Mozos I, Vergara-Irigaray M, Segura V, Villanueva M, Bitarte N, Saramago M, Domingues S, Arraiano CM, Fechter P, Romby P, Valle J, Solano C, Lasa I, Toledo-Arana A. 2013. Base pairing interaction between 5'- and 3'-UTRs controls *icaR* mRNA translation in *Staphylococcus aureus*. *PLoS Genet* **9:**e1004001. doi:10.1371/journal.pgen.1004001.

272. Lopez-Garrido J, Puerta-Fernandez E, Casadesus J. 2014. A eukaryotic-like 3' untranslated region in *Salmonella enterica hilD* mRNA. *Nucleic Acids Res* **42:**5894–5906.

273. Miyakoshi M, Chao Y, Vogel J. 2015. Cross talk between ABC transporter mRNAs via a target mRNA-derived sponge of the GcvB small RNA. *EMBO J* **34:**1478–1492.

274. Liu N, Niu G, Xie Z, Chen Z, Itzek A, Kreth J, Gillaspy A, Zeng L, Burne R, Qi F, Merritt J. 2015. The *Streptococcus mutans irvA* gene encodes a trans-acting riboregulatory mRNA. *Mol Cell* **57:**179–190.

275. Bossi L, Schwartz A, Guillemardet B, Boudvillain M, Figueroa-Bossi N. 2012. A

role for Rho-dependent polarity in gene regulation by a noncoding small RNA. *Genes Dev* **26**:1864–1873.

276. **Figueroa-Bossi N, Valentini M, Malleret L, Fiorini F, Bossi L.** 2009. Caught at its own game: regulatory small RNA inactivated by an inducible transcript mimicking its target. *Genes Dev* **23**:2004–2015.

277. **Rasmussen AA, Johansen J, Nielsen JS, Overgaard M, Kallipolitis B, Valentin-Hansen P.** 2009. A conserved small RNA promotes silencing of the outer membrane protein YbfM. *Mol Microbiol* **72**:566–577.

278. **Overgaard M, Johansen J, Moller-Jensen J, Valentin-Hansen P.** 2009. Switching off small RNA regulation with trap-mRNA. *Mol Microbiol* **73**:790–800.

279. **Sterzenbach T, Nguyen KT, Nuccio SP, Winter MG, Vakulskas CA, Clegg S, Romeo T, Baumler AJ.** 2013. A novel CsrA titration mechanism regulates fimbrial gene expression in *Salmonella typhimurium*. *EMBO J* **32**:2872–2883.

280. **Lalaouna D, Carrier MC, Semsey S, Brouard JS, Wang J, Wade JT, Masse E.** 2015. A 3′ external transcribed spacer in a tRNA transcript acts as a sponge for small RNAs to prevent transcriptional noise. *Mol Cell* **58**:393–405.

281. **Rutherford ST, Bassler BL.** 2012. Bacterial quorum sensing: its role in virulence and possibilities for its control. *Cold Spring Harbor Perspect Med* **2**(11).

282. **Moore S, Thomson N, Mutreja A, Piarroux R.** 2014. Widespread epidemic cholera caused by a restricted subset of *Vibrio cholerae* clones. *Clin Microbiol Infect* **20**:373–379.

283. **Nelson EJ, Harris JB, Morris JG Jr, Calderwood SB, Camilli A.** 2009. Cholera transmission: the host, pathogen and bacteriophage dynamic. *Nat Rev Microbiol* **7**:693–702.

284. **Fu Y, Waldor MK, Mekalanos JJ.** 2013. Tn-Seq analysis of *Vibrio cholerae* intestinal colonization reveals a role for T6SS-mediated antibacterial activity in the host. *Cell Host Microbe* **14**:652–663.

285. **Teschler JK, Zamorano-Sanchez D, Utada AS, Warner CJ, Wong GC, Linington RG, Yildiz FH.** 2015. Living in the matrix: assembly and control of *Vibrio cholerae* biofilms. *Nat Rev Microbiol* **13**:255–268.

286. **Borgeaud S, Metzger LC, Scrignari T, Blokesch M.** 2015. The type VI secretion system of *Vibrio cholerae* fosters horizontal gene transfer. *Science* **347**:63–67.

287. **Krukonis ES, DiRita VJ.** 2003. From motility to virulence: sensing and responding to environmental signals in *Vibrio cholerae*. *Curr Opin Microbiol* **6**:186–190.

288. **Matson JS, Withey JH, DiRita VJ.** 2007. Regulatory networks controlling *Vibrio cholerae* virulence gene expression. *Infect Immun* **75**:5542–5549.

289. **Weber GG, Kortmann J, Narberhaus F, Klose KE.** 2014. RNA thermometer controls temperature-dependent virulence factor expression in *Vibrio cholerae*. *Proc Natl Acad Sci USA* **111**:14241–14246.

290. **Richard AL, Withey JH, Beyhan S, Yildiz F, DiRita VJ.** 2010. The *Vibrio cholerae* virulence regulatory cascade controls glucose uptake through activation of TarA, a small regulatory RNA. *Mol Microbiol* **78**:1171–1181.

291. **Song T, Sabharwal D, Wai SN.** 2010. VrrA mediates Hfq-dependent regulation of OmpT synthesis in *Vibrio cholerae*. *J Mol Biol* **400**: 682–688.

292. **Sabharwal D, Song T, Papenfort K, Wai SN.** 2015. The VrrA sRNA controls a stationary phase survival factor Vrp of *Vibrio cholerae*. *RNA Biol* **12**:186–196.

293. **Song T, Mika F, Lindmark B, Liu Z, Schild S, Bishop A, Zhu J, Camilli A, Johansson J, Vogel J, Wai SN.** 2008. A new *Vibrio cholerae* sRNA modulates colonization and affects release of outer membrane vesicles. *Mol Microbiol* **70**:100–111.

294. **Zhu J, Miller MB, Vance RE, Dziejman M, Bassler BL, Mekalanos JJ.** 2002. Quorum-sensing regulators control virulence gene expression in *Vibrio cholerae*. *Proc Natl Acad Sci USA* **99**:3129–3134.

295. **Rutherford ST, van Kessel JC, Shao Y, Bassler BL.** 2011. AphA and LuxR/HapR reciprocally control quorum sensing in vibrios. *Genes Dev* **25**:397–408.

296. **Yang M, Frey EM, Liu Z, Bishar R, Zhu J.** 2010. The virulence transcriptional activator AphA enhances biofilm formation by *Vibrio cholerae* by activating expression of the biofilm regulator VpsT. *Infect Immun* **78**:697–703.

297. **Lenz DH, Mok KC, Lilley BN, Kulkarni RV, Wingreen NS, Bassler BL.** 2004. The small RNA chaperone Hfq and multiple small RNAs control quorum sensing in *Vibrio harveyi* and *Vibrio cholerae*. *Cell* **118**:69–82.

298. **Caswell CC, Oglesby-Sherrouse AG, Murphy ER.** 2014. Sibling rivalry: related bacterial small RNAs and their redundant and non-redundant roles. *Front Cell Infect Microbiol* **4**:151.

299. **Shao Y, Bassler BL.** 2012. Quorum-sensing non-coding small RNAs use unique pairing regions to differentially control mRNA targets. *Mol Microbiol* **83**:599–611.

300. **Shao Y, Feng L, Rutherford ST, Papenfort K, Bassler BL.** 2013. Functional determinants of

the quorum-sensing non-coding RNAs and their roles in target regulation. *EMBO J* **32:**2158–2171.

301. **Zhao X, Koestler BJ, Waters CM, Hammer BK.** 2013. Post-transcriptional activation of a diguanylate cyclase by quorum sensing small RNAs promotes biofilm formation in *Vibrio cholerae*. *Mol Microbiol* **89:**989–1002.

302. **Shao Y, Bassler BL.** 2014. Quorum regulatory small RNAs repress type VI secretion in *Vibrio cholerae*. *Mol Microbiol* **92:**921–930.

303. **Waters CM, Lu W, Rabinowitz JD, Bassler BL.** 2008. Quorum sensing controls biofilm formation in *Vibrio cholerae* through modulation of cyclic di-GMP levels and repression of *vpsT*. *J Bacteriol* **190:**2527–2536.

304. **Svenningsen SL, Waters CM, Bassler BL.** 2008. A negative feedback loop involving small RNAs accelerates *Vibrio cholerae*'s transition out of quorum-sensing mode. *Genes Dev* **22:**226–238.

305. **Tu KC, Long T, Svenningsen SL, Wingreen NS, Bassler BL.** 2010. Negative feedback loops involving small regulatory RNAs precisely control the *Vibrio harveyi* quorum-sensing response. *Mol Cell* **37:**567–579.

306. **Lenz DH, Miller MB, Zhu J, Kulkarni RV, Bassler BL.** 2005. CsrA and three redundant small RNAs regulate quorum sensing in *Vibrio cholerae*. *Mol Microbiol* **58:**1186–1202.

307. **Romilly C, Caldelari I, Parmentier D, Lioliou E, Romby P, Fechter P.** 2012. Current knowledge on regulatory RNAs and their machineries in *Staphylococcus aureus*. *RNA Biol* **9:**402–413.

308. **Ji G, Beavis RC, Novick RP.** 1995. Cell density control of staphylococcal virulence mediated by an octapeptide pheromone. *Proc Natl Acad Sci USA* **92:**12055–12059.

309. **Novick RP.** 2003. Autoinduction and signal transduction in the regulation of staphylococcal virulence. *Mol Microbiol* **48:**1429–1449.

310. **Janzon L, Lofdahl S, Arvidson S.** 1989. Identification and nucleotide sequence of the delta-lysin gene, *hld*, adjacent to the accessory gene regulator (*agr*) of *Staphylococcus aureus*. *Mol Gen Genet* **219:**480–485.

311. **Verdon J, Girardin N, Lacombe C, Berjeaud JM, Hechard Y.** 2009. delta-hemolysin, an update on a membrane-interacting peptide. *Peptides* **30:**817–823.

312. **Felden B, Vandenesch F, Bouloc P, Romby P.** 2011. The *Staphylococcus aureus* RNome and its commitment to virulence. *PLoS Pathog* **7:** e1002006. doi:10.1371/journal.ppat.1002006.

313. **Monteiro C, Papenfort K, Hentrich K, Ahmad I, Le Guyon S, Reimann R, Grantcharova N,** Romling U. 2012. Hfq and Hfq-dependent small RNAs are major contributors to multicellular development in *Salmonella enterica* serovar Typhimurium. *RNA Biol* **9:**489–502.

314. **Geisinger E, Adhikari RP, Jin R, Ross HF, Novick RP.** 2006. Inhibition of *rot* translation by RNAIII, a key feature of *agr* function. *Mol Microbiol* **61:**1038–1048.

315. **Chabelskaya S, Bordeau V, Felden B.** 2014. Dual RNA regulatory control of a *Staphylococcus aureus* virulence factor. *Nucleic Acids Res* **42:**4847–4858.

316. **Chabelskaya S, Gaillot O, Felden B.** 2010. A *Staphylococcus aureus* small RNA is required for bacterial virulence and regulates the expression of an immune-evasion molecule. *PLoS Pathog* **6:** e1000927. doi:10.1371/journal.ppat.1000927.

317. **Romilly C, Lays C, Tomasini A, Caldelari I, Benito Y, Hammann P, Geissmann T, Boisset S, Romby P, Vandenesch F.** 2014. A non-coding RNA promotes bacterial persistence and decreases virulence by regulating a regulator in *Staphylococcus aureus*. *PLoS Pathog* **10:**e1003979. doi:10.1371/journal.ppat.1003979.

318. **Sayed N, Jousselin A, Felden B.** 2012. A *cis*-antisense RNA acts in *trans* in *Staphylococcus aureus* to control translation of a human cytolytic peptide. *Nat Struct Mol Biol* **19:**105–112.

319. **Miyakoshi M, Chao Y, Vogel J.** 2015. Cross talk between ABC transporter mRNAs via a target mRNA-derived sponge of the GcvB small RNA. *EMBO J* **34:**1478–1492.

320. **Weiberg A, Wang M, Lin FM, Zhao H, Zhang Z, Kaloshian I, Huang HD, Jin H.** 2013. Fungal small RNAs suppress plant immunity by hijacking host RNA interference pathways. *Science* **342:**118–123.

321. **Oldenburg M, Kruger A, Ferstl R, Kaufmann A, Nees G, Sigmund A, Bathke B, Lauterbach H, Suter M, Dreher S, Koedel U, Akira S, Kawai T, Buer J, Wagner H, Bauer S, Hochrein H, Kirschning CJ.** 2012. TLR13 recognizes bacterial 23S rRNA devoid of erythromycin resistance-forming modification. *Science* **337:**1111–1115.

322. **Abdullah Z, Schlee M, Roth S, Mraheil MA, Barchet W, Bottcher J, Hain T, Geiger S, Hayakawa Y, Fritz JH, Civril F, Hopfner KP, Kurts C, Ruland J, Hartmann G, Chakraborty T, Knolle PA.** 2012. RIG-I detects infection with live *Listeria* by sensing secreted bacterial nucleic acids. *EMBO J* **31:**4153–4164.

323. **Barrangou R, Marraffini LA.** 2014. CRISPR-Cas systems: prokaryotes upgrade to adaptive immunity. *Mol Cell* **54:**234–244.

324. **Ratner HK, Sampson TR, Weiss DS.** 2015. I can see CRISPR now, even when phage are gone: a view on alternative CRISPR-Cas

functions from the prokaryotic envelope. *Curr Opin Infect Dis* **28:**267–274.

325. **Westra ER, Buckling A, Fineran PC.** 2014. CRISPR-Cas systems: beyond adaptive immunity. *Nat Rev Microbiol* **12:**317–326.

326. **Palmer KL, Gilmore MS.** 2010. Multidrug-resistant enterococci lack CRISPR-*cas*. *MBio* **1:** e00227-10. doi:10.1128/mBio.00227-10.

327. **Bikard D, Hatoum-Aslan A, Mucida D, Marraffini LA.** 2012. CRISPR interference can prevent natural transformation and virulence acquisition during *in vivo* bacterial infection. *Cell Host Microbe* **12:**177–186.

328. **Sampson TR, Napier BA, Schroeder MR, Louwen R, Zhao J, Chin CY, Ratner HK, Llewellyn AC, Jones CL, Laroui H, Merlin D, Zhou P, Endtz HP, Weiss DS.** 2014. A CRISPR-Cas system enhances envelope integrity mediating antibiotic resistance and inflammasome evasion. *Proc Natl Acad Sci USA* **111:**11163–11168.

329. **Sampson TR, Saroj SD, Llewellyn AC, Tzeng YL, Weiss DS.** 2013. A CRISPR/Cas system mediates bacterial innate immune evasion and virulence. *Nature* **497:**254–257.

330. **Gunderson FF, Mallama CA, Fairbairn SG, Cianciotto NP.** 2015. Nuclease activity of *Legionella pneumophila* Cas2 promotes intracellular infection of amoebal host cells. *Infect Immun* **83:**1008–1018.

331. **Gunderson FF, Cianciotto NP.** 2013. The CRISPR-associated gene *cas2* of *Legionella pneumophila* is required for intracellular infection of amoebae. *MBio* **4:**e00074-13. doi:10.1128/mBio.00074-13.

332. **Ingolia NT, Ghaemmaghami S, Newman JR, Weissman JS.** 2009. Genome-wide analysis *in vivo* of translation with nucleotide resolution using ribosome profiling. *Science* **324:**218–223.

333. **Guo MS, Updegrove TB, Gogol EB, Shabalina SA, Gross CA, Storz G.** 2014. MicL, a new σ_E-dependent sRNA, combats envelope stress by repressing synthesis of Lpp, the major outer membrane lipoprotein. *Genes Dev* **28:**1620–1634.

334. **Westermann AJ, Gorski SA, Vogel J.** 2012. Dual RNA-seq of pathogen and host. *Nat Rev Microbiol* **10:**618–630.

335. **Humphrys MS, Creasy T, Sun Y, Shetty AC, Chibucos MC, Drabek EF, Fraser CM, Farooq U, Sengamalay N, Ott S, Shou H,** **Bavoil PM, Mahurkar A, Myers GS.** 2013. Simultaneous transcriptional profiling of bacteria and their host cells. *PLoS One* **8:**e80597. doi:10.1371/journal.pone.0080597.

336. **Saliba AE, Westermann AJ, Gorski SA, Vogel J.** 2014. Single-cell RNA-seq: advances and future challenges. *Nucleic Acids Res* **42:**8845–8860.

337. **Van Roosbroeck K, Pollet J, Calin GA.** 2013. miRNAs and long noncoding RNAs as biomarkers in human diseases. *Expert Rev Mol Diagn* **13:**183–204.

338. **Wright PR, Richter AS, Papenfort K, Mann M, Vogel J, Hess WR, Backofen R, Georg J.** 2013. Comparative genomics boosts target prediction for bacterial small RNAs. *Proc Natl Acad Sci USA* **110:**E3487–E3496.

339. **Howe JA, Wang H, Fischmann TO, Balibar CJ, Xiao L, Galgoci AM, Malinverni JC, Mayhood T, Villafania A, Nahvi A, Murgolo N, Barbieri CM, Mann PA, Carr D, Xia E, Zuck P, Riley D, Painter RE, Walker SS, Sherborne B, de Jesus R, Pan W, Plotkin MA, Wu J, Rindgen D, Cummings J, Garlisi CG, Zhang R, Sheth PR, Gill CJ, Tang H, Roemer T.** 2015. Selective small-molecule inhibition of an RNA structural element. *Nature* **526:**672–677.

340. **Dorr T, Vulic M, Lewis K.** 2010. Ciprofloxacin causes persister formation by inducing the TisB toxin in *Escherichia coli*. *PLoS Biol* **8:** e1000317. doi:10.1371/journal.pbio.1000317.

341. **Ortega AD, Gonzalo-Asensio J, Garcia-del Portillo F.** 2012. Dynamics of *Salmonella* small RNA expression in non-growing bacteria located inside eukaryotic cells. *RNA Biol* **9:**469–488.

342. **Sesto N, Touchon M, Andrade JM, Kondo J, Rocha EP, Arraiano CM, Archambaud C, Westhof E, Romby P, Cossart P.** 2014. A PNPase dependent CRISPR system in *Listeria*. *PLoS Genet* **10:**e1004065. doi:10.1371/journal. pgen.1004065.

343. **Hagblom P, Segal E, Billyard E, So M.** 1985. Intragenic recombination leads to pilus antigenic variation in *Neisseria gonorrhoeae*. *Nature* **315:**156–158.

344. **Westermann AJ, Förstner KU, Amman F, Barquist L, Chao Y, Schulte LN, Müller L, Reinhardt R, Stadler PF, Vogel J.** 2016. Dual RNA-seq unveils noncoding RNA functions in host-pathogen interactions. *Nature* **529:**496–501.

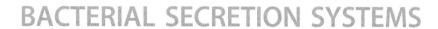

BACTERIAL SECRETION SYSTEMS

Bacterial Secretion Systems: An Overview

8

ERIN R. GREEN[1] and JOAN MECSAS[1,2]

INTRODUCTION

One essential prokaryotic cell function is the transport of proteins from the cytoplasm into other compartments of the cell, the environment, and/or other bacteria or eukaryotic cells—a process known as protein secretion. Prokaryotes have developed numerous ways of transporting protein cargo between locations, which largely involve the assistance of dedicated protein secretion systems. Protein secretion systems are essential for the growth of bacteria and are used in an array of processes. Some secretion systems are found in almost all bacteria and secrete a wide variety of substrates, while others have been identified in only a small number of bacterial species or are dedicated to secreting only one or a few proteins. In certain cases, these dedicated secretion systems are used by bacterial pathogens to manipulate the host and establish a replicative niche. Other times, they are required to take advantage of an environmental niche, perhaps by secreting proteins that help bacteria to compete with nearby microorganisms. There are several different classes of bacterial secretion systems, and their designs can differ based on whether their protein substrates cross a single phospholipid membrane,

[1]Program in Molecular Microbiology, Sackler School of Graduate Biomedical Sciences, Tufts University, Boston, MA 02111; [2]Department of Molecular Biology and Microbiology, Tufts University School of Medicine, Boston, MA 02111.
Virulence Mechanisms of Bacterial Pathogens, 5th edition
Edited by Indira T. Kudva, Nancy A. Cornick, Paul J. Plummer, Qijing Zhang, Tracy L. Nicholson, John P. Bannantine, and Bryan H. Bellaire
© 2016 American Society for Microbiology, Washington, DC
doi:10.1128/microbiolspec.VMBF-0012-2015

two membranes, or even three membranes, where two are bacterial and one is a host membrane. Due to the specificity of expression of some of these secretion systems in bacterial pathogens, antimicrobials are being developed against these systems to augment our current repertoire of antibiotics. This topic is discussed in Section VII, "Targeted Therapies".

Five secretion systems will be discussed in depth in subsequent chapters in this section: the type III secretion system (T3SS), T4SS, T5SS, T6SS, and T7SS. In this overview, we provide a brief introduction to several protein secretion systems, including those that are not discussed in depth in other chapters, to highlight the structural and functional similarities and differences between these systems. Our discussions will focus on the canonical features of each system rather than the multitude of variations (Table 1). In addition, we will briefly review recent findings that indicate that the innate immune system of the host can detect and respond to the presence of protein secretion systems during mammalian infection.

SECRETION ACROSS THE CYTOPLASMIC MEMBRANE

A major focus of this chapter is the use of dedicated secretion systems to transport proteins out of the bacterial cell and into the environment or into a recipient cell. However, protein secretion from the bacterial cytoplasmic compartment into other compartments of the cell, particularly into or across the cytoplasmic membrane, also occurs. The general secretion (Sec) and twin arginine translocation (Tat) pathways are the bacterial secretion systems most commonly used to transport proteins across the cytoplasmic membrane (1). The Sec and Tat pathways are the most highly conserved mechanisms of protein secretion and have been identified in all domains of life (bacteria, archaea, and eukarya) (2, 3). Most proteins transported by the Sec and Tat pathways remain inside the cell, in either the periplasm or the inner membrane. However, in Gram-negative bacteria, proteins delivered to the cytoplasmic membrane or periplasm of the cell by the Sec or Tat pathway can either stay in those compartments or may be transported outside of the cell with the help of another secretion system. While the Sec and Tat systems have several common elements, they transport proteins by fundamentally different mechanisms.

The Sec Secretion Pathway

The Sec pathway primarily translocates proteins in their unfolded state. This system consists of three parts: a protein targeting

TABLE 1 Classes of bacterial protein secretion systems

Secretion apparatus	Secretion signal	Steps in secretion	Folded substrates?	Number of membranes	Gram (+) or Gram (−)
Sec	N-terminus	1	No	1	Both
Tat	N-terminus	1	Yes	1	Both
T1SS	C-terminus	1	No	2	Gram (−)
T2SS	N-terminus	2	Yes	1	Gram (−)
T3SS	N-terminus	1-2	No	2–3	Gram (−)
T4SS	C-terminus	1	No	2–3	Gram (−)
T5SS	N-terminus	2	No	1	Gram (−)
T6SS	No known secretion signal	1	Unknown	2–3	Gram (−)
SecA2	N-terminus	1	No	1	Gram (+)
Sortase	N-terminus (Sec)C-terminus (cell wall sorting)	2	Yes	1	Gram (+)
Injectosome	N-terminus	2	Yes	1	Gram (+)
T7SS	C-terminus	1	Yes	1–3	Gram (+)

component, a motor protein, and a membrane integrated conducting channel, called the SecYEG translocase (2). Additionally, several Gram-positive bacteria produce Sec accessory proteins that serve important roles in the secretion of specific proteins. While proteins secreted by the Sec apparatus can serve many roles, a number of proteins that promote virulence of bacterial pathogens are transported through this pathway. Pathogens that use Sec-dependent secretion to transport virulence factors across the cytoplasmic membrane include the Gram-negative bacteria *Vibrio cholerae*, *Klebsiella pneumoniae*, and *Yersinia enterocolitica* (4). Examples of Gram-positive pathogens that employ Sec accessory systems include *Staphylococcus aureus* and *Listeria monocytogenes* (5–8). The use of Sec accessory proteins in secretion by Gram-positive bacteria will be covered in more detail later in this chapter.

Export by the Sec pathway relies on a hydrophobic signal sequence at the N-terminus of the secreted protein, which is typically 20 amino acids in length and contains three regions: a positively charged amino terminal, a hydrophobic core, and a polar carboxyl-terminal (2). Proteins that will be secreted into the periplasm or outside of the cell by the Sec pathway contain SecB-specific signal sequences, while proteins meant to remain in the inner membrane contain a signal recognition particle (SRP)–specific signal sequence. The differences between these two pathways are outlined below (2).

The SecB pathway

In many Gram-negative bacteria, proteins destined for transport to the periplasm or outside of the cell contain a removable signal sequence recognized by the SecB protein (Fig. 1A). This protein serves as a chaperone, binding to presecretory proteins and preventing them from folding (9). SecB then delivers its substrates to SecA, a multifunctional protein that both guides proteins to the SecYEG channel and serves as the ATPase that provides the energy for protein translocation

(10). Prior to transport through the channel, a protease protein cleaves off the SecB signal sequence from the protein, and the secreted protein is then is folded upon delivery to the periplasm (11). While many proteins delivered by the SecB system remain in the periplasm, some will ultimately become extracellular. Once these proteins are delivered to the periplasm, they can be transported across the outer membrane with the help of the T2SS and T5SS. We will discuss these Sec-dependent mechanisms of protein secretion in detail later in this chapter.

The SRP pathway

The Sec system can also transport proteins that are meant to remain in the inner membrane by way of the SRP pathway (Fig 1B). Transmembrane proteins often contain hydrophobic domains and thus are unstable when cytoplasmic. Therefore, secretion by the SRP pathway utilizes a cotranslational mechanism of export that couples translation of the protein by the ribosome with secretion through the SecYEG channel (12). The SRP pathway relies on the SRP particle, which contains a small, 4.5S RNA bound to a protein called Ffh (12). During protein secretion by this pathway, the SRP first binds the transmembrane domain of proteins as they emerge from the ribosome (13). The SRP then binds the docking protein FtsY, which delivers the ribosome-protein complex to the SecYEG channel (2). Translation of the protein then drives the secretion of the nascent protein through the channel. During this process, the transmembrane domain of the protein escapes through the side of the channel into the membrane, where it remains attached (14). The mechanism of this final step is not yet known.

The Tat Secretion Pathway

In contrast to the Sec pathway, the Tat pathway primarily secretes folded proteins (3) (Fig. 2). This pathway is critical because not all proteins can be secreted in their unfolded

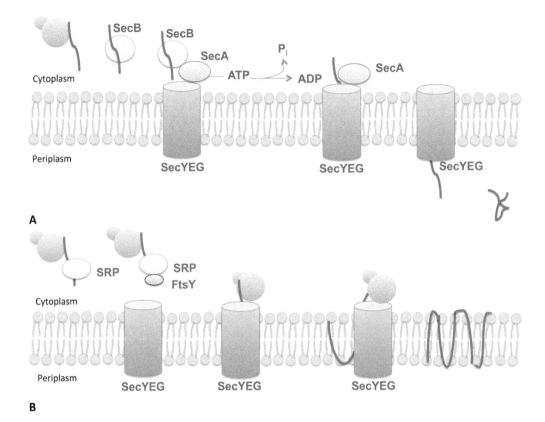

FIGURE 1 Export through the Sec pathway. In bacteria, the Sec pathway transports unfolded proteins across the cytoplasmic membrane. Proteins secreted by this pathway may either become embedded in the inner membrane or will be released into the periplasm. In Gram-negative organisms, these periplasmic proteins may be released extracellularly with the help of an additional secretion system. (A) Proteins destined for the periplasm (or extracellular release) are translocated by a posttranslational mechanism and contain a removable signal sequence recognized by the SecB protein. SecB binds presecretory proteins and prevents them from folding while also delivering its substrates to SecA. SecA both guides proteins to the SecYEG channel and serves as the ATPase that provides the energy for protein translocation. Following transport through the SecYEG channel, proteins are folded in the periplasm. (B) The Sec pathway utilizes a cotranslational mechanism of export to secrete proteins destined for the inner membrane. These proteins contain a signal sequence recognized by the signal recognition particle (SRP). During translation, the SRP binds target proteins as they emerge from the ribosome and recruits the docking protein FtsY. FtsY delivers the ribosome-protein complex to the SecYEG channel, which translocates the nascent protein across the cytoplasmic membrane. During translocation across the channel, the transmembrane domain is able to escape through the side of the channel into the membrane, where the protein remains attached.

state. For example, certain proteins that contain posttranslational modifications, such as redox factors, which are synthesized in the cytoplasm (15). Because the materials required for these modifications would not be available extracellularly or in the periplasm and, these proteins must be folded and

modified in the cytoplasm prior to secretion in their three-dimensional state.

The Tat pathway of protein secretion consists of two or three subunits: TatA, TatB, and TatC (in Gram-positive bacteria, TatA and TatB are combined into one multifunctional protein) (16, 17). The Tat signal

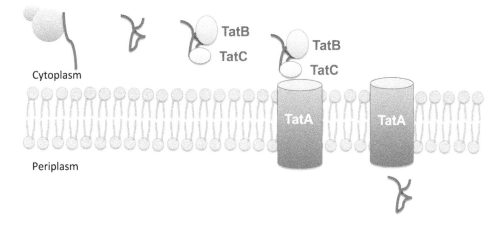

FIGURE 2 **Secretion through the Tat pathway. Bacteria secrete folded proteins across the cytoplasmic membrane using the Tat secretion pathway. This pathway consists of two or three components (TatA, TatB, and TatC). In Gram-negative bacteria, TatB and TatC bind a specific N-terminal signal peptide containing a "twin" arginine motif on folded Tat secretion substrates. TatB and TatC then recruit TatA to the cytoplasmic membrane, where it forms a channel. Folded proteins are then translocated across the channel and into the periplasm. In Gram-negative bacteria, these proteins may remain in the periplasm or can be exported out of the cell by the T2SS.**

sequence contains a pair of "twin" arginines in the motif S-R-R at the N-terminus of the folded protein (18). In *Escherichia coli*, TatB and TatC bind the signal peptide of Tat-secreted proteins and then recruit TatA, which forms the membrane-spanning channel (18). Whereas most proteins secreted by the Tat apparatus in Gram-positive bacteria are released extracellularly, Tat-secreted proteins in Gram-negative bacteria can either remain periplasmic or are transported out of the cell by the T2SS through a mechanism that will be reviewed later in this chapter.

While the Tat pathway is important for the physiology and survival of both pathogenic and nonpathogenic bacteria, several pathogenic bacteria, including *Pseudomonas aeruginosa* (19), *Yersinia pseudotuberculosis* (20), and *E. coli* O157:H7 (21), require a functional Tat pathway for full virulence in animal infection models. Phospholipase C enzymes are a notable example of Tat-secreted proteins that serve as virulence factors for a number of pathogens, including *P. aeruginosa* (19), *Legionella pneumophila* (22), and *Myco-*

bacterium tuberculosis (23). These enzymes, which cleave phospholipids immediately before their phosphate group, can serve a variety of functions during infection, including suppression of immune cell activity and promotion of intracellular survival (24).

PROTEIN SECRETION BY GRAM-NEGATIVE BACTERIA

Several Gram-negative bacteria rely on dedicated secretion systems to transport virulence proteins outside of the cell and, in some cases, directly into the cytoplasm of a eukaryotic or prokaryotic target cell. Extracellular protein secretion can be a challenge for Gram-negative bacteria, because these secreted proteins must cross two (and in some cases three) phospholipid membranes to reach their final destination (Fig. 3). Some secreted proteins in Gram-negative bacteria traverse these membranes in two separate steps, where they are first delivered to the periplasm through the Sec or Tat secretion

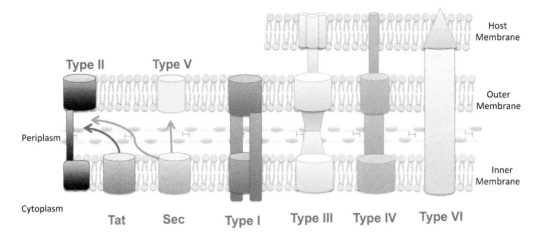

FIGURE 3 Secretion systems in Gram-negative bacteria. Gram-negative bacteria utilize a number of dedicated protein secretion systems to transport proteins across one, two, or three phospholipid membranes. Some proteins are secreted in a two-step, Sec- or Tat-dependent mechanism. These proteins cross the inner membrane with the help of either the Sec or Tat secretion pathways and are then transported across the outer membrane using a second secretion system. The T2SS and T5SS secrete proteins in this manner. Because it secretes folded substrates, the T2SS translocates proteins initially transported by either the Tat or Sec pathway (where Sec substrates are folded in the periplasm). In contrast, autotransporters of the T5SS must be unfolded prior to outer membrane transport and thus must be secreted across the inner membrane by the Sec pathway. Additionally, several Gram-negative protein secretion systems transport their substrates across both bacterial membranes in a one-step, Sec- or Tat-independent process. These include the T1SS, T3SS, T4SS, and T6SS. All of these pathways contain periplasm-spanning channels and secrete proteins from the cytoplasm outside the cell, but their mechanisms of protein secretion are quite different. Three of these secretion systems, the T3SS, T4SS, and T6SS, can also transport proteins across an additional host cell membrane, delivering secreted proteins directly to the cytosol of a target cell.

systems, as discussed in the preceding section, and are then transferred across the outer membrane by a second transport system. This process is known as Sec- or Tat-dependent protein secretion. Additionally, many other proteins are secreted through channels that span both the inner and outer bacterial membranes through a process known as Sec- or Tat-independent protein secretion. The dedicated secretion systems in Gram-negative bacteria are numbered type I through type VI, with each system transporting a specific subset of proteins. These systems all rely on β-barrel channels that form a ring in the outer membrane of the bacterial cell, but otherwise they exhibit a fair amount of diversity in their structures and mechanistic functions, as will be outlined below.

The T1SS

T1SSs have been found in a large number of Gram-negative bacteria, including pathogens of plants and animals, where they transport their substrates in a one-step process (as demonstrated in Fig. 3) across both the inner and outer bacterial membranes (recently reviewed in reference 25). Unlike other protein transport systems found in Gram-negative bacteria, T1SSs closely resemble a large family of ATP-binding cassette (ABC) transporters, which export small molecules such as antibiotics and toxins out of the cell (26). Some bacteria may have several T1SSs, each of which is dedicated to transporting one or a few unfolded substrates (27). These substrates range in function and include digestive enzymes, such as proteases and lipases, as well as adhesins, heme-binding proteins, and proteins with repeats-in-toxins (RTX) motifs. T1SS substrates are generally Sec-independent and typically, but not always, contain a C-terminal signal sequence that is recognized by the T1SS and remains uncleaved (see below).

T1SSs have three essential structural components: (i) an ABC transporter protein in the inner membrane and (ii) a membrane fusion protein (MFP) that crosses the inner membrane and bridges it to the outer membrane, and (iii) the outer membrane factor (OMF) in the outer membrane (25). The ABC transporter component associated with the T1SS has several critical functions: it catalyzes ATP to provide the energy to transport the substrate, interacts with the MFP, and participates in substrate recognition (28). The MFP associates with the ABC transporter in the inner membrane and spans the periplasm to associate with the OMF (29–31). In addition, the cytoplasmically located N-terminus of the MFP is believed to play a role in substrate selection (30, 32). The OMF generates a pore in the outer membrane, through which the substrate passes in an unfolded state. Interestingly, T1SSs often use the multipurpose protein TolC as their OMF (27). This pore-forming protein is also used to export molecules and other compounds and is recruited to the MFP after the ABC transporter and MFP have contacted a substrate (32).

The T1SS ABC transporters have been furher divided into three groups based on their N-terminal sequences (reviewed in reference 28). One class of ABC transporters contains a C39 peptidase domain, which belongs to the papain superfamily structural motif. The C39-peptidase-containing ABC-transporters are critical for recognizing and cleaving the N-termini of substrates. An example of a T1SS substrate with a C39 peptidase domain is Colicin V of *E. coli* (33). A second class of ABC transporters contains a C39-like peptidase domain that lacks pro-

teolytic activity and therefore does not cleave its designated substrates (34). Substrates of C39-like peptidase domain–containing ABC transporters generally contain RTX motifs and are much larger than those secreted by a C39-containing peptidase ABC transporter. Interestingly, RTX motifs bind to calcium at extracellular, but not intracellular, levels. Because calcium binding promotes the folding of these proteins, these large substrates are able to remain unfolded inside the cell (35). Finally, a third class of T1SS ABC transporters lacks any additional sequences in the N-terminal domain. Their substrates may or may not contain RTX motifs but are smaller in size than substrates transported by C39-like peptidase domain–containing ABC transporters and contain secretion signals at their C-termini (27).

T1SS substrates contribute to virulence in a variety of bacterial pathogens, including *V. cholerae*, which uses its T1SS to secrete the MARTX toxin (36), and *Serratia marcescens*, which secretes the hemophore HasA via the T1SS pathway (29). One of the best-studied T1SS substrates is the HlyA hemolysin protein of uropathogenic *E. coli* (37–39). This RTX-family toxin inserts into the membranes of both erythrocytes and nucleated eukaryotic cells, causing them to rupture (37). Rupture of host cells by HlyA can help the bacteria to cross mucosal barriers and, additionally, can damage effector immune cells, which prevents clearance of the infection.

The T2SS

T2SSs are conserved in most Gram-negative bacteria, where they transport folded proteins from the periplasm into the extracellular environment. Because the T2SS channel is found only in the outer membrane (Fig. 3), proteins secreted through this apparatus must first be delivered to the periplasm via the Sec or Tat secretion pathways, which transfer protein substrates across the inner membrane, as described above. This secretion system was originally called the main terminal branch of the Sec secretion pathway due to its ability to export proteins transported across the inner membrane by the Sec secretion system (4). However, this nomenclature has since been updated to the T2SS to reflect the ability of these secretion systems to transport Tat-secreted proteins as well (40). Because proteins destined for secretion by the T2SS apparatus must first pass through the Sec or Tat inner membrane transporters, T2SS substrates must have a Sec- or Tat-type cleavable signal sequence at their N-termini (4). Additionally, because the T2SS secretes folded substrates, proteins transported across the cytoplasmic membrane by the Sec pathway must be folded in the periplasm prior to export through the T2SS.

T2SSs have a broad specificity and are capable of secreting a diverse array of substrates outside of the bacterial cell, some of which contribute to the virulence of bacterial pathogens (4). In some bacterial species, the T2SS is required for the secretion of multiple substrates, while in others, it is only used to transport a single protein (41). These secreted proteins have a range of biological functions but are generally enzymes, such as proteases, lipases, and phosphatases, as well as several proteins that process carbohydrates (4).

T2SSs are complex and consist of as many as 15 proteins, which can be broken down into four subassemblies: the outer-membrane complex, the inner-membrane platform, the secretion ATPase, and the pseudopilus (4). As its name suggests, the outer-membrane complex resides in the outer membrane, where it serves as the channel through which folded periplasmic T2SS substrates are translocated (42). This channel is composed of a multimeric protein called the secretin. The secretin has a long N-terminus, which is believed to extend all the way to the periplasm to make contact with other T2SS proteins in the inner membrane (42). The inner-membrane platform, which is composed of multiple copies of at least four proteins, is embedded in the inner membrane and extends into the periplasm, contacting the secretin. This platform plays a crucial role in the secretion process by communicating with the secretin, pseudopilus, and ATPase to coordinate export of substrates (4). The ATPase is located in the cytoplasm and provides the energy to power the system. As its name implies, the T2SS pseudopilus is evolutionarily related and structurally similar to proteins that comprise type IV pili on bacterial cell surfaces, as well as some bacterial competence systems (43). Therefore, one model for secretion through the T2SS channel proposes that these pseudopili retract to push the folded T2SS substrate through the outer membrane channel. In this "piston" model, "secretion-competent" proteins in the periplasm contact the periplasmic domain of the secretin. This interaction is believed to stimulate the cytoplasmic ATPase to drive retraction of the T2SS pseudopili, which push proteins through the secretin channel (4, 44, 45).

A number of bacterial pathogens employ T2SSs to transport virulence factors outside of the cell. Examples of T2SS substrates that are important for virulence in a mammalian host include the cholera toxin of *V. cholerae* (46), which causes the watery diarrhea associated with the disease cholera, and exotoxin A of *P. aeruginosa* (47), which blocks protein synthesis in host cells, leading to lethal infection by this bacterium. Still other pathogens use their T2SSs to secrete enzymes that help them adapt to their environment, which can include plant and animal hosts. These pathogens include *L. pneumophila* (48), enterotoxigenic and enterohemorrhagic *E. coli* (49–51), *K. pneumoniae* (52), *Aeromonas hydrophila* (53), and *Dickeya dadantii* (54).

The T3SSs

T3SSs are found in a large number of Gram-negative bacterial pathogens and symbionts (reviewed in reference 55). T3SSs have been described as "injectisomes" and "needle and syringe"–like apparatuses because of their structure (see Fig. 3). They secrete a wide variety of proteinaceous substrates across both the inner and outer bacterial membranes. In addition, most T3SSs also transport substrates across a target eukaryotic cell membrane in the same step and, therefore, actually transport proteins across three membranes. Secretion of T3SS substrates is generally thought to be a one-step process, although recently this notion has been challenged in *Yersinia* (discussed below). T3SS substrates are generically called effector proteins. Pathogens may secrete only a few effector proteins, as in the cases of *Pseudomonas* and *Yersinia*, or several dozen, as in the cases of *Shigella* and enterohemorrhagic *E. coli*. Secretion signals are embedded within the N-termini of T3SS substrates and are not cleaved. Many, but not all, T3SS effectors have chaperones that guide them to the T3SS base, where they are secreted in an ATP-dependent, unfolded state.

The T3SS has a core of nine proteins that are highly conserved among all known systems (reviewed in references 56, 57). They share eight of these proteins with the flagellar apparatus found in many bacteria and are evolutionarily related to flagellin (58). In addition to these 9 core proteins, T3SSs have an additional 10 to 20 proteins that play either essential or important roles in their function. The structural components of T3SSs are typically encoded in a few operons, which can be found either in pathogenicity islands in the bacterial chromosome or on plasmids. Because T3SSs are typically horizontally acquired, bacteria that are evolutionarily distinct may have closely related systems and vice versa (58). For example, the genomes of *Shigella* and *E. coli* are highly homologous, yet the *Shigella* T3SS is more similar to the *Salmonella* T3SS than it is to systems found in the pathogens enterohemorrhagic *E. coli* and enteropathogenic *E. coli*. Seven families of T3SSs have been proposed, primarily based on the homology of their extracellularly elaborated needles, tips, and translocons (58).

The T3SS can be broken down into three main components: a base complex or basal body, the needle component, and the translocon (56). The base complex contains cytoplasmic components and spans the inner and outer membrane, forming a socket-like structure consisting of several rings with a center rod (59). In most systems it is comprised of at least 15 proteins (56, 57). Encased by and emanating from this socket and rod-like structure is a filament called the needle, which extends through the secretin and into the extracellular space (59). The T3SS needle has an inner hollow core that is wide enough to permit an unfolded effector to traverse (60, 61). Excitingly, recent work has visualized a "trapped" effector protein by cryo–electron microscopy and single particle analysis, supporting the model in which substrates can traverse through the needle (62, 63).

The T3SS tip complex, which resides on the outer end of the needle, is critical for sensing contact with host cells and regulating secretion of effectors (64, 65). It is also necessary for insertion of the translocon into host cell membranes (65, 66). The T3SS translocon is essential for passage of effectors through host cell membranes, but not for secretion of effectors outside of the bacterium (67, 68). Translocons are assembled upon contact with host cells and form a pore that is essential for effector delivery (66). Recently, however, an alternative two-step model of translocation of type 3 effectors was proposed, where effectors and translocon components are secreted prior to host cell contact and remain associated with the bacteria, perhaps in lipid vesicles (69, 70). After contact with host cells, perhaps sensed through the needle, the translocon and tip proteins form a pore through which the effectors pass. Additional experiments are needed to determine the mechanism by which translocation occurs.

Translocation of T3SS effectors into host cells is essential for the virulence of many pathogens, including pathogenic species of *Yersinia*, *Salmonella*, and *Shigella* (55). Over the past 25 years, much work has focused on understanding the functions of T3SS effector proteins. Their functions vary widely among different pathogens, and how they jointly orchestrate their effects on host cells is still being elucidated (71–74). Many of these effectors remodel normal cellular functions to enable the pathogen to establish an infectious niche either within the host cell or in mammalian tissue sites. Impressively, the study of these effectors has provided fundamental insights into several facets of eukaryotic cell biology.

The T4SS

T4SSs are ancestrally related to bacterial DNA conjugation systems and can secrete a variety of substrates, including single proteins and protein–protein and DNA–protein complexes (75). T4SSs secrete substrates into a wide range of target cells, including other bacteria (of the same or different species) and eukaryotic cells. These macromolecular complexes are largely found in Gram-negative bacteria, where they transport substrates across both the inner and outer membranes (Fig. 3). Like T3SSs, T4SSs can span an additional host cell membrane, allowing for direct transfer of substrates into the cytoplasm of the recipient cell. Because T4SSs are capable of transferring both DNA and proteins, they can serve a variety of functions, including conjugative transfer of DNA, DNA uptake and release, and translocation of effector proteins or DNA/protein complexes directly into recipient cells.

Despite the diversity in their substrates and functions, all T4SSs are evolutionarily related, sharing common components and operating in a similar manner (76). Therefore, the remainder of this section will focus on the VirB/D system of *Agrobacterium tumeficans* as a model of type IV secretion. *A. tumeficans* uses its T4SS to transport oncogenic transfer DNA into plant cells and has served as the paradigm for studying T4SS assembly and function (77). The VirB/D T4SS

contains 12 proteins: VirB1 to VirB11 and VirD4 (78). Most of these proteins are membrane-associated and multicopy, interacting with themselves and each other. The VirB6 to VirB10 proteins are found in the periplasm and inner and outer membranes and form the secretion channel as well as its accessory proteins. VirB4, VirB11, and VirD4 localize to the inner membrane and serve as the ATPases that power the system. VirD4 also functions as a coupling protein, binding proteins prior to secretion through the channel. Generally, T4SSs also include an extracellular pilus, composed of a major (VirB2) and minor (VirB5) subunit.

The process of substrate secretion through the T4SS apparatus is still an active area of investigation. However, it is believed that substrate DNA or protein first makes contact with VirD4, which functions as a molecular "gate" at the base of the secretion apparatus (79). VirD4 then transfers the substrate to VirB11, which delivers the substrate to the inner membrane channel complex. Finally, the substrate is transferred across the periplasm to the outer membrane protein complex. It is not currently known what role the T4SS pilus plays in the secretion process. Some believe that the pilus may serve merely as an attachment device, allowing bacteria to come into tight contact with target cells (78). Others have predicted that the pilus may actually serve as the conduit for substrate translocation, particularly into target cells (80). Work to determine which of these two models is correct is currently ongoing.

T4SSs play pivotal roles in the pathogenesis of a wide range of bacteria. Notable examples of bacterial pathogens that employ T4SSs for virulence are *Neisseria gonorrhoeae*, which uses its T4SS to mediate DNA uptake (which promotes virulence gene acquisition) (81), and *L. pneumophila*, *Brucella suis*, and *Helicobacter pylori*, which use their T4SSs to translocate effector proteins into host cells during infection to disrupt their defense strategies (82). These effector proteins have a wide range of functions. For example, the intracellular pathogen *L. pneumophila* uses its T4SS to translocate more than 200 effector proteins into the host cell, where they play important roles in remodeling the host cell architecture to create a vacuole suitable for bacterial replication (83). A major focus in the T4SS field is now on understanding how these effector proteins affect host cell functions. In addition to enhancing our understanding of host–pathogen interactions, these studies have also led to novel insights into eukaryotic cellular biology.

The T5SS

T5SS substrates are unique in that, unlike other secreted substrates, which cross the bacterial membrane with the help of a dedicated secretion apparatus or membrane channel, they secrete themselves. These proteins or groups of proteins carry their own β-barrel domain, which inserts into the outer membrane and forms a channel through which either the remainder of the protein or a separate protein is transported (84, 85). Because protein secretion by T5SSs occurs only in the outer membrane, these proteins must first be translocated across the inner membrane and into the periplasm in an unfolded state by the Sec apparatus (Fig. 3). Therefore, T5SS proteins carry an N-terminal Sec signal sequence that is cleaved off as they pass into the periplasm (86).

Most well-known T5SS substrates are virulence proteins, serving as toxins and receptor-binding proteins. Some examples of T5SS substrates that play important roles in pathogenesis include the immunoglobulin A protease of *N. gonorrhoeae*, which cleaves host antibodies (87), the IcsA protein of *Shigella flexneri* (88), which promotes actin-based intracellular motility and also serves as an adhesin (89), and YadA of *Y. enterocolitica* (90), which helps to promote translocation of T3SS substrates into host cells and assists in mediating resistance to attack by the host complement system (91). T5SSs can be sep-

arated into three classes, depending on the number of proteins involved in the secretion process. These classes include autotransporter secretion, two-partner secretion, and chaperone-usher secretion (92).

Autotransporter secretion

The simples form of type V secretion is known as the autotransporter system. As the name implies, autotransporters contain components that allow them to secrete themselves (92). More specifically, autotransporters contain three or four domains: a translocator domain at the C-terminus that forms the outer membrane channel, a linker domain, a passenger domain that contains the functional part of the autotransporter protein, and sometimes a protease domain that cleaves off the passenger domain once it passes through the channel (85).

Following secretion of the unfolded autotransporter protein through the inner membrane, the translocator domain assembles in the outer membrane, forming a 12-stranded β-barrel, usually with the help of several accessory factors, including the periplasmic chaperone Skp and the Bam complex (93, 94). The flexible linker domain then leads the passenger domain through the channel to the outside of the cell. Once the transporter domain has reached the outside of the cell, it is either released by its own protease domain or remains attached to the translocator domain and protrudes outside the cell (85).

Two-partner secretion

While the majority of T5SS substrates are secreted via the autotransporter mechanism, a few rely on different polypeptides for transport outside of the cells. In a process called two-partner secretion, a pair of proteins participates in the secretion process, in which one partner carries the β-barrel domain while the other partner serves as the secreted protein (95). Two-partner secretion has been observed in a large variety of Gram-negative bacteria and is primarily responsible for transporting large virulence proteins, such as the filamentous hemagglutinin of *Bordetella pertussis* and the high-molecular-weight adhesins HWM1 and HWM2 of *Haemophilus influenzae* (96, 97).

Chaperone–usher secretion

A third subcategory of T5SSs involves proteins secreted with the help of two other proteins: the usher protein, which forms the β-barrel channel in the outer membrane, and the chaperone, a periplasmic protein that facilitates folding of the secreted protein prior to delivery to the channel (98). Chaperone–usher systems are commonly used to assemble pilins on the surface of Gram-negative bacteria, such as the P. pilus of uropathogenic *E. coli* (98).

The T6SS

T6SSs are the most recent bacterial secretion systems to be discovered (99), and therefore, there is still much to learn about their structure and functions. T6SSs translocate proteins into a variety of recipient cells, including eukaryotic cell targets and, more commonly, other bacteria (100). These systems are fairly well conserved in a wide-range of Gram-negative bacterial species, with nearly a quarter of sequenced genomes containing genes for T6SS components (101). Unlike many of the other characterized Gram-negative secretion systems, T6SSs are capable of transporting effector proteins from one bacterium to another in a contact-dependent manner, which is believed to play a role in bacterial communication and interactions in the environment (100).

T6SSs are very large, with up to 21 proteins encoded within a contiguous gene cluster (100). Thirteen of these proteins appear to be conserved in all T6SSs and are thought to play a structural role in the secretion apparatus. Intriguingly, T6SSs share structural homology to phage tails, and it has been hypothesized that T6SSs may have arisen from inverted phage tails that eject proteins outside of the bacterial cell rather than injecting

them inside the cell (Fig. 3) (102). It has been proposed that some structural components of the T6SS apparatus may also serve as effector proteins, though other T6SS effector proteins have also been identified. These effectors have many forms and functions, with many directed against the bacterial cell wall and membrane, which supports a role for this secretion apparatus in promoting interspecies bacterial competition (100, 101). Lending further credence to this hypothesis, many T6SS effectors are encoded alongside a gene that provides immunity to the effector, thereby preventing self-intoxication (100).

T6SSs are hypothesized to contribute to the virulence of some bacterial pathogens, both through delivery of protein substrates to host cells and by secreting substrates into neighboring bacteria that may be competing to exploit a specific host niche. While we know that many bacterial pathogens, including *P. aeruginosa*, *V. cholerae*, and *S. marcescens* are able to use their T6SSs under laboratory conditions (101–103), the mechanisms of how these T6SSs contribute to survival in the environment (and in mammalian infection) have not been determined.

PROTEIN SECRETION BY GRAM-POSITIVE BACTERIA

Thus far, our discussion of protein secretion has primarily focused on Gram-negative bacteria, which possess two phospholipid membranes separated by a periplasm compartment containing a thin layer of peptidoglycan. In contrast, as demonstrated in Fig. 4, Gram-positive bacteria contain only one lipid bilayer and are surrounded by a very thick cell wall (considerably thicker than that of Gram-negative bacteria). Additionally, some species of Gram-positive bacteria, most notably the *Mycobacteria*, contain a cell wall that is heavily modified by lipids, called a mycomembrane (Fig. 5). Because of these differences in basic cell structure, it is not surprising that Gram-positive bacteria differ from Gram-negative

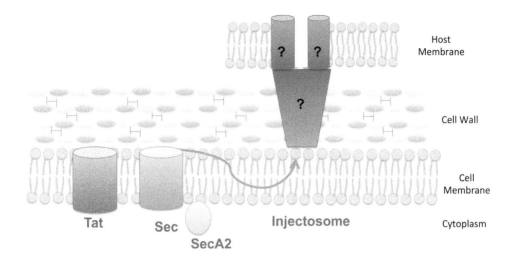

FIGURE 4 **Four secretion systems in Gram-positive bacteria. Gram-positive bacteria contain a single cytoplasmic membrane surrounded by a very thick cell wall. These organisms can secrete proteins across the membrane using the Tat and Sec secretion systems. In contrast to Gram-negative organisms, many Gram-positive bacteria use an additional factor for Sec secretion of a smaller subset of proteins, called SecA2. Additionally, there is evidence that some Gram-positive bacteria may use dedicated secretion apparatuses, called "injectosomes" to transport proteins from the bacterial cytoplasm into the cytoplasm of a host cell in a two-step process. The specific mechanism of this process has not been determined, though it has been proposed that the injectosome may utilize a protected channel to transport proteins across the cell wall during export.**

organisms in their mechanisms of extracellular protein secretion. Like Gram-negative organisms, Gram-positive bacteria employ both the Tat and Sec pathways to transport proteins across the cytoplasmic membrane. However, in many cases, this transport is not sufficient to deliver proteins to their final destinations. In the following section, we review conserved mechanisms of protein secretion in Gram-positive bacteria including *Mycobacteria*, many of which are used by pathogens to transport important virulence factors out of the cell during mammalian infection.

SecA2 Secretion

As discussed above, the Sec secretion pathway is one of the most conserved mechanisms of protein export and is found in all classes of bacteria. An essential component of posttranslational Sec export (through the SecB pathway) is the targeting and ATPase protein SecA. For years, it was thought that all bacteria contained a single SecA protein; however, recent discoveries have shown that many Gram-positive organisms, including *L. monocytogenes*, *Bacillus subtilis*, *Clostridium difficile*, *M. tuberculosis*, and *Corynebacteria glutamicum*, contain two SecA homologues, called SecA1 and SecA2 (reviewed in references 104, 105) (Fig. 4). In these organisms, SecA1 is essential and aids in the secretion of proteins via the canonical Sec pathway, as described above. In contrast, SecA2 is seldom required for growth under standard laboratory conditions and is used to export a smaller set of proteins. Generally, SecA2 substrates are involved in stress responses and/or cell wall modifications, repair, and metabolism. While SecA2 is often not essential for growth under normal laboratory conditions, it is required under specific stress conditions and has also been linked to virulence.

It is currently thought that the SecYEG core transporter transports SecA2 substrates and that SecA2 provides an additional means

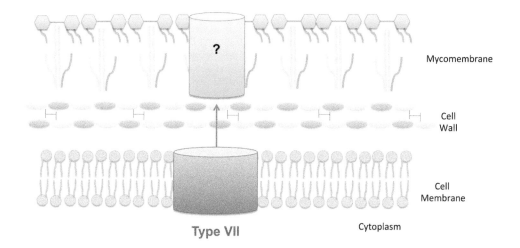

Mycomembrane

Cell
Wall

Cell
Membrane

Cytoplasm

Type VII

FIGURE 5 The T7SS. Certain Gram-positive organisms, including members of the genus *Mycobacteria*, contain a cell wall layer that is heavily modified by lipids, called a mycomembrane. These organisms contain a distinct protein secretion apparatus called a T7SS. T7SSs contain several core inner membrane proteins that interact with cytosolic chaperones and form a channel through which proteins are secreted. Additionally, it has been proposed that T7SSs may contain an additional, mycomembrane-spanning channel that aids in extracellular secretion of substrates, though this model has not been experimentally proven.

of regulation of specific substrates. The SecA2 protein, like SecA, contains two nucleotide-binding domains, a preprotein cross-linking domain, a helical wing and helical scaffold domain, and a C-terminal domain (106). However, most SecA2 proteins are smaller than their corresponding SecA homologs, because they have small deletions in one of these domains (107). These deletions may alter the rate of ATP hydrolysis, the interaction with the rest of the Sec apparatus, and/or the location of SecA2 molecules (108, 109). For these reasons, secretion of the substrates associated with SecA2 molecules may be regulated differently compared to secretion of SecA substrates.

Although some information has been gleaned from studies of SecA2 in various bacteria, there are a number of unanswered questions about SecA2 systems. While it appears most likely that SecA2 substrates are secreted through the normal SecYEG secretion system, SecA2 interactions with other transporters cannot be ruled out. Likewise, it is unclear how SecA2 interacts

with SecYEG and how SecA versus SecA2 substrates are selected for secretion, if indeed both are directed to the same core apparatus. Finally, how SecA2 discriminates among potential substrates is poorly understood.

A number of *Streptococci* and *Staphylococci* express a second Sec secretion system called aSec or SecA2-SecY2. These systems not only contain SecA2, but also have other proteins that serve to transport SecA2 substrates, including SecY2 and at least three accessory Sec transport proteins. aSec systems typically transport large, highly glycosylated cell-wall anchor proteins with serine-rich repeats (110, 111). These serine-rich repeat glycosylated proteins function as adhesins in several *Streptococcus* and *Staphylococcus* species and can contribute to virulence in these pathogens.

In contrast to bacteria that only express SecA1, bacteria expressing aSec are thought to transport substrates through a channel called SecY2. SecY2 lacks the cytoplasmic loops in SecY that normally interact with SecA1, and therefore SecA1-bound substrates are unlikely to interact with SecY2 transporters (107). In addition, there are three accessory proteins in this system, whose roles are not yet understood, although they are essential for secretion of these glycoproteins (112). All of these proteins localize to the membrane and cytosol and may help deliver the SecA2-substrate complex to SecY2, open the pore, assist in transport of the substrate, and participate in complete glycosylation of these substrates.

Sortases

Like their Gram-negative counterparts, many Gram-positive pathogens express proteins on their outer surfaces that assist in survival during infection of a mammalian host. Because Gram-positive bacteria lack an outer membrane, these proteins must embed themselves into the Gram-positive cell wall to be retained on the outer surface of the bacterium. To fulfill this function, Gram-positive bacteria encode a class of enzymes, called sortases, which covalently attach proteins to the cell wall following secretion across the cytoplasmic membrane (reviewed in references 113, 114).

Most Gram-positive bacteria express a variety of sortases, which can range in specificity. For example, the general, "housekeeping" sortase, SrtA, can attach as many as 40 proteins to the cell wall, while other sortases are specific for only one or two proteins (114). Sortases carry out covalent linkages of proteins to the cell wall in a catalytic reaction called transpeptidation. Targets of SrtA typically contain an N-terminal signal peptide, as well as a 30- to 40-residue C-terminal cell wall sorting signal, which is composed of a pentapeptide cleavage site, LPXTG, and a hydrophobic domain (114, 115). Proteins destined for cell wall attachment by SrtA are first targeted to the Sec translocase by their N-terminal signal sequences and are translocated across the membrane through the canonical Sec pathway. Next, the sorting signals of these proteins are processed by

SrtA, which cuts between the threonine and glycine residues of their LPXTG sites (114, 115). The carboxyl group of the threonine is then covalently linked to a cysteine residue on the C-terminus of the sortase, effectively cleaving off the C-terminus of the original protein (114, 115). Finally, this intermediate is covalently attached to the amino group on the cell wall precursor lipid II. This modified lipid II is then incorporated into peptidoglycan during cell wall synthesis, effectively embedding the SrtA substrate into the cell wall. Other sortases attach their substrates via a similar catalytic reaction to that used by SrtA, but they have specificities for different LPXTG motifs and amino groups.

Sortases are found in nearly all Gram-positive bacteria and, as mentioned above, process some proteins that contribute to the virulence of many pathogens. Pili are a classical example of cell surface proteins in Gram-positive bacteria (113, 114). These filamentous protein structures are often involved in adhering to and invading host tissue sites during infection. Pili are typically composed of a major subunit, called pilin, and one or more minor subunits, which are usually assembled sequentially using specialized sortases (113, 114). Pathogens that are known to utilize pili during infection include *Streptococcus pneumoniae*, *Streptococcus pyogenes*, and *S. aureus* (113, 114).

Extracellular Protein Secretion In Gram-Positive Bacteria

Not all secreted proteins in Gram-positive bacteria remain embedded in the cell wall. Rather, many proteins exported across the cytoplasmic membrane by the Sec or Tat pathways are eventually released into the extracellular environment, often through passive diffusion through the peptidoglycan layer. Additionally, some Gram-positive organisms use a separate secretion apparatus (named the T7SS) to export certain proteins across the cytoplasmic membrane and, potentially, through the cell wall.

Like the T3SS and T4SS effectors of Gram-negative bacteria, some proteins secreted by Gram-positive pathogens are delivered to the cytoplasmic compartments of eukaryotic host cells. The mechanisms by which Gram-positive effector proteins reach the cytoplasm of eukaryotic cells are varied and are in large part exemplified by the self-translocating AB toxin model of delivery. However, recent evidence suggests that some Gram-positive organisms may use a protein secretion apparatus to directly deliver certain effector proteins to eukaryotic cells (116).

Gram-positive injectosomes: a model for effector transport into host cells

One secretion apparatus in Gram-positive organisms, coined the "injectosome" (note the difference in spelling from the Gram-negative T3SS injectisome), is proposed to be functionally analogous (but structurally unrelated) to the T4SSs and T3SSs of Gram-negative bacteria. This model of protein secretion has been observed in the Gram-positive pathogen *S. pyogenes*, which injects at least one virulence factor, NAD glycohydrolase (SPN), into the cytoplasm of keratinocytes by this mechanism (116, 117). To create the pore required for SPN translocation, another protein, SLO, is first secreted via the Sec pathway. SLO is a member of a class of toxins called cholesterol-dependent cytolysins, which bind cholesterol on the surface of eukaryotic cells and insert into their membranes, creating pores (118). Following pore formation by SLO, SPN is translocated across the plasma membrane by Sec and into the eukaryotic cell through the pore (119). Once it reaches the cytosol of host cells, SPN cleaves the glycosidic bond of β-NAD$^+$ to produce nicotinamide and ADP-ribose, a potent second messenger, thereby disrupting normal cell functions (120). For this reason, SPN serves as a major virulence factor for *S. pyogenes*, particularly during severe infections with this bacterium.

Interestingly, there is some evidence that SPN translocation is not simply the result of diffusion of effectors through the pore (116, 121). Rather, some have speculated that a protected channel is formed between the bacterium and the translocation apparatus, similar to the T3SS (see Fig. 4). However, much more work still needs to be done to determine whether this model is accurate.

The T7SS

Certain Gram-positive organisms, including species of *Mycobacteria* and *Corynebacteria*, contain a heavily lipidated cell wall layer called a mycomembrane. These lipids form a very dense, waxy, hydrophobic layer on the outer surface of the bacteria, which serves as an effective barrier against a number of environmental stresses and antimicrobial therapies. However, as one might imagine, this layer makes extracellular protein transport more difficult for these species of bacteria. Therefore, these bacteria utilize specialized mechanisms for protein transport across their inner and mycomembranes, called T7SSs (reviewed in references 105, 122, 123) (see Fig. 5). T7SSs were originally identified in *M. tuberculosis* in 2003 (124), where they are called ESX systems. These systems have now been identified in a number of bacteria in the order *Corynebacteriales*. In addition, analogous substrates and some components of these systems have also been identified in several Gram-positive organisms that lack mycomembranes, including the pathogens *S. aureus*, *Bacillus anthracis*, and *L. monocytogenes* (125–127).

The core structural components of T7SSs, and frequently their substrates, are typically encoded in linked gene clusters (123). In general, five core structural proteins appear in most of these gene clusters. These core components, called EccB, EccC, EccD, EccE, and MycP in the ESX systems, are all membrane proteins (128). All except EccD have hydrophobic domains, and thus all may interact with various other accessory components in the cytoplasm or peptidoglycan layer, such as chaperones or the cytosolic protein, EccA, which may supply the source of energy for substrate transport (129). The four membrane-associated Ecc proteins from ESX-5 form a large inner membrane complex, which presumably contains a channel through which the substrates traverse (128). The fifth component, MycP, is a mycosin or subtilisin-like protease. The role of MycP in protein translocation through the T7SS is not completely understood, but it is believed to play an important role in the regulation of secretion (130). T7SSs also have a variable number of additional proteins that are important for the function of specific systems. For instance, some systems may derive energy from the EccA cytosolic protein, an ATPase associated with diverse cellular activities (129). Other T7SSs may use energy generated by EccCb1, a protein that forms a SpoIIIE-type ATPase with the integral membrane component EccCa1 (131). Additionally, in *Mycobacteria*, chaperones are used to recognize specific substrates and target them to specific ESX systems (132).

While a tremendous amount of work has been done to understand the mechanism of protein translocation through the T7SS since its discovery 12 years ago, we do not yet understand how substrates navigate through the mycomembrane. The mycomembrane has been likened to the outer membrane of Gram-negative bacteria based on electron microscopy studies, so presumably there should be factors required for passage through this layer (133, 134). It remains to be seen whether some of the already recognized components of the T7SS, or other not yet identified factors, are critical for passage through this barrier.

T7SSs play a variety of roles in bacterial physiology and pathogenesis. The first system identified, ESX-1, is a major virulence factor in *M. tuberculosis* (135, 136). To date, five T7SSs have been identified in *Mycobacteria*, named ESX-1 to ESX-5, although not all *Mycobacteria* harbor all five systems (137). In fact, only ESX-3 and ESX-4 are found in all *Mycobacteria* species. Curiously, although

ESX-4 appears to be the most ancient system, secretion from ESX-4 has not yet been demonstrated, and it lacks several genes found in most other systems. Secretion from ESX-2 has also not been demonstrated.

While some T7SSs can contribute to virulence, as outlined above, not all of these systems function in virulence or even in secretion of substrates. For example, the T7SS in *Listeria* does not appear essential for virulence (126). Likewise, the ESX-1, which is essential for the virulence of *M. tuberculosis*, is also present in the nonpathogenic *Mycobacterium smegmatis*, where it functions in conjugation of DNA substrates (reminiscent of some T4SSs) (138). In *M. tuberculosis*, ESX-3-secreted substrates are critical in iron acquisition and growth *in vitro* (139), whereas ESX-1 and ESX-5 are essential for virulence but not for growth in medium (124, 140). Thus, these systems apparently play diverse roles depending on the species of *Mycobacteria*. This diversity of function is likely to exist also in their roles in other bacteria.

HOST IMMUNE RECOGNITION OF BACTERIAL SECRETION SYSTEMS

A recent area of active investigation in the fields of bacterial pathogenesis and innate immunity has been the study of how the mammalian immune system discriminates between pathogenic and commensal bacteria. One way in which innate immune systems recognize pathogens is through the utilization of specific receptors and immune cell proteins that sense mechanisms, or patterns, of bacterial pathogenesis (141). This is in contrast to simply sensing molecules carried by both pathogens and commensals, such as lipopolysaccharide or peptidoglycan. One hallmark of bacterial infection for many pathogens is the use of dedicated protein secretion systems to directly deposit effector proteins or toxins into mammalian tissue sites and/or host cells. For this reason, the mammalian innate immune system has developed strategies to detect the use of bacterial secretion systems and/or their secreted substrates during infection (141). Because bacterial secretion of virulence proteins can occur by many different mechanisms, the host immune system has developed multiple methods of sensing these processes (Fig. 6).

One mechanism by which the innate immune response can detect bacterial secretion systems is by sensing the cytosolic access of bacterial products. These products are often small molecules, such as peptidoglycan, flagellin, and lipopolysaccharide, which can be aberrantly translocated into the bacterial cytoplasm through bacterial secretion systems. Because these receptors are limited to the bacterial cytosol, their activation would be indicative of the specific use of a secretion system by an invading pathogen. One such example is the family of cytoplasmic receptors called Nod-like receptors, which can directly sense cytosolic molecules, including lipopolysaccharide and flagellin (141). Activation of these receptors leads to a cascade of signaling that ultimately induces the production of inflammatory cytokines. Additionally,

the immune system has developed methods to directly sense the translocation of secreted effectors. For example, recent findings have shown that macrophages can sense manipulation of Rho GTPases by the *Yersinia* T3SS effector YopE (142). Following detection of this signal, macrophages mount (through an unknown mechanism) a response that ultimately results in clearance of intracellular bacteria.

The mammalian innate immune system can also detect the disruption of membranes by pore-forming proteins, such as the translocons of T3SSs or the cholesterol-dependent cytolysins of Gram-positive pathogens, which are often secreted or inserted by bacterial secretion systems that directly deliver effector proteins to target cells. For example, pore formation by SLO of *S. pyogenes* has been shown to activate the Nod-like receptor family receptor NLRP3 (143). This activation eventually stimulates the production of inflammatory cytokines that help the host to respond to and clear the infection.

Finally, there is some evidence that the host immune system can detect components of secretion channels that protrude out of the

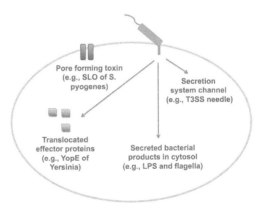

FIGURE 6 Mechanisms of innate immune recognition of bacterial secretion systems. To distinguish between pathogenic and commensal bacteria, the mammalian innate immune system has developed methods to directly recognize patterns unique to bacterial pathogens, such as the use of protein secretion apparatuses. The immune system can sense several facets of bacterial protein secretion. These include the pore formation by secretion systems or secreted proteins, aberrant translocation of bacterial molecules into the cytosol, the presence of effector proteins and/or their activities, as well as the components of the secretion systems themselves.

bacterial membrane, such as the T3SS needle and components of the translocon. Recently, it has been shown that recognition of several T3SS needle proteins, including YscF of *Yersinia* and MxiH from *Shigella*, can induce proinflammatory cytokine production in host cells (144).

CONCLUSIONS

Bacterial pathogens utilize a multitude of methods to invade mammalian hosts, damage tissue sites, and thwart the immune system from responding. One essential component of these strategies for many bacterial pathogens is the secretion of proteins across phospholipid membranes. Secreted proteins can play many roles in promoting bacterial virulence, from enhancing attachment to eukaryotic cells, to scavenging resources in an environmental niche, to directly intoxicating target cells and disrupting their functions. As we discussed in this chapter, these proteins may be transferred out of the bacterial cytoplasm through a variety of mechanisms, usually involving the use of dedicated protein secretion systems. For this reason, the study of protein secretion systems has been an important focus in the field of bacterial pathogenesis. The remaining chapters in this section will offer a more detailed focus on the molecular and functional characteristics of some of these secretion systems.

ACKNOWLEDGMENTS

This work is funded by NIH/National Institute of Allergy and Infectious Diseases (NIAID) grant AI113166.

CITATION

Green ER, Mecsas J. 2016. Bacterial secretion systems: an overview. Microbiol Spectrum 4(1):VMBF-0012-2015.

REFERENCES

1. **Natale P, Bruser T, Driessen AJ.** 2008. Sec- and Tat-mediated protein secretion across the bacterial cytoplasmic membrane: distinct translocases and mechanisms. *Biochim Biophys Acta* **1778:**1735–1756.
2. **Papanikou E, Karamanou S, Economou A.** 2007. Bacterial protein secretion through the translocase nanomachine. *Nat Rev Microbiol* **5:**839–851.
3. **Robinson C, Bolhuis A.** 2004. Tat-dependent protein targeting in prokaryotes and chloroplasts. *Biochim Biophys Acta Mol Cell Res* **1694:** 135–147.
4. **Korotkov KV, Sandkvist M, Hol WGH.** 2012. The type II secretion system: biogenesis, molecular architecture and mechanism. *Nat Rev Microbiol* **10:**336–351.
5. **Lenz LL, Mohammadi S, Geissler A, Portnoy DA.** 2003. SecA2-dependent secretion of autolytic enzymes promotes *Listeria monocytogenes* pathogenesis. *Proc Natl Acad Sci USA* **100:**12432–12437.
6. **Braunstein M, Espinosa BJ, Chan J, Belisle JT, Jacobs WR.** 2003. SecA2 functions in the secretion of superoxide dismutase A and in the virulence of *Mycobacterium tuberculosis*. *Mol Microbiol* **48:**453–464.
7. **Lenz LL, Portnoy DA.** 2002. Identification of a second *Listeria* secA gene associated with protein secretion and the rough phenotype. *Mol Microbiol* **45:**1043–1056.
8. **Bensing BA, Sullam PM.** 2002. An accessory sec locus of *Streptococcus gordonii* is required for export of the surface protein GspB and for normal levels of binding to human platelets. *Mol Microbiol* **44:**1081–1094.
9. **Randall LL, Hardy SJ.** 2002. SecB, one small chaperone in the complex milieu of the cell. *Cell Mol Life Sci* **59:**1617–1623.
10. **Hartl FU, Lecker S, Schiebel E, Hendrick JP, Wickner W.** 1990. The binding cascade of SecB to SecA to SecY/E mediates preprotein targeting to the *E. coli* plasma membrane. *Cell* **63:**269–279.
11. **Mogensen JE, Otzen DE.** 2005. Interactions between folding factors and bacterial outer membrane proteins. *Mol Microbiol* **57:**326–346.
12. **Luirink J, Sinning I.** 2004. SRP-mediated protein targeting: structure and function revisited. *Biochim Biophys Acta Mol Cell Res* **1694:**17–35.
13. **Sijbrandi R, Urbanus ML, ten Hagen-Jongman CM, Bernstein HD, Oudega B, Otto BR, Luirink J.** 2003. Signal recognition particle (SRP)-mediated targeting and

sec-dependent translocation of an extracellular *Escherichia coli* protein. *J Biol Chem* **278:** 4654–4659.

14. **Paetzel M, Karla A, Strynadka NCJ, Dalbey RE.** 2002. Signal peptidases. *Chem Rev* **102:** 4549–4579.

15. **Berks BC, Palmer T, Sargent F.** 2005. Protein targeting by the bacterial twin-arginine translocation (Tat) pathway. *Curr Opin Microbiol* **8:**174–181.

16. **Sargent F, Stanley NR, Berks BC, Palmer T.** 1999. Sec-independent protein translocation in *Escherichia coli*: a distinct and pivotal role for the TatB protein. *J Biol Chem* **274:**36073–36082.

17. **Pop O, Martin U, Abel C, Muller JP.** 2002. The twin-arginine signal peptide of PhoD and the TatA(d)/C-d proteins of *Bacillus subtilis* form an autonomous tat translocation system. *J Biol Chem* **277:**3268–3273.

18. **Müller M.** 2005. Twin-arginine-specific protein export in *Escherichia coli*. *Res Microbiol* **156:**131–136.

19. **Ochsner UA, Snyder A, Vasil AI, Vasil ML.** 2002. Effects of the twin-arginine translocase on secretion of virulence factors, stress response, and pathogenesis. *Proc Natl Acad Sci USA* **99:**8312–8317.

20. **Lavander M, Ericsson SK, Broms JE, Forsberg A.** 2006. The twin arginine translocation system is essential for virulence of *Yersinia pseudotuberculosis*. *Infect Immun* **74:** 1768–1776.

21. **Pradel N, Ye CY, Livrelli V, Xu HG, Joly B, Wu LF.** 2003. Contribution of the twin arginine translocation system to the virulence of enterohemorrhagic *Escherichia coli* O157:H7. *Infect Immun* **71:**4908–4916.

22. **Rossier O, Cianciotto NP.** 2005. The *Legionella pneumophila* tatB gene facilitates secretion of phospholipase C, growth under iron-limiting conditions, and intracellular infection. *Infect Immun* **73:**2020–2032.

23. **McDonough JA, McCann JR, Tekippe EM, Silverman JS, Rigel NW, Braunstein M.** 2008. Identification of functional Tat signal sequences in *Mycobacterium tuberculosis* proteins. *J Bacteriol* **190:**6428–6438.

24. **Songer JG.** 1997. Bacterial phospholipases and their role in virulence. *Trends Microbiol* **5:**156–161.

25. **Thomas S, Holland IB, Schmitt L.** 2014. The type 1 secretion pathway: the hemolysin system and beyond. *Biochim Biophys Acta* **1843:** 1629–1641.

26. **Symmons MF, Bokma E, Koronakis E, Hughes C, Koronakis V.** 2009. The assembled structure of a complete tripartite bacterial multidrug efflux pump. *Proc Natl Acad Sci USA* **106:**7173–7178.

27. **Delepelaire P.** 2004. Type I secretion in Gram-negative bacteria. *Biochim Biophys Acta* **1694:** 149–161.

28. **Kanonenberg K, Schwarz CK, Schmitt L.** 2013. Type I secretion systems: a story of appendices. *Res Microbiol* **164:**596–604.

29. **Letoffe S, Delepelaire P, Wandersman C.** 1996. Protein secretion in Gram-negative bacteria: assembly of the three components of ABC protein-mediated exporters is ordered and promoted by substrate binding. *EMBO J* **15:**5804–5811.

30. **Pimenta AL, Young J, Holland IB, Blight MA.** 1999. Antibody analysis of the localisation, expression and stability of HlyD, the MFP component of the *E. coli* haemolysin translocator. *Mol Gen Genet* **261:**122–132.

31. **Lee M, Jun SY, Yoon BY, Song S, Lee K, Ha NC.** 2012. Membrane fusion proteins of type I secretion system and tripartite efflux pumps share a binding motif for TolC in Gram-negative bacteria. *PLoS One* **7:**e40460. doi:10.1371/journal.pone.0040460.

32. **Balakrishnan L, Hughes C, Koronakis V.** 2001. Substrate-triggered recruitment of the TolC channel-tunnel during type I export of hemolysin by *Escherichia coli*. *J Mol Biol* **313:** 501–510.

33. **Wu KH, Tai PC.** 2004. Cys32 and His105 are the critical residues for the calcium-dependent cysteine proteolytic activity of CvaB, an ATP-binding cassette transporter. *J Biol Chem* **279:**901–919.

34. **Lecher J, Schwarz CK, Stoldt M, Smits SH, Willbold D, Schmitt L.** 2012. An RTX transporter tethers its unfolded substrate during secretion via a unique N-terminal domain. *Structure* **20:**1778–1787.

35. **Linhartova I, Bumba L, Masin J, Basler M, Osicka R, Kamanova J, Prochazkova K, Adkins I, Hejnova-Holubova J, Sadilkova L, Morova J, Sebo P.** 2010. RTX proteins: a highly diverse family secreted by a common mechanism. *FEMS Microbiol Rev* **34:**1076–1112.

36. **Dolores JS, Agarwal S, Egerer M, Satchell KJ.** 2015. *Vibrio cholerae* MARTX toxin heterologous translocation of beta-lactamase and roles of individual effector domains on cytoskeleton dynamics. *Mol Microbiol* **95:**590–604.

37. **Welch RA, Dellinger EP, Minshew B, Falkow S.** 1981. Haemolysin contributes to virulence of extra-intestinal *E. coli* infections. *Nature* **294:**665–667.

38. **Hughes C, Muller D, Hacker J, Goebel W.** 1982. Genetics and pathogenic role of *Escherichia coli* haemolysin. *Toxicon* **20:**247–252.

39. **Mackman N, Holland IB.** 1984. Functional characterization of a cloned haemolysin determinant from *E. coli* of human origin, encoding information for the secretion of a 107K polypeptide. *Mol Gen Genet* **196:**129–134.

40. **Voulhoux R, Ball G, Ize B, Vasil ML, Lazdunski A, Wu LF, Filloux A.** 2001. Involvement of the twin-arginine translocation system in protein secretion via the type II pathway. *EMBO J* **20:**6735–6741.

41. **Cianciotto NP.** 2005. Type II secretion: a protein secretion system for all seasons. *Trends Microbiol* **13:**581–588.

42. **Korotkov KV, Gonen T, Hol WGJ.** 2100. Secretins: dynamic channels for protein transport across membranes. *Trends Biochem Sci* **36:**433–443.

43. **Sauvonnet N, Vignon G, Pugsley AP, Gounon P.** 2000. Pilus formation and protein secretion by the same machinery in *Escherichia coli*. *EMBO J* **19:**2221–2228.

44. **Hobbs M, Mattick JS.** 1993. Common components in the assembly of type-4 fimbriae, DNA transfer systems, filamentous phage and protein-secretion apparatus: a general system for the formation of surface-associated protein complexes. *Mol Microbiol* **10:**233–243.

45. **Shevchik VE, Robert-Baudouy J, Condemine G.** 1997. Specific interaction between OutD, an *Erwinia chrysanthemi* outer membrane protein of the general secretory pathway, and secreted proteins. *EMBO J* **16:**3007–3016.

46. **Sandkvist M, Michel LO, Hough LP, Morales VM, Bagdasarian M, Koomey M, DiRita VJ, Bagdasarian M.** 1997. General secretion pathway (eps) genes required for toxin secretion and outer membrane biogenesis in *Vibrio cholerae*. *J Bacteriol* **179:**6994–7003.

47. **Lu HM, Lory S.** 1996. A specific targeting domain in mature exotoxin A is required for its extracellular secretion from *Pseudomonas aeruginosa*. *EMBO J* **15:**429–436.

48. **Cianciotto NP.** 2013. Type II secretion and *Legionella* virulence. *Curr Topics Microbiol Immunol* **376:**81–102.

49. **Kulkarni R, Dhakal BK, Slechta ES, Kurtz Z, Mulvey MA, Thanassi DG.** 2009. Roles of putative type II secretion and type IV pilus systems in the virulence of uropathogenic *Escherichia coli*. *Plos One* **4:**e4752. doi:10.1371/journal.pone.0004752.

50. **Tauschek M, Gorrell RJ, Strugnell RA, Robins-Browne RM.** 2002. Identification of a protein secretory pathway for the secretion of heat-labile enterotoxin by an enterotoxigenic strain of *Escherichia coli*. *Proc Natl Acad Sci USA* **99:**7066–7071.

51. **Lathem WW, Grys TE, Witowski SE, Torres AG, Kaper JB, Tarr PI, Welch RS.** 2002. StcE, a metalloprotease secreted by *Escherichia coli* O157:H7, specifically cleaves C1 esterase inhibitor. *Mol Microbiol* **45:**277–288.

52. **Pugsley AP, Chapon C, Schwartz M.** 1986. Extracellular pullulanase of *Klebsiella pneumoniae* is a lipoprotein. *J Bacteriol* **166:**1083–1088.

53. **Jiang B, Howard SP.** 1992. The aeromonas-hydrophila exeE gene, required both for protein secretion and normal outer-membrane biogenesis, is a member of a general secretion pathway. *Mol Microbiol* **6:**1351–1361.

54. **He SY, Lindeberg M, Chatterjee AK, Collmer A.** 1991. Cloned *Erwinia chrysanthemi out* genes enable *Escherichia coli* to selectively secrete a diverse family of heterologous proteins to its milieu. *Proc Natl Acad Sci USA* **88**:1079–1083.

55. **Buttner D.** 2012. Protein export according to schedule: architecture, assembly, and regulation of type III secretion systems from plant- and animal-pathogenic bacteria. *Microbiol Mol Biol Rev* **76:**262–310.

56. **Abrusci P, McDowell MA, Lea SM, Johnson S.** 2014. Building a secreting nanomachine: a structural overview of the T3SS. *Curr Opin Struct Biol* **25:**111–117.

57. **Burkinshaw BJ, Strynadka NC.** 2014. Assembly and structure of the T3SS. *Biochim Biophys Acta* **1843:**1649–1663.

58. **Troisfontaines P, Cornelis GR.** 2005. Type III secretion: more systems than you think. *Physiology (Bethesda)* **20:**326–339.

59. **Kubori T, Matsushima Y, Nakamura D, Uralil J, Lara-Tejero M, Sukhan A, Galan JE, Aizawa SI.** 1998. Supramolecular structure of the *Salmonella typhimurium* type III protein secretion system. *Science* **280:**602–605.

60. **Deane JE, Cordes FS, Roversi P, Johnson S, Kenjale R, Picking WD, Picking WL, Lea SM, Blocker S.** 2006. Expression, purification, crystallization and preliminary crystallographic analysis of MxiH, a subunit of the *Shigella flexneri* type III secretion system needle. *Acta Crystallogr Sect F Struct Biol Cryst Commun* **62** (Pt 3):302–305.

61. **Demers JP, Habenstein B, Loquet A, Kumar Vasa S, Giller K, Becker S, Baker D, Lange A, Sgourakis NG.** 2014. High-resolution structure of the *Shigella* type-III secretion needle by solid-state NMR and cryo-electron microscopy. *Nat Commun* **5:**4976.

62. **Dohlich K, Zumsteg AB, Goosmann C, Kolbe M.** 2014. A substrate-fusion protein is trapped inside the type III secretion system channel in *Shigella flexneri*. *PLoS Pathog* **10:**e1003881. doi:10.1371/journal.ppat.1003881.

63. **Radics J, Konigsmaier L, Marlovits TC.** 2014. Structure of a pathogenic type 3 secretion system in action. *Nat Struct Mol Biol* **21:**82–87.

64. **Price SB, Cowan C, Perry RD, Straley SC.** 1991. The *Yersinia pestis* V antigen is a regulatory protein necessary for Ca2(+)-dependent growth and maximal expression of low-Ca2+ response virulence genes. *J Bacteriol* **173:**2649–2657.

65. **Picking WL, Nishioka H, Hearn PD, Baxter MA, Harrington AT, Blocker A, Picking WD.** 2005. IpaD of *Shigella flexneri* is independently required for regulation of Ipa protein secretion and efficient insertion of IpaB and IpaC into host membranes. *Infect Immun* **73:**1432–1440.

66. **Holmstrom A, Olsson J, Cherepanov P, Maier E, Nordfelth R, Pettersson J, Benz R, Wolf-Watz H, Forsberg S.** 2001. LcrV is a channel size-determining component of the Yop effector translocon of *Yersinia*. *Mol Microbiol* **39:**620–632.

67. **Hakansson S, Bergman T, Vanooteghem JC, Cornelis G, Wolf-Watz H.** 1993. YopB and YopD constitute a novel class of *Yersinia* Yop proteins. *Infect Immun* **61:**71–80.

68. **Hakansson S, Schesser K, Persson C, Galyov EE, Rosqvist R, Homble F, Wolf-Watz H.** 1996. The YopB protein of *Yersinia pseudotuberculosis* is essential for the translocation of Yop effector proteins across the target cell plasma membrane and displays a contact-dependent membrane disrupting activity. *EMBO J* **15:**5812–5823.

69. **Akopyan K, Edgren T, Wang-Edgren H, Rosqvist R, Fahlgren A, Wolf-Watz H, Fallman M.** 2011. Translocation of surface-localized effectors in type III secretion. *Proc Natl Acad Sci USA* **108:**1639–1644.

70. **Edgren T, Forsberg A, Rosqvist R, Wolf-Watz H.** 2012. Type III secretion in *Yersinia*: injectisome or not? *PLoS Pathog* **8:**e1002669. doi:10.1371/journal.ppat.1002669.

71. **Angot A, Vergunst A, Genin S, Peeters N.** 2007. Exploitation of eukaryotic ubiquitin signaling pathways by effectors translocated by bacterial type III and type IV secretion systems. *PLoS Pathog* **3:**e3. doi:10.1371/journal.ppat.0030003.

72. **Ham H, Sreelatha A, Orth K.** 2011. Manipulation of host membranes by bacterial effectors. *Nat Rev Microbiol* **9:**635–646.

73. **Spano S, Galan JE.** 2013. A novel antimicrobial function for a familiar Rab GTPase. *Small GTPases* **4:**252–254.

74. **Tosi T, Pflug A, Discola KF, Neves D, Dessen A.** 2013. Structural basis of eukaryotic cell targeting by type III secretion system (T3SS) effectors. *Res Microbiol* **164:**605–619.

75. **Cascales E, Christie PJ.** 2003. The versatile bacterial type IV secretion systems. *Nat Rev Microbiol* **1:**137–149.

76. **Lessl M, Lanka E.** 1994. Common mechanisms in bacterial conjugation and Ti-mediated T-DNA transfer to plant cells. *Cell* **77:**321–324.

77. **Bundock P, den Dulk-Ras A, Beijersbergen A, Hooykaas PJ.** 1995. Trans-kingdom T-DNA transfer from *Agrobacterium tumefaciens* to *Saccharomyces cerevisiae*. *EMBO J* **14:**3206–3214.

78. **Fronzes R, Christie PJ, Waksman G.** 2009. The structural biology of type IV secretion systems. *Nat Rev Microbiol* **7:**703–714.

79. **Atmakuri K, Cascales E, Christie PJ.** 2004. Energetic components VirD4, VirB11 and VirB4 mediate early DNA transfer reactions required for bacterial type IV secretion. *Mol Microbiol* **54:**1199–1211.

80. **Babic A, Lindner AB, Vulic M, Stewart EJ, Radman M.** 2008. Direct visualization of horizontal gene transfer. *Science* **319:**1533–1536.

81. **Hamilton HL, Dillard JP.** 2006. Natural transformation of *Neisseria gonorrhoeae*: from DNA donation to homologous recombination. *Mol Microbiol* **59:**376–385.

82. **Backert S, Meyer TF.** 2006. Type IV secretion systems and their effectors in bacterial pathogenesis. *Curr Opin Microbiol* **9:**207–217.

83. **Isberg RR, O'Connor TJ, Heidtman M.** 2009. The *Legionella pneumophila* replication vacuole: making a cosy niche inside host cells. *Nat Rev Microbiol* **7:**13–24.

84. **Pohlner J, Halter R, Beyreuther K, Meyer TF.** 1987. Gene structure and extracellular secretion of *Neisseria gonorrhoeae* IgA protease. *Nature* **325:**458–462.

85. **Leyton DL, Rossiter AE, Henderson IR.** 2012. From self sufficiency to dependence: mechanisms and factors important for autotransporter biogenesis. *Nat Rev Microbiol* **10:**213–225.

86. **van Ulsen P, Rahman SU, Jong WSP, Daleke-Schermerhorn MH, Luirink J.** 2014. Type V secretion: from biogenesis to biotechnology. *Biochim Biophys Acta Mol Cell Res* **1843:**1592–1611.

87. **Pohlner J, Halter R, Meyer TF.** 1987. *Neisseria gonorrhoeae* IgA protease. Secretion and implications for pathogenesis. *Antonie Van Leeuwenhoek* **53:**479–484.

88. **Brandon LD, Goehring N, Janakiraman A, Yan AW, Wu T, Beckwith J, Goldberg MB.** 2003. IcsA, a polarly localized autotransporter with an atypical signal peptide, uses the Sec apparatus for secretion, although the Sec apparatus is circumferentially distributed. *Mol Microbiol* **50:**45–60.

89. **Zumsteg AB, Goosmann C, Brinkmann V, Morona R, Zychlinsky A.** 2014. IcsA is a *Shigella flexneri* adhesion regulated by the type III secretion system and required for pathogenesis. *Cell Host Microbe* **15:**435–445.

90. **Roggenkamp A, Ackermann N, Jacobi CA, Truelzsch K, Hoffmann H, Heesemann H.** 2003. Molecular analysis of transport and oligomerization of the *Yersinia enterocolitica* adhesin YadA. *J Bacteriol* **185:**3735–3744.

91. **Mikula KM, Kolodziejczyk R, Goldman A.** 2013. *Yersinia* infection tools: characterization of structure and function of adhesins. *Front Cell Infect Microbiol* **2:**169.

92. **Leyton DL, Rossiter AE, Henderson IR.** 2012. From self sufficiency to dependence: mechanisms and factors important for autotransporter biogenesis. *Nat Rev Microbiol* **10:**213–225.

93. **Wagner JK, Heindl JE, Gray AN, Jain S, Goldberg MB.** 2009. Contribution of the periplasmic chaperone Skp to efficient presentation of the autotransporter IcsA on the surface of *Shigella flexneri*. *J Bacteriol* **191:**815–821.

94. **Ruiz-Perez F, Henderson IR, Leyton DL, Rossiter AE, Zhang Y, Nataro JP.** 2009. Roles of periplasmic chaperone proteins in the biogenesis of serine protease autotransporters of *Enterobacteriaceae*. *J Bacteriol* **191:** 6571–6583.

95. **Henderson IR, Navarro-Garcia F, Desvaux M, Fernandez RC, Ala'Aldeen D.** 2004. Type V protein secretion pathway: the autotransporter story. *Microbiol Mol Biol Rev* **68:**692–744.

96. **Lambert-Buisine C, Willery E, Locht C, Jacob-Dubuisson F.** 1998. N-terminal characterization of the *Bordetella pertussis* filamentous haemagglutinin. *Mol Microbiol* **28:** 1283–1293.

97. **McCann JR, St Geme JW 3rd.** 2014. The HMW1C-like glycosyltransferases: an enzyme family with a sweet tooth for simple sugars. *PLoS Pathog* **10:**e1003977. doi:10.1371/journal. ppat.1003977.

98. **Waksman G, Hultgren SJ.** 2009. Structural biology of the chaperone-usher pathway of pilus biogenesis. *Nat Rev Microbiol* **7:**765–774.

99. **Mougous JD, Cuff ME, Raunser S, Shen A, Zhou M, Gifford CA, Goodman AL, Joachimiak G, Ordoñez CL, Lory S, Walz T, Joachimiak A, Mekalanos JJ.** 2006. A virulence locus of *Pseudomonas aeruginosa* encodes a protein secretion apparatus. *Science* **312:**1526–1530.

100. **Russell AB, Peterson SB, Mougous JD.** 2014. Type VI secretion system effectors: poisons with a purpose. *Nat Rev Microbiol* **12:**137–148.

101. **Russell AB, Hood RD, Bui NK, LeRoux M, Vollmer W, Mougous JD.** 2011. Type VI secretion delivers bacteriolytic effectors to target cells. *Nature* **475:**343–347.

102. **Pukatzki S, Ma AT, Revel AT, Sturtevant D, Mekalanos JJ.** 2007. Type VI secretion system translocates a phage tail spike-like protein into target cells where it cross-links actin. *Proc Natl Acad Sci USA* **104:**15508–15513.

103. **English G, Trunk K, Rao VA, Srikannathasan V, Hunter WN, Coulthurst SJ.** 2012. New secreted toxins and immunity proteins encoded within the type VI secretion system gene cluster of *Serratia marcescens*. *Mol Microbiol* **86:**921–936.

104. **Feltcher ME, Braunstein M.** 2012. Emerging themes in SecA2-mediated protein export. *Nat Rev Microbiol* **10:**779–789.

105. **Freudl R.** 2013. Leaving home ain't easy: protein export systems in Gram-positive bacteria. *Res Microbiol* **164:**664–674.

106. **Rigel NW, Braunstein M.** 2008. A new twist on an old pathway: accessory Sec [corrected] systems. *Mol Microbiol* **69:**291–302.

107. **Bensing BA, Seepersaud R, Yen YT, Sullam PM.** 2014. Selective transport by SecA2: an expanding family of customized motor proteins. *Biochim Biophys Acta* **1843:**1674–1686.

108. **Hou JM, D'Lima NG, Rigel NW, Gibbons HS, McCann JR, Braunstein M, Teschke CM.** 2008. ATPase activity of *Mycobacterium tuberculosis* SecA1 and SecA2 proteins and its importance for SecA2 function in macrophages. *J Bacteriol* **190:**4880–4887.

109. **Fagan RP, Fairweather NF.** 2011. *Clostridium difficile* has two parallel and essential Sec secretion systems. *J Biol Chem* **286:**27483–27493.

110. **Siboo IR, Chaffin DO, Rubens CE, Sullam PM.** 2008. Characterization of the accessory Sec system of *Staphylococcus aureus*. *J Bacteriol* **190:**6188–6196.

111. **Mistou MY, Dramsi S, Brega S, Poyart C, Trieu-Cuot P.** 2009. Molecular dissection of the secA2 locus of group B *Streptococcus* reveals that glycosylation of the Srr1 LPXTG protein is required for full virulence. *J Bacteriol* **191:**4195–4206.

112. **Seepersaud R, Bensing BA, Yen YT, Sullam PM.** 2010. Asp3 mediates multiple protein-protein interactions within the accessory Sec system of *Streptococcus gordonii*. *Mol Microbiol* **78:**490–505.

113. **Telford JL, Barocchi MA, Margarit I, Rappuoli R, Grandi G.** 2006. Pili in Gram-positive pathogens. *Nat Rev Microbiol* **4:**509–519.

114. **Hendrickx AP, Budzik JM, Oh SY, Schneewind O.** 2011. Architects at the bacterial surface: sortases and the assembly of pili with isopeptide bonds. *Nat Rev Microbiol* **9:**166–176.

115. **Mazmanian SK, Liu G, Hung TT, Schneewind O.** 1999. *Staphylococcus aureus* sortase, an enzyme that anchors surface proteins to the cell wall. *Science* **285:**760–763.

116. **Madden JC, Ruiz N, Caparon M.** 2001. Cytolysin-mediated translocation (CMT): A functional equivalent of type III secretion in Gram-positive bacteria. *Cell* **104:**143–152.

117. **Ghosh J, Caparon MG.** 2006. Specificity of *Streptococcus pyogenes* NAD(+) glycohydrolase in cytolysin-mediated translocation. *Mol Microbiol.* **62:**1203–1214.

118. **Tweten RK.** 2005. Cholesterol-dependent cytolysins, a family of versatile pore-forming toxins. *Infect Immun* **73:**6199–6209.

119. **Madden JC, Ruiz N, Caparon M.** 2001. Cytolysin-mediated translocation (CMT): a functional equivalent of type III secretion in Gram-positive bacteria. *Cell* **104:**143–152.

120. **Ghosh J, Anderson PJ, Chandrasekaran S, Caparon MG.** 2010. Characterization of *Streptococcus pyogenes* beta-NAD(+) glycohydrolase re-evaluation of enzymatic properties associated with pathogenesis. *J Biol Chem* **285:**5683–5694.

121. **Magassa NG, Chandrasekaran S, Caparon MG.** 2010. *Streptococcus pyogenes* cytolysin-mediated translocation does not require pore formation by streptolysin O. *EMBO Rep* **11:**400–405.

122. **Simeone R, Bottai D, Brosch R.** 2009. ESX/type VII secretion systems and their role in host-pathogen interaction. *Curr Opin Microbiol* **12:**4–10.

123. **Houben EN, Korotkov KV, Bitter W.** 2014. Take five: type VII secretion systems of *Mycobacteria*. *Biochim Biophys Acta* **1843:**1707–1716.

124. **Stanley SA, Raghavan S, Hwang WW, Cox JS.** 2003. Acute infection and macrophage subversion by *Mycobacterium tuberculosis* require a specialized secretion system. *Proc Natl Acad Sci USA* **100:**13001–13006.

125. **Burts ML, Williams WA, DeBord K, Missiakas DM.** 2005. EsxA and EsxB are secreted by an ESAT-6-like system that is required for the pathogenesis of *Staphylococcus aureus* infections. *Proc Natl Acad Sci USA* **102:**1169–1174.

126. **Way SS, Wilson CB.** 2005. The *Mycobacterium tuberculosis* ESAT-6 homologue in *Listeria monocytogenes* is dispensable for growth *in vitro* and *in vivo*. *Infect Immun* **73:**6151–6153.

127. **Baptista C, Barreto HC, Sao-Jose C.** 2013. High levels of DegU-P activate an Esat-6-like secretion system in *Bacillus subtilis*. *PLoS One* **8:**e67840. doi:10.1371/journal.pone.0067840.

128. **Houben EN, Bestebroer J, Ummels R, Wilson L, Piersma SR, Jimenez CR, Ottenhoff TH, Luirink J, Bitter W.** 2012. Composition of the type VII secretion system membrane complex. *Mol Microbiol* **86:**472–484.

129. **Luthra A, Mahmood A, Arora A, Ramachandran R.** 2008. Characterization of Rv3868, an essential hypothetical protein of the ESX-1 secretion system in *Mycobacterium tuberculosis*. *J Biol Chem* **283:**36532–36541.

130. **Ohol YM, Goetz DH, Chan K, Shiloh MU, Craik CS, Cox JS.** 2010. *Mycobacterium tuberculosis* MycP1 protease plays a dual role in regulation of ESX-1 secretion and virulence. *Cell Host Microbe* **7:**210–220.

131. **Champion PAD, Stanley SA, Champion MM, Brown EJ, Cox JS.** 2006. C-terminal signal sequence promotes virulence factor secretion in *Mycobacterium tuberculosis*. *Science* **313:** 1632–1636.

132. **Daleke MH, van der Woude AD, Parret AH, Ummels R, de Groot AM, Watson D, Piersma SR, Jimenez CR, Luirink J, Bitter W, Houben EN.** 2012. Specific chaperones for the type VII protein secretion pathway. *J Biol Chem* **287:** 31939–31947.

133. **Hoffmann C, Leis A, Niederweis M, Plitzko JM, Engelhardt H.** 2008. Disclosure of the mycobacterial outer membrane: cryo-electron tomography and vitreous sections reveal the lipid bilayer structure. *Proc Natl Acad Sci USA* **105:**3963–3967.

134. **Zuber B, Chami M, Houssin C, Dubochet J, Griffiths G, Daffe M.** 2008. Direct visualization of the outer membrane of *Mycobacteria* and *Corynebacteria* in their native state. *J Bacteriol* **190:**5672–5680.

135. **Pym AS, Brodin P, Brosch R, Huerre M, Cole ST.** 2002. Loss of RD1 contributed to the attenuation of the live tuberculosis vaccines *Mycobacterium bovis* BCG and *Mycobacterium microti*. *Mol Microbiol* **46:**709–717.

136. **Lewis KN, Liao R, Guinn KM, Hickey MJ, Smith S, Behr MA, Sherman DR.** 2003. Deletion of RD1 from *Mycobacterium tuberculosis* mimics bacille Calmette-Guerin attenuation. *J Infect Dis* **187:**117–123.

137. **Gey Van Pittius NC, Gamieldien J, Hide W, Brown GD, Siezen RJ, Beyers AD.** 2001. The ESAT-6 gene cluster of *Mycobacterium tuberculosis* and other high G+C Gram-positive bacteria. *Genome Biol* **2**:RESEARCH0044.

138. **Coros A, Callahan B, Battaglioli E, Derbyshire KM.** 2008. The specialized secretory apparatus ESX-1 is essential for DNA transfer in *Mycobacterium smegmatis*. *Mol Microbiol* **69**:794–808.

139. **Siegrist MS, Unnikrishnan M, McConnell MJ, Borowsky M, Cheng TY, Siddiqi N, Fortune SM, Moody DB, Rubin EJ.** 2009. Mycobacterial Esx-3 is required for mycobactin-mediated iron acquisition. *Proc Natl Acad Sci USA* **106**:18792–18797.

140. **Ekiert DC, Cox JS.** 2014. Structure of a PE-PPE-EspG complex from *Mycobacterium tuberculosis* reveals molecular specificity of ESX protein secretion. *Proc Natl Acad Sci USA* **111**:14758–14763.

141. **Vance RE, Isberg RR, Portnoy DA.** 2009. Patterns of pathogenesis: discrimination of pathogenic and nonpathogenic microbes by the innate immune system. *Cell Host Microbe* **6**:10–21.

142. **Wang X, Parashar K, Sitaram A, Bliska JB.** 2014. The GAP activity of type III effector YopE triggers killing of *Yersinia* in macrophages. *PLoS Pathog* **10**:e1004346. doi:10.1371/journal.ppat.1004346.

143. **Harder J, Franchi L, Munoz-Planillo R, Park JH, Reimer T, Nunez G.** 2009. Activation of the Nlrp3 inflammasome by *Streptococcus pyogenes* requires streptolysin O and NF-kappa B activation but proceeds independently of TLR signaling and P2X7 receptor. *J Immunol* **183**:5823–5829.

144. **Osei-Owusu P, Jessen DL, Toosky M, Roughead W, Bradley DS, Nilles ML.** 2015. The N-terminus of the type III secretion needle protein YscF from *Yersinia pestis* functions to modulate innate immune responses. *Infect Immun* **83**:1507–1522.

The Structure and Function of Type III Secretion Systems

9

RYAN Q. NOTTI[1,2] and C. EREC STEBBINS[1]

INTRODUCTION

Type III secretion systems (T3SSs) afford Gram-negative bacteria an intimate means of altering the biology of their eukaryotic hosts—the direct delivery of effector proteins from the bacterial cytoplasm to that of the eukaryote (1, 2). T3SSs utilize a conserved set of homologous gene products to assemble the nanosyringe "injectisomes" capable of traversing the three plasma membranes, peptidoglycan layer, and extracellular space that form a barrier to the direct delivery of proteins from bacterium to host. While the injectisome is architecturally similar across disparate Gram-negative organisms, its applications are a study in diversity: T3SSs are employed by both symbionts and pathogens; they target animals, plants, and protists; and they are used to manipulate a wide array of cellular activities and pathways.

T3SSs have attracted intense scientific interest since the seminal work documenting their discovery was published over two decades ago (3–5). Given their role in the virulence of several human and plant pathogens (e.g., *Salmonella enterica*, *Shigella flexneri*, *Yersinia* spp., pathogenic *Escherichia coli*, *Vibrio* spp., *Pseudomonas* spp., *Chlamydia* spp.), T3SSs are attractive targets for the discovery or design of novel anti-infective agents and vaccine approaches.

[1]Laboratory of Structural Microbiology, Rockefeller University, New York, NY 10065; [2]Tri-Institutional Medical Scientist Training Program, Weill Cornell Medical College, New York, NY, 10021.
Virulence Mechanisms of Bacterial Pathogens, 5th edition
Edited by Indira T. Kudva, Nancy A. Cornick, Paul J. Plummer, Qijing Zhang, Tracy L. Nicholson, John P. Bannantine, and Bryan H. Bellaire
© 2016 American Society for Microbiology, Washington, DC
doi:10.1128/microbiolspec.VMBF-0004-2015

Conversely, because T3SSs accomplish the biophysical feat of protein transduction across multiple membranes, their re-engineering for *in vivo* delivery of therapeutic proteins or *in vitro* production of protein reagents provides an exciting prospect for future biomedical application. In either case, the manipulation of T3SSs for human benefit will require highly refined mechanistic models of T3SS function. Drawing on research from multiple disciplines and employing complementary techniques, such models are beginning to emerge. In particular, the application of structural biochemical approaches to the T3SS has provided numerous insights into the assembly and function of this system.

The focus of this chapter will be on T3SS function at the structural level; we will summarize the core findings that have shaped our understanding of the structure and function of these systems and highlight recent developments in the field. In turn, we will describe the T3SS secretory apparatus, consider its engagement with secretion substrates, and discuss the posttranslational regulation of secretory function. Lastly, we close with a discussion of the future prospects for the interrogation of structure-function relationships in the T3SS.

ARCHITECTURE OF A NANOSYRINGE

The genomic islands and virulence plasmids that support the T3SS encode proteins of four broad classes: the components of the secretory system itself, the effector substrates, their chaperones, and transcriptional regulators. Working in concert, these components form a complete secretory system that dechaperones and secretes substrates in a defined hierarchy and delivers them to the host cytoplasm. The repertoire of effector proteins secreted by a given T3SS is species-specific, as is the transcriptional network regulating T3SS expression (6). A discussion of these elements is beyond the scope of this review and has been expertly reviewed

elsewhere (7–16). In contrast to the diverse, species-specific catalog of effector proteins and transcriptional regulators, the nanosyringe-like secretory machinery is well conserved across species, and advances in our mechanistic understanding of one species' injectisome are often applicable to others.

The core secretion machinery of the T3SS is comprised of a homologous set of approximately two-dozen gene products. Because of the high degree of homology of some components of the system, a universal nomenclature was previously suggested to facilitate cross-species comparisons (17), and recently others in the field have endorsed this naming system (18, 19). Similarly, we will employ this nomenclature (Table 1) wherever possible. Additionally, a subset of these proteins have conserved homologues in the flagellar apparatus (Table 1), which uses its own T3SS machine to assemble the flagellar filament (20). Given that these T3SS subtypes appear to have diverged from a common ancestor some hundreds of millions of years ago (21), their conservation is noteworthy. While the focus of this review is the injectisome T3SS subtype, we will draw on the flagellar literature where it offers insights into injectisome function.

The core conserved proteins of the T3SS form a double-membrane-spanning syringe-like structure (22, 23), including its extracellular needle-like appendage, and the associated cytoplasmic and membrane-integral secretion machinery (Fig. 1). It is these components that are collectively responsible for the delivery of effector proteins into the cytosol of the eukaryotic host cell (24, 25). While our mechanistic model of this cytoplasm-to-cytoplasm secretion system continues to evolve, (ultra-)structural and biochemical characterization of its core components has yielded significant insights.

The Basal Body

The bacterial double membrane and peptidoglycan layer are spanned by a stack of

TABLE 1 A unified nomenclature for the homologous core components of the T3SS[a]

Notes	Universal nomenclature	Salmonella SPI-1	Shigella	Enteropathogenic Escherichia. coli	Yersinia spp.	Pseudomonas aeruginosa	Flagellar apparatus
Basal body	SctC	InvG	MxiD	EscC	YscC	PscC	
	SctD	PrgH	MxiG	EscD	YscD	PscD	
	SctJ	PrgK	MxiJ	EscJ	YscJ	PscJ	
Pilotin		InvH	MxiM		YscW	ExsB	
Inner rod	SctI	PrgJ	Mxil	Escl	Yscl	Pscl	
Needle filament	SctF	PrgI	MxiH	EscF	YscF	PscF	
Needle length regulator	SctP	InvJ	Spa32	EscP (Orf16)	YscP	PscP	FliK
Inner membrane machinery	SctV	InvA	MxiA	EscV	YscV (LcrD)	PcrD	FlhA
	SctR	SpaP	Spa24	EscR	YscR	PscR	FliP
	SctS	SpaQ	Spa9	EscS	YscS	PscS	FliQ
	SctT	SpaR	Spa29	EscT	YscT	PscT	FliR
	SctU	SpaS	Spa40	EscU	YscU	PscU	FlhB
Needle tip and translocon		SipB	IpaB	EspD	YopB	PopB	
		SipC	IpaC	EspB	YopD	PopD	
		SipD	IpaD	EspA	LcrV	PcrV	
ATPase	SctN	InvC	Spa47	EscN	YscN	PscN	Flil
Coiled coil linker	SctO	Invl	Spa13	EscO (Orf15, EscA)	YscO	PscO	FliJ
Sorting platform	SctQ	SpaO	Spa33	SepQ	YscQ	PscQ	FliM/FliN
	SctK	OrgA	MxiK		YscK		
	SctL	OrgB	MxiN	EscL	YscL	PscL	FliH
Needle length regulator	SctP	InvJ	Spa32	EscP (Orf16)	YscP	PscP	FliK
Export regulator	SctW	InvE	MxiC	SepL/SepD	YopN/TyeA	PopN	

[a]Based on the nomenclature proposed by Hueck (17), with modifications and additions from others (16, 18, 19, 90).

protein annuli known as the basal body (Fig. 1). This is comprised of an outer membrane-anchored layer (SctC) and an inner membrane-anchored layer (SctD and SctJ) that interface at a "neck" (26, 27). In electron microscopic (EM) reconstructions of the injectisome, SctC forms two distinct outer rings (OR1 and OR2), SctD and SctJ together form the distal inner ring (IR1), and the cytoplasmic amino-terminus of SctD forms the innermost ring (IR2) (26). The highest-resolution cryo-EM models of the *Salmonella* basal body reveal an overall 3-fold rotational symmetry, with a resultant symmetry mismatch between the inner and outer layers: each basal body contains 24 SctD molecules, 24 SctJ molecules, and 15 SctC molecules (27). While the 24-fold symmetry of the inner membrane rings appears conserved across T3SSs (28, 29), the stoichiometry of the SctC outer membrane ring may vary between species (12 to 15 molecules per basal body), such that some systems have an overall 12-fold rotational symmetry (29, 30).

SctC is homologous to the type II secretion system secretins (5, 31), and like other secretin family members requires a pilotin lipoprotein for its optimal localization and assembly (32–34). The membrane-embedded, β-rich region at the SctC carboxy-terminus can be isolated and has been visualized by EM (30), but it has yet to be characterized at moderate or high resolution. The periplasmic amino-terminus of SctC contains a modular

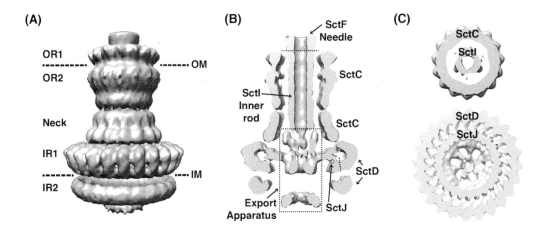

FIGURE 1 **Gross architecture of the T3SS. Cryo-EM reconstruction of the *Salmonella enterica* serovar Typhimurium injectisome basal body at subnanometer resolution reveals its overall architecture. (A) Surface representation of the highest resolution cryo-EM map (EMD 1875, contour level 0.0233) published by Schraidt and Marlovits (27). Dashed lines indicate the positions of bacterial membranes *in vivo*. Abbreviations: OR, outer ring; IR, inner ring; OM, outer membrane; IM, inner membrane. (B) An axial section through the map in (A). (C) Transverse sections through the map in (A) at the level of the neck (top) and IR1 (bottom).**

domain architecture (35) that interacts with the inner membrane ring (36, 37).

SctD and SctJ form the inner membrane rings (26). Each is anchored to the membrane by a single transmembrane helix, and SctJ is additionally lipidated near its aminoterminus (38). Like the amino-terminal periplasmic region of SctC, the periplasmic domains of SctD and SctJ are comprised of a modular multidomain architecture (35). Despite differences in connectivity and little sequence homology, the mixed α/β domains of SctC, SctD, and SctJ show a similar three-dimensional structure: two α-helices pack against the same face of a three-strand β-sheet (35, 39). Superhelical crystal packing of the *E. coli* SctJ periplasmic region provided initial insights into the mechanism of inner membrane ring assembly (38), and the modular arrangement of these domains seems to promote oligomerization (40); however, none of these domains have been shown to clearly form annuli in solution, suggesting that additional constraints (e.g., protein-protein interactions or lipid membrane planarity) are critical for ring forma-

tion. Similarly, despite their 1:1 stoichiometry in the basal body, the periplasmic domains of SctD and SctJ have not been crystallized in complex.

Might there be a specific functional advantage for the modular domain architecture common to the SctCDJ periplasmic regions? Recent *in situ* electron tomography of the *Yersinia* and *Shigella* injectisomes shows that the basal body has the ability to stretch in response to osmotic expansion of the periplasmic space (29). This resilience could be of potential importance for the maintenance of intact T3SS injectisomes under physiologic stresses and membrane deformations (29). Molecular dynamic simulations suggest that relative motions of the SctD periplasmic domains could account in part for this flexibility (29), but this hypothesis requires empiric support.

The amino-terminal cytoplasmic domain of SctD forms the innermost ring of the T3SS basal body. High-resolution structural analyses have determined this domain to have a forkhead-associated fold that interacts with cytoplasmic components of the T3SS (41–44).

Forkhead-associated domains are β-sandwiches that typically serve as phosphothreonine-binding scaffolds, suggesting a means of signal-dependent recruitment of the cytoplasmic secretory apparatus to the basal body. However, the potential phosphopeptide-binding residues are not conserved among T3SSs, and the precise nature of the interactions between SctD and the cytoplasmic apparatus remains to be determined.

Within the central lumen of the basal body annuli, SctI is believed to form a cylindrical "inner rod" (26) structure that may support the extracellular needle filament. Computational methods have suggested a predominantly α-helical structure for SctI similar to that of the needle filament protomer (below); however, structural analyses of *Salmonella* and *Shigella* SctI in solution showed little secondary or tertiary structure (45). It remains to be determined whether SctI can adopt a stable fold within the confines of the basal body. The functional significance of the inner rod in the regulation of needle length and secretion substrate switching will be discussed below.

Direct structural characterization of the T3SS basal body epitomizes the challenges associated with the interrogation of high-molecular-weight macromolecular machines: the assembly spans two membranes and a layer of peptidoglycan, and *in situ* electron tomographic analyses suggest that the basal body is capable of substantial conformational dynamism (29). Because direct, high-resolution structural characterization of the assembled T3SS basal body has not yet been possible, a multidisciplinary approach integrating cryo-EM maps, x-ray crystallographic domain structures, biochemical analyses, and computer modeling has yielded a high-probability static model for injectisome architecture (46) (Fig. 2). Such "hybrid" models will allow the testing of molecular-level hypotheses about ring assembly until the structure of the T3SS basal body has been determined at high-resolution *in toto*.

The Inner Membrane Machinery

Five highly conserved inner membrane proteins (SctRSTUV) are necessary for the function of the pathogenic T3SS; however their individual functions are unclear. It is worth noting that these proteins show a high degree of sequence homology to components of the evolutionarily related flagellar T3SS (Table 1) and may represent a functional core, serving critical chemical roles in initiating or powering protein secretion.

Among the SctRSTUV cohort, SctU and SctV possess cytoplasmic domains in addition to their transmembrane helices, and these domains have been best characterized to date. The cytoplasmic region of SctV contains a modular array of small domains (47–49), and crystallographic data suggest SctV may nonamerize (49). Intriguingly, such an oligomer is well suited to fit in a torus of SctV-associated density observed 5 to 10 nm beneath the basal body in EM reconstructions of the T3SS (29, 49). Lea and colleagues (49) have forwarded the hypothesis that this SctV homo-oligomer may serve as a "cage" to facilitate the complete unfolding of folded or partially unfolded secretion substrates, but this possibility has not yet been experimentally validated. The cytoplasmic region of SctU is considerably smaller than that of SctV and contains an autoprotease (50); its potential role in the regulation of secretion will be discussed below.

SctRSTUV are important in the organized, stepwise assembly of the T3SS basal body. Galan and colleagues (51) employed a combination of genetic and structural approaches to show that SctRSTUV help to organize the SctDJ inner membrane rings. Subsequently, the SctC ring and cytoplasmic machinery (below) are recruited, and the inner rod and needle polymers assembled (19). While SctRSTUV are individually not strictly necessary for the formation of the SctCDJ basal body, the efficiency of basal body assembly is significantly ameliorated in their absence (51).

(A)

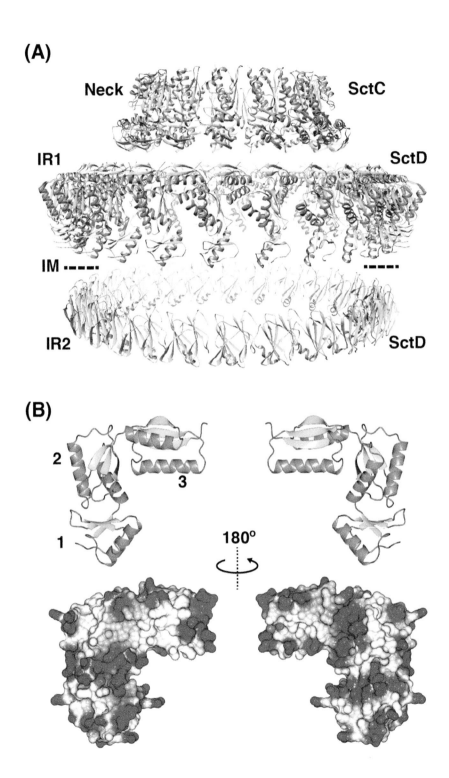

(B)

The Needle Filament

A needle-like filament tens of nanometers in length protrudes from the extracellular face of the T3SS basal body (22, 52). The needle is formed by a helical assembly of the protein SctF, with an outer diameter of 8 nm and an inner pore diameter of 2.5 nm (53). The apparent similarity of the T3SS basal body and needle filament to a macroscopic syringe makes it tempting to speculate that the T3SS directly injects its substrates into the host cell cytoplasm, with the needle filament serving as a conduit for the passage of partially unfolded effector proteins. Until recently, this hypothesis lacked direct empirical support, and alternative "noninjectisome" models for T3SS effector delivery had been proposed (54). Analyzing substrate-trapped injectisomes by cryo-EM, Marlovits and colleagues (55) and Kolbe and colleagues (56) demonstrated the presence of additional density in the lumen of the T3SS needle filament, consistent with the passage of partially unfolded substrate molecules through the needle.

High-resolution structures of monomeric SctF mutants (57) or chaperone-bound SctF (58, 59) have allowed the characterization of the needle protomer fold. SctF is a hairpin of alpha helices with an intervening conserved PXXP motif. The oligomeric nature of the needle filament had posed a practical barrier to high-resolution structure determination for the intact assembly. Recent hybrid approaches combining cryo-EM with solid-state nuclear magnetic resonance spectroscopy (NMR) and computational modeling have since afforded such a model for both the *Salmonella* (53) and *Shigella* (60) needle filaments. In these models, the SctF amino-terminus is oriented toward the convex needle exterior, the carboxy-terminus points toward the lumen, and the apex loop connecting the two alpha helices points away from the bacterium. It should be noted that this arrangement is in contrast to prior lower-resolution models (61), which oriented the SctF amino-terminus toward the needle lumen. This correction is significant: the orientation of SctF protomers in the solid state NMR models is such that the lumen walls are formed by highly conserved residues, consistent with the passage of secretion substrates through the lumen (53, 60).

Assembly of needle filaments of a given length is necessary for the proper infectivity of T3SS-bearing pathogens, possibly matching the dimensions of host-pathogen adhesion complexes (62). How, though, is the length of the needle filament controlled? SctP regulates the length of the needle filament in several species (63–65). In *Yersinia* spp., the number of residues in SctP correlates with needle filament length, leading to the hypothesis that SctP functions as a "molecular ruler" (65). That is, SctP might attach at one end to the basal body or cytoplasmic apparatus and at the other end to the growing needle filament, and once SctP was stretched beyond a given length, it would signal to the secretion apparatus to change substrates.

In contrast to the molecular ruler model, work with *Salmonella* suggests that SctP regulates needle length through control of inner rod assembly (52). *Salmonella* organisms lacking SctP show decreased density in the inner rod-supporting socket region, lack a polymerized inner rod, and generate long needles (52, 66). Accordingly, Galan and colleagues hypothesized that SctI and SctF are secreted simultaneously and that completion

---

FIGURE 2 **Hybrid models of basal body structure. (A) Computational modeling of the neck (SctC, PDB 3J1V), IR1 (SctD, PDB 3J1X), and IR2 (SctD, PDB 3J1W) annuli of the *Salmonella enterica* serovar Typhimurium basal body. No high-resolution structural information is available for the basal body above the neck. (B) In this model, complementary electrostatic surfaces support ring building, as shown for the SctD periplasmic domains. Note the modular domain architecture (enumerated 1, 2, 3) for SctD_{periplasmic}.**

of inner rod assembly terminates needle growth in an SctP-dependent fashion. Consistent with this "timer" model of length control (19), overexpression of SctF or SctI leads to longer or shorter needles, respectively (52). Moreover, alanine-scanning mutagenesis analyses of the inner rod protein SctI in *Salmonella* revealed numerous point mutations that increased needle length without compromising secretory function, perhaps by slowing the rate of inner rod polymerization (66). Intriguingly, the elongate needles generated by most of these mutants remained attached to the basal body (66), in contrast to those produced by *sctP* deletion mutants, which are easily sheered off (52). This observation is consistent with the hypothesis that the polymerized inner rod joins with the needle filament, anchoring it to the basal body (66).

The Needle Tip and Translocon Pore

At the tip of the T3SS needle filament is a pentameric cap formed by the hydrophilic translocator protein (67, 68). The needle tip is believed to interact directly with the host cell surface to facilitate the insertion of a multimeric pore (69, 70), thus completing the cytoplasm-to-cytoplasm protein conduit. The structure and function of the needle tip is of particular biomedical interest, because the hydrophilic translocator protein is a protective antigen in anti-*Yersinia* vaccine formulations (71) and is targeted by a recently developed passive immunization strategy for the treatment of *Pseudomonas aeruginosa* infections (72).

X-ray crystallographic analysis of the monomeric tip protein from several species reveals some conserved architectural features (73, 74): the tips of all species show an elongate coiled-coil region and a central mixed α/β subdomain. The overall structure of the tip protein shows some interspecies variation, though, with *Salmonella*/*Shigella* SipD/IpaD possessing an amino-terminal autochaperoning subdomain (74) lacked by

the *Yersinia/Pseudomonas* LcrV/PcrV tip proteins (19, 70). High-resolution models of the pentameric needle tip are not available, but low-resolution negative stain EM models have offered some insight into its gross architecture. While both appear pentameric, the *Shigella* tip complex is narrow and elongated relative to that of the *Yersinia* tip (67, 68), and fitting the *Shigella* IpaD monomeric crystal structure into the EM map required a significant rearrangement of the mixed α/β domain (68).

Attempts to model the tip protein–needle filament interaction at high resolution using NMR or x-ray crystallographic data have so far proven challenging, with incompatibilities arising between the proposed models and other data sets (75–77). The crystal structure of a *Salmonella* SctF-SipD fusion protein identified a potential binding mode for the tip with the needle (75); however, modeling the fusion structure onto the solid state NMR model of the needle filament (53) resulted in steric clashes, suggesting that artifactual constraints imposed by the protein fusion strategy biased the architecture of the complex (77). Regardless, a synthesis of the available data shows that the needle filament interacts with the tip protein at least in part through its elongate coiled-coil, a motif observed in all T3SS tip proteins described to date.

EM and biochemical analyses have shown that the *Shigella* tip complex is actually a heteropentamer containing four copies of the hydrophilic translocator IpaD and one copy of the hydrophobic translocator IpaB (76). A refined tip model incorporating this insight is similar to previous models, in that the amino- and carboxy-termini of IpaD are oriented toward the needle filament, with portions of the coiled-coil region contacting the needle. However, the refined model presents an IpaD orientation consistent with antibody binding data, and the heteropentameric architecture explains the transition from a helical needle filament to a nearly flat-topped tip complex (76).

In contrast to the annular, pentameric tip complexes observed for other T3SSs, entero-pathogenic *E. coli* possess a long filamentous needle accessory comprised of EspA, the SipD/IpaD/LcrV/PcrV homologue (78). EspA forms a helical filament similar to the SctF needle, with an internal diameter of approximately 2.5 nm (79), suggesting that it functions to extend the T3SS transport conduit. Filling a functional niche similar to needle filament length control in other T3SSs, *E. coli* EspA polymers may adapt the injectisome to reach the target cell membrane beneath the intestinal glycocalyx (70).

The translocon permeating the host cell membrane is formed by the hydrophobic translocators SipB and SipC in *Salmonella* and their homologues (Table 1). Experiments in red blood cell membranes have shown that the needle tip is crucial for the insertion of the hydrophobic translocators into the host membrane and/or the organization of inserted translocators into functional pores (69, 80). While numerous experimental approaches have been employed to characterize the pore diameter and structure of the translocon (70), direct structural interrogation of native translocons is lacking. Intriguingly, the amino-termini of *Salmonella* SipB and *Shigella* IpaB contain extended coiled-coils reminiscent of the colicin family of bacteriocins (81), which are known to function in the delivery of protein toxins across bacterial membranes. However, the precise mechanisms of host cell recognition, membrane insertion, pore formation, and protein translocation remain unclear for the T3SS translocon.

SUBSTRATE RECRUITMENT AND SECRETION

T3SSs secrete only a small fraction of the proteins present in the bacterial cytosol (82), and do so in a defined hierarchy. How does the T3SS select its substrates, how is its secretion hierarchy maintained, and what is the mechanism of secretion? A combination of genetic, biochemical, and structural data provide insight into the role of cytoplasmic injectisome-associated proteins in these processes.

Secretion Chaperones

The amino-terminal ~100 amino acids of T3SS substrates possess two secretion signals: an unstructured extreme amino-terminus followed by a chaperone-binding region. While the extreme amino-termini of T3SS substrates are highly variable, computational approaches have identified commonalities in the chemical composition of this secretion signal (83–85): the first ~15 amino acids in an effector sequence are enriched in serine, threonine, isoleucine, and proline. Indeed, an effector with a synthetic, amphipathic poly-serine/isoleucine secretion signal was secreted by *Yersinia* even in the absence of the second secretion signal (its secretion chaperone) (86). However, other studies have shown that chaperone-substrate interactions are necessary for targeting substrates specifically to the injectisome T3SS, because the extreme amino-terminal secretion signal sequence can facilitate injectisome substrate export through the flagellar apparatus in the absence of a chaperone-binding domain. This finding suggests that the extreme amino-terminal secretion signal is evolutionarily "ancient" and shared by both types of T3SS (87).

Downstream of the amino-terminal secretion signal, each secretion substrate is recognized by a specific chaperone protein that maintains the bound region of the substrate in a partially unfolded state (88). It is hypothesized that this nonglobular conformation primes the substrate for secretion through the narrow aperture of the T3SS conduit (89). Chaperones can be classified by their structure and substrate type (90), as follows: class IA chaperones are mixed α/β homodimers that bind to one effector; class IB chaperones are structurally similar to IA but bind multiple effectors; class II chaperones are alpha helical tetratricopeptide repeat (TPR) proteins that bind to translocon proteins; and class III chaperones are heterodimeric TPR proteins that bind SctF needle filament protomers. It should be noted that while the premature polymerization of SipD/IpaD tip proteins is prevented by their autochaperoning domain (74), tip proteins in *Yersinia* and *Pseudomonas* utilize a unique chaperone (LcrG/PcrG) to stabilize their tip protein monomers (91).

Like the extreme amino-terminal secretion signal, the chaperone-binding sequences of secretion substrates are variable. However, class I chaperone recognition of a conserved β-strand(s) is a common feature of a diverse array of T3SS effectors (92), and it is conserved from animal to plant pathogens (93) (Fig. 3). Indeed, the sparse sequence conservation associated with the "β-motif" (92) can be used to recognize previously unknown T3SS effector proteins (94). In contrast, class II and III TPR chaperones can recognize substrate sequences in either extended unstructured or α-helical conformations; the commonality here is that the TPR concavity is used to bind the substrate (90) (Fig. 3).

The aforementioned substrate secretion signals are not only necessary for protein secretion through the T3SS; they are sufficient. Fusion of the secretion signal and chaperone-binding domain from endogenous T3SS substrates to heterologously expressed

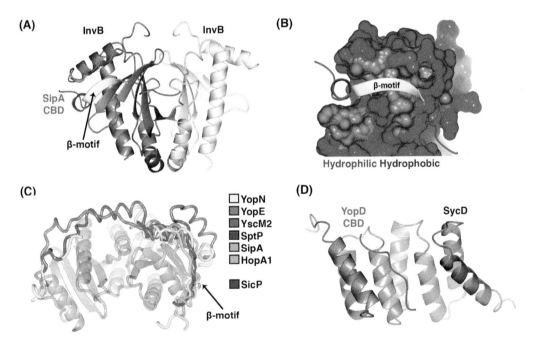

FIGURE 3 **Chaperone-substrate interactions. Structural distinctions between effector-chaperone and translocator-chaperone complexes. (A) The structure of the *Salmonella* effector SipA chaperone-binding domain (CBD, red and yellow) in complex with the class IB chaperone InvB (dark gray, light gray). PDB 2FM8 (47). The structurally conserved β-motif is highlighted in yellow. (B) The SipA β-motif is bound by a hydrophobic (gray) patch on the InvB surface (blue/gray). (C) Superposition of the CBDs from effectors from multiple species shows a common binding mode marked by the structurally conserved β-motif. The prototypical class I chaperone SicP is shown in place of the various chaperones. PDB codes: YopN, 1XKP (153); YopE, 1L2W (170); YscM2, 1TTW (171); SptP-SicP, 1JYO (88); SipA, 2FM8 (47); HopA1, 4G6T (93). (D) The *Yersinia* translocator YopD CBD (red) lacks secondary structure and is bound by the concave cleft of the class II chaperone SycD (gray). Protein Data bank ID number 4AM9 (PDB 4AM9) (172).**

proteins results in their secretion through the T3SS (95), provided they can be properly unfolded for transit through the needle (55, 56). While this observation is noteworthy for its mechanistic insight into the targeting of virulence factors for secretion, it has allowed the benevolent re-engineering of the system to deliver protective antigens in vaccine design (96) and the large-scale production of challenging protein reagents, such as spider silk (97).

The ATPase

Both the injectisome and flagellar T3SS include an ATPase with notable sequence homology to the β subunit of the F_0F_1 ATPase (98). For the injectisome, this ATPase is SctN; for the flagellar apparatus, it is FliI (Table 1). High-resolution structural analysis of the *E. coli* SctN catalytic domain showed similarities to V- and F-type ATPases and confirmed that SctN hexamerization would be required for efficient ATP hydrolysis (99). Both FliI (100, 101) and SctN (98, 102) form such oligomers, but neither has been characterized structurally as a catalytically active hexamer.

Interaction of chaperone-substrate complexes with the T3SS ATPase SctN causes the dechaperoning and unfolding of the substrate in an ATP hydrolysis-dependent fashion (103). Given that disruption of the tertiary structure is necessary to fit protein substrates in the 2.5-nm conduit of the needle filament (55, 56), it is not surprising that loss of function mutations in SctN cause the near complete abrogation of T3SS function (98, 103). Similarly, genomic deletion of *fliI* severely compromises flagellar filament assembly (104–107). Consistent with the role of SctN in preparing substrates for export, SctN/FliI-dependent density is observed directly beneath the T3SS basal body by EM (108, 109). The partial structural similarity of SctO/FliJ with the γ-subunit of F-type ATPases and the ability of FliJ to stimulate FliI hexamerization (101) has led to the hypothesis that this

coiled-coil-containing protein (110) might connect oligomeric SctN to the SctV export gate, thus linking the subbasal body toruses of electron density (49). However, the mere presence of a coiled-coil is insufficient evidence to ascribe a γ-like function to SctO (19), and its precise role remains to be determined.

Given the ATPase activity of SctN/FliI, it is tempting to speculate that ATP hydrolysis provides the free energy for protein secretion; however, chemical and genetic analyses show that SctN/FliI is not the sole energizer of the T3SS. Experiments with the protonophore CCCP have shown that the inner membrane proton motive force is necessary for secretion by both injectisome (111) and flagellar (104, 105) T3SSs. Additionally, the flagellar assembly defect of ATPase deletion mutants can be at least partially corrected by mutations that alter the export apparatus, increase substrate levels, or increase the magnitude of the proton motive force (104–106). A similar result was recently reported for SPI-1 T3SS in *Salmonella* (106). These results suggest that under sufficiently permissive conditions, the actual transit of substrates into and/or through the conduit is powered by the proton motive force. However, one must interpret these results with some caution, because ionophores can significantly perturb cellular physiology (112), and SctN-independent injectisome secretion of a substrate requiring dechaperoning has not yet been demonstrated (106). A reasonable synthesis of the available data might suggest that both ATP hydrolysis and the proton motive force are important for energizing T3SSs: the SctN/FliI ATPase functions to dechaperone and begin unfolding the secretion substrates with optimal efficiency under (nonideal) physiologic conditions, while the proton motive force is responsible for the apical transit of the nonglobular substrate (106).

Regardless of the quantitative contributions of either energy source, the mechanics of secretion remain poorly understood. There are no available high-resolution structural models of the interaction between chaperone-substrate complexes and the SctN ATPase. One computational model suggests a mode of ATPase-chaperone interaction based on structural similarities between class I chaperones and the F-type ATPase γ-subunit (113). While this model and the accompanying biochemical data are consistent with the observation that relatively carboxy-terminal residues of SctN interact with chaperones (113), its structural accuracy lacks empiric support. Recent small-angle x-ray scattering (SAXS) data suggest an alternative model for the interaction of substrates, chaperones, and the ATPase. Complexes of the *Salmonella* effector-chaperone pair SopB-SigE are able to hexamerize in a concentration dependent manner with dimensions comparable to the hexameric models of the ATPase (114). While it is too early to say whether other chaperone-effector complexes can oligomerize (115), whether these oligomers can interact with SctN, or whether such interactions—even if possible—are physiologically relevant, these results raise the possibility of alternative ATPase-cargo stoichiometries.

Recent solution NMR analyses suggest an interesting role for chaperone structure in the targeting of substrates to the T3SS. In solution, the *E. coli* chaperone CesAB is a partially folded molten globule (116) that does not interact with the hexameric SctN (117). However, upon binding to its substrate—the EspA tip filament protein—CesAB becomes fully structured and is able to bind SctN (117). The binding site for SctN was mapped onto the CesAB-EspA heterodimer, where it covered regions of CesAB unstructured in the absence of substrate (117). Consistent with the hypothesis that substrate-induced folding of the chaperone allows for targeting to the ATPase, a mutation-stabilized, structured CesAB homodimer was able to bind SctN in the absence of substrate (117). While it remains to be determined whether similar disorder-to-order transitions effect SctN binding for other chaperone classes, these

results are consistent with the role of chaperone-substrate interactions in targeting substrates for secretion. Additionally, the observation that substrate-chaperone complexes are recognized by hexameric SctN, but not its amino-terminally truncated monomeric form, suggests that ATPase hexamerization is critical for both hydrolytic catalysis and substrate recognition (117).

The Sorting Platform

Located at the peripheral cytoplasmic face of the flagellar basal body is a ring of robust density in EM reconstructions (109). Known as the "C-ring," this annulus is composed of the flagellar proteins FliM, FliN, and FliG, and it plays a role in flagellar motor function (torque generation) and rotational switching (20). FliM and FliN have an injectisome homologue with some conserved domains (SctQ), but torque generation by the injectisome is controversial (118), and a robust C-ring is absent in tomographic reconstructions of the injectisome basal body (29, 109). However, immuno-EM analysis of purified *Shigella* injectisomes shows localization of SctQ to the cytoplasmic face (119), suggesting that it plays some role in protein secretion or the regulation of the secretory process. Indeed, recent cryo-electron tomographic analyses of the *Shigella* injectisome have identified six SctQ-dependent "pods" of density proximal to the cytoplasmic face of the basal body, forming a structure distinct from that of the flagellar C-ring (120).

Seminal biochemical and genetics work by Galan and colleagues revealed that SctQ forms a critical "sorting platform" for the T3SS (121). Affinity purification of SctQ from secretion-competent *Salmonella* produces high-molecular-weight complexes containing the SctN ATPase, regulatory proteins, chaperones, and secretion substrates (121). Most notably, the sorting platform plays a role in the hierarchical secretion of substrates, queuing substrates in their appropriate order. For example, in *Salmonella* with assembled injectisomes, the sorting platform is predominantly occupied by translocon proteins, but genomic deletion of the translocators allows the next tier of substrates (effector proteins) to access the sorting platform (121).

In addition to SctQ, formation of the sorting platform requires the proteins SctK and SctL (121). While the role of SctK is at present unclear, biochemical analyses of the flagellar apparatus shed light on the potential function of SctL. SctL is a homologue of the flagellar protein FliH (Table 1). The SctL/FliH family is predicted to have a conserved domain architecture: an amino-terminal disordered region is followed by a coiled-coil and then a mixed α/β domain (122). The carboxy-terminus of FliH interacts with the amino-terminal oligomerization domain of FliI (122), inhibiting its ATPase activity (123). While sequence similarities between the FliH carboxy-terminal domain and the F-type ATPase δ-subunit suggest a role for FliH as a "stator" (124), it is not obvious that FliH interacts with oligomeric FliI, and the structural details of this interaction are not yet known. The amino-terminus of FliH interacts with FliN (125), and this FliH-FliN interaction is important (126)—if not absolutely necessary (127)—for the recruitment of FliI to the export apparatus. Given that the homologous injectisome complex (SctQ-SctL-SctN) forms a portion of the sorting platform and that chaperone-substrate complexes interact with the ATPase, these data suggest that one function of the SctQ sorting platform could be to localize chaperone-effector-ATPase complexes to the injectisome export apparatus. Indeed, Minamino, Namba, and colleagues have hypothesized that the FliI ATPase exists in two forms: an ATP-hydrolyzing hexamer and a dynamic substrate-carrying monomer bound to FliH and the C-ring (128). Similarly, SctQ-injectisome interactions are dynamic in *Yersinia*, because injectisome-associated SctQ exchanges with a cytoplasmic pool with a half-time of approximately 1 minute (129).

Structural models of SctQ are a work in progress and have focused to date on the carboxy-terminus of the molecule. In *Pseudomonas syringae*, SctQ is spread over two open reading frames (*hrcQA* and *hrcQB*), much like FliM and FliN in the flagellar system. The structure of the carboxy-terminal domain of HrcQB is quite similar to that of the carboxy-terminal domain of FliN (130, 131); both domains are homodimers of the "surface presentation of antigens" (SpoA) fold. The folded core of each protomer is an antiparallel β-sheet, and a loop from each protomer containing a β-strand and α-helix wraps around the β-sheet core of the other protomer. In *Yersinia*, SctQ is the product of a single open reading frame (as in most injectisomes), but the carboxy-terminal SpoA domain is duplicitously translated from an internal translation start site (132). The homodimer produced by this translation product is able to interact with full-length SctQ and, at least in the *Yersinia* system, is necessary for secretion *in vivo*. In both the flagellar (133, 134) and injectisome (135) systems, this SpoA domain tetramerizes as a dimer of dimers but appears to do so in different orientations in each system. Cross-linking analyses suggest that the FliN SpoA tetramers form a "doughnut" at the base of the C-ring (133), but high-resolution support for this arrangement is lacking.

Despite the progress that has been made, numerous structural questions remain unanswered for the SctQ sorting platform. The function of the SpoA domain is unclear, SctQ-SctQ(SpoA) interactions have yet to be structurally characterized, and the structural basis for the interaction of SctL with SctQ has not yet been determined. Moreover, while the amino-terminal domains of FliM have well-characterized functions in the regulation of flagellar rotation switching (136, 137), these motor functions are likely flagella-specific and involve interactions with partners not conserved from the flagellar apparatus to the injectisome (e.g., FliG, CheY). Thus, the function of the SctQ amino-terminus is also unclear. Lastly, how and when SctQ or its soluble interaction partners interface with the basal body or export apparatus remains to be determined.

Substrate Switching

T3SS substrates are secreted in a defined order that is necessary for the proper assembly and function of the system (138, 139): secretion of the needle filament (SctF) and inner rod (SctI) is followed by secretion of the needle tip protein and translocon pore proteins, which is followed by the secretion of effector proteins. Thus, it seems that there are several sequential substrate "switching" events that must occur for the hierarchical secretion of substrates to be maintained (139).

The first such switching event halts the extension of the growing needle filament upon completion of the inner rod and allows for secretion of the needle tip protein and translocators. As discussed above, the length of the needle filament is controlled by the assembly of the inner rod in an SctP-dependent fashion (52, 66). Full deletion of *sctP* locks the T3SS into a mode of exclusive SctF filament secretion; that is, deletion of *sctP* results not only in elongate needles, but in a lack of translocon and effector secretion (63, 65, 140, 141). Indeed, deletion of *sctP* results in the absence of translocon components from the SctQ sorting platform (121). However, small deletions in the amino-terminal regions of SctP alter needle length without compromising translocon secretion, suggesting that some portion of SctP performs a crucial switching function (141). Deletions within the conserved mixed α/β region at the carboxy-terminus of the protein compromise translocon secretion (in addition to disrupting needle length regulation), and this presumptive domain has been termed the "type III secretion substrate specificity switch" (T3S4) domain (141).

The three-dimensional structure of an injectisome T3S4 domain has not yet been determined, but the flagellar FliK T3S4 domain has been solved by NMR (142). The carboxy-terminal domain of FliK possesses two α-helices folded against a four-strand β-sheet (142), and the predicted structural conservation of these secondary structural elements in SctP suggests that this model may be generalizable to the injectisome. While it is still unclear at the molecular level how SctP functions to promote specificity switching, its interaction partners suggest some viable hypotheses. For example, the SctP T3S4 domain interacts with the SctO protein (143), suggesting that it may be able to transmit regulatory information to the SctN ATPase or the SctV export gate. Moreover, the T3S4 domain interacts with the cytoplasmic autoprotease domain of SctU (144). Like SctP, SctU regulates the secretion of the inner rod protein (145). The interaction between these two proteins is intriguing given that SctU interacts with components of the SctQ sorting platform and the SctV export apparatus (146), again suggesting mechanisms for the relay of switching information throughout the secretory apparatus.

The second major switching event distinguishes between translocon components and effector proteins (121). Deletion of translocon components allows for the localization of effector proteins to the sorting platform, consistent with a model where a gradient of substrate and/or chaperone affinities for the sorting platform controls the hierarchy of secretion (121). The identification of several classes of secretion apparatus mutants that can secrete effectors but not translocon proteins offers some insights into the establishment of secretion hierarchy. Deletion of *sctW* in *Salmonella* results in the specific loss of translocon component secretion (138). SctW binds the translocon proteins and their chaperone in *Salmonella* (SicA) (138), and it is necessary for translocator binding to the SctQ sorting platform (121). These observations are consistent with SctW enhancing the affinity of translocon-containing complexes for the sorting platform. However, recent genetics data suggest the mechanism of hierarchy control for SctW may be more complex. A subset of the SctI alanine mutants identified by Lefebre and Galan (66) have normal needle lengths but phenocopy *sctW* deletion, and an interaction between SctW and SctI was recently reported in *Shigella* (147). Together, these data raise the possibility of SctW binding not only the sorting platform but also portions of the basal body.

Further clouding the role of SctW in the T3SS is the observation of species-specific effects of *sctW* mutation. In *Yersinia* and *Shigella*, SctW is secreted and *sctW* deletion does not specifically impair translocon protein secretion (148, 149). Moreover, the *Yersinia* SctW protein pair YopN/TyeA is part of a complex calcium response apparatus in the bacterial cytosol (150) that involves several *Yersinia*-specific proteins (151, 152). While the structures of the *Shigella* and *Yersinia* SctW homologues have been determined (153, 154), a fuller understanding of SctW function (and its species-specific nuances) will require structural characterization in complex with other injectisome components.

In addition to its role in the first switching event, SctU is also involved in the second switch. The cytoplasmic domain of the SctU family autocatalyzes cleavage between the asparagine and proline residues of its conserved asparagine-proline-threonine-histidine (NPTH) motif cleavage site (139). Alanine mutations on either side of the cleavage site cause aberrant specificity switching: translocon proteins are no longer secreted, but effector secretion remains intact (50, 148). An amphipathic linker connects the SctU transmembrane region to the cytoplasmic autoprotease, and this linker undergoes a disorder-to-order transition in the presence of anionic lipids (155). Introducing charge-altering mutations in the linker impaired T3SS function, suggesting that the ordering of the SctU linker against the bacterial inner membrane is crucial, perhaps favorably orienting the autoprotease domain for interactions with other

members of the export apparatus (155). As mentioned above, SctU interacts with multiple members of the sorting platform, but the bases for these interactions—and the mechanisms by which they would effect specificity switching—are unclear.

Control of Secretion

The T3SS can assemble a basal body, needle, and tip and then pause in a "primed" state until the relevant stimulus arrives and secretion resumes. This strategy prevents the wanton waste of translocon and effector proteins. Exploring this additional level of complexity is important to our full understanding of the pathobiology of the T3SS and may suggest routes to antivirulence compounds that prevent the activation of otherwise structurally competent injectisomes.

Bile salts play a regulatory role in the T3SSs used by several enteric pathogens. The interaction of bile salts with the *Shigella* tip complex promotes IpaB recruitment to the tip, forming the heteropentameric tip complex described above (76, 156). In contrast, bile salts suppress *Salmonella* SPI-1 T3SS function (157). These observations provide an intriguing correlation between host gastrointestinal physiology and pathogen virulence that ties environmental factors to the species-specific adaptation of the T3SS. Despite reports describing the interaction of bile salts with monomeric *Shigella* IpaD (158) and *Salmonella* SipD (75, 159), the structural basis for bile salt interaction with the intact tip complex has yet to be determined in either species, so the mechanism of its regulatory activity remains unclear.

Contact with host cells stimulates the activation of the T3SS in several species (160–162). In *Salmonella*, contact with target cells stimulates the secretion of the translocon proteins SipB and SipC (163), and in *Shigella*, interaction of the IpaD-IpaB tip with liposomes resembling host cell membranes induces IpaC secretion (164). It is tempting to speculate that contact of the needle tip with the host cell sends a mechanical signal to the basal body and/or export apparatus that reinitiates secretion (6, 19, 165). As the connecting factor between the host cell surface and the basal body, the needle filament itself is a promising candidate for force transduction. Specific needle filament protein mutations can trap the *Shigella* T3SS in a constitutively active secretion mode, and one might hypothesize that these mutations stabilize needle filaments in a postcontact activated conformation (166). However, the filaments formed by these mutants do not exhibit the gross conformational changes one might expect if the needle filament architecture were transducing this signal (166). Alternatively, local changes in the tip environment may permit the secretion of substrates trapped within the needle by a closed tip, restarting secretion without requiring signal transduction to the bacterial cytoplasm or basal body (165).

Work with the *Salmonella* SPI-2 T3SS suggests a tantalizing third (and nonmutually exclusive) possibility, that the needle is not only a conduit for protein secretion, but a passageway for the diffusion of chemical signals (167). *Salmonella* makes use of two T3SSs: broadly, the SPI-1 T3SS promotes cell invasion, and subsequently, the SPI-2 T3SS facilitates the formation of the *Salmonella*-containing vacuole, an intracellular environment for *Salmonella* survival and replication (168). Holden and colleagues noted that priming of the SPI-2 T3SS requires exposure of the bacteria to low pH (as would be experienced in the endosomal compartment) but that triggering of effector secretion required a return to neutral pH (167). It is noteworthy that the SPI-2 SctW protein was required for this transition (167), consistent with the apparent role of SctW in translocon-to-effector specificity switching in other systems (above). However, it is most intriguing that this switch required intact translocon components, suggesting that the neutral pH signal may be transduced from the host cell cytosol, through the translocon and needle, to the basal body and/or export apparatus (167).

In light of these findings from *Salmonella* SPI-2, one wonders whether the needle conduit could serve as a channel for other small molecule signals from the host cytosol: perhaps the needle of *Yersinia* spp. transmits the decreased calcium ion concentration of the eukaryotic cytosol, resulting in T3SS reactivation. Intriguingly, Plano and colleagues have shown that point mutations in the *Yersinia* needle filament protein result in calcium-independent, constitutive T3SS (169); however, the mechanism of this altered calcium response is unclear. One might hypothesize that these mutant needles are unable to associate with tip or translocator proteins, preventing access to—and transmission of—the low-calcium environment of the host cytosol. Consistent with this hypothesis, a subset of the constitutively secreting mutants were deficient in delivery of T3SS substrates to the host (169). Alternatively, extracellular calcium might regulate T3SS by altering the conformation of the needle filament protein (akin to the aforementioned force transduction hypothesis), and these mutants might simply be unable to assume some putative calcium-dependent conformations.

FUTURE PROSPECTS

In the past 20 years, our models of T3SS structure and function have evolved substantially, from the first visualization of the injectisome architecture to the high-resolution structural interrogation of many of its individual components. Combining these insights with a plethora of genetic and biochemical data, the molecular mechanics of this astounding secretory nanomachine are coming into focus. However, numerous questions remain—the answers to which are critical to our understanding of bacterial virulence, the design of new therapeutics, and the imaginative re-engineering of the system.

Despite the improvements in cryo-EM models of the injectisome, the precise architecture of the membrane-embedded components of the T3SS is still unclear, as is the structural basis for their interactions with the soluble components of the system. The native structures of the filament-bound needle tip and the translocon in the host membrane must be determined to understand how the extracellular environment regulates secretion, how proteins penetrate to the host cytosol, and how to rationally design secretion-blocking vaccines. Although the constituents of the cytoplasmic sorting platform have been identified, the structural bases for their interactions are unknown: how the sorting platform assembles, how substrate-chaperone complexes engage the system, and how the numerous regulatory elements interact to govern a secretory hierarchy all remain to be determined.

Answering these questions is likely to require a hybrid approach, characterizing local interactions and large assemblies alike, and employing a range of structural and molecular techniques. However, it is clear that high-resolution models of intact macromolecular assemblies (e.g., basal body, needle tip, translocon pore) would greatly advance the field. Much like the role that atomic models of the ribosome have played in the interrogation of its multiple functional states, one can imagine the watershed of insight that would come from successful visualization of the injectisome or sorting platform in each of their several forms: needle-assembling, translocator-secreting, and effector-secreting. Ideally, these mechanistic insights will allow the uncoupling of some pathogenic Gram-negative bacteria from virulence and the re-engineering of the nanosyringe for the benefit of biotechnology.

ACKNOWLEDGMENTS

Work in the laboratory of C.E.S. is funded in part by the NIH and research funds from the Rockefeller University. R.Q.N. was supported by the Hearst Foundation and by a Medical Scientist Training Program grant from the National Institute of General Medical Sciences of the National Institutes of Health under award number T32GM07739 to the Weill Cornell/Rockefeller/Sloan-Kettering Tri-Institutional MD-PhD Program.

CITATION

Notti RQ, Stebbins CE. 2016. The structure and function of type III secretion systems. Microbiol Spectrum 4(1):VMBF-0004-2015.

REFERENCES

1. **Galan JE, Collmer A.** 1999. Type III secretion machines: bacterial devices for protein delivery into host cells. *Science* **284**:1322–1328.
2. **Gauthier A, Thomas NA, Finlay BB.** 2003. Bacterial injection machines. *J Biol Chem* **278**:25273–25276.
3. **Galan JE, Curtiss R 3rd.** 1989. Cloning and molecular characterization of genes whose products allow *Salmonella typhimurium* to penetrate tissue culture cells. *Proc Natl Acad Sci USA* **86**:6383–6387.
4. **Michiels T, Wattiau P, Brasseur R, Ruysschaert JM, Cornelis G.** 1990. Secretion of Yop proteins by *Yersiniae. Infect Immun* **58**:2840–2849.
5. **Michiels T, Vanooteghem JC, Lambert de Rouvroit C, China B, Gustin A, Boudry P, Cornelis GR.** 1991. Analysis of virC, an operon involved in the secretion of Yop proteins by *Yersinia enterocolitica. J Bacteriol* **173**:4994–5009.
6. **Galan JE, Wolf-Watz H.** 2006. Protein delivery into eukaryotic cells by type III secretion machines. *Nature* **444**:567–573.
7. **Cornelis GR.** 2002. *Yersinia* type III secretion: send in the effectors. *J Cell Biol* **158**:401–408.
8. **Francis MS, Wolf-Watz H, Forsberg A.** 2002. Regulation of type III secretion systems. *Curr Opin Microbiol* **5**:166–172.
9. **Waterman SR, Holden DW.** 2003. Functions and effectors of the *Salmonella* pathogenicity island 2 type III secretion system. *Cell Microbiol* **5**:501–511.
10. **Stebbins CE.** 2004. Structural insights into bacterial modulation of the host cytoskeleton. *Curr Opin Struct Biol* **14**:731–740.
11. **Yahr TL, Wolfgang MC.** 2006. Transcriptional regulation of the *Pseudomonas aeruginosa* type III secretion system. *Mol Microbiol* **62**:631–640.

12. **Bhavsar AP, Guttman JA, Finlay BB.** 2007. Manipulation of host-cell pathways by bacterial pathogens. *Nature* **449:**827–834.

13. **Ellermeier JR, Slauch JM.** 2007. Adaptation to the host environment: regulation of the SPI1 type III secretion system in *Salmonella enterica* serovar Typhimurium. *Curr Opin Microbiol* **10:**24–29.

14. **Galan JE.** 2007. SnapShot: effector proteins of type III secretion systems. *Cell* **130:**192.

15. **Buttner D.** 2012. Protein export according to schedule: architecture, assembly, and regulation of type III secretion systems from plant- and animal-pathogenic bacteria. *Microbiol Mol Biol Rev* **76:**262–310.

16. **Burkinshaw BJ, Strynadka NC.** 2014. Assembly and structure of the T3SS. *Biochim Biophys Acta* **1843:**1649–1663.

17. **Hueck CJ.** 1998. Type III protein secretion systems in bacterial pathogens of animals and plants. *Microbiol Mol Biol Rev* **62:**379–433.

18. **Abrusci P, McDowell MA, Lea SM, Johnson S.** 2014. Building a secreting nanomachine: a structural overview of the T3SS. *Curr Opin Struct Biol* **25:**111–117.

19. **Galan JE, Lara-Tejero M, Marlovits TC, Wagner S.** 2014. Bacterial type III secretion systems: specialized nanomachines for protein delivery into target cells. *Annu Rev Microbiol* **68:**415–438.

20. **Macnab RM.** 2003. How bacteria assemble flagella. *Annu Rev Microbiol* **57:**77–100.

21. **Gophna U, Ron EZ, Graur D.** 2003. Bacterial type III secretion systems are ancient and evolved by multiple horizontal-transfer events. *Gene* **312:**151–163.

22. **Kubori T, Matsushima Y, Nakamura D, Uralil J, Lara-Tejero M, Sukhan A, Galan JE, Aizawa SI.** 1998. Supramolecular structure of the *Salmonella typhimurium* type III protein secretion system. *Science* **280:**602–605.

23. **Blocker A, Jouihri N, Larquet E, Gounon P, Ebel F, Parsot C, Sansonetti P, Allaoui A.** 2001. Structure and composition of the *Shigella flexneri* "needle complex", a part of its type III secreton. *Mol Microbiol* **39:**652–663.

24. **Schlumberger MC, Muller AJ, Ehrbar K, Winnen B, Duss I, Stecher B, Hardt WD.** 2005. Real-time imaging of type III secretion: *Salmonella* SipA injection into host cells. *Proc Natl Acad Sci USA* **102:**12548–12553.

25. **Van Engelenburg SB, Palmer AE.** 2010. Imaging type-III secretion reveals dynamics and spatial segregation of *Salmonella* effectors. *Nat Methods* **7:**325–330.

26. **Marlovits TC, Kubori T, Sukhan A, Thomas DR, Galan JE, Unger VM.** 2004. Structural insights into the assembly of the type III secretion needle complex. *Science* **306:**1040–1042.

27. **Schraidt O, Marlovits TC.** 2011. Three-dimensional model of *Salmonella*'s needle complex at subnanometer resolution. *Science* **331:**1192–1195.

28. **Hodgkinson JL, Horsley A, Stabat D, Simon M, Johnson S, da Fonseca PC, Morris EP, Wall JS, Lea SM, Blocker AJ.** 2009. Three-dimensional reconstruction of the *Shigella* T3SS transmembrane regions reveals 12-fold symmetry and novel features throughout. *Nat Struct Mol Biol* **16:**477–485.

29. **Kudryashev M, Stenta M, Schmelz S, Amstutz M, Wiesand U, Castano-Diez D, Degiacomi MT, Munnich S, Bleck CK, Kowal J, Diepold A, Heinz DW, Dal Peraro M, Cornelis GR, Stahlberg H.** 2013. *In situ* structural analysis of the *Yersinia enterocolitica* injectisome. *Elife* **2:**e00792. doi:10.7554/eLife.00792.

30. **Kowal J, Chami M, Ringler P, Muller SA, Kudryashev M, Castano-Diez D, Amstutz M, Cornelis GR, Stahlberg H, Engel A.** 2013. Structure of the dodecameric *Yersinia enterocolitica* secretin YscC and its trypsin-resistant core. *Structure* **21:**2152–2161.

31. **Kaniga K, Bossio JC, Galan JE.** 1994. The *Salmonella typhimurium* invasion genes invF and invG encode homologues of the AraC and PulD family of proteins. *Mol Microbiol* **13:**555–568.

32. **Crago AM, Koronakis V.** 1998. *Salmonella* InvG forms a ring-like multimer that requires the InvH lipoprotein for outer membrane localization. *Mol Microbiol* **30:**47–56.

33. **Daefler S, Russel M.** 1998. The *Salmonella typhimurium* InvH protein is an outer membrane lipoprotein required for the proper localization of InvG. *Mol Microbiol* **28:**1367–1380.

34. **Burghout P, Beckers F, de Wit E, van Boxtel R, Cornelis GR, Tommassen J, Koster M.** 2004. Role of the pilot protein YscW in the biogenesis of the YscC secretin in *Yersinia enterocolitica. J Bacteriol* **186:**5366–5375.

35. **Spreter T, Yip CK, Sanowar S, Andre I, Kimbrough TG, Vuckovic M, Pfuetzner RA, Deng W, Yu AC, Finlay BB, Baker D, Miller SI, Strynadka NC.** 2009. A conserved structural motif mediates formation of the periplasmic rings in the type III secretion system. *Nat Struct Mol Biol* **16:**468–476.

36. **Sanowar S, Singh P, Pfuetzner RA, Andre I, Zheng H, Spreter T, Strynadka NC, Gonen T, Baker D, Goodlett DR, Miller SI.** 2010. Interactions of the transmembrane polymeric rings of the *Salmonella enterica* serovar

Typhimurium type III secretion system. *MBio* 1:e00158-10. doi:10.1128/mBio.00158-10.

37. **Schraidt O, Lefebre MD, Brunner MJ, Schmied WH, Schmidt A, Radics J, Mechtler K, Galan JE, Marlovits TC.** 2010. Topology and organization of the *Salmonella typhimurium* type III secretion needle complex components. *PLoS Pathog* 6:e1000824. doi:10.1371/journal.ppat.1000824.

38. **Yip CK, Kimbrough TG, Felise HB, Vuckovic M, Thomas NA, Pfuetzner RA, Frey EA, Finlay BB, Miller SI, Strynadka NC.** 2005. Structural characterization of the molecular platform for type III secretion system assembly. *Nature* 435:702–707.

39. **Marlovits TC, Stebbins CE.** 2010. Type III secretion systems shape up as they ship out. *Curr Opin Microbiol* 13:47–52.

40. **Bergeron JR, Worrall LJ, De S, Sgourakis NG, Cheung AH, Lameignere E, Okon M, Wasney GA, Baker D, McIntosh LP, Strynadka NC.** 2015. The modular structure of the inner-membrane ring component PrgK facilitates assembly of the type III secretion system basal body. *Structure* 23:161–172.

41. **McDowell MA, Johnson S, Deane JE, Cheung M, Roehrich AD, Blocker AJ, McDonnell JM, Lea SM.** 2011. Structural and functional studies on the N-terminal domain of the *Shigella* type III secretion protein MxiG. *J Biol Chem* 286:30606–30614.

42. **Barison N, Lambers J, Hurwitz R, Kolbe M.** 2012. Interaction of MxiG with the cytosolic complex of the type III secretion system controls *Shigella* virulence. *FASEB J* 26:1717–1726.

43. **Gamez A, Mukerjea R, Alayyoubi M, Ghassemian M, Ghosh P.** 2012. Structure and interactions of the cytoplasmic domain of the Yersinia type III secretion protein YscD. *J Bacteriol* 194:5949–5958.

44. **Lountos GT, Tropea JE, Waugh DS.** 2012. Structure of the cytoplasmic domain of *Yersinia pestis* YscD, an essential component of the type III secretion system. *Acta Crystallogr D Biol Crystallogr* 68:201–209.

45. **Zhong D, Lefebre M, Kaur K, McDowell MA, Gdowski C, Jo S, Wang Y, Benedict SH, Lea SM, Galan JE, De Guzman RN.** 2012. The *Salmonella* type III secretion system inner rod protein PrgJ is partially folded. *J Biol Chem* 287:25303–25311.

46. **Bergeron JR, Worrall LJ, Sgourakis NG, DiMaio F, Pfuetzner RA, Felise HB, Vuckovic M, Yu AC, Miller SI, Baker D, Strynadka NC.** 2013. A refined model of the prototypical *Salmonella* SPI-1 T3SS basal body reveals the molecular basis for its assembly. *PLoS Pathog* 9:e1003307. doi:10.1371/journal.ppat.1003307.

47. **Lilic M, Quezada CM, Stebbins CE.** 2010. A conserved domain in type III secretion links the cytoplasmic domain of InvA to elements of the basal body. *Acta Crystallogr D Biol Crystallogr* 66:709–713.

48. **Worrall LJ, Vuckovic M, Strynadka NC.** 2010. Crystal structure of the C-terminal domain of the *Salmonella* type III secretion system export apparatus protein InvA. *Protein Sci* 19:1091–1096.

49. **Abrusci P, Vergara-Irigaray M, Johnson S, Beeby MD, Hendrixson DR, Roversi P, Friede ME, Deane JE, Jensen GJ, Tang CM, Lea SM.** 2013. Architecture of the major component of the type III secretion system export apparatus. *Nat Struct Mol Biol* 20:99–104.

50. **Zarivach R, Deng W, Vuckovic M, Felise HB, Nguyen HV, Miller SI, Finlay BB, Strynadka NC.** 2008. Structural analysis of the essential self-cleaving type III secretion proteins EscU and SpaS. *Nature* 453:124–127.

51. **Wagner S, Konigsmaier L, Lara-Tejero M, Lefebre M, Marlovits TC, Galan JE.** 2010. Organization and coordinated assembly of the type III secretion export apparatus. *Proc Natl Acad Sci USA* 107:17745–17750.

52. **Marlovits TC, Kubori T, Lara-Tejero M, Thomas D, Unger VM, Galan JE.** 2006. Assembly of the inner rod determines needle length in the type III secretion injectisome. *Nature* 441:637–640.

53. **Loquet A, Sgourakis NG, Gupta R, Giller K, Riedel D, Goosmann C, Griesinger C, Kolbe M, Baker D, Becker S, Lange A.** 2012. Atomic model of the type III secretion system needle. *Nature* 486:276–279.

54. **Edgren T, Forsberg A, Rosqvist R, Wolf-Watz H.** 2012. Type III secretion in *Yersinia*: injectisome or not? *PLoS Pathog* 8:e1002669. doi:10.1371/journal.ppat.1002669.

55. **Radics J, Konigsmaier L, Marlovits TC.** 2014. Structure of a pathogenic type 3 secretion system in action. *Nat Struct Mol Biol* 21:82–87.

56. **Dohlich K, Zumsteg AB, Goosmann C, Kolbe M.** 2014. A substrate-fusion protein is trapped inside the type III secretion system channel in *Shigella flexneri*. *PLoS Pathog* 10:e1003881. doi:10.1371/journal.ppat.1003881.

57. **Deane JE, Roversi P, Cordes FS, Johnson S, Kenjale R, Daniell S, Booy F, Picking WD, Picking WL, Blocker AJ, Lea SM.** 2006. Molecular model of a type III secretion system needle: implications for host-cell sensing. *Proc Natl Acad Sci USA* 103:12529–12533.

58. **Cordes FS, Komoriya K, Larquet E, Yang S, Egelman EH, Blocker A, Lea SM.** 2003. Helical structure of the needle of the type III

secretion system of *Shigella flexneri*. *J Biol Chem* **278:**17103–17107.

59. **Poyraz O, Schmidt H, Seidel K, Delissen F, Ader C, Tenenboim H, Goosmann C, Laube B, Thunemann AF, Zychlinsky A, Baldus M, Lange A, Griesinger C, Kolbe M.** 2010. Protein refolding is required for assembly of the type three secretion needle. *Nat Struct Mol Biol* **17:**788–792.

60. **Demers JP, Habenstein B, Loquet A, Kumar Vasa S, Giller K, Becker S, Baker D, Lange A, Sgourakis NG.** 2014. High-resolution structure of the *Shigella* type-III secretion needle by solid-state NMR and cryo-electron microscopy. *Nat Commun* **5:**4976. doi:10.1038/ncomms5976.

61. **Fujii T, Cheung M, Blanco A, Kato T, Blocker AJ, Namba K.** 2012. Structure of a type III secretion needle at 7-A resolution provides insights into its assembly and signaling mechanisms. *Proc Natl Acad Sci USA* **109:**4461–4466.

62. **Mota LJ, Journet L, Sorg I, Agrain C, Cornelis GR.** 2005. Bacterial injectisomes: needle length does matter. *Science* **307:**1278.

63. **Kubori T, Sukhan A, Aizawa SI, Galan JE.** 2000. Molecular characterization and assembly of the needle complex of the *Salmonella typhimurium* type III protein secretion system. *Proc Natl Acad Sci USA* **97:**10225–10230.

64. **Tamano K, Katayama E, Toyotome T, Sasakawa C.** 2002. *Shigella* Spa32 is an essential secretory protein for functional type III secretion machinery and uniformity of its needle length. *J Bacteriol* **184:**1244–1252.

65. **Journet L, Agrain C, Broz P, Cornelis GR.** 2003. The needle length of bacterial injectisomes is determined by a molecular ruler. *Science* **302:**1757–1760.

66. **Lefebre MD, Galan JE.** 2014. The inner rod protein controls substrate switching and needle length in a *Salmonella* type III secretion system. *Proc Natl Acad Sci USA* **111:**817–822.

67. **Mueller CA, Broz P, Muller SA, Ringler P, Erne-Brand F, Sorg I, Kuhn M, Engel A, Cornelis GR.** 2005. The V-antigen of *Yersinia* forms a distinct structure at the tip of injectisome needles. *Science* **310:**674–676.

68. **Epler CR, Dickenson NE, Bullitt E, Picking WL.** 2012. Ultrastructural analysis of IpaD at the tip of the nascent MxiH type III secretion apparatus of *Shigella flexneri*. *J Mol Biol* **420:**29–39.

69. **Goure J, Broz P, Attree O, Cornelis GR, Attree I.** 2005. Protective anti-V antibodies inhibit *Pseudomonas* and *Yersinia* translocon assembly within host membranes. *J Infect Dis* **192:**218–225.

70. **Mueller CA, Broz P, Cornelis GR.** 2008. The type III secretion system tip complex and translocon. *Mol Microbiol* **68:**1085–1095.

71. **Lawton WD, Surgalla MJ.** 1963. Immunization against plague by a specific fraction of *Pasteurella pseudotuberculosis*. *J Infect Dis* **113:**39–42.

72. **DiGiandomenico A, Keller AE, Gao C, Rainey GJ, Warrener P, Camara MM, Bonnell J, Fleming R, Bezabeh B, Dimasi N, Sellman BR, Hilliard J, Guenther CM, Datta V, Zhao W, Gao C, Yu XQ, Suzich JA, Stover CK.** 2014. A multifunctional bispecific antibody protects against *Pseudomonas aeruginosa*. *Sci Transl Med* **6:**262ra155.

73. **Derewenda U, Mateja A, Devedjiev Y, Routzahn KM, Evdokimov AG, Derewenda ZS, Waugh DS.** 2004. The structure of *Yersinia pestis* V-antigen, an essential virulence factor and mediator of immunity against plague. *Structure* **12:**301–306.

74. **Johnson S, Roversi P, Espina M, Olive A, Deane JE, Birket S, Field T, Picking WD, Blocker AJ, Galyov EE, Picking WL, Lea SM.** 2007. Self-chaperoning of the type III secretion system needle tip proteins IpaD and BipD. *J Biol Chem* **282:**4035–4044.

75. **Lunelli M, Hurwitz R, Lambers J, Kolbe M.** 2011. Crystal structure of PrgI-SipD: insight into a secretion competent state of the type three secretion system needle tip and its interaction with host ligands. *PLoS Pathog* **7:**e1002163. doi:10.1371/journal.ppat.1002163.

76. **Cheung M, Shen DK, Makino F, Kato T, Roehrich AD, Martinez-Argudo I, Walker ML, Murillo I, Liu X, Pain M, Brown J, Frazer G, Mantell J, Mina P, Todd T, Sessions RB, Namba K, Blocker AJ.** 2015. Three-dimensional electron microscopy reconstruction and cysteine-mediated crosslinking provide a model of the type III secretion system needle tip complex. *Mol Microbiol* **95:**31–50.

77. **Rathinavelan T, Lara-Tejero M, Lefebre M, Chatterjee S, McShan AC, Guo DC, Tang C, Galan JE, De Guzman RN.** 2014. NMR model of PrgI-SipD interaction and its implications in the needle-tip assembly of the *Salmonella* type III secretion system. *J Mol Biol* **426:**2958–2969.

78. **Knutton S, Rosenshine I, Pallen MJ, Nisan I, Neves BC, Bain C, Wolff C, Dougan G, Frankel G.** 1998. A novel EspA-associated surface organelle of enteropathogenic *Escherichia coli* involved in protein translocation into epithelial cells. *EMBO J* **17:**2166–2176.

79. **Daniell SJ, Kocsis E, Morris E, Knutton S, Booy FP, Frankel G.** 2003. 3D structure of EspA filaments from enteropathogenic *Escherichia coli*. *Mol Microbiol* **49:**301–308.

80. **Picking WL, Nishioka H, Hearn PD, Baxter MA, Harrington AT, Blocker A, Picking WD.** 2005. IpaD of *Shigella flexneri* is independently required for regulation of Ipa protein secretion and efficient insertion of IpaB and IpaC into host membranes. *Infect Immun* **73:**1432–1440.

81. **Barta ML, Dickenson NE, Patil M, Keightley A, Wyckoff GJ, Picking WD, Picking WL, Geisbrecht BV.** 2012. The structures of coiled-coil domains from type III secretion system translocators reveal homology to pore-forming toxins. *J Mol Biol* **417:**395–405.

82. **Mizusaki H, Takaya A, Yamamoto T, Aizawa S.** 2008. Signal pathway in salt-activated expression of the *Salmonella* pathogenicity island 1 type III secretion system in *Salmonella enterica* serovar Typhimurium. *J Bacteriol* **190:**4624–4631.

83. **Arnold R, Brandmaier S, Kleine F, Tischler P, Heinz E, Behrens S, Niinikoski A, Mewes HW, Horn M, Rattei T.** 2009. Sequence-based prediction of type III secreted proteins. *PLoS Pathog* **5:**e1000376. doi:10.1371/journal.ppat.1000376.

84. **Samudrala R, Heffron F, McDermott JE.** 2009. Accurate prediction of secreted substrates and identification of a conserved putative secretion signal for type III secretion systems. *PLoS Pathog* **5:**e1000375. doi:10.1371/journal.ppat.1000375.

85. **McDermott JE, Corrigan A, Peterson E, Oehmen C, Niemann G, Cambronne ED, Sharp D, Adkins JN, Samudrala R, Heffron F.** 2011. Computational prediction of type III and IV secreted effectors in Gram-negative bacteria. *Infect Immun* **79:**23–32.

86. **Lloyd SA, Norman M, Rosqvist R, Wolf-Watz H.** 2001. *Yersinia* YopE is targeted for type III secretion by N-terminal, not mRNA, signals. *Mol Microbiol* **39:**520–531.

87. **Lee SH, Galan JE.** 2004. *Salmonella* type III secretion-associated chaperones confer secretion-pathway specificity. *Mol Microbiol* **51:**483–495.

88. **Stebbins CE, Galan JE.** 2001. Maintenance of an unfolded polypeptide by a cognate chaperone in bacterial type III secretion. *Nature* **414:**77–81.

89. **Stebbins CE, Galan JE.** 2003. Priming virulence factors for delivery into the host. *Nat Rev Mol Cell Biol* **4:**738–743.

90. **Izore T, Job V, Dessen A.** 2011. Biogenesis, regulation, and targeting of the type III secretion system. *Structure* **19:**603–612.

91. **DeBord KL, Lee VT, Schneewind O.** 2001. Roles of LcrG and LcrV during type III targeting of effector Yops by *Yersinia enterocolitica*. *J Bacteriol* **183:**4588–4598.

92. **Lilic M, Vujanac M, Stebbins CE.** 2006. A common structural motif in the binding of virulence factors to bacterial secretion chaperones. *Mol Cell* **21:**653–664.

93. **Janjusevic R, Quezada CM, Small J, Stebbins CE.** 2013. Structure of the HopA1(21-102)-ShcA chaperone-effector complex of *Pseudomonas syringae* reveals conservation of a virulence factor binding motif from animal to plant pathogens. *J Bacteriol* **195:**658–664.

94. **Costa SC, Schmitz AM, Jahufar FF, Boyd JD, Cho MY, Glicksman MA, Lesser CF.** 2012. A new means to identify type 3 secreted effectors: functionally interchangeable class IB chaperones recognize a conserved sequence. *MBio* **3:**e00243-11. doi:10.1128/mBio.00243-11.

95. **Michiels T, Cornelis GR.** 1991. Secretion of hybrid proteins by the *Yersinia* Yop export system. *J Bacteriol* **173:**1677–1685.

96. **Chen LM, Briones G, Donis RO, Galan JE.** 2006. Optimization of the delivery of heterologous proteins by the *Salmonella enterica* serovar Typhimurium type III secretion system for vaccine development. *Infect Immun* **74:**5826–5833.

97. **Widmaier DM, Tullman-Ercek D, Mirsky EA, Hill R, Govindarajan S, Minshull J, Voigt CA.** 2009. Engineering the *Salmonella* type III secretion system to export spider silk monomers. *Mol Syst Biol* **5:**309.

98. **Akeda Y, Galan JE.** 2004. Genetic analysis of the *Salmonella enterica* type III secretion-associated ATPase InvC defines discrete functional domains. *J Bacteriol* **186:**2402–2412.

99. **Zarivach R, Vuckovic M, Deng W, Finlay BB, Strynadka NC.** 2007. Structural analysis of a prototypical ATPase from the type III secretion system. *Nat Struct Mol Biol* **14:**131–137.

100. **Claret L, Calder SR, Higgins M, Hughes C.** 2003. Oligomerization and activation of the FliI ATPase central to bacterial flagellum assembly. *Mol Microbiol* **48:**1349–1355.

101. **Ibuki T, Imada K, Minamino T, Kato T, Miyata T, Namba K.** 2011. Common architecture of the flagellar type III protein export apparatus and F- and V-type ATPases. *Nat Struct Mol Biol* **18:**277–282.

102. **Pozidis C, Chalkiadaki A, Gomez-Serrano A, Stahlberg H, Brown I, Tampakaki AP, Lustig A, Sianidis G, Politou AS, Engel A, Panopoulos NJ, Mansfield J, Pugsley AP, Karamanou S, Economou A.** 2003. Type III protein translocase: HrcN is a peripheral ATPase that is activated by oligomerization. *J Biol Chem* **278:**25816–25824.

103. **Akeda Y, Galan JE.** 2005. Chaperone release and unfolding of substrates in type III secretion. *Nature* **437:**911–915.

104. **Minamino T, Namba K.** 2008. Distinct roles of the FliI ATPase and proton motive force in bacterial flagellar protein export. *Nature* **451:**485–488.

105. **Paul K, Erhardt M, Hirano T, Blair DF, Hughes KT.** 2008. Energy source of flagellar type III secretion. *Nature* **451:**489–492.

106. **Erhardt M, Mertens ME, Fabiani FD, Hughes KT.** 2014. ATPase-independent type-III protein secretion in *Salmonella enterica*. *PLoS Genet* **10:**e1004800. doi:10.1371/journal.pgen.1004800.

107. **Minamino T, Morimoto YV, Kinoshita M, Aldridge PD, Namba K.** 2014. The bacterial flagellar protein export apparatus processively transports flagellar proteins even with extremely infrequent ATP hydrolysis. *Sci Rep* **4:**7579. doi:10.1038/srep07579.

108. **Chen S, Beeby M, Murphy GE, Leadbetter JR, Hendrixson DR, Briegel A, Li Z, Shi J, Tocheva EI, Muller A, Dobro MJ, Jensen GJ.** 2011. Structural diversity of bacterial flagellar motors. *EMBO J* **30:**2972–2981.

109. **Kawamoto A, Morimoto YV, Miyata T, Minamino T, Hughes KT, Kato T, Namba K.** 2013. Common and distinct structural features of *Salmonella* injectisome and flagellar basal body. *Sci Rep* **3:**3369. doi:10.1038/srep03369.

110. **Lorenzini E, Singer A, Singh B, Lam R, Skarina T, Chirgadze NY, Savchenko A, Gupta RS.** 2010. Structure and protein-protein interaction studies on *Chlamydia trachomatis* protein CT670 (YscO Homolog). *J Bacteriol* **192:**2746–2756.

111. **Wilharm G, Lehmann V, Krauss K, Lehnert B, Richter S, Ruckdeschel K, Heesemann J, Trulzsch K.** 2004. *Yersinia enterocolitica* type III secretion depends on the proton motive force but not on the flagellar motor components MotA and MotB. *Infect Immun* **72:**4004–4009.

112. **Galan JE.** 2008. Energizing type III secretion machines: what is the fuel? *Nat Struct Mol Biol* **15:**127–128.

113. **Allison SE, Tuinema BR, Everson ES, Sugiman-Marangos S, Zhang K, Junop MS, Coombes BK.** 2014. Identification of the docking site between a type III secretion system ATPase and a chaperone for effector cargo. *J Biol Chem* **289:**23734–23744.

114. **Roblin P, Dewitte F, Villeret V, Biondi EG, Bompard C.** 2015. A *Salmonella* type three secretion effector/chaperone complex adopts a hexameric ring-like structure. *J Bacteriol* **197:**688–698.

115. **Tsai CL, Burkinshaw BJ, Strynadka NC, Tainer JA.** 2015. The *Salmonella* type III secretion system virulence effector forms a new hexameric chaperone assembly for export of effector/chaperone complexes. *J Bacteriol* **197:**672–675.

116. **Chen L, Balabanidou V, Remeta DP, Minetti CA, Portaliou AG, Economou A, Kalodimos CG.** 2011. Structural instability tuning as a regulatory mechanism in protein-protein interactions. *Mol Cell* **44:**734–744.

117. **Chen L, Ai X, Portaliou AG, Minetti CA, Remeta DP, Economou A, Kalodimos CG.** 2013. Substrate-activated conformational switch on chaperones encodes a targeting signal in type III secretion. *Cell Rep* **3:**709–715.

118. **Ohgita T, Hayashi N, Hama S, Tsuchiya H, Gotoh N, Kogure K.** 2013. A novel effector secretion mechanism based on proton-motive force-dependent type III secretion apparatus rotation. *FASEB J* **27:**2862–2872.

119. **Morita-Ishihara T, Ogawa M, Sagara H, Yoshida M, Katayama E, Sasakawa C.** 2006. Shigella Spa33 is an essential C-ring component of type III secretion machinery. *J Biol Chem* **281:**599–607.

120. **Hu B, Morado DR, Margolin W, Rohde JR, Arizmendi O, Picking WL, Picking WD, Liu J.** 2015. Visualization of the type III secretion sorting platform of *Shigella flexneri*. *Proc Natl Acad Sci USA* **112:**1047–1052.

121. **Lara-Tejero M, Kato J, Wagner S, Liu X, Galan JE.** 2011. A sorting platform determines the order of protein secretion in bacterial type III systems. *Science* **331:**1188–1191.

122. **Gonzalez-Pedrajo B, Fraser GM, Minamino T, Macnab RM.** 2002. Molecular dissection of *Salmonella* FliH, a regulator of the ATPase FliI and the type III flagellar protein export pathway. *Mol Microbiol* **45:**967–982.

123. **Minamino T, MacNab RM.** 2000. FliH, a soluble component of the type III flagellar export apparatus of *Salmonella*, forms a complex with FliI and inhibits its ATPase activity. *Mol Microbiol* **37:**1494–1503.

124. **Lane MC, O'Toole PW, Moore SA.** 2006. Molecular basis of the interaction between the flagellar export proteins FliI and FliH from *Helicobacter pylori*. *J Biol Chem* **281:**508–517.

125. **Minamino T, Yoshimura SD, Morimoto YV, Gonzalez-Pedrajo B, Kami-Ike N, Namba K.** 2009. Roles of the extreme N-terminal region of FliH for efficient localization of the FliH-FliI complex to the bacterial flagellar type III export apparatus. *Mol Microbiol* **74:**1471–1483.

126. **McMurry JL, Murphy JW, Gonzalez-Pedrajo B.** 2006. The FliN-FliH interaction mediates localization of flagellar export ATPase FliI to the C ring complex. *Biochemistry* **45:**11790–11798.

127. **Minamino T, Gonzalez-Pedrajo B, Kihara M, Namba K, Macnab RM.** 2003. The ATPase FliI can interact with the type III flagellar protein export apparatus in the absence of its regulator, FliH. *J Bacteriol* **185:**3983–3988.

128. **Bai F, Morimoto YV, Yoshimura SD, Hara N, Kami-Ike N, Namba K, Minamino T.** 2014. Assembly dynamics and the roles of FliI ATPase of the bacterial flagellar export apparatus. *Sci Rep* **4:**6528. doi:10.1038/srep06528.

129. **Diepold A, Kudryashev M, Delalez NJ, Berry RM, Armitage JP.** 2015. Composition, formation, and regulation of the cytosolic c-ring, a dynamic component of the type III secretion injectisome. *PLoS Biol* **13:**e1002039. doi:10.1371/journal.pbio.1002039.

130. **Fadouloglou VE, Tampakaki AP, Glykos NM, Bastaki MN, Hadden JM, Phillips SE, Panopoulos NJ, Kokkinidis M.** 2004. Structure of HrcQB-C, a conserved component of the bacterial type III secretion systems. *Proc Natl Acad Sci USA* **101:**70–75.

131. **Brown PN, Mathews MA, Joss LA, Hill CP, Blair DF.** 2005. Crystal structure of the flagellar rotor protein FliN from *Thermotoga maritima*. *J Bacteriol* **187:**2890–2902.

132. **Bzymek KP, Hamaoka BY, Ghosh P.** 2012. Two translation products of *Yersinia* yscQ assemble to form a complex essential to type III secretion. *Biochemistry* **51:**1669–1677.

133. **Paul K, Blair DF.** 2006. Organization of FliN subunits in the flagellar motor of *Escherichia coli*. *J Bacteriol* **188:**2502–2511.

134. **Paul K, Harmon JG, Blair DF.** 2006. Mutational analysis of the flagellar rotor protein FliN: identification of surfaces important for flagellar assembly and switching. *J Bacteriol* **188:**5240–5248.

135. **Fadouloglou VE, Bastaki MN, Ashcroft AE, Phillips SE, Panopoulos NJ, Glykos NM, Kokkinidis M.** 2009. On the quaternary association of the type III secretion system HrcQB-C protein: experimental evidence differentiates among the various oligomerization models. *J Struct Biol* **166:**214–225.

136. **Lee SY, Cho HS, Pelton JG, Yan D, Henderson RK, King DS, Huang L, Kustu S, Berry EA, Wemmer DE.** 2001. Crystal structure of an activated response regulator bound to its target. *Nat Struct Biol* **8:**52–56.

137. **Vartanian AS, Paz A, Fortgang EA, Abramson J, Dahlquist FW.** 2012. Structure of flagellar motor proteins in complex allows for insights into motor structure and switching. *J Biol Chem* **287:**35779–35783.

138. **Kubori T, Galan JE.** 2002. *Salmonella* type III secretion-associated protein InvE controls translocation of effector proteins into host cells. *J Bacteriol* **184:**4699–4708.

139. **Deane JE, Abrusci P, Johnson S, Lea SM.** 2010. Timing is everything: the regulation of type III secretion. *Cell Mol Life Sci* **67:**1065–1075.

140. **Magdalena J, Hachani A, Chamekh M, Jouihri N, Gounon P, Blocker A, Allaoui A.** 2002. Spa32 regulates a switch in substrate specificity of the type III secreton of *Shigella flexneri* from needle components to Ipa proteins. *J Bacteriol* **184:**3433–3441.

141. **Agrain C, Callebaut I, Journet L, Sorg I, Paroz C, Mota LJ, Cornelis GR.** 2005. Characterization of a type III secretion substrate specificity switch (T3S4) domain in YscP from *Yersinia enterocolitica*. *Mol Microbiol* **56:**54–67.

142. **Mizuno S, Amida H, Kobayashi N, Aizawa S, Tate S.** 2011. The NMR structure of FliK, the trigger for the switch of substrate specificity in the flagellar type III secretion apparatus. *J Mol Biol* **409:**558–573.

143. **Mukerjea R, Ghosh P.** 2013. Functionally essential interaction between *Yersinia* YscO and the T3S4 domain of YscP. *J Bacteriol* **195:**4631–4638.

144. **Botteaux A, Sani M, Kayath CA, Boekema EJ, Allaoui A.** 2008. Spa32 interaction with the inner-membrane Spa40 component of the type III secretion system of *Shigella flexneri* is required for the control of the needle length by a molecular tape measure mechanism. *Mol Microbiol* **70:**1515–1528.

145. **Wood SE, Jin J, Lloyd SA.** 2008. YscP and YscU switch the substrate specificity of the *Yersinia* type III secretion system by regulating export of the inner rod protein YscI. *J Bacteriol* **190:**4252–4262.

146. **Botteaux A, Kayath CA, Page AL, Jouihri N, Sani M, Boekema E, Biskri L, Parsot C, Allaoui A.** 2010. The 33 carboxyl-terminal residues of Spa40 orchestrate the multi-step assembly process of the type III secretion needle complex in *Shigella flexneri*. *Microbiology* **156:**2807–2817.

147. **Cherradi Y, Schiavolin L, Moussa S, Meghraoui A, Meksem A, Biskri L, Azarkan M, Allaoui A, Botteaux A.** 2013. Interplay between predicted inner-rod and gatekeeper in controlling substrate specificity of the type III secretion system. *Mol Microbiol* **87:**1183–1199.

148. **Sorg I, Wagner S, Amstutz M, Muller SA, Broz P, Lussi Y, Engel A, Cornelis GR.** 2007. YscU recognizes translocators as export substrates of the *Yersinia* injectisome. *EMBO J* **26:**3015–3024.

149. **Botteaux A, Sory MP, Biskri L, Parsot C, Allaoui A.** 2009. MxiC is secreted by and controls the substrate specificity of the *Shigella flexneri* type III secretion apparatus. *Mol Microbiol* **71:**449–460.

150. **Cheng LW, Kay O, Schneewind O.** 2001. Regulated secretion of YopN by the type III machinery of *Yersinia enterocolitica. J Bacteriol* **183:**5293–5301.

151. **Rimpilainen M, Forsberg A, Wolf-Watz H.** 1992. A novel protein, LcrQ, involved in the low-calcium response of *Yersinia pseudotuberculosis* shows extensive homology to YopH. *J Bacteriol* **174:**3355–3363.

152. **Skrzypek E, Straley SC.** 1993. LcrG, a secreted protein involved in negative regulation of the low-calcium response in *Yersinia pestis. J Bacteriol* **175:**3520–3528.

153. **Schubot FD, Jackson MW, Penrose KJ, Cherry S, Tropea JE, Plano GV, Waugh DS.** 2005. Three-dimensional structure of a macromolecular assembly that regulates type III secretion in *Yersinia pestis. J Mol Biol* **346:**1147–1161.

154. **Deane JE, Roversi P, King C, Johnson S, Lea SM.** 2008. Structures of the *Shigella flexneri* type 3 secretion system protein MxiC reveal conformational variability amongst homologues. *J Mol Biol* **377:**985–992.

155. **Weise CF, Login FH, Ho O, Grobner G, Wolf-Watz H, Wolf-Watz M.** 2014. Negatively charged lipid membranes promote a disorder-order transition in the *Yersinia* YscU protein. *Biophys J* **107:**1950–1961.

156. **Stensrud KF, Adam PR, La Mar CD, Olive AJ, Lushington GH, Sudharsan R, Shelton NL, Givens RS, Picking WL, Picking WD.** 2008. Deoxycholate interacts with IpaD of *Shigella flexneri* in inducing the recruitment of IpaB to the type III secretion apparatus needle tip. *J Biol Chem* **283:**18646–18654.

157. **Prouty AM, Gunn JS.** 2000. *Salmonella enterica* serovar Typhimurium invasion is repressed in the presence of bile. *Infect Immun* **68:**6763–6769.

158. **Barta ML, Guragain M, Adam P, Dickenson NE, Patil M, Geisbrecht BV, Picking WL, Picking WD.** 2012. Identification of the bile salt binding site on IpaD from *Shigella flexneri* and the influence of ligand binding on IpaD structure. *Proteins* **80:**935–945.

159. **Chatterjee S, Zhong D, Nordhues BA, Battaile KP, Lovell S, De Guzman RN.** 2011. The crystal structures of the *Salmonella* type III secretion system tip protein SipD in complex with deoxycholate and chenodeoxycholate. *Protein Sci* **20:**75–86.

160. **Menard R, Sansonetti P, Parsot C.** 1994. The secretion of the *Shigella flexneri* Ipa invasins is activated by epithelial cells and controlled by IpaB and IpaD. *EMBO J* **13:**5293–5302.

161. **Rosqvist R, Magnusson KE, Wolf-Watz H.** 1994. Target cell contact triggers expression and polarized transfer of *Yersinia* YopE cytotoxin into mammalian cells. *EMBO J* **13:**964–972.

162. **Zierler MK, Galan JE.** 1995. Contact with cultured epithelial cells stimulates secretion of *Salmonella typhimurium* invasion protein InvJ. *Infect Immun* **63:**4024–4028.

163. **Lara-Tejero M, Galan JE.** 2009. *Salmonella enterica* serovar typhimurium pathogenicity island 1-encoded type III secretion system translocases mediate intimate attachment to nonphagocytic cells. *Infect Immun* **77:**2635–2642.

164. **Epler CR, Dickenson NE, Olive AJ, Picking WL, Picking WD.** 2009. Liposomes recruit IpaC to the *Shigella flexneri* type III secretion apparatus needle as a final step in secretion induction. *Infect Immun* **77:**2754–2761.

165. **Blocker AJ, Deane JE, Veenendaal AK, Roversi P, Hodgkinson JL, Johnson S, Lea SM.** 2008. What's the point of the type III secretion system needle? *Proc Natl Acad Sci USA* **105:**6507–6513.

166. **Cordes FS, Daniell S, Kenjale R, Saurya S, Picking WL, Picking WD, Booy F, Lea SM, Blocker A.** 2005. Helical packing of needles from functionally altered *Shigella* type III secretion systems. *J Mol Biol* **354:**206–211.

167. **Yu XJ, McGourty K, Liu M, Unsworth KE, Holden DW.** 2010. pH sensing by intracellular *Salmonella* induces effector translocation. *Science* **328:**1040–1043.

168. **Figueira R, Holden DW.** 2012. Functions of the *Salmonella* pathogenicity island 2 (SPI-2) type III secretion system effectors. *Microbiology* **158:**1147–1161.

169. **Torruellas J, Jackson MW, Pennock JW, Plano GV.** 2005. The *Yersinia pestis* type III secretion needle plays a role in the regulation of Yop secretion. *Mol Microbiol* **57:**1719–1733.

170. **Birtalan SC, Phillips RM, Ghosh P.** 2002. Three-dimensional secretion signals in chaperone-effector complexes of bacterial pathogens. *Mol Cell* **9:**971–980.

171. **Phan J, Tropea JE, Waugh DS.** 2004. Structure of the *Yersinia pestis* type III secretion chaperone SycH in complex with a stable fragment of YscM2. *Acta Crystallogr D Biol Crystallogr* **60:**1591–1599.

172. **Schreiner M, Niemann HH.** 2012. Crystal structure of the *Yersinia enterocolitica* type III secretion chaperone SycD in complex with a peptide of the minor translocator YopD. *BMC Struct Biol* **12:**13.

Mechanism and Function of Type IV Secretion During Infection of the Human Host

10

CHRISTIAN GONZALEZ-RIVERA,[1] MINNY BHATTY,[1] and PETER J. CHRISTIE[1]

INTRODUCTION

Bacterial type IV secretion systems (T4SSs) are widely distributed among Gram-negative and Gram-positive bacteria. These systems contribute in various ways to infection processes among clinically important pathogens, including *Helicobacter pylori*, *Brucella* and *Bartonella* species, *Bordetella pertussis*, and *Legionella pneumophila* (1–3). The list of pathogens employing T4SSs to subvert host cellular pathways for establishment of a replication niche continues to expand, making these machines an important subject of study for defining critical features of disease progression and development of strategies aimed at suppressing T4SS function (4). Also of importance, studies of T4SSs and effector functions have coincidentally and appreciably augmented our understanding of basic cellular processes in the human host.

The T4SSs are a highly diverse translocation superfamily in terms of (i) overall machine architecture, (ii) the secretion substrates translocated, and (iii) target cell types, which can be bacteria, amoebae, fungal, plant, or human (5). Several classification schemes have emerged to describe the T4SSs, the most widely used being based on overall machine function (1). Accordingly, one subfamily existing within nearly all species of bacteria and even some

[1]Department of Microbiology and Molecular Genetics, University of Texas Medical School at Houston, Houston, TX 77030.

Virulence Mechanisms of Bacterial Pathogens, 5th edition
Edited by Indira T. Kudva, Nancy A. Cornick, Paul J. Plummer, Qijing Zhang, Tracy L. Nicholson, John P. Bannantine, and Bryan H. Bellaire
© 2016 American Society for Microbiology, Washington, DC
doi:10.1128/microbiolspec.VMBF-0024-2015

Archaea are the conjugation systems (Fig. 1) (5). These systems mediate the transfer of mobile genetic elements in the form of conjugative plasmids or chromosomally located integrative and conjugative elements to other bacteria by a mechanism requiring direct cell-to-cell contact (6–8). These systems are highly important vehicles for the widespread and rapid transmission of antibiotic resistance genes and virulence traits among medically important pathogens. In a context of the recent emergence of multiply drug-resistant "superbugs," the dissemination of mobile genetic elements via conjugation represents a huge threat to human health and an enormous financial burden to society (9).

The second subfamily, the "effector translocator" systems, evolved from the conjugation systems but have acquired a different substrate repertoire composed mainly but not

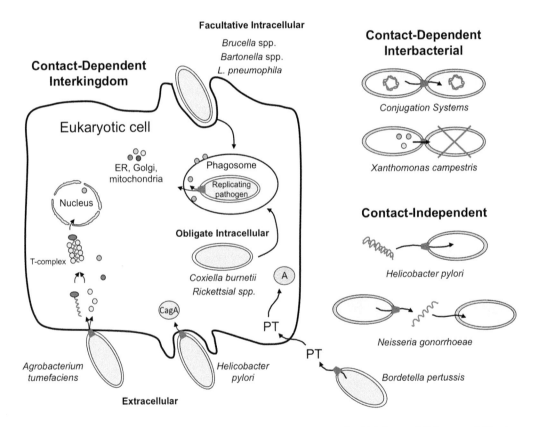

FIGURE 1 Bacterial pathogens employing type IV secretion systems (T4SSs) for establishment within the human host, acquisition of DNA encoding virulence traits, or out-competition of other bacteria for niche occupation. Extracellular pathogens deliver substrates to human or plant cells by contact-dependent or -independent mechanisms. These pathogens deliver diverse substrates including oncogenic T-DNA, monomeric CagA, and multimeric pertussis toxin. Facultative intracellular pathogens enter the host cell from an environmental sample, whereas obligate intracellular pathogens enter directly from another host cell. The intracellular pathogens employ T4SSs to deliver a myriad of effectors whose collective function is to subvert host cellular processes principally for establishment of replicative niches. Shown are T4SSs on the bacterial cell envelope (red trapezoids), effectors (proteins: multicolor circles; tDNA: red wavy line), and various target organelles/sites of effector action within the host cell. T4SSs also mediate interbacterial transfer by contact-dependent mechanisms for conjugative DNA transfer or to kill neighboring bacteria (red X), or by contact-independent mechanisms to exchange DNA with the environment.

exclusively of proteins (1). Thus far, these systems have been identified only in Gram-negative pathogens, but recent work suggests that a number of medically important Gram-positive species also rely on T4SSs for colonization through mechanisms not exclusively related to gene transfer (4, 10). The effector translocator systems deliver their cargoes into the eukaryotic cell cytosol usually by a cell-contact-dependent mechanism (Fig. 1). Upon translocation, the effector proteins target specific physiological pathways or biochemical processes with a variety of biological consequences that benefit survival, colonization, and transmission of the invading pathogens (3, 11, 12).

A third T4SS subfamily, the "DNA release and uptake systems," currently is composed of a *Neisseria gonorrhoeae* T4SS that delivers substrate DNA to the extracellular milieu and an *H. pylori* competence system used for DNA uptake by the bacterium (1). Both systems are closely functionally related to conjugation systems but adapted for DNA translocation in the absence of direct recipient cell contact (13, 14).

T4SSs alternatively have been designated as types IVA, IVB, and recently, IVC (10, 15, 16). The type IVA systems are composed of a dozen or so subunits homologous to components of the paradigmatic *Agrobacterium tumefaciens* VirB/VirD4 T4SS (17). This subfamily includes the well-characterized conjugation machines encoded by plasmids R388, pKM101, RP4, and F, as well as effector translocators employed by *H. pylori*, *B. pertussis*, *Bartonella* and *Brucella* spp., and *Rickettsia* spp. (5). The type IVB systems, exemplified by the *L. pneumophila* Dot/Icm system, bear little sequence relatedness to the type IVA systems and are composed of over 25 subunits (16, 18). Other members of this family include the plasmid ColIb-P9 conjugation system and the *Coxiella burnetii* Dot/Icm effector translocator. The type IVC systems, found almost exclusively in Gram-positive species, are composed of as few as five subunits and thus are also termed

"minimized" T4SSs (4, 10). Subunits of the type IVC systems exhibit sequence similarities to a subset of the type IVA components, and results of phylogenetic analyses suggest that the type IVC systems arose from the type IVA systems (19).

An inherent difficulty in classifying T4SSs on the basis of function, structure, or phylogeny is that these are highly versatile and adaptive machines. A prominent example is the *A. tumefaciens* VirB/VirD4 T4SS, which functions as both a conjugation machine and an effector translocator and, while its target is plant cells in nature, it can also deliver substrates to other bacteria as well as various fungal and human cells (20). Many T4SSs also are highly mosaic in their subunit composition. For example, although the type IVA systems are built from homologs of VirB and VirD4 subunits, many systems have evolved specialized functions through loss of certain components or acquisition of others from unrelated ancestries (5, 19).

This article will summarize our recent progress in understanding the mechanism of action of T4SSs and their contributions to pathogenesis. We will focus the discussion mainly on contributions of the effector translocators to infection. To further highlight mechanistic themes and variations, we will group these systems according to the invasive mechanism of the pathogen, e.g., extracellular, facultative intracellular, obligate intracellular, as illustrated in Fig. 1. To further orient the reader, the pathogens discussed herein and some relevant properties relating to infection are presented in Table 1.

T4SS ARCHITECTURES AND ADAPTATIONS

By way of introducing these fascinating and complex machines, we will first summarize recent exciting progress in structure–function studies of the paradigmatic *A. tumefaciens* VirB/VirD4 T4SS and related conjugation systems, and then briefly describe some of

TABLE 1 Type IV secretion systems and disease manifestations

Bacteria	T4SS	Diseases	Substrates	References
Interkingdom transfer				
Extracellular pathogens				
Agrobacterium tumefaciens	VirB/VirD4	Crown gall	Oncogenic T-DNA VirE2, VirE3, VirF	20
Bordetella pertussis	Ptl	Whooping cough	Pertussis toxin	47
Helicobacter pylori	Cag	Gastritis, peptic ulcer, cancer	CagA	65, 66, 90
Facultative intracellular				
Bartonella spp.	VirB/VirD4 Trw	Cat-scratch, angiomatosis	BepA-BepG None	95, 105
Brucella spp.	VirB	Brucellosis	~14	95, 121, 222
Legionella pneumophila	Dot/Icm	Legionnaire's pneumonia	~300	18, 127, 135, 137
Obligate intracellular				
Coxiella burnetii	Dot/Icm	Q fever	~130	169, 223
Anaplasma phagocytophilum	VirB/VirD4	Granulocytic anaplasmosis	AnkA, Ats-1, APH_0455	190, 224
Anaplasma marginale	VirB/VirD4	Anaplasmosis	AM185, AM1141, AM470, AM705[AnkA]	196
Ehrlichia spp.	VirB/VirD4	Ehrlichiosis	ECH0825	202
Rickettsia spp.	VirB/VirD4	Epidemic typhus, Mediterranean spotted fever	Unknown	179, 188
Wolbachia spp.	VirB/VirD4	Endosymbiont of filarial nematodes and arthropods	Unknown	187
Interbacterial transfer				
Conjugation machines	Tra	Virulence and antibiotic resistance gene transfer Genome plasticity	Mobile DNA elements	5, 8, 9
A. tumefaciens	VirB/VirD4	Conjugation	IncQ plasmid	35
Bartonella spp.	VirB/VirD4	Conjugation	IncW plasmid, Bartonella plasmid	111
L. pneumophila	Dot/Icm	Conjugation	IncQ plasmid	129
Neisseria gonorrhoeae	Tra	DNA release	Chromosomal DNA	14
H. pylori	Com	DNA uptake	Exogenous DNA	13
Xanthomonas campestris	Xac	Killing: interbacterial competition	Xac toxins	219

the structural adaptations acquired by T4SSs for specialized functions in pathogenic settings.

The Paradigmatic *A. tumefaciens* VirB/VirD4 T4SS

The T4SSs of Gram-negative bacteria are composed of four distinct machine subassemblies: (i) the type IV coupling protein (T4CP), a hexameric ATPase related to the SpoIIIE/FtsK DNA translocases that recruits secretion substrates to the translocation machinery, (ii) an inner membrane complex (IMC)

responsible for substrate transfer across the inner membrane, (iii) an envelope-spanning outer membrane complex (OMC) required for substrate passage across the periplasm and outer membrane, and (iv) the conjugative pilus, an extracellular organelle that initiates contact with potential recipient cells (Fig. 2) (8, 21, 22).

A. tumefaciens is a phytopathogen that uses the VirB/VirD4 system to deliver oncogenic transfer DNA (T-DNA) and effector proteins to plants (Fig. 1) (20). A combination of structural and functional studies of the VirB/VirD4 T4SS and of closely related

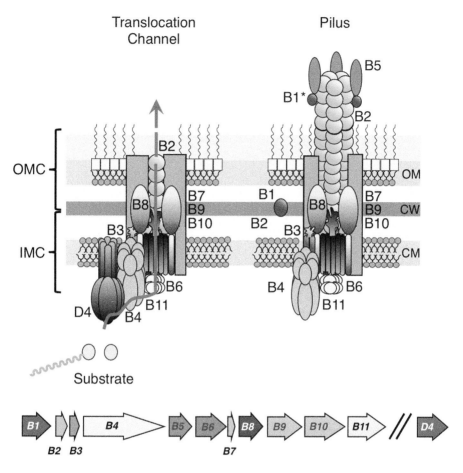

FIGURE 2 Schematic of the *Agrobacterium* VirB/VirB type IV secretion system (T4SS). (Lower) *virB* genes are expressed from the same *virB* promoter, and *virD4* from a separate promoter (indicated by two slashes). (Upper) The VirB and VirD4 subunits assemble as the translocation channel, which presents as two subcomplexes termed the outer membrane complex (OMC), composed of VirB7, VirB9, VirB10, and VirB2, and the inner membrane complex (IMC), composed of VirB3, VirB4, VirB6, VirB8, VirB11, and VirD4. VirB2, VirB5, and a proteolytic fragment of VirB1 (B1*) also assemble as the conjugative pilus without a requirement for VirD4. The physical and functional relationships between the translocation channel and the conjugative pilus are not yet known. OM, outer membrane; CW, cell wall; CM, cytoplasmic membrane. See references 24, 25, and 237 for recent structures of related T4SSs. Adapted from Bhatty M, Laverde Gomez JA, Christie PJ. 2013. The expanding bacterial type IV secretion lexicon. Res Microbiol 164:620–629. Copyright 2013, Institut Pasteur, published by Elsevier Masson SAS. All rights reserved.

systems encoded by *Escherichia coli* conjugative plasmids, e.g., pKM101 and R388, have generated for the first time a view of how the VirB/VirD4 T4SSs are architecturally arranged and function to convey secretion substrates across the Gram-negative cell envelope (Fig. 2). In studies carried out over a decade ago, the route of transfer of the oncogenic T-DNA substrate through the *A. tumefaciens* VirB/VirD4 T4SS was mapped with a formaldehyde-cross-linking assay termed transfer DNA immunoprecipitation (TrIP) (23). Results of the TrIP studies showed that the DNA substrate engages sequentially with VirD4, which then transfers it to the VirB11 ATPase. VirB11 in turn delivers the substrate to a putative translocation channel composed of VirB6 and VirB8 for delivery across the inner membrane. The substrate then passes through the periplasm and across the outer membrane via a channel minimally composed of VirB2 and VirB9.

More recent structural work has generated high-resolution structures of T4SS complexes, the latest of the near entire VirB/VirD4-like T4SS encoded by the conjugative plasmid R388 (24). Although the VirD4 and VirB11 ATPase subunits as well as the extracellular pilus were missing from this structure, the large ~3.2-MDa structure identified two VirB4 hexamers as part of a larger substructure the authors termed the IMC. Other IMC components include VirB3, VirB6, and VirB8. In the periplasm, the IMC is connected by a narrow stalk to the so-called OMC (also called the core complex). The OMC of the closely related *E. coli* pKM101-encoded T4SS is configured as a large barrel composed of 14 copies each of homologs of VirB7, VirB9, and VirB10 that extends across the entire cell envelope (25). Combining the results of the TrIP studies and the recent R388 structure, a cohesive model can thus be presented depicting the route(s) of substrate transfer across the Gram-negative bacterial cell envelope (Fig. 2) (22). Interestingly, in the pKM101 and R388 structures, the C-terminal regions of the VirB10-like scaffold proteins are predicted to form a channel across the outer membrane. While this might correspond to the pore through which substrates pass, it is likely that this region of the channel is structurally more complex than currently depicted. This is because the structures solved to date lacked the pilin subunit and the conjugative pilus, which is also part of many T4SS structures (24, 25). In the TrIP studies, the DNA substrate did not cross-link with *A. tumefaciens* VirB10, but rather, with the VirB2 pilin and VirB9. Conceivably, the distal portion of the translocation channel consists of a pilus-like structure that protrudes through the pore formed by the C terminus of VirB10 (Fig. 2) (17).

The *A. tumefaciens* VirB/VirD4 T4SS elaborates a conjugative pilus to mediate attachment to target cells. Assembly of the pilus does not require the VirD4 T4CP but does require the VirB1 lytic transglycosylase (17, 26). This pilus is composed of the pilin subunit VirB2 and the pilus-tip adhesin VirB5 (Fig. 2) (26). Its physical relationship to the VirB/VirD4 T4SS is not yet defined. However, in view of its role as an attachment organelle, it is interesting to speculate that the T4SS initially elaborates a pilus structure to establish contact with target cells. Then, once productive mating junctions are formed, the T4SS recruits the VirD4 T4CP for activation of the channel and subsequent substrate transfer. In such a model, the T4SS would function sequentially, first for elaboration of the pilus and second for biogenesis of the transfer channel.

Structure/Function Adaptations Among T4SSs

While the R388 IMC/OMC complex can be viewed as a structural unit conserved among most if not all Gram-negative T4SSs, a large body of evidence now establishes that this structural unit has undergone extensive adaptation during establishment of pathogen–host relationships. Generally, the adaptations allow for (i) substrate-specific trafficking and spatiotemporal control of translocation during infection and (ii) elaboration of novel and potentially antigenically variable pili or other surface structures. Examples of such adaptations are described briefly here and in Table 2 and are discussed in more detail in subsequent sections.

Substrate recruitment and translocation across the inner membrane

With a few notable exceptions, the T4SSs employ a T4CP receptor to recruit cognate substrates to the transfer channel. For docking with the T4CP, secretion substrates carry either translocation signals located C terminally and composed of clusters of positively

TABLE 2 T4SS machine adaptations enabling specialized functions

Bacteria	T4SS	T4SS machine adaptation(s)	Specialized functions	References
Agrobacterium tumefaciens	VirB/VirD4	VirB1-VirB11, VirD4	Transfer channel, Conjugative pilus; Translocates DNA and protein substrates	35, 57
Bordetella pertussis	Ptl	No VirD4, VirB1, VirB5 homologs	Two-step translocation: PT subunits cross IM via GSP, PT crosses OM via Ptl T4SS; No extracellular pilus	47
Helicobacter pylori	Cag	VirB7-like CagT VirB10-like CagY have surface-exposed variable or repeat sequences CagY; VirB5-like CagL RGD motif; CagA substrate at pilus tip	Phenotypic variation: Binding to different cell types, immune evasion; $\beta1$ integrin binding; $\beta1$ integrin binding; $\beta1$ integrin binding; translocation intermediate	40, 60, 69
Bartonella spp.	VirB/VirD4	None	Translocates effectors and DNA substrate to human cells	105, 110
	Trw	No VirD4 homolog; Multiple copies of VirB2 and VirB5 homologs	No substrate transfer; Variant forms of surface-exposed pilus for binding to different erythrocyte receptors?	42, 96
Brucella spp.	VirB	Multiple copies of VirB6 & VirB7 homologs; No VirD4 homolog VirB12, *orf13* gene product	Unknown; One-(?) and two-step translocation via GSP and VirB systems; Serological marker, surface-exposed?	114, 118, 225
A. phagocytophilum *E. chaffeensis* *Rickettsia* spp. *Wolbachia*	VirB/VirD4	No VirB1, VirB5 homologs, but carries multiple copies of VirB2 paralogs and of "extended VirB6" subunits	Variable pilus? Binding of different host cell/receptors?; Immune modulation?	41, 43, 187, 226, 227
Legionella pneumophila *Coxiella burnetii*	Dot/Icm	Unrelated to VirB/VirD4 system; VirB7 lipoprotein: N0 domain; Fibrous surface mesh	Translocates effectors and DNA substrate (to bacteria); Novel OMC structure; Host cell binding?; Immune modulation?	18, 44, 130, 131
N. gonorrhoeae	Tra	No VirB11 homolog Additional subunits related to F plasmid T4SS; Variant forms of TraA pilin	DNA release to milieu	228
H. pylori	Com	No VirD4, VirB5, VirB11; Com: DNA uptake across OM; ComEC: DNA uptake across IM	Unknown; Natural transformation	14 / 13
X. campestris	Xac	VirB/VirD4 T4SS; VirB7 ortholog has N0 domain	Interbacterial delivery of Xac toxins for killing	219

charged or hydrophobic residues, one or more internal signals of unspecified composition, or a combination of C-terminal and internal signals (27–31). Substrates also can have distinct translocation signals for docking with different T4SSs, providing another example of the functional versatility of these systems (30). In addition to these intrinsic translocation signals, T4SSs employ various chaperones or adaptor proteins for conferring substrate specificity and maintaining the substrate in a translocation-competent form (32, 33). In the *A. tumefaciens* T4SS system, for example, translocation of the VirF effector proceeds independently of other known factors, whereas translocation of VirE2 requires cosynthesis of the VirE1 chaperone (34, 35). VirE2 is a single-stranded DNA binding protein that, upon transfer to plant cells interacts with the cotranslocated T-DNA to protect the DNA substrate and facilitate its delivery to the plant nucleus (Fig. 1). VirE1 shares several features of the specialized chaperones associated with type III secretion systems (T3SSs), including a small size, acidic pI, and an amphipathic helix. As discussed further below, the *L. pneumophila* Dot/Icm T4SS translocates hundreds of effectors to mammalian cells during infection. A subset of these is dependent on four accessory proteins residing in the cytoplasm or inner membrane. These include DotM, DotN, IcmS, and IcmW, which interact with each other in different combinations to mediate binding and recruitment of different substrates to the DotL T4CP (32). Thus, in *L. pneumophila*, a combination of C-terminal and internal translocation signals, together with a complex network of chaperone/adaptor/substrate interactions, regulates delivery of specific subsets of effector proteins through the Dot/Icm T4SS to host cells during *L. pneumophila* infection (32, 33).

T4SS structural and surface organelle variations

Many VirB/VirD4-like systems also have appropriated novel domains of functional importance (Table 2) (36). For example, some VirB6 subunits possess >30-kDa domains located at their C termini that have been shown or are proposed to localize at the cell surface (37, 38). Some VirB7-like lipoproteins and VirB10-like structural scaffolds also carry novel surface-localized motifs. Most notably, *H. pylori* CagT and CagY are classified as VirB7- and VirB10-like, respectively, but both subunits are considerably larger than their VirB counterparts and both localize extracellularly as a component of a large sheathed filament produced by the Cag T4SS (39). CagT and CagY also possess repeat regions that differ in size and composition among Cag systems of different *H. pylori* isolates (5, 40). Additionally, several systems including the *Bartonella* Trw system and VirB/VirD4 T4SSs carried by species in the order *Rickettsiales* carry multiple pilin genes in tandem array in their genomes, suggesting that variable pilus structures are elaborated through differential expression or intergenic recombination (41–43). Other T4SSs lack pilin genes or genes encoding the pilus tip protein VirB5, which is essential for elaboration of pili. These systems therefore probably do not elaborate pili but might still display surface structures, as exemplified by the *L. pneumophila* Dot/Icm, which encodes a fibrous structure on the cell surface (44). Collectively, the novel surface-variable proteins or structures acquired by various T4SSs during evolution are thought to contribute to the establishment of pathogen–host cell interactions, e.g., by mediating attachment to different host cells or host cell receptors or through modulation of the immune response.

T4SS EFFECTORS AND THEIR ROLES IN PATHOGENESIS

Besides appropriating novel structural motifs for specialized functions, the versatility of T4SSs is reflected in the diversity of substrates translocated to bacterial or eukaryotic target cells. Among the effector translocators employed by pathogens during infection, some translocate a single substrate, most deliver a restricted number of a half dozen or so, and a few highly promiscuous systems are estimated to translocate from 50 to several hundred effectors (Fig. 1, Table 1). In the following sections, we will review recent information about these systems, focusing mainly on the biochemical and cellular activities of effectors upon delivery to the host. Over the past decade, as studies have progressed on the T4SSs as well as the functionally (but not ancestrally) related T3SSs, it has become clear that common themes have emerged in the evolutionary design of many effectors. Most prominently, many effectors carry eukaryotic-like domains and thus exert their effects on various cellular processes or signaling pathways by mimicking activities of endogenous cellular proteins. For both the T4SSs and T3SSs, molecular mimicry has evolved predominantly to "fine-tune" specific cellular functions to the advantage of the invading pathogen rather than irreversibly blocking cellular homeostasis. Indeed, recent work shows that both of these dedicated secretion pathways often target apoptotic pathways with the aim of inhibiting premature death of the host cell in which the pathogen is attempting to establish a replicative niche.

Extracellular Pathogens

B. pertussis

B. pertussis is the causative agent of whooping cough, a respiratory illness spread mainly through aerosolization (45). Vaccination initiated in the 1940s led to a decline in incidence, but since the 1990s the number of cases of whooping cough has increased worldwide (46). The reasons underlying the resurgence are not clear but are generally attributed to the waning of protective immunity from vaccination or natural infection, low vaccination coverage, transmission from individuals vaccinated with the currently used acellular vaccines, or genetic changes

in *B. pertussis* to resistance against current vaccines (46). *B. pertussis* has several virulence factors of importance to infection and human-to-human spread, including pertussis toxin (PT) which is the sole substrate of the Ptl T4SS (47). PT is an ADP-ribosylating toxin composed of the catalytic A subunit and five B subunits required for translocation of the A subunit across eukaryotic cell membranes (48–51). Genes encoding PT subunits and the Ptl T4SS are genetically linked and coexpressed from the same promoter (52, 53).

Although the Ptl T4SS was recognized over 20 years ago to be closely related in overall gene order and subunit composition to the *A. tumefaciens* VirB/VirD4 T4SS and conjugation machines (54), it has several important distinctions that impart novel structural and functional features (Table 2). First, it lacks a homolog for the VirD4 substrate receptor, implying that an alternative mechanism has evolved for recruitment of the PT substrate to the transfer machine. In fact, the A and B subunits each carry a classical *sec* signal sequence and are translocated across the inner membrane via the general secretory pathway (GSP), completely independently of the Ptl system (55). Once in the periplasm, the subunits associate with the outer membrane and then assemble as the holotoxin, a process requiring extensive folding and disulfide bond formation. Mature holotoxin no longer associates with the outer membrane, but instead is released to periplasm and becomes available for recruitment to the Ptl T4SS (47). The signal(s) mediating toxin recruitment to the T4SS is currently unspecified, although a domain of the A subunit may comprise part of it. Upon recruitment, the Ptl T4SS delivers PT across the outer membrane and to the extracellular milieu (56). Thus, two distinct machines, the Sec translocase and the Ptl T4SS, export PT in a two-step translocation reaction, in contrast to the one-step translocation route envisioned for the T4CP-dependent T4SSs (Fig. 2) (57).

Also in contrast to other T4SSs, which translocate partially or completely unfolded substrates, the Ptl system exports PT as a large, tightly folded multimer. The most recent structures obtained for VirB/VirD4 conjugation systems show no obvious portals of entry or outer membrane channels of a size sufficient to accommodate PT (24, 25, 58). This suggests that the Ptl T4SS must have acquired a novel outer membrane architecture for exporting this AB_5-type toxin. Finally, the Ptl system lacks homologs for VirB1 and VirB5, two subunits required for biogenesis of pili (54). Accordingly, the Ptl system releases its cargo to the milieu, dispensing with a need for pilus-dependent contacts with the host cell.

Once PT is released to the milieu, it can interact with various mammalian cells, predominantly respiratory epithelial cells (Fig. 3) (45). The B oligomer of the toxin mediates binding to cell surface receptors, predominantly glycosylated proteins or lipids, which can induce host cellular responses such as T cell mitogenicity and hemagglutination independently of the biological activities attributable to the catalytic function of the A subunit within the host cell (59). Entry of PT into the host cell occurs by receptor-mediated endocytosis. PT trafficking follows the retrograde transport system sequentially through the endosomal compartment, Golgi apparatus, and endoplasmic reticulum (ER). Independently of the B moiety, the A moiety translocates through the ER into the cytosol to its target protein, membrane-associated trimeric G proteins. Upon binding, the A subunit catalyzes ADP-ribosylation of Cys residues

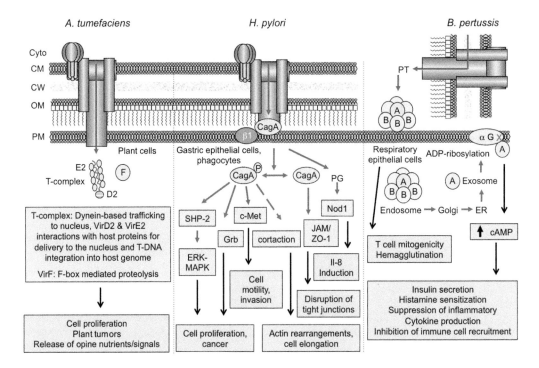

FIGURE 3 Type IV secretion system effectors and cellular consequences of translocation by extracellular pathogens. *Agrobacterium tumefaciens* and *Helicobacter pylori* deliver substrates through direct cell–cell contact, and *Bordetella pertussis* does so by a contact-independent mechanism. Pathogens target the host cell types listed. Translocated effectors interact (red arrows; dash denotes indirect interaction) with host cell proteins (light green boxes) to modulate various cellular processes and signaling pathways. Cellular consequences of the effector–host protein interactions (black arrows) are listed (aqua boxes).

in the C-terminal part of the α subunit of trimeric G proteins. ADP-ribosylation of Giα locks the protein in an inactive state, resulting in a loss of inhibition of adenylate cyclase activity and an increase in intracellular concentration of cyclic AMP (cAMP). Increased cAMP levels disrupt many cellular processes, accounting for the majority of pathological consequences of *B. pertussis* infection. Common effects are increased insulin secretion, sensitization to histamine, and inhibition of immune cell recruitment (Fig. 3) (45, 47).

Overall, the *B. pertussis* Ptl system represents a fascinating and, to date, novel example of a T4SS that evolved through loss of conserved subunits from an ancestral machine as a two-step translocation pathway capable of delivering a folded multimeric toxin to eukaryotic cells independently of direct cell-cell contact.

H. pylori

H. pylori is an extracellular pathogen that colonizes the gastric epithelium. It is the principal cause of chronic active gastritis and peptic ulcer disease and a risk factor for the development of gastric carcinoma and mucosa-associated lymphoid tissue (MALT) lymphoma (Table 1) (60, 61). Virulent strains of *H. pylori* associated with the enhanced risk of developing peptic ulcers or adenocarcinoma harbor a 37-kilobase (kb) pathogenicity island encoding the cytotoxin-associated gene (Cag) T4SS (62, 63). Also present on this pathogenicity island is a gene encoding CagA, the only known protein substrate of this T4SS (64). CagA is an ~120- to 145-kDa protein that shows no significant homology with other known proteins. Its size variation is due to structural diversity in its C-terminal region (65). In contrast to the *B. pertussis* Ptl system, the Cag T4SS recruits CagA from the bacterial cytoplasm via the Cagβ substrate receptor for transfer in one step across the *H. pylori* cell envelope and into mammalian target cells (Fig. 3).

The Cag T4SS is related to the *A. tumefaciens* VirB/VirD4 system but is also considerably more complex, as evidenced by the appropriation of more than a half dozen subunits and subdomains from unknown ancestries (66). As mentioned earlier, CagT and CagY are, respectively, classified as VirB7- and VirB10-like, yet both subunits are considerably larger than their VirB counterparts. These subunits comprise part of an OMC that is probably similar in overall structure to those solved for conjugation machines, while their additional domains localize extracellularly as a component of an extracellular pilus or large sheathed filament associated with the Cag T4SS (Table 2) (39). Importantly, these domains are composed of repeat regions that differ in size and composition among the various *H. pylori* strains (67, 68). Functions of these repeat regions are not yet defined, but are postulated to affect binding of *H. pylori* cells to mammalian cells through modulation of host β1 integrin interactions (69). There is also evidence that passage of *H. pylori* in mouse models results in variant forms of VirB10-like CagY, originally prompting the suggestion that CagY undergoes antigenic variation through homologous recombination within its repeat regions to evade the host immune response while maintaining T4SS function (67, 68). However, very recent work showed that immune-driven DNA rearrangements in CagY serve not so much to evade the host immune response altogether, but rather to fine-tune the response to establish the optimal homeostatic conditions of inflammation for persistent infection (40).

The Cag T4SS reportedly elaborates two types of surface structures: a large sheathed structure and pili, both implicated in interactions with host cells (39, 70, 71). The sheathed structures are 70 nm in diameter and are composed of pilin-like proteins CagC and CagL, as well as extracellular domains of CagY, CagT, and CagX (39). CagY and CagL bind β1 integrins, consistent with a role for this structure in attachment to host cells (69). More recent work has focused on the much narrower (~13 nm wide) pilus-like structures

(71, 72). These pili are detected only when *H. pylori* cells are cocultured with gastric epithelial cells, in an abundance of 3 to 4 pili per adherent *H. pylori* cell. Most of the Cag T4SS subunits are required for pilus assembly, although strikingly not the VirB2 pilin-like CagC subunit or VirB10-like CagY, even though both of these subunits are required for T4SS function as monitored by induction of IL-8 production and CagA translocation (72). Together, these observations raise the interesting possibility that the Cag T4SS elaborates distinct organelles for different purposes in relation to the infection process. Although specific functions of these T4SS structures await further definition, it is noteworthy that CagL, a homolog of the VirB5 pilus tip protein in *A. tumefaciens*, clearly plays a role in mediating interaction with host cell β1 integrins via its RGD motif (73). Through its RGD-dependent integrin-binding activities, purified CagL has been shown to elicit several responses in human cells, including cell adhesion, cell spreading, activation of host cell tyrosine kinases, and secretion of IL-8 (74, 75).

The importance of Cag T4SS-encoded pili to the *H. pylori* infection process is further underscored by the finding that strains that fail to produce pili are defective in Cag T4SS-dependent IL-8 induction in gastric epithelial cells (71, 76). Furthermore, changes in environmental conditions, such as reduced iron concentration, result in correlative increases in pilus production and Cag T4SS-associated activities (77). Also of interest, the sole protein substrate, CagA, of this T4SS is detectable on the *H. pylori* cell surface, particularly at the tips of pili (Fig. 3) (40, 69, 73). Both the surface display and pilus association of CagA are unique features among other known T4SS secretion substrates, and at least two lines of evidence support the notion that CagA surface accessibility is a biologically relevant entity. First, CagA binds phosphatidylserine at the outer leaflet of the host cell cytoplasmic membrane, which in turn induces its uptake into the cell (78). Second, as noted above, CagA translocation depends on the presence of β1 integrins as receptors for binding by the T4SS components CagL, CagY, and CagI. However, CagA itself also binds strongly to β1 integrins, suggesting that the pilus-tip bound form is a translocation intermediate (69).

Several recent studies have explored the underlying mechanisms responsible for recruitment and passage of CagA through the Cag T4SS. Docking of CagA with the T4SS requires three proteins: a chaperone CagF, the VirD4 homolog Cagβ, and CagZ (79, 80). CagA is highly labile in *H. pylori* cells unless it is coproduced and forms a complex in a 1:1 stoichiometry with the CagF chaperone. CagF differs from other T4SS or T3SS secretion chaperones, e.g., *A. tumefaciens* VirE1. Besides being much larger (32 kDa) than the other (<5 kDa) chaperones, CagF is highly hydrophobic and recently was shown to bind all five domains of CagA, presumably forming a broad interaction surface that protects the entire protein from degradation (81). CagF binding is also thought to prevent CagA intramolecular interactions of importance for protein function upon translocation to mammalian cells but might block CagA docking with the Cagβ receptor in *H. pylori*. While the nature of the CagA–Cagβ docking reaction remains to be defined, it is evident that the Cag T4SS has appropriated a novel CagF accessory factor to promote stabilization of the large, multidomain CagA substrate and docking with the Cagβ receptor (81).

Upon delivery into gastric epithelial cells, CagA is localized to the inner leaflet of the plasma membrane, where it undergoes tyrosine phosphorylation (Fig. 3). The phosphorylated protein interacts with SH2-domain-containing protein tyrosine phosphatase (SHP2) (82). CagA resembles the Gab family of scaffold proteins, which also form a complex with SHP2 in a tyrosine phosphorylation dependent manner in juxtaposition to the plasma membrane. Thus, partly through Gab mimicry, CagA exerts its many effects in host cells through promiscuous binding of a variety of human proteins by both phosphorylation-dependent and -independent mechanisms (Table 3) (83).

TABLE 3 Molecular mimicry: eukaryotic protein domains carried by T4SS effectors

Motif	Biochemical function	T4SS effector	References
EPIYA	Tyrosine phosphorylation	*Helicobacter pylori* CagA *Bartonella henselae* BepD, BepE, BepF *Anaplasma phagocytophilum* AnkA	87–89, 229
Ank	Protein-protein interaction	*A. phagocytophilum, Ehrlichia chaffeensis,* *Rickettsia rickettsii* AnkA *E. chaffeensis* p200 *Legionella pneumophila* AnkB, AnkX, AnkH, AnkJ, 7 others *Coxiella burnetii* AnkA,B, D*,F,G *Wolbachia wPip*: 60 Ank proteins *Orientia tsutsugamushi*: 50 Ank proteins *Rickettsia felis*: 22 Ank proteins	198, 199, 230, 231
F box	Interaction with SCF ubiquitination complexes	*Agrobacterium tumefaciens* VirF *L. pneumophila* AnkB, LicA, LegU1, PpgA, Lpg2525 *C. burnetii* AnkD, CBU0814, CBU0014 *O. tsutsugamushi* Anklu9	158, 159, 232, 233
Farnesylation/ prenylation	Posttranslational modification for protein–protein, protein–membrane interactions	*L. pneumophila* AnkB *L. pneumophila* Lpg2525, LegU1?	234, 235
FIC	AMPylation, phosphorylation, UMPylation, phosphocholination	*L. pneumophila* AnkX *B. henselae* BepA, BepB, BepC	96, 102
Gab	Family of scaffold protein	*H. pylori* CagA	83
ARF-, Ras-GEF	Guanine nucleotide exchange	*L. pneumophila* RalF, LegG2	152, 236
SREBPs	Sterol regulatory element binding proteins	*Anaplasma marginale* APH_0455	197

CagA is phosphorylated by Src family kinases at Tyr residues in the Glu-Pro-Ile-Tyr-Ala (EPIYA) motifs that resemble c-Src consensus phosphorylation sites and are located in variable numbers in the C-terminal region of the protein (Table 3) (84). Binding of phosphorylated CagA (CagA-P) to SHP2 causes aberrant activation of SHP2 and consequently of the ERK-MAPK (mitogen-activated protein kinase) pathway, which reportedly contributes to carcinogenesis by inducing mitogenic responses (Fig. 3) (65). CagA-activated SHP2 also dephosphorylates focal adhesion kinase, causing impaired focal adhesions that are associated with an elongated cell shape known as the hummingbird phenotype (85). Interestingly, East Asian CagA and Western CagA are, respectively, characterized by the presence of an EPIYA-D segment and an EPIYA-C segment to which SHP2 binds in a phosphorylation-dependent manner. The EPIYA-D segment binds SHP2 more strongly than the EPIYA-C segment,

and it is speculated that *H. pylori* carrying the biologically more active East Asian CagA variant is responsible for the propensity of these strains to induce severe gastric atrophy and gastric cancers in infected patients (86).

Since the discovery of the CagA EPIYA motif, at least nine other T4SS or T3SS effectors were shown to carry such eukaryotic-like motifs with similar biochemical activities upon translocation to host cells. Among the T4SSs discussed in more detail below, the *Bartonella henselae* VirB/VirD4 T4SS translocates three effectors (BepD, PepE, and BepF), each with one or more EPIYA or EPIYA-like motifs (87). The *Anaplasma phagocytophilum* AnkA effector also bears multiple EPIYA motifs that display variations in number and subtypes among different bacterial strains (88). Other pathogens employing T3SSs to translocate EPIYA-bearing effectors during infection include *Chlamydia trachomatis* (the Tarp effector, induces cytoskeletal rearrangements) and enteropathogenic *E. coli* (Tir, triggers actin pedestal formation). *Haemophilus ducreyi* also delivers two EPIYA-containing effectors, LspA1 and LspA2, via a two-partner secretion system to eukaryotic cells, whereupon inhibition of Src family kinase functions blocks Fcγ-mediated triggering of phagocytosis (Table 3) (89).

In addition to the SHP2 interaction, an array of other CagA-binding partners has been described, including carboxy-terminal Src kinase (Csk), growth factor receptor-bound protein 2 (Grb2), tight junction protein zonula occludens 1 (ZO-1), scatter factor receptor c-Met, and phospholipase C-γ. This plethora of CagA phosphorylation-dependent and -independent interactions modulates pathways involved in the innate immune response, cell shape regulation, and signal transduction (Fig. 3) (see references 90, 91). There is also compelling evidence that the Cag T4S machine, through receptor-dependent activation or translocation of fragments of peptidoglycan or another unidentified effector (s), operates independently of CagA and of VirD4-like Cagβ to elicit stress-response pathways that result in induction of IL-8 secretion (Fig. 3) (92).

Facultative Intracellular Pathogens

Bartonella

Bartonella spp. reside in erythrocytes and cause long-lasting bacteremic infections in diverse mammalian hosts. They are transmitted by blood-sucking arthropods, usually through dermal inoculation. Upon reaching the blood stream, *Bartonella* spp. invade erythrocytes and persist intracellularly for the lifetime of the red blood cell. Adaptation to the reservoir host causes no or mild disease symptoms, whereas infection of incidental hosts can cause a spectrum of diseases including cat-scratch disease, Carrion's disease, chronic lymphadenopathy, trench fever, chronic bacteremia, endocarditis, bacillary angiomatosis, peliosis hepatis, and neurological disorder. Without treatment, *Bartonella* infections are associated with high mortality

and the potential for relapse due to the existence of an intraerythrocytic phase that may provide a protective niche for the bacteria (93–95).

Bartonella spp. employ two T4SSs for different purposes relating to the infection process (Table 2) (96). The Trw T4SS shares strong sequence similarities with the Trw system encoded by the IncW plasmid R388, with the exception that it lacks a homolog for the VirD4-like substrate receptor (97). The Trw homologs of the two systems share 20 to 80% sequence identities, and interestingly, the *Bartonella tribocorum* Trw genes encoding VirB5-like TrwH, VirB10-like TrwE, and VirB11-like TrwD substitute for their homologs in the Trw$_{R388}$ system (97, 98). This finding underscores the conservation of machine architecture between two T4SSs that have evolved for completely different functions. However, since the *Bartonella* Trw system lacks a VirD4-like T4CP, it is postulated not to function as a translocation system, but rather to mediate attachment to host cells. In line with such a function, the Trw locus possesses tandem copies of genes encoding homologs of the VirB2 and VirB5 pilin proteins, suggesting that this system is specifically adapted for the production of antigenically variable pili through intergenic recombination (97). The adaptation of a T4SS for elaboration of a variable surface structure aligns this system with the *H. pylori* Cag system, which elaborates variant forms of surface-exposed channel subunits, as well as rickettsial systems discussed later in this chapter.

Studies have shown that the Trw system is required for establishing intraerythrocytic infection in a *B. tribocorum* rat model (93, 97). A signature-tagged mutagenesis screen further identified mutations in the *trw* locus that severely impaired adhesion of *Bartonella birtlesii* to erythrocytes (99). Based on the postulated surface location of the Trw components, this T4SS might directly interact with the erythrocyte surface, thereby restricting the host range of the erythrocyte infection. A role for this system in host specificity was confirmed through a demonstration that swapping of Trw from rat-specific *B. ribocorum* for that of cat-specific *B. henselae* and human-specific *Bartonella quintana* shifted the host ranges of these latter species for erythrocyte infection toward rats (42). The further observation that the Trw pilin subunits exist in multiple copies suggests that the *trw* locus encodes variant forms of surface-exposed pilus which might facilitate the specific interaction with polymorphic erythrocyte receptors either within the reservoir host population or among different reservoir hosts (42).

The second T4SS, designated VirB/VirD4, is composed of a complete set of homologs of the *A. tumefaciens* VirB and VirD4 subunits (100, 101). It contributes to pathogenicity by delivering up to seven effector proteins termed Beps (*Bartonella* effector proteins) into nucleated cells (Fig. 4). The Beps were identified originally by the presence of an ~140-residue domain near their C termini that was termed BID (Bep intracellular delivery). This domain and a positively charged C-terminal tail sequence correspond to a bipartite translocation signal required for delivery of several of the Beps through the VirB/VirD4 T4SS (28). For a few Beps, the BID domain is not required for translocation but, rather, contributes to effector function in the host cell.

Once inside the host cells, Beps target host components and modulate cellular processes to the benefit of the bacteria. A deletion of all seven *bep* genes (*bepA* to *bepG*) abolishes all VirB/VirD4-dependent cellular phenotypes, including cell invasion, proinflammatory activation, and the inhibition of apoptosis (Fig. 4) (28). The Beps have a modular architecture that includes one or more BID domains. BepA, BepB, and BepC also carry a FIC (filamentation induced by cAMP) domain, which is present in many bacteria and eukaryotes including mammals (Table 3) (96). FIC enzymes posttranslationally modify proteins through AMPylation, UMPylation,

phosphorylation, or phosphocholination. All FIC enzymes catalyze the transfer of a part of a metabolite upon cleavage of a pyrophosphate bond (102). Besides their presence in *Bartonella* Beps, FIC domains have been identified in effectors translocated by the *L. pneumophila* Dot/Icm system (AnkX) as well as T3SSs employed by *Pseudomonas syringae* (AvrB), *Vibrio parahaemolyticus* (VopS), and *Xanthomonas campestris* (AvrAC) (102). At this point, however, the contributions of Bep FIC domains to *Bartonella* infection processes have not been defined. As mentioned earlier, some Beps also carry EPIYA motifs serving as sites of tyrosine phosphorylation upon delivery into the mammalian host (Table 3) (28, 103).

Considerable progress has been made toward defining specific contributions of the Bep proteins to stages of the infection cycle (Fig. 4). In brief, upon deposition on the skin by a blood-sucking arthropod, one or a few *Bartonella* cells are taken up by endocytosis into a vacuole called the *Bartonella*-containing vacuole (104, 105). The process of endocytosis is arrested by Beps (BepC, BepF, BepG) delivered into the host cytoplasm by the VirB/VirD4 T4SS (106, 107). Bacterial aggregates form at the cell surface, and these bacteria then invade the endothelial cells via F-actin-dependent invasome-mediated internalization (105). *Bartonella* then colonizes the "dermal niche," most likely within dendritic cells, which are considered important for dissemination to the "blood-seeding niche." BepE is essential for invasion of cells in the dermal niche and for subsequent spread to the bloodstream. Recently, it was reported that the BID domains of BepE contribute to endothelial cell migration and prevent cell fragmentation through interference of the RhoA signaling pathway (108). Furthermore, BepA mediates protection of endothelial cells from apoptosis through binding of a BID domain to host cell adenylyl cyclase with a consequence of elevated cAMP production and inhibition of apoptosis (109).

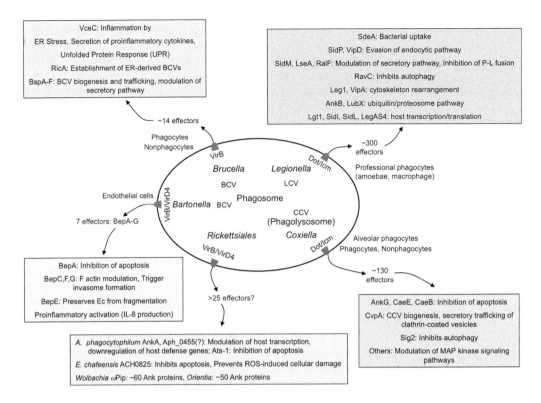

FIGURE 4 **Type IV secretion system (T4SS) effectors and cellular consequences of translocation by intracellular pathogens.** The pathogens listed deliver effector proteins to establish a replicative niche within phagosomal compartments. Associated with each organism is the name of the T4SS, the replicative niche (e.g., LCV for *Legionella*-containing vacuole), the host cell type(s) targeted, and the current number of known or estimated effectors. Also for each organism is a list of representative effectors and cellular consequences of their activity within the host cell (colored boxes).

In sum, investigations to date point to essential contributions of the VirB/VirD4 T4SS and Bep effectors to the primary stages of infection. All Bep-dependent phenotypes have been shown to rely on the different BID domains, which collectively exert their effects on different physiological or signaling pathways in the human host and also serve as translocation signals in the bacterium, presumably for productive binding with the VirD4 receptor. At this time, nothing is known of how the FIC and EPIYA domains contribute to the Bep-dependent phenotypes, despite evidence for tyrosine-phosphorylation of BepE's EPIYA motif and binding of phosphorylated BepE to SHP2 and Csk, two well-characterized binding targets

of *H. pylori* CagA. Of final note, the *B. henselae* VirB/VirD4 T4SS was shown to be capable of delivering DNA into vascular endothelial cells (110). This T4SS is closely related in subunit composition to conjugation systems, underscoring both the common ancestry and functional similarities of effector translocator and conjugation systems (111). Whether DNA transfer is a natural substrate that *Bartonella* delivers to eukaryotic cells during the infection process is an intriguing question for further study.

Brucella

Brucella spp. cause abortion in their natural animal hosts (e.g., swine, goats, sheep, cattle, bison) and are responsible for human brucellosis. *Brucella* infects and replicates in phagocytic and nonphagocytic cells. The bacteria can persist for years in the reticuloendothelial system of their natural hosts as well as incidental human hosts (112). Human brucellosis is characterized by undulant fevers and constitutional symptoms including malaise, myalgia, and enlarged spleen and liver. Chronic infection can progress to severe complications including arthritis and endocarditis. Factors mediating uptake are not completely defined, but once endocytosed, *Brucella* resides initially in the *Brucella*-containing vacuole (BCV). The BCV interacts sequentially with early and late endosomes and lysosomes, finally establishing an intracellular replicative niche derived from the ER. Subsequent to replication, *Brucella* exits host cells to reinfect adjacent cells (113).

The VirB T4SS of *Brucella* plays a critical role in establishment of the ER-derived replicative BCVs and is an essential virulence factor in a mouse model of infection (114–116). It is also essential for persistence of the bacteria in a mouse model and goat host (115, 117). While the *Brucella* T4SS gene cluster contains homologs of all of the *A. tumefaciens* VirB genes, there is no VirD4-like receptor, and the operon contains two additional genes, *virB12* and *orf13* (Table 2) (114). The absence of a VirD4-like receptor suggests either that an alternative routing mechanism exists for substrate transfer across the inner membrane (as shown for *B. pertussis* PT translocation) or that this machine does not translocate substrates but provides another function, e.g., attachment, of importance for infection (as proposed for the *Bartonella* Trw system). Confirming the former model, several *Brucella* effectors are now known to be translocated by a VirB-dependent mechanism to host cells (see below). Intriguingly, only a subset of the effectors carry a classical *sec* signal suggestive of a two-step translocation route reminiscent of the PT export system (118). The mechanism(s) by which other *Brucella* effectors engage with the VirB machine, and in which cellular compartment

(e.g., cytoplasm, periplasm), remains to be determined.

Acidification of the phagosome is required for induction of the *virB* operon encoding the *Brucella* VirB T4SS during infection of macrophages (119). Production of the T4SS and effector translocation allows for evasion of lysosomal fusion with the BCV and association with the ER-derived intracellular compartment (120). Effector candidates were identified by bioinformatics screens for eukaryotic-like domains, genes that are coregulated with the *virB* operon, and genes whose products interact with human ER exit site–associated proteins. At this time, 14 effectors have been identified, although in most cases their functions during infection are not yet established (Fig. 4). Interestingly, an additional six candidate effectors also appear to be translocated to human cells independently of the T4SS (121).

The first-identified effectors were VceA and VceE, and VceE is currently the best characterized among all *Brucella* effectors (118). VceC has been shown to induce ER stress and secretion of proinflammatory cytokines (Fig. 4). Ectopically expressed VceC binds the ER in HeLa cells via an interaction with the ER chaperone BiP/Grp78, and VceC production is correlated with reorganization of ER structures (122). Furthermore, in macrophages, VceC triggers the unfolded protein response, resulting in the induction of inflammation by *Brucella abortus* (122). Whether VceC exerts its activity on the unfolded protein response through binding of BiP remains to be determined. VceC is not thought to be involved in establishment of the BCV, but rather, contributes to long-term colonization and overall fitness of the infecting *Brucella* organisms. However, another effector, termed RicA (Rab2 interacting conserved protein A), binds the GDP-bound form of Rab2, a host GTPase shown to be essential for *Brucella* intracellular replication through binding of BCVs. Correspondingly, *ricA* mutants show a decrease in Rab2 recruitment to BCVs (123). These findings led the authors to postulate that T4SS-mediated translocation of RicA is important for establishment of the ER-derived replicative BCVs by enabling precise interactions with secretory pathway organelles (Fig. 4).

Two effectors, BrpA and BtpB, share a conserved TIR (toll/interleukin-1 receptor)–containing domain, and both are essential for virulence (124, 125). BtpA exerts its effects through inhibition of NF-kB and the toll-like receptor signaling pathway, whereas BtpB activates NF-kB and the toll-like receptor pathway. TIR-containing adaptors are widely present in mammals, where the associated proteins regulate the signaling cascades of innate immune recognition. However, many bacteria besides *Brucella* employ TIR domain–containing proteins for modulation of the toll-like receptor signaling cascade, thus providing another example of molecular mimicry by pathogens for subversion of host cellular processes.

Finally, by use of a reporter assay for translocation, five candidate effectors designated BspA-F were identified whose delivery to human cells was dependent on the VirB T4SS (121). Importantly, several of these effectors were shown to localize to compartments of the secretory pathway when ectopically expressed in HeLa cells. Furthermore, ectopically expressed BsbA, BspB, and BspF were found to specifically inhibit host protein secretion and membrane trafficking along the secretory pathway, in line with observations that such perturbations are also observed during *Brucella* infection. Additionally, evidence was presented that these Bsps contribute to the biogenesis of BCVs and to bacterial replication in macrophages, as well as to long-term persistence in the liver of chronically infected mice. These new findings establish a possible link between BCV trafficking and VirB T4SS-dependent modulation of the secretory pathway (Fig. 4) (121).

L. pneumophila

L. pneumophila is ubiquitous in the environment, preferentially thriving in water systems.

It colonizes a variety of ecological niches, including various amoebae and other protozoa in which it can grow and replicate (126). *Legionella* enters the human lung via inhalation of *Legionella*-containing aerosols. The bacteria replicate in alveolar macrophages and can cause a potentially fatal pneumonia termed Legionnaires' disease. The *L. pneumophila* infection cycle involves host-cell entry by phagocytosis, creation of a specialized vacuole termed the *Legionella*-containing vacuole (LCV) for replication, macrophage lysis, and infection of neighboring cells (127). Creation of the LCV requires the Dot/Icm T4SS, which has the amazing capacity to translocate an estimated 300 effector proteins, approximately 10% of this organism's proteome, into target cells (18, 128). Like the *Bartonella* spp. and *A. tumefaciens* VirB/VirD4 systems, the Dot/Icm T4SS has retained a functional vestige of its ancestral conjugation system in being able to mobilize transfer of IncQ plasmids to bacterial recipients, although the functional significance of DNA transfer during the infection process is not known (129).

As mentioned earlier, the Dot/Icm systems are only weakly related to the VirB/VirD4 systems and thus were termed type IVB systems (15). The Dot/Icm systems are composed of at least 25 to 27 proteins, many of which localize to the cytoplasm or inner membrane (32). A number of these are chaperones or adaptors that fulfill the complex task of delivering the multitude of effectors to the host cell at appropriate times during the infection cycle. Recent structural work has shown that the cell envelope–spanning channel consists in part of a ring-shaped OMC similar to that of the VirB/VirD4 T4SSs (130). A notable variation from the latter systems is that DotD, a lipoprotein thought to provide a stabilizing function similar to that of VirB7, possesses a large domain structurally similar to N0 domains (131). Such domains are also found associated with secretins in the type II and III secretion systems and might serve as a structural scaffold or for recruitment of substrates in the periplasm (see 131). The Dot/Icm T4SS is thought to translocate substrates in one step across the cell envelope, but this model has not been rigorously tested, so a role for the N0 domain of DotD in substrate binding remains a possibility. Another difference with the VirB/VirD4 T4SSs is that the Dot/Icm system elaborates not an extracellular pilus, but rather a fibrous mesh on the bacterial cell surface composed at least in part of the DotH and DotO proteins (44).

Most of the candidate effectors were identified through a combination of bioinformatics screens and assays for translocation using reporter protein fusions (132). Efforts to establish the importance of given effectors to the infection process, however, have been hampered by the fact that many effectors have redundant functions (133). In some cases, mutant strains lacking a single effector show intracellular growth defects upon depletion of specific host factors or are outcompeted by wild-type bacteria in competition assays (127, 134). Functions have been assigned for about 50 of the candidate effectors, which can be grouped based on their major cellular target pathway(s) during the infection cycle (135). A full description of the biochemical activities of the Dot/Icm T4SS effectors is beyond the scope of this article, and the interested reader is referred to several excellent reviews (127, 135–137). Here, we will identify and describe activities of a subset of the effectors shown to affect specific secretory pathways and cellular functions relevant to the infection process.

L. pneumophila replicates in "professional" phagocytes such as amoebae and macrophages (133, 138). It employs the Dot/Icm T4SS to deliver effector proteins as soon as it contacts the cell (Fig. 4). One effector, SdeA, is implicated as being important for bacterial adherence and uptake, although further work is needed to confirm this function (139). However, the internalization process activates T4SS function, resulting in the translocation of presynthesized effector molecules (140, 141). Effector translocation enables

L. pneumophila to evade endocytic (lysosome) fusion and intercept ER-to-Golgi vesicular traffic to remodel its phagosome into an ER-derived vacuole that serves as a proliferation niche (133). Internalization progresses to formation of the LCV, which communicates extensively with the endosomal trafficking route largely through acquisition of host molecules and effectors on the LCV membrane. For example, the LCV acquires two types of molecules, phosphoinositide lipid phosphatidylinositol-3-phosphate [PtdIns(3)P] and Rab GTPases, that are key regulators of the early endocytic pathway (135). Several Dot/Icm substrates including LidA, LptD, RidL, and SetA have been shown to bind PtdIns(3)P, possibly as an LCV membrane anchor (142–145). The effector SidP is a phosphoinositide 3-phosphatase that hydrolyses PtdIns(3)P and thus might contribute to evasion of the endocytic pathway (146). A number of Rab GTPases (Rab5A, Rab7, Rab14, Rab21) are recruited to the LCV, and several effectors interact with these GTPases. One of these, VipD, is activated by Rab5, and one of its functions is to remove PtdIns(3)P from the LCV membrane (147). Thus, like SidP, VipD is thought to promote LCV evasion of the endocytic pathway. Other effectors acting on the endocytic pathway include SidK, which binds one of the subunits of V-type H+-ATPase (a late endosomal marker that also binds the LCV) and inhibits ATP hydrolysis, proton translocation, and LCV acidification (148).

The LCV compartment also modulates the secretory pathway by intercepting early secretory vesicles released from ER exit sites toward the Golgi apparatus. The Dot/Icm effectors SidM and LseA have been shown to modulate this secretory pathway by promoting the fusion of LCVs with ER-derived vesicles through effects on SNARE (soluble N-ethylmaleimide-sensitive factor attachment protein receptor) complex formation (149, 150). SNARES are responsible for the docking and fusion of many different vesicle-mediated transport events. Another phosphatidylinositol, PtdIns(4)P, as well as the GTPase Rab1 are major regulators of Golgi-bound, secretory vesicle trafficking. PtdIns(4)P is formed on the LCV membrane through the actions of SidF (151) and other effectors. Several Dot/Icm effectors bind the LCV via PtdIns(4)P or Rab1. These effectors collectively modulate the secretory pathway through their various biochemical activities including AMPylation, deAMPylation, ubiquitination, phosphocholination, and guanine nucleotide exchange (see 135). For example, RalF, the first identified Dot/Icm effector, functions as a guanine nucleotide exchange factor that mediates LCV fusion with ER-derived secretory vesicles and the ER by recruiting and activating Arf1, another small GTPase involved in vesicle trafficking from the ER to the Golgi (152).

Besides altering the endocytic and secretory pathways, *L. pneumophila* uses the Dot/Icm T4SS to translocate numerous other effectors that act on a plethora of other host cellular processes to benefit survival in the host cell (Fig. 4). In brief, effectors such as RavZ are known to inhibit autophagy (153), and RidL, to modulate the retrograde pathway (145). Others such as Legs2 associate with mitochondria, possibly disrupting host cell bioenergetics (154), VipA with actin to effect cytoskeleton remodeling (155, 156), and AnkB with the ubiquitin/proteasome pathway (157–159). Others modulate programmed cell death in several ways that include modulation of host transcription and translation (see 135).

Studies over the past decade have generated an extensive literature about the *L. pneumophila* T4SS and contributions of effectors to the infection process. Equally importantly, these studies have identified novel features of fundamental biochemical and cellular processes in the host cell. Given that only a small subset of the candidate effectors have been characterized so far, future studies will assuredly continue to unveil new mechanistic insights at many levels into the fascinating *L. pneumophila*– host cell relationship.

Obligate Intracellular Pathogens

C. burnetii

C. burnetii is an intracellular bacterium that causes the zoonotic disease Q fever. It is transmitted by inhalation of contaminated aerosols and can cause life-threatening illness with vague symptoms similar to those described above for *Rickettsia* infections that can progress to pneumonia, hepatitis, myocarditis, or central nervous system complications (160). *C. burnetii* can also cause long-term chronic disease that can manifest as endocarditis years after the initial infection (161). Ruminants are the natural reservoir for *Coxiella*, and infections of these animals can cause abortion and subsequent contamination of the environment. As for the *Rickettsia* species, studies of *C. burnetii* pathogenesis have been hampered by the obligate intracellular lifestyle of the bacterium. However, an axenic culture condition was described in 2009, which has revolutionized studies of this pathogen that have supplied important new information about the bacterial factors, particularly its Dot/Icm T4SS and translocated effectors, to virulence (162).

Coxiella has the capacity to enter both phagocytic and nonphagocytic cells, where it replicates to high numbers inside a specialized vacuole termed the *Coxiella*-containing vacuole (CCV) (163). The CCV undergoes normal endocytic trafficking through early and late endosomes to a lysosome. In contrast to the LCV, which subverts the endocytic trafficking to avoid lysosome fusion, however, the CCV fuses with the lysosome. Within this acidic environment, *Coxiella* then differentiates from an environmentally stable small cell variant into a replicating large cell variant. The CCV then undergoes expansion by recruitment of cellular vesicles that fuse with the vacuole membrane, during which time *Coxiella* replicates to large numbers (164).

The Dot/Icm system was discovered by genome sequencing and was shown to be essential for virulence through construction and analysis of *dot/icm* transposon insertion or deletion mutations (165–168). As discussed above, the *L. pneumophila* T4SS assembles prior to host cell uptake and delivers effectors upon initial contact to subvert the endocytic pathway and promote fusion with secretory vesicles. By contrast, the *Coxiella* T4SS translocates effectors only several hours after infection, following CCV-lysosome fusion, with the overall objective of remodeling this vacuole to facilitate replication.

To date, over 130 candidate effectors have been identified for this system, through bioinformatics screens to identify proteins with eukaryotic-like motifs and experimental verification by use of reporter protein translocation assays (see 169). Interestingly, a large number of the candidate effectors were classified as pseudogenes in some strains that can block synthesis or translocation or alter the protein's activity in the host through loss of one or more domains. Such genetic alterations have been postulated to contribute to the evolution of different *Coxiella* variants (170).

Although biochemical characterization of *Coxiella* effectors is still in its infancy, a variety of screens and approaches have identified effectors that contribute to CCV biogenesis and intracellular growth and that modulate different cellular processes and pathways (Fig. 4). The host cell must remain viable to support *Coxiella* replication, and several effectors have been shown to inhibit the host cell death pathway. AnkG, for example, blocks apoptosis by interacting first with the host mitochondrial protein p32 and subsequently with the nucleus, where it exerts its antiapoptotic effects by an unknown mechanism (171, 172). Other antiapoptotic effectors include CaeA and CaeB, which bind, respectively, to the mitochondria and nucleus, where they are thought to interfere with apoptotic signaling (173). A number of other effectors, identified through large-scale transposon mutagenesis screens, have been shown to be important for intracellular replication. This list now includes

CirA-E (*Coxiella* effector for intracellular replication) as well as Cig57, CoxCC8, CBU1754, and CvpA-CvpE (174, 175). Identification of CvpA was of interest in view of evidence that clathrin-mediated vesicular trafficking is important for CCV biogenesis. Clathrin was shown to be present on the CCV membrane, and reduction in the level of CCV-bound clathrin was correlated with diminished *Coxiella* replication. Further studies showed that CvpA interacts with the clathrin-adaptor complex AP2, leading to a proposal that this effector contributes to CCV biogenesis and intracellular replication through recruitment of host cell clathrin transport machinery and possibly other factors to the CCV (176). Another effector, Cig2, was shown to contribute to establishment of the replicative niche by blocking autophagy, a process used by the host cell to remove misfolded proteins, damaged organelles, and intracellular pathogens through targeting to the lysosome (175). Finally, several effectors have been shown to modulate MAP kinase signaling pathways in yeast, possibly through disruption of the phosphorylation state of proapoptotic proteins (166, 177, 178).

At this time, studies of effector function have identified important contributions to establishment of the CCV and intracellular replication through effects on autophagy, secretory trafficking of clathrin-coated vesicles, apoptosis, and signal transduction. The challenges for the future are to define the specific biochemical functions of these effectors. Another important goal is to define the contributions of the Dot/Icm system and other virulence factors to the unique capacity of this bacterium to survive and replicate in the acidic, proteolytic and oxidative environment of the lysosome-derived CCV.

Rickettsia

Rickettsia spp. are obligate intracellular pathogens or endosymbionts. The major genera include *Anaplasma*, *Ehrlichia*, *Orientia*, *Rickettsia*, and *Wolbachia* (179). The *Rickettsiales*

associate with diverse eukaryotic hosts in pathogenic or symbiotic relationships. *Rickettsia* species are responsible for major human diseases including Rocky Mountain spotted fever (*Rickettsia rickettsii*), epidemic typhus (*Rickettsia prowazekii*), and zoonotic diseases of granulocytic anaplasmosis (*A. phagocytophilum*) and monocytic ehrlichiosis (*Ehrlichia chaffeensis*) (179, 180). *Orientia tsutsugamushi is* the causative agent of scrub typhus (181). Clinical signs of these diseases are similar and include fever, headache, myalgia, anorexia, and chills, frequently accompanied by leukopenia. Diseases can progress to meningitis and disseminated intravascular coagulation, which if left untreated can progress to multiple organ failure. Transmission is generally by a tick, mite, or other insect vector from animal reservoirs (179, 180).

Wolbachia are endosymbionts or parasites associated with numerous invertebrates including arthropods and nematodes. In filarial nematodes, *Wolbachia* are essential for survival and replication of their host (182). In arthropods, *Wolbachia* are mostly parasites that affect reproduction of their hosts in ways that enhance their own transmission through maternal inheritance from infected females to progeny (183). Strikingly, there is evidence for widespread horizontal gene transfer of *Wolbachia* chromosomal fragments into many species of arthropods and nematodes, and in the latter for expression of the integrated genes (184). These findings raise the intriguing possibility that *Wolbachia* might employ their T4SSs to translocate chromosomal DNA for establishment of symbiotic or parasitic relationships with their hosts.

All characterized members of the *Rickettsiales* carry genes for T4SSs, although the genes typically are not clustered in a single operon but rather in two or three operons scattered around the genome (43, 185–188). *O. tsutsugamushi* offers the most extreme known example of the fragmentation of T4SS genes around the chromosome (189).

The chromosomes of these bacteria are themselves highly fragmented, presumably as a result of extensive recombination at the 4,197 identical repeat sequences shown to be distributed around the genome. The *O. tsutsugamushi* genome also carries over 1,100 mobile genetic elements, which is especially intriguing in view of the fact that mobile elements are only rarely present in the genomes of other *Rickettsia* species (189). These findings provide compelling evidence that conjugative transfer has played an important role in the shaping of the *O. tsutsugamushi* genome throughout evolution.

Besides the unusual distribution of T4SS genes around the chromosome, the *Rickettsia* T4SSs possess a number of variations from the archetypal VirB/VirD4 T4SSs (Table 2). First, these systems lack the pilus-associated proteins (VirB1, VirB5) thought to be involved in intercellular attachment processes, possibly reflecting the intracellular lifestyle of these bacteria (41, 43, 190). Another novel adaptation is the presence of multiple copies of genes encoding several of the VirB homologs. The genomes typically carry genes in single copy for the structural subunits VirB8, VirB9, and VirB10, as well as the ATPases VirB11 and VirD4. However, multiple copies exist for genes encoding inner membrane channel subunits VirB3 and the VirB4 ATPase as well as polytopic VirB6 (43, 190). Most noteworthy, the multiple VirB6 subunits display considerable variability in length and sequence composition, particularly in their hydrophilic C-terminal regions (5). There is evidence for surface exposure of VirB6 homologs in *E. chaffeensis* and *Wolbachia*, leading to the suggestion that these variable proteins promote survival in the host through binding of host cell receptors or evasion of host immune defenses (37, 191–193). Additionally, multiple copies exist of genes encoding sequence-variable VirB2 pilin-like subunits, reminiscent of the *Bartonella* Trw T4SS (Table 2) (41). How these T4SS-encoded surface structures contribute to the infection processes of these intracellular pathogens is an intriguing question for further study.

Identification of T4SS effectors functioning in *Rickettsia* species has been challenging given a lack of genetic systems for mutant strain constructions and the inability to culture these bacteria axenically. However, a number of candidate or confirmed effectors have been identified through a combination of bioinformatics screens, two-hybrid assays for protein interactions with the VirD4-like substrate receptors, and use of surrogate T4SSs, e.g., the *A. tumefaciens* VirB/VirD4 and *Legionella* Dot/Icm systems, to assay for translocation (194–197). In bioinformatics screens, the ankyrin repeat (Ank) is a particularly prominent eukaryotic-like domain identified in the genomes of various members of the *Rickettsiales*. *Wolbachia* strain ωPip and *O. tsutsugamushi*, respectively, carry an astonishing 60 and 50 *ank* genes, the most identified to date for any bacterial species (198).

The Ank repeat is a 33-residue motif, often in tandem arrays, that cooperatively folds into structures that mediate molecular recognition via protein-protein interactions (Table 2). These are widespread interaction motifs in eukaryotes, and they are also features of T4SS as well as T3SS effectors, and there is evidence that such proteins play important roles in pathogenesis by mimicking or interfering with host cell functions (199). Indeed, the first T4SS effector identified among the *Rickettsiales* was AnkA, which was shown to be a secretion substrate of the *A. phagocytophilum* T4SS (Fig. 4) (194). AnkA contains 11 Ank repeat motifs and a positively charged C-terminal tail similar to those carried by secretion substrates of the *A. tumefaciens* VirB/VirD4 T4SS. Accordingly, AnkA was shown to be translocated through the *A. tumefaciens* VirB/VirD4 T4SS to plant cells (194). In its natural mammalian host cell, AnkA is phosphorylated by the Abl-1 and Src kinases, and phospho-AnkA then binds the host protein Src homology phosphatase-1

(SHP-1) (88). Interestingly, AnkA binds nuclear proteins and forms complexes with AT-rich DNA sequences, resulting in modulation of host gene transcription (200). Recently, AnkA was found to downregulate expression of multiple host defense genes, including the NADH oxidase component, CYBB. AnkA also binds the histone deacetylase 1 (HDAC1), which is critical for AnkA-mediated CYBB repression. The consequence of CYBB downregulation is a decrease in superoxide anion production by the NADH oxidase, which is a key mechanism of pathogen killing for neutrophils (201). Given the observation that AnkA binds to numerous sites in the host genome and histone deacetylation is frequently observed at host promoters of host defense genes, it is likely that AnkA broadly impacts the host transcriptional response to *A. phagocytophilum* infection (Fig. 4).

A second confirmed *A. phagocytophilum* effector, termed Ats-1 (*Anaplasma* translocated substrate), was identified through a two-hybrid screen for binding partners of the VirD4 receptor (195). Ats-1 also has a positively charged C terminus but was not translocated through the *A. tumefaciens* VirB/VirD4 T4SS. Nevertheless, it is a *bona fide* substrate of the *A. phagocytophilum* T4SS, as shown by its abundant secretion into mammalian cells, where a large proportion localizes to the *A. phagocytophilum* inclusion. Ats-1 lacks known protein motifs, but it does carry an N-terminal mitochondria-targeting presequence. This translocation signal directs Ats-1 into the mitochondrial matrix of infected human neutrophils, HeLa cells, and even yeast cells (195). Consequently, Ats-1 passes through a total of five membranes—bacterial inner and outer membranes, the inclusion membrane, and the mitochondrial membranes—en route to its postulated site of action. One of the hallmarks of this infection process is the inhibition of spontaneous induced apoptosis of human neutrophils. Although several cellular mechanisms have been described by which *A. phagocytophilum* inhibits apoptosis (inhibition of the loss of mitochondrial membrane potential, inhibition of Bax translocation to the mitochondria, inhibition of activation of caspase 3), the role of Ats-1 in one or more of these processes is not yet known (Fig. 4).

Several candidate effectors of the *E. chaffeensis* T4SS also have been identified. The best characterized, ECH0825, carries a positively charged C terminus and interacts with the VirD4$_{Ec}$ receptor. ECH0825 is highly upregulated during infection, translocated to the host cell cytoplasm and, reminiscent of Ats-1, localizes to the mitochondria (202). Ectopically expressed ECH0825 inhibits apoptosis in response to etoposide treatment, and also inhibits Bax-induced apoptosis. ECH0825 production also was correlated with upregulation of mitochondrial manganese superoxide dismutase (MnSOD) and reduced reactive oxygen species. By preventing reactive oxygen species–induced cellular damage and apoptosis, ECH0825 thus might promote intracellular infection (Fig. 4) (202).

Although no other effectors have been confirmed for *Rickettsia* T4SSs, a bioinformatics screen identified 21 possible effectors for *A. marginale*, of which four (AM185, AM1141, AM470, AM705[AnkA]) were shown to be translocated through the surrogate *L. pneumophila* Dot/Icm T4SS (196). More recently, a study seeking to identify potential *A. phagocytophilum*–derived nuclear-transported proteins that could impact host cell transcription identified 50 candidate proteins through a combination of bioinformatics and iTRAQ protein profiling (197). Nuclear localization was confirmed for six of these candidate effectors through ectopic expression, but only one (APH_0455) was translocated through a surrogate *C. burnetii* Dot/Icm T4SS at detectable levels. APH_0455 is of interest because it carries domains resembling those found in sterol regulatory element binding proteins (SREBPs), which in humans can modulate chromatin structure and gene transcription (Table 3, Fig. 4) (197).

INTERBACTERIAL SYSTEMS

The effector translocator systems clearly play important and varied roles in establishment of the replicative niches of many extracellular and intracellular pathogens. As mentioned earlier, conjugation systems also play important roles in promoting growth of bacterial pathogens in clinical settings. It is becoming increasingly evident, however, that bacteria have adapted the T4SSs in ways not limited to conjugative DNA transfer to enhance their growth potential. Below, we describe T4SSs functioning in novel ways to facilitate colonization and proliferation of invading pathogens.

Conjugation Machines

It is well established that conjugation provides a selective advantage for growth and colonization of invading pathogens through rapid intra- and interspecies dissemination of antibiotic resistance genes and virulence determinants in clinical settings (9). Even without gene transfer, however, the conjugation machines mediate functions of importance for virulence. Most notably, they promote bacterial attachment to biotic and abiotic surfaces, interbacterial aggregation, and development of biofilms in the human host (203–205). Among the Gram-negative species, these processes are mediated largely by conjugative pili (203, 204). The Gram-positive bacteria lack such pili, but their conjugation systems typically encode one or more surface adhesins as functional substitutes (5). The *Enterococcus faecalis* pCF10 conjugation system, for example, codes for three surface adhesins, of which one, termed aggregation substance, was shown to play an important role in intercellular aggregation, formation of robust biofilms, and bacterial attachment to heart tissues and endocarditis development in animal models (205, 206). The Gram-positive conjugation systems also code for multidomain cell wall hydrolases that are possibly involved in autolysis and release of extracellular DNA or other matrix components, as well as release of cell wall fragments, all of which could serve as potentiators of inflammatory responses in the human host (38). Conjugation machines are widely distributed among the medically important pathogens, and their multifaceted contributions to the infection process cannot be overstated.

Additionally, although the Gram-positive bacterial T4SSs currently are known to function only as conjugation machines, there is accumulating evidence that T4SSs might also be employed for effector translocation. It was recently shown that clusters of T4SS genes are much more widely distributed among the genomes of Gram-positive species than previously thought, largely because gene functions were misannotated during genomic sequence analyses (4). Typically, the T4SS gene clusters code for homologs of subunits that in the Gram-negative systems comprise the inner membrane translocase, e.g., VirB3, VirB4, VirB6, VirB8, and VirD4, as well as a VirB1-like cell wall hydrolase. These Gram-positive T4SSs lack genes encoding the OMCs and pili of the Gram-negative systems, which is consistent with the lack of an outer membrane or evidence for elaboration of conjugative pili. The Gram-positive T4SSs were designated as type IVC or "minimized" T4SSs, the latter reflecting the fact that these are the simplest known T4SSs in terms of subunit composition (4, 10). The Gram-positive T4SSs are therefore excellent subjects for detailed structure-function studies of the cytoplasmic membrane translocase stripped of other T4SS adaptations acquired over evolutionary time.

Whether these minimized systems translocate effector proteins during the course of infection is still not known. However, there is some experimental support for an effector function by a T4SS encoded by the 89K pathogenicity island of *Streptococcus suis* strain 05ZYH33, which was the cause of a recent outbreak of streptococcal toxic shock in China (207–209). Mutations introduced into the *virB4-* or *virD4*-like genes abolished virulence of strain 05ZYH33, and the mutant strains also failed to trigger a host immune response in a mouse infection model (10). Based on these findings, it was proposed that this pathogen utilizes the 89K T4SS to deliver an unknown effector protein(s) to the cell surface or into eukaryotic target cells. Whether Gram-positive T4SSs function in effector translocation and immune modulation remains an intriguing question for future investigation.

H. pylori Competence System

H. pylori carries a second T4SS adapted for the novel purpose of importing DNA from the extracellular milieu (210, 211). While not directly related to virulence, the ability to acquire foreign DNA imparts plasticity to the genome and genetic diversity of potential benefit for the invading pathogen in changing environmental settings. Natural transformation or competence (Com), for example, allows for recombinogenic alteration of surface antigens, enabling both attachment to different cell types and immune evasion. The *H. pylori* Com system consists of homologs of most VirB/VirD4 proteins with the exception of the pilus assembly factors VirB1 and VirB5, VirD4 T4CP, and VirB11 ATPase (211, 212). Additionally, the VirB machinery functionally interfaces with an inner membrane channel protein ComEC (13). Thus, in a unique two-step translocation reaction, the VirB complex is postulated to take up double-stranded DNA from the milieu into the periplasm and then deliver the substrate to ComEC, which degrades one strand while importing the second across the inner membrane (13). The importance of the *H. pylori* Com system to infection is underscored by a recent study showing that mutations of the Com machine resulted in reduced persistence in a mouse model, suggesting that DNA exchange between genetically heterogeneous *H. pylori* contributes to establishment of chronic infection (213).

N. gonorrhoeae DNA Release System

N. gonorrhoeae is the causative agent of gonorrhoeae. It is an exclusively human pathogen transmitted by sexual contact. Approximately 80% of gonococcal strains carry a 57-kb gonococcal genetic island (GGI), which is thought to be disseminated through release of genomic DNA to the milieu followed by acquisition by gonococci in the vicinity via a natural competence system (214). Gonococci naturally undergo autolysis, which represents one source for DNA uptake by transformation. Additionally, the GGI encodes a T4SS with the novel capacity to deliver DNA to the milieu (215). This DNA release system strikingly contrasts with the mechanism of conjugation, which requires a signal(s) transduced by recipient cell contact to activate the process of intercellular DNA transfer (216).

The GGI-encoded DNA release system is closely related in subunit composition, and probably architecture, to the *E. coli* F plasmid conjugation system (214). Both of these systems are assembled from homologs of the 12 VirB/VirD4 subunits, plus another subset of proteins unique to F-like T4SSs. One striking difference between the GGI- and F-encoded T4SSs, however, is that, while the TraA pilin is required for F plasmid transfer, the GGI system carries variant alleles of the TraA pilin subunits. Indeed, TraA is completely dispensable for DNA release by the GGI T4SS, as shown through mutational analyses (14). Conjugative pili are thought to initiate contacts with recipient cells, and the F-encoded pilus dynamically extends and retracts to bring donors and recipients into close apposition. However, *N. gonorrhoeae* does not require a target cell contact for GGI-dependent DNA release, thus dispensing with the need for a conjugative pilus. Besides their roles in attachment processes, conjugative pili or pilin subunits might contribute to recipient-stimulated DNA transfer through conformational effects on the OMC channel, thus ensuring substrate transfer only upon establishment of productive mating junctions. In *N. gonorrhoeae*, the lack of a TraA pilin requirement suggests the possibility that this F-like system evolved as a nonspecific DNA release system through loss of a critical gating activity. While the GGI T4SS is the only system known to mediate DNA release, as mentioned above there is some evidence that T4SSs of Gram-positive bacteria contribute directly or indirectly to the release of extracellular DNA, thereby stimulating colonization, biofilm formation, and infection (205).

Xanthomonas: a T4SS Killing Machine

Xanthomonas citri is a gammaproteobacterial phytopathogen that causes citrus canker, a disease that affects all citrus plants. Genome sequencing identified a *virB/virD4* locus closely resembling the *A. tumefaciens* locus with the exception that the *virB7* homolog encodes a much larger (139 residues) lipoprotein than *A. tumefaciens* VirB7 (4.5 kDa) (217). An X-ray structure revealed a N0 structural fold, which as described above is also present in DotD of the *L. pneumophila* Dot/Icm system and other outer membrane secretins (218). This domain is postulated to form an extra ring in the OMC, which might be a functionally important motif in view of recent work showing that the *Xanthomonas* T4SS functions not as a conjugation system or an effector translocator—at least in the classical sense (219). This system does translocate proteins, but to bacterial recipients with the goal of killing them. The effectors are toxins that were originally identified in a two-hybrid screen for VirD4-interacting proteins (220). All of the 13 candidate effectors carry a conserved motif (XVIPCD) near their C termini that is implicated as a potential translocation signal and VirD4 interaction domain. These proteins also carry toxin motifs with peptidoglycan binding or hydrolase, lipase, or nuclease activities. Recent work confirmed that *Xanthomonas* employs its T4SS to kill neighboring bacteria and that donors are themselves immune to killing by virtue of a coproduced cognate antitoxin (219). This killing activity increases competitiveness of *Xanthomonas* over coresident bacteria, presumably yielding a growth advantage through access to limiting nutrients in the environment. This striking new finding functionally aligns the T4SSs with the type VI secretion systems, which also have been exploited by bacteria for the specialized purpose of killing their neighbors (221).

SUMMARY AND FUTURE DIRECTIONS

In the past decade, there has been striking progress in our understanding of the structural diversity and functional versatility of the T4SSs. In this article, we have highlighted the principal ways pathogens have adapted T4SSs for specialized purposes geared toward establishment of replicative niches, proliferation, and spread in the human host. Studies of the paradigmatic T4SSs have generated detailed views of how T4SSs are architecturally arranged and how they recruit and mediate the transfer of DNA and protein substrates across the bacterial cell envelope. Corresponding work on the T4SSs employed by many medically important pathogens has further generated important insights into how the ancestral conjugation systems were adapted through appropriation of novel structural features. These structural modifications have endowed invading pathogens with the capacity to translocate a specific substrate repertoire—ranging from one to many hundreds of effectors—to host cells during the infection process. Structural adaptations also arm the pathogen with the ability to attach to specific host cells or, alternatively through intra- or intergenic recombination of variant T4SS genes, to a range of different host cell types. The display of surface-variable antigens also potentially cloaks the invading pathogen, allowing evasion of the host immune response.

The explosion of interest in T4SS effectors in recent years has yielded an extensive body of new information about the infection processes of many medically important pathogens. The known extracellular pathogens employ T4SSs primarily for delivery of one or a few effectors that target major cellular pathways with a variety of physiological consequences. The intracellular pathogens, on the other hand, appear to use their T4SSs for delivery of a number of effectors ranging from a half dozen to many hundreds, some acting on specific biochemical functions and others more generally on a number of cellular targets. Several themes have been identified in the evolutionary design of the T4SS effectors. Most widespread is the concept of molecular mimicry, which enables the pathogen essentially to fly below the radar of host cellular and immune responses. Also, in line with the overarching aim of a pathogen to survive and replicate within an established niche, effectors often exert subtle and modulatory effects on cellular processes as opposed to blocking cellular functions and activating cell death pathways. Two other themes are evident among intracellular pathogens such as *L. pneumophila* that employ their T4SSs to deliver many hundreds of effectors to the host. First, many effectors target similar pathways and carry out redundant activities which, for interested scientists, has unfortunately thwarted efforts to assign their functional importance. From the pathogen's perspective, however, functional redundancy can serve as a useful strategy for maintaining a broad host range of infection and for minimizing the number of effectors that are absolutely required for growth of the pathogen within the human host (127). Second, it is increasingly recognized that effectors often work in concert with other effectors to modulate complex biochemical pathways. With respect to the T4SS, this requires precise delivery in space and time of coordinately acting effectors and, hence, the evolution of recruitment mechanisms, e.g., chaperones/adaptors, to achieve such spatiotemporal control (11).

Finally, although the list of pathogens shown to employ T4SSs for delivery of effector proteins during infection continues to expand, it is still small compared to the number of bacteria that carry mobile genetic elements capable of elaborating conjugation systems. Most if not all members of the human microbiota carry such elements, many of which can become serious opportunistic pathogens in immunocompromised hosts or individuals suffering microbial dysbiosis as a result of antibiotic therapy or various illnesses. In such settings, conjugation systems can contribute significantly to establishment of infection not just through genetic exchange, but also by the elaboration of surface pili or adhesins capable of promoting attachment, colonization, and biofilm formation. Also of considerable interest is the recent discovery that a T4SS was adapted to deliver toxins interbacterially. This expanded feature of the T4SS arsenal enables invading bacteria to kill members of the normal flora, thus gaining access to space and resources for establishment of a replicative niche.

Clearly, there are many exciting avenues for further exploration toward the ultimate goal of gaining a comprehensive understanding of how T4SSs contribute to infection processes. While considerable headway has been made for the paradigmatic conjugation machines, fundamental questions remain about the architectures and mechanisms of action of T4SSs employed by pathogens. In particular, it is imperative to determine the structures of T4SS surface organelles and proteins, identify the basis for surface variability, and understand how these surface components mediate host cell binding and immune evasion. Studies of the effectors will assuredly continue to add detail to our understanding of various infection processes and of the mechanistic themes and variations associated with T4SS-mediated effector translocation. In particular, studies aimed at defining the T4SS effectors translocated by the obligate intracellular *Rickettsia* species appear poised to make significant progress over the next few years. Finally, as evident from the recent work and explosion of interest, we can anticipate that studies of specific pathogen–host cell interactions will not only define the functions of new T4SS effectors but also yield a broader understanding of basic biological processes of human host cells.

ACKNOWLEDGMENTS

We thank members of the Christie laboratory for helpful discussions. We also thank reviewers of this chapter for insightful comments.

Studies in the Christie laboratory were supported by NIH R01GM48476 and R21AI105454. C. G.-R. was supported in part by NRSA fellowship F32 AI114182.

CITATION

Gonzalez-Rivera C, Bhatty M, Christie PJ. 2016. Mechanism and function of type IV secretion during infection of the human host. Microbiol Spectrum 4(3):VMBF-0024-2015.

REFERENCES

1. **Cascales E, Christie PJ.** 2003. The versatile bacterial type IV secretion systems. *Nat Rev Microbiol* **1:**137–150.
2. **Backert S, Meyer TF.** 2006. Type IV secretion systems and their effectors in bacterial pathogenesis. *Curr Opin Microbiol* **9:**207–217.
3. **Asrat S, Davis KM, Isberg RR.** 2015. Modulation of the host innate immune and inflammatory response by translocated bacterial proteins. *Cell Microbiol* **17:**785–795.
4. **Bhatty M, Laverde Gomez JA, Christie PJ.** 2013. The expanding bacterial type IV secretion lexicon. *Res Microbiol* **164:**620–639.
5. **Alvarez-Martinez CE, Christie PJ.** 2009. Biological diversity of prokaryotic type IV secretion systems. *Microbiol Mol Biol Rev* **73:**775–808.
6. **Juhas M, van der Meer JR, Gaillard M, Harding RM, Hood DW, Crook DW.** 2009. Genomic islands: tools of bacterial horizontal gene transfer and evolution. *FEMS Microbiol Rev* **33:**376–393.

7. **Guglielmini J, Quintais L, Garcillan-Barcia MP, de la Cruz F, Rocha EP.** 2011. The repertoire of ICE in prokaryotes underscores the unity, diversity, and ubiquity of conjugation. *PLoS Genet* **7:**e1002222. doi:10.1371/journal.pgen.1002222.

8. **Cabezon E, Ripoll-Rozada J, Pena A, de la Cruz F, Arechaga I.** 2014. Towards an integrated model of bacterial conjugation. *FEMS Microbiol Rev* **39:**81–95.

9. **Juhas M.** 2015. Horizontal gene transfer in human pathogens. *Crit Rev Microbiol* **41:**101–108.

10. **Zhang W, Rong C, Chen C, Gao GF.** 2012. Type-IVC secretion system: a novel subclass of type IV secretion system (T4SS) common existing in Gram-positive genus *Streptococcus*. *PLoS One* **7:**e46390. doi:10.1371/journal.pone.0046390.

11. **Galán JE.** 2009. Common themes in the design and function of bacterial effectors. *Cell Host Microbe* **5:**571–579.

12. **Llosa M, Roy C, Dehio C.** 2009. Bacterial type IV secretion systems in human disease. *Mol Microbiol* **73:**141–51.

13. **Stingl K, Muller S, Scheidgen-Kleyboldt G, Clausen M, Maier B.** 2010. Composite system mediates two-step DNA uptake into *Helicobacter pylori*. *Proc Nat Acad Sci USA* **107:**1184–1189.

14. **Ramsey ME, Woodhams KL, Dillard JP.** 2011. The gonococcal genetic island and type IV secretion in the pathogenic *Neisseria*. *Front Microbiol* **2:**61.

15. **Christie PJ, Vogel JP.** 2000. Bacterial type IV secretion: conjugation systems adapted to deliver effector molecules to host cells. *Trends Microbiol* **8:**354–360.

16. **Sexton JA, Vogel JP.** 2002. Type IVB secretion by intracellular pathogens. *Traffic* **3:**178–185.

17. **Christie PJ, Atmakuri K, Krishnamoorthy V, Jakubowski S, Cascales E.** 2005. Biogenesis, architecture, and function of bacterial type IV secretion systems. *Annu Rev Microbiol* **59:**451–485.

18. **Nagai H, Kubori T.** 2011. Type IVB secretion systems of *Legionella* and other Gram-negative bacteria. *Front Microbiol* **2:**136.

19. **Guglielmini J, de la Cruz F, Rocha EP.** 2012. Evolution of conjugation and type IV secretion systems. *Mol Biol Evol* **30:**315–331.

20. **Tzfira T, Citovsky V.** 2008. *Agrobacterium*: from Biology to Biotechnology. Springer, New York, NY.

21. **Gomis-Ruth FX, Sola M, de la Cruz F, Coll M.** 2004. Coupling factors in macromolecular type-IV secretion machineries. *Curr Pharm Des* **10:**1551–1565.

22. **Trokter M, Felisberto-Rodrigues C, Christie PJ, Waksman G.** 2014. Recent advances in the structural and molecular biology of type IV secretion systems. *Curr Opin Struct Biol* **27:**16–23.

23. **Cascales E, Christie PJ.** 2004. Definition of a bacterial type IV secretion pathway for a DNA substrate. *Science* **304:**1170–1173.

24. **Low HH, Gubellini F, Rivera-Calzada A, Braun N, Connery S, Dujeancourt A, Lu F, Redzej A, Fronzes R, Orlova EV, Waksman G.** 2014. Structure of a type IV secretion system. *Nature* **508:**550–553.

25. **Fronzes R, Schafer E, Wang L, Saibil HR, Orlova EV, Waksman G.** 2009. Structure of a type IV secretion system core complex. *Science* **323:**266–268.

26. **Aly KA, Baron C.** 2007. The VirB5 protein localizes to the T-pilus tips in *Agrobacterium tumefaciens*. *Microbiol* **153:**3766–3775.

27. **Vergunst AC, van Lier MC, den Dulk-Ras A, Grosse Stuve TA, Ouwehand A, Hooykaas PJ.** 2005. Positive charge is an important feature of the C-terminal transport signal of the VirB/D4-translocated proteins of *Agrobacterium*. *Proc Natl Acad Sci USA* **102:**832–837.

28. **Schulein R, Guye P, Rhomberg TA, Schmid MC, Schroder G, Vergunst AC, Carena I, Dehio C.** 2005. A bipartite signal mediates the transfer of type IV secretion substrates of *Bartonella henselae* into human cells. *Proc Natl Acad Sci USA* **102:**856–861.

29. **Hohlfeld S, Pattis I, Puls J, Plano GV, Haas R, Fischer W.** 2006. A C-terminal translocation signal is necessary, but not sufficient for type IV secretion of the *Helicobacter pylori* CagA protein. *Mol Microbiol* **59:**1624–1637.

30. **Alperi A, Larrea D, Fernandez-Gonzalez E, Dehio C, Zechner EL, Llosa M.** 2013. A translocation motif in relaxase TrwC specifically affects recruitment by its conjugative type IV secretion system. *J Bacteriol* **195:**4999–5006.

31. **Redzej A, Ilangovan A, Lang S, Gruber CJ, Topf M, Zangger K, Zechner EL, Waksman G.** 2013. Structure of a translocation signal domain mediating conjugative transfer by type IV secretion systems. *Mol Microbiol* **89:**324–333.

32. **Sutherland MC, Nguyen TL, Tseng V, Vogel JP.** 2012. The *Legionella* IcmSW complex directly interacts with DotL to mediate translocation of adaptor-dependent substrates. *PLoS Pathog* **8:**e1002910. doi:10.1371/journal.ppat.1002910.

33. **Jeong KC, Sutherland MC, Vogel JP.** 2015. Novel export control of a *Legionella* Dot/Icm

substrate is mediated by dual, independent signal sequences. *Mol Microbiol* **96**:175–188.

34. **Sundberg CD, Ream W.** 1999. The *Agrobacterium tumefaciens* chaperone-like protein, VirE1, interacts with VirE2 at domains required for single-stranded DNA binding and cooperative interaction. *J Bacteriol* **181**:6850–6855.

35. **Christie PJ, Whitaker N, Gonzalez-Rivera C.** 2014. Mechanism and structure of the bacterial type IV secretion systems. *Biochim Biophys Acta* **1843**:1578–1591.

36. **Thanassi DG, Bliska JB, Christie PJ.** 2012. Surface organelles assembled by secretion systems of Gram-negative bacteria: diversity in structure and function. *FEMS Microbiol Rev* **36**:1046–1082.

37. **Bao W, Kumagai Y, Niu H, Yamaguchi M, Miura K, Rikihisa Y.** 2009. Four VirB6 paralogs and VirB9 are expressed and interact in *Ehrlichia chaffeensis*-containing vacuoles. *J Bacteriol* **191**:278–286.

38. **Marrero J, Waldor MK.** 2005. Interactions between inner membrane proteins in donor and recipient cells limit conjugal DNA transfer. *Dev Cell* **8**:963–970.

39. **Rohde M, Puls J, Buhrdorf R, Fischer W, Haas R.** 2003. A novel sheathed surface organelle of the *Helicobacter pylori cag* type IV secretion system. *Mol Microbiol* **49**:219–234.

40. **Barrozo RM, Cooke CL, Hansen LM, Lam AM, Gaddy JA, Johnson EM, Cariaga TA, Suarez G, Peek RM Jr, Cover TL, Solnick JV.** 2013. Functional plasticity in the type IV secretion system of *Helicobacter pylori*. *PLoS Pathog* **9**:e1003189. doi:10.1371/journal.ppat.1003189.

41. **Gillespie JJ, Ammerman NC, Dreher-Lesnick SM, Rahman MS, Worley MJ, Setubal JC, Sobral BS, Azad AF.** 2009. An anomalous type IV secretion system in *Rickettsia* is evolutionarily conserved. *PLoS One* **4**:e4833. doi:10.1371/journal.pone.0004833.

42. **Vayssier-Taussat M, Le Rhun D, Deng HK, Biville F, Cescau S, Danchin A, Marignac G, Lenaour E, Boulouis HJ, Mavris M, Arnaud L, Yang H, Wang J, Quebatte M, Engel P, Saenz H, Dehio C.** 2010. The Trw type IV secretion system of *Bartonella* mediates host-specific adhesion to erythrocytes. *PLoS Pathog* **6**:e1000946. doi:10.1371/journal.ppat.1000946.

43. **Al-Khedery B, Lundgren AM, Stuen S, Granquist EG, Munderloh UG, Nelson CM, Alleman AR, Mahan SM, Barbet AF.** 2012. Structure of the type IV secretion system in different strains of *Anaplasma phagocytophilum*. *BMC Genomics* **13**:678.

44. **Watarai M, Andrews HL, Isberg R.** 2000. Formation of a fibrous structure on the surface of *Legionella pneumophila* associated with exposure of DotH and DotO proteins after intracellular growth. *Mol Microbiol* **39**:313–329.

45. **Melvin JA, Scheller EV, Miller JF, Cotter PA.** 2014. *Bordetella pertussis* pathogenesis: current and future challenges. *Nat Rev Microbiol* **12**:274–288.

46. **Althouse BM, Scarpino SV.** 2015. Asymptomatic transmission and the resurgence of *Bordetella pertussis*. *BMC Med* **13**:146.

47. **Locht C, Coutte L, Mielcarek N.** 2011. The ins and outs of pertussis toxin. *FEBS J* **278**:4668–4682.

48. **Katada T, Ui M.** 1982. Direct modification of the membrane adenylate cyclase system by islet-activating protein due to ADP-ribosylation of a membrane protein. *Proc Natl Acad Sci USA* **79**:3129–3133.

49. **Tamura M, Nogimori K, Murai S, Yajima M, Ito K, Katada T, Ui M, Ishii S.** 1982. Subunit structure of islet-activating protein, pertussis toxin, in conformity with the A-B model. *Biochemistry* **21**:5516–5522.

50. **Burns DL, Hewlett EL, Moss J, Vaughan M.** 1983. Pertussis toxin inhibits enkephalin stimulation of GTPase of NG108-15 cells. *J Biol Chem* **258**:1435–1438.

51. **Stein PE, Boodhoo A, Armstrong GD, Cockle SA, Klein MH, Read RJ.** 1994. The crystal structure of pertussis toxin. *Structure* **2**:45–57.

52. **Weiss AA, Johnson FD, Burns DL.** 1993. Molecular characterization of an operon required for pertussis toxin secretion. *Proc Natl Acad Sci USA* **90**:2970–2974.

53. **Burns DL.** 2003. Type IV transporters of pathogenic bacteria. *Curr Opin Microbiol* **6**:29–34.

54. **Winans SC, Burns DL, Christie PJ.** 1996. Adaptation of a conjugal transfer system for the export of pathogenic macromolecules. *Trends Microbiol* **4**:64–68.

55. **Nicosia A, Perugini M, Franzini C, Casagli MC, Borri MG, Antoni G, Almoni M, Neri P, Ratti G, Rappuoli R.** 1986. Cloning and sequencing of the pertussis toxin genes: operon structure and gene duplication. *Proc Natl Acad Sci USA* **83**:4631–4635.

56. **Farizo KM, Huang T, Burns DL.** 2000. Importance of holotoxin assembly in Ptl-mediated secretion of pertussis toxin from *Bordetella pertussis*. *Infect Immun* **68**:4049–4054.

57. **Christie PJ.** 2004. Bacterial type IV secretion: The *Agrobacterium* VirB/D4 and related conjugation systems. *Biochim Biophys Acta* **1694**:219–234.

58. Rivera-Calzada A, Fronzes R, Savva CG, Chandran V, Lian PW, Laeremans T, Pardon E, Steyaert J, Remaut H, Waksman G, Orlova EV. 2013. Structure of a bacterial type IV secretion core complex at subnanometre resolution. *EMBO J* **32**:1195–1204.

59. Witvliet MH, Burns DL, Brennan MJ, Poolman JT, Manclark CR. 1989. Binding of pertussis toxin to eucaryotic cells and glycoproteins. *Infect Immun* **57**:3324–3330.

60. Covacci A, Telford JL, Del Giudice G, Parsonnet J, Rappuoli R. 1999. *Helicobacter pylori* virulence and genetic geography. *Science* **284**:1328–1333.

61. Parsonnet J, Friedman GD, Vandersteen DP, Chang Y, Vogelman JH, Orentreich N, Sibley RK. 1991. *Helicobacter pylori* infection and the risk of gastric carcinoma. *N Engl J Med* **325**:1127–1131.

62. Censini S, Lange C, Xiang Z, Crabtree JE, Ghiara P, Borodovsky M, Rappuoli R, Covacci A. 1997. *cag*, a pathogenicity island of *Helicobacter pylori*, encodes type I-specific and disease-associated virulence factors. *Proc Natl Acad Sci USA* **93**:14648–14653.

63. Akopyants NS, Clifton SW, Kersulyte D, Crabtree JE, Youree BE, Reece CA, Bukanov NO, Drazek ES, Roe BA, Berg DE. 1998. Analyses of the cag pathogenicity island of *Helicobacter pylori*. *Mol Microbiol* **28**:37–53.

64. Backert S, Ziska E, Brinkmann V, Zimny-Arndt U, Fauconnier A, Jungblut PR, Naumann M, Meyer TF. 2000. Translocation of the *Helicobacter pylori* CagA protein in gastric epithelial cells by a type IV secretion apparatus. *Cell Microbiol* **2**:155–164.

65. Hatakeyama M. 2014. *Helicobacter pylori* CagA and gastric cancer: a paradigm for hit-and-run carcinogenesis. *Cell Host Microbe* **15**:306–316.

66. Fischer W. 2011. Assembly and molecular mode of action of the *Helicobacter pylori* Cag type IV secretion apparatus. *FEBS J* **278**:1203–1212.

67. Aras RA, Fischer W, Perez-Perez GI, Crosatti M, Ando T, Haas R, Blaser MJ. 2003. Plasticity of repetitive DNA sequences within a bacterial (type IV) secretion system component. *J Exp Med* **198**:1349–1360.

68. Delahay RM, Balkwill GD, Bunting KA, Edwards W, Atherton JC, Searle MS. 2008. The highly repetitive region of the *Helicobacter pylori* CagY protein comprises tandem arrays of an alpha-helical repeat module. *J Mol Biol* **377**:956–971.

69. Jimenez-Soto LF, Kutter S, Sewald X, Ertl C, Weiss E, Kapp U, Rohde M, Pirch T, Jung K, Retta SF, Terradot L, Fischer W, Haas R. 2009. *Helicobacter pylori* type IV secretion apparatus exploits beta1 integrin in a novel RGD-independent manner. *PLoS Pathog* **5**: e1000684. doi:10.1371/journal.ppat.1000684.

70. Tanaka J, Suzuki T, Mimuro H, Sasakawa C. 2003. Structural definition on the surface of *Helicobacter pylori* type IV secretion apparatus. *Cell Microbiol* **5**:395–404.

71. Shaffer CL, Gaddy JA, Loh JT, Johnson EM, Hill S, Hennig EE, McClain MS, McDonald WH, Cover TL. 2011. *Helicobacter pylori* exploits a unique repertoire of type IV secretion system components for pilus assembly at the bacteria-host cell interface. *PLoS Pathog* **7**: e1002237. doi:10.1371/journal.ppat.1002237.

72. Johnson EM, Gaddy JA, Voss BJ, Hennig EE, Cover TL. 2014. Genes required for assembly of pili associated with the *Helicobacter pylori* cag type IV secretion system. *Infect Immun* **82**:3457–3470.

73. Kwok T, Zabler D, Urman S, Rohde M, Hartig R, Wessler S, Misselwitz R, Berger J, Sewald N, Konig W, Backert S. 2007. *Helicobacter* exploits integrin for type IV secretion and kinase activation. *Nature* **449**:862–866.

74. Tegtmeyer N, Hartig R, Delahay RM, Rohde M, Brandt S, Conradi J, Takahashi S, Smolka AJ, Sewald N, Backert S. 2010. A small fibronectin-mimicking protein from bacteria induces cell spreading and focal adhesion formation. *J Biol Chem* **285**:23515–23526.

75. Gorrell RJ, Guan J, Xin Y, Tafreshi MA, Hutton ML, McGuckin MA, Ferrero RL, Kwok T. 2013. A novel NOD1- and CagA-independent pathway of interleukin-8 induction mediated by the *Helicobacter pylori* type IV secretion system. *Cell Microbiol* **15**:554–570.

76. Fischer W, Puls J, Buhrdorf R, Gebert B, Odenbreit S, Haas R. 2001. Systematic mutagenesis of the *Helicobacter pylori* cag pathogenicity island: essential genes for CagA translocation in host cells and induction of interleukin-8. *Mol Microbiol* **42**:1337–1348.

77. Noto JM, Gaddy JA, Lee JY, Piazuelo MB, Friedman DB, Colvin DC, Romero-Gallo J, Suarez G, Loh J, Slaughter JC, Tan S, Morgan DR, Wilson KT, Bravo LE, Correa P, Cover TL, Amieva MR, Peek RM Jr. 2013. Iron deficiency accelerates *Helicobacter pylori*-induced carcinogenesis in rodents and humans. *J Clin Invest* **123**:479–492.

78. Murata-Kamiya N, Kikuchi K, Hayashi T, Higashi H, Hatakeyama M. 2010. *Helicobacter pylori* exploits host membrane phosphatidylserine for delivery, localization, and pathophysiological action of the CagA oncoprotein. *Cell Host Microbe* **7**:399–411.

79. Couturier MR, Tasca E, Montecucco C, Stein M. 2006. Interaction with CagF is required for translocation of CagA into the host via the *Helicobacter pylori* type IV secretion system. *Infect Immun* **74**:273–281.

80. Jurik A, Hausser E, Kutter S, Pattis I, Prassl S, Weiss E, Fischer W. 2010. The coupling protein Cagbeta and its interaction partner CagZ are required for type IV secretion of the *Helicobacter pylori* CagA protein. *Infect Immun* **78**:5244–5251.

81. Bonsor DA, Weiss E, Iosub-Amir A, Reingewertz TH, Chen TW, Haas R, Friedler A, Fischer W, Sundberg EJ. 2013. Characterization of the translocation-competent complex between the *Helicobacter pylori* oncogenic protein CagA and the accessory protein CagF. *J Biol Chem* **288**:32897–32909.

82. Higashi H, Tsutsumi R, Muto S, Sugiyama T, Azuma T, Asaka M, Hatakeyama M. 2002. SHP-2 tyrosine phosphatase as an intracellular target of *Helicobacter pylori* CagA protein. *Science* **295**:683–686.

83. Hatakeyama M. 2003. *Helicobacter pylori* CagA: a potential bacterial oncoprotein that functionally mimics the mammalian Gab family of adaptor proteins. *Microbes Infect* **5**:143–150.

84. Hatakeyama M. 2004. Oncogenic mechanisms of the *Helicobacter pylori* CagA protein. *Nat Rev Cancer* **4**:688–694.

85. Selbach M, Moese S, Hauck CR, Meyer TF, Backert S. 2002. Src is the kinase of the *Helicobacter pylori* CagA protein *in vitro* and *in vivo*. *J Biol Chem* **277**:6775–6778.

86. Higashi H, Tsutsumi R, Fujita A, Yamazaki S, Asaka M, Azuma T, Hatakeyama M. 2002. Biological activity of the *Helicobacter pylori* virulence factor CagA is determined by variation in the tyrosine phosphorylation sites. *Proc Natl Acad Sci USA* **99**:14428–14433.

87. Selbach M, Paul FE, Brandt S, Guye P, Daumke O, Backert S, Dehio C, Mann M. 2009. Host cell interactome of tyrosine-phosphorylated bacterial proteins. *Cell Host Microbe* **5**:397–403.

88. JW IJ, Carlson AC, Kennedy EL. 2007. *Anaplasma phagocytophilum* AnkA is tyrosine-phosphorylated at EPIYA motifs and recruits SHP-1 during early infection. *Cell Microbiol* **9**:1284–1296.

89. Hayashi T, Morohashi H, Hatakeyama M. 2013. Bacterial EPIYA effectors: where do they come from? What are they? Where are they going? *Cell Microbiol* **15**:377–385.

90. Backert S, Tegtmeyer N, Selbach M. 2010. The versatility of *Helicobacter pylori* CagA effector protein functions: The master key hypothesis. *Helicobacter* **15**:163–176.

91. Suzuki N, Murata-Kamiya N, Yanagiya K, Suda W, Hattori M, Kanda H, Bingo A, Fujii Y, Maeda S, Koike K, Hatakeyama M. 2015. Mutual reinforcement of inflammation and carcinogenesis by the *Helicobacter pylori* CagA oncoprotein. *Sci Rep* **5**:10024

92. Viala J, Chaput C, Boneca IG, Cardona A, Girardin SE, Moran AP, Athman R, Memet S, Huerre MR, Coyle AJ, DiStefano PS, Sansonetti PJ, Labigne A, Bertin J, Philpott DJ, Ferrero RL. 2004. Nod1 responds to peptidoglycan delivered by the *Helicobacter pylori* cag pathogenicity island. *Nat Immunol* **5**:1166–1174.

93. Dehio C. 2004. Molecular and cellular basis of *Bartonella* pathogenesis. *Annu Rev Microbiol* **58**:365–390.

94. Pulliainen AT, Dehio C. 2009. *Bartonella henselae*: subversion of vascular endothelial cell functions by translocated bacterial effector proteins. *Int J Biochem Cell Biol* **41**:507–510.

95. Ben-Tekaya H, Gorvel JP, Dehio C. 2013. *Bartonella* and *Brucella*: weapons and strategies for stealth attack. *Cold Spring Harbor Perspect Med* **3**(8). doi:10.1101/cshperspect.a010231.

96. Dehio C. 2008. Infection-associated type IV secretion systems of *Bartonella* and their diverse roles in host cell interaction. *Cell Microbiol* **10**:1591–1598.

97. Seubert A, Hiestand R, de la Cruz F, Dehio C. 2003. A bacterial conjugation machinery recruited for pathogenesis. *Mol Microbiol* **49**:1253–1266.

98. de Paz HD, Sangari FJ, Bolland S, Garcia-Lobo JM, Dehio C, de la Cruz F, Llosa M. 2005. Functional interactions between type IV secretion systems involved in DNA transfer and virulence. *Microbiol* **151**:3505–3516.

99. Saenz HL, Dehio C. 2005. Signature-tagged mutagenesis: technical advances in a negative selection method for virulence gene identification. *Curr Opin Microbiol* **8**:612–619.

100. Padmalayam I, Karem K, Baumstark B, Massung R. 2000. The gene encoding the 17-kDa antigen of *Bartonella henselae* is located within a cluster of genes homologous to the *virB* virulence operon. *DNA Cell Biol* **19**:377–382.

101. Saenz HL, Engel P, Stoeckli MC, Lanz C, Raddatz G, Vayssier-Taussat M, Birtles R, Schuster SC, Dehio C. 2007. Genomic analysis of *Bartonella* identifies type IV secretion systems as host adaptability factors. *Nat Genet* **39**:1469–1476.

102. Garcia-Pino A, Zenkin N, Loris R. 2014. The many faces of Fic: structural and functional

aspects of Fic enzymes. *Trends Biochem Sci* **39:**121–129.

103. **Backert S, Selbach M.** 2005. Tyrosine-phosphorylated bacterial effector proteins: the enemies within. *Trends Microbiol* **13:**476–484.

104. **Schulein R, Seubert A, Gille C, Lanz C, Hansmann Y, Piemont Y, Dehio C.** 2001. Invasion and persistent intracellular colonization of erythrocytes. A unique parasitic strategy of the emerging pathogen *Bartonella. J Exp Med* **193:**1077–1086.

105. **Siamer S, Dehio C.** 2015. New insights into the role of *Bartonella* effector proteins in pathogenesis. *Curr Opin Microbiol* **23:**80–85.

106. **Eicher SC, Dehio C.** 2012. *Bartonella* entry mechanisms into mammalian host cells. *Cell Microbiol* **14:**1166–1173.

107. **Truttmann MC, Rhomberg TA, Dehio C.** 2011. Combined action of the type IV secretion effector proteins BepC and BepF promotes invasome formation of *Bartonella henselae* on endothelial and epithelial cells. *Cell Microbiol* **13:**284–299.

108. **Okujava R, Guye P, Lu YY, Mistl C, Polus F, Vayssier-Taussat M, Halin C, Rolink AG, Dehio C.** 2014. A translocated effector required for *Bartonella* dissemination from derma to blood safeguards migratory host cells from damage by co-translocated effectors. *PLoS Pathog* **10:** e1004187. doi:10.1371/journal.ppat.1004187.

109. **Pulliainen AT, Pieles K, Brand CS, Hauert B, Bohm A, Quebatte M, Wepf A, Gstaiger M, Aebersold R, Dessauer CW, Dehio C.** 2012. Bacterial effector binds host cell adenylyl cyclase to potentiate Galphas-dependent cAMP production. *Proc Natl Acad Sci USA* **109:**9581–9586.

110. **Schroder G, Schuelein R, Quebatte M, Dehio C.** 2011. Conjugative DNA transfer into human cells by the VirB/VirD4 type IV secretion system of the bacterial pathogen *Bartonella henselae. Proc Natl Acad Sci USA* **108:**14643–14648.

111. **Llosa M, Schroder G, Dehio C.** 2012. New perspectives into bacterial DNA transfer to human cells. *Trends Microbiol* **20:**355–359.

112. **von Bargen K, Gorvel JP, Salcedo SP.** 2012. Internal affairs: investigating the *Brucella* intracellular lifestyle. *FEMS Microbiol Rev* **36:**533–562.

113. **Atluri VL, Xavier MN, de Jong MF, den Hartigh AB, Tsolis RM.** 2011. Interactions of the human pathogenic *Brucella* species with their hosts. *Annu Rev Microbiol* **65:**523–541.

114. **O'Callaghan D, Cazevieille C, Allardet-Servent A, Boschiroli ML, Bourg G, Foulongne V, Frutos P, Kulakov Y, Ramuz M.** 1999. A homologue of the *Agrobacterium tumefaciens* VirB and *Bordetella pertussis* Ptl type IV secretion systems is essential for intracellular survival of *Brucella suis. Mol Microbiol* **33:**1210–1220.

115. **Hong PC, Tsolis RM, Ficht TA.** 2000. Identification of genes required for chronic persistence of *Brucella abortus* in mice. *Infect Immun* **68:**4102–4107.

116. **Celli J, de Chastellier C, Franchini DM, Pizarro-Cerda J, Moreno E, Gorvel JP.** 2003. *Brucella* evades macrophage killing via VirB-dependent sustained interactions with the endoplasmic reticulum. *J Exp Med* **198:**545–556.

117. **Kahl-McDonagh MM, Elzer PH, Hagius SD, Walker JV, Perry QL, Seabury CM, den Hartigh AB, Tsolis RM, Adams LG, Davis DS, Ficht TA.** 2006. Evaluation of novel *Brucella melitensis* unmarked deletion mutants for safety and efficacy in the goat model of brucellosis. *Vaccine* **24:**5169–5177.

118. **de Jong MF, Sun YH, den Hartigh AB, van Dijl JM, Tsolis RM.** 2008. Identification of VceA and VceC, two members of the VjbR regulon that are translocated into macrophages by the *Brucella* type IV secretion system. *Mol Microbiol* **70:**1378–1396.

119. **Boschiroli ML, Ouahrani-Bettache S, Foulongne V, Michaux-Charachon S, Bourg G, Allardet-Servent A, Cazevieille C, Liautard JP, Ramuz M, O'Callaghan D.** 2002. The *Brucella suis virB* operon is induced intracellularly in macrophages. *Proc Natl Acad Sci USA* **99:**1544–1549.

120. **Comerci DJ, Martinez-Lorenzo MJ, Sieira R, Gorvel JP, Ugalde RA.** 2001. Essential role of the VirB machinery in the maturation of the *Brucella abortus*-containing vacuole. *Cell Microbiol* **3:**159–168.

121. **Myeni S, Child R, Ng TW, Kupko JJ 3rd, Wehrly TD, Porcella SF, Knodler LA, Celli J.** 2013. *Brucella* modulates secretory trafficking via multiple type IV secretion effector proteins. *PLoS Pathog* **9:**e1003556. doi:10.1371/journal.ppat.1003556.

122. **de Jong MF, Starr T, Winter MG, den Hartigh AB, Child R, Knodler LA, van Dijl JM, Celli J, Tsolis RM.** 2013. Sensing of bacterial type IV secretion via the unfolded protein response. *MBio* **4:**e00418-12. doi:10.1128/mBio.00418-12.

123. **de Barsy M, Jamet A, Filopon D, Nicolas C, Laloux G, Rual JF, Muller A, Twizere JC, Nkengfac B, Vandenhaute J, Hill DE, Salcedo SP, Gorvel JP, Letesson JJ, De Bolle X.** 2011. Identification of a *Brucella* spp. secreted effector specifically interacting with human small GTPase Rab2. *Cell Microbiol* **13:**1044–1058.

124. **Salcedo SP, Marchesini MI, Lelouard H, Fugier E, Jolly G, Balor S, Muller A, Lapaque N, Demaria O, Alexopoulou L, Comerci DJ, Ugalde RA, Pierre P, Gorvel JP.** 2008. *Brucella* control of dendritic cell maturation is dependent on the TIR-containing protein Btp1. *PLoS Pathog* 4:e21. doi:10.1371/journal. ppat.0040021.

125. **Salcedo SP, Marchesini MI, Degos C, Terwagne M, Von Bargen K, Lepidi H, Herrmann CK, Santos Lacerda TL, Imbert PR, Pierre P, Alexopoulou L, Letesson JJ, Comerci DJ, Gorvel JP.** 2013. BtpB, a novel *Brucella* TIR-containing effector protein with immune modulatory functions. *Front Cell Infect Microbiol* 3:28.

126. **Barbaree JM, Fields BS, Feeley JC, Gorman GW, Martin WT.** 1986. Isolation of protozoa from water associated with a legionellosis outbreak and demonstration of intracellular multiplication of *Legionella pneumophila*. *Appl Environ Microbiol* 51:422–424.

127. **Isaac DT, Isberg R.** 2014. Master manipulators: an update on *Legionella pneumophila* Icm/Dot translocated substrates and their host targets. *Future Microbiol* 9:343–359.

128. **Hubber A, Roy CR.** 2010. Modulation of host cell function by *Legionella pneumophila* type IV effectors. *Annu Rev Cell Dev Biol* 26:261–283.

129. **Vogel JP, Andrews HL, Wong SK, Isberg RR.** 1998. Conjugative transfer by the virulence system of *Legionella pneumophila*. *Science* 279:873–876.

130. **Kubori T, Koike M, Bui XT, Higaki S, Aizawa S, Nagai H.** 2014. Native structure of a type IV secretion system core complex essential for *Legionella* pathogenesis. *Proc Natl Acad Sci USA* 111:11804–11809.

131. **Nakano N, Kubori T, Kinoshita M, Imada K, Nagai H.** 2010. Crystal structure of *Legionella* DotD: insights into the relationship between type IVB and type II/III secretion systems. *PLoS Pathog* 6:e1001129. doi:10.1371/journal.ppat.1001129.

132. **Zhu W, Banga S, Tan Y, Zheng C, Stephenson R, Gately J, Luo ZQ.** 2011. Comprehensive identification of protein substrates of the Dot/Icm type IV transporter of *Legionella pneumophila*. *PLoS One* 6:e17638. doi:10.1371/journal. pone.0017638.

133. **Isberg RR, O'Connor TJ, Heidtman M.** 2009. The *Legionella pneumophila* replication vacuole: making a cosy niche inside host cells. *Nat Rev Microbiol* 7:13–24.

134. **O'Connor TJ, Boyd D, Dorer MS, Isberg RR.** 2012. Aggravating genetic interactions allow a solution to redundancy in a bacterial pathogen. *Science* 338:1440–1444.

135. **Finsel I, Hilbi H.** 2015. Formation of a pathogen vacuole according to *Legionella pneumophila*: how to kill one bird with many stones. *Cell Microbiol* 17:935–950.

136. **Gomez-Valero L, Rusniok C, Cazalet C, Buchrieser C.** 2011. Comparative and functional genomics of *Legionella* identified eukaryotic like proteins as key players in host-pathogen interactions. *Front Microbiol* 2:208.

137. **Prashar A, Terebiznik MR.** 2015. *Legionella pneumophila*: homeward bound away from the phagosome. *Curr Opin Microbiol* 23:86–93.

138. **Hoffmann C, Harrison CF, Hilbi H.** 2014. The natural alternative: protozoa as cellular models for *Legionella* infection. *Cell Microbiol* 16:15–26.

139. **Bardill JP, Miller JL, Vogel JP.** 2005. IcmS-dependent translocation of SdeA into macrophages by the *Legionella pneumophila* type IV secretion system. *Mol Microbiol* 56:90–103.

140. **Nagai H, Cambronne ED, Kagan JC, Amor JC, Kahn RA, Roy CR.** 2005. A C-terminal translocation signal required for Dot/Icm-dependent delivery of the *Legionella* RalF protein to host cells. *Proc Natl Acad Sci USA* 102:826–831.

141. **Chen J, Reyes M, Clarke M, Shuman HA.** 2007. Host cell-dependent secretion and translocation of the LepA and LepB effectors of *Legionella pneumophila*. *Cell Microbiol* 9:1660–1671.

142. **Brombacher E, Urwyler S, Ragaz C, Weber SS, Kami K, Overduin M, Hilbi H.** 2009. Rab1 guanine nucleotide exchange factor SidM is a major phosphatidylinositol 4-phosphate-binding effector protein of *Legionella pneumophila*. *J Biol Chem* 284:4846–4856.

143. **Hilbi H, Weber S, Finsel I.** 2011. Anchors for effectors: subversion of phosphoinositide lipids by legionella. *Front Microbiol* 2:91.

144. **Jank T, Bohmer KE, Tzivelekidis T, Schwan C, Belyi Y, Aktories K.** 2012. Domain organization of *Legionella effector* SetA. *Cell Microbiol* 14:852–868.

145. **Finsel I, Ragaz C, Hoffmann C, Harrison CF, Weber S, van Rahden VA, Johannes L, Hilbi H.** 2013. The *Legionella* effector RidL inhibits retrograde trafficking to promote intracellular replication. *Cell Host Microbe* 14:38–50.

146. **Toulabi L, Wu X, Cheng Y, Mao Y.** 2013. Identification and structural characterization of a *Legionella* phosphoinositide phosphatase. *J Biol Chem* 288:24518–24527.

147. **Gaspar AH, Machner MP.** 2014. VipD is a Rab5-activated phospholipase A1 that protects *Legionella pneumophila* from endosomal fusion. *Proc Natl Acad Sci USA* 111:4560–4565.

148. Xu L, Shen X, Bryan A, Banga S, Swanson MS, Luo ZQ. 2010. Inhibition of host vacuolar H+-ATPase activity by a *Legionella pneumophila* effector. *PLoS Pathog* **6**:e1000822. doi:10.1371/journal.ppat.1000822.

149. Arasaki K, Toomre DK, Roy CR. 2012. The *Legionella pneumophila* effector DrrA is sufficient to stimulate SNARE-dependent membrane fusion. *Cell Host Microbe* **11**:46–57.

150. King NP, Newton P, Schuelein R, Brown DL, Petru M, Zarsky V, Dolezal P, Luo L, Bugarcic A, Stanley AC, Murray RZ, Collins BM, Teasdale RD, Hartland EL, Stow JL. 2015. Soluble NSF attachment protein receptor molecular mimicry by a *Legionella pneumophila* Dot/Icm effector. *Cell Microbiol* **17**:767–784.

151. Hsu F, Zhu W, Brennan L, Tao L, Luo ZQ, Mao Y. 2012. Structural basis for substrate recognition by a unique *Legionella* phosphoinositide phosphatase. *Proc Natl Acad Sci USA* **109**:13567–13572.

152. Nagai H, Kagan JC, Zhu X, Kahn RA, Roy CR. 2002. A bacterial guanine nucleotide exchange factor activates ARF on *Legionella* phagosomes. *Science* **295**:679–682.

153. Choy A, Dancourt J, Mugo B, O'Connor TJ, Isberg RR, Melia TJ, Roy CR. 2012. The *Legionella* effector RavZ inhibits host autophagy through irreversible Atg8 deconjugation. *Science* **338**:1072–1076.

154. Degtyar E, Zusman T, Ehrlich M, Segal G. 2009. A *Legionella* effector acquired from protozoa is involved in sphingolipids metabolism and is targeted to the host cell mitochondria. *Cell Microbiol* **11**:1219–1235.

155. Shohdy N, Efe JA, Emr SD, Shuman HA. 2005. Pathogen effector protein screening in yeast identifies *Legionella* factors that interfere with membrane trafficking. *Proc Natl Acad Sci USA* **102**:4866–4871.

156. Franco IS, Shohdy N, Shuman HA. 2012. The *Legionella pneumophila* effector VipA is an actin nucleator that alters host cell organelle trafficking. *PLoS Pathog* **8**:e1002546. doi:10.1371/journal.ppat.1002546.

157. Al-Khodor S, Price CT, Habyarimana F, Kalia A, Abu Kwaik Y. 2008. A Dot/Icm-translocated ankyrin protein of *Legionella pneumophila* is required for intracellular proliferation within human macrophages and protozoa. *Mol Microbiol* **70**:908–923.

158. Price CT, Al-Khodor S, Al-Quadan T, Santic M, Habyarimana F, Kalia A, Kwaik YA. 2009. Molecular mimicry by an F-box effector of *Legionella pneumophila* hijacks a conserved polyubiquitination machinery within macro-phages and protozoa. *PLoS Pathog* **5**:e1000704. doi:10.1371/journal.ppat.1000704.

159. Lomma M, Dervins-Ravault D, Rolando M, Nora T, Newton HJ, Sansom FM, Sahr T, Gomez-Valero L, Jules M, Hartland EL, Buchrieser C. 2010. The *Legionella pneumophila* F-box protein Lpp2082 (AnkB) modulates ubiquitination of the host protein parvin B and promotes intracellular replication. *Cell Microbiol* **12**:1272–1291.

160. Raoult D, Marrie T, Mege J. 2005. Natural history and pathophysiology of Q fever. *Lancet Infect Dis* **5**:219–226.

161. Mazokopakis EE, Karefilakis CM, Starakis IK. 2010. Q fever endocarditis. *Infect Disord Drug Targets* **10**:27–31.

162. Omsland A, Cockrell DC, Howe D, Fischer ER, Virtaneva K, Sturdevant DE, Porcella SF, Heinzen RA. 2009. Host cell-free growth of the Q fever bacterium *Coxiella burnetii*. *Proc Natl Acad Sci USA* **106**:4430–4434.

163. Voth DE, Heinzen RA. 2007. Lounging in a lysosome: the intracellular lifestyle of *Coxiella burnetii*. *Cell Microbiol* **9**:829–840.

164. Coleman SA, Fischer ER, Howe D, Mead DJ, Heinzen RA. 2004. Temporal analysis of *Coxiella burnetii* morphological differentiation. *J Bacteriol* **186**:7344–7352.

165. Beare PA, Gilk SD, Larson CL, Hill J, Stead CM, Omsland A, Cockrell DC, Howe D, Voth DE, Heinzen RA. 2011. Dot/Icm type IVB secretion system requirements for *Coxiella burnetii* growth in human macrophages. *MBio* **2**:e00175-11. doi:10.1128/mBio.00175-11.

166. Carey KL, Newton HJ, Luhrmann A, Roy CR. 2011. The *Coxiella burnetii* Dot/Icm system delivers a unique repertoire of type IV effectors into host cells and is required for intracellular replication. *PLoS Pathog* **7**:e1002056. doi:10.1371/journal.ppat.1002056.

167. Beare PA, Sandoz KM, Omsland A, Rockey DD, Heinzen RA. 2011. Advances in genetic manipulation of obligate intracellular bacterial pathogens. *Front Microbiol* **2**:97.

168. Beare PA, Larson CL, Gilk SD, Heinzen RA. 2012. Two systems for targeted gene deletion in *Coxiella burnetii*. *Appl Environ Microbiol* **78**:4580–4589.

169. Moffatt JH, Newton P, Newton HJ. 2015. *Coxiella burnetii*: turning hostility into a home. *Cell Microbiol* **17**:621–631.

170. Beare PA, Unsworth N, Andoh M, Voth DE, Omsland A, Gilk SD, Williams KP, Sobral BW, Kupko JJ 3rd, Porcella SF, Samuel JE, Heinzen RA. 2009. Comparative genomics reveal extensive transposon-mediated genomic plasticity and diversity among potential

effector proteins within the genus *Coxiella*. *Infect Immun* **77**:642–656.

171. **Luhrmann A, Nogueira CV, Carey KL, Roy CR.** 2010. Inhibition of pathogen-induced apoptosis by a *Coxiella burnetii* type IV effector protein. *Proc Natl Acad Sci USA* **107**:18997–19001.

172. **Eckart RA, Bisle S, Schulze-Luehrmann J, Wittmann I, Jantsch J, Schmid B, Berens C, Luhrmann A.** 2014. Antiapoptotic activity of *Coxiella burnetii* effector protein AnkG is controlled by p32-dependent trafficking. *Infect Immun* **82**:2763–2771.

173. **Klingenbeck L, Eckart RA, Berens C, Luhrmann A.** 2013. The *Coxiella burnetii* type IV secretion system substrate CaeB inhibits intrinsic apoptosis at the mitochondrial level. *Cell Microbiol* **15**:675–687.

174. **Martinez E, Cantet F, Fava L, Norville I, Bonazzi M.** 2014. Identification of OmpA, a *Coxiella burnetii* protein involved in host cell invasion, by multi-phenotypic high-content screening. *PLoS Pathog* **10**:e1004013. doi:10.1371/journal.ppat.1004013.

175. **Newton HJ, Kohler LJ, McDonough JA, Temoche-Diaz M, Crabill E, Hartland EL, Roy CR.** 2014. A screen of *Coxiella burnetii* mutants reveals important roles for Dot/Icm effectors and host autophagy in vacuole biogenesis. *PLoS Pathog* **10**:e1004286. doi:10.1371/journal.ppat.1004286.

176. **Larson CL, Beare PA, Howe D, Heinzen RA.** 2013. *Coxiella burnetii* effector protein subverts clathrin-mediated vesicular trafficking for pathogen vacuole biogenesis. *Proc Natl Acad Sci USA* **110**:E4770–E4779.

177. **Weber MM, Chen C, Rowin K, Mertens K, Galvan G, Zhi H, Dealing CM, Roman VA, Banga S, Tan Y, Luo ZQ, Samuel JE.** 2013. Identification of *Coxiella burnetii* type IV secretion substrates required for intracellular replication and *Coxiella*-containing vacuole formation. *J Bacteriol* **195**:3914–3924.

178. **Lifshitz Z, Burstein D, Schwartz K, Shuman HA, Pupko T, Segal G.** 2014. Identification of novel *Coxiella burnetii* Icm/Dot effectors and genetic analysis of their involvement in modulating a mitogen-activated protein kinase pathway. *Infect Immun* **82**:3740–3752.

179. **Renvoise A, Merhej V, Georgiades K, Raoult D.** 2011. Intracellular *Rickettsiales*: insights into manipulators of eukaryotic cells. *Trends Mol Med* **17**:573–583.

180. **Rikihisa Y.** 2010. *Anaplasma phagocytophilum* and *Ehrlichia chaffeensis*: subversive manipulators of host cells. *Nat Rev Microbiol* **8**:328–339.

181. **Ge Y, Rikihisa Y.** 2011. Subversion of host cell signaling by *Orientia tsutsugamushi*. *Microbes Infect* **13**:638–648.

182. **Bandi C, McCall JW, Genchi C, Corona S, Venco L, Sacchi L.** 1999. Effects of tetracycline on the filarial worms *Brugia pahangi* and *Dirofilaria immitis* and their bacterial endosymbionts *Wolbachia*. *Int J Parasitol* **29**:357–364.

183. **Werren JH.** 1997. Biology of *Wolbachia*. *Annu Rev Entomol* **42**:587–609.

184. **Hotopp JC, Clark ME, Oliveira DC, Foster JM, Fischer P, Torres MC, Giebel JD, Kumar N, Ishmael N, Wang S, Ingram J, Nene RV, Shepard J, Tomkins J, Richards S, Spiro DJ, Ghedin E, Slatko BE, Tettelin H, Werren JH.** 2007. Widespread lateral gene transfer from intracellular bacteria to multicellular eukaryotes. *Science* **317**:1753–1756.

185. **Andersson SG, Zomorodipour A, Andersson JO, Sicheritz-Ponten T, Alsmark UC, Podowski RM, Naslund AK, Eriksson AS, Winkler HH, Kurland CG.** 1998. The genome sequence of *Rickettsia prowazekii* and the origin of mitochondria. *Nature* **396**:133–140.

186. **Ohashi N, Zhi N, Lin Q, Rikihisa Y.** 2002. Characterization and transcriptional analysis of gene clusters for a type IV secretion machinery in human granulocytic and monocytic ehrlichiosis agents. *Infect Immun* **70**:2128–2138.

187. **Pichon S, Bouchon D, Cordaux R, Chen L, Garrett RA, Greve P.** 2009. Conservation of the type IV secretion system throughout *Wolbachia* evolution. *Biochem Biophys Res Commun* **385**:557–562.

188. **Gillespie JJ, Kaur SJ, Rahman MS, Rennoll-Bankert K, Sears KT, Beier-Sexton M, Azad AF.** 2015. Secretome of obligate intracellular *Rickettsia*. *FEMS Microbiol Rev* **39**:47–80.

189. **Cho NH, Kim HR, Lee JH, Kim SY, Kim J, Cha S, Kim SY, Darby AC, Fuxelius HH, Yin J, Kim JH, Kim J, Lee SJ, Koh YS, Jang WJ, Park KH, Andersson SG, Choi MS, Kim IS.** 2007. The *Orientia tsutsugamushi* genome reveals massive proliferation of conjugative type IV secretion system and host-cell interaction genes. *Proc Natl Acad Sci USA* **104**:7981–7986.

190. **Rikihisa Y, Lin M, Niu H.** 2010. Type IV secretion in the obligatory intracellular bacterium *Anaplasma phagocytophilum*. *Cell Microbiol* **12**:1213–1221.

191. **Niu H, Rikihisa Y, Yamaguchi M, Ohashi N.** 2006. Differential expression of VirB9 and VirB6 during the life cycle of *Anaplasma phagocytophilum* in human leucocytes is associated

with differential binding and avoidance of lysosome pathway. *Cell Microbiol* **8:**523–534.

192. **Ge Y, Rikihisa Y.** 2007. Surface-exposed proteins of *Ehrlichia chaffeensis*. *Infect Immun* **75:**3833–3841.

193. **Ge Y, Rikihisa Y.** 2007. Identification of novel surface proteins of *Anaplasma phagocytophilum* by affinity purification and proteomics. *J Bacteriol* **189:**7819–7828.

194. **Lin M, den Dulk-Ras A, Hooykaas PJ, Rikihisa Y.** 2007. *Anaplasma phagocytophilum* AnkA secreted by type IV secretion system is tyrosine phosphorylated by Abl-1 to facilitate infection. *Cell Microbiol* **9:**2644–2657.

195. **Niu H, Kozjak-Pavlovic V, Rudel T, Rikihisa Y.** 2010. *Anaplasma phagocytophilum* Ats-1 is imported into host cell mitochondria and interferes with apoptosis induction. *PLoS Pathog* **6:**e1000774. doi:10.1371/journal.ppat.1000774.

196. **Lockwood S, Voth DE, Brayton KA, Beare PA, Brown WC, Heinzen RA, Broschat SL.** 2011. Identification of *Anaplasma marginale* type IV secretion system effector proteins. *PLoS One* **6:**e27724. doi:10.1371/journal.pone.0027724.

197. **Sinclair SH, Garcia-Garcia JC, Dumler JS.** 2015. Bioinformatic and mass spectrometry identification of *Anaplasma phagocytophilum* proteins translocated into host cell nuclei. *Front Microbiol* **6:**55.

198. **Al-Khodor S, Price CT, Kalia A, Abu Kwaik Y.** 2010. Functional diversity of ankyrin repeats in microbial proteins. *Trends Microbiol* **18:**132–139.

199. **Voth DE.** 2011. ThANKs for the repeat: intracellular pathogens exploit a common eukaryotic domain. *Cell Logist* **1:**128–132.

200. **Garcia-Garcia JC, Rennoll-Bankert KE, Pelly S, Milstone AM, Dumler JS.** 2009. Silencing of host cell CYBB gene expression by the nuclear effector AnkA of the intracellular pathogen *Anaplasma phagocytophilum*. *Infect Immun* **77:**2385–2391.

201. **Rennoll-Bankert KE, Garcia-Garcia JC, Sinclair SH, Dumler JS.** 2015. Chromatin-bound bacterial effector ankyrin A recruits histone deacetylase 1 and modifies host gene expression. *Cell Microbiol* **17:**1640–1652.

202. **Liu H, Bao W, Lin M, Niu H, Rikihisa Y.** 2012. *Ehrlichia* type IV secretion effector ECH0825 is translocated to mitochondria and curbs ROS and apoptosis by upregulating host MnSOD. *Cell Microbiol* **14:**1037–1050.

203. **Ghigo JM.** 2001. Natural conjugative plasmids induce bacterial biofilm development. *Nature* **412:**442–445.

204. **Reisner A, Holler BM, Molin S, Zechner EL.** 2006. Synergistic effects in mixed *Escherichia coli* biofilms: conjugative plasmid transfer drives biofilm expansion. *J Bacteriol* **188:**3582–3588.

205. **Bhatty M, Cruz MR, Frank KL, Gomez JA, Andrade F, Garsin DA, Dunny GM, Kaplan HB, Christie PJ.** 2015. *Enterococcus faecalis* pCF10-encoded surface proteins PrgA, PrgB (aggregation substance) and PrgC contribute to plasmid transfer, biofilm formation and virulence. *Mol Microbiol* **95:**660–677.

206. **Schlievert PM, Gahr PJ, Assimacopoulos AP, Dinges MM, Stoehr JA, Harmala JW, Hirt H, Dunny GM.** 1998. Aggregation and binding substances enhance pathogenicity in rabbit models of *Enterococcus faecalis* endocarditis. *Infect Immun* **66:**218–223.

207. **Chen C, Tang J, Dong W, Wang C, Feng Y, Wang J, Zheng F, Pan X, Liu D, Li M, Song Y, Zhu X, Sun H, Feng T, Guo Z, Ju A, Ge J, Dong Y, Sun W, Jiang Y, Wang J, Yan J, Yang H, Wang X, Gao GF, Yang R, Wang J, Yu J.** 2007. A glimpse of streptococcal toxic shock syndrome from comparative genomics of *S. suis* 2 Chinese isolates. *PLoS One* **2:**e315. doi:10.1371/journal.pone.0000315.

208. **Zhang A, Yang M, Hu P, Wu J, Chen B, Hua Y, Yu J, Chen H, Xiao J, Jin M.** 2011. Comparative genomic analysis of *Streptococcus suis* reveals significant genomic diversity among different serotypes. *BMC Genomics* **12:**523.

209. **Li M, Shen X, Yan J, Han H, Zheng B, Liu D, Cheng H, Zhao Y, Rao X, Wang C, Tang J, Hu F, Gao GF.** 2011. GI-type T4SS-mediated horizontal transfer of the 89K pathogenicity island in epidemic *Streptococcus suis* serotype 2. *Mol Microbiol* **79:**1670–1683.

210. **Hofreuter D, Odenbreit S, Puls J, Schwan D, Haas R.** 2000. Genetic competence in *Helicobacter pylori*: mechanisms and biological implications. *Res Microbiol* **151:**487–491.

211. **Hofreuter D, Odenbreit S, Haas R.** 2001. Natural transformation competence in *Helicobacter pylori* is mediated by the basic components of a type IV secretion system. *Mol Microbiol* **41:**379–391.

212. **Karnholz A, Hoefler C, Odenbreit S, Fischer W, Hofreuter D, Haas R.** 2006. Functional and topological characterization of novel components of the comB DNA transformation competence system in *Helicobacter pylori*. *J Bacteriol* **188:**882–893.

213. **Dorer MS, Cohen IE, Sessler TH, Fero J, Salama NR.** 2013. Natural competence promotes *Helicobacter pylori* chronic infection. *Infect Immun* **81:**209–215.

214. **Dillard JP, Seifert HS.** 2001. A variable genetic island specific for *Neisseria gonorrhoeae* is involved in providing DNA for natural transfor-

mation and is found more often in disseminated infection isolates. *Mol Microbiol* **41**:263–277.

215. Hamilton HL, Dominguez NM, Schwartz KJ, Hackett KT, Dillard JP. 2005. *Neisseria gonorrhoeae* secretes chromosomal DNA via a novel type IV secretion system. *Mol Microbiol* **55**:1704–1721.

216. Lang S, Kirchberger PC, Gruber CJ, Redzej A, Raffl S, Zellnig G, Zangger K, Zechner EL. 2011. An activation domain of plasmid R1 TraI protein delineates stages of gene transfer initiation. *Mol Microbiol* **82**:1071–1085.

217. da Silva AC, Ferro JA, Reinach FC, Farah CS, Furlan LR, Quaggio RB, Monteiro-Vitorello CB, Van Sluys MA, Almeida NF, Alves LM, do Amaral AM, Bertolini MC, Camargo LE, Camarotte G, Cannavan F, Cardozo J, Chambergo F, Ciapina LP, Cicarelli RM, Coutinho LL, Cursino-Santos JR, El-Dorry H, Faria JB, Ferreira AJ, Ferreira RC, Ferro MI, Formighieri EF, Franco MC, Greggio CC, Gruber A, Katsuyama AM, Kishi LT, Leite RP, Lemos EG, Lemos MV, Locali EC, Machado MA, Madeira AM, Martinez-Rossi NM, Martins EC, Meidanis J, Menck CF, Miyaki CY, Moon DH, Moreira LM, Novo MT, Okura VK, Oliveira MC, Oliveira VR, Pereira HA, Rossi A, Sena JA, Silva C, de Souza RF, Spinola LA, Takita MA, Tamura RE, Teixeira EC, Tezza RI, Trindade dos Santos M, Truffi D, Tsai SM, White FF, Setubal JC, Kitajima JP. 2002. Comparison of the genomes of two *Xanthomonas* pathogens with differing host specificities. *Nature* **417**:459–463.

218. Souza DP, Andrade MO, Alvarez-Martinez CE, Arantes GM, Farah CS, Salinas RK. 2011. A component of the *Xanthomonadaceae* type IV secretion system combines a VirB7 motif with a N0 domain found in outer membrane transport proteins. *PLoS Pathog* **7**:e1002031. doi:10.1371/journal.ppat.1002031.

219. Souza DP, Oka GU, Alvarez-Martinez CE, Bisson-Filho AW, Dunger G, Hobeika L, Cavalcante NS, Alegria MC, Barbosa LR, Salinas RK, Guzzo CR, Farah CS. 2015. Bacterial killing via a type IV secretion system. *Nat Commun* **6**:6453.

220. Alegria MC, Docena C, Khater L, Ramos CHI, da Silva ACR, Farah CS. 2004. Identification of new protein-protein interactions involving products of the chromosome- and plasmid-encoded type IV secretion loci of the phytopathogen *Xanthomonas axonopodis* pv. citri. *J Bacteriol* **187**:2315–2325.

221. Russell AB, Hood RD, Bui NK, LeRoux M, Vollmer W, Mougous JD. 2011. Type VI secretion delivers bacteriolytic effectors to target cells. *Nature* **475**:343–347.

222. Lacerda TL, Salcedo SP, Gorvel JP. 2013. *Brucella* T4SS: the VIP pass inside host cells. *Curr Opin Microbiol* **16**:45–51.

223. Voth DE, Heinzen RA. 2009. *Coxiella* type IV secretion and cellular microbiology. *Curr Opin Microbiol* **12**:74–80.

224. Rikihisa Y, Lin M. 2010. *Anaplasma phagocytophilum* and *Ehrlichia chaffeensis* type IV secretion and Ank proteins. *Curr Opin Microbiol* **13**:59–66.

225. Rolan HG, den Hartigh AB, Kahl-McDonagh M, Ficht T, Adams LG, Tsolis RM. 2008. VirB12 is a serological marker of *Brucella* infection in experimental and natural hosts. *Clin Vacc Immun* **15**:208–214.

226. Rances E, Voronin D, Tran-Van V, Mavingui P. 2008. Genetic and functional characterization of the type IV secretion system in *Wolbachia*. *J Bacteriol* **190**:5020–5030.

227. Gillespie JJ, Joardar V, Williams KP, Driscoll T, Hostetler JB, Nordberg E, Shukla M, Walenz B, Hill CA, Nene VM, Azad AF, Sobral BW, Caler E. 2012. A *Rickettsia* genome overrun by mobile genetic elements provides insight into the acquisition of genes characteristic of an obligate intracellular lifestyle. *J Bacteriol* **194**:376–394.

228. Pachulec E, Siewering K, Bender T, Heller EM, Salgado-Pabon W, Schmoller SK, Woodhams KL, Dillard JP, van der Does C. 2014. Functional analysis of the gonococcal genetic island of *Neisseria gonorrhoeae*. *PLoS One* **9**:e109613. doi:10.1371/journal.pone.0109613.

229. Stein M, Bagnoli F, Halenbeck R, Rappuoli R, Fantl WJ, Covacci A. 2002. c-Src/Lyn kinases activate *Helicobacter pylori* CagA through tyrosine phosphorylation of the EPIYA motifs. *Mol Microbiol* **43**:971–980.

230. VieBrock L, Evans SM, Beyer AR, Larson CL, Beare PA, Ge H, Singh S, Rodino KG, Heinzen RA, Richards AL, Carlyon JA. 2014. *Orientia tsutsugamushi* ankyrin repeat-containing protein family members are type 1 secretion system substrates that traffic to the host cell endoplasmic reticulum. *Front Cell Infect Microbiol* **4**:186.

231. Voth DE, Howe D, Beare PA, Vogel JP, Unsworth N, Samuel JE, Heinzen RA. 2009. The *Coxiella burnetii* ankyrin repeat domain-containing protein family is heterogeneous, with C-terminal truncations that influence Dot/Icm-mediated secretion. *J Bacteriol* **191**:4232–4242.

232. Schrammeijer B, Risseeuw E, Pansegrau W, Regensburg-Tuink TJ, Crosby WL, Hooykaas PJ. 2001. Interaction of the virulence protein

VirF of *Agrobacterium tumefaciens* with plant homologs of the yeast Skp1 protein. *Curr Biol* **11**:258–262.

233. **Hubber A, Kubori T, Nagai H.** 2013. Modulation of the ubiquitination machinery by *Legionella. Curr Top Microbiol Immunol* **376**:227–247.

234. **Price CT, Jones SC, Amundson KE, Kwaik YA.** 2010. Host-mediated post-translational prenylation of novel dot/icm-translocated effectors of *Legionella pneumophila. Front Microbiol* **1**:131.

235. **Price CT, Al-Quadan T, Santic M, Jones SC, Abu Kwaik Y.** 2010. Exploitation of conserved eukaryotic host cell farnesylation machinery by an F-box effector of *Legionella pneumophila. J Exp Med* **207**:1713–1726.

236. **de Felipe KS, Pampou S, Jovanovic OS, Pericone CD, Ye SF, Kalachikov S, Shuman HA.** 2005. Evidence for acquisition of *Legionella* type IV secretion substrates via interdomain horizontal gene transfer. *J Bacteriol* **187**:7716–7726.

237. **Chandran V, Fronzes R, Duquerroy S, Cronin N, Navaza J, Waksman G.** 2009. Structure of the outer membrane complex of a type IV secretion system. *Nature* **462**:1011–1015.

Type V Secretion Systems
in Bacteria

11

ENGUO FAN,[1] NANDINI CHAUHAN,[2] D. B. R. K. GUPTA UDATHA,[2]
JACK C. LEO,[2] and DIRK LINKE[2]

INTRODUCTION

Gram-negative bacteria are surrounded by two membranes, called the outer and inner membranes. The space between these membranes, the periplasm, is spanned by a polymeric glycopeptide network, the peptidoglycan. This net has a closely defined mesh size and is attached to the outer and inner membranes by various proteins in the different Gram-negative organisms, leading to an even distance between the two membranes. Proteins that are to be transported to the outer membrane or the extracellular space thus have to cross various obstacles on their way; this process is mediated by a number of highly specialized secretion systems, mostly classified by Roman numerals from type I to type VII (see other chapters in this book for a comprehensive review of these systems). More secretion systems, or new variations of the ones previously described, are still found on a regular basis, making a comprehensive listing almost impossible. The major systems that are either well described and/or widely present in many Gram-negative species can be classified into two general architectures: those that span both membranes and the

[1]Institute of Biochemistry and Molecular Biology, University of Freiburg, Freiburg D-79104, Germany;
[2]Department of Biosciences, University of Oslo, Blindern, 0316 Oslo, Norway.
Virulence Mechanisms of Bacterial Pathogens, 5th edition
Edited by Indira T. Kudva, Nancy A. Cornick, Paul J. Plummer, Qijing Zhang, Tracy L. Nicholson,
John P. Bannantine, and Bryan H. Bellaire
© 2016 American Society for Microbiology, Washington, DC
doi:10.1128/microbiolspec.VMBF-0009-2015

periplasm as one large secretion complex and those where the individual membranes are crossed using independent (i.e., not physically connected) secretion machineries. Type V secretion systems are part of the latter systems.

Type V secretion systems come in different "flavors," currently classified as types Va to Ve (1). They share a common principle that distinguishes them from other secretion systems: in type V secretion, the secretion pore (called the translocation domain) through the outer membrane is typically part of the same polypeptide chain as the payload (called the passenger domain) that is to be secreted to the cell surface (Fig. 1). This makes type V secretion a very simple system in terms of primary structure and its minimalist number of components but raises complicated questions when it comes to the actual mechanism of secretion, as described throughout this chapter. It is this seemingly self-sufficient export mechanism within one polypeptide chain that gave rise to the term "autotransporter" (2)—commonly used at least for the type Va, Vc, and Ve secretion systems.

It is well established that type V–secreted proteins cross the inner membrane through

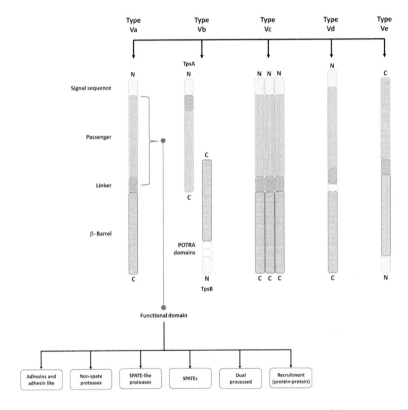

FIGURE 1 **Schematic domain organization among the five subcategories of known type V bacterial autotransporter proteins. The overall organization is labeled according to four major and common features (175): signal sequence, passenger, linker, and β-barrel. Note that similar features are based only on functional considerations in this context; they are not necessarily homologous. An example is the linker depicted for TpsA proteins here, which is the TPS domain that targets TpsA proteins for secretion by its TpsB partner. For a detailed discussion of the various linker regions and their function(s) see reference 175. The figure also shows the major families of the functional domains in the type Va autotransporter sequences of bacterial species that were defined through hidden Markov model–based phylogenetic analysis of 1,210 bacterial genomes (19).**

the Sec system, using cleavable N-terminal signal peptides. Then, the translocation domain forms a pore in the outer membrane through which the passenger domain is secreted. What distinguishes the different subtypes of type V secretion systems is their domain organization (Fig. 1) and the resulting variations in the transport mechanism(s).

Type Va systems are the prototypical ("classical") autotransporters. The first autotransporter described was IgA1 protease from *Neisseria gonorrhoeae* (3). In type Va systems, the pore is formed by the C-terminus of the polypeptide, while the N-terminus is exported to the cell surface. In many cases, including IgA1 protease, the passenger domain is cleaved off in an autocatalytic process after translocation is complete, releasing the passenger into the extracellular medium but leaving the translocation domain in the outer membrane. Other type Va systems are not autoprocessed in this way and thus keep the passenger domain anchored to the cell surface via the translocation domain. Typically, the passengers of noncleavable type Va systems function as adhesins, while the cleavable ones have enzymatic (protease or lipase) activities (1).

Type Vb systems, on first sight, seem like a split variant of type Va systems: the passenger domain and translocation domain are two separate protein chains but are expressed from the same operon structure. Type Vb systems are thus also called two-partner secretion (Tps) systems. The translocator proteins of type Vb systems are collectively called TpsB proteins, and the transported proteins (corresponding to the passenger domains of type Va autotransporters) are referred to as TpsA proteins. Notably, the TpsB protein that forms the translocation pore contains additional periplasmic domains not present in classical autotransporters. While the splitting of transport and passenger function would in principle allow for multiple passengers being secreted by the same TpsB protein, there are many cases where the TpsA is retained on the surface attached to

the TpsB, leading again to a 1:1 transport stoichiometry. It is mostly this observation that has led to the classification of two-partner secretion systems as part of type V secretion (1, 4), although there might be significant differences in the actual transport process compared to classical autotransporters (5).

Type Vc systems are probably the most complex autotransporter systems. They are obligate trimers, and the fact that most if not all of them function as bacterial adhesins has led to their alternative name, trimeric autotransporter adhesins (TAAs) (6). The passenger domains of the type Vc secretion systems are highly diverse and modular, while their translocation domain is highly conserved. Type Vc systems are the only type V systems in which the translocation pore is an oligomeric structure.

Type Vd systems were only recently described in the literature, and only a few exemplars have been studied in detail. Their general setup is very similar to type Va systems, with a C-terminal translocation domain and an N-terminal passenger domain. In contrast to the classical autotransporters, though, these domains are connected via an additional, periplasmic domain homologous to the periplasmic domains of the type Vb translocation pores.

Type Ve systems are also called inverse autotransporters, based on the fact that the domain order is reversed and that it is the C-terminal part that comprises the passenger domain, while the N-terminal part forms the translocation pore (7). The passenger domains are typically Ig-like and lectin-like domains that are not found in other type V secretion systems but that are widespread in adhesins from Gram-positive bacteria and in many other cell surface and periplasmic proteins (8, 9). An additional, small periplasmic domain is present at the N-terminus of the polypeptide chain, but this is not homologous to the periplasmic domains in Vb and Vd systems; instead, it in some cases contains a peptidoglycan-binding motif (10).

It is a matter of continuing debate whether the secretion mechanisms of all type V systems are indeed homologous and thus justify their classification as variations of the "same" theme. The intention of this chapter is to review the data on the different systems, obtained from various computational and experimental methods, to advance this discussion.

IN SILICO ANALYSIS: FROM SEQUENCE TO STRUCTURE

Few of the type V secretion systems have been studied experimentally in detail, and these model systems are typically limited to exemplars from medically important species. In silico analysis shows that a wide variety of type V system genes are also in nonpathogenic organisms and in environmental sequence datasets. Here, we review what information has been obtained on the diversity of type V secretion systems using various bioinformatics tools.

Sequence Alignment and Phylogenetic Analysis

Currently, our knowledge of the diversity of type V secretion systems is mostly based on similarity searches. The most popular in silico sequence analysis algorithm is BLAST, the Basic Local Alignment Search Tool (11–13), which has been widely used for identifying type V systems and other adhesins (1, 6, 7, 14–34). The standard protein-protein BLAST (blastp) has been used routinely for identifying adhesin or autotransporter sequences in genomes and in protein databases. The more sensitive Position-Specific Iterated (PSI)-BLAST has also been used for finding more distantly related type V-secreted proteins from the sequence databases or to identify the new members in a type V secretion system family. The sequences of type V–secreted proteins share high similarities in their respective subgroups due to their domain organization (35, 36) and thus, the cutoffs in the BLAST programs were generally set to the E-value 1×10^{-10} to detect as few false-positive hits as possible.

Many sequence analysis methods and applications in bioinformatics (e.g., evolutionary analysis, protein secondary structure predictions, phylogenetic analysis, etc.) rely on multiple sequence alignments as an input. Clustal Omega has been employed in a recent study to identify the prevalence of 18 different type Va autotransporters in 111 publicly available genomes of Escherichia coli (36). Clustal Omega uses seeded guide trees and hidden Markov model (HMM) profile-profile techniques to generate alignments between three or more sequences (37, 38).

It is generally accepted that when the pair-wise sequence identity is greater than 40% for continuous, long alignments, the corresponding protein pair will have a similar structure (39). The diverse and multidomain nature of type V secretion systems imposes strong limitations to such inferences: in most type V secretion systems, domains can be small and can occur in different orders. The need to detect individual, small domains with sometimes very high sequence diversity led to the implementation of HMMs for the detection and classification of bacterial type V secretion systems through bioinformatics analysis (19).

The HMM search strategy resulted in the identification of more than 1,500 putative type Va autotransporter sequences from 1,210 bacterial genomes. Only three broad functional classes (esterases, proteases, and adhesins) of autotransporters are recognized in the literature based on the type of passenger domain, whereas the phylogenetic analysis of autotransporters through HMM search strategies resulted in six major families (Fig. 1) based on the function of the autotransported domains. Further cluster analysis of conserved motifs in the β-barrel domain resulted in 14 distinct groups of type Va autotransporter sequences among the proteobacterial species (19).

A distinct feature of the conventional type Va autotransporter sequences is the size of the β-barrel domain which consists of approximately 300 amino acids that forms the 12 transmembrane β-strand pore with a transmembrane α-helix spanning the pore (40). The sequence composition of the β-barrel domain is different in trimeric or type Vc autotransporter proteins, where it is formed from three polypeptide chains. Each subunit contributes four β-strands that oligomerize to form the transmembrane pore of the type Vc autotransporters. It is self-evident that the sequence alignments of type Va and type Vc autotransporter β-barrel domains will result into two distinct clades in a phylogenetic tree, as shown by Cotter et al. (41). In a study of outer membrane β-barrel proteins in general, Remmert et al. found evidence that that all major groups of outer membrane β-barrels (including all type V secretion systems) from Gram-negative bacteria are homologous and evolved from an ancestral ββ hairpin sequence (42, 43). Taking this analysis one step further, using the combination of sequence analysis tools and secondary structure prediction tools, an HMM search strategy has been developed for the annotation of various domain regions in the trimeric or type Vc autotransporters (31). The domain annotation of TAAs is available as an online server called daTAA (http://toolkit.tuebingen.mpg.de/dataa).

Posttranslational Modification Analysis

As membrane proteins in the outer membrane of Gram-negative bacteria, type V secretion systems generally possess signal peptides for translocation across the inner membrane. The algorithms to identify these secretion signals use specific sequence features present in the short N-terminal signal peptides. The most widely used tool for the identification of signal peptides is SignalP, which is based on a combination of several artificial neural networks (44). According to Dautin and Bernstein, approximately 10% of the known type Va autotransporters possess an unusually long signal sequence of more than 50 amino acid residues (45). Generally, the N-terminal signal sequences in proteins show a tripartite organization of *n, h, c*, referring to the regions of N-terminal, hydrophobic, and cleavage site (46). Several studies showed variations (*n1-h1-n2-h2; n2-h2*) of the signal peptide tripartite organization in type V systems (4, 47) and called the region the extended signal peptide region (ESPR), which might have additional functions besides targeting or protein translocation (48–50). It is important to note that using simple sequence analysis tools such as BLAST and ClustalX, Desvaux and his colleagues showed that the ESPR sequence pattern is phylogenetically restricted among the Gram-negative bacterial type V–secreted proteins from the classes of β- and γ-*Proteobacteria* (47). Later on, several studies analyzing the function of ESPRs of type Vc autotransporters in Gram-negative bacteria showed that the amino acids of the ESPR are required for protein stability and the proper assembly of the monomers to form functional proteins (49, 51, 52). In contrast, the work by Leyton et al. on a serine protease autotransporter (SPATE subgroup of autotransporters of type Va shown in Fig. 1) indicates that ESPR is not essential for the secretion and the function of SPATEs in the *Enterobacteriaceae*, which makes the role of ESPR in targeting of the autotransporter protein contentious or controversial (48, 51, 52).

Glycosylation, one of the most common protein modification processes, plays an important role in the interaction of the bacterium with its environment via secreted or surface-exposed proteins (53). In addition to the proper delivery of the proteins onto the bacterial surface via type V secretion systems, glycosylation is required for proper molecular and cellular adhesion properties of some autotransporters in bacteria (54, 55). A recent study by Lu et al. (56) shows that heptosylation of bacterial autotransporters by autotransporter adhesin heptosyltransferase proteins can modify the adhesion property of type Va transporters to host cells. The combination of *in vitro* and *in silico* methods has increased our understanding of the complex structure-function mechanism of the autotransporter glycosylation process. Homology modeling of autotransporter adhesin heptosyltransferase protein structure using MODELLER in combination with CHARMM force field–based molecular dynamics simulation helped in gaining insights into the simultaneous hyperglycosylation of six autotransporter protein substrates by autotransporter adhesin heptosyltransferase via dodecamer enzyme complex (56). Glycosylation has also been shown in a type Vc autotransporter, EmaA from *Aggregatibacter actinomycetemcomitans* (57), suggesting that this might be a more widespread mechanism that modulates type V secretion.

STRUCTURAL BIOLOGY OF TYPE V SECRETION SYSTEMS

X-ray crystallography has been the method most widely applied to studying the structure of type V secretion systems (58, 59), and almost all the high-resolution structures currently available have been solved by crystallography. These have confirmed a number of hypotheses concerning autotransport and have been the starting point for new hypotheses. However, crystal structures only give snapshots of the final structures. Furthermore, almost all the available structures are fragments. There is only one complete structure of a classical, type Va autotransporter, the esterase EstA (60), but modeling efforts have produced plausible structures for several type Vc systems (16, 20, 61) and for the type Vb-secreted filamentous hemagglutinin FHA (62). More dynamic data might be obtained using nuclear magnetic resonance (NMR) spectroscopy, but to date NMR has hardly been used to probe autotransporter structures, probably because of the large size, oligomeric nature (for TAAs), and aggrega-

tion behavior of these proteins. However, NMR has been used to determine the structure of domains from inverse autotransporters (10, 63), and recently the structure of the translocation domain of the TAA YadA was solved using solid-state NMR (17). Electron microscopy and small-angle X-ray scattering have been used for low-resolution structural analysis, particularly of type Vc systems (64–68).

Passenger Domains

The passenger domains of type V secretion systems display a number of common features. Most passenger domains, regardless of type V subclass, are long, fibrous structures, in many cases well over 1,000 residues in length. Although in x-ray structures these fibers appear to be rigid rods, other methods have shown that they contain regions of at least limited flexibility that may be of functional significance (16, 27, 63, 65, 67). Another common theme is the prevalence of β-solenoids in passenger domains (69). β-solenoids are supersecondary structures, where the polypeptide chain winds around a central axis in a helical manner (70). The structure is formed by 2 to 4 parallel β-sheets aligned along the central axis; the corresponding β-strands of each coil contribute to the long β-sheets (Fig. 2). The interior of β-solenoids is usually hydrophobic and tightly packed, which contributes to the overall stability of the structure. β-solenoids are found in the vast majority of type Va, Vb, and Vc proteins (69, 71), though it should be noted that completely different passenger domain folds also exist, as exemplified by the all-α, globular passenger domain of EstA (60) (Fig. 3). In contrast, the passenger domains of type Ve autotransporters typically consist of tandemly repeated immunoglobulin (Ig)-like domains, often capped by a C-type lectin-like domain at the C-terminus of the protein (63, 72, 73) (Fig. 2). To date, there is no experimental structural information on type Vd passenger domains.

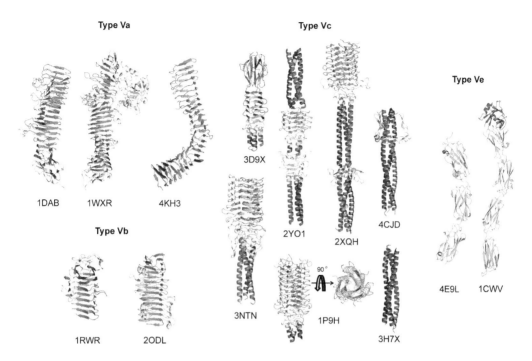

Type Va

1DAB   1WXR   4KH3

Type Vb

1RWR   2ODL

Type Vc

3D9X

2YO1   2XQH   4CJD

3NTN   1P9H   3H7X

90°

Type Ve

4E9L   1CWV

FIGURE 2 Experimental structures of passenger domains from type V secretion systems. Examples from type Va (classical autotransporters), type Vb (TpsA proteins), type Vc (trimeric autotransporter adhesins), and type Ve (inverse autotransporters) are included. Structures are shown in cartoon representation. β-solenoid structures are orange, with extrahelical domains and elements in yellow. β-prism domains are purple and coiled coils are red; connector elements are cyan. For type Vc proteins, each chain is colored with a slightly different hue. Chloride ions within coiled-coil stalks are represented by green spheres. Immunoglobulin-like domains are green, and C-type lectin-like domains blue. The structures representing type Va passengers are the pertactin passenger domain (PDB ID: 1DAB), the Hbp passenger (1WXR), and a fragment of the antigen 43 passenger (4KH3). TpsA proteins are represented by the FHA and HMW1 Tps domains (1RWR and 2ODL, respectively). Trimeric autotransporter adhesin passenger domains are represented by large fragments from EibD (2XQH) and SadA (2YO1), the Trp ring and GIN domains of the BadA head (3DX9), the head domains of YadA (1P9H), UspA1 (3NTN) and NadA (4CJD), and the region of the YadA stalk transitioning from right-handed (at the top) to left-handed (at the bottom) supercoiling. Fragments from the FdeC (4E9L) and invasin (1CWV) passenger domains represent type Ve passengers. The structures are oriented so that the portion of passenger domains distal to the outer membrane is pointing toward the top of the page. Note that for types Va, Vb, and Vc, the distal end is the N-terminus, whereas for type Ve passengers the C-terminus is distal.

The first type Va autotransporter passenger domain structure to be solved was that of pertactin from *Bordetella pertussis*, an important component of whooping cough vaccines (74). The pertactin structure can be considered prototypical of type Va passenger domains. It is a simple, right-handed β-helix with 16 rungs (Fig. 2). β-helices are a subclass of β-solenoids with three axial β-sheets. Though the β-helix of pertactin is continuous in the sense that it is not interrupted by any other kinds of domains, several of the turns connecting adjacent β-strands are extended into loops projecting out of the β-helical core, including the loop with the RGD motif presumed to be important for binding to host receptors (74). In other type Va autotransporters, these loops extend even further and form extrahelical domains bulging out of the β-helical scaffold, as exemplified by the subtilisin-like and chitinase-like domains in the hemoglobin protease Hbp

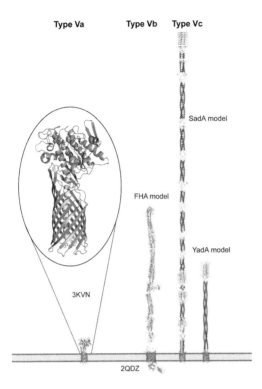

FIGURE 3 Full-length structures of type V–secreted proteins. The only experimental structure of a complete autotransporter is that of EstA (PDB ID: 3KVN). Efforts using experimental structures of fragments, homology, and *ab initio* modeling have generated models for full-length fibers of TpsA proteins (exemplified here as the FHA model with a total length of ~46 nm [117]) and trimeric autotransporter adhesins, exemplified by the long SadA fiber (total length ~108 nm) (16), and the much shorter YadA fiber (~35 nm) (61). In addition, the structure of FhaC (2QDZ) is shown. The structures of the different type V subclasses are to approximate scale, and in addition, the EstA structure is shown in close-up. β-barrel domains are blue, linkers are yellow, the lipase domain of EstA is pink, β-solenoids are orange, extrahelical extensions are yellow, connector elements are cyan, coiled coils are red, and periplasmic domains are green. The approximate span of the outer membrane is shown as a gray bar.

(75). In contrast to the relatively straight β-helices of pertactin and Hpb, a β-helical fragment from the antigen 43 (Ag43) passenger domain adopts a bent form resembling the letter L (76) (Fig. 2). β-helices are also found in the crystal structures of the passenger domains of Hap, EspP, and Pet and the p55 fragment of VacA (77–80).

The TpsA proteins of type Vb systems are also predicted to be rich in β-solenoid structures (62, 70). These predictions were confirmed when the structure of the TPS domain of the *B. pertussis* TpsA protein FHA was solved (81). The TPS domain of TpsA proteins is required for targeting to the TpsB protein and secretion; its function could therefore be considered analogous to that of the linker regions of type Va, Vc, and Ve autotransporters (Fig. 1). The FHA TPS domain structure shows a right-handed β-helix with several extrahelical elements protruding from the β-helical core (Fig. 2). The structure of the TPS domain from the *Haemophilus influenzae* adhesin HMW1 is remarkably similar to the FHA TPS domain, though there are some differences at the very N-termini of the structures (82).

In contrast to both type Va and type Vb, type Vc–secreted proteins are obligate homotrimers that form highly intertwined structures. When viewed in electron micrographs, these proteins resemble lollipops, having a globular "head" domain distal from the cell, followed by an elongated "stalk" (27, 64). However, though many type Vc systems follow this relatively simple architecture, it is now clear that they are modular in structure and can have several head domains interspersed by regions of stalk (16, 27) (Fig. 2, Fig. 3). The stalk regions of type Vc autotransporters consist largely of α-helical parallel coiled coils. Though type Vc autotransporters, such as UspA1 (66), contain regions of canonical coiled coil, i.e. a left-handed superhelix, they typically have a significant amount of right-handed coiled coil (20, 83) (Fig. 2, Fig. 3). In contrast to most coiled coils, where the core is hydrophobic, the interior of the coiled coils of type Vc autotransporters can contain a large proportion of hydrophilic residues. In some cases, these residues coordinate the binding of anions such as chloride or nitrate within the core (20, 66, 68, 84). The stalks also often contain large cavities, which have been postulated as sites that would allow deformation of the coiled coil and thus enable bending of the fiber (20). Some connector elements (discussed below) can also confer limited local flexibility (16).

In addition to often lengthy coiled-coil segments, stalks can contain connector regions that mediate transitions from one type of supercoil to another or the transition from head domain to coiled coil or vice versa. Another feature of connectors is to displace the polypeptide chain by 120°, usually in the direction opposite to the handedness of the preceding segment (16). These connectors include necks (31, 85), saddles (20), KG domains (86), and HANS, DALL, and FGG elements (16, 31); the somewhat cryptic names of the domains refer to short sequence motifs typically found in them. It should be noted that transitions of handedness do not necessarily require a connector, as shown by the YadA stalk (83) (Fig. 2).

The type Vc autotransporters also contain β-solenoids, but these structures are limited to the globular head domains. The first such structure to be solved was the head of the *Yersinia* adhesin YadA. Each monomer of the structure forms a left-handed β-roll (a subclass of β-solenoids with two axially stacked β-sheets). The trimeric structure is stabilized by a shared, tightly packed hydrophobic core and a "lock-nut" structure, where the polypeptide chain from one monomer crosses over to connect with the next monomer at both the N- and C-termini (Fig. 2). At the C-terminus, this crossover is mediated by a neck element, which leads the polypeptide into the right-handed coiled-coil stalk. YadA-like β-roll domains are found in a number of type Vc autotransporters, though not all have the highly stable lock-nut configuration (20, 67, 87) (Fig. 2). Other kinds of head domain also exist, as exemplified by the Trp ring and GIN domains of Hia and BadA (27, 88). Both domain types are rich in β-structure and are formally variations of a β-prism fold (Fig. 2). Unlike the β-rolls and

β-prisms of type Vc autotransporters, which form intricately intertwining structures, the very recently solved NadA head structure is formed of three wing-like protrusions from the coiled-coil stalk that neither interconnect nor introduce a 120° twist into the chain (68) (Fig. 2).

Translocation Domains

The translocation domains of type V systems formally consist of two components: the transmembrane β-barrel domain, embedded in the outer membrane, and the linker region connecting the β-barrel to the passenger domain. This is the configuration seen for type Va, Vc, and Ve translocation domains (Fig. 4). In contrast, for type Vb, the β-barrel domain and the passenger domain are separate polypeptides, so there is no linker region in the classical sense, though the periplasmic polypeptide transport-associated POTRA domains of TpsB proteins and the TPS domain of TpsAs might play analogous roles to the linker region of the other classes.

In type Va, Vc, and Ve proteins, the translocation domain comprises a 12-stranded β-barrel (Fig. 4). In type Va and type Ve autotransporters, the β-barrel is formed by a single polypeptide chain, whereas in type Vc systems, like the passenger domain, the β-barrel consists of three polypeptide chains. The β-barrels of all three classes are very similar in size, with a pore diameter of approximately 10 Å (17, 89–92).

A remarkable feature of type Va translocation domains is the position of the linker within the β-barrel pore. In the first structure of a translocation domain from a type Va autotransporter, NalP, the linker traverses the pore of the β-barrel from the periplasmic side to the extracellular side and adopts an α-helical conformation (92). Because this structure was obtained from protein refolded from inclusion bodies, the question was raised of whether the position of the α-helical linker within the β-barrel pore might be an artifact of refolding or

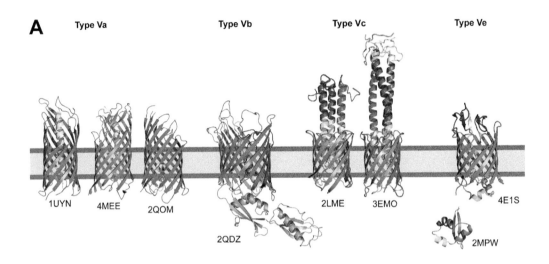

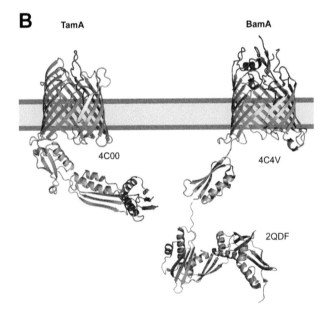

crystallization. However, other type Va translocation domain structures, including those from EspP and AIDA-I, show the linker positioned similarly in the pore (89, 93) (Fig. 4). The structure of a full-length type Va autotransporter, EstA, with the α-helical linker clearly residing inside the β-barrel, has laid to rest any remaining controversy about the position of the linker (60) (Fig. 3).

Though the linker is clearly inside the β-barrel pore in all type Va translocation domain structures, there are differences in the size and orientation of the α-helical linker. In NalP, Hbp, AIDA-I, and the full-length EstA, the linker traverses the entire length of the pore and extends some way into the extracellular space (60, 92, 93). In EspP, an autocatalytic reaction within the β-barrel leads to cleavage of the linker and release of the passenger domain into the extracellular medium (89). The remaining stub of the linker forms a short α-helix, but this lies perpendicular to the axis of the pore (Fig. 4).

To date, there are only structures from two type Vc translocation domains. These are the crystal structure of the Hia translocation domain and the solid-state NMR structure of the YadA membrane anchor (17, 91). The structures are almost completely superimposable, showing the high degree of structural conservation in the domains. They are also similar in general appearance to the type Va translocation domains, the major difference being the trimeric quaternary structure of the β-barrel and the three chains of the linker passing through the pore of the barrel. Like the linkers of type Va translocation domains, the linkers of type Vc systems also adopt a mostly helical conformation, which forms a canonical left-handed coiled coil when exiting the pore (17, 94). Interestingly, the residues at the transition point into the left-handed coiled coil (termed the ASSA region) show a marked drop in α-helical propensity (17).

In type Va and type Vc autotransporters, the linker is immediately N-terminal to the β-barrel domain. In the type Ve autotransporters intimin and invasin, the linker is C-terminal to the β-barrel, i.e., the topology is inverted (90). In addition, there is a short periplasmically located α-helical stretch between the linker region and the β-barrel. In contrast to type Va and type Vc autotransporters, the linker is not in an α-helical conformation but is an extended chain traversing the β-barrel pore (Fig. 4).

FIGURE 4 (A) Experimental structures of translocation units of type V secretion systems. Examples from type Va (classical autotransporters), type Vb (TpsB proteins), type Vc (trimeric autotransporter adhesins), and type Ve (inverse autotransporters) are included. Structures are shown in cartoon representation. β-barrel domains are blue, linker regions or intrabarrel α-helices are yellow, significant extracellular loops are brown, periplasmically located domains and extensions are green, coiled-coil stalks are red, and connector elements are cyan. For type Vc proteins, each chain is colored with a slightly different hue. All proteins are oriented such that the extracellular face of the β-barrel is pointing toward the top of the page, and the approximate positioning of the outer membrane is shown in gray. Note that for type Va and type Vc translocation domains, the N-termini of the proteins are extracellular, whereas for types Vb and Ve, the N-termini are periplasmic. Type Va translocation domains are represented by structures from NalP (PDB ID: 1UYN), EspP (2QOM), and AIDA-I (4MEE). TpsB proteins are represented by FhaC (2QDZ), with two POTRA domains. Type Vc translocation domains are exemplified by the YadA (2LME) and Hia (3EMO) structures. The intimin translocation domain (4E1S) and LysM (2MPW, with additional α-helix highlighted) represent type Ve translocation and periplasmic domains. (B) β-barrel proteins involved in the biogenesis of type V–secreted proteins, BamA and TamA. The structures of TamA (4C00) and BamA (4C4V) from *E. coli* are also shown, with the unstable β-strand 16 highlighted (the coloring otherwise corresponds to panel A). TamA has three N-terminal periplasmic POTRA domains. The *E. coli* BamA has five POTRA domains; one is part of the β-barrel structure and the other four have been crystallized separately (2QDF). The approximate span of the outer membrane is shown as a gray bar.

In contrast to the 12-stranded β-barrels of type Va, Vc, and Ve autotransporters, the TpsB proteins of type Vb secretion systems consist of a 16-stranded β-barrel and associated periplasmic POTRA domains. The only TpsB protein structure to have been solved to date is FhaC, the transporter partner of FHA (95) (Fig. 4). In the structure, the pore of the FhaC β-barrel is occluded by the large extracellular loop L6, which reaches inside the pore and extends almost to the periplasmic face of the β-barrel. In addition, an N-terminal α-helix (H1) inserts into the pore from the periplasmic side, thus plugging it. However, H1 is mobile and probably moves out of the pore during FHA secretion (96, 97). FhaC contains two periplasmic POTRA domains, discussed below. The transmembrane domain of type Vd secretion systems is predicted to be a 16-stranded β-barrel, like it is for type Vb systems. In addition, these proteins are predicted to contain a single periplasmic POTRA domain (98); however, no structural verification of these predictions is yet available.

The TpsB proteins are homologous to BamA, the central component of a multiprotein complex, the β-barrel assembly machinery or Bam complex, responsible for the insertion of all transmembrane β-barrel proteins into the outer membrane (99, 100). Because BamA has been implicated in the biogenesis of autotransporter proteins (25, 101–105), we include a short discussion on the structure of this protein. Like FhaC, BamA consists of a 16-stranded β-barrel (106–108) (Fig. 4). Unlike in FhaC, the large L6 loop does not penetrate deep into the pore of the β-barrel but, rather, covers the extracellular side of the pore by forming a dome-like structure with the other extracellular loops. Another notable feature is that β-strand 16 of the barrel is destabilized in two of the four available structures, leading to a shortened hydrophobic sheet on one side of the β-barrel (Fig. 4). This may lead to perturbation of the outer membrane. In addition, the destabilized β-strand may serve as a lateral gate that

allows insertion of nascent β-barrel proteins into the outer membrane, possibly involving a hybrid barrel intermediate, but the details of the insertion mechanism remain under debate (106, 109). Enterobacteria encode an additional BamA homologue referred to as TamA, which together with an inner membrane protein TamB forms a complex implicated in the biogenesis of a subset of type Va autotransporters (110). The structure of TamA has been solved, and the 16-stranded β-barrel structure resembles BamA in both the extracellular dome and the potential for lateral opening via a destabilized C-terminal β-strand (111).

Periplasmic Domains

Most type Va and type Vc autotransporters have the translocation unit at their C-terminus; thus, they do not contain any appreciable periplasmic regions. However, some type Vc systems are predicted to have extensions C-terminal to the translocation unit, which would form coiled coils in the periplasm (31). Currently, there are no structures of these putative periplasmic regions. In contrast to type Va and type Vc autotransporters, where periplasmic domains are rare, all type Ve proteins appear to have periplasmic extensions (10, 112). These are usually quite short (<50 residues) and comprise only two predicted α-helices. Some proteins from the *Enterobacteriaceae* have larger periplasmic regions containing a lysin motif (LysM), a peptidoglycan-binding minidomain. The structure of the LysM from intimin was recently solved by NMR; it contains two α-helices packed against an antiparallel β-sheet, common to other LysMs, but in addition the intimin LysM has a third short α-helix preceding the C-terminal β-strand (10) (Fig. 4).

TpsB proteins and type Vd autotransporters contain periplasmic POTRA domains, as do their homologues BamA and TamA. POTRA domains are small, globular domains of approximately 80 residues (113). The fold consists of a three-stranded β-sheet packed against two α-helices with the topology β-α-α-β-β (Fig. 4). POTRA domains from different proteins and even the same protein share only low sequence similarity, and conserved regions are mostly limited to the hydrophobic core of the fold (114). The number of POTRA domains in different BamA homologues varies; in enterobacteria, BamA has five POTRA domains, but the number can vary from three to seven in other phyla (114). TamA has three POTRA domains, TpsBs such as FhaC have two, and type Vd proteins have a single POTRA domain (95, 98, 111). POTRA domains are often connected by linkers that can confer flexibility to the domains (115). POTRA domains interact with substrate proteins (nascent outer membrane proteins in the case of BamA, TpsAs for TpsBs), possibly through β-augmentation (115, 116), but it is worth noting that the detailed function of the POTRA domains is under debate.

Full-Length Fibers

The only extant experimental structure of a full-length autotransporter is that of EstA (60) (Fig. 3). EstA is an unusually small type Va autotransporter, and its passenger domain is not a β-solenoid structure, but adopts an all-α fold similar to GDSL lipases.

Although no experimental structures of other complete autotransporters are available, the existing structures of fragments have allowed modeling of several fibers. This has been particularly successful for the trimeric autotransporters (type Vc systems), whose modular nature has allowed crystallizing fragments and connecting these later *in silico* in combination with homology modeling. Using this approach, the group of Andrei Lupas has provided complete models for the relatively short prototypical TAA YadA and for the much longer and architecturally more complex TAA SadA from *Salmonella* and its two *E. coli* orthologues, EhaG

and UpaG (16, 61). The YadA model shows the simple lollipop-like shape of the molecule, with the globular head projected away from the outer membrane by the coiled-coil stalk. The C-terminal β-barrel domain anchors the protein in the outer membrane (Fig. 3). In contrast, the model for the SadA fiber is much more elaborate, with two head domains connected by coiled-coil regions interrupted by connectors (Fig. 3). This exemplifies the modular make-up of many of the larger type Vc autotransporters.

In the case of TPS proteins, a full-length structure containing both the translocation unit and the passenger domain is not possible, because the two functional domains are separate polypeptides that interact only transiently during export. In this sense, a full-length structure of the TpsB moiety does exist, represented by FhaC. Sequence analysis has allowed modeling of the entire FHA structure, which forms a long, parallel β-helix (62, 117) (Fig. 3).

MOLECULAR BIOLOGY ANALYSIS: POINT MUTATIONS AND DELETIONS OF GENES

Mutagenesis is widely used to decipher parts of genomes and to understand the function of individual genes and proteins. A better understanding of the type V secretion systems has been obtained by introducing insertions, deletions, and point mutations into genes encoding these proteins.

Gene Inactivation and Plasmid Complementation

Reverse genetics is an approach to studying the function of a gene by studying the phenotypic effect of specific known DNA sequences. It has been used to characterize many type V secretion genes in various Gram-negative bacteria. This approach involves inactivation of the putative gene followed by a number of assays to study phenotypic changes. The following paragraphs discuss examples of various type V systems studied by this method, to show the potential of the method to study mainly the function of these systems.

BcaA (type Va) of *Burkholderia pseudomallei* was characterized by creating large in-frame deletions in the gene. Plasmid complementation is a method in which a functional copy of a gene is encoded on a plasmid that is transformed into cells where the gene was deleted, to check if the function is fully restored. This is considered the "gold standard" in deletion analysis, because it helps to distinguish direct from indirect effects of the deletion of a gene. In the case of BcaA, plasmid complementation showed that it is required for efficient plaque formation. *In vivo* studies indicated that BcaA is also required for efficient dissemination and survival of bacteria in spleen (118). In a less targeted approach, transposon mutagenesis with TnphoA was used to identify potential genes encoding surface-exposed virulence factors in enterotoxigenic *E. coli*. TnphoA is a derivative of the Tn5 transposon, which also contains a modified alkaline phosphatase gene lacking a promoter and signal sequence. This construct, when inserted in a frame, leads to chimeric proteins, and if the fused protein has a signal sequence, then the alkaline phosphatase activity is restored in the periplasm. Thus, it helps in localizing export signals within a protein and also in identifying secreted proteins or transmembrane proteins (119). Using this approach, the virulence factor EatA belonging to the serine protease family of type Va transporters was identified in *E. coli* (120). Similarly, random transposon mutagenesis was used to create a mutant library in *Fusobacteria* species followed by phenotypic screening and identification of virulence traits. Mutants were screened for loss of hemagglutination, and the gene responsible was identified as *fap2*, an autotransporter protein (121).

The Pdt two-partner secretion system (type Vb) of *Pseudomonas aeruginosa* was characterized by creating deletion mutants of *pdtA* and *pdtB* genes. It was found that the translocation of PdtA across the outer membrane does not occur in the absence of PdtB (122). Similarly, a two-partner secretion system was characterized in *Moraxella catarrhalis*. MchA1 and MchA2 were found to be secreted into the outer membrane, and some amount was found in the culture medium. Deletion of *mchB* completely abolished extracellular secretion of both MchA1 and MchA2 (123).

A genomic knockout of the type Vc transporter hemagglutinin of *Avibacterium paragallinarum* was created to study the function of the gene which is involved in hemagglutination, cell adherence, and biofilm formation (124). To study the mechanism of biofilm formation in *Veillonella* species, insertional inactivation of eight putative hemagglutinin genes was carried out using a tetracycline cassette. The *hag1* gene encodes a YadA-like type Vc transporter that is involved in coaggregation with other colonizing bacteria and helps in adherence to cells (125).

The product of the *eaeA* gene of *E. coli* is also called intimin. It was shown to be membrane-localized and surface-exposed. An intimin-negative mutant still adhered to epithelial cells but failed to form actin pedestals (126). Later studies have shown that intimin belongs to the type Ve class of autotransporters (7).

Fusions and Exchange of Domains

Fusion and exchange of domains in autotransporters has been useful in studying the translocation mechanism of autotransporters and also has biotechnological applications, because it can be used for surface display of recombinant proteins (127). The fusion partner size can vary from small peptides to whole proteins. Either the complete autotransporter or just the translocation domain can be used for the fusion, as long as an N-terminal signal peptide is present. Most of such fusion studies have been carried out in type Va autotransporters, though some have also been performed on type Ve (128, 129).

Fusion of the translocation domain of IgA protease (type Va) with cholera toxinB (CtxB) subunit showed outer membrane integration of these fusion proteins as well as surface exposure of ctxB moieties (130). Again using cholera toxin as a fusion partner, AIDA-I-ctxB fusions were designed to identify the minimal unit that would translocate the passenger domain. By stepwise introduction of N-terminal deletions in the passenger domain of AIDA-I, it was found that a minimum linker region between 28 and 48 amino acids is essential for successful translocation (40). Taken together, both studies showed that the N- terminal region of the passenger domain does not play a role in initiating translocation.

The ability of another type Va autotransporter, Pet, to mediate secretion of heterologous proteins was tested by creating fusions with a fluorescent protein (mCherry) and E-SAT6, a diagnostic marker of *Mycobacterium tuberculosis*. It was shown that the heterologous fusions were expressed and actively translocated to the cell surface. The Pet construct used for expression consisted of the β-barrel, the α-helical linker, and the so-called autochaperone domain, a C-terminal part of the passenger domain essential for proper folding of the complete secreted passenger domain (131). Several type Va autotransporters contain such a folding core in the C-terminus of the passenger domain, which has been referred to as an autochaperone (132–134). In some instances, the autochaperone can even promote autotransporter folding and secretion when added in *trans* (132, 135).

The minimum construct length required for translocation was also determined in the Pet study, and it was shown that the autochaperone domain is not required for secretion, but only for folding (131). Following the unfolding of the pertactin passenger domain with circular dichroism spectroscopy revealed a two-step process, where a part of the passenger domain was significantly more stable than the rest of the protein (71). A similar study in the autotransporter Hbp was carried out, again using E-SAT6 as a fusion partner. Substitution of parts of the Hbp passenger domain still gives high-level expression and secretion of the fused protein. It was also found that the Hbp passenger β-helix is not essential for secretion but that its presence improves secretion and stability of the chimera (136). Likewise, β-lactamase and maltose-binding protein were fused with either the full-length type Va *Shigella flexneri* transporter, IcsA, or only with its translocation domain. The fused proteins were tested for expression, surface localization, and folding. Fusion of exogenous proteins to full-length IcsA improved expression and surface exposure of the chimeric protein compared to the ones directly fused to IcsA translocation domain, again indirectly suggesting a role of parts of the passenger in proper surface display (137).

Insertion of a calmodulin moiety into the type Va transporter Hbp completely blocks passenger domain translocation in the presence of calcium because it forms a rigid and stable structure (132), indicating that a more or less flexible passenger domain is required for the translocation to be successful. Similar results were observed when calmodulin replaced part of the intimin passenger domain, a type Ve transporter, where calmodulin could only be exported in the presence of a chelator (129). For type Vc transporters, it was shown that heterologous translocation domains can be used for surface display of other trimeric passengers, using, e.g., the *Yersinia* YadA membrane anchor for export of passengers from *Bartonella* (133) or the *Haemophilus* Hia, *Moraxella* UspA, or *E. coli* Eib translocators to export the YadA passenger domain (134, 135). Similarly, the passenger domains can be swapped between the two type Ve transporters intimin and invasin, keeping the binding functions intact (138).

Hybrid constructs for surface display have many possible applications in biotechnology.

As an example, a complete protein with a binding function, the lectin moiety of FimH, was surface-displayed and was found to be functionally active after expression. It is worth noting that this domain has two disulfide bridges which did not interfere with the translocation process. (139). Similarly, constructs consisting of the translocation domain of the *N. gonorrhoeae* type Va transporter IgA and leucine zippers of eukaryotic transcription factors Fos and Jun were expressed in *E. coli*. The *E. coli* cells showed a novel adherence trait that resulted in clumping and self-association of cells in liquid media. This and other studies showed that the biotechnological possibilities of autotransporter surface display are not limited to prokaryotic proteins (140). Ag43 of *E. coli* was used to display immunogenic epitope tags such as CTP3, a conformational loop of CtxB, and Chlam12, a 12-residue epitope of the *Chlamydia trachomatis* DnaK protein. The site of fusion was within the passenger domain of Ag43. The immunogenic tags were found to be correctly folded and well displayed. In the same way, epitopes but also complete proteins can be displayed on the surface via type Ve secretion systems such as *E. coli* intimin and *Yersinia* invasin (7, 128). Thus, type V systems in general are useful for the surface expression of both small peptides and larger proteins.

Insertional Mutagenesis and Point Mutations

To study the contribution of specific amino acids or small subdomains toward the function or structure of a protein, point mutations or short stretches of additional residues can be deliberately introduced in the gene encoding the protein. These approaches have been widely used to study the function of autotransporter passengers but also to study the transport mechanism as such.

An insertion is the addition of nucleotide base pairs into the DNA sequence of a gene and has been useful in studying the structure-function relationship in autotransporters. In a technique called linker scanning mutagenesis the gene is systematically scanned by inserting a linker in various regions (141). A study of the type Va autotransporter, Pet, using a transposon-based in-frame insertion kit which randomly inserts a 19-amino-acid linker into the gene, revealed that linker insertions in the N-terminal half of the passenger domain resulted in lower levels of secretion and aberrantly folded protein, whereas insertions in the C-terminal half of the passenger domain abolished secretion. This study helped in predicting regions of the passenger domain with functions such as protease activity or cell-binding activity but also identified a region essential for the secretion of the passenger domain (142). A penta-peptide linker scanning mutagenesis of another type Va autotransporter, IcsA, showed similar results: insertions in the C-terminal half of the passenger domain led to aberrant production of the protein compared to the wild type. For some mutants, the protein level was restored to wild type when expressed in protease-deficient *E. coli* UT5600, indicating that the protein may be susceptible to degradation by an endogenous outer membrane protease (143).

Insertions of immunogenic tags can also obstruct the transport process in various type V systems, e.g., in the type Va autotransporter Pet, where a hemagglutinin (HA) tag was used. Although the tag is small in length, the obstruction probably occurs due to the bulky and rigid nature of the tag (144). Similarly, an HA tag introduced after position 453 in the type Ve autotransporter intimin resulted in a stalled translocation intermediate. It was shown that the β-barrel was well inserted into the membrane while the passenger domain was unfolded. The HA tag was accessible by antibodies in unpermeabilized cells, whereas the C-terminus of the passenger domain was not. The C-terminus was in turn stained with antibodies only upon permeabilization of cells with detergent. This strongly suggests the presence of a hairpin-like conformation of the stalled translocation inter- mediate (105).

Point mutations in the C-terminal segment of the EspP passenger domain are predicted to disrupt the packing of the hydrophobic core and obstruct folding and completion of translocation (145), whereas point muta- tions introduced in the other segments of the EspP passenger domain do not signifi- cantly affect the translocation efficiency or structure of the protein, indicating that the C-terminal region of the passenger domain is more important—if not essential—for folding (146), at least in this case, and it has been sug- gested that this region has an autochaperone function, similar to that in the type Va system Pet mentioned above (131). In another study of Pet, paired cysteine residues were system- atically introduced, and the result indicated an inverse relationship between secretion efficiency and size of the disulfide-bonded loop. The longest disulfide bond that did not interfere with secretion consisted of 18 resi- dues, and a loop consisting of 20 or more amino acids stalled the translocation process, indicating that large covalently constrained elements do interfere with the translocation process (144). In the case of the type Va auto- transporter Hbp, a disulfide bond between closely spaced cysteine residues also did not interfere with translocation efficiency, whereas distantly placed cysteine residues resulted in a stalled translocation intermediate (132).

A number of residues are conserved in the translocation domain(s) of type V secretion systems. In a study of the type Va transporter Tsh, highly conserved residues among the SPATE family of autotransporters were mu- tated: nonaromatic hydrophobic residues were changed to tyrosine or alanine. Some of the mutations impaired secretion of the passenger domain into the culture medium and resulted in the accumulation of unpro- cessed protein in the bacterial outer mem- brane. It was noticed that the side chains of these residues face the interior of the barrel and therefore might be involved in passenger cleavage or proper positioning of

the α-helical linker for cleavage (147). When periplasmic fractions of mutants showing this defective phenotype were screened, only the processed form of Tsh was observed, which according to the authors suggests that the β-barrel already obtains a certain folded conformation before insertion into the outer membrane. Based on these results, a model has been proposed where a proto-β-barrel like structure forms in the periplasm and is stabilized by the formation of α-helical linker in the β-barrel (147). In another study sup- porting such a proto-β-barrel model, tomato etch virus sites and single cysteine residues were introduced in the junction between the translocation domain and passenger do- main of the *E. coli* type Va autotransporter EspP. Tomato etch virus protease acces- sibility and accessibility toward a cysteine- specific biotinylation agent were measured, and no differences in accessibility were observed between stalled transport inter- mediates and fully assembled (wild-type) protein. Cell fractionation experiments sug- gested that the assembly intermediate forms in the periplasm (148).

Mutation of a conserved glycine residue to larger residues in the type Vc autotrans- porter YadA resulted in decreased stability of the protein and degradation by DegP protease. When the mutants were grown in a DegP-deficient strain, YadA could reach the cell surface, indicating that the highly conserved glycine is important for efficient transport, probably by providing enough space in the translocation pore (32). In the type Ve transporter invasin and intimin, the same conserved glycine residue was found, and mutations disrupted surface display of the passenger in a similar way, but no sig- nificant degradation of the protein was evi- dent (7). Inside the pore of the translocation domain of autotransporters, conserved pairs of aromatic residues and glycine residues are perfectly positioned in neighboring β-strands so that the large aromatic residue can in- tercalate in the space made available by the small glycine residue. Such motifs are known as mortise-tenon motifs. Mutation of such conserved glycines (mortise motifs) to alanine in the type Va transporter Pet resulted in a slower rate of surface exposure as well as a decreased rate of autocatalytic processing. The results indicate that these motifs allow correct and efficient folding of autotransporters (149). Mutations of hydrophobic residues in the lumen of the translocation domain β-barrel of the type Va transporter BrkA to charged residues such as aspartate or lysine resulted in decreased translocation efficiency without affecting the ability of BrkA to localize in the outer membrane (150). The results of this study support a hairpin model of translocation for a passenger domain, where the presence of hydrophobic patches would provide a suitable environment for anchoring a hairpin-like hydrophobic structural motif.

Additional Factors Involved in Autotransporter Assembly

Type V secretion systems, and especially the classical type Va autotransporters, were previously believed to be self-sufficient for their secretion and insertion into the outer membrane. Later studies showed the involvement of a number of proteins which aid in the assembly of autotransporters, many of them periplasmic chaperones. Double (deletion) mutants of the periplasmic chaperone factors *skp*, *degP*, and *surA* can be created in all possible combinations, but a triple mutant resulted in a synthetic lethal phenotype (151). Depletion of SurA resulted in reduced levels of the outer membrane proteins LamB and OmpA, whereas depletion of Skp and DegP did not cause these effects, suggesting that SurA plays a major role in the assembly of outer membrane proteins, whereas Skp and DegP act in a rescue pathway for proteins that did not assemble normally (152).

The *S. flexneri* type Va transporter IcsA was found to be less accessible on the surface when expressed in a *degP* mutant, although the amount of IcsA in the outer membrane

was comparable to the wild-type levels, indicating a defect in proper insertion of the protein in the outer membrane (153). Yeast two-hybrid analysis and surface plasmon resonance analysis have shown SurA, Skp, and DegP to directly interact with the type Va autotransporter EspP (102, 154). However, *in vitro* studies indicate that chaperones are not always required for type Va autotransporter biogenesis. In the case of *E. coli* AIDA-I, refolding of the translocation domain was not enhanced upon transfer from urea to refolding conditions with chaperones such as Skp, DegP, and SurA (155). Note also that although the IcsA passenger domain was less efficiently translocated in *surA*, *skp*, and *degP* mutants, the protein still localized to the outer membrane (153, 156). Similarly, the secretion of the EspP passenger domain was reduced in *surA*, *degP*, and *skp* mutants, but the translocation domain levels in the outer membrane were comparable to the wild type (154). Involvement of the same periplasmic factors has to some extent also been shown for type Vc and type Ve autotransporters. The type Vc transporter YadA is degraded by the chaperone/protease DegP under overexpression conditions when the passenger translocation is impaired (32), and YadA interacts with periplasmic chaperones as well as with the Bam complex during its biogenesis (25). The same is true to some extent for the type Ve systems invasin and intimin (7, 105). The type Vc transporter SadA from *Salmonella* requires an additional, specific export factor, SadB, for its biogenesis. The genes *sadA* and *sadB* are organized in an operon structure. SadB is a trimeric, inner membrane lipoprotein, suggesting that it helps in trimerization of the type Vc system before translocation of the passenger (15).

IN VITRO ASSAYS TO STUDY MEMBRANE TRANSLOCATION

The *in vitro* reconstitution of protein translocation pathways is a powerful tool to identify the components required for a specific translocation mechanism and to study the details of the translocation process. In principle, four distinct types of model membrane systems exist for such reconstitution assays: lipid monolayers, supported lipid bilayers, liposomes, and lipid nanodiscs (157). Until today, only the type Va and Vb secretion pathways have been reconstituted successfully using liposomes (Fig. 5), solid-supported membranes, and nanodiscs (104, 158–160), while the reconstitution of type Vc, Vd, and Ve pathways has not been reported yet.

The C-terminal translocation domain of type Va secretion systems was originally believed to be the sole mediator of outer membrane translocation of its N-terminal passenger domain, which led to the term "autotransporter." However, this concept was challenged by the findings that only 12 β-strands form the β-barrel of the translocation domain, and the diameter of the formed pore is only ≈10 Å according to the available crystal structures (89, 92). It has been suggested that this pore is too narrow to accommodate type Va-secreted, folded domains (132, 161, 162). Further investigations showed that BamA depletion in *S. flexneri* interferes with the secretion of the passenger domains of type Va systems (101), suggesting that the Bam complex is involved in the biogenesis of type Va systems, a concept that was further supported by the observation that

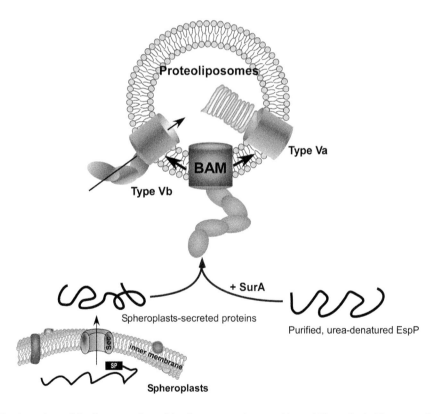

FIGURE 5 Overview of the liposome-based *in vitro* system for type Va and Vb analysis. The test substrates are prepared as urea-denatured, purified proteins or by using spheroplasts. Translocation may need additional factors added to the proteoliposome mix, such as chaperone(s) for urea-denatured substrates. The success of the translocation is then monitored either by protease accessibility assays or by checking heat-modifiability (a unique feature of bacterial β-barrels).

Bam complex components could be photo-cross-linked to type Va transporters *in vivo* (102). However, it remains unknown if the secretion defect caused by BamA depletion is a direct or an indirect effect.

To complicate the matter, a recently identified translocation and assembly module (TAM or Tam complex) seems to be involved in the secretion of some type Va proteins in proteobacteria (110, 160). It is still unclear if the Tam and Bam complexes function individually or have to cooperate with each other to mediate the secretion of all or only a subset of autotransporters, but *in vitro* biochemical reconstitution assays have shed some light on the matter. With the help of reconstituted liposomes containing the complete, purified *E. coli* Bam complex, it was demonstrated that two type Va systems, EspP and Ag43, depend on the presence of Bam to be successfully translocated through the membrane *in vitro* (104, 159). Furthermore, though the exact function of each Bam component during type Va translocation is unknown, at least BamB and BamC are not essential for the process, because the lack of both components in the reconstituted liposomes merely resulted in a less efficient transport of EspP (104). Further analysis using a nanodisc-based strategy demonstrated that a single copy of the Bam complex can mediate the biogenesis of EspP and that the translocation domain assembly seems to be the rate-limiting step in the whole process (104).

In a similar approach, liposomes were used to analyze the translocation mechanism of type Vb secretion systems, using the filamentous hemagglutinin FHA of *B. pertussis* as a model system. When the type Vb translocation component of FHA (FhaC) was reconstituted into liposomes to perform swelling assays, it formed a channel. The swelling rate correlated positively with the amount of reconstituted FhaC but negatively with the size of the sugars, suggesting that the reconstituted pore is at least large enough to transport sugar molecules (163). In a similar study, the calculated pore diameter

of the type Vb translocator protein HMW1B *H. influenzae* was ~1.9 nm (164). In single-channel conductance measurements using planar lipid bilayers to determine the electrophysiological properties of the channel, a comparable channel conductance in 1 M KCl was observed both for FhaC (1,200 pS) and HMW1B (1,400 pS) (96, 165). In agreement with liposome swelling analysis, these electrophysiological measurements show that the translocator proteins of type Vb are able to form conductive pores, but with low open probability. It is interesting to mention that for purified translocator domains of type Va proteins, including Hbp (166), NalP (92), and IgA (167), liposome swelling assay and electrophysiological measurements suggest that these translocator domains have pore activity as well. Assuming these domains form perfect cylinders, their pore diameters can be calculated to be ~0.8 nm or ~2.1 nm depending on the method used, in line with the diameter of regular β-barrel outer membrane proteins (166, 168).

In a cell-free *in vitro* system, in which purified FhaC was reconstituted into liposomes and combined with a fragment of the FHA passenger that was previously produced in and secreted from spheroplasts, FHA was translocated without the addition of any other protein component. Even fragments of FHA that contained all the necessary information required for outer membrane translocation *in vivo* (81) were successfully translocated into the lumen of liposomes by reconstituted FhaC (159). Likewise, it was shown that for a well-studied heterologous yet complementary type Vb pair—a passenger protein called HpmA (a hemolysin from *Proteus mirabilis*) and a translocator protein called ShlB from *Serratia marcescens*—full translocation could be reproduced using this liposome strategy (159). Taken together, these *in vitro* reconstitution assays of type Vb secretion systems clearly demonstrate that a single TpsB outer membrane protein is sufficient to enable the outer membrane translocation of its cognate TpsA substrates.

In vitro reconstitution systems not only provide the opportunity for in-depth analysis of the molecular details of the processes of β-barrel assembly and the passenger domain translocation of type V secretion pathways, but also make it possible to address the functions of chaperones and other more peripheral components in type V secretion. The assembly of urea-denatured EspP from *E. coli* can only be successfully reconstructed *in vitro* in the presence of the periplasmic chaperone SurA, while another chaperone, Skp, seems to inhibit the biogenesis of EspP under the reported experimental conditions (104). This is somewhat in contrast to earlier reports that Skp prevents misfolding, while SurA promotes the folding of β-barrel outer membrane proteins (169, 170).

DISCUSSION

What Drives the Transport Process?

The outer membrane of Gram-negative bacteria has no direct access to cytosolic energy sources such as ATP, and it lacks an electrochemical gradient of protons or other ions, simply because it is full of pore proteins that allow free diffusion of small substrates into and out of the periplasm. The most probable driving force for type V secretion is thus the free energy gained by folding the passenger domain on the cell surface, which probably also includes entropic effects that are based on molecular crowding in the periplasm. It has been shown that passenger domains of various type V systems are slow-folding entities (171), presumably to avoid premature folding in the periplasm. At the same time, they do not seem to aggregate easily when unfolded, which would be an advantage for slow-folding proteins and would give enough time for a complex transport process. The overall negatively charged nature of passenger domains has been implicated as an additional factor (172).

Is Type V Secretion a Uniform Mechanism that Just Comes in Different Flavors (from Type Va to Type Ve)?

To be able to answer this question, it is important to understand the hairpin model for the transport process (Fig. 6). When looking at monomeric autotransporters of type Va, there are in principle two ways of pushing an attached polypeptide chain through the pore: (i) the attached chain can go into the pore "head-first," with the advantage that only one unfolded polypeptide chain is in the translocation pore at any given time but with the disadvantage that finding the entrance to the pore is probably difficult for a passenger that can be hundreds—or even thousands—of residues long. (ii) The attached chain can enter the translocation pore as a hairpin ("tail-first"): in this case, two unfolded polypeptide chains are in the translocation pore at any given time until the transport process is concluded and the head reaches the cell surface, leading to potential problems with space in the very small pore but solving the problem of how the passenger finds the entrance to the translocation domain in the first place. Both of these models work under the assumption that the translocation pore is formed first and that transport of the passenger proceeds after this step.

The hairpin model is strongly favored based on several lines of evidence. The passenger domains in type Va systems have their folding core at their C-terminus, strongly suggesting that folding proceeds from the C- to N-terminus. This was demonstrated for various exemplars of type Va systems, including pertactin (71), Hbp (173), and EspP (145). Moreover, the so-called autochaperone domain of many type Va autotransporters at the very C-terminus of the passenger domain catalyzes (or at least initiates) the folding of the rest of the passenger (174, 175), again speaking for a stepwise process that starts at the C-terminus. Cysteine scanning mutations leading to stalled autotransport intermediates

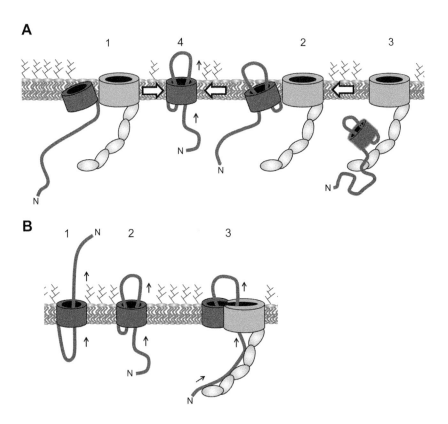

FIGURE 6 Models of outer membrane insertion and passenger secretion in type Va autotransporters. (A) Models of membrane insertion. Membrane insertion of autotransporters (and other outer membrane β-barrel proteins) depends on BamA (depicted in light gray). The autotransporter itself is shown in dark gray. Currently, three models are envisaged to explain membrane insertion and initiation of autotransport. In model 1, BamA catalyzes the insertion of the β-barrel domain of the autotransporter, after which hairpin formation and passenger domain secretion proceed autonomously. In model 2, membrane insertion and hairpin formation happen concomitantly. A third model (model 3) has been proposed, where a semifolded "protobarrel" already containing the hairpin is formed in the periplasm. This is then inserted into the outer membrane by BamA. All three models lead to the autotransporter β-barrel being folded and inserted into the outer membrane and passenger secretion proceeding via a hairpin from the C- to the N-terminus (model 4). Note that BamA may also be involved in passenger secretion (see panel B). Small black arrows depict the direction of secretion; large light arrows depict the flow of events. The N-terminus of the autotransporter is denoted by an N for clarity. (B) Models of passenger secretion. Two models exist where passenger secretion is autonomous, i.e., genuine autotransport (models 1 and 2). In the threading model (model 1), the passenger is secreted through the pore of the autotransporter β-barrel (in dark gray) N-terminus first. The hairpin model (model 2) is preferred over this because it is more in line with current biochemical evidence (see text); here, the C-terminus of the passenger domain (the linker region) forms a hairpin within the pore of the autotransporter β-barrel. Secretion then proceeds C to N. In the third model of passenger secretion, a secondary protein (BamA or TamA, in light gray) assists in passenger secretion, possibly by forming a hybrid barrel with the autotransporter as depicted here. Small gray arrows depict the direction of secretion; the N-terminus of the autotransporter is denoted by an N for clarity.

showed that the C-terminal part of the passenger domain passes the autotransporter pore first (161). On top of this, the unusually long signal peptides observed in many type V–secreted proteins function as a retention signal at the Sec machinery, presumably to allow the passenger domain to initiate translocation—and possibly to initiate folding on the cell surface—prior to cleavage of the signal and release from the inner membrane (52). Taken together, all of this biochemical evidence strongly favors the hairpin over the threading model for type Va autotransport (Fig. 6).

Based on the fact that all type V translocation domains are homologous to the larger family of outer membrane β-barrel proteins (42), it is safe to assume that they follow the same route of outer membrane insertion, by interacting with the Bam complex. The question is whether the translocation pore—after membrane insertion—can autonomously transport the passenger or whether this process is also mediated by BamA (or TamA). While the hairpin model described above might still be valid (and seems proven at least for type Va systems), the direct interaction of autotransporters with different parts of the Bam complex has thus added a different level of complexity to the system. Current models of transport range from autotransport to the insertion of a hairpin intermediate by BamA to a complete process run by BamA (or its paralogue TamA), where a larger, fused pore is formed as an intermediate (Fig. 6).

In this context, it is interesting to look at type V systems other than just the well-studied type Va ones. The membrane insertion of the type Vb translocator protein requires the Bam complex (159), but at the same time, translocation of the passenger is independent of the Bam complex when the translocation pore is already present (158). On the one hand, this could suggest that the only requirement for type V secretion is a membrane-inserted pore, in line with a unifying model for autotransport in which the Bam complex inserts the pore, but the passenger translocation is an autonomous process. On the other hand, type Vb translocation pores themselves are very similar to BamA: they include POTRA domains, and they are 16-stranded barrels and thus have larger pores compared to the 12-stranded barrels of type Va or Ve systems. Some models suggest that the Bam complex creates a fused pore with the Va and Ve translocation domains to achieve a larger pore. But space is even more scarce in type Vc translocation domains, where three polypeptide chains need to be transported in parallel through the 12-stranded barrel. In these highly intertwined structures, it is hard to see how one or, alternatively, three Bam complexes could assemble the type Vc trimeric barrel after individual passenger transport of three such fused pores is completed.

The physical connection of the passenger domain with the translocation domain in Va systems might relieve the requirements for a molecular recognition event such as by the POTRA domains, which is essential in type Vb systems. But if this is true, what is the function of the POTRA domain present in type Vd secretion systems, which are in principle a fusion of a 16-stranded TpsB (the translocation pore), a POTRA linker, and a TpsA (passenger) domain?

There might be a unifying model that explains type V secretion. There seems to be no doubt that all systems (with the possible exception of type Vb or at least some of its variants [5]) use a hairpin intermediate to initiate translocation of the passenger domain and that the Bam complex (or its paralogue, the Tam complex) plays a role in membrane insertion of the translocation pore. An open question in the field of type V secretion is whether there are significant differences between the involvement of Bam or Tam in the biogenesis of the various subclasses and whether Bam or Tam are also directly involved in the later steps of passenger secretion.

CITATION

Fan E, Chauhan N, Gupta Udatha DBRK, Leo JC, Linke D. 2016. Type V secretion systems in bacteria. Microbiol Spectrum 4(1):VMBF-0009-2015.

REFERENCES

1. **Leo JC, Grin I, Linke D.** 2012. Type V secretion: mechanism(s) of autotransport through the bacterial outer membrane. *Philos Trans R Soc Lond B Biol Sci* **367**:1088–1101.

2. **Jose J, Jahnig F, Meyer TF.** 1995. Common structural features of IgA1 protease-like outer membrane protein autotransporters. *Mol Microbiol* **18**:378–380.

3. **Pohlner J, Halter R, Beyreuther K, Meyer TF.** 1987. Gene structure and extracellular secretion of *Neisseria gonorrhoeae* IgA protease. *Nature* **325**:458–462.

4. **Henderson IR, Navarro-Garcia F, Desvaux M, Fernandez RC, Ala'Aldeen D.** 2004. Type V protein secretion pathway: the autotransporter story. *Microbiol Mol Biol Rev* **68**:692–744.

5. **Jacob-Dubuisson F, Guerin J, Baelen S, Clantin B.** 2013. Two-partner secretion: as simple as it sounds? *Res Microbiol* **164**:583–595.

6. **Linke D, Riess T, Autenrieth IB, Lupas A, Kempf VA.** 2006. Trimeric autotransporter adhesins: variable structure, common function. *Trends Microbiol* **14**:264–270.

7. **Oberhettinger P, Schutz M, Leo JC, Heinz N, Berger J, Autenrieth IB, Linke D.** 2012. Intimin and invasin export their C-terminus to the bacterial cell surface using an inverse mechanism compared to classical autotransport. *PLoS One* **7**:e47069.

8. **Bateman A, Eddy SR, Chothia C.** 1996. Members of the immunoglobulin superfamily in bacteria. *Protein Sci* **5**:1939–1941.

9. **Bodelon G, Palomino C, Fernandez LA.** 2013. Immunoglobulin domains in *Escherichia coli* and other enterobacteria: from pathogenesis to applications in antibody technologies. *FEMS Microbiol Rev* **37**:204–250.

10. **Leo JC, Oberhettinger P, Chaubey M, Schutz M, Kuhner D, Bertsche U, Schwarz H, Gotz F, Autenrieth IB, Coles M, Linke D.** 2015. The intimin periplasmic domain mediates dimerisation and binding to peptidoglycan. *Mol Microbiol* **95**:80–100.

11. **Matsuda F, Tsugawa H, Fukusaki E.** 2013. Method for assessing the statistical significance of mass spectral similarities using basic local alignment search tool statistics. *Anal Chem* **85**:8291–8297.

12. **Mount DW.** 2007. Using the Basic Local Alignment Search Tool (BLAST). *CSH Protoc* **2007**:pdb.top17.

13. **Altschul SF, Gish W, Miller W, Myers EW, Lipman DJ.** 1990. Basic local alignment search tool. *J Mol Biol* **215**:403–410.

14. **Ulrich T, Oberhettinger P, Schutz M, Holzer K, Ramms AS, Linke D, Autenrieth IB, Rapaport D.** 2014. Evolutionary conservation in biogenesis of beta-barrel proteins allows mitochondria to assemble a functional bacterial trimeric autotransporter protein. *J Biol Chem* **289**:29457–29470.

15. **Grin I, Hartmann MD, Sauer G, Hernandez Alvarez B, Schutz M, Wagner S, Madlung J, Macek B, Felipe-Lopez A, Hensel M, Lupas A, Linke D.** 2014. A trimeric lipoprotein assists in trimeric autotransporter biogenesis in enterobacteria. *J Biol Chem* **289**:7388–7398.

16. **Hartmann MD, Grin I, Dunin-Horkawicz S, Deiss S, Linke D, Lupas AN, Hernandez Alvarez B.** 2012. Complete fiber structures of complex trimeric autotransporter adhesins conserved in enterobacteria. *Proc Natl Acad Sci USA* **109**:20907–20912.

17. **Shahid SA, Bardiaux B, Franks WT, Krabben L, Habeck M, van Rossum BJ, Linke D.** 2012. Membrane-protein structure determination by solid-state NMR spectroscopy of microcrystals. *Nat Methods* **9**:1212–1217.

18. **Kaiser PO, Linke D, Schwarz H, Leo JC, Kempf VA.** 2012. Analysis of the BadA stalk from *Bartonella henselae* reveals domain-specific and domain-overlapping functions in the host cell infection process. *Cell Microbiol* **14**:198–209.

19. **Celik N, Webb CT, Leyton DL, Holt KE, Heinz E, Gorrell R, Kwok T, Naderer T, Strugnell RA, Speed TP, Teasdale RD, Likic VA, Lithgow T.** 2012. A bioinformatic strategy for the detection, classification and analysis of bacterial autotransporters. *PLoS One* **7**:e43245. doi:10.1371/journal.pone.0043245.

20. **Leo JC, Lyskowski A, Hattula K, Hartmann MD, Schwarz H, Butcher SJ, Linke D, Lupas AN, Goldman A.** 2011. The structure of *E. coli* IgG-binding protein D suggests a general model for bending and binding in trimeric autotransporter adhesins. *Structure* **19**:1021–1030.

21. **Wagner C, Polke M, Gerlach RG, Linke D, Stierhof YD, Schwarz H, Hensel M.** 2011. Functional dissection of SiiE, a giant non-fimbrial adhesin of *Salmonella enterica*. *Cell Microbiol* **13**:1286–1301.

22. **O'Rourke F, Schmidgen T, Kaiser PO, Linke D, Kempf VA.** 2011. Adhesins of *Bartonella* spp. *Adv Exp Med Biol* **715**:51–70.

23. **Muller NF, Kaiser PO, Linke D, Schwarz H, Riess T, Schafer A, Eble JA, Kempf VA.** 2011. Trimeric autotransporter adhesin-dependent adherence of *Bartonella henselae*, *Bartonella quintana*, and *Yersinia enterocolitica* to matrix components and endothelial cells under static

and dynamic flow conditions. *Infect Immun* **79:**2544–2553.

24. **Muller JE, Papic D, Ulrich T, Grin I, Schutz M, Oberhettinger P, Tommassen J, Linke D, Dimmer KS, Autenrieth IB, Rapaport D.** 2011. Mitochondria can recognize and assemble fragments of a beta-barrel structure. *Mol Biol Cell* **22:**1638–1647.

25. **Lehr U, Schutz M, Oberhettinger P, Ruiz-Perez F, Donald JW, Palmer T, Linke D, Henderson IR, Autenrieth IB.** 2010. C-terminal amino acid residues of the trimeric autotransporter adhesin YadA of *Yersinia enterocolitica* are decisive for its recognition and assembly by BamA. *Mol Microbiol* **78:**932–946.

26. **Schutz M, Weiss EM, Schindler M, Hallstrom T, Zipfel PF, Linke D, Autenrieth IB.** 2010. Trimer stability of YadA is critical for virulence of *Yersinia enterocolitica. Infect Immun* **78:**2677–2690.

27. **Szczesny P, Linke D, Ursinus A, Bar K, Schwarz H, Riess TM, Kempf VA, Lupas AN, Martin J, Zeth K.** 2008. Structure of the head of the *Bartonella adhesin* BadA. *PLoS Pathog* **4:**e1000119. doi:10.1371/journal.ppat.1000119.

28. **Kaiser PO, Riess T, Wagner CL, Linke D, Lupas AN, Schwarz H, Raddatz G, Schafer A, Kempf VA.** 2008. The head of *Bartonella* adhesin A is crucial for host cell interaction of *Bartonella henselae. Cell Microbiol* **10:**2223–2234.

29. **Wagner CL, Riess T, Linke D, Eberhardt C, Schafer A, Reutter S, Maggi RG, Kempf VA.** 2008. Use of *Bartonella* adhesin A (BadA) immunoblotting in the serodiagnosis of *Bartonella henselae* infections. *Int J Med Microbiol* **298:**579–590.

30. **Hernandez Alvarez B, Hartmann MD, Albrecht R, Lupas AN, Zeth K, Linke D.** 2008. A new expression system for protein crystallization using trimeric coiled-coil adaptors. *Protein Eng Des Sel* **21:**11–18.

31. **Szczesny P, Lupas A.** 2008. Domain annotation of trimeric autotransporter adhesins: daTAA. *Bioinformatics* **24:**1251–1256.

32. **Grosskinsky U, Schutz M, Fritz M, Schmid Y, Lamparter MC, Szczesny P, Lupas AN, Autenrieth IB, Linke D.** 2007. A conserved glycine residue of trimeric autotransporter domains plays a key role in *Yersinia* adhesin A autotransport. *J Bacteriol* **189:**9011–9019.

33. **Riess T, Raddatz G, Linke D, Schafer A, Kempf VA.** 2007. Analysis of *Bartonella* adhesin A expression reveals differences between various *B. henselae* strains. *Infect Immun* **75:**35–43.

34. **Wollmann P, Zeth K, Lupas AN, Linke D.** 2006. Purification of the YadA membrane anchor for secondary structure analysis and crystallization. *Int J Biol Macromol* **39:**3–9.

35. **Tapader R, Chatterjee S, Singh AK, Dayma P, Haldar S, Pal A, Basu S.** 2014. The high prevalence of serine protease autotransporters of *Enterobacteriaceae* (SPATEs) in *Escherichia coli* causing neonatal septicemia. *Eur J Clin Microbiol Infect Dis* **33:**2015–2024.

36. **Zude I, Leimbach A, Dobrindt U.** 2014. Prevalence of autotransporters in *Escherichia coli:* what is the impact of phylogeny and pathotype? *Int J Med Microbiol* **304:**243–256.

37. **Sievers F, Higgins DG.** 2014. Clustal Omega, accurate alignment of very large numbers of sequences. *Methods Mol Biol* **1079:**105–116.

38. **Sievers F, Wilm A, Dineen D, Gibson TJ, Karplus K, Li W, Lopez R, McWilliam H, Remmert M, Soding J, Thompson JD, Higgins DG.** 2011. Fast, scalable generation of high-quality protein multiple sequence alignments using Clustal Omega. *Mol Syst Biol* **7:**539.

39. **Rost B.** 1999. Twilight zone of protein sequence alignments. *Protein Eng* **12:**85–94.

40. **Maurer J, Jose J, Meyer TF.** 1999. Characterization of the essential transport function of the AIDA-I autotransporter and evidence supporting structural predictions. *J Bacteriol* **181:**7014–7020.

41. **Cotter SE, Surana NK, St Geme JW 3rd.** 2005. Trimeric autotransporters: a distinct subfamily of autotransporter proteins. *Trends Microbiol* **13:**199–205.

42. **Remmert M, Biegert A, Linke D, Lupas AN, Soding J.** 2010. Evolution of outer membrane beta-barrels from an ancestral beta beta hairpin. *Mol Biol Evol* **27:**1348–1358.

43. **Remmert M, Linke D, Lupas AN, Soding J.** 2009. HHomp: prediction and classification of outer membrane proteins. *Nucleic Acids Res* **37:**W446–W451.

44. **Emanuelsson O, Brunak S, von Heijne G, Nielsen H.** 2007. Locating proteins in the cell using TargetP, SignalP and related tools. *Nature Protocols* **2:**953–971.

45. **Dautin N, Bernstein HD.** 2007. Protein secretion in Gram-negative bacteria via the autotransporter pathway. *Annu Rev Microbiol* **61:**89–112.

46. **von Heijne G.** 1985. Signal sequences: the limits of variation. *J Mol Biol* **184:**99–105.

47. **Desvaux M, Cooper LM, Filenko NA, Scott-Tucker A, Turner SM, Cole JA, Henderson IR.** 2006. The unusual extended signal peptide region of the type V secretion system is phylogenetically restricted. *FEMS Microbiol Lett* **264:**22–30.

48. **Leyton DL, de Luna M, Sevastsyanovich YR, Tveen Jensen K, Browning DF, Scott-Tucker A, Henderson IR.** 2010. The unusual extended signal peptide region is not required for secretion and function of an *Escherichia coli* autotransporter. *FEMS Microbiol Lett* **311:**133–139.

49. **Desvaux M, Scott-Tucker A, Turner SM, Cooper LM, Huber D, Nataro JP, Henderson IR.** 2007. A conserved extended signal peptide region directs posttranslational protein translocation via a novel mechanism. *Microbiology* **153:**59–70.

50. **Hiss JA, Resch E, Schreiner A, Meissner M, Starzinski-Powitz A, Schneider G.** 2008. Domain organization of long signal peptides of single-pass integral membrane proteins reveals multiple functional capacity. *PLoS One* **3:**e2767. doi:10.1371/journal.pone.0002767.

51. **Jiang X, Ruiz T, Mintz KP.** 2011. The extended signal peptide of the trimeric autotransporter EmaA of *Aggregatibacter actinomycetemcomitans* modulates secretion. *J Bacteriol* **193:**6983–6994.

52. **Szabady RL, Peterson JH, Skillman KM, Bernstein HD.** 2005. An unusual signal peptide facilitates late steps in the biogenesis of a bacterial autotransporter. *Proc Natl Acad Sci USA* **102:**221–226.

53. **Schmidt MA, Riley LW, Benz I.** 2003. Sweet new world: glycoproteins in bacterial pathogens. *Trends Microbiol* **11:**554–561.

54. **Reidl S, Lehmann A, Schiller R, Salam Khan A, Dobrindt U.** 2009. Impact of O-glycosylation on the molecular and cellular adhesion properties of the *Escherichia coli* autotransporter protein Ag43. *Int J Med Microbiol* **299:**389–401.

55. **Tang GY, Ruiz T, Mintz KP.** 2012. O-polysaccharide glycosylation is required for stability and function of the collagen adhesin EmaA of *Aggregatibacter actinomycetemcomitans*. *Infect Immun* **80:**2868–2877.

56. **Yao Q, Lu QH, Wan XB, Song F, Xu Y, Hu M, Zamyatina A, Liu XY, Huang N, Zhu P, Shao F.** 2014. A structural mechanism for bacterial autotransporter glycosylation by a dodecameric heptosyltransferase family. *Elife* **3:**e03714.

57. **Tang G, Mintz KP.** 2010. Glycosylation of the collagen adhesin EmaA of *Aggregatibacter actinomycetemcomitans* is dependent upon the lipopolysaccharide biosynthetic pathway. *J Bacteriol* **192:**1395–1404.

58. **Nishimura K, Tajima N, Yoon YH, Park SY, Tame JR.** 2010. Autotransporter passenger proteins: virulence factors with common structural themes. *J Mol Med (Berl)* **88:**451–458.

59. **Lyskowski A, Leo JC, Goldman A.** 2011. Structure and biology of trimeric autotransporter adhesins. *Adv Exp Med Biol* **715:**143–158.

60. **van den Berg B.** 2010. Crystal structure of a full-length autotransporter. *J Mol Biol* **396:**627–633.

61. **Koretke KK, Szczesny P, Gruber M, Lupas AN.** 2006. Model structure of the prototypical non-fimbrial adhesin YadA of *Yersinia enterocolitica*. *J Struct Biol* **155:**154–161.

62. **Kajava AV, Cheng N, Cleaver R, Kessel M, Simon MN, Willery E, Jacob-Dubuisson F, Locht C, Steven AC.** 2001. Beta-helix model for the filamentous haemagglutinin adhesin of *Bordetella pertussis* and related bacterial secretory proteins. *Mol Microbiol* **42:**279–292.

63. **Kelly G, Prasannan S, Daniell S, Fleming K, Frankel G, Dougan G, Connerton I, Matthews S.** 1999. Structure of the cell-adhesion fragment of intimin from enteropathogenic *Escherichia coli*. *Nat Struct Biol* **6:**313–318.

64. **Hoiczyk E, Roggenkamp A, Reichenbecher M, Lupas A, Heesemann J.** 2000. Structure and sequence analysis of *Yersinia* YadA and *Moraxella* UspAs reveal a novel class of adhesins. *EMBO J* **19:**5989–5999.

65. **Yu C, Mintz KP, Ruiz T.** 2009. Investigation of the three-dimensional architecture of the collagen adhesin EmaA of *Aggregatibacter actinomycetemcomitans* by electron tomography. *J Bacteriol* **191:**6253–6261.

66. **Conners R, Hill DJ, Borodina E, Agnew C, Daniell SJ, Burton NM, Sessions RB, Clarke AR, Catto LE, Lammie D, Wess T, Brady RL, Virji M.** 2008. The *Moraxella* adhesin UspA1 binds to its human CEACAM1 receptor by a deformable trimeric coiled-coil. *EMBO J* **27:**1779–1789.

67. **Agnew C, Borodina E, Zaccai NR, Conners R, Burton NM, Vicary JA, Cole DK, Antognozzi M, Virji M, Brady RL.** 2011. Correlation of *in situ* mechanosensitive responses of the *Moraxella catarrhalis* adhesin UspA1 with fibronectin and receptor CEACAM1 binding. *Proc Natl Acad Sci USA* **108:**15174–15178.

68. **Malito E, Biancucci M, Faleri A, Ferlenghi I, Scarselli M, Maruggi G, Lo Surdo P, Veggi D, Liguori A, Santini L, Bertoldi I, Petracca R, Marchi S, Romagnoli G, Cartocci E, Vercellino I, Savino S, Spraggon G, Norais N, Pizza M, Rappuoli R, Masignani V, Bottomley MJ.** 2014. Structure of the meningococcal vaccine antigen NadA and epitope mapping of a bactericidal antibody. *Proc Natl Acad Sci USA* **111:**17128–17133.

69. **Kajava AV, Steven AC.** 2006. The turn of the screw: variations of the abundant beta-

solenoid motif in passenger domains of type V secretory proteins. *J Struct Biol* **155**:306–315.

70. **Kajava AV, Steven AC.** 2006. Beta-rolls, beta-helices, and other beta-solenoid proteins. *Adv Protein Chem* **73**:55–96.

71. **Junker M, Schuster CC, McDonnell AV, Sorg KA, Finn MC, Berger B, Clark PL.** 2006. Pertactin beta-helix folding mechanism suggests common themes for the secretion and folding of autotransporter proteins. *Proc Natl Acad Sci USA* **103**:4918–4923.

72. **Hamburger ZA, Brown MS, Isberg RR, Bjorkman PJ.** 1999. Crystal structure of invasin: a bacterial integrin-binding protein. *Science* **286**:291–295.

73. **Nesta B, Spraggon G, Alteri C, Moriel DG, Rosini R, Veggi D, Smith S, Bertoldi I, Pastorello I, Ferlenghi I, Fontana MR, Frankel G, Mobley HL, Rappuoli R, Pizza M, Serino L, Soriani M.** 2012. FdeC, a novel broadly conserved *Escherichia coli* adhesin eliciting protection against urinary tract infections. *MBio* **3**:e00010-12. doi:10.1128/mBio.00010-12.

74. **Emsley P, Charles IG, Fairweather NF, Isaacs NW.** 1996. Structure of *Bordetella pertussis* virulence factor P.69 pertactin. *Nature* **381**:90–92.

75. **Otto BR, Sijbrandi R, Luirink J, Oudega B, Heddle JG, Mizutani K, Park SY, Tame JR.** 2005. Crystal structure of hemoglobin protease, a heme binding autotransporter protein from pathogenic *Escherichia coli*. *J Biol Chem* **280**:17339–17345.

76. **Heras B, Totsika M, Peters KM, Paxman JJ, Gee CL, Jarrott RJ, Perugini MA, Whitten AE, Schembri MA.** 2014. The antigen 43 structure reveals a molecular Velcro-like mechanism of autotransporter-mediated bacterial clumping. *Proc Natl Acad Sci USA* **111**:457–462.

77. **Meng G, Spahich N, Kenjale R, Waksman G, St Geme JW 3rd.** 2011. Crystal structure of the *Haemophilus influenzae* Hap adhesin reveals an intercellular oligomerization mechanism for bacterial aggregation. *EMBO J* **30**:3864–3874.

78. **Domingo Meza-Aguilar J, Fromme P, Torres-Larios A, Mendoza-Hernandez G, Hernandez-Chinas U, Arreguin-Espinosa de Los Monteros RA, Eslava Campos CA, Fromme R.** 2014. X-ray crystal structure of the passenger domain of plasmid encoded toxin(Pet), an autotransporter enterotoxin from enteroaggregative *Escherichia coli* (EAEC). *Biochem Biophys Res Commun* **445**:439–444.

79. **Khan S, Mian HS, Sandercock LE, Chirgadze NY, Pai EF.** 2011. Crystal structure of the passenger domain of the *Escherichia coli* autotransporter EspP. *J Mol Biol* **413**:985–1000.

80. **Gangwer KA, Mushrush DJ, Stauff DL, Spiller B, McClain MS, Cover TL, Lacy DB.** 2007. Crystal structure of the *Helicobacter pylori* vacuolating toxin p55 domain. *Proc Natl Acad Sci USA* **104**:16293–16298.

81. **Clantin B, Hodak H, Willery E, Locht C, Jacob-Dubuisson F, Villeret V.** 2004. The crystal structure of filamentous hemagglutinin secretion domain and its implications for the two-partner secretion pathway. *Proc Natl Acad Sci USA* **101**:6194–6199.

82. **Yeo HJ, Yokoyama T, Walkiewicz K, Kim Y, Grass S, Geme JW 3rd.** 2007. The structure of the *Haemophilus influenzae* HMW1 pro-piece reveals a structural domain essential for bacterial two-partner secretion. *J Biol Chem* **282**:31076–31084.

83. **Alvarez BH, Gruber M, Ursinus A, Dunin-Horkawicz S, Lupas AN, Zeth K.** 2010. A transition from strong right-handed to canonical left-handed supercoiling in a conserved coiled-coil segment of trimeric autotransporter adhesins. *J Struct Biol* **170**:236–245.

84. **Hartmann MD, Ridderbusch O, Zeth K, Albrecht R, Testa O, Woolfson DN, Sauer G, Dunin-Horkawicz S, Lupas AN, Alvarez BH.** 2009. A coiled-coil motif that sequesters ions to the hydrophobic core. *Proc Natl Acad Sci USA* **106**:16950–16955.

85. **Nummelin H, Merckel MC, Leo JC, Lankinen H, Skurnik M, Goldman A.** 2004. The *Yersinia* adhesin YadA collagen-binding domain structure is a novel left-handed parallel beta-roll. *EMBO J* **23**:701–711.

86. **Meng G, St Geme JW 3rd, Waksman G.** 2008. Repetitive architecture of the *Haemophilus influenzae* Hia trimeric autotransporter. *J Mol Biol* **384**:824–836.

87. **Edwards TE, Phan I, Abendroth J, Dieterich SH, Masoudi A, Guo W, Hewitt SN, Kelley A, Leibly D, Brittnacher MJ, Staker BL, Miller SI, Van Voorhis WC, Myler PJ, Stewart LJ.** 2010. Structure of a *Burkholderia pseudomallei* trimeric autotransporter adhesin head. *PLoS One* **5**:e12803. doi:10.1371/journal.pone.0012803.

88. **Yeo HJ, Cotter SE, Laarmann S, Juehne T, St Geme JW 3rd, Waksman G.** 2004. Structural basis for host recognition by the *Haemophilus influenzae* Hia autotransporter. *EMBO J* **23**:1245–1256.

89. **Barnard TJ, Dautin N, Lukacik P, Bernstein HD, Buchanan SK.** 2007. Autotransporter structure reveals intra-barrel cleavage followed by conformational changes. *Nat Struct Mol Biol* **14**:1214–1220.

90. **Fairman JW, Dautin N, Wojtowicz D, Liu W, Noinaj N, Barnard TJ, Udho E, Przytycka TM, Cherezov V, Buchanan SK.** 2012. Crystal structures of the outer membrane domain of intimin and invasin from enterohemorrhagic *E. coli* and enteropathogenic *Y. pseudotuberculosis. Structure* **20:**1233–1243.

91. **Meng G, Surana NK, St Geme JW 3rd, Waksman G.** 2006. Structure of the outer membrane translocator domain of the *Haemophilus influenzae* Hia trimeric autotransporter. *EMBO J* **25:**2297–2304.

92. **Oomen CJ, van Ulsen P, van Gelder P, Feijen M, Tommassen J, Gros P.** 2004. Structure of the translocator domain of a bacterial autotransporter. *EMBO J* **23:**1257–1266.

93. **Gawarzewski I, DiMaio F, Winterer E, Tschapek B, Smits SH, Jose J, Schmitt L.** 2014. Crystal structure of the transport unit of the autotransporter adhesin involved in diffuse adherence from *Escherichia coli. J Struct Biol* **187:**20–29.

94. **Shahid SA, Markovic S, Linke D, van Rossum BJ.** 2012. Assignment and secondary structure of the YadA membrane protein by solid-state MAS NMR. *Sci Rep* **2:**803.

95. **Clantin B, Delattre AS, Rucktooa P, Saint N, Meli AC, Locht C, Jacob-Dubuisson F, Villeret V.** 2007. Structure of the membrane protein FhaC: a member of the Omp85-TpsB transporter superfamily. *Science* **317:**957–961.

96. **Meli AC, Hodak H, Clantin B, Locht C, Molle G, Jacob-Dubuisson F, Saint N.** 2006. Channel properties of TpsB transporter FhaC point to two functional domains with a C-terminal protein-conducting pore. *J Biol Chem* **281:**158–166.

97. **Guerin J, Baud C, Touati N, Saint N, Willery E, Locht C, Vezin H, Jacob-Dubuisson F.** 2014. Conformational dynamics of protein transporter FhaC: large-scale motions of plug helix. *Mol Microbiol* **92:**1164–1176.

98. **Salacha R, Kovacic F, Brochier-Armanet C, Wilhelm S, Tommassen J, Filloux A, Voulhoux R, Bleves S.** 2010. The *Pseudomonas aeruginosa* patatin-like protein PlpD is the archetype of a novel type V secretion system. *Environ Microbiol* **12:**1498–1512.

99. **Knowles TJ, Scott-Tucker A, Overduin M, Henderson IR.** 2009. Membrane protein architects: the role of the BAM complex in outer membrane protein assembly. *Nat Rev Microbiol* **7:**206–214.

100. **Voulhoux R, Bos MP, Geurtsen J, Mols M, Tommassen J.** 2003. Role of a highly conserved bacterial protein in outer membrane protein assembly. *Science* **299:**262–265.

101. **Jain S, Goldberg MB.** 2007. Requirement for YaeT in the outer membrane assembly of autotransporter proteins. *J Bacteriol* **189:**5393–5398.

102. **Ieva R, Bernstein HD.** 2009. Interaction of an autotransporter passenger domain with BamA during its translocation across the bacterial outer membrane. *Proc Natl Acad Sci USA* **106:**19120–19125.

103. **Bodelon G, Marin E, Fernandez LA.** 2009. Role of periplasmic chaperones and BamA (YaeT/Omp85) in folding and secretion of intimin from enteropathogenic *Escherichia coli* strains. *J Bacteriol* **191:**5169–5179.

104. **Roman-Hernandez G, Peterson JH, Bernstein HD.** 2014. Reconstitution of bacterial autotransporter assembly using purified components. *Elife* **3:**e04234.

105. **Oberhettinger P, Leo JC, Linke D, Autenrieth IB, Schutz MS.** 2015. The inverse autotransporter intimin exports its passenger domain via a hairpin intermediate. *J Biol Chem* **290:**1837–1849.

106. **Noinaj N, Kuszak AJ, Gumbart JC, Lukacik P, Chang H, Easley NC, Lithgow T, Buchanan SK.** 2013. Structural insight into the biogenesis of beta-barrel membrane proteins. *Nature* **501:**385–390.

107. **Ni D, Wang Y, Yang X, Zhou H, Hou X, Cao B, Lu Z, Zhao X, Yang K, Huang Y.** 2014. Structural and functional analysis of the beta-barrel domain of BamA from *Escherichia coli. FASEB J* **28:**2677–2685.

108. **Albrecht R, Schutz M, Oberhettinger P, Faulstich M, Bermejo I, Rudel T, Diederichs K, Zeth K.** 2014. Structure of BamA, an essential factor in outer membrane protein biogenesis. *Acta Crystallogr D Biol Crystallogr* **70:**1779–1789.

109. **van den Berg B.** 2013. Lateral gates: beta-barrels get in on the act. *Nat Struct Mol Biol* **20:**1237–1239.

110. **Selkrig J, Mosbahi K, Webb CT, Belousoff MJ, Perry AJ, Wells TJ, Morris F, Leyton DL, Totsika M, Phan MD, Celik N, Kelly M, Oates C, Hartland EL, Robins-Browne RM, Ramarathinam SH, Purcell AW, Schembri MA, Strugnell RA, Henderson IR, Walker D, Lithgow T.** 2012. Discovery of an archetypal protein transport system in bacterial outer membranes. *Nat Struct Mol Biol* **19:**506–510, S501.

111. **Gruss F, Zahringer F, Jakob RP, Burmann BM, Hiller S, Maier T.** 2013. The structural basis of autotransporter translocation by TamA. *Nat Struct Mol Biol* **20:**1318–1320.

112. **Tsai JC, Yen MR, Castillo R, Leyton DL, Henderson IR, Saier MH Jr.** 2011. The bacterial intimins and invasins: a large and

novel family of secreted proteins. *PLoS One* **5:** e14403.

113. **Kim S, Malinverni JC, Sliz P, Silhavy TJ, Harrison SC, Kahne D.** 2007. Structure and function of an essential component of the outer membrane protein assembly machine. *Science* **317:**961–964.

114. **Arnold T, Zeth K, Linke D.** 2010. Omp85 from the thermophilic cyanobacterium *Thermosynechococcus elongatus* differs from proteobacterial Omp85 in structure and domain composition. *J Biol Chem* **285:**18003–18015.

115. **Knowles TJ, Jeeves M, Bobat S, Dancea F, McClelland D, Palmer T, Overduin M, Henderson IR.** 2008. Fold and function of polypeptide transport-associated domains responsible for delivering unfolded proteins to membranes. *Mol Microbiol* **68:**1216–1227.

116. **Delattre AS, Saint N, Clantin B, Willery E, Lippens G, Locht C, Villeret V, Jacob-Dubuisson F.** 2011. Substrate recognition by the POTRA domains of TpsB transporter FhaC. *Mol Microbiol* **81:**99–112.

117. **Alsteens D, Martinez N, Jamin M, Jacob-Dubuisson F.** 2013. Sequential unfolding of beta helical protein by single-molecule atomic force microscopy. *PLoS One* **8:**e73572. doi:10.1371/journal.pone.0073572.

118. **Campos CG, Borst L, Cotter PA.** 2013. Characterization of BcaA, a putative classical autotransporter protein in *Burkholderia pseudomallei*. *Infect Immun* **81:**1121–1128.

119. **Manoil C, Beckwith J.** 1985. TnphoA: a transposon probe for protein export signals. *Proc Natl Acad Sci USA* **82:**8129–8133.

120. **Patel SK, Dotson J, Allen KP, Fleckenstein JM.** 2004. Identification and molecular characterization of EatA, an autotransporter protein of enterotoxigenic *Escherichia coli*. *Infect Immun* **72:**1786–1794.

121. **Coppenhagen-Glazer S, Sol A, Abed J, Naor R, Zhang X, Han YW, Bachrach G.** 2015. Fap2 of *Fusobacterium nucleatum* is a galactose inhibitable adhesin, involved in coaggregation, cell adhesion and preterm birth. *Infect Immun* **83:**1104–1113.

122. **Faure LM, Garvis S, de Bentzmann S, Bigot S.** 2014. Characterization of a novel two-partner secretion system implicated in the virulence of *Pseudomonas aeruginosa*. *Microbiology* **160:** 1940–1952.

123. **Plamondon P, Luke NR, Campagnari AA.** 2007. Identification of a novel two-partner secretion locus in *Moraxella catarrhalis*. *Infect Immun* **75:**2929–2936.

124. **Wang YP, Hsieh MK, Tan DH, Shien JH, Ou SC, Chen CF, Chang PC.** 2014. The haemagglutinin of *Avibacterium paragallinarum* is a trimeric autotransporter adhesin that confers haemagglutination, cell adherence and biofilm formation activities. *Vet Microbiol* **174:**474–482.

125. **Zhou P, Liu J, Merritt J, Qi F.** 2014. A YadA-like autotransporter, Hag1 in *Veillonella atypica* is a multivalent hemagglutinin involved in adherence to oral streptococci, *Porphyromonas gingivalis*, and human oral buccal cells. *Mol Oral Microbiol* doi:10.1111/omi.12091.

126. **Louie M, de Azavedo JC, Handelsman MY, Clark CG, Ally B, Dytoc M, Sherman P, Brunton J.** 1993. Expression and characterization of the eaeA gene product of *Escherichia coli* serotype O157:H7. *Infect Immun* **61:**4085–4092.

127. **Rutherford N, Mourez M.** 2006. Surface display of proteins by Gram-negative bacterial autotransporters. *Microb Cell Fact* **5:**22.

128. **Wentzel A, Christmann A, Adams T, Kolmar H.** 2001. Display of passenger proteins on the surface of *Escherichia coli* K-12 by the enterohemorrhagic *E. coli* intimin EaeA. *J Bacteriol* **183:**7273–7284.

129. **Adams TM, Wentzel A, Kolmar H.** 2005. Intimin-mediated export of passenger proteins requires maintenance of a translocation-competent conformation. *J Bacteriol* **187:** 522–533.

130. **Klauser T, Pohlner J, Meyer TF.** 1990. Extracellular transport of cholera toxin B subunit using *Neisseria* IgA protease beta-domain: conformation-dependent outer membrane translocation. *EMBO J* **9:**1991–1999.

131. **Sevastsyanovich YR, Leyton DL, Wells TJ, Wardius CA, Tveen-Jensen K, Morris FC, Knowles TJ, Cunningham AF, Cole JA, Henderson IR.** 2012. A generalised module for the selective extracellular accumulation of recombinant proteins. *Microb Cell Fact* **11:**69.

132. **Jong WS, ten Hagen-Jongman CM, den Blaauwen T, Slotboom DJ, Tame JR, Wickstrom D, de Gier JW, Otto BR, Luirink J.** 2007. Limited tolerance towards folded elements during secretion of the autotransporter Hbp. *Mol Microbiol* **63:**1524–1536.

133. **Schmidgen T, Kaiser PO, Ballhorn W, Franz B, Gottig S, Linke D, Kempf VA.** 2014. Heterologous expression of *Bartonella* Adhesin A in *Escherichia coli* by exchange of trimeric autotransporter adhesin domains results in enhanced adhesion properties and a pathogenic phenotype. *J Bacteriol* **196:**2155–2165.

134. **Ackermann N, Tiller M, Anding G, Roggenkamp A, Heesemann J.** 2008. Contribution of trimeric

autotransporter C-terminal domains of oligomeric coiled-coil adhesin (Oca) family members YadA, UspA1, EibA, and Hia to translocation of the YadA passenger domain and virulence of *Yersinia enterocolitica*. *J Bacteriol* **190**:5031–5043.

135. **Mikula KM, Leo JC, Lyskowski A, Kedracka-Krok S, Pirog A, Goldman A.** 2012. The translocation domain in trimeric autotransporter adhesins is necessary and sufficient for trimerization and autotransportation. *J Bacteriol* **194**:827–838.

136. **Jong WS, Soprova Z, de Punder K, ten Hagen-Jongman CM, Wagner S, Wickstrom D, de Gier JW, Andersen P, van der Wel NN, Luirink J.** 2012. A structurally informed autotransporter platform for efficient heterologous protein secretion and display. *Microb Cell Fact* **11**:85.

137. **Lum M, Morona R.** 2012. IcsA autotransporter passenger promotes increased fusion protein expression on the cell surface. *Microb Cell Fact* **11**:20.

138. **Liu H, Magoun L, Luperchio S, Schauer DB, Leong JM.** 1999. The Tir-binding region of enterohaemorrhagic *Escherichia coli* intimin is sufficient to trigger actin condensation after bacterial-induced host cell signalling. *Mol Microbiol* **34**:67–81.

139. **Kjaergaard K, Hasman H, Schembri MA, Klemm P.** 2002. Antigen 43-mediated autotransporter display, a versatile bacterial cell surface presentation system. *J Bacteriol* **184**:4197–4204.

140. **Veiga E, de Lorenzo V, Fernandez LA.** 2003. Autotransporters as scaffolds for novel bacterial adhesins: surface properties of *Escherichia coli* cells displaying Jun/Fos dimerization domains. *J Bacteriol* **185**:5585–5590.

141. **McKnight SL, Kingsbury R.** 1982. Transcriptional control signals of a eukaryotic protein-coding gene. *Science* **217**:316–324.

142. **Dutta PR, Sui BQ, Nataro JP.** 2003. Structure-function analysis of the enteroaggregative *Escherichia coli* plasmid-encoded toxin autotransporter using scanning linker mutagenesis. *J Biol Chem* **278**:39912–39920.

143. **May KL, Morona R.** 2008. Mutagenesis of the *Shigella flexneri* autotransporter IcsA reveals novel functional regions involved in IcsA biogenesis and recruitment of host neural Wiscott-Aldrich syndrome protein. *J Bacteriol* **190**:4666–4676.

144. **Leyton DL, Sevastsyanovich YR, Browning DF, Rossiter AE, Wells TJ, Fitzpatrick RE, Overduin M, Cunningham AF, Henderson IR.** 2011. Size and conformation limits to secretion of disulfide-bonded loops in auto-transporter proteins. *J Biol Chem* **286**:42283–42291.

145. **Peterson JH, Tian P, Ieva R, Dautin N, Bernstein HD.** 2010. Secretion of a bacterial virulence factor is driven by the folding of a C-terminal segment. *Proc Natl Acad Sci USA* **107**:17739–17744.

146. **Kang'ethe W, Bernstein HD.** 2013. Stepwise folding of an autotransporter passenger domain is not essential for its secretion. *J Biol Chem* **288**:35028–35038.

147. **Yen YT, Tsang C, Cameron TA, Ankrah DO, Rodou A, Stathopoulos C.** 2010. Importance of conserved residues of the serine protease autotransporter beta-domain in passenger domain processing and beta-barrel assembly. *Infect Immun* **78**:3516–3528.

148. **Ieva R, Skillman KM, Bernstein HD.** 2008. Incorporation of a polypeptide segment into the beta-domain pore during the assembly of a bacterial autotransporter. *Mol Microbiol* **67**:188–201.

149. **Leyton DL, Johnson MD, Thapa R, Huysmans GH, Dunstan RA, Celik N, Shen HH, Loo D, Belousoff MJ, Purcell AW, Henderson IR, Beddoe T, Rossjohn J, Martin LL, Strugnell RA, Lithgow T.** 2014. A mortise-tenon joint in the transmembrane domain modulates autotransporter assembly into bacterial outer membranes. *Nat Commun* **5**:4239.

150. **Zhai Y, Zhang K, Huo Y, Zhu Y, Zhou Q, Lu J, Black I, Pang X, Roszak AW, Zhang X, Isaacs NW, Sun F.** 2011. Autotransporter passenger domain secretion requires a hydrophobic cavity at the extracellular entrance of the beta-domain pore. *Biochem J* **435**:577–587.

151. **Rizzitello AE, Harper JR, Silhavy TJ.** 2001. Genetic evidence for parallel pathways of chaperone activity in the periplasm of *Escherichia coli*. *J Bacteriol* **183**:6794–6800.

152. **Sklar JG, Wu T, Kahne D, Silhavy TJ.** 2007. Defining the roles of the periplasmic chaperones SurA, Skp, and DegP in *Escherichia coli*. *Genes Dev* **21**:2473–2484.

153. **Purdy GE, Fisher CR, Payne SM.** 2007. IcsA surface presentation in *Shigella flexneri* requires the periplasmic chaperones DegP, Skp, and SurA. *J Bacteriol* **189**:5566–5573.

154. **Ruiz-Perez F, Henderson IR, Leyton DL, Rossiter AE, Zhang Y, Nataro JP.** 2009. Roles of periplasmic chaperone proteins in the biogenesis of serine protease autotransporters of *Enterobacteriaceae*. *J Bacteriol* **191**:6571–6583.

155. **Mogensen JE, Kleinschmidt JH, Schmidt MA, Otzen DE.** 2005. Misfolding of a bacterial autotransporter. *Protein Sci* **14**:2814–2827.

156. **Wagner JK, Heindl JE, Gray AN, Jain S, Goldberg MB.** 2009. Contribution of the periplasmic chaperone Skp to efficient presentation of the autotransporter IcsA on the surface of *Shigella flexneri*. *J Bacteriol* **191:**815–821.

157. **Shen HH, Lithgow T, Martin L.** 2013. Reconstitution of membrane proteins into model membranes: seeking better ways to retain protein activities. *Int J Mol Sci* **14:**1589–1607.

158. **Fan E, Fiedler S, Jacob-Dubuisson F, Muller M.** 2012. Two-partner secretion of Gram-negative bacteria: a single beta-barrel protein enables transport across the outer membrane. *J Biol Chem* **287:**2591–2599.

159. **Norell D, Heuck A, Tran-Thi TA, Gotzke H, Jacob-Dubuisson F, Clausen T, Daley DO, Braun V, Muller M, Fan E.** 2014. Versatile *in vitro* system to study translocation and functional integration of bacterial outer membrane proteins. *Nat Commun* **5:**5396.

160. **Shen HH, Leyton DL, Shiota T, Belousoff MJ, Noinaj N, Lu J, Holt SA, Tan K, Selkrig J, Webb CT, Buchanan SK, Martin LL, Lithgow T.** 2014. Reconstitution of a nanomachine driving the assembly of proteins into bacterial outer membranes. *Nat Commun* **5:**5078.

161. **Junker M, Besingi RN, Clark PL.** 2009. Vectorial transport and folding of an autotransporter virulence protein during outer membrane secretion. *Mol Microbiol* **71:**1323–1332.

162. **Skillman KM, Barnard TJ, Peterson JH, Ghirlando R, Bernstein HD.** 2005. Efficient secretion of a folded protein domain by a monomeric bacterial autotransporter. *Mol Microbiol* **58:**945–958.

163. **Jacob-Dubuisson F, El-Hamel C, Saint N, Guedin S, Willery E, Molle G, Locht C.** 1999. Channel formation by FhaC, the outer membrane protein involved in the secretion of the *Bordetella pertussis* filamentous hemagglutinin. *J Biol Chem* **274:**37731–37735.

164. **Surana NK, Buscher AZ, Hardy GG, Grass S, Kehl-Fie T, St Geme JW 3rd.** 2006. Translocator proteins in the two-partner secretion family have multiple domains. *J Biol Chem* **281:**18051–18058.

165. **Duret G, Szymanski M, Choi KJ, Yeo HJ, Delcour AH.** 2008. The TpsB translocator HMW1B of *haemophilus influenzae* forms a large conductance channel. *J Biol Chem* **283:**15771–15778.

166. **Roussel-Jazede V, Van Gelder P, Sijbrandi R, Rutten L, Otto BR, Luirink J, Gros P, Tommassen J, Van Ulsen P.** 2011. Channel properties of the translocator domain of the autotransporter Hbp of *Escherichia coli*. *Mol Membr Biol* **28:**158–170.

167. **Veiga E, Sugawara E, Nikaido H, de Lorenzo V, Fernandez LA.** 2002. Export of autotransported proteins proceeds through an oligomeric ring shaped by C-terminal domains. *EMBO J* **21:**2122–2131.

168. **Arnold T, Poynor M, Nussberger S, Lupas AN, Linke D.** 2007. Gene duplication of the eight-stranded beta-barrel OmpX produces a functional pore: a scenario for the evolution of transmembrane beta-barrels. *J Mol Biol* **366:**1174–1184.

169. **Bos MP, Robert V, Tommassen J.** 2007. Biogenesis of the Gram-negative bacterial outer membrane. *Annu Rev Microbiol* **61:**191–214.

170. **Walther DM, Rapaport D, Tommassen J.** 2009. Biogenesis of beta-barrel membrane proteins in bacteria and eukaryotes: evolutionary conservation and divergence. *Cell Mol Life Sci* **66:**2789–2804.

171. **Junker M, Clark PL.** 2010. Slow formation of aggregation-resistant beta-sheet folding intermediates. *Proteins* **78:**812–824.

172. **Kang'ethe W, Bernstein HD.** 2013. Charge-dependent secretion of an intrinsically disordered protein via the autotransporter pathway. *Proc Natl Acad Sci USA* **110:**E4246–E4255.

173. **Soprova Z, Sauri A, van Ulsen P, Tame JR, den Blaauwen T, Jong WS, Luirink J.** 2010. A conserved aromatic residue in the autochaperone domain of the autotransporter Hbp is critical for initiation of outer membrane translocation. *J Biol Chem* **285:**38224–38233.

174. **Oliver DC, Huang G, Fernandez RC.** 2003. Identification of secretion determinants of the *Bordetella pertussis* BrkA autotransporter. *J Bacteriol* **185:**489–495.

175. **Drobnak I, Braselmann E, Chaney JL, Leyton DL, Bernstein HD, Lithgow T, Luirink J, Nataro JP, Clark PL.** 2015. Of linkers and autochaperones: an unambiguous nomenclature to identify common and uncommon themes for autotransporter secretion. *Mol Microbiol* **95:**1–16.

The Versatile Type VI Secretion System

12

CHRISTOPHER J. ALTERI[1] and HARRY L.T. MOBLEY[1]

INTRODUCTION

The type VI secretion system (T6SS), a Gram-negative secretion pathway (1, 2), delivers effectors upon direct contact with a target cell (3, 4). Death of the target cell is the primary outcome that follows the delivery of the lethal effectors, which are translocated from the attacker cell cytoplasm into the periplasm of the target cell via a T6S apparatus in a contact-dependent process (5, 6). It is well known that bacteria release bactericidal agents such as bacteriocins and antibiotics into the extracellular environment as a means to indiscriminately eliminate bacterial competitors (7). In addition, it is now understood that many Gram-negative bacteria also use the T6SS to directly antagonize bacteria in close proximity (5). Direct antagonism of neighboring cells can provide a selective advantage for bacteria in their natural habitat in dense biofilm communities or during a multicellular lifestyle that requires direct contact and cooperation (8, 9). As a consequence, bacteria benefit from a specific mechanism that depends on cell–cell contact to discriminate between one another and eliminate nonself bacteria, potential cheaters, or competitors from the population. In particular, lethal action of the T6

[1]Department of Microbiology and Immunology, University of Michigan Medical School, Ann Arbor, MI 48109.
Virulence Mechanisms of Bacterial Pathogens, 5th edition
Edited by Indira T. Kudva, Nancy A. Cornick, Paul J. Plummer, Qijing Zhang, Tracy L. Nicholson, John P. Bannantine, and Bryan H. Bellaire
© 2016 American Society for Microbiology, Washington, DC
doi:10.1128/microbiolspec.VMBF-0026-2015

contractile puncturing device provides a specific advantage for bacteria that possess the T6SS to discriminate, recognize, and kill competitors.

Many secretion systems that function to translocate proteins are present in Gram-negative bacteria. The T6SS is the most recently identified secretion system; the gene clusters that encode the system were named the T6SS following a genetic screen in *Vibrio cholerae* (2). Interestingly, genes or proteins that belong to or are dependent on the T6SS had been previously identified, mainly as virulence (or symbiosis) factors (10–13). In *Rhizobium leguminosarum*, a gene cluster later to be appreciated as encoding a T6SS was identified that played a role in symbiosis and was required for protein secretion (11). A proteomics study examining secreted proteins of *Edwardsiella tarda* also identified a large conserved gene cluster with noted similarity to the one identified in *R. leguminosarum* that was proposed to encode a novel protein secretion system (13). The widespread presence of T6SS genes was also noted prior to functional classification and discovery of the actual T6SS machinery (14–16). The T6SS has now been studied extensively in numerous organisms. Here, we consider much of what has been well characterized since the T6SS was discovered nearly a decade ago.

T6SS STRUCTURAL COMPONENTS

Hcp and VgrG

The first discovered and most studied components of the T6SS are Hcp and VgrG (2), which are both secreted and required for T6SS activity (1, 2). These two components comprise the hollow tube and puncturing tip that is delivered by the action of the T6SS. Bioinformatics analysis (3) and structural analysis show that VgrG is an excellent match with the cell-puncturing T4 bacteriophage tail spike (17). This structural study provides compelling evidence that Hcp and VgrG assemble to form a membrane-puncturing device. While direct evidence that VgrG is indeed the puncturing tip is lacking, work on Hcp has demonstrated that it forms a tube made of hexameric "stacked rings" (1, 18). Additional studies have predicted that the Hcp tube would form a complex with a trimeric VgrG tip (17, 19, 20). It is now apparent that the T6SS functions in a manner analogous to an inverted phage tail and tube (21).

VipA and VipB

As predicted, the T6SS is known to contain proteins that assemble to form a sheath structure. The sheath proteins, VipA and VipB (or TssBC), have been shown to form tube structures or polysheaths (22, 23). It was also noted that the VipA and VipB polysheaths appeared to disassemble, an event dependent on ClpV-mediated ATP hydrolysis (22). The appearance of these tubules is remarkably consistent with T4 phage tail sheaths and suggests a common molecular mechanism between bacteriophage and T6SS function (24–26). When the bacteriophage tail or a T6SS make contact with target cells, contraction of the respective sheath delivers a puncturing device that facilitates delivery of phage DNA or T6SS effectors, respectively (Fig. 1). The contraction event is presumed to coincide with effector secretion into target cells (27–30).

Effector Delivery Module

The structure of the contractile sheath of the T6SS has been particularly well characterized. Cryo-electron microscopy and reconstruction of contracted VipA/B tubules have shown that the tubule is constructed of six protofilaments arranged in a right-handed helical arrangement (31). This symmetry has been described as an assembly of stacked hexameric rings analogous to the T4 tail sheath (31–33). An insightful result from these structural studies has shown that the ClpV recognition motif of VipB is buried in the protofilament of the elongated sheath and becomes exposed in the contracted sheath structure (31, 33). This distinct outer layer of the T6SS sheath is a key difference from the architecture of the bacteriophage tail sheath and facilitates interactions with the ClpV ATPase, which enables multiple rounds of sheath extension and contraction via a contraction-state-specific recycling mechanism (31, 33). This ability of the T6SS sheath to be reused is in contrast to the bacteriophage tail sheath, which can be contracted only once. In support of this, T6SS sheath recycling and activity have been visualized in real time using fluorescent reporters fused to VipA (Fig. 2) (8, 29). Collectively, evidence has led to a parallel assembly pathway between T6SS and bacteriophage morphogenesis. A proposed mechanism to form the T6SS effector delivery module is that VgrG attracts Hcp, which forms a hollow inner tube of stacked hexamers, and Hcp tube formation then recruits and facilitates assembly of the outer tubule sheath structure (34).

Envelope-Spanning Complex

The phage-like T6SS tail or effector delivery module is anchored to the cell membrane by a trans envelope complex (35). These additional structural components of the T6SS are TssL, TssM, and TssJ, which form the envelope-spanning complex (36, 37). The minimal core set of conserved membrane proteins required for T6SS function are the inner membrane proteins TssL and TssM as well as the outer membrane lipoprotein TssJ (35–38). These proteins are connected by interactions between TssM and TssL and between TssM and TssJ (35, 36, 39, 40). This envelope-spanning complex has been shown to be assembled by the sequential addition of the three subunits, TssJ, TssM, and TssL (41). The structure of the fully assembled envelope complex was determined by

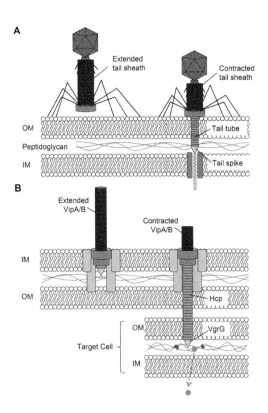

FIGURE 1 **Comparison of bacteriophage and the T6SS. (A) Bacteriophage possess tail fibers that attach to lipopolysaccharides of target bacterial cells. During reversible binding, the tail fibers bring the base plate in contact with the cell surface. Once in contact, irreversible binding is initiated, the tail sheath contracts and the rigid tail tube and spike are forced though the outer membrane (OM), proteins of the spike degrade the peptidoglycan, and final interaction with the inner membrane (IM) initiates translocation of viral DNA into the cell. (B) The T6SS functions much like a bacteriophage with several proteins being structurally similar, depicted here in the same color. Formation of the T6SS base plate complex, which spans the IM, peptidoglycan, and OM, initiates Hcp tube polymerization and sheath formation of VipA and VipB heterodimers. Upon contact with a target bacterial cell, this "ready to fire" state is triggered, causing the sheath to contract and the Hcp tube and VgrG spike to deploy into the target cell. Effector proteins are delivered into the periplasm, possibly degrading peptidoglycan for cytoplasmic effectors to gain further access into the cell. OM, outer membrane; IM, inner membrane.**

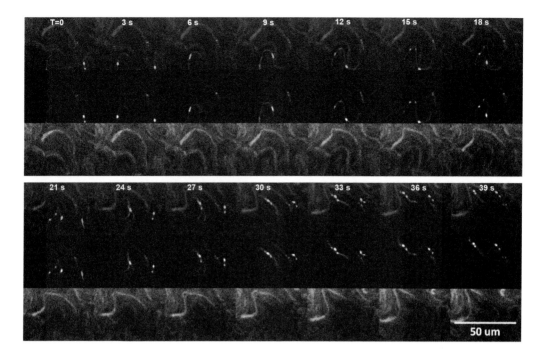

FIGURE 2 Infiltration of resistant and sensitive opposing swarms by *Proteus mirabilis* HI4320 expressing VipA::sfGFP. Agar plate inoculated with *P. mirabilis* HI4320 VipA::sfGFP opposing strains HI4320 or mutant 9C1 (mutation in immunity protein PefE) expressing dsRED. Infiltrating *P. mirabilis* HI4320 expressing VipA::sfGFP opposing strains HI4320 or mutant 9C1 expressing dsRED. Elapsed time (T) is indicated in seconds. Reprinted from reference 8, with permission.

negative-stain electron microscopy and was shown to form a large base in the cytoplasm (41). The envelope-spanning complex was also observed to extend into the periplasm to form a double ring structure containing the carboxy-terminal domain of TssM and TssJ, which is anchored in the outer membrane (41). This structural study of the T6SS envelope complex suggests that conformational changes allow passage of the puncturing device made of the Hcp tube and VgrG spike through a transient pore in the outer membrane (41). Additionally, the cytoplasmic protein TssK has been shown to interact with Hcp, TssL, and TssC and is proposed to link the sheath-Hcp-VgrG complex to the envelope-spanning complex (42). Thus, it is not unreasonable that the assembled effector delivery module interacts with the membrane-spanning complex via TssK.

T6SS EFFECTORS

The delivery module of the T6SS can translocate a diversity of protein effectors into the target cell. It is notable that the core T6SS genes, which encode structural components, are highly conserved across bacterial species (Fig. 3), in contrast to the clear diversity among effectors identified from these same organisms. These T6SS effectors have been identified using a number of techniques, and the toxic activities for many of the identified effectors have been biochemically characterized. T6SS effectors include VgrG, PAAR (proline alanine alanine arginine) domain–containing proteins that associate with VgrG, Rhs repeat proteins, and effector proteins that may be delivered within the hollow Hcp inner tube. The known and suspected activities of T6SS effectors include

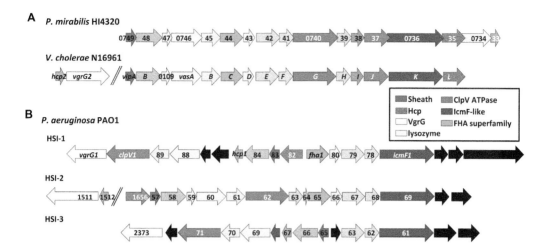

FIGURE 3 **Conservation of the T6SS effector operons among** *Proteus mirabilis, Vibrio cholerae,* **and** *Pseudomonas aeruginosa.* **(A) The 17 genes that encode the** *P. mirabilis* **HI4320 T6SS are highly conserved with the well-characterized T6SS genes from** *V. cholerae* **N16961 and have identical gene order in their respective chromosome. (B) Comparison to the three known T6SSs (HSI-1, HSI-2, HSI-3) encoded by the genome of** *P. aeruginosa* **PA01. The arrows are color-coded based upon known or predicted gene function. Black arrows represent genes that are not found in either the** *P. mirabilis* **HI4320 or** *V. cholerae* **N16961 T6SS gene locus. Reprinted from reference 8, with permission.**

amidases, lipases, nucleases, and chaperone functions.

Identification of Effectors

Both biochemical and bioinformatics approaches have been successfully used to identify T6SS effectors. One such study used bioinformatics analyses based on known *Pseudomonas aeruginosa* effectors; this heuristic approach led to the identification of a superfamily of amidase effectors, which has greatly expanded the known diversity of effectors exhibiting amidase activity (43). This work also noted a potential for substantial diversity among T6SS effectors because these analyses failed to identify effectors that have been identified in other bacteria. (43). An alternative bioinformatics strategy to identify T6SS effectors is to scan the genome in areas immediately downstream of orphan *hcp-vgrG* gene pairs (8, 44, 45). Genes downstream of these *hcp-vgrG* pairs likely encode effectors in other organisms.

Biochemical approaches have also been employed to identify T6SS effectors. One key approach that led to the discovery of the first nonstructural effectors is to compare proteins secreted by wild-type and T6SS mutant bacteria (5). The use of whole-cell proteomics to identify proteins destabilized in the absence of Hcp has also been a successful approach to discover T6SS effectors (46).

VgrG Family

The first T6SS effectors to be appreciated are members of the VgrG family, which are thought to act as a puncturing tip of the delivered Hcp tube. In *V. cholerae* (3) and *P. aeruginosa* (20), there is evidence that VgrG forms a trimer. It is notable that some organisms have only a single copy of VgrG, while other bacteria can have upward of 30 distinct VgrG proteins. This indicates that delivery of different effectors may require a specifically adapted VgrG protein (18). These findings suggest that heterotrimeric VgrG complexes could be loaded and deliver multiple effectors in the context of a single puncturing tip. Aside from the proposed role as a structural component of the effector delivery module, VgrG can also be classified as an effector because some VgrG proteins contain additional functional domains beyond the minimal trimeric structure required for T6SS function. In *V. cholerae*, the carboxyterminus of VgrG3 has muramidase activity (47), and VgrG-1 contains an actin crosslinking domain (3).

PAAR Proteins

Another group of gene products, PAAR domain–containing proteins, has been shown to be T6SS effectors. It has been shown that PAAR proteins can interact with the tip of the VgrG trimer (48). PAAR proteins are associated with a myriad of predicted effector functions, suggesting that numerous PAAR proteins encoded within bacterial genomes are likely T6SS effectors (48). It has been speculated that PAAR proteins might complex with any given VgrG trimer; however, other data suggest specific interactions between VgrG proteins and effectors (20). One example of a PAAR effector is the nuclease RhsA, which has been identified as T6SS-dependent in *Dickeya dadantii* (44). This nuclease requires one of two VgrG genes, demonstrating that this PAAR domain effector can be delivered by T6SS effector tubes capped with different VgrG puncturing tips. As mentioned, there are often multiple PAAR domain–containing proteins in bacteria that also encode a T6SS.

Rhs-Repeat Proteins

As noted above, another group of T6SS effectors are members of the Rhs-repeat-containing protein family (44). Structural analysis has shown that the Rhs-repeat domain forms a structure that completely encloses and protects the folded enzymatically active effector domain (49). Many Rhs-repeat proteins also contain PAAR domains in addition to effector domains (48). In *P. aeruginosa* PA14, the H2-T6SS encodes an Rhs effector protein that may contribute to internalization by eukaryotic cells (50). In addition, this group also found that VgrG1 of the H1-T6SS is responsible for delivering an Rhs effector protein to target cells (51). It is noteworthy that Rhs domain proteins function as antibacterial toxins in contact-dependent inhibition systems (44), which suggests that Rhs proteins have evolved to be delivered by both the T6SS and two-partner secretion systems.

Non-VgrG Effectors

The T6SS also delivers effectors that lack PAAR domains. This could suggest that the Hcp/VgrG puncturing tube may act as a conduit through which effectors are delivered to target cells (1, 52). Since the inner diameter of the Hcp tube is approximately 40 Å (1), this requires that many effector proteins would have to be delivered in an unfolded state (53). Consistent with this notion, there is one example of a T6SS effector operon that encodes a small molecular mass thioredoxin that could presumably function to fold effector proteins upon delivery to the target cell (8). Alternatively, or in addition, a thioredoxin protein could also serve to maintain effectors in an unfolded state prior to being loaded into an Hcp/VgrG puncturing tube.

Hcp tubes may also serve a chaperone function during delivery of T6SS effectors. Hcp–effector interactions were initially noted during biochemical analysis of the T6SS in *E. tarda* that showed that the secreted effector EvpP interacted with Hcp (54). Additional biochemical approaches have shown that T6SS effectors can bind to residues exposed on the inner face of the tube forming Hcp hexamers and can even stabilize effectors; thus, Hcp could be considered a molecular chaperone for effectors (55). Collectively, these experiments suggest that effectors can be loaded into the puncturing tube during assembly of the T6SS structure and may be delivered into target cells concomitantly with the puncturing device.

Numerous non-VgrG effectors have been identified, and the list of these effectors is continually growing (5, 43). In fact, T6SS effectors exhibit a broad range of functions capable of targeting both eukaryotic and prokaryotic cells. Effector activities include actin cross-linking (3, 56), muramidases and peptidases that hydrolyze peptidoglycan (5, 6, 43, 57–59), nucleases (44), and lipases (60). In *Proteus mirabilis*, there are numerous effectors that exhibit lethal activity through an unknown mechanism (8). In all cases, bacteria that produce these T6SS effectors also encode immunity proteins to protect against their cognate effectors (5, 8, 47, 58, 61).

Peptidoglycan-Degrading Effectors

One class of T6SS effectors targets the cell wall peptidoglycan. In *P. aeruginosa*, Tse1 and Tse3, among the first T6SS effectors to be characterized, both exhibit lytic activity (6). These effectors target peptide and sugar portions of the peptidoglycan. Characterization of Tse1 by several groups revealed crystal structures that indicate an amidase with a common cysteine protease fold (53, 57, 62). Peptidoglycan is a polymer composed of alternating *N*-acetylmuramic acid and *N*-acetylglucosamine residues. The muramic acid residues are modified with peptides that provide structural integrity by cross-linking with adjacent peptides. Tse1 cleaves between the second and third residues of the peptide modification (6). The specificity of Tse1 suggests that the effector could attack at sites of peptidoglycan synthesis (57). This is consistent with the observation that Tse1 is required for the *P. aeruginosa* T6SS-dependent lysis of target bacteria (63).

It is now appreciated that Tse1 belongs to a group of effectors that has been termed the type VI amidase effector (Tae) superfamily (43). Tae effectors appear to belong to four

divergent groups of cell wall–degrading enzymes (64). Further evidence indicates that the Tae proteins are functional analogs, because *tae* genes are located adjacent to genes encoding immunity determinants. It appears that all members of the Tae family function as amidases that hydrolyze peptidoglycan of Gram-negative bacteria (64). Studies examining effectors of these Tae family members have shown that T6SS activity is required for their action on target cells (6, 43, 58).

In contrast to Tse1, Tse3 acts on the sugar backbone rather than on the peptide bonds contained within peptidoglycan (6). The β1,4 bonds between muramic acid and *N*-acetylglucosamine are common targets of a multitude of bacteriocidal enzymes, including lysozyme. Indeed, these enzymes share the lysozyme muramidase fold but have an active site tyrosine residue and exhibit *N*-acetylglucosaminidase activity (6, 65). The VgrG protein of the puncturing device can also exhibit peptidoglycan-degrading activity. The C-terminal domain of *V. cholerae* VgrG3 has a predicted muramidase fold, can degrade peptidoglycan, and can cause lysis when expressed in the periplasm (47). Furthermore, the presence of a cognate immunity gene suggests that the VgrG3 protein is itself a T6SS effector (61).

Lipases

T6SS effectors can also act as lipases to disrupt cell membranes. A group of phospholipase effectors have been identified that hydrolyze plasma membrane lipids (60). These lipase effectors degrade membranes by attacking different bonds in phospholipids (64). T6SS lipase effectors have been experimentally demonstrated to cleave phospholipids at three bonds (60). Certain lipase effectors demonstrate preference for specific head group moieties. One lipase effector in *P. aeruginosa* exhibits specificity for phosphatidylethanolamine, which is a primary phospholipid found in the bacterial membrane (60). Because phospholipids are ubiquitous in nature, that is, are found in both bacterial and eukaryotic membranes, this raises the obvious possibility that T6SS lipase effectors would target both bacterial and host cell membranes. Consistent with this notion, genetic disruption of lipase effector-encoding genes in *P. aeruginosa* and *V. cholerae* creates fitness defects in infection models (60, 61).

Nucleases

Nucleases are another class of T6SS-dependent effectors. Recent studies of Rhs domain proteins showed that subsets of these proteins are also T6SS nuclease effectors (44, 66). In *D. dadantii*, RhsA and RhsB contain endonuclease effector domains that are dependent on neighboring VgrG proteins for delivery to target cells. When produced in target cells, these domains result in DNA degradation, growth inhibition, and a loss of nucleic acid staining (44). *Agrobacterium tumefaciens*, a soil bacterium that triggers tumorigenesis in plants, produces a family of T6SS DNase effectors that are distinct from previously known polymorphic toxins and nucleases. These effectors exhibit an antibacterial DNase activity that relies on a conserved motif and can be counteracted by a cognate immunity protein (67).

T6SS REGULATION

It is assumed that elaboration and usage of the T6SS nanomachine is energetically costly to the bacterial cell. It follows that expression and assembly of this structure would be tightly regulated. In some cases, there is evidence for transcriptional regulation of the T6SS via quorum sensing (68–70). In other cases, T6SS expression is regulated during biofilm formation (71, 72) by iron limitation (73, 74), is temperature-dependent (70, 75), and may react to both osmolarity changes (70) and stress responses (76). There is also evidence for independent regulation for the expression of the structural components of the T6SS and the expression of effectors.

RpoN and VasH

In *V. cholerae*, the primary T6SS gene cluster encodes a regulator, VasH, which acts as an activator via effects on RpoN. In *V. cholerae*, both RpoN and VasH are required for T6SS activity (2, 77, 78); environmental cues likely stimulate the transcription of the major cluster so that VasH is produced, which subsequently activates the transcription of the *hcp* operons by RpoN (18, 79). However, this control is limited to the transcription of two *hcp* effector operons and not the T6SS itself (79). The finding that RpoN and VasH only control the *hcp* operons suggests that additional regulators of the T6SS remain to be elucidated (18). The *hcp* operons encode the secreted T6SS effectors, while the main T6SS locus encodes structural components of the apparatus itself. This has been postulated as evidence for two-tiered regulation that may be important for maintaining different levels of expression for components that can be recycled versus those that are released to target cells (18). It is notable that pandemic *V. cholerae* strains tightly regulate the expression of the T6SS (68), while non-pandemic serotype O37 strain V52 and environmental isolates constitutively express the T6SS (80). It is possible that this difference results from increased interbacterial competition in the environment and/or as a defense mechanism against predation.

Quorum Sensing

Differences in quorum sensing–mediated transcriptional control expression of *vas* genes could be partially responsible for T6SS variability among *V. cholerae* strains. There is evidence for a strong link between HapR and Hcp expression among a number of pandemic isolates (81). Further work showed that a deletion of *luxO* was able to induce T6SS expression in two O1 serotype strains (68, 81). It was also noted that T6SS activity was not fully induced despite transcriptional activation in the absence of LuxO (68). Thus, while quorum sensing represses T6SS expression, it appears that complete T6SS activation in pandemic *V. cholerae* involves additional inputs such as high osmolarity and possibly low temperature (82).

Iron Regulation

Iron limitation controls the expression of the T6SS in *Edwardsiella* spp. and enteroaggregative *Escherichia coli*. In these bacteria, the T6SS is repressed directly at the transcriptional level by Fur (73, 74). It was shown that Fur confers iron-dependent repression of production and export of an Hcp homolog (EvpC) in *E. tarda* and that the Fur protein binds directly to a Fur box sequence upstream of *evpP*, the first gene in the T6SS gene cluster (74). In enteroaggregative *E. coli*, the Sci-1 T6SS is required for biofilm formation and is regulated by iron availability through a pathway involving Dam methylation and Fur repression (73). Two Fur binding sites and three Dam methylation sites reside upstream of the Sci-1 T6SS gene cluster. Further, one of the Fur binding sites overlaps a Dam methylation site. In the absence of iron, Fur dissociates and allows RNA polymerase to bind and initiate transcription. Similarly, the loss of Fur also permits methylation at the site, which inhibits the binding by Fur (73). Thus, iron limitation results in stable expression of the T6SS.

H-NS Regulation

Regulation of T6SS gene clusters by members of the H-NS family of regulators has also been reported. These repressor proteins function as global regulators by controlling the expression of a large number of genes throughout the genome (83). Many genes and entire gene clusters that have been horizontally acquired are silenced by H-NS (84, 85). Indeed, this is what occurs for several T6SS gene clusters, like that in *Salmonella enterica* (86). In *P. aeruginosa*, the H-NS-like protein MvaT represses the HSI-2 and HSI-3 T6SS gene clusters (87).

RetS Signaling Pathway

Control of T6SS activity in *P. aeruginosa* is well characterized, but much of what is described is based upon studies involving bacteria harboring a *retS* mutation, which leads to constitutive expression of the T6SS. The RetS regulon controls a range of virulence and fitness factors and is involved in the reciprocal control of traits important during the acute and chronic phases of lung infection (88, 89). RetS is a hybrid sensor kinase that acts upstream of the Gac/Rsm pathway in *P. aeruginosa* (88). Along with regulation of the T6SS, this regulatory pathway controls numerous traits related to antagonism or social behavior in pseudomonads (90). It should be noted that wild-type *P. aeruginosa* poorly expresses the T6SS in liquid medium, but the T6SS is expressed by wild-type bacteria during surface growth (91) and in response to cell lysate (92).

Posttranslational Control of T6SS Activity

P. aeruginosa also controls its T6SS through a posttranslational regulatory system termed the threonine phosphorylation pathway (93). In this system, the T6SS requires a T6SS-encoded forkhead-associated protein, Fha, to be phosphorylated by the kinase PpkA (93). The activity of the kinase requires the lipoprotein TagQ and an outer membrane protein termed TagR (91). Studies have shown that TagQ is required for proper localization of TagR, and TagR likely interacts directly with the periplasmic domain of PpkA (94, 95). It has also been shown that two proteins, TagS and TagT, form a membrane-associated complex that is required for full activation of PpkA (95). In this scheme, the T6SS is shut down following dephosphorylation of Fha by the phosphatase PppA (93). Consistent with this, phosphatase mutants exhibit greater levels of T6SS activity (27, 93).

Studies aimed at dissecting the posttranslational regulation of the T6SS in *P. aeruginosa* have led to a defensive T6SS hypothesis (27). This work, using a *retS* mutant strain, showed that when cultured on a solid surface, a *P. aeruginosa* bacterium that is attacked by a neighboring cell will strike back with a retaliatory T6SS counterattack (18, 27). This phenomenon has been named "T6SS dueling" (28). The threonine phosphorylation pathway plays a role in this dueling phenomenon (27). Despite finding that bacteria lacking PppA have high levels of T6SS activity, the dueling response appeared defective (27). This result suggested that dephosphorylation of Fha might somehow control the positioning of the T6SS in this scenario (18, 27). This would be consistent with the observation that surface growth, with greater numbers of neighboring cells in contact, correlates with increased PpkA activity (95).

T6SS ACTIVITY AND ACTIONS

Mechanisms to Trigger T6SS-Mediated Killing

The defensive nature of the T6SS activity in *P. aeruginosa* is supported by other studies. When cocultured with T6SS$^+$ *V. cholerae* and *Acinetobacter baylyi*, *P. aeruginosa* killed both species in a TagT-dependent manner (27). This killing was not observed when the attacking bacteria were lacking a functional T6SS. A similar differentiation between T6SS$^+$ and T6SS$^-$ *Burkholderia thailandensis* has also been observed (63). Using the *retS* background in *P. aeruginosa*, it has also been shown that a variety of conditions that mimic direct antagonistic contact can trigger firing of the T6SS. For example, during conjugation, *E. coli* cells expressing the plasmid RP4 T4SS were highly sensitive to killing by *P. aeruginosa* (30). These studies further showed that DNA transfer

was not required, but genes involved in pilus and mating pair formation were (30). The antimicrobial peptide polymyxin B also was shown to induce T6SS activity (30). These observations suggested that membrane perturbation may be the elusive signal that triggers defensive T6SS counterattacks in *P. aeruginosa* (18).

Recent work from the Mougous laboratory has provided a more complete understanding of *P. aeruginosa* response to antagonism (92). Their findings demonstrate that the response does not require the threonine phosphorylation pathway and involves the release of a diffusible signal from lysed *P. aeruginosa* sibling bacteria (92). This work goes on to show that the signal from lysed cells leads to posttranscriptional upregulation of the T6SS via the aforementioned Gac/Rsm pathway (92). Future studies are needed to better understand why *P. aeruginosa* would use the T6SS solely as a defensive weapon, or to identify the natural conditions under which the bacteria might deploy the T6SS in a preemptive manner. Other species such as *P. mirabilis* and *Serratia marcescens* do not require an attack by neighboring cells to stimulate the T6SS (8, 96). In enteroaggregative *E. coli*, it has been shown that a similar diffusible signal and counterattack mechanism might exist (97). This T6SS activity observed in *E. coli* appeared to spread within a population of cells (97).

P. mirabilis Swarming and Dienes Line Formation

The opportunistic pathogen *P. mirabilis* undergoes a characteristic developmental process to coordinate multicellular swarming behavior and discriminates itself from another *Proteus* isolate during swarming, resulting in a visible boundary termed a Dienes line (98, 99). The formation of this demarcation is dependent on the activity of the T6SS (8) (Fig. 4). Further experiments using the *P. mirabilis* model to study the T6SS demonstrated that all five identified T6SS *hcp/vgrG*

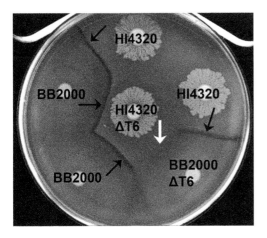

FIGURE 4 Contact-dependent preemptive antagonism is dependent on the T6SS in *Proteus mirabilis*. A Dienes line (black arrows) forms between two different wild-type isolates, HI4320 and BB2000 (strain A and B kill each other). Loss of the T6SS (ΔT6) in either isolate by disruption of PMI0742 does not affect the discriminatory Dienes line (strain A kills strain B or strain B kills strain A). Loss of the T6SS in both isolates allows nonidentical swarms to merge, and the lack of T6SS-dependent killing appears as "recognition" (white arrow). Reprinted from reference 8, with permission.

effector operons, found in the single prototype strain, were transcriptionally active only during active swarming (8). The regulatory pathways that control this specific regulation of the T6SS in *P. mirabilis* could involve the regulator MrpJ (100). The observation that *P. mirabilis* T6SS is controlled by swarming was also observed for the identity-of-self (*ids*) effector operon (8, 101). The implication from these studies is that *P. mirabilis* preemptively deploys the T6SS during a growth phase, swarming, that requires close and direct contact across a large population of bacteria.

Interbacterial Antagonism

The T6SS is a macromolecular machine that delivers protein effectors into both prokaryotic and eukaryotic cells, thus playing important roles during interbacterial competition and virulence in the host (102). In addition

to the versatility, the genes encoding the T6SS are widely distributed and found in approximately one-third of sequenced Gram-negative bacterial genomes (103). Numerous studies have revealed that the activity of the T6SS is important in bacterial communities, either by promoting biofilm formation or by competing with neighboring bacteria (64). It is now appreciated that the T6SS is used to deliver antibacterial toxins directly inside neighboring bacterial cells. The role for the T6SS during interbacterial competition was first noted in *P. aeruginosa* (5). Subsequently, a similar function has been shown in *B. thailandensis*, *V. cholerae*, *S. marcescens*, enteroaggregative *E. coli*, *Citrobacter rodentium*, *Acinetobacter baumannii*, and *P. mirabilis* (8, 76, 104–107). The T6SS also plays an important role in intraspecies competition, that is, different isolates of the same species produce different sets of toxin effectors (8, 108). As noted, this intraspecies warfare is responsible for the formation of macroscopic boundaries between nonisogenic strains in several species, most notably in swarming *P. mirabilis* (8, 109).

Biofilm Formation

Several bacterial species use the T6SS during biofilm formation. Mutations in the enteroaggregative *E. coli* Sci-1 T6SS or avian pathogenic *E. coli* T6SS genes decrease the ability to form biofilms (38). Additionally, a second T6SS gene cluster in enteroaggregative *E. coli*, Sci-2 T6SS, and the *P. aeruginosa* H1-T6SS are upregulated under biofilm-forming conditions (93). Much like during cooperative swarming motility in *P. mirabilis*, coordination of T6SS production with biofilm determinants may help to promote formation of monospecies biofilms or create a protective isogenic zone within a mixed community.

Host–Microbe Interactions

There are also studies demonstrating that the T6SS is expressed during interactions with host cells (110–113). Closer inspection reveals a limited number of studies that show a direct role for the T6SS in bacterial pathogenesis. The *V. cholerae* T6SS is required to escape predation and for toxicity toward phagocytes (2). In a mouse model of infection, *V. cholerae* causes inflammation and increased recovery of bacteria from the intestine (4). The *P. aeruginosa* H1- and H3-T6SS may influence interactions with host cells through enhanced invasion (113–115). It is important to note that most of the T6SS effectors characterized to date are antimicrobial. Thus, it must be considered that the observed upregulation of the T6SS in the host, or fitness defects of T6SS mutant bacteria in infection models, reflects an indirect relation to pathogenesis. For example, T6SS antibacterial antagonism was recently revealed to contribute to efficient colonization of *V. cholerae* in an animal model (116). That study clearly showed that bacteria lacking immunity against sister cells had a significant fitness defect during infection. Collectively, the limited numbers of studies that show a direct role for the T6SS in bacterial pathogenesis suggest that the T6SS has evolved as a weapon used during interbacterial competition.

Competition in the Host

Often, for bacteria to establish an infection, pathogens must be able to overcome colonization resistance created by the natural microbiome. This could be important for enteric bacteria that compete against the intestinal microbiome community (117). In support of this, a number of pathogens that colonize the intestine produce a T6SS, including *S. enterica*, *C. rodentium*, *Aeromonas hydrophila*, and enteroaggregative *E. coli* (38, 118–120). The T6SS can be envisioned to provide bacteria with a competitive advantage in other host sites. For example, opportunistic pathogens that cause wound infections, such as *A. baumannii*, *P. aeruginosa*, *S. marcescens*, and *P. mirabilis*, all are known to produce at

least one T6SS with antibacterial activity (5, 8, 106, 107). Once these opportunistic pathogens establish tissue colonization, the T6SS could provide a mechanism to prevent colonization by another strain or species. For *P. aeruginosa*, it is known that diversity within the cystic fibrosis lung decreases over time (121). Indeed, isolates of *P. aeruginosa* from cystic fibrosis patients have an active T6SS, and these patients produce antibodies against Hcp (64, 72).

Additionally, there is a substantial amount of genomic evidence to support the primary role for the T6SS during interbacterial warfare. Immunity proteins are maintained in the genomes of bacteria that lack cognate T6SS effector proteins (43). The presence of orphan immunity proteins suggests that there is positive selection imposed by T6SS attacks (43). The observation that effector proteins are accompanied by immunity proteins is evidence for the selection against self-intoxication. This highlights the fitness cost that is associated with effector intoxication in the absence of immunity. It also appears that bacteria with a lifestyle that precludes interbacterial competition tend to lack a T6SS. For example, in *Burkholderia mallei*, the loss of interbacterial T6SS has been proposed to coincide with the evolution from a free-living opportunistic pathogen to an obligate pathogen (104).

Intraspecies Antagonism

Bacteria that are closely related, for example, the same species or close relatives, are most likely to directly compete with one another for the same niche or resources. Although strains will cooperate and form mixed communities, in many cases, growth of one strain precludes growth of another (8, 98, 122–124). Antagonism between isolates has been well studied, and the most obvious example is bacteriocin production and targeting of closely related competitors (7). Another mechanism of intraspecies antagonism that has been recently characterized is known as contact-dependent inhibition and requires direct contact like the T6SS (125, 126).

Intraspecies competition using the T6SS has been shown for many bacterial species. T6SS-mediated antagonism was observed between isolates of *S. marcescens* and in *V. cholerae* (80, 106). Additionally, bacteria such as *P. aeruginosa*, *V. cholerae*, and *P. mirabilis* all possess variable complements of T6SS effector and immunity pairs, which would result in competition between isolates of the species (8, 108). An exceptionally clear example of intraspecies antagonism using the T6SS can be observed between swarming populations of *P. mirabilis*. Macroscopic boundaries form between nonidentical isolates upon contact during swarming (Fig. 4). Upon initiation of swarming differentiation, the T6SS is assembled and appears to fire when opposing swarms meet (8). Boundary formation, underlying killing, and immunity to killing, can be assigned to specific T6SS genes and effector proteins. It is now becoming clear that the ability of *P. mirabilis* to self-recognize is a result of being immune to T6SS attack (8) (Fig. 5). Indeed, the *P. mirabilis*

recognition system appears to depend largely on diversity of *hcp/vgrG* effector operons and variation between otherwise identical effector operons (8, 127).

Intraspecies competition is consistent with the presence of diverse repertoires of T6SS effector and immunity pairs in many other bacterial species. Selection to maintain diversity could occur when a bacterium that lacks immunity to a specific T6SS effector that is present in its neighbor is rapidly killed (64). This further provides an explanation for why a given organism would translocate closely related effector proteins, which can differ in immune recognition and, thus, would be nonredundant in antagonistic function (58, 122). Studying bacterial antagonism has led to the hypothesis that antibacterial activities could be preferentially produced in response to competition-induced stress (128). As discussed for *P. aeruginosa* and the Fha phosphorylation cascade, both intra- and interbacterial interactions of the T6SS in one cell can stimulate the system in neighboring cells (27, 63). This recognition is sufficiently integral to the activity of the *P. aeruginosa* H1-T6SS that

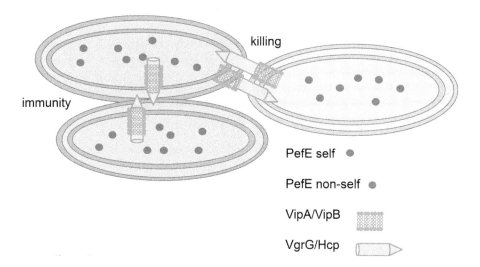

FIGURE 5 Immunity against T6SS is the basis for self-recognition. If two strains of *Proteus mirabilis* synthesize the same immunity protein, then both strains are immune to killing by the T6SS and recognize as "self." However, if two strains have divergent immunity proteins, then both strains are subject to killing by each of the other strain's T6SS.

inactivation of the T6SS of a competitor organism confers resistance to intoxication (27, 28).

The conditions that control T6SS activity can provide valuable insights into the physiological relevance of T6SS function. As noted, the H1-T6SS of *P. aeruginosa* and the T6SS of *V. cholerae* O1 serotypes are repressed by quorum sensing (81, 129). Repression of the T6SS by quorum sensing indicates that these systems are active when cells are at relatively low cell density and may function to displace unrelated or more distantly related bacteria in a densely populated mixed community. Other systems, such as the H2-T6SS of *P. aeruginosa*, are induced under conditions of high cell density (72, 129). This might indicate a role for that T6SS during high cell density of an isogenic population or a role during intraspecies antagonism. As discussed, other bacteria control their T6SS in response to environmental cues such as temperature, pH, or iron availability (47, 70–77). These cues may indicate the movement of bacteria into a condition where competitor bacteria are likely to be encountered.

CONCLUDING REMARKS

Remarkable progress has been made toward understanding the T6SS and its role in numerous bacterial species. The structural details of T6SS assembly and the effector delivery module have been elucidated. The diversity of effectors that elicit numerous antagonistic activities upon interaction with target cells are now appreciated. Studies by many research groups have provided substantial clues to answer the question of why bacteria would use contact-dependent delivery of effectors to eliminate their neighbors. It is becoming clear that bacteria can benefit from the T6SS to discriminate, "recognize," and kill competitors rather than indiscriminately secrete bactericidal agents when competing for resources in their natural habitats. It is evident that T6SS-dependent interac-

tions are involved in developmental processes such as multicellularity or organized communities (8). For bacteria that cooperate to achieve a behavior such as swarming, the T6SS could prevent cheaters from benefiting from the cooperative behavior (130, 131). In other instances, T6SS killing of neighboring cells can facilitate the release of genetic material for horizontal gene transfer between closely related species (132). Studies like these are likely to focus greater attention on the biological relevance of the T6SS in bacteria. As community behaviors of microbes are beginning to be more thoroughly appreciated, it is expected that the T6SS will be a key determinant in shaping these microbial communities.

ACKNOWLEDGMENTS

We thank Stephanie Himpsl for many helpful discussions and for assistance in creating figures.

Our work on the T6SS in *P. mirabilis* is supported by grant AI059722 from the National Institute of Allergy and Infectious Disease.

CITATION

Alteri CJ, Mobley HLT. 2016. The versatile type VI secretion system. Microbiol Spectrum 4(2):VMBF-0026-2015.

REFERENCES

1. **Mougous JD, Cuff ME, Raunser S, Shen A, Zhou M, Gifford CA, Goodman AL, Joachimiak G, Ordonez CL, Lory S, Walz T, Joachimiak A, Mekalanos JJ.** 2006. A virulence locus of *Pseudomonas aeruginosa* encodes a protein secretion apparatus. *Science* **312:**1526–1530.

2. **Pukatzki S, Ma AT, Sturtevant D, Krastins B, Sarracino D, Nelson WC, Heidelberg JF, Mekalanos JJ.** 2006. Identification of a conserved bacterial protein secretion system in *Vibrio cholerae* using the *Dictyostelium* host model system. *Proc Natl Acad Sci USA* **103:**1528–1533.

3. **Pukatzki S, Ma AT, Revel AT, Sturtevant D, Mekalanos JJ.** 2007. Type VI secretion system translocates a phage tail spike-like protein into target cells where it cross-links actin. *Proc Natl Acad Sci USA* **104:**15508–15513.

4. **Ma AT, Mekalanos JJ.** 2010. *In vivo* actin cross-linking induced by *Vibrio cholerae* type VI secretion system is associated with intestinal inflammation. *Proc Natl Acad Sci USA* **107:** 4365–4370.

5. **Hood RD, Singh P, Hsu F, Guvener T, Carl MA, Trinidad RR, Silverman JM, Ohlson BB, Hicks KG, Plemel RL, Li M, Schwarz S, Wang WY, Merz AJ, Goodlett DR, Mougous JD.** 2010. A type VI secretion system of *Pseudomonas aeruginosa* targets a toxin to bacteria. *Cell Host Microbe* **7:**25–37.

6. **Russell AB, Hood RD, Bui NK, LeRoux M, Vollmer W, Mougous JD.** 2011. Type VI secretion delivers bacteriolytic effectors to target cells. *Nature* **475:**343–347.

7. **Riley MA, Wertz JE.** 2002. Bacteriocins: evolution, ecology, and application. *Annu Rev Microbiol* **56:**117–137.

8. **Alteri CJ, Himpsl SD, Pickens SR, Lindner JR, Zora JS, Miller JE, Arno PD, Straight SW, Mobley HL.** 2013. Multicellular bacteria deploy the type VI secretion system to preemptively strike neighboring cells. *PLoS Pathog* **9:** e1003608. doi:10.1371/journal.ppat.1003608.

9. **Cotter P.** 2011. Microbiology: molecular syringes scratch the surface. *Nature* **475:**301–303.

10. **Folkesson A, Lofdahl S, Normark S.** 2002. The *Salmonella enterica* subspecies I specific centisome 7 genomic island encodes novel protein families present in bacteria living in close contact with eukaryotic cells. *Res Microbiol* **153:**537–545.

11. **Bladergroen MR, Badelt K, Spaink HP.** 2003. Infection-blocking genes of a symbiotic *Rhizobium leguminosarum* strain that are involved in temperature-dependent protein secretion. *Mol Plant Microbe Interact* **16:**53–64.

12. **Nano FE, Zhang N, Cowley SC, Klose KE, Cheung KK, Roberts MJ, Ludu JS, Letendre GW, Meierovics AI, Stephens G, Elkins KL.** 2004. A *Francisella tularensis* pathogenicity island required for intramacrophage growth. *J Bacteriol* **186:**6430–6436.

13. **Rao PS, Yamada Y, Tan YP, Leung KY.** 2004. Use of proteomics to identify novel virulence determinants that are required for *Edwardsiella tarda* pathogenesis. *Mol Microbiol* **53:** 573–586.

14. **Das S, Chaudhuri K.** 2003. Identification of a unique IAHP (IcmF associated homologous proteins) cluster in *Vibrio cholerae* and other

proteobacteria through *in silico* analysis. *In Silico Biol* **3:**287–300.

15. **Pallen M, Chaudhuri R, Khan A.** 2002. Bacterial FHA domains: neglected players in the phospho-threonine signalling game? *Trends Microbiol* **10:**556–563.

16. **Schlieker C, Zentgraf H, Dersch P, Mogk A.** 2005. ClpV, a unique Hsp100/Clp member of pathogenic proteobacteria. *Biol Chem* **386:**1115–1127.

17. **Leiman PG, Basler M, Ramagopal UA, Bonanno JB, Sauder JM, Pukatzki S, Burley SK, Almo SC, Mekalanos JJ.** 2009. Type VI secretion apparatus and phage tail-associated protein complexes share a common evolutionary origin. *Proc Natl Acad Sci USA* **106:**4154–4159.

18. **Ho BT, Dong TG, Mekalanos JJ.** 2014. A view to a kill: the bacterial type VI secretion system. *Cell Host Microbe* **15:**9–21.

19. **Ballister ER, Lai AH, Zuckermann RN, Cheng Y, Mougous JD.** 2008. *In vitro* self-assembly of tailorable nanotubes from a simple protein building block. *Proc Natl Acad Sci USA* **105:** 3733–3738.

20. **Hachani A, Lossi NS, Hamilton A, Jones C, Bleves S, Albesa-Jove D, Filloux A.** 2011. Type VI secretion system in *Pseudomonas aeruginosa*: secretion and multimerization of VgrG proteins. *J Biol Chem* **286:**12317–12327.

21. **Pell LG, Kanelis V, Donaldson LW, Howell PL, Davidson AR.** 2009. The phage lambda major tail protein structure reveals a common evolution for long-tailed phages and the type VI bacterial secretion system. *Proc Natl Acad Sci USA* **106:**4160–4165.

22. **Bonemann G, Pietrosiuk A, Diemand A, Zentgraf H, Mogk A.** 2009. Remodelling of VipA/VipB tubules by ClpV-mediated threading is crucial for type VI protein secretion. *EMBO J* **28:**315–325.

23. **Lossi NS, Manoli E, Forster A, Dajani R, Pape T, Freemont P, Filloux A.** 2013. The HsiB1C1 (TssB-TssC) complex of the *Pseudomonas aeruginosa* type VI secretion system forms a bacteriophage tail sheathlike structure. *J Biol Chem* **288:**7536–7548.

24. **Bonemann G, Pietrosiuk A, Mogk A.** 2010. Tubules and donuts: a type VI secretion story. *Mol Microbiol* **76:**815–821.

25. **Filloux A.** 2009. The type VI secretion system: a tubular story. *EMBO J* **28:**309–310.

26. **Records AR.** 2011. The type VI secretion system: a multipurpose delivery system with a phage-like machinery. *Mol Plant Microbe Interact* **24:**751–757.

27. **Basler M, Ho BT, Mekalanos JJ.** 2013. Tit-for-tat: type VI secretion system counterattack

during bacterial cell-cell interactions. *Cell* **152:** 884–894.

28. **Basler M, Mekalanos JJ.** 2012. Type 6 secretion dynamics within and between bacterial cells. *Science* **337:**815.

29. **Basler M, Pilhofer M, Henderson GP, Jensen GJ, Mekalanos JJ.** 2012. Type VI secretion requires a dynamic contractile phage tail-like structure. *Nature* **483:**182–186.

30. **Ho BT, Basler M, Mekalanos JJ.** 2013. Type 6 secretion system-mediated immunity to type 4 secretion system-mediated gene transfer. *Science* **342:**250–253.

31. **Kube S, Kapitein N, Zimniak T, Herzog F, Mogk A, Wendler P.** 2014. Structure of the VipA/B type VI secretion complex suggests a contraction-state-specific recycling mechanism. *Cell Rep* **8:**20–30.

32. **Clemens DL, Ge P, Lee BY, Horwitz MA, Zhou ZH.** 2015. Atomic structure of T6SS reveals interlaced array essential to function. *Cell* **160:**940–951.

33. **Kudryashev M, Wang RY, Brackmann M, Scherer S, Maier T, Baker D, DiMaio F, Stahlberg H, Egelman EH, Basler M.** 2015. Structure of the type VI secretion system contractile sheath. *Cell* **160:**952–962.

34. **Brunet YR, Henin J, Celia H, Cascales E.** 2014. Type VI secretion and bacteriophage tail tubes share a common assembly pathway. *EMBO Rep* **15:**315–321.

35. **Aschtgen MS, Gavioli M, Dessen A, Lloubes R, Cascales E.** 2010. The SciZ protein anchors the enteroaggregative *Escherichia coli* type VI secretion system to the cell wall. *Mol Microbiol* **75:**886–899.

36. **Felisberto-Rodrigues C, Durand E, Aschtgen MS, Blangy S, Ortiz-Lombardia M, Douzi B, Cambillau C, Cascales E.** 2011. Towards a structural comprehension of bacterial type VI secretion systems: characterization of the TssJ-TssM complex of an *Escherichia coli* pathovar. *PLoS Pathog* **7:**e1002386. doi:10.1371/journal.ppat.1002386.

37. **Zoued A, Brunet YR, Durand E, Aschtgen MS, Logger L, Douzi B, Journet L, Cambillau C, Cascales E.** 2014. Architecture and assembly of the type VI secretion system. *Biochim Biophys Acta* **1843:**1664–1673.

38. **Aschtgen MS, Bernard CS, De Bentzmann S, Lloubes R, Cascales E.** 2008. SciN is an outer membrane lipoprotein required for type VI secretion in enteroaggregative *Escherichia coli.* *J Bacteriol* **190:**7523–7531.

39. **Ma LS, Narberhaus F, Lai EM.** 2012. IcmF family protein TssM exhibits ATPase activity and energizes type VI secretion. *J Biol Chem* **287:**15610–15621.

40. **Ma LS, Lin JS, Lai EM.** 2009. An IcmF family protein, ImpLM, is an integral inner membrane protein interacting with ImpKL, and its walker a motif is required for type VI secretion system-mediated Hcp secretion in *Agrobacterium tumefaciens.* *J Bacteriol* **191:**4316–4329.

41. **Durand E, Nguyen VS, Zoued A, Logger L, Pehau-Arnaudet G, Aschtgen MS, Spinelli S, Desmyter A, Bardiaux B, Dujeancourt A, Roussel A, Cambillau C, Cascales E, Fronzes R.** 2015. Biogenesis and structure of a type VI secretion membrane core complex. *Nature* **523:**555–560.

42. **Zoued A, Durand E, Bebeacua C, Brunet YR, Douzi B, Cambillau C, Cascales E, Journet L.** 2013. TssK is a trimeric cytoplasmic protein interacting with components of both phage-like and membrane anchoring complexes of the type VI secretion system. *J Biol Chem* **288:**27031–27041.

43. **Russell AB, Singh P, Brittnacher M, Bui NK, Hood RD, Carl MA, Agnello DM, Schwarz S, Goodlett DR, Vollmer W, Mougous JD.** 2012. A widespread bacterial type VI secretion effector superfamily identified using a heuristic approach. *Cell Host Microbe* **11:**538–549.

44. **Koskiniemi S, Lamoureux JG, Nikolakakis KC, t'Kint de Roodenbeke C, Kaplan MD, Low DA, Hayes CS.** 2013. Rhs proteins from diverse bacteria mediate intercellular competition. *Proc Natl Acad Sci USA* **110:**7032–7037.

45. **Miyata ST, Kitaoka M, Brooks TM, McAuley SB, Pukatzki S.** 2011. *Vibrio cholerae* requires the type VI secretion system virulence factor VasX to kill *Dictyostelium discoideum.* *Infect Immun* **79:**2941–2949.

46. **Whitney JC, Beck CM, Goo YA, Russell AB, Harding BN, De Leon JA, Cunningham DA, Tran BQ, Low DA, Goodlett DR, Hayes CS, Mougous JD.** 2014. Genetically distinct pathways guide effector export through the type VI secretion system. *Mol Microbiol* **92:**529–542.

47. **Brooks TM, Unterweger D, Bachmann V, Kostiuk B, Pukatzki S.** 2013. Lytic activity of the *Vibrio cholerae* type VI secretion toxin VgrG-3 is inhibited by the antitoxin TsaB. *J Biol Chem* **288:**7618–7625.

48. **Shneider MM, Buth SA, Ho BT, Basler M, Mekalanos JJ, Leiman PG.** 2013. PAAR-repeat proteins sharpen and diversify the type VI secretion system spike. *Nature* **500:**350–353.

49. **Busby JN, Panjikar S, Landsberg MJ, Hurst MR, Lott JS.** 2013. The BC component of ABC toxins is an RHS-repeat-containing protein encapsulation device. *Nature* **501:**547–550.

50. **Jones C, Hachani A, Manoli E, Filloux A.** 2014. An rhs gene linked to the second type VI secretion cluster is a feature of the *Pseudomonas aeruginosa* strain PA14. *J Bacteriol* **196:** 800–810.

51. **Hachani A, Allsopp LP, Oduko Y, Filloux A.** 2014. The VgrG proteins are "a la carte" delivery systems for bacterial type VI effectors. *J Biol Chem* **289:**17872–17884.

52. **Silverman JM, Brunet YR, Cascales E, Mougous JD.** 2012. Structure and regulation of the type VI secretion system. *Annu Rev Microbiol* **66:**453–472.

53. **Benz J, Sendlmeier C, Barends TR, Meinhart A.** 2012. Structural insights into the effector-immunity system Tse1/Tsi1 from *Pseudomonas aeruginosa*. *PLoS One* **7:**e40453. doi:10.1371/journal.pone.0040453.

54. **Zheng J, Leung KY.** 2007. Dissection of a type VI secretion system in *Edwardsiella tarda*. *Mol Microbiol* **66:**1192–1206.

55. **Silverman JM, Agnello DM, Zheng H, Andrews BT, Li M, Catalano CE, Gonen T, Mougous JD.** 2013. Haemolysin coregulated protein is an exported receptor and chaperone of type VI secretion substrates. *Mol Cell* **51:** 584–593.

56. **Suarez G, Sierra JC, Erova TE, Sha J, Horneman AJ, Chopra AK.** 2010. A type VI secretion system effector protein, VgrG1, from *Aeromonas hydrophila* that induces host cell toxicity by ADP ribosylation of actin. *J Bacteriol* **192:**155–168.

57. **Chou S, Bui NK, Russell AB, Lexa KW, Gardiner TE, LeRoux M, Vollmer W, Mougous JD.** 2012. Structure of a peptidoglycan amidase effector targeted to Gram-negative bacteria by the type VI secretion system. *Cell Rep* **1:**656–664.

58. **English G, Trunk K, Rao VA, Srikannathasan V, Hunter WN, Coulthurst SJ.** 2012. New secreted toxins and immunity proteins encoded within the type VI secretion system gene cluster of *Serratia marcescens*. *Mol Microbiol* **86:**921–936.

59. **Whitney JC, Chou S, Russell AB, Biboy J, Gardiner TE, Ferrin MA, Brittnacher M, Vollmer W, Mougous JD.** 2013. Identification, structure, and function of a novel type VI secretion peptidoglycan glycoside hydrolase effector-immunity pair. *J Biol Chem* **288:** 26616–26624.

60. **Russell AB, LeRoux M, Hathazi K, Agnello DM, Ishikawa T, Wiggins PA, Wai SN, Mougous JD.** 2013. Diverse type VI secretion phospholipases are functionally plastic antibacterial effectors. *Nature* **496:**508–512.

61. **Dong TG, Ho BT, Yoder-Himes DR, Mekalanos JJ.** 2013. Identification of T6SS-dependent effector and immunity proteins by Tn-seq in *Vibrio cholerae*. *Proc Natl Acad Sci USA* **110:** 2623–2628.

62. **Ding J, Wang W, Feng H, Zhang Y, Wang DC.** 2012. Structural insights into the *Pseudomonas aeruginosa* type VI virulence effector Tse1 bacteriolysis and self-protection mechanisms. *J Biol Chem* **287:**26911–26920.

63. **LeRoux M, De Leon JA, Kuwada NJ, Russell AB, Pinto-Santini D, Hood RD, Agnello DM, Robertson SM, Wiggins PA, Mougous JD.** 2012. Quantitative single-cell characterization of bacterial interactions reveals type VI secretion is a double-edged sword. *Proc Natl Acad Sci USA* **109:**19804–19809.

64. **Russell AB, Peterson SB, Mougous JD.** 2014. Type VI secretion system effectors: poisons with a purpose. *Nat Rev Microbiol* **12:**137–148.

65. **Li L, Zhang W, Liu Q, Gao Y, Gao Y, Wang Y, Wang DZ, Li Z, Wang T.** 2013. Structural insights on the bacteriolytic and self-protection mechanism of muramidase effector Tse3 in *Pseudomonas aeruginosa*. *J Biol Chem* **288:** 30607–30613.

66. **Poole SJ, Diner EJ, Aoki SK, Braaten BA, de Roodenbeke CT, Low DA, Hayes CS.** 2011. Identification of functional toxin/immunity genes linked to contact-dependent growth inhibition (CDI) and rearrangement hotspot (Rhs) systems. *Plos Genetics* **7:**e1002217. doi:10.1371/journal.pgen.1002217.

67. **Ma LS, Hachani A, Lin JS, Filloux A, Lai EM.** 2014. *Agrobacterium tumefaciens* deploys a superfamily of type VI secretion DNase effectors as weapons for interbacterial competition *in planta*. *Cell Host Microbe* **16:**94–104.

68. **Zheng J, Shin OS, Cameron DE, Mekalanos JJ.** 2010. Quorum sensing and a global regulator TsrA control expression of type VI secretion and virulence in *Vibrio cholerae*. *Proc Natl Acad Sci USA* **107:**21128–21133.

69. **Kitaoka M, Miyata ST, Brooks TM, Unterweger D, Pukatzki S.** 2011. VasH is a transcriptional regulator of the type VI secretion system functional in endemic and pandemic *Vibrio cholerae*. *J Bacteriol* **193:**6471–6482.

70. **Salomon D, Gonzalez H, Updegraff BL, Orth K.** 2013. *Vibrio parahaemolyticus* type VI secretion system 1 is activated in marine conditions to target bacteria, and is differentially regulated from system 2. *PLoS One* **8:**e61086. doi:10.1371/journal.pone.0061086.

71. **Aubert DF, Flannagan RS, Valvano MA.** 2008. A novel sensor kinase-response regulator

hybrid controls biofilm formation and type VI secretion system activity in *Burkholderia cenocepacia*. *Infect Immun* **76**:1979–1991.

72. **Moscoso JA, Mikkelsen H, Heeb S, Williams P, Filloux A.** 2011. The *Pseudomonas aeruginosa* sensor RetS switches type III and type VI secretion via c-di-GMP signalling. *Environ Microbiol* **13**:3128–3138.

73. **Brunet YR, Bernard CS, Gavioli M, Lloubes R, Cascales E.** 2011. An epigenetic switch involving overlapping fur and DNA methylation optimizes expression of a type VI secretion gene cluster. *PLoS Genet* **7**:e1002205. doi:10.1371/journal.pgen.1002205.

74. **Chakraborty S, Sivaraman J, Leung KY, Mok YK.** 2011. Two-component PhoB-PhoR regulatory system and ferric uptake regulator sense phosphate and iron to control virulence genes in type III and VI secretion systems of *Edwardsiella tarda*. *J Biol Chem* **286**:39417–39430.

75. **Pieper R, Huang ST, Robinson JM, Clark DJ, Alami H, Parmar PP, Perry RD, Fleischmann RD, Peterson SN.** 2009. Temperature and growth phase influence the outer-membrane proteome and the expression of a type VI secretion system in *Yersinia pestis*. *Microbiology* **155**:498–512.

76. **Gueguen E, Durand E, Zhang XY, d'Amalric Q, Journet L, Cascales E.** 2013. Expression of a type VI secretion system is responsive to envelope stresses through the OmpR transcriptional activator. *PLoS One* **8**:e66615. doi:10.1371/journal.pone.0066615.

77. **Bernard CS, Brunet YR, Gavioli M, Lloubes R, Cascales E.** 2011. Regulation of type VI secretion gene clusters by sigma54 and cognate enhancer binding proteins. *J Bacteriol* **193**:2158–2167.

78. **Zheng J, Ho B, Mekalanos JJ.** 2011. Genetic analysis of anti-amoebae and anti-bacterial activities of the type VI secretion system in *Vibrio cholerae*. *PLoS One* **6**:e23876. doi:10.1371/journal.pone.0023876.

79. **Dong TG, Mekalanos JJ.** 2012. Characterization of the RpoN regulon reveals differential regulation of T6SS and new flagellar operons in *Vibrio cholerae* O37 strain V52. *Nucleic Acids Res* **40**:7766–7775.

80. **Unterweger D, Kitaoka M, Miyata ST, Bachmann V, Brooks TM, Moloney J, Sosa O, Silva D, Duran-Gonzalez J, Provenzano D, Pukatzki S.** 2012. Constitutive type VI secretion system expression gives *Vibrio cholerae* intra- and interspecific competitive advantages. *PLoS One* **7**:e48320. doi:10.1371/journal.pone.0048320.

81. **Ishikawa T, Rompikuntal PK, Lindmark B, Milton DL, Wai SN.** 2009. Quorum sensing regulation of the two hcp alleles in *Vibrio cholerae* O1 strains. *PLoS One* **4**:e6734. doi:10.1371/journal.pone.0006734.

82. **Ishikawa T, Sabharwal D, Broms J, Milton DL, Sjostedt A, Uhlin BE, Wai SN.** 2012. Pathoadaptive conditional regulation of the type VI secretion system in *Vibrio cholerae* O1 strains. *Infect Immun* **80**:575–584.

83. **Navarre WW, McClelland M, Libby SJ, Fang FC.** 2007. Silencing of xenogeneic DNA by H-NS-facilitation of lateral gene transfer in bacteria by a defense system that recognizes foreign DNA. *Genes Dev* **21**:1456–1471.

84. **Grainger DC, Hurd D, Goldberg MD, Busby SJ.** 2006. Association of nucleoid proteins with coding and non-coding segments of the *Escherichia coli* genome. *Nucleic Acids Res* **34**:4642–4652.

85. **Navarre WW, Porwollik S, Wang Y, McClelland M, Rosen H, Libby SJ, Fang FC.** 2006. Selective silencing of foreign DNA with low GC content by the H-NS protein in *Salmonella*. *Science* **313**:236–238.

86. **Lucchini S, Rowley G, Goldberg MD, Hurd D, Harrison M, Hinton JC.** 2006. H-NS mediates the silencing of laterally acquired genes in bacteria. *PLoS Pathog* **2**:e81. doi:10.1371/journal.ppat.0020081.

87. **Castang S, McManus HR, Turner KH, Dove SL.** 2008. H-NS family members function coordinately in an opportunistic pathogen. *Proc Natl Acad Sci USA* **105**:18947–18952.

88. **Goodman AL, Kulasekara B, Rietsch A, Boyd D, Smith RS, Lory S.** 2004. A signaling network reciprocally regulates genes associated with acute infection and chronic persistence in *Pseudomonas aeruginosa*. *Dev Cell* **7**:745–754.

89. **Ventre I, Goodman AL, Vallet-Gely I, Vasseur P, Soscia C, Molin S, Bleves S, Lazdunski A, Lory S, Filloux A.** 2006. Multiple sensors control reciprocal expression of *Pseudomonas aeruginosa* regulatory RNA and virulence genes. *Proc Natl Acad Sci USA* **103**:171–176.

90. **Lapouge K, Schubert M, Allain FH, Haas D.** 2008. Gac/Rsm signal transduction pathway of gamma-proteobacteria: from RNA recognition to regulation of social behaviour. *Mol Microbiol* **67**:241–253.

91. **Silverman JM, Austin LS, Hsu F, Hicks KG, Hood RD, Mougous JD.** 2011. Separate inputs modulate phosphorylation-dependent and -independent type VI secretion activation. *Mol Microbiol* **82**:1277–1290.

92. **LeRoux M, Kirkpatrick RL, Montauti EI, Tran BQ, Peterson SB, Harding BN, Whitney**

JC, Russell AB, Traxler B, Goo YA, Goodlett DR, Wiggins PA, Mougous JD. 2015. Kin cell lysis is a danger signal that activates antibacterial pathways of *Pseudomonas aeruginosa*. *Elife* **4**. doi:10.7554/eLife.05701.

93. **Mougous JD, Gifford CA, Ramsdell TL, Mekalanos JJ.** 2007. Threonine phosphorylation post-translationally regulates protein secretion in *Pseudomonas aeruginosa*. *Nat Cell Biol* **9**:797–803.

94. **Hsu F, Schwarz S, Mougous JD.** 2009. TagR promotes PpkA-catalysed type VI secretion activation in *Pseudomonas aeruginosa*. *Mol Microbiol* **72**:1111–1125.

95. **Casabona MG, Silverman JM, Sall KM, Boyer F, Coute Y, Poirel J, Grunwald D, Mougous JD, Elsen S, Attree I.** 2013. An ABC transporter and an outer membrane lipoprotein participate in posttranslational activation of type VI secretion in *Pseudomonas aeruginosa*. *Environ Microbiol* **15**:471–486.

96. **Fritsch MJ, Trunk K, Diniz JA, Guo M, Trost M, Coulthurst SJ.** 2013. Proteomic identification of novel secreted antibacterial toxins of the *Serratia marcescens* type VI secretion system. *Mol Cell Proteomics* **12**:2735–2749.

97. **Brunet YR, Espinosa L, Harchouni S, Mignot T, Cascales E.** 2013. Imaging type VI secretion-mediated bacterial killing. *Cell Rep* **3**:36–41.

98. **Dienes L.** 1946. Reproductive processes in *Proteus* cultures. *Proc Soc Exp Biol Med* **63**:265–270.

99. **Dienes L.** 1947. Further observations on the reproduction of bacilli from large bodies in *Proteus* cultures. *Proc Soc Exp Biol Med* **66**:97.

100. **Bode NJ, Debnath I, Kuan L, Schulfer A, Ty M, Pearson MM.** 2015. Transcriptional analysis of the MrpJ network: modulation of diverse virulence-associated genes and direct regulation of mrp fimbrial and flhDC flagellar operons in *Proteus mirabilis*. *Infect Immun* **83**:2542–2556.

101. **Gibbs KA, Wenren LM, Greenberg EP.** 2011. Identity gene expression in *Proteus mirabilis*. *J Bacteriol* **193**:3286–3292.

102. **Schwarz S, Hood RD, Mougous JD.** 2010. What is type VI secretion doing in all those bugs? *Trends Microbiol* **18**:531–537.

103. **Durand E, Cambillau C, Cascales E, Journet L.** 2014. VgrG, Tae, Tle, and beyond: the versatile arsenal of type VI secretion effectors. *Trends Microbiol* **22**:498–507.

104. **Schwarz S, West TE, Boyer F, Chiang WC, Carl MA, Hood RD, Rohmer L, Tolker-Nielsen T, Skerrett SJ, Mougous JD.** 2010. *Burkholderia* type VI secretion systems have distinct roles in eukaryotic and bacterial cell interactions. *PLoS Pathog* **6**:e1001068. doi:10.1371/journal.ppat.1001068.

105. **MacIntyre DL, Miyata ST, Kitaoka M, Pukatzki S.** 2010. The *Vibrio cholerae* type VI secretion system displays antimicrobial properties. *Proc Natl Acad Sci USA* **107**:19520–19524.

106. **Murdoch SL, Trunk K, English G, Fritsch MJ, Pourkarimi E, Coulthurst SJ.** 2011. The opportunistic pathogen *Serratia marcescens* utilizes type VI secretion to target bacterial competitors. *J Bacteriol* **193**:6057–6069.

107. **Carruthers MD, Nicholson PA, Tracy EN, Munson RS Jr.** 2013. *Acinetobacter baumannii* utilizes a type VI secretion system for bacterial competition. *PLoS One* **8**:e59388. doi:10.1371/journal.pone.0059388.

108. **Unterweger D, Miyata ST, Bachmann V, Brooks TM, Mullins T, Kostiuk B, Provenzano D, Pukatzki S.** 2014. The *Vibrio cholerae* type VI secretion system employs diverse effector modules for intraspecific competition. *Nat Commun* **5**:3549.

109. **Wenren LM, Sullivan NL, Cardarelli L, Septer AN, Gibbs KA.** 2013. Two independent pathways for self-recognition in *Proteus mirabilis* are linked by type VI-dependent export. *MBio* **4**:e00374-13. doi:10.1128/mBio.00374-13.

110. **Bernard CS, Brunet YR, Gueguen E, Cascales E.** 2010. Nooks and crannies in type VI secretion regulation. *J Bacteriol* **192**:3850–3860.

111. **Shalom G, Shaw JG, Thomas MS.** 2007. *In vivo* expression technology identifies a type VI secretion system locus in *Burkholderia pseudomallei* that is induced upon invasion of macrophages. *Microbiology* **153**:2689–2699.

112. **Parsons DA, Heffron F.** 2005. sciS, an icmF homolog in *Salmonella enterica* serovar Typhimurium, limits intracellular replication and decreases virulence. *Infect Immun* **73**:4338–4345.

113. **Chugani S, Greenberg EP.** 2007. The influence of human respiratory epithelia on *Pseudomonas aeruginosa* gene expression. *Microb Pathog* **42**:29–35.

114. **Sana TG, Hachani A, Bucior I, Soscia C, Garvis S, Termine E, Engel J, Filloux A, Bleves S.** 2012. The second type VI secretion system of *Pseudomonas aeruginosa* strain PAO1 is regulated by quorum sensing and Fur and modulates internalization in epithelial cells. *J Biol Chem* **287**:27095–27105.

115. **Jiang F, Waterfield NR, Yang J, Yang G, Jin Q.** 2014. A *Pseudomonas aeruginosa* type VI secretion phospholipase D effector targets both prokaryotic and eukaryotic cells. *Cell Host Microbe* **15**:600–610.

116. **Fu Y, Waldor MK, Mekalanos JJ.** 2013. Tn-Seq analysis of *Vibrio cholerae* intestinal colonization reveals a role for T6SS-mediated antibacterial activity in the host. *Cell Host Microbe* **14**:652–663.

117. **Yurist-Doutsch S, Arrieta MC, Vogt SL, Finlay BB.** 2014. Gastrointestinal microbiota-mediated control of enteric pathogens. *Annu Rev Genet* **48:**361–382.

118. **Blondel CJ, Jimenez JC, Contreras I, Santiviago CA.** 2009. Comparative genomic analysis uncovers 3 novel loci encoding type six secretion systems differentially distributed in *Salmonella* serotypes. *BMC Genomics* **10:**354.

119. **Petty NK, Bulgin R, Crepin VF, Cerdeno-Tarraga AM, Schroeder GN, Quail MA, Lennard N, Corton C, Barron A, Clark L, Toribio AL, Parkhill J, Dougan G, Frankel G, Thomson NR.** 2010. The *Citrobacter rodentium* genome sequence reveals convergent evolution with human pathogenic *Escherichia coli. J Bacteriol* **192:**525–538.

120. **Suarez G, Sierra JC, Sha J, Wang S, Erova TE, Fadl AA, Foltz SM, Horneman AJ, Chopra AK.** 2008. Molecular characterization of a functional type VI secretion system from a clinical isolate of *Aeromonas hydrophila. Microb Pathog* **44:**344–361.

121. **Zhao J, Schloss PD, Kalikin LM, Carmody LA, Foster BK, Petrosino JF, Cavalcoli JD, VanDevanter DR, Murray S, Li JZ, Young VB, LiPuma JJ.** 2012. Decade-long bacterial community dynamics in cystic fibrosis airways. *Proc Natl Acad Sci USA* **109:**5809–5814.

122. **Gibbs KA, Urbanowski ML, Greenberg EP.** 2008. Genetic determinants of self identity and social recognition in bacteria. *Science* **321:**256–259.

123. **Strassmann JE, Gilbert OM, Queller DC.** 2011. Kin discrimination and cooperation in microbes. *Annu Rev Microbiol* **65:**349–367.

124. **Vos M, Velicer GJ.** 2009. Social conflict in centimeter-and global-scale populations of the bacterium *Myxococcus xanthus. Curr Biol* **19:**1763–1767.

125. **Aoki SK, Diner EJ, de Roodenbeke CT, Burgess BR, Poole SJ, Braaten BA, Jones AM, Webb JS, Hayes CS, Cotter PA, Low DA.** 2010. A widespread family of polymorphic contact-dependent toxin delivery systems in bacteria. *Nature* **468:**439–442.

126. **Aoki SK, Pamma R, Hernday AD, Bickham JE, Braaten BA, Low DA.** 2005. Contact-dependent inhibition of growth in *Escherichia coli. Science* **309:**1245–1248.

127. **Cardarelli L, Saak C, Gibbs KA.** 2015. Two proteins form a heteromeric bacterial self-recognition complex in which variable subdomains determine allele-restricted binding. *MBio* **6:**e00251.

128. **Cornforth DM, Foster KR.** 2013. Competition sensing: the social side of bacterial stress responses. *Nat Rev Microbiol* **11:**285–293.

129. **Lesic B, Starkey M, He J, Hazan R, Rahme LG.** 2009. Quorum sensing differentially regulates *Pseudomonas aeruginosa* type VI secretion locus I and homologous loci II and III, which are required for pathogenesis. *Microbiology* **155:**2845–2855.

130. **West SA, Gardner A.** 2010. Altruism, spite, and greenbeards. *Science* **327:**1341–1344.

131. **Hamilton WD.** 1964. The genetical evolution of social behaviour. I. *J Theor Biol* **7:**1–16.

132. **Borgeaud S, Metzger LC, Scrignari T, Blokesch M.** 2015. The type VI secretion system of *Vibrio cholerae* fosters horizontal gene transfer. *Science* **347:**63–67.

Type VII Secretion: A Highly Versatile Secretion System

13

LOUIS S. ATES,[1] EDITH N. G. HOUBEN,[2] and WILBERT BITTER[1,2]

Bacterial secretion systems were initially studied in the Gram-negative bacterium *Escherichia coli* K-12. When researchers started to explore protein secretion in different Gram-negative bacteria and especially in bacterial pathogens, it was clear that *E. coli* K-12 was not able to present us with a complete picture of protein secretion systems. Type II, type III, and type IV secretion systems were quickly discovered and revolutionized host-pathogen interaction studies. Gram-negative bacteria need these specialized secretion systems to transport proteins across two membranes (also called a diderm cell envelope). The presence of this complex cell envelope not only means that two membranes have to be crossed, but an additional problem is that there is no energy source at the outer membrane. This means that alternative mechanisms for protein transport need to be present, such as coupling the energy of the inner membrane to protein transport across the outer membrane or crossing the entire cell envelope in a single step. Although the discovery of different secretion systems in Gram-negative bacteria was a major breakthrough, the downside has been that secretion systems in other bacteria have been neglected. It was generally thought that secretion in other bacteria, which are generally monoderm, would completely depend on the universal Sec or

[1]Department of Medical Microbiology and Infection Control, VU University Medical Center, Amsterdam, The Netherlands; [2]Section Molecular Microbiology, Amsterdam Institute of Molecules, Medicine and Systems, Vrije Universiteit Amsterdam, 1081 BT Amsterdam, The Netherlands.

Virulence Mechanisms of Bacterial Pathogens, 5th edition
Edited by Indira T. Kudva, Nancy A. Cornick, Paul J. Plummer, Qijing Zhang, Tracy L. Nicholson, John P. Bannantine, and Bryan H. Bellaire
© 2016 American Society for Microbiology, Washington, DC
doi:10.1128/microbiolspec.VMBF-0011-2015

Tat system. Only in recent years has this idea begun shifting, and again it started by studying pathogens, i.e., the pathogenic mycobacteria.

The genus *Mycobacterium* contains a number of important pathogens, including *Mycobacterium tuberculosis* and *Mycobacterium leprae*. These pathogens are generally slow growing and have a distinctive growth pattern, known as cording. Although these bacteria genetically belong to the high-GC Gram-positive bacteria, they produce a second membrane composed of unique and complex lipids (1, 2). The cell envelope of these bacteria is therefore diderm, and protein secretion is as problematic as for Gram-negative bacteria. Among the first identified secreted proteins of *M. tuberculosis* were two

small proteins, known as ESAT-6 and CFP-10 (3). Later they were renamed EsxA and EsxB (4). These proteins lack any obvious canonical secretion signal (Sec or Tat) and therefore seemed to depend on a new secretion system. Detailed analysis of the tuberculosis vaccine strain *Mycobacterium bovis* BCG indicated that this strain had lost not only both the *esxAB* genes, but also several surrounding genes responsible for EsxAB secretion (5, 6). Subsequent research showed that many of the genes surrounding *esxAB* are indeed part of this secretion system (7). This region is now known as the *esx-1* locus and contains 20 genes (Fig. 1). With these genes identified, it quickly became clear that mycobacteria have several of these secretion

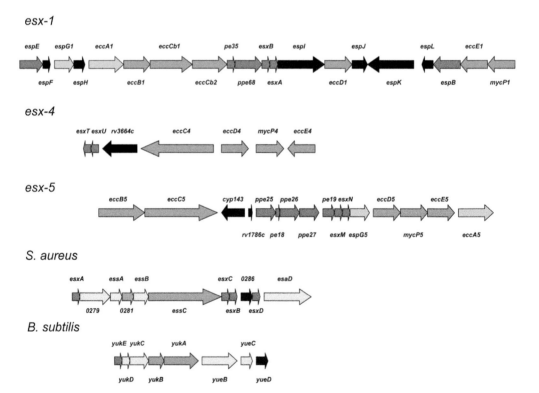

FIGURE 1 Genetic loci of different T7S (and T7S-like) systems. Depicted are the T7S loci, *esx-1*, *esx-4*, and *esx-5* of *M. tuberculosis* H37Rv (101), as well the T7S-like systems of *S. aureus* (strain USA300, annotation based on Anderson et al. [63]) and *B. subtilis* subsp. *subtilis* (strain 168, annotation based on Huppert et al. [12]). Color coding represents conserved T7S membrane components (dark blue), (putative) substrates of the systems (green), cytosolic chaperones (yellow), and *Firmicutes*-specific T7S-like membrane components (light blue).

systems. In fact, up to five different *esx*-loci can be present on the chromosome of mycobacterial species. Recently, additional ESX systems have been identified on conjugative mycobacterial plasmids (8). On these plasmids, the *esx* clusters are located adjacent to a type IV-like secretion cluster, and together they are required for the conjugation process (8).

To emphasize that these ESX systems are required for secretion over the diderm mycobacterial cell envelope, they were named type VII secretion (T7S) (4, 9). In the literature the terms Wss (for WxG100 secretion system) and ESX have been infrequently used, but in this chapter we will use T7S as a general term for these secretion systems and ESX for the different mycobacterial secretion systems. T7S systems are not specific for pathogenic mycobacteria; they are also present in nonpathogenic mycobacteria, and many other bacteria have homologous systems. Most of these bacteria, such as *Rhodococcus*, *Corynebacterium*, and *Nocardia* species, are closely related to mycobacteria and have a similar diderm cell envelope. Probably, the T7S systems of these species are involved in protein secretion as well, although currently there is no data supporting this. An interesting group of T7S homologs is present in several *Firmicutes* species, including many *Bacillus* and *Staphylococcus* species (10). However, these systems are only distantly related since only a homolog of the EccC membrane component (see below) and homolog(s) of the EsxA substrates are present in these bacteria. These latter systems have recently been shown to function as active secretion systems (11, 12). Clearly, there is an evolutionary link between the diderm T7S systems and the newly identified *Firmicutes* secretion systems, but nomenclature could be an issue. Previously, we suggested that they might be called type VIIb systems, analogous to the type IV secretion systems where similar heterogeneity occurs (9). We will comprehensively discuss the mycobacterial T7S systems, which have been studied most intensively, and give an over-view of the similarities with the *Firmicutes* T7S-like secretion systems, with a focus on the nature of the substrates and the conserved secretion signal.

COMPOSITION AND FUNCTIONING OF T7S IN MYCOBACTERIA

T7S gene clusters of *M. tuberculosis* usually share a number of conserved genes that belong to 10 gene families. A general nomenclature for these proteins was agreed on in an early phase (4); the name ESX-conserved component (Ecc) is used for components that are present in most systems, and ESX-1-specific components (Esp) for components that are (mostly) unique for the best-studied secretion system, ESX-1. Finally, for some conserved proteins the old and well-established names were kept, i.e., mycosins (MycP), Esx, and PE and PPE proteins. Within the *esx* loci we can find genes that encode both substrates and structural components. In addition to the Esx proteins, PE and PPE proteins and most Esp proteins are probably substrates. Thus far, there seem to be seven conserved genes that are required for the secretion process and can therefore be considered as core components of the secretion machinery. Two of these core components (EspG and EccA) are localized to the mycobacterial cytosol, while the other five (EccB, EccC, EccD, EccE, and MycP) contain transmembrane domains (TMDs) and reside in the mycobacterial cell envelope (Fig. 2). All *esx* gene clusters contain members of these 10 conserved gene families, except for the most archaic cluster, i.e., *esx-4*, which lacks the *pe*, *ppe*, *espG*, *eccA*, and *eccE* genes (Fig. 1). We will first discuss the two cytosolic conserved components of mycobacterial T7S systems and then the membrane components.

EspG

EspG was initially not considered a T7S core component (4), because these proteins share

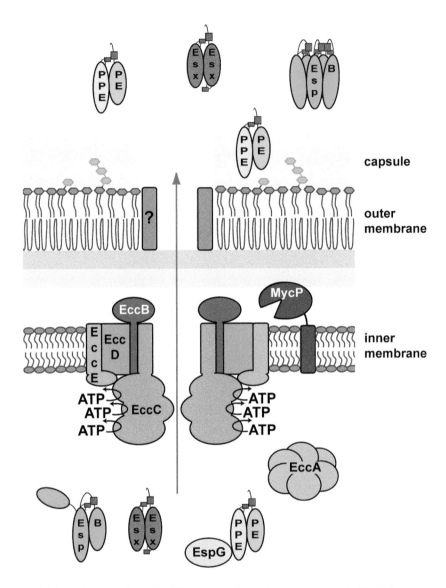

FIGURE 2 Model for T7S in mycobacteria. The conserved membrane components (blue) form a complex in which the EccC homolog is the ATPase possibly providing energy for the secretion process. The mycosin (MycP) is not part of the core complex but is essential for successful secretion. The T7S substrates (green) are secreted dependently on the conserved signals YxxxD/E and WxG (red). Secretion of PE-PPE dimers is dependent on the cytosolic chaperones EspG and EccA (yellow). While EspG binds to the substrate pair in the cytosol, EccA might be involved in releasing this chaperone from the PE-PPE dimer upon contact with the membrane complex. In contrast, Esx proteins are not recognized by EspG, and their dependence on the cytosolic chaperones might be indirect due to interdependence of Esx and PE-PPE for secretion. The EspB monomer has a similar fold to PE-PPE dimers and contains the putative secretion signal. Upon translocation, EspB is processed and forms a heptamer with a barrel-like structure. Whether PE-PPE dimers adopt a similar quaternary structure is yet unknown. Secreted substrates can localize to the culture supernatant or remain attached in the capsular layer. Whether the secretion process is a one- or two-step process is not known, so a putative outer membrane component (gray) is indicated by a question mark.

relative low sequence identity (20 to 25%). However, recent experiments have clearly shown that these proteins are structural and functional equivalents. To acknowledge this, it would be more appropriate to rename this component Esx conserved component, but we realize that the current name is already established and should be kept. The first indication of a role for EspG in secretion was a study describing that EspG$_5$ is required for the secretion of PE-PPE proteins via the ESX-5 system (13, 14). Subsequently, immunoprecipitation experiments showed that EspG$_5$ specifically interacts with the heterodimeric model substrates PE25 and PPE41 (15) (for dimer formation of T7S substrates see below). Additional biophysical analysis of the EspG$_5$-PE25/PPE41 complex showed a tight interaction. Because EspG$_5$ is located in the cytosol and could not be identified in the culture supernatant, it probably dissociates from the substrate pair upon contacting the secretion machinery. Interestingly, the interaction of EspG with PE-PPE proteins shows considerable system specificity, because

EspG$_5$ does not interact with the PE35/PPE68_1 protein pair that is secreted via ESX-1 (15). Conversely, EspG$_1$ of the ESX-1 system does not bind the ESX-5-dependent PE25/PPE41 but does interact with the ESX-1 protein pair PE35/PPE68_1. This suggests that EspG proteins are cytosolic chaperones that specifically recognize their cognate PE-PPE substrates. This component might therefore determine through which T7S system these substrates are transported. The discovery that EspG proteins are PE-PPE-specific chaperones also explains why the *esx-4* locus is lacking *espG*, in addition to *pe* and *ppe* genes.

Recently, crystal structures of EspG$_5$ in complex with PE25/PPE41 were obtained (Fig. 3C) (16, 17). The structures reveal that the EspG$_5$ protein has a novel mixed α/β-fold. The crystal structure of EspG$_3$ of the ESX-3 system was solved in one of these studies (16). Despite the low similarity on the sequence level, EspG$_3$ has a highly similar fold, confirming that these proteins have a similar function. The structure of the EspG$_5$-PE25/

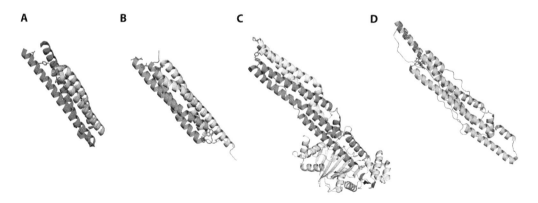

FIGURE 3 Crystal structures of T7S substrates. **(A)** Structure of the heterodimer EsxB (dark blue) and EsxA (light blue) of *M. tuberculosis* (3FAV). The two proteins form a four-helix bundle. The Tyr of the YxxxD motif and the Gly and Trp residues of the WxG motif that are postulated to together constitute the T7S signal are shown in red (54). **(B)** The EsxA protein of *S. aureus* forms a homodimer that results in two putative secretion signals (VxxxD) on each end of the four-helix bundle (red) (2VRZ) (139). **(C)** Crystal structure of PE25 (light blue) and PPE41 (dark blue) of *M. tuberculosis* in complex with the chaperone EspG$_5$ (yellow). EspG interacts with the PPE protein through hydrophobic interactions but not directly with the PE protein. The WxG motif on the PPE and the YxxxE motif on the PE protein together form a putative T7S signal (red residues) (4KXR) (17). **(D)** Crystal structure of monomeric EspB visualizing an extended secretion signal that includes the YxxxD/E and WxG motif (red residues) (3J83) (18).

PPE41 complex shows that EspG$_5$ binds to the tip of the PPE protein, which is not involved in the interaction with the PE protein. This tip region of PPE contains some hydrophobic residues that are now buried in a hydrophobic groove formed by a central β-sheet and C-terminal α-helical bundle of EspG$_5$. Subsequent mutagenesis in the EspG$_5$-recognition motif of various ESX-5 dependent PPE proteins showed that mutations that abolish EspG$_5$ binding *in vitro* usually affect substrate secretion (17). Additionally, coexpression of EspG proteins increased the *in vitro* solubility of PE-PPE pairs, which suggests a role of EspG in keeping these protein pairs soluble. Recently published x-ray diffraction and electron microscopy data of the ESX-1 substrate EspB shows not only that this protein has a highly similar fold as PE-PPE heterodimers (see below, Fig. 3D), but also that it can form pore-like quaternary structures (18). Modeling suggests that EspB could be organized as a heptamer and that the multimerization is mediated by its putative EspG-binding domain. Therefore, the EspG proteins could be responsible for preventing this multimerization from occurring intracellularly. Together, these data suggest that EspG proteins are chaperones involved in substrate recognition and perhaps in preventing their aggregation in the cytosol.

Although the EspG proteins seem to play a central role in recognition of the PE and PPE substrates in the cytosol, they do not interact with the Esx proteins (15). Perhaps the intrinsic solubility of Esx protein pairs makes a role for the EspG chaperone superfluous. EspG might therefore be a dedicated chaperone of PE-PPE proteins (and perhaps several Esp proteins such as EspB) that are more prone to aggregate.

EccA

EccA is the second cytosolic protein encoded by most mycobacterial T7S systems. EccA belongs to the AAA+ (ATPases associated

with various cellular activities) protein family, members of which are involved in diverse processes, including protein degradation, signal transduction, and (dis)assembly of protein complexes. AAA+ proteins typically form ring-shaped hexamers with a central pore. EccA$_1$ also forms oligomers, possibly hexamers, upon overexpression in *E. coli* (19). ATP hydrolysis by these hexamers usually induces a conformational change in the complex that is transferred to the bound substrate(s). All EccA homologs are composed of two conserved domains joined by a linker region. The C-terminal domain of EccA is the ATPase domain and contains all the motifs that are characteristic for AAA+ proteins. In line with this, *in vitro* ATPase activity of EccA$_1$ can be pinpointed to this C-terminal domain (20). The N-terminus of EccA contains six tetratricopeptide repeat motifs, which are known for mediating protein-protein interactions in other proteins (21). The structure of this N-terminal domain of *M. tuberculosis* EccA$_1$ has recently been solved, showing an arrangement of these motifs in a right-handed superhelix (19). Interestingly, the structure of this N-terminal domain of EccA$_1$ resembles the structure of PilF, which is involved in the assembly of the type IV pili system in *Pseudomonas aeruginosa* (19).

EccA is important for T7S, because disruption of *eccA* genes in *esx-1* and *esx-5* clusters results in the loss of secretion of Esx and PE-PPE proteins (22–24). In addition, a mutation in the ATPase domain of EccA$_1$ disrupts secretion (25), and EccA$_3$ is, similar to other core components of the ESX-3 system, essential for viability (26). However, EccA-independent secretion through ESX-1 and ESX-5 (27, 28) (Houben and Bitter, unpublished results) has been observed. These results suggest either that EccA plays different roles in different mycobacterial species/strains or that the function of EccA is redundant in specific cases. Interestingly, EccA is, like EspG, not present in ESX-4. This protein therefore could also play a role in the secretion of specific substrates, such as the PE and PPE proteins. Perhaps analogous to the AAA+ protein in the type VI secretion system, EccA could be involved in the disassembly of EspG chaperones from the PE-PPE dimers (16).

THE T7S MEMBRANE COMPLEX

After synthesis and folding in the cytosol, the T7S substrates should be guided to the inner membrane, where their transport across the mycobacterial cell envelope is initiated. For the other specialized secretion systems, a complex machinery is involved in the actual secretion process. In line with this, all five conserved T7S membrane components (EccB, EccC, EccD, EccE, and MycP) have been shown to be essential for protein secretion by ESX-1 (27, 29, 30), ESX-5, and ESX-3 (22, 27, 31). Most of these membrane components have large N- or C-terminal hydrophilic domains and only one or two predicted TMDs. EccD is the exception. This protein is highly hydrophobic, usually having 11 predicted TMDs and only a relatively small N-terminal hydrophilic part. Based solely on this characteristic, EccD has been postulated to form the membrane pore through which substrates are transported (30), although there is no functional proof of this. The first evidence of the composition of the transport channel was provided by the observation that four of the conserved components of the ESX-5 system (i.e., EccB, EccC, EccD, and EccE) form a stable membrane complex of ~1.5 MDa (27). It is highly likely that this large complex forms the channel through which substrates are transported, although evidence of channel activity has not yet been provided. Because the substrates are probably secreted as (hetero)dimers, the translocation pore should be relatively large to allow passage of these folded structures. Of the four components of the membrane complex, only EccE is not present in all T7S systems; again, ESX-4 lacks this component. This could suggest that this protein is located at the periphery of the complex, which is supported by the observation that EccE is highly sensitive to proteolytic degradation when the membrane complex is treated with trypsin (27).

The presence of classical TMDs with high hydrophobicity predicts that all the Ecc components are inserted in the inner membrane of the mycobacterial cell envelope. Because substrates also need to cross the outer membrane to end up in the extracellular environment, the question remains whether the observed membrane complex also inserts into the outer membrane. The identification of an outer membrane channel is complicated by the fact that our knowledge of mycobacterial outer membrane proteins is limited (32). The only mycobacterial outer membrane protein that has been studied in detail, MspA, does show structural similarity to the outer membrane proteins of Gram-negative bacteria, because MspA spans the outer membrane using short β-sheet transmembrane domains that are organized in a so-called β-barrel. Although the size of the T7S membrane complex would allow it to span both the inner and the outer membrane, none of the subunits have a substantial domain with predicted β-sheets that could form a β-barrel. Perhaps outer membrane transport is mediated by other (unidentified) proteins that more loosely associate with the T7S membrane complex. Of course, other structures, like amphipathic α-helices, such as those involved in formation of the type IV secretion complex (33), could play a role. However, these latter unusual structures are more difficult to predict *in silico*.

Another option is that the T7S system is involved only in transport across the inner membrane and that outer membrane transport depends on a separate transport system, which would mean a two-step process. Although hard evidence for a one-step secretion process across the complex mycobacterial cell envelope is still missing, there is currently also no data showing that the T7S substrates are exposed to the mycobacterial periplasm at any point during the translocation process (34).

EccC

Of the four subunits of the T7S membrane complex, only EccC has predicted functional domains; it contains three conserved nucleotide binding domains (NBDs). EccC is one of the most conserved T7S components; it is not only present in all mycobacterial T7S systems, but is also the only protein that is present in T7S-like systems in *Firmicutes*. Apparently, EccC homologs are central players in these secretion systems. While EccC is usually encoded by a single gene, the homolog in the ESX-1 system of *M. tuberculosis* is composed of two distinct proteins. However, it is most likely that these two EccC subunits together form a functional unit (30) and originated from a single gene. All three predicted NBDs of EccC show homology to members of the FtsK/SpoIIIE family of ATPases. This large protein family consists of ATPases that are involved in a wide range of cellular processes, of which FtsK and SpoIIIE, which are involved in DNA transport (35), are the best studied. Similar to the AAA+ ATPases, FtsK/SpoIIIE-like ATPases usually form ring-like hexamers, which suggests that EccC is functional as a hexameric complex as well. However, because EccC has three successive FtsK/SpoIIIE-like ATP-binding domains instead of one, this protein could have different characteristics.

Other type IV secretion systems also contain a member of the FtsK/SpoIIIE protein family, the type IV coupling protein. This protein plays a key role in substrate recognition and protein transport (36). Possibly, EccC performs similar functions in T7S by recognizing chaperone-substrate complexes at the membrane. Accordingly, EccC of the ESX-1 system was shown to interact with the substrate EsxB in both immunoprecipitation and yeast two-hybrid experiments. This interaction was dependent on the presence of the C-terminal secretion signal of EsxB (37).

Although EccC proteins have three NBDs (38), mutational analysis of individual NBDs of EccC molecules of both mycobacteria and *Firmicutes* suggests distinct roles of each domain in secretion; while ATP binding to the first domain is essential for secretion, the other two domains are not strictly required for protein transport (39). In addition, ATP binding to any of the three NBDs of $EccC_5$ does not seem to be required for formation of the ESX-5 membrane complex (39), suggesting that ATP hydrolysis by EccC is not involved in complex assembly, but that it is dedicated to substrate recognition and/or transport.

Recent structural analysis of EccC from the thermophilic actinobacterium *Thermomonospora curvata* (*Tc*) with and without bound substrate *Tc*EsxB provides important insight to the role of the individual NBDs in substrate recognition and transport (40). In this study, Rosenberg et al. described the structure of *Tc*EccC in complex with a peptide representing the *Tc*EsxB secretion signal, revealing that the signal binds to a hydrophobic pocket of NBD3, while both NBD2 and NBD3 were bound to ATP (Fig. 4). In contrast, NBD1 is visualized in a nucleotide-free state, suggesting that NBD2 and NBD3 are relatively inefficient ATPases. The hydrophobic binding pockets of NBD1 and NBD2 do not bind the secretion signal but are filled by a linker region of the adjacent NBD3. Mutating the linker of NBD2 that binds NBD1 (R543A) subsequently activated ATPase activity by NBD1, and this activity is increased upon binding of *Tc*EsxB to NBD3. These results suggest that substrate binding activates a chain of events leading to ATPase activation. In line with the previously obtained data in mycobacteria and *Bacillus subtilis* (38, 39), the authors showed that mutations in catalytic residues of NBD1 completely abolished ATP hydrolysis, while similar mutations in NBD2 and NBD3 only reduced this activity. Rosenberg et al. provide evidence that *Tc*EccC (R543A) multimerizes *in vitro* upon binding of *Tc*EsxB, indicating that this substrate triggers both ATPase

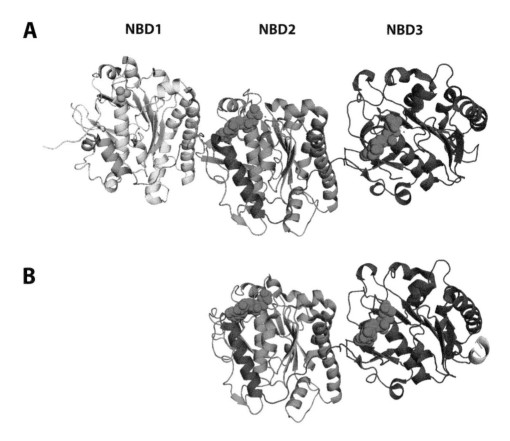

A   NBD1   NBD2   NBD3

B

FIGURE 4 **Crystal structures of EccC of *Thermomonospora curvata*. C-terminal domains of *Tc*EccC containing all three NBDs (A) or containing only NBD2 and NBD3 and with a bound secretion signal of *Tc*EsxB (B) are shown as described by Rosenberg et al. (40). The secretion signal (in green) is bound to a hydrophobic pocket of NBD3. While NBD2 and NBD3 have a bound ATP molecule (red), NBD1 has a sulfate ion at the ATP binding site instead (in orange). NBD1 activity is inhibited by a linker domain of NBD2. This inhibition can be alleviated by changing arginine 543 (the orange residue) to an alanine.**

activity and multimerization. However, addition of *Tc*EsxA, most likely the binding partner of *Tc*EsxB, abolishes both multimerization and ATPase activity of this *Tc*EccC construct. How the *in vitro* multimerization of EccC correlates with the settings in the bacterial cell, where EccC is already multimeric as part of a large membrane complex (27), remains to be investigated.

Mycosin

The only conserved membrane protein of T7S systems that is not part of the ESX-5 membrane complex is mycosin (MycP). Mycosins are subtilisin-like proteases with

a classical signal sequence that presumably directs the protease domain to the periplasm. In addition, mycosins have a putative C-terminal TMD to anchor the protein in the membrane (41, 42). Although mycosins are essential for T7S, their role in secretion is still an enigma. The only known substrate for any mycosin is the ESX-1 substrate EspB, which is an ESX-1 secreted protein cleaved by $MycP_1$ (43). In addition, structural analysis of EspB with and without the C-terminus that is cleaved by $MycP_1$ shows that $MycP_1$ might be involved in inducing a conformational change of the EspB quaternary structure (18). Although this finding suggests that mycosins are involved in substrate processing, the proteolytic activity of MycP$_1$ seems to be dispensable for the secretion process (43). Similarly, MycP$_5$ of the ESX-5 system is essential for ESX-5-dependent secretion, but its protease activity is not (van Winden, Houben, and Bitter, unpublished results). This surprising observation suggests that mycosins have a second role in secretion, besides their function as a protease. Further research is needed to understand this crucial additional role of mycosins in T7S.

Recently, the structures of both *Mycobacterium smegmatis* and *Mycobacterium thermoresistibile* MycP$_1$ were solved, which show a typical subtilisin core domain decorated with several extended loops (44, 45). The most distinctive structural feature of mycosins is the presence of an N-terminal extension. Many subtilisins are produced with an N-terminal extension, called a propeptide, that prevents premature substrate access to the active site (46). However, classical subtilisin propeptides form a tightly folded structure near the active site, and this propeptide is usually degraded by the subtilisin-like proteases after folding and/or transport. The N-terminal extension of mycosins does not display homology with subtilisin propeptides and is structurally different as well, because it is wrapped around the protease domain and does not block the active site (44, 45). In addition, MycP$_1$ with an intact N-terminal extension is able to cleave EspB *in vitro* (44, 45). Therefore, the term "propeptide" for this N-terminal extension of mycosins is probably incorrect. Interestingly, the structure of *M. smegmatis* MycP$_3$ was solved, revealing a very similar fold of the protease domain to the MycP$_1$ structure, including the N-terminal extension (45). The properties of the active site clefts are quite distinct between these two mycosins, suggesting different substrate specificities.

T7S SUBSTRATES

Although the different T7S systems that have been studied in detail secrete different classes of substrates, most of these substrates belong to the EsxAB clan (Pfam CL0352) (47). This clan contains six protein families: Esx (WxG100), PE, PPE, LXG, DUF2563, and DUF2580. The best known of these is the Esx family. The first Esx protein that was discovered is the EsxA (ESAT-6) protein of *M. tuberculosis*, which is secreted as a heterodimer together with EsxB (CFP-10). Since then, members of this protein family have been described over a wide range of species, mostly in the phyla *Actinobacteria* and *Firmicutes* (11, 48), but have also been found in *Verrucomicrobia*, *Lentisphaerae*, *Planctomycetes*, *Chloroflexi*, and even some in *Proteobacteria* (47). Esx proteins are also called WxG100 proteins (10), based on a short conserved motif, tryptophan-X-glycine (WxG), in the middle of the protein and their typical size of approximately 100 amino acids (Fig. 3A). Esx proteins form two helices separated by a turn, which contains the conserved WxG motif. Although most Esx proteins are small, some contain an extended C-terminal domain. The C-terminal domains of these extended WxG100 proteins are highly variable and, although largely uncharacterized, are predicted to have highly divergent functions. Esx proteins of mycobacteria, such as EsxA and EsxB, are secreted as antiparallel heterodimers (49, 50). These cosecreted dimers are usually encoded by adjacent genes and are part of the same operon (51). In contrast, some Esx proteins from *Streptococcus* (52) and *Staphylococcus* (53) exclusively form homodimers and are encoded by genes that are generally monocistronic (Fig. 3B). It has been suggested that the bicistronic heterodimers evolved after a duplication event, which suggests that the original substrates were homodimers (54).

The structure of the EsxAB complex (55) shows that the N- and C-termini of both EsxA and EsxB are predominantly unstructured. The longest of these unordered stretches, the C-terminus of EsxB, merits special attention since this region has been shown to contain a secretion motif that is required for secretion (see below). The overall structure of Esx dimers is also observed for other Esx proteins, such as EsxGH (56) and EsxRS (57).

PE and PPE Proteins

Two other major classes of the T7S substrates belonging to the EsxAB clan are the PE and PPE proteins. Although they belong to different protein families, these proteins form secreted heterodimers and, similar to the mycobacterial Esx substrates, their genes are often located adjacently on the genome. Therefore, they will be discussed together in this section. PE proteins are named for their conserved proline-glutamic acid motifs at positions 8 and 9 of the N-terminus of these proteins, whereas PPE proteins are defined by a proline-proline-glutamic acid motif at positions 7 to 9. PE and PPE proteins have only been described in members of the phylum *Actinobacteria* and are most widespread in the slow-growing species of mycobacteria (58). The structure of PE25 of *M. tuberculosis* in complex with PPE41 has been solved by Strong and colleagues (59) and shows an antiparallel dimer forming a four-helix bundle, similar to that of the Esx proteins. The recently solved crystal structure of EspB has revealed that this protein is similar to a PE-PPE dimer (Fig. 3D) (18). Interestingly, this protein multimerizes as a heptamer, indicating that a similar confirmation could be formed by PE-PPE dimers.

PE proteins are characterized by a conserved N-terminal PE domain of approximately 110 amino acids, which forms a helix-turn-helix structure similar to the Esx proteins, but the turn is less defined compared to the Esx proteins and does not contain the WxG motif. The PE domain interacts with a PPE domain through conserved apolar residues that establish strong hydrophobic interactions (59). A secretion motif in the mostly unstructured C-terminal domain of PE proteins is, similar to EsxB, essential for secretion (54, 60). While the genes coding for the most ancient PE

proteins are located within the *esx* loci and mostly consist of only the PE domain, more recently evolved members of this protein family have (large) extended C-terminal domains. For instance, *M. tuberculosis* contains 99 genes encoding PE proteins, of which 69 belong to the PE_PGRS group, named after polymorphic GC-rich repetitive sequences that code for the C-terminal domains. These C-terminal domains are composed of glycine-rich repeats and can be up to 1,550 residues long. These long PE proteins are secreted to the cell surface by a T7S system (i.e., the ESX-5 system) as well.

The PPE domain, with approximately 180 amino acids, is slightly larger than the PE domain and contains five α-helices. The three N-terminal α-helices interact with the PE partner protein. A typical WxG motif is present in the turn between the second and the third α-helix, similar to that of the ESX proteins. The fourth and fifth α-helices also pair together to form an extension of the PE-PPE dimer. This extended region forms the interaction site for the EspG chaperone (15, 17). Similar to PE proteins, PPE proteins can have (largely) extended C-terminal domains.

As mentioned previously, the interaction of the PPE41 protein with EspG$_5$ is mediated by the conserved hydrophobic tip of the PPE proteins, mostly formed by α-4 and α-5. Bioinformatic analysis suggests that PPE proteins secreted by the different ESX systems in mycobacteria can be grouped on the basis of these conserved residues in the hydrophobic patch (17), and this phenomenon could explain how the EspG chaperones establish system specificity (15). Thus far, the PE and PPE proteins are the only T7S substrates shown to require such a specific chaperone.

Other T7S Substrates

The EsxAB clan also contains the DUF2563, DUF2580, and LxG families. The first of these is a small *Mycobacterium*-specific protein family about which not much is known.

Members of the second family, DUF2580, are restricted to the mycobacteria as well, but some members of this family are T7S substrates: both the ESX-1 substrates EspC and EspF belong to this family. Interestingly, the genes encoding these substrates are located in an operon with genes encoding other T7S substrates, i.e., EspA and EspE, respectively. Although EspA and EspE do not officially belong to the EsxAB clan, the structure prediction program (Phyre2) (61) predicts with high confidence a helix-turn-helix domain at the N-terminus of these proteins, with Esx proteins as the best template. Therefore, these proteins possibly form heterodimers with EspC and EspF. Another known ESX-1 substrate is EspB. Recently, the structure of this protein was elucidated, which showed that it has an N-terminal helix-turn-helix motif followed by a T7S signal motif (see below and Fig. 3D) (60). The major surprise was that the adjacent region of this domain showed structural homology to PPE proteins, which means that this protein forms a four-helix bundle by itself and therefore could be secreted as a monomer. The study by Solomonson et al. (18) further shows that these monomeric structures multimerize as a heptamer with a barrel-shaped structure. This suggests that PE-PPE dimers could form similar quaternary structures, which might have important implications to predict their functions.

Firmicutes have different T7S substrates as well, both EsxAB-like proteins and proteins that do not seem to belong to the EsxAB clan. Recently, in *Staphylococcus aureus* two new substrates were identified with the somewhat misleading names EsxC and EsxD. Although they officially do not belong to the EsxAB clan (and therefore also not to the Esx family), again structure prediction indicates a helix-turn-helix motif.

The final and perhaps most intriguing protein family within the EsxAB clan is LxG. This recently described extended protein family contains diverse proteins, including (putative) endonucleases and toxins (62). These members have an N-terminal LxG domain and a nuclease domain (SUKH family) at the C-terminus. Members of this family are mainly found in the *Firmicutes*. Unfortunately, secretion of these proteins has not been studied. However, because they belong to the EsxAB clan, secretion via T7S seems likely. Supporting this prediction is the observation that homologs of SUKH endonucleases in other bacteria have different N-terminal domains that are linked to secretion; in *Proteobacteria* they are predicted to be secreted via the two-step secretion pathway, and in *Actinobacteria*, via a classical (Sec/Tat) secretion pathway.

T7S Signal

How are the T7S substrates recognized, and what determines system specificity? The first indication of a secretion signal was identified for the EsxAB dimer. Deletion of the unstructured C-terminal tail of EsxB completely blocked secretion (37). Furthermore, in the same study it was shown that in yeast two-hybrid experiments the C-terminal tail of EsxB interacts with the EccC protein of ESX-1. This first study could not identify crucial residues within this C-terminal tail, but later it was shown that there was indeed a conserved consensus, albeit slightly more upstream (60). The presence of a C-terminal secretion signal was also shown for other T7S substrates, including EspC and PE25. Detailed analysis showed that two residues within the C-terminal tail of PE25 are crucial and that the spacing between these residues is important as well. The identified signal, YxxxD/E, is crucial for the secretion of Esx, PE, and Esp proteins in mycobacteria (60). If we look at all T7S substrates from different organisms, a broader consensus must be used, as described by Poulsen *et al.* (54). Interestingly, although the secretion signal was first identified in the unstructured C-terminal tail of T7S substrates, more recent structural studies of Esx, PE, and EspB proteins showed that this signal is part of the elongated second helix. In these structures the two crucial residues, i.e., tyrosine and the acidic amino acid, are located on the same side of the helix (54). Furthermore, the tyrosine is positioned close to the conserved tryptophan residue of the WxG motif in the turn region of the dimer partner. It has been suggested that this tryptophan residue is therefore also part of the secretion signal (54). Because the deletion of several C-terminal residues beyond the YxxxD/E motif is already enough to block secretion, the signal probably extends at least 10 amino acids further than the consensus sequence, but without any clear conserved features.

Recent data (40) indicate that this unstructured tail is recognized by the C-terminal domain of EccC and is responsible for the multimerization of EccC. Probably, a similar secretion signal is present for T7S substrates in *Firmicutes*, but the role in secretion has not been studied in the same detail. Although the C-terminus was shown to be important for these *Firmicutes* substrates, the wrong amino acids were examined (i.e., an erroneous YxxxD/E motif), without any effect (54, 63).

One puzzling observation is that exchange of the secretion signal between an ESX-1 and an ESX-5 substrate restores secretion but does not redirect the substrate to another secretion system. Therefore, this secretion signal does not seem to determine system specificity. Apparently, a second signal is required for this. For the PE-PPE heterodimeric complex this second signal is probably provided by the chaperone EspG, which was shown to specifically recognize substrates of the cognate secretion system. However, it is still unknown what characteristic of the Esx dimers determines their systems' specificity.

Other major questions concerning substrates and substrate specificity remain. For instance, the large majority of PE and PPE proteins in mycobacteria seem to be without an obvious partner protein. Are they secreted as single proteins, or are they also secreted as a heterodimer with an unknown partner? Furthermore, many of these PE and PPE proteins contain large C-terminal extensions. A good example is LipY, one of the few PE-PPE proteins with a known function. This protein contains a PE domain in *M. tuberculosis*, a PPE domain in *Mycobacterium marinum*, and a classical signal peptide in the fast-growing *Mycobacterium gilvum* (13). Interestingly, whereas both the PE and PPE domain were shown to be interchangeable for secretion to the cell surface via T7S, exchange for a classical signal sequence did not result in surface localization. What is interesting to note is that many of the WxG (and LxG) proteins in *Actinobacteria* and *Firmicutes* have C-terminal protein domains with described functions as well, indicating that there might be overlapping structural and mechanistic similarities between these proteins and the PE-PPE proteins. Unfortunately, no protein structures are known for these putative substrates, and therefore many questions about the folding, chaperones, secretion partners, and functions of these proteins remain.

THE ROLE OF T7S SYSTEMS IN VIRULENCE

ESX-1 System of Pathogenic Mycobacteria

The specific roles of T7S systems and their substrates have been best described in mycobacteria. The ESX-1 system of *M. tuberculosis* was the first T7S system identified; this region was lost when *M. bovis* was cultured for 11 years by Calmette and Guerin to create the live attenuated-vaccine strain *M. bovis* BCG (51, 64). It was named region of difference 1 (RD1), and Pym et al. showed that this region is (mainly) responsible for the attenuation of *M. bovis* BCG and the vole bacillus *Mycobacterium microti* (65).

Since then, the importance of the ESX-1 system for the virulence of mycobacteria has been strongly established (29, 66–68), but the role of the individual secreted substrates has been more difficult to investigate. The first ESX-1 substrates that were identified were EsxA and EsxB (3), which are major secreted proteins and dominant T-cell antigens. As such, they were regarded as the principle substrates and responsible for the attenuation of *M. bovis* BCG. The EsxA protein seemed to be the prime candidate for mediating phagosomal escape (see below). Later it was shown that more proteins are secreted via this system; these proteins are known as ESX-1-associated proteins (Esp). EspA and EspB, in particular, seem to be involved in virulence as well (18, 69–71). A complicating factor in determining the role of individual components in virulence is their codependence for secretion. Secretion of EspA and possibly EspB is shown to be linked to functional secretion of EsxAB and vice versa (68). Redirection of ESX-1 substrates through other T7S systems could help to solve this conundrum.

Virulence

Although the interdependence of ESX-1 substrates makes the study of individual substrates difficult, major steps have been taken to elucidate the function of ESX-1 and its substrates in virulence. The ESX-1 system plays an important role in the macrophage infection cycle of pathogenic mycobacteria. Several species of *Mycobacteria*, including *M. tuberculosis*, *M. marinum*, and *M. leprae*, have been shown to translocate from the phagosome to the cytosol in late stages of the macrophage infection cycle (72). Upon translocation to the cytosol, bacteria start to replicate and ultimately induce a necrosis-like cell death. After necrosis of the host cell the bacteria can spread to neighboring macrophages within the host (73). Therefore, escape into the cytosol is essential for full virulence. This crucial step is dependent on a functional ESX-1 system (72), since phagosomal escape is not observed for *M. bovis* BCG or *esx-1* mutants of *M. tuberculosis* and *M. marinum* (72, 74). Furthermore, it has also

been shown that mycobacteria can lyse erythrocytes in an ESX-1- and contact-dependent manner (24, 75). This phenomenon is seen as a direct effect of the membrane-disrupting potential of ESX-1 substrates (75, 76). Several studies have implicated EsxA as the main membrane-disrupting protein of the ESX-1 system (76, 77), although some questions remain. Most importantly, EsxA and EsxB are present in nonpathogenic mycobacteria as well as pathogenic mycobacteria and seem to have similar functions (78). Furthermore, *Mycobacterium kansasii* has several subtypes, of which only one shows phagosomal escape and a concomitant increased virulence. Avirulent subtypes of *M. kansasii* do efficiently secrete EsxA (74). Perhaps different ESX-1-dependent substrates are together required for phagosome escape. EspA would be an important candidate for this, since this protein is highly upregulated within the phagosomal environment. Another important substrate is EspB, which was shown to be crucial for the virulence of *M. marinum*. Interestingly, this protein forms ring-shaped heptamers with a hydrophobic domain (18). As such, it could be involved in perturbation of host cell membranes.

In *M. marinum*, ESX-1 proteins have been shown to localize in the capsular layer at the cell surface (2). This surface localization of ESX-1 substrates would be in line with the membrane-disrupting capacities of mycobacteria (79). Whether this phenomenon is the same for *M. tuberculosis* remains to be established. Furthermore, the components of the ESX-1 machinery have been shown to be localized to the cell poles of multiple species of mycobacteria (80, 81). The ESX-1 system and its substrates seem to be enriched in new cell poles with active peptidoglycan synthesis, indicating that there might be a role for the ESX-1 system in cell wall growth (81).

ESX-1 Regulation

The ESX-1 system is active in culture medium but is upregulated when mycobacteria encounter host cells. This process is regulated by multiple transcriptional regulators. The best-described transcriptional regulator is the two-component sensor kinase PhoPR system. The PhoPR system is activated by a decrease in pH (82), as well as increased Cl⁻ concentration (83), which are conditions that occur in maturing phagosomes. The avirulent *M. tuberculosis* strain H37Ra contains a single point mutation in the DNA binding domain of PhoP, which abrogates DNA binding and results in reduced virulence (84). PhoP was later shown to regulate secretion of ESX-1 indirectly through regulation of the *espACD* locus (85).

Another gene that is part of the PhoP regulon is *whiB6* (*Rv3862c*), which is a transcriptional regulator situated in close genetic proximity to the *esx-1* gene cluster (86). In clinical *M. tuberculosis* strains, PhoP binds to the promoter region of *whiB6*, which induces transcription. Increased production of WhiB6 positively regulates the expression of several *esx-1* genes and in that way is able to increase ESX-1 secretion. Point mutations in the promoter region of *whiB6* in laboratory strains H37Rv and H37Ra result in an inverted regulation of *whiB6* by PhoP, making PhoP a negative regulator of ESX-1 secretion (86).

The *espACD* operon is also regulated by other factors, one of which is EspR. This protein was discovered as a regulator of ESX-1 secretion and was first hypothesized to be an ESX-1 substrate itself (87) but was later confirmed to be a more general nucleoid-associated protein that is not secreted (88). EspR is a transcriptional regulator with a unique helix-turn-helix structure and a C-terminal domain that is essential for dimerization. In its dimerized form it binds two specific operator sites situated 177 bp apart, thereby probably creating a loop in the promoter region of e*spACD* (89).

Finally, the *espACD* operon is also regulated by the two-component regulator MprAB (69) and the regulator Lsr2 (90). Altogether, a picture is emerging of a secretion system that is tightly regulated by multiple layers of regulation adapted to different conditions. These networks can be highly relevant for the virulence capacities of clinical strains, since small mutations in regulators or promoter regions can have significant effects on virulence (84, 91).

Role of ESX-1 and T7S in Horizontal Gene Transfer

Although the role of the ESX-1 system in pathogenic mycobacteria is tightly linked with intracellular routing and host cell death, a completely different role has been described in *M. smegmatis*. This bacterium is capable of horizontal gene transfer, in which large genomic fragments are exchanged between different strains (reviewed in reference 92). This process is an atypical form of conjugation and is called distributive conjugal transfer. Interestingly, this process is dependent on ESX-1 in different and opposing ways: *esx-1* mutants of donor strains are shown to be hyperconjugative (78), whereas *esx-1* mutants in the recipient strains are hypoconjugative (93). This paradoxical dual role of ESX-1 in mycobacteria has not been mechanistically explained yet, but it will be interesting to discover if DNA is transported through this T7S system or if secreted proteins located at the cell surface play a role in cell-cell adhesion. An interesting observation is that the hyperconjugative phenotype of the *M. smegmatis esx-1* mutants can be complemented with its *M. tuberculosis* counterparts. However, distributive conjugal transfer has not been described in *M. tuberculosis* or other slow-growing mycobacteria (94, 95).

The ESX-1 system of *M. smegmatis* is not the only ESX system that has been linked to DNA transport. Recently, a conjugative plasmid (pRAW) was discovered in *M. marinum* (8). This plasmid efficiently conjugated between different slow-growing species of *Mycobacteria*, including *M. tuberculosis*. No conjugation to fast-growing mycobacteria was observed, indicating specific genetic requirements for recipient strains. The pRAW plasmid was shown to contain a newly identified T7S system called ESX-P1. This ESX system was shown to be essential for conjugal transfer of pRAW. ESX-P1 has the highest homology with the ESX-5 system (8).

ESX-3

The ESX-3 system is essential for the growth of *M. tuberculosis*, as was shown by both directed mutagenesis and saturated transposon mutagenesis (26, 96). ESX-3 is regulated by iron- and zinc-dependent transcription regulators ideR (97) and Zur (FurB) (98). Siegrist et al. have shown that expression of the *esx-3* system is highly upregulated when iron chelators are added to the growth medium (99). Additionally, several groups have reported that ESX-3 is essential for growth only under iron-limiting conditions (99, 100). It is postulated that a functional ESX-3 system is crucial for the uptake of iron via mycobactin, a siderophore produced by mycobacteria, but a mechanism for this phenomenon remains to be elucidated. In conditions of high zinc availability, the essentiality of ESX-3 can be rescued as well. The most efficient complementation of ESX-3 essentiality is achieved by supplementing both iron and zinc, which suggests that mycobactin uptake is not the only function of the ESX-3 system (100). There seems to be only a partial correlation of functional ESX-3 secretion and mycobactin uptake, indicating that the role of ESX-3 is probably broader than metal ion acquisition. It is somewhat counterintuitive that a protein secretion system should be involved in the uptake of metal ions, but perhaps ESX-3 substrates play a role in the uncoupling of the Fe-mycobactin complex or in the actual binding of this siderophore at the cell surface.

The only known substrates of the ESX-3 system are EsxG and EsxH, which are both encoded by the *esx3* locus itself. These two proteins are secreted as a heterodimer, just like their ESX-1 homologs EsxAB. Two other putative ESX-3 substrates are PE5 and PPE4,

which are encoded by the *esx-3* cluster and which are also essential. However, experimental evidence for the secretion of these proteins via ESX-3 is lacking.

ESX-5

The ESX-5 system is probably the most recently evolved T7S system in mycobacteria and is only present in slow-growing species (58). The slow-growing mycobacteria include most pathogenic species, such as *M. tuberculosis*, *M. leprae*, *M. marinum*, *Mycobacterium ulcerans*, and *Mycobacterium avium*. The evolution of the ESX-5 system, probably through a duplication of the *esx-2* gene cluster, was followed by a large expansion of the *pe* and *ppe* genes in species such as *M. tuberculosis* (101) and *M. marinum*. Genomic analysis suggests that ESX-5 could be responsible for the secretion of most PE and PPE proteins and that the ESX-5 system plays an important role in virulence and/or the slow-growing phenotype of mycobacteria. Different biochemical methods have experimentally validated the first hypothesis; indeed, many PE and PPE proteins of *M. marinum* and *M. tuberculosis* are secreted via ESX-5, especially the recently evolved subclasses of PE and PPE proteins, such as the PE-PGRS and PPE-MPTR proteins (14).

After secretion these proteins can be identified mainly at the cell surface but also in the culture filtrate (14, 22, 102). There are indications that a number of these surface-localized PE-PPE proteins play a direct role in virulence by interacting with host immune receptors, such as Toll-like receptor (TLR) 2 and the inflammasome (reviewed in reference 103), but recent data indicate that there could be an important second role for ESX-5 substrates. Just like for ESX-3, the membrane components of the ESX-5 system are essential for the *in vitro* growth of *M. bovis* BCG, *M. marinum* (39), and *M. tuberculosis* H37Rv on culture plate or broth (96, 104). However, this essentiality is not observed in all *M. tuberculosis* strains; for instance, in CDC1551 *esx-5* mutations can be readily identified (22, 27). Recent data could explain this apparent discrepancy; the essentiality of *esx-5* is linked to the permeability of the outer membrane. The ESX-5 system is no longer essential when outer membrane permeability is increased, either by mutations in lipid biosynthesis or by the introduction of the pore-forming protein MspA from *M. smegmatis*. Slow-growing mycobacteria do not produce MspA-like pores and as such probably need alternative mechanisms for nutrient transport over the outer membrane. The ESX-5 system and its substrates are responsible for the uptake of fatty acids and probably other nutrients (39). The expression of MspA-like pores makes mycobacteria more vulnerable to defense systems of the host (105), which suggests that the slow-growing mycobacteria utilize ESX-5 substrates to acquire nutrients while maintaining resistance against bactericidal host factors.

In *M. marinum*, *esx-5* mutants with a strongly reduced secretion phenotype (recall that knock-out mutants are not viable) are attenuated in cell-infection experiments and show delayed phagosomal escape. The ESX-5 system also seems to be involved in inducing cell death through inflammasome activation via an unknown mechanism (106). An *espG₅* transposon mutant of *M. marinum* is attenuated in zebra fish embryo experiments, but surprisingly, this mutant is hypervirulent in adult zebra fish (107). This hypervirulence is characterized by increased bacterial numbers in the organs, an altered pro-inflammatory cytokine response, and more severe immunopathology (107). This suggests that the ESX-5 system might be responsible for manipulation of the adaptive immune response, which is not developed in zebra fish embryos. However, the same effect was observed in $rag^{-/-}$ zebra fish that lacked B-cells and T-cells, indicating that antigen-specific adaptive immune responses are probably not responsible for the hypervirulence of the *esx-5* mutant. Additionally, expression of dormancy-related genes was not clearly

affected in the *esx-5* mutant strain, indicating that hypervirulence is not due to an inability to enter the dormant phase of infection (107). In contrast to these results, Bottai et al. (22) showed that an *eccD₅* mutant of *M. tuberculosis* has reduced cell wall integrity and is significantly attenuated in a SCID mouse model.

One of the few ESX-5 substrates with a well-studied and -defined function is the LipY protein. This protein is a PE protein in *M. tuberculosis* but a PPE protein in *M. marinum*, illustrating that the PE-PPE domains are probably not involved in the function of these proteins but are responsible for the secretion (13, 102). LipY is a lipase, which can efficiently degrade long chain triacylglycerols that are present in the host cell or stored inside the mycobacteria (108, 109). Utilization of triacylglycerols is important during latent infection, and expression of LipY is upregulated in *in vitro* models of dormancy (109). *M. bovis* BCG overexpressing *lipY* was shown to lose its capacity to induce protection against *M. tuberculosis* (110), and an *M. tuberculosis* strain which overexpressed LipY was hypervirulent in a mouse model (111). These data indicate that LipY is an important virulence factor in *M. tuberculosis*.

PE_PGRS

As mentioned previously, the major group of PE proteins is the so-called PE_PGRS proteins, which are characterized by a long C-terminal region with glycine-rich repeats. Notably, PE_PGRS proteins are not present in all ESX-5-containing mycobacteria. *M. avium* and *Mycobacterium xenopi*, fo instance, do not contain any PE_PGRS protein (58). PE_PGRS proteins have been hypothesized to be involved in several pathogenesis-related or immunological mechanisms. The PE_PGRS wag22 was proposed to contain a C-terminal fragment with fibronectin binding properties (112). In a subsequent study the *wag22* gene was shown to be a vaccine candidate that prevents reactivation of *M. tuberculosis* infection in a mouse model (113). PE-PGRS proteins have also been proposed to protect against proteasomal degradation and therefore reduced activation of CD8$^+$ T-cells (114, 115). The glycine-alanine-rich repeat regions of PE_PGRS proteins are similar in composition to the EBNA1 protein of the human Epstein-Barr virus. The EBNA1 protein was shown to be a virulence factor of Epstein-Barr virus that is able to block its own proteasomal processing (116), and the same phenomenon was shown for PE_PGRS proteins, suggesting a role in immune evasion for these proteins (114, 115). However, in recent publications it has been shown that repetitive protein sequences of EBNA1 are not involved in preventing antigenic presentation. Instead, expression of these proteins seems to be self-limited by the mRNA sequence coding for these proteins, which is very rich in purines. These unstructured, purine-rich mRNA sequences make translation efficiencies high enough to create sufficient protein levels for infection but low enough to avoid immune recognition (117, 118). These results question the function of PE_PGRS proteins in blocking epitope processing.

The PE_PGRS proteins have also been hypothesized to be a source of antigenic variation in mycobacteria (119). However, a conserved hierarchy of immune recognition of various PE-PPE proteins suggests that differential immune responses are driven not by antigenic variation but by infection-stage-specific expression of these proteins (120). Additionally, sequencing of multiple clinical strains and their *pe_pgrs* sequences has led to the observation that *pe_pgrs* diversity as a whole is not driven by antigenic pressure (121, 122). In fact, bio-informatic analysis indicates that the PE_PGRS proteins contain very few epitopes. Of the 1,649 known epitopes of *M. tuberculosis*, only 3 are situated in the PGRS domain of PE_PGRS proteins (121). Nonetheless, there seems to be antigenic pressure on some of the *pe_pgrs*

genes, while others seem to evolve neutrally. This suggests that the group of PE_PGRS proteins may not be as homogenous as sometimes thought and that individual genes or subgroups of these genes and proteins of these groups need to be examined for their biological roles.

One of the PE_PGRS proteins that has been studied in more detail is PE_PGRS33 (*Rv1818c*). Polymorphisms in *pe_pgrs33*, including large insertions, deletions, or truncations, correlate with an absence of lung cavities in patients (123). As shown for other PE proteins, the PE domain of PE_PGRS33 is necessary for the surface localization of this protein (124, 125). The PGRS domain of PE_PGRS33 is shown to localize to the mitochondria of the host cell and is able to induce apoptosis (126). Surprisingly, the full-length PE_PGRS33 was also able to induce necrosis, showing that the PE and linker domains can perform additional functions in this mechanism. Another study showed that PE_PGRS33 was able to induce host-cell apoptosis by specifically binding to the TLR2 (127).

Together, these data show that the PE_PGRS proteins are important manipulators of the host immune response. However, the role of the PE_PGRS proteins remains to be fully elucidated. Understanding the role of these proteins will be a major step in increasing our knowledge of *M. tuberculosis* and will most likely contribute to our understanding of disease pathogenesis as well as vaccine design.

TYPE VII(-LIKE) SECRETION IN MONODERM BACTERIAL SPECIES

T7S systems are widely present in mycobacteria and closely related bacteria. Mycobacteria are characterized by a diderm cell envelope, the outer membrane of which is characterized by the presence of unusual lipids known as mycolic acids. These mycolic acids are partially linked to the arabinogalactan layer and partially coupled to treha-lose molecules. Mycolic acids are not unique for mycobacteria; they can also be found in several close relatives, including *Coryne-bacteria* and *Rhodococcus* species. These bacteria therefore have a diderm envelope similar to mycobacteria and usually have a locus potentially coding for a T7S system (128). Unfortunately, T7S systems have not been analyzed in these bacteria.

Interestingly, a number of monoderm bac-teria also have T7S(-like) systems, and some of these have been studied in more detail. The first one we will discuss is the T7S system present in streptomycetes. Although these bacteria are monoderm and do not produce mycolic acids, they do belong to the same taxonomic order (*Actinomycetales*) as myco-bacteria and have a well-conserved T7S sys-tem; in *Streptomyces* species all genes coding for the five conserved membrane proteins, i.e., homologs of EccBCDE and MycP, are usually present (128, 129). Several substrates seem to be present in these loci, of which the two small Esx proteins have indeed been shown to be secreted by *Streptomyces coelicolor* (129). In two species of *Streptomy-ces*, i.e., *S. coelicolor* and *Streptomyces scabies* (129, 130), deletion of genes coding for the Esx-like T7S substrates resulted in abnormal spore formation and/or altered timing of spore formation. Surprisingly, absence of the T7S components did not show the same effect as the substrates, which seems to suggest that these Esx proteins have an intracellular effect on spore formation.

A number of *Firmicutes* species have a T7S-like system that contains only two of the original genes, i.e., an *eccC* homolog and one or more of the *esx* genes. In addition, there are usually a variable number of other (membrane) proteins required for secretion (discussed below). In contrast to the T7S sys-tems in mycolic-acid-containing bacteria, the T7S-like systems in *Firmicutes* were probably acquired relatively recently, be-cause their composition and distribution are highly variable. For instance, *Streptococcus*

agalactiae is the only species in the *Strepto-coccaceae* family that has an intact T7S-like system, and the T7S-like system of *Bacillus cereus* is more similar in composition and homology to that of *Listeria* species than those of other *Bacillus* species. Most data on T7S-like systems in *Firmicutes* has been ob-tained for *B. subtilis* and *S. aureus*, so these systems will be discussed in more detail.

Although protein secretion in *B. subtilis* has been studied for decades, only recently, a T7S-like system (Fig. 1) was shown to be functional, which seems to be due to de-fective regulation in domesticated *Bacillus* strains (53). In undomesticated strains se-cretion could be readily observed in late log phase. The secreted substrate is an Esx-like protein known as YukE (53). Proteomic analysis showed that, under normal labora-tory conditions, this is the only T7S-like substrate (12). YukE is secreted as a dimer and, in analogy to the mycobacterial T7S sub-strates, the C-terminal tail is required for secretion. Unfortunately, the extracellular function of YukE is currently unknown. De-tailed mutational analysis has shown that, in addition to the EccC-homolog (called YukB or YukBA), YukCD and YueBC are also re-quired (12, 53). Apart from YukD, these pro-teins are all membrane proteins. Of these membrane proteins, YueB is the one with most potential TMDs (6). Because this pro-tein probably forms a dimer (131), this com-plex could be somewhat similar to EccD of mycobacteria. YueB-like proteins therefore could form a central component in T7S-like systems. In contrast to EccD, the YueB pro-tein has a very substantial extracellular domain of more than 800 amino acids. This extracellular domain is a receptor for the bacteriophage SPP1 (131). The only cytosolic protein that is essential for secretion, YukD, has a ubiquitin-like fold (132). Despite this structural similarity, YukD does not seem to be conjugated, either to itself or to other proteins (132). For the YukD homolog of *S. aureus* (SAUSA300_0281, also described as EsaB [11] [Fig. 1]), it has been shown that this protein is involved in intracellular posttranscriptional regulation of a specific substrate of the T7S-like system (133). Therefore, this ubiquitin-like protein perhaps functions as a specific chaperone or regulator.

The T7S-like system of *S. aureus* is called Ess and contains the same elements as the T7S-like system in *B. subtilis*, but the gene order is different (Fig. 1). The only difference is that in *S. aureus* an additional gene is identified that might be required for secretion, i.e., *esaD* (134). However, the effect of an *esaD* deletion on secretion is not absolute; a major reduction of protein secretion is observed when this gene is deleted, but not a complete blockade. Moreover, in other species *esaD* homologs are not always linked to this secretion system, and the C-terminal domain of EsaD is predicted to form a nuclease/hydrolase. Therefore, more research is needed to substantiate this component. Another feature of T7S-like systems that is conserved between *B. subtilis* and *S. aureus* is the variability in secretion between strains. Both the amount and timing of secretion is highly strain dependent for *S. aureus* (135), which indicates that this system is controlled by a complex and variable regulation system. Some of these regulators have been identified; the production of the main substrate EsxA, in particular, seems to be controlled by several regulators (63, 136).

The most important difference between the T7S-like systems in *S. aureus* and *B. subtilis* is the number of substrates that are secreted. Whereas *B. subtilis* secretes only a single substrate, four substrates have been identified thus far for *S. aureus*. Two Esx proteins are secreted, as well as two proteins that do not officially belong to the EsxAB clan (63) but are predicted to form an N-terminal helix-turn-helix motif. These new substrates are unfortunately called EsxC and EsxD. All these substrates are encoded by genes within the T7S-like locus.

Ess secretion is important for both colonization and persistence of *S. aureus* (11, 135). Disruption of this T7S-like system or deletion of the substrates results in significantly reduced bacterial numbers and reduced pathology in a mouse model. Interestingly, a recent report indicates that this secretion system is involved in the intracellular survival of *S. aureus* in epithelial cells by blocking apoptosis and promoting escape (137). If substantiated, this would be highly similar to the function of the ESX-1 system in pathogenic mycobacteria. In line with this function, close homologs of the *S. aureus* Ess system are present in other pathogens, such as *Listeria monocytogenes* and *B. cereus*.

CONCLUDING REMARKS

In approximately one decade of research on T7S, major advances have been made to elucidate the mechanism of T7S and its role in pathogenesis. However, many questions remain about the functioning and structure of T7S systems. Is the T7S membrane channel in mycolic-acid-containing bacteria a double membrane-spanning complex, mediating transport in a one-step mechanism, or are there unidentified outer membrane components of T7S systems that are responsible for transport over the specific outer membrane? Solving the structure of the mycobacterial T7S membrane complex will answer many of these questions and would be a major breakthrough in this field. Another topic that needs to be addressed is the function of individual T7S substrates. Unfortunately, the interdependence of substrates for secretion and complex regulatory and posttranslational networks complicates research on this topic. The observed roles of T7S systems and their substrates in virulence and in nutrient acquisition show that these systems are promising targets for future drug development. Recently, the first T7S inhibitors have been identified and could be the front-runners of new classes of drugs against pathogenic mycobacteria (138). A more detailed understanding of T7S systems and their substrates could lead to new concepts for treatment of mycobacterial diseases but might also shed light on novel potential virulence factors secreted by other *Actinobacteria* and *Firmicutes*.

CITATION

Ates LS, Houben ENG, Bitter W. 2016. Type VII secretion: a highly versatile secretion system. Microbiol Spectrum 4(1):VMBF-0011-2015.

REFERENCES

1. **Zuber B, Chami M, Houssin C, Dubochet J, Griffiths G, Daffé M.** 2008. Direct visualization of the outer membrane of mycobacteria and corynebacteria in their native state. *J Bacteriol* **190**:5672–5680.

2. **Sani M, Houben ENG, Geurtsen J, Pierson J, de Punder K, van Zon M, Wever B, Piersma SR, Jiménez CR, Daffé M, Appelmelk BJ, Bitter W, van der Wel N, Peters PJ.** 2010. Direct visualization by cryo-EM of the mycobacterial capsular layer: a labile structure containing ESX-1-secreted proteins. *PLoS Pathog* **6**:e1000794. doi:10.1371/journal.ppat.1000794.

3. **Andersen P, Andersen AB, Sørensen AL, Nagai S.** 1995. Recall of long-lived immunity to *Mycobacterium tuberculosis* infection in mice. *J Immunol* **154**:3359–3372.

4. **Bitter W, Houben ENG, Bottai D, Brodin P, Brown EJ, Cox JS, Derbyshire K, Fortune SM, Gao L-Y, Liu J, Gey van Pittius NC, Pym AS, Rubin EJ, Sherman DR, Cole ST, Brosch R.** 2009. Systematic genetic nomenclature for type VII secretion systems. *PLoS Pathog* **5**:e1000507. doi:10.1371/journal.ppat.1000507.

5. **Mahairas GG, Sabo PJ, Hickey MJ, Singh DC, Stover CK.** 1996. Molecular analysis of genetic differences between *Mycobacterium bovis* BCG and virulent *M. bovis*. *J Bacteriol* **178**:1274–1282.

6. **Pym AS, Brodin P, Majlessi L, Brosch R, Demangel C, Williams A, Griffiths KE, Marchal G, Leclerc C, Cole ST.** 2003. Recombinant BCG exporting ESAT-6 confers enhanced protection against tuberculosis. *Nat Med* **9**:533–539.

7. **Gey Van Pittius NC, Gamieldien J, Hide W, Brown GD, Siezen RJ, Beyers AD.** 2001. The ESAT-6 gene cluster of *Mycobacterium tuberculosis* and other high G+C Gram-positive bacteria. *Genome Biol* **2**:RESEARCH0044.

8. **Ummels R, Abdallah AM, Kuiper V, Aâjoud A, Sparrius M, Naeem R, Spaink HP, van D, Pain A, Bitter W.** 2014. Identification of a novel conjugative plasmid in mycobacteria that requires both type IV and type VII secretion. *MBio* **5**:e01744-14. doi:10.1128/mBio.01744-14.

9. **Abdallah AM, Gey van Pittius NC, Champion PAD, Cox J, Luirink J, Vandenbroucke-Grauls CMJE, Appelmelk BJ, Bitter W.** 2007. Type VII secretion: mycobacteria show the way. *Nat Rev Microbiol* **5**:883–891.

10. **Pallen MJ.** 2002. The ESAT-6/WXG100 superfamily: and a new Gram-positive secretion system? *Trends Microbiol* **10**:209–212.

11. **Burts ML, Williams WA, DeBord K, Missiakas DM.** 2005. EsxA and EsxB are secreted by an ESAT-6-like system that is required for the pathogenesis of *Staphylococcus aureus* infections. *Proc Natl Acad Sci USA* **102**:1169–1174.

12. **Huppert LA, Ramsdell TL, Chase MR, Sarracino DA, Fortune SM, Burton BM.** 2014. The ESX system in *Bacillus subtilis* mediates protein secretion. *PLoS One* **9**:e96267. doi:10.1371/journal.pone.0096267.

13. **Daleke MH, Cascioferro A, de Punder K, Ummels R, Abdallah AM, van der Wel N, Peters PJ, Luirink J, Manganelli R, Bitter W.** 2011. Conserved Pro-Glu (PE) and Pro-Pro-Glu (PPE) protein domains target LipY lipases of pathogenic mycobacteria to the cell surface via the ESX-5 pathway. *J Biol Chem* **286**:19024–19034.

14. **Abdallah AM, Verboom T, Weerdenburg EM, Gey van Pittius NC, Mahasha PW, Jiménez C, Parra M, Cadieux N, Brennan MJ, Appelmelk BJ, Bitter W.** 2009. PPE and PE_PGRS proteins of *Mycobacterium marinum* are transported via the type VII secretion system ESX-5. *Mol Microbiol* **73**:329–340.

15. **Daleke MH, van der Woude AD, Parret AH, Ummels R, de Groot AM, Watson D, Piersma SR, Jiménez CR, Luirink J, Bitter W, Houben ENG.** 2012. Specific chaperones for the type VII protein secretion pathway. *J Biol Chem* **287**:31939–31947.

16. **Ekiert DC, Cox JS.** 2014. Structure of a PE-PPE-EspG complex from *Mycobacterium tuberculosis* reveals molecular specificity of ESX protein secretion. *Proc Natl Acad Sci USA* **111**:14758–14763.

17. **Korotkova N, Freire D, Phan TH, Ummels R, Creekmore CC, Evans TJ, Wilmanns M, Bitter W, Parret AHA, Houben ENG, Korotkov KV.** 2014. Structure of the *Mycobacterium tuberculosis* type VII secretion system chaperone EspG5 in complex with PE25-PPE41 dimer. *Mol Microbiol* **94**:367–382.

18. **Solomonson M, Setiaputra D, Makepeace KAT, Lameignere E, Petrotchenko EV, Conrady DG, Bergeron JR, Vuckovic M, DiMaio F, Borchers CH, Yip CK, Strynadka NCJ.** 2015. Structure of EspB from the ESX-1 type VII secretion system and insights into its export mechanism. *Structure* **23**:571–583.

19. **Wagner JM, Evans TJ, Korotkov KV.** 2014. Crystal structure of the N-terminal domain of EccA$_5$ ATPase from the ESX-1 secretion system of *Mycobacterium tuberculosis*. *Proteins* **82**:159–163.

20. **Luthra A, Mahmood A, Arora A, Ramachandran R.** 2008. Characterization of Rv3868, an essential hypothetical protein of the ESX-1 secretion system in *Mycobacterium tuberculosis*. *J Biol Chem* **283**:36532–36541.

21. **Cerveny L, Straskova A, Dankova V, Hartlova A, Ceckova M, Staud F, Stulik J.** 2013. Tetraricopeptide repeat motifs in the world of bacterial pathogens: role in virulence mechanisms. *Infect Immun* **81**:629–635.

22. **Bottai D, Di Luca M, Majlessi L, Frigui W, Simeone R, Sayes F, Bitter W, Brennan MJ, Leclerc C, Batoni G, Campa M, Brosch R, Esin S.** 2012. Disruption of the ESX-5 system of *Mycobacterium tuberculosis* causes loss of PPE protein secretion, reduction of cell wall integrity and strong attenuation. *Mol Microbiol* **83**:1195–1209.

23. **Abdallah AM, Verboom T, Hannes F, Safi M, Strong M, Eisenberg D, Musters RJP, Vandenbroucke-Grauls CMJE, Appelmelk BJ, Luirink J, Bitter W.** 2006. A specific secretion system mediates PPE41 transport in pathogenic mycobacteria. *Mol Microbiol* **62**:667–679.

24. **Gao L-Y, Guo S, McLaughlin B, Morisaki H, Engel JN, Brown EJ.** 2004. A mycobacterial virulence gene cluster extending RD1 is required for cytolysis, bacterial spreading and ESAT-6 secretion. *Mol Microbiol* **53**:1677–1693.

25. **Joshi SA, Ball DA, Sun MG, Carlsson F, Watkins BY, Aggarwal N, McCracken JM, Huynh KK, Brown EJ.** 2012. EccA1, a component of the *Mycobacterium marinum* ESX-1 protein virulence factor secretion pathway, regulates mycolic acid lipid synthesis. *Chem Biol* **19**:372–380.

26. **Sassetti CM, Boyd DH, Rubin EJ.** 2003. Genes required for mycobacterial growth defined by high density mutagenesis. *Mol Microbiol* **48**:77–84.

27. **Houben ENG, Bestebroer J, Ummels R, Wilson L, Piersma SR, Jiménez CR, Ottenhoff THM, Luirink J, Bitter W.** 2012. Composition of the type VII secretion system membrane complex. *Mol Microbiol* **86**:472–484.

28. **Converse SE, Cox JS.** 2005. A protein secretion pathway critical for *Mycobacterium tuberculosis* virulence is conserved and functional in *Mycobacterium smegmatis*. *J Bacteriol* **187**:1238–1245.

29. **Brodin P, Majlessi L, Marsollier L, de Jonge MI, Bottai D, Demangel C, Hinds J, Neyrolles O, Butcher PD, Leclerc C, Cole ST, Brosch R.** 2006. Dissection of ESAT-6 system 1 of *Mycobacterium tuberculosis* and impact on immunogenicity and virulence. *Infect Immun* **74**:88–98.

30. **Stanley SA, Raghavan S, Hwang WW, Cox JS.** 2003. Acute infection and macrophage subversion by *Mycobacterium tuberculosis* require a specialized secretion system. *Proc Natl Acad Sci USA* **100**:13001–13006.

31. **Siegrist MS, Steigedal M, Ahmad R, Mehra A, Dragset MS, Schuster BM, Philips JA, Carr SA, Rubin EJ.** 2014. Mycobacterial Esx-3 requires multiple components for iron acquisition. *MBio* **5**:e01073-14. doi:10.1128/mBio.01073-14.

32. **Niederweis M, Danilchanka O, Huff J, Hoffmann C, Engelhardt H.** 2010. Mycobacterial outer membranes: in search of proteins. *Trends Microbiol* **18**:109–116.

33. **Chandran V, Fronzes R, Duquerroy S, Cronin N, Navaza J, Waksman G.** 2009. Structure of the outer membrane complex of a type IV secretion system. *Nature* **462**:1011–1015.

34. **Rosenberger T, Brülle JK, Sander P.** 2013. Correction: A β-lactamase based reporter system for ESX dependent protein translocation in mycobacteria. *PLoS One* **8**. doi:10.1371/annotation/f03f7456-0e04-4c4b-a606-51f262900e8d.

35. **Burton B, Dubnau D.** 2010. Membrane-associated DNA transport machines. *Cold Spring Harbor Perspect Biol* **2**:a000406.

36. **Atmakuri K, Cascales E, Christie PJ.** 2004. Energetic components VirD4, VirB11 and VirB4 mediate early DNA transfer reactions required for bacterial type IV secretion. *Mol Microbiol* **54**:1199–1211.

37. **Champion PAD, Stanley SA, Champion MM, Brown EJ, Cox JS.** 2006. C-terminal signal sequence promotes virulence factor secretion in *Mycobacterium tuberculosis*. *Science* **313**:1632–1636.

38. **Ramsdell TL, Huppert LA, Sysoeva TA, Fortune SM, Burton BM.** 2014. Linked domain architectures allow for specialization of function in the FtsK/SpoIIIE ATPases of ESX secretion systems. *J Mol Biol* **427**:1119–1132.

39. **Ates LS, Ummels R, Commandeur S, van der Weerd R, Sparrius M, Weerdenburg E, Alber**

M, Kalscheuer R, Piersma SR, Abdallah AM, Abd El Ghany M, Abdel-Haleem AM, Pain A, Jiménez CR, Bitter W, Houben ENG. 2015. Essential role of the ESX-5 secretion system in outer membrane permeability of pathogenic mycobacteria. *PLOS Genet* **11:**e1005190. doi:10.1371/journal.pgen.1005190.

40. Rosenberg OS, Dovala D, Li X, Connolly L, Bendebury A, Finer-Moore J, Holton J, Cheng Y, Stroud RM, Cox JS. 2015. Substrates control multimerization and activation of the multi-domain ATPase motor of type VII secretion. *Cell* **161:**501–512.

41. Brown GD, Dave JA, Gey NC, Stevens L, Ehlers MR, Beyers AD. 2000. The mycosins of *Mycobacterium tuberculosis* H37Rv: a family of subtilisin-like serine proteases. *Gene* **254:**147–155.

42. Dave JA, Gey van Pittius NC, Beyers AD, Ehlers MRW, Brown GD. 2002. Mycosin-1, a subtilisin-like serine protease of *Mycobacterium tuberculosis*, is cell wall-associated and expressed during infection of macrophages. *BMC Microbiol* **2:**30.

43. Ohol YM, Goetz DH, Chan K, Shiloh MU, Craik CS, Cox JS. 2010. *Mycobacterium tuberculosis* MycP1 protease plays a dual role in regulation of ESX-1 secretion and virulence. *Cell Host Microbe* **7:**210–220.

44. Solomonson M, Huesgen PF, Wasney GA, Watanabe N, Gruninger RJ, Prehna G, Overall CM, Strynadka NCJ. 2013. Structure of the mycosin-1 protease from the mycobacterial ESX-1 protein type VII secretion system. *J Biol Chem* **288:**17782–17790.

45. Wagner JM, Evans TJ, Chen J, Zhu H, Houben ENG, Bitter W, Korotkov KV. 2013. Understanding specificity of the mycosin proteases in ESX/type VII secretion by structural and functional analysis. *J Struct Biol* **184:**115–128.

46. Shinde U, Inouye M. 1995. Folding mediated by an intramolecular chaperone: autoprocessing pathway of the precursor resolved via a substrate assisted catalysis mechanism. *J Mol Biol* **247:**390–395.

47. Finn RD, Bateman A, Clements J, Coggill P, Eberhardt RY, Eddy SR, Heger A, Hetherington K, Holm L, Mistry J, Sonnhammer ELL, Tate J, Punta M. 2014. Pfam: the protein families database. *Nucleic Acids Res* **42:**D222–D230.

48. Garufi G, Butler E, Missiakas D. 2008. ESAT-6-like protein secretion in *Bacillus anthracis*. *J Bacteriol* **190:**7004–7011.

49. Renshaw PS, Panagiotidou P, Whelan A, Gordon SV, Hewinson RG, Williamson RA, Carr MD. 2002. Conclusive evidence that the major T-cell antigens of the *Mycobacterium tuberculosis* complex ESAT-6 and CFP-10 form a tight, 1:1 complex and characterization of the structural properties of ESAT-6, CFP-10, and the ESAT-6*CFP-10 complex. Implications for pathogenesis and virulence. *J Biol Chem* **277:**21598–21603.

50. Lightbody KL, Renshaw PS, Collins ML, Wright RL, Hunt DM, Gordon SV, Hewinson RG, Buxton RS, Williamson RA, Carr MD. 2004. Characterisation of complex formation between members of the *Mycobacterium tuberculosis* complex CFP-10/ESAT-6 protein family: towards an understanding of the rules governing complex formation and thereby functional flexibility. *FEMS Microbiol Lett* **238:**255–262.

51. Berthet FX, Rasmussen PB, Rosenkrands I, Andersen P, Gicquel B. 1998. A *Mycobacterium tuberculosis* operon encoding ESAT-6 and a novel low-molecular-mass culture filtrate protein (CFP-10). *Microbiology* **144:**3195–3203.

52. Shukla A, Pallen M, Anthony M, White SA. 2010. The homodimeric GBS1074 from *Streptococcus agalactiae*. *Acta Crystallogr Sect F Struct Biol Cryst Commun* **66:**1421–1425.

53. Baptista C, Barreto HC, São-José C. 2013. High levels of DegU-P activate an Esat-6-like secretion system in *Bacillus subtilis*. *PLoS One* **8:**e67840. doi:10.1371/journal.pone.0067840.

54. Poulsen C, Panjikar S, Holton SJ, Wilmanns M, Song Y-H. 2014. WXG100 protein superfamily consists of three subfamilies and exhibits an α-helical C-terminal conserved residue pattern. *PLoS One* **9:**e89313. doi:10.1371/journal.pone.0089313.

55. Renshaw PS, Lightbody KL, Veverka V, Muskett FW, Kelly G, Frenkiel TA, Gordon SV, Hewinson RG, Burke B, Norman J, Williamson RA, Carr MD. 2005. Structure and function of the complex formed by the tuberculosis virulence factors CFP-10 and ESAT-6. *EMBO J* **24:**2491–2498.

56. Ilghari D, Lightbody KL, Veverka V, Waters LC, Muskett FW, Renshaw PS, Carr MD. 2011. Solution structure of the *Mycobacterium tuberculosis* EsxG·EsxH complex: functional implications and comparisons with other *M. tuberculosis* Esx family complexes. *J Biol Chem* **286:**29993–30002.

57. Arbing MA, Kaufmann M, Phan T, Chan S, Cascio D, Eisenberg D. 2010. The crystal structure of the *Mycobacterium tuberculosis* Rv3019c-Rv3020c ESX complex reveals a domain-swapped heterotetramer. *Protein Sci* **19:**1692–1703.

58. Gey van Pittius NC, Sampson SL, Lee H, Kim Y, van Helden PD, Warren RM. 2006.

Evolution and expansion of the *Mycobacterium tuberculosis* PE and PPE multigene families and their association with the duplication of the ESAT-6 (esx) gene cluster regions. *BMC Evol Biol* **6**:95.

59. **Strong M, Sawaya MR, Wang S, Phillips M, Cascio D, Eisenberg D.** 2006. Toward the structural genomics of complexes: crystal structure of a PE/PPE protein complex from *Mycobacterium tuberculosis*. *Proc Natl Acad Sci USA* **103**:8060–8065.

60. **Daleke MH, Ummels R, Bawono P, Heringa J, Vandenbroucke-Grauls CMJE, Luirink J, Bitter W.** 2012. General secretion signal for the mycobacterial type VII secretion pathway. *Proc Natl Acad Sci USA* **109**:11342–11347.

61. **Kelley LA, Sternberg MJE.** 2009. Protein structure prediction on the Web: a case study using the Phyre server. *Nat Protoc* **4**:363–371.

62. **Zhang D, Iyer LM, Aravind L.** 2011. A novel immunity system for bacterial nucleic acid degrading toxins and its recruitment in various eukaryotic and DNA viral systems. *Nucleic Acids Res* **39**:4532–4552.

63. **Anderson M, Aly KA, Chen Y-H, Missiakas D.** 2013. Secretion of atypical protein subtrates by the ESAT-6 secretion system of *Staphylococcus aureus*. *Mol Microbiol* **90**:734–743.

64. **Philipp WJ, Nair S, Guglielmi G, Lagranderie M, Gicquel B, Cole ST.** 1996. Physical mapping of *Mycobacterium bovis* BCG pasteur reveals differences from the genome map of *Mycobacterium tuberculosis* H37Rv and from *M. bovis*. *Microbiology* **142**:3135–3145.

65. **Pym AS, Brodin P, Brosch R, Huerre M, Cole ST.** 2002. Loss of RD1 contributed to the attenuation of the live tuberculosis vaccines *Mycobacterium bovis* BCG and *Mycobacterium microti*. *Mol Microbiol* **46**:709–717.

66. **Hsu T, Hingley-Wilson SM, Chen B, Chen M, Dai AZ, Morin PM, Marks CB, Padiyar J, Goulding C, Gingery M, Eisenberg D, Russell RG, Derrick SC, Collins FM, Morris SL, King CH, Jacobs WR.** 2003. The primary mechanism of attenuation of bacillus Calmette-Guerin is a loss of secreted lytic function required for invasion of lung interstitial tissue. *Proc Natl Acad Sci USA* **100**:12420–12425.

67. **Lewis KN, Liao R, Guinn KM, Hickey MJ, Smith S, Behr MA, Sherman DR.** 2003. Deletion of RD1 from *Mycobacterium tuberculosis* mimics bacille Calmette-Guérin attenuation. *J Infect Dis* **187**:117–123.

68. **Fortune SM, Jaeger A, Sarracino DA, Chase MR, Sassetti CM, Sherman DR, Bloom BR, Rubin EJ.** 2005. Mutually dependent secretion of proteins required for mycobacterial virulence. *Proc Natl Acad Sci USA* **102**:10676–10681.

69. **Pang X, Samten B, Cao G, Wang X, Tvinnereim AR, Chen X-L, Howard ST.** 2013. MprAB regulates the espA operon in *Mycobacterium tuberculosis* and modulates ESX-1 function and host cytokine response. *J Bacteriol* **195**:66–75.

70. **Hunt DM, Sweeney NP, Mori L, Whalan RH, Comas I, Norman L, Cortes T, Arnvig KB, Davis EO, Stapleton MR, Green J, Buxton RS.** 2012. Long-range transcriptional control of an operon necessary for virulence-critical ESX-1 secretion in *Mycobacterium tuberculosis*. *J Bacteriol* **194**:2307–2320.

71. **Garces A, Atmakuri K, Chase MR, Woodworth JS, Krastins B, Rothchild AC, Ramsdell TL, Lopez MF, Behar SM, Sarracino DA, Fortune SM.** 2010. EspA acts as a critical mediator of ESX1-dependent virulence in *Mycobacterium tuberculosis* by affecting bacterial cell wall integrity. *PLoS Pathog* **6**:e1000957. doi:10.1371/journal.ppat.1000957.

72. **Van N, Hava D, Houben D, Fluitsma D, van Zon M, Pierson J, Brenner M, Peters PJ.** 2007. *M. tuberculosis* and *M. leprae* translocate from the phagolysosome to the cytosol in myeloid cells. *Cell* **129**:1287–1298.

73. **Simeone R, Bobard A, Lippmann J, Bitter W, Majlessi L, Brosch R, Enninga J.** 2012. Phagosomal rupture by *Mycobacterium tuberculosis* results in toxicity and host cell death. *PLoS Pathog* **8**:e1002507. doi:10.1371/journal.ppat.1002507.

74. **Houben D, Demangel C, van Ingen J, Perez J, Baldeón L, Abdallah AM, Caleechurn L, Bottai D, van Zon M, de Punder K, van der Laan T, Kant A, Bossers-de Vries R, Willemsen P, Bitter W, van Soolingen D, Brosch R, van der Wel N, Peters PJ.** 2012. ESX-1-mediated translocation to the cytosol controls virulence of mycobacteria. *Cell Microbiol* **14**:1287–1298.

75. **Koo IC, Wang C, Raghavan S, Morisaki JH, Cox JS, Brown EJ.** 2008. ESX-1-dependent cytolysis in lysosome secretion and inflammasome activation during mycobacterial infection. *Cell Microbiol* **10**:1866–1878.

76. **Smith J, Manoranjan J, Pan M, Bohsali A, Xu J, Liu J, McDonald KL, Szyk A, LaRonde-LeBlanc N, Gao L-Y.** 2008. Evidence for pore formation in host cell membranes by ESX-1-secreted ESAT-6 and its role in *Mycobacterium marinum* escape from the vacuole. *Infect Immun* **76**:5478–5487.

77. **De Jonge MI, Pehau-Arnaudet G, Fretz MM, Romain F, Bottai D, Brodin P, Honoré N, Marchal G, Jiskoot W, England P, Cole ST, Brosch R.** 2007. ESAT-6 from *Mycobacterium*

tuberculosis dissociates from its putative chaperone CFP-10 under acidic conditions and exhibits membrane-lysing activity. *J Bacteriol* **189:**6028–6034.

78. **Flint JL, Kowalski JC, Karnati PK, Derbyshire KM.** 2004. The RD1 virulence locus of *Mycobacterium tuberculosis* regulates DNA transfer in *Mycobacterium smegmatis*. *Proc Natl Acad Sci USA* **101:**12598–12603.

79. **Kennedy GM, Hooley GC, Champion MM, Mba Medie F, Champion PAD.** 2014. A novel ESX-1 locus reveals that surface-associated ESX-1 substrates mediate virulence in *Mycobacterium marinum*. *J Bacteriol* **196:**1877–1888.

80. **Wirth SE, Krywy JA, Aldridge BB, Fortune SM, Fernandez-Suarez M, Gray TA, Derbyshire KM.** 2012. Polar assembly and scaffolding proteins of the virulence-associated ESX-1 secretory apparatus in mycobacteria. *Mol Microbiol* **83:**654–664.

81. **Carlsson F, Joshi SA, Rangell L, Brown EJ.** 2009. Polar localization of virulence-related Esx-1 secretion in mycobacteria. *PLoS Pathog* **5:**e1000285. doi:10.1371/journal.ppat.1000285.

82. **Abramovitch RB, Rohde KH, Hsu F-F, Russell DG.** 2011. aprABC: a *Mycobacterium tuberculosis* complex-specific locus that modulates pH-driven adaptation to the macrophage phagosome. *Mol Microbiol* **80:**678–694.

83. **Tan S, Sukumar N, Abramovitch RB, Parish T, Russell DG.** 2013. *Mycobacterium tuberculosis* responds to chloride and pH as synergistic cues to the immune status of its host cell. *PLoS Pathog* **9:**e1003282. doi:10.1371/journal.ppat.1003282.

84. **Lee JS, Krause R, Schreiber J, Mollenkopf H-J, Kowall J, Stein R, Jeon B-Y, Kwak J-Y, Song M-K, Patron JP, Jorg S, Roh K, Cho S-N, Kaufmann SHE.** 2008. Mutation in the transcriptional regulator PhoP contributes to avirulence of *Mycobacterium tuberculosis* H37Ra strain. *Cell Host Microbe* **3:**97–103.

85. **Frigui W, Bottai D, Majlessi L, Monot M, Josselin E, Brodin P, Garnier T, Gicquel B, Martin C, Leclerc C, Cole ST, Brosch R.** 2008. Control of *M. tuberculosis* ESAT-6 secretion and specific T cell recognition by PhoP. *PLoS Pathog* **4:**e33. doi:10.1371/journal.ppat.0040033.

86. **Solans L, Aguiló N, Samper S, Pawlik A, Frigui W, Martín C, Brosch R, Gonzalo-Asensio J.** 2014. A specific polymorphism in *Mycobacterium tuberculosis* H37Rv causes differential ESAT-6 expression and identifies WhiB6 as a novel ESX-1 component. *Infect Immun* **82:**3446–3456.

87. **Raghavan S, Manzanillo P, Chan K, Dovey C, Cox JS.** 2008. Secreted transcription factor controls *Mycobacterium tuberculosis* virulence. *Nature* **454:**717–721.

88. **Blasco B, Chen JM, Hartkoorn R, Sala C, Uplekar S, Rougemont J, Pojer F, Cole ST.** 2012. Virulence regulator EspR of *Mycobacterium tuberculosis* is a nucleoid-associated protein. *PLoS Pathog* **8:**e1002621. doi:10.1371/journal.ppat.1002621.

89. **Rosenberg OS, Dovey C, Tempesta M, Robbins RA, Finer-Moore JS, Stroud RM, Cox JS.** 2011. EspR, a key regulator of *Mycobacterium tuberculosis* virulence, adopts a unique dimeric structure among helix-turn-helix proteins. *Proc Natl Acad Sci USA* **108:**13450–13455.

90. **Gordon BRG, Li Y, Wang L, Sintsova A, van Bakel H, Tian S, Navarre WW, Xia B, Liu J.** 2010. Lsr2 is a nucleoid-associated protein that targets AT-rich sequences and virulence genes in *Mycobacterium tuberculosis*. *Proc Natl Acad Sci USA* **107:**5154–5159.

91. **Gonzalo-Asensio J, Malaga W, Pawlik A, Astarie-Dequeker C, Passemar C, Moreau F, Laval F, Daffé M, Martin C, Brosch R, Guilhot C.** 2014. Evolutionary history of tuberculosis shaped by conserved mutations in the PhoPR virulence regulator. *Proc Natl Acad Sci USA* **111:**11491–11496.

92. **Derbyshire KM, Gray TA.** 2014. Distributive conjugal transfer: new insights into horizontal gene transfer and genetic exchange in mycobacteria. *Microbiol Spectrum* **2**(1). doi:10.1128/microbiolspec.MGM2-0022-2013.

93. **Coros A, Callahan B, Battaglioli E, Derbyshire KM.** 2008. The specialized secretory apparatus ESX-1 is essential for DNA transfer in *Mycobacterium smegmatis*. *Mol Microbiol* **69:**794–808.

94. **Gray TA, Krywy JA, Harold J, Palumbo MJ, Derbyshire KM.** 2013. Distributive conjugal transfer in mycobacteria generates progeny with meiotic-like genome-wide mosaicism, allowing mapping of a mating identity locus. *PLoS Biol* **11:**e1001602. doi:10.1371/journal.pbio.1001602.

95. **Gutierrez MC, Brisse S, Brosch R, Fabre M, Omaïs B, Marmiesse M, Supply P, Vincent V.** 2005. Ancient origin and gene mosaicism of the progenitor of *Mycobacterium tuberculosis*. *PLoS Pathog* **1:**e5. doi:10.1371/journal.ppat.0010005.

96. **Griffin JE, Gawronski JD, Dejesus MA, Ioerger TR, Akerley BJ, Sassetti CM.** 2011. High-resolution phenotypic profiling defines genes essential for mycobacterial growth and cholesterol catabolism. *PLoS Pathog* **7:**e1002251. doi:10.1371/journal.ppat.1002251.

97. **Rodriguez GM, Voskuil MI, Gold B, Schoolnik GK, Smith I.** 2002. ideR, an essential gene in *Mycobacterium tuberculosis*: role

of IdeR in iron-dependent gene expression, iron metabolism, and oxidative stress response. *Infect Immun* **70:**3371–3381.

98. **Maciag A, Dainese E, Rodriguez GM, Milano A, Provvedi R, Pasca MR, Smith I, Palù G, Riccardi G, Manganelli R.** 2007. Global analysis of the *Mycobacterium tuberculosis* Zur (FurB) regulon. *J Bacteriol* **189:**730–740.

99. **Siegrist MS, Unnikrishnan M, McConnell MJ, Borowsky M, Cheng T-Y, Siddiqi N, Fortune SM, Moody DB, Rubin EJ.** 2009. Mycobacterial Esx-3 is required for mycobactin-mediated iron acquisition. *Proc Natl Acad Sci USA* **106:**18792–18797.

100. **Serafini A, Boldrin F, Palù G, Manganelli R.** 2009. Characterization of a *Mycobacterium tuberculosis* ESX-3 conditional mutant: essentiality and rescue by iron and zinc. *J Bacteriol* **191:**6340–6344.

101. **Cole ST, Brosch R, Parkhill J, Garnier T, Churcher C, Harris D, Gordon SV, Eiglmeier K, Gas S, Barry CE, Tekaia F, Badcock K, Basham D, Brown D, Chillingworth T, Connor R, Davies R, Devlin K, Feltwell T, Gentles S, Hamlin N, Holroyd S, Hornsby T, Jagels K, Krogh A, McLean J, Moule S, Murphy L, Oliver K, Osborne J, Quail MA, Rajandream MA, Rogers J, Rutter S, Seeger K, Skelton J, Squares R, Squares S, Sulston JE, Taylor K, Whitehead S, Barrell BG.** 1998. Deciphering the biology of *Mycobacterium tuberculosis* from the complete genome sequence. *Nature* **393:**537–544.

102. **Mishra KC, de Chastellier C, Narayana Y, Bifani P, Brown AK, Besra GS, Katoch VM, Joshi B, Balaji KN, Kremer L.** 2008. Functional role of the PE domain and immunogenicity of the *Mycobacterium tuberculosis* triacylglycerol hydrolase LipY. *Infect Immun* **76:**127–140.

103. **Sampson SL.** 2011. Mycobacterial PE/PPE proteins at the host-pathogen interface. *Clin Dev Immunol* **2011:**497203.

104. **Di Luca M, Bottai D, Batoni G, Orgeur M, Aulicino A, Counoupas C, Campa M, Brosch R, Esin S.** 2012. The ESX-5 associated eccB-EccC locus is essential for *Mycobacterium tuberculosis* viability. *PLoS One* **7:**e52059. doi:10.1371/journal.pone.0052059.

105. **Lamrabet O, Ghigo E, Mège J-L, Lepidi H, Nappez C, Raoult D, Drancourt M.** 2014. MspA-*Mycobacterium tuberculosis*-transformant with reduced virulence: the "unbirthday paradigm". *Microb Pathog* **76:**10–18.

106. **Abdallah AM, Bestebroer J, Savage NDL, de Punder K, van Zon M, Wilson L, Korbee CJ, van der Sar AM, Ottenhoff THM,**

van der Wel NN, Bitter W, Peters PJ. 2011. Mycobacterial secretion systems ESX-1 and ESX-5 play distinct roles in host cell death and inflammasome activation. *J Immunol* **187:**4744–4753.

107. **Weerdenburg EM, Abdallah AM, Mitra S, de Punder K, van der Wel NN, Bird S, Appelmelk BJ, Bitter W, van der Sar AM.** 2012. ESX-5-deficient *Mycobacterium marinum* is hypervirulent in adult zebrafish. *Cell Microbiol* **14:**728–739.

108. **Daniel J, Maamar H, Deb C, Sirakova TD, Kolattukudy PE.** 2011. *Mycobacterium tuberculosis* uses host triacylglycerol to accumulate lipid droplets and acquires a dormancy-like phenotype in lipid-loaded macrophages. *PLoS Pathog* **7:**e1002093. doi:10.1371/journal.ppat. 1002093.

109. **Deb C, Daniel J, Sirakova TD, Abomoelak B, Dubey VS, Kolattukudy PE.** 2006. A novel lipase belonging to the hormone-sensitive lipase family induced under starvation to utilize stored triacylglycerol in *Mycobacterium tuberculosis*. *J Biol Chem* **281:**3866–3875.

110. **Singh VK, Srivastava V, Singh V, Rastogi N, Roy R, Shaw AK, Dwivedi AK, Srivastava R, Srivastava BS.** 2011. Overexpression of Rv3097c in *Mycobacterium bovis* BCG abolished the efficacy of BCG vaccine to protect against *Mycobacterium tuberculosis* infection in mice. *Vaccine* **29:**4754–4760.

111. **Singh VK, Srivastava M, Dasgupta A, Singh MP, Srivastava R, Srivastava BS.** 2014. Increased virulence of *Mycobacterium tuberculosis* H37Rv overexpressing LipY in a murine model. *Tuberculosis(Edinb)* **94:**252–261.

112. **Espitia C, Laclette JP, Mondragón-Palomino M, Amador A, Campuzano J, Martens A, Singh M, Cicero R, Zhang Y, Moreno C.** 1999. The PE-PGRS glycine-rich proteins of *Mycobacterium tuberculosis*: a new family of fibronectin-binding proteins? *Microbiology* **145:**3487–3495.

113. **Campuzano J, Aguilar D, Arriaga K, León JC, Salas-Rangel LP, González-y-Merchand J, Hernández-Pando R, Espitia C.** 2007. The PGRS domain of *Mycobacterium tuberculosis* PE_PGRS Rv1759c antigen is an efficient subunit vaccine to prevent reactivation in a murine model of chronic tuberculosis. *Vaccine* **25:**3722–3729.

114. **Koh KW, Lehming N, Seah GT.** 2009. Degradation-resistant protein domains limit host cell processing and immune detection of mycobacteria. *Mol Immunol* **46:**1312–1318.

115. **Brennan MJ, Delogu G.** 2002. The PE multigene family: a "molecular mantra" for mycobacteria. *Trends Microbiol* **10:**246–249.

116. Levitskaya J, Coram M, Levitsky V, Imreh S, Steigerwald-Mullen PM, Klein G, Kurilla MG, Masucci MG. 1995. Inhibition of antigen processing by the internal repeat region of the Epstein-Barr virus nuclear antigen-1. *Nature* **375**:685–688.

117. Tellam J, Smith C, Rist M, Webb N, Cooper L, Vuocolo T, Connolly G, Tscharke DC, Devoy MP, Khanna R. 2008. Regulation of protein translation through mRNA structure influences MHC class I loading and T cell recognition. *Proc Natl Acad Sci USA* **105**:9319–9324.

118. Tellam JT, Lekieffre L, Zhong J, Lynn DJ, Khanna R. 2012. Messenger RNA sequence rather than protein sequence determines the level of self-synthesis and antigen presentation of the EBV-encoded antigen, EBNA1. *PLoS Pathog* **8**:e1003112. doi:10.1371/journal.ppat.1003112.

119. Banu S, Honoré N, Saint-Joanis B, Philpott D, Prévost M-C, Cole ST. 2002. Are the PE-PGRS proteins of *Mycobacterium tuberculosis* variable surface antigens? *Mol Microbiol* **44**:9–19.

120. Vordermeier HM, Hewinson RG, Wilkinson RJ, Wilkinson KA, Gideon HP, Young DB, Sampson SL. 2012. Conserved immune recognition hierarchy of mycobacterial PE/PPE proteins during infection in natural hosts. *PLoS One* **7**:e40890. doi:10.1371/journal.pone.0040890.

121. Copin R, Coscollá M, Seiffert SN, Bothamley G, Sutherland J, Mbayo G, Gagneux S, Ernst JD. 2014. Sequence diversity in the pe_pgrs genes of *Mycobacterium tuberculosis* is independent of human T cell recognition. *MBio* **5**:e00960-13. doi:10.1128/mBio.00960-13.

122. McEvoy CRE, Cloete R, Müller B, Schürch AC, van Helden PD, Gagneux S, Warren RM, Gey NC. 2012. Comparative analysis of *Mycobacterium tuberculosis pe* and *ppe* genes reveals high sequence variation and an apparent absence of selective constraints. *PLoS One* **7**:e30593. doi:10.1371/journal.pone.0030593.

123. Talarico S, Cave MD, Foxman B, Marrs CF, Zhang L, Bates JH, Yang Z. 2007. Association of *Mycobacterium tuberculosis* PE PGRS33 polymorphism with clinical and epidemiological characteristics. *Tuberculosis (Edinb)* **87**:338–346.

124. Cascioferro A, Daleke MH, Ventura M, Donà V, Delogu G, Palù G, Bitter W, Manganelli R. 2011. Functional dissection of the PE domain responsible for translocation of PE_PGRS33 across the mycobacterial cell wall. *PLoS One* **6**:e27713. doi:10.1371/journal.pone.0027713.

125. Delogu G, Pusceddu C, Bua A, Fadda G, Brennan MJ, Zanetti S. 2004. Rv1818c-encoded PE_PGRS protein of *Mycobacterium tuberculosis* is surface exposed and influences bacterial cell structure. *Mol Microbiol* **52**:725–733.

126. Cadieux N, Parra M, Cohen H, Maric D, Morris SL, Brennan MJ. 2011. Induction of cell death after localization to the host cell mitochondria by the *Mycobacterium tuberculosis* PE_PGRS33 protein. *Microbiology* **157**:793–804.

127. Basu S, Pathak SK, Banerjee A, Pathak S, Bhattacharyya A, Yang Z, Talarico S, Kundu M, Basu J. 2007. Execution of macrophage apoptosis by PE_PGRS33 of *Mycobacterium tuberculosis* is mediated by Toll-like receptor 2-dependent release of tumor necrosis factor-alpha. *J Biol Chem* **282**:1039–1050.

128. Houben ENG, Korotkov KV, Bitter W. 2013. Take five: type VII secretion systems of mycobacteria. *Biochim Biophys Acta* **1843**:1707–1716.

129. Akpe San Roman S, Facey PD, Fernandez-Martinez L, Rodriguez C, Vallin C, Del Sol R, Dyson P. 2010. A heterodimer of EsxA and EsxB is involved in sporulation and is secreted by a type VII secretion system in *Streptomyces coelicolor*. *Microbiology* **156**:1719–1729.

130. Fyans JK, Bignell D, Loria R, Toth I, Palmer T. 2013. The ESX/type VII secretion system modulates development, but not virulence, of the plant pathogen *Streptomyces scabies*. *Mol Plant Pathol* **14**:119–130.

131. São-José C, Baptista C, Santos MA. 2004. *Bacillus subtilis* operon encoding a membrane receptor for bacteriophage SPP1. *J Bacteriol* **186**:8337–8346.

132. Van den Ent F, Löwe J. 2005. Crystal structure of the ubiquitin-like protein YukD from *Bacillus subtilis*. *FEBS Lett* **579**:3837–3841.

133. Burts ML, DeDent AC, Missiakas DM. 2008. EsaC substrate for the ESAT-6 secretion pathway and its role in persistent infections of *Staphylococcus aureus*. *Mol Microbiol* **69**:736–746.

134. Anderson M, Chen Y-H, Butler EK, Missiakas DM. 2011. EsaD, a secretion factor for the Ess pathway in *Staphylococcus aureus*. *J Bacteriol* **193**:1583–1589.

135. Kneuper H, Cao ZP, Twomey KB, Zoltner M, Jäger F, Cargill JS, Chalmers J, van der Kooi-Pol MM, van Dijl JM, Ryan RP, Hunter WN, Palmer T. 2014. Heterogeneity in ess transcriptional organization and variable contribution of the Ess/type VII protein secretion system to virulence across closely related *Staphylocccus aureus* strains. *Mol Microbiol* **93**:928–943.

136. **Schulthess B, Bloes DA, Berger-Bächi B.** 2012. Opposing roles of σB and σB-controlled SpoVG in the global regulation of esxA in *Staphylococcus aureus*. *BMC Microbiol* **12:**17.

137. **Korea CG, Balsamo G, Pezzicoli A, Merakou C, Tavarini S, Bagnoli F, Serruto D, Unnikrishnan M.** 2014. Staphylococcal Esx proteins modulate apoptosis and release of intracellular *Staphylococcus aureus* during infection in epithelial cells. *Infect Immun* **82:**4144–4153.

138. **Rybniker J, Chen JM, Sala C, Hartkoorn RC, Vocat A, Benjak A, Boy-Röttger S, Zhang M, Székely R, Greff Z, Orfi L, Szabadkai I, Pató J, Kéri G, Cole ST.** 2014. Anticytolytic screen identifies inhibitors of mycobacterial virulence protein secretion. *Cell Host Microbe* **16:**538–548.

139. **Sundaramoorthy R, Fyfe PK, Hunter WN.** 2008. Structure of *Staphylococcus aureus* EsxA suggests a contribution to virulence by action as a transport chaperone and/or adaptor protein. *J Mol Biol* **383:**603–614.

BACTERIAL DEFENSES

Stress Responses, Adaptation, and Virulence of Bacterial Pathogens During Host Gastrointestinal Colonization

14

ANNIKA FLINT,[1] JAMES BUTCHER,[1] and ALAIN STINTZI[1]

STRESS RESPONSE AND ADAPTATION

Bacterial pathogens are exposed to a variety of stressful conditions while spreading to and colonizing new hosts to cause infection. Gastrointestinal pathogens such as *Campylobacter*, *Escherichia*, *Helicobacter*, *Listeria*, *Salmonella*, and *Shigella* species encounter numerous stresses during host colonization and infection. During transit through the gastrointestinal tract these pathogens are exposed to physical stresses (pH and osmotic stresses) as well as noxious substances (reactive oxygen and nitrosative species). Bacteria respond to these stresses by altering their transcriptome/proteome in an adaptive manner to either overcome the stress or resist the stress long enough to transition to more favorable conditions. The following sections will present the current state of knowledge for each stress response mentioned above and how these defenses contribute to bacterial virulence.

[1]Ottawa Institute of Systems Biology, Department of Biochemistry, Microbiology and Immunology, Faculty of Medicine, University of Ottawa, Ottawa, Ontario, Canada K1H 8M5.
Virulence Mechanisms of Bacterial Pathogens, 5th edition
Edited by Indira T. Kudva, Nancy A. Cornick, Paul J. Plummer, Qijing Zhang, Tracy L. Nicholson, John P. Bannantine, and Bryan H. Bellaire
© 2016 American Society for Microbiology, Washington, DC
doi:10.1128/microbiolspec.VMBF-0007-2015

PH STRESS RESPONSE

Following ingestion, bacteria must passage through the stomach. The pH of the stomach can range from as low as pH 2 (during fasting state) up to pH 7 (during meal intake) (1). Injury to the outer bacterial membrane and/ or disruption of the cytoplasmic pH due to H^+ ion exposure and influx can result in damage to DNA and enzymes, leading to cell death (2, 3). The detrimental effects of acid exposure necessitate expression of acid defense, adaptation, and repair mechanisms to facilitate bacterial survival during passage through the stomach.

Direct Defenses Against Acid Stress

Direct defense mechanisms for acid stress survival have been well studied in enteric pathogens such as *Listeria monocytogenes* (4), *Salmonella enterica* (5), and *Helicobacter pylori* (6, 7), which are the causative agents of listeriosis, salmonellosis, and gastric ulcers, respectively. Upon exposure to acidic conditions, these bacteria upregulate expression of defense enzymes such as amino acid carboxylases (4, 5), deiminases (4), ureases (7), and F1F0 ATPase pumps (7) to help maintain pH homeostasis within the cell. *S. enterica* strains encode for several decarboxylase enzymes including lysine and arginine decarboxylases. The lysine decarboxylase system consists of CadA, a lysine decarboxylase enzyme, and CadB, a lysine-cadaverine antiporter (5). The conversion of lysine to cadaverine by CadA within the cytoplasm requires a proton to be consumed. The CadB antiporter then exports the newly synthesized cadaverine out of the cell while importing lysine to begin the process anew (5). Overall, the enzymatic activity of CadA and the transport function of CadB help increase intracellular pH levels via consumption of H^+ ions. *S. enterica* also encodes for a second amino acid decarboxylase system involving an arginine carboxylase, AdiA, and an arginine-agmatine antiporter, AdiC (8). Similar to the lysine decarboxylase system, the AdiAC system also functions to consume H^+ ions during the enzymatic conversion of arginine to agmatine via AdiA and thus lowers the acidity within the cytoplasmic space. The AdiC antiporter subsequently exchanges the intracellular agmatine for extracellular arginine. The importance of these amino acid decarboxylase systems has been highlighted using *in vivo* experiments with BALB/c mice, which demonstrated upregulation of *cadBC* expression during infection (9). *cadBC* were similarly found to be induced when introduced into macrophages (10).

L. monocytogenes likewise encodes for a glutamate amino acid decarboxylase system which consists of GadD1, GadD2, GadD3, GadT1, and GadT2. *gadD1*, *gadD2*, and *gadD3* encode for glutamate decarboxylase enzymes, whereas *gadT1* and *gadT2* encode for glutamate/aminobutyric acid antiporters. Notably, not all strains of *L. monocytogenes* encode for the GadD1/GadT1 decarboxylase system (11). The consumption of protons during the enzymatic production of γ-aminobutyric acid from glutamate contributes to raising the pH within the cell. Colonization of gnotobiotic mice with *L. monocytogenes* resulted in significant upregulation of the glutamate decarboxylase system genes, suggesting the importance of this system for acid survival during colonization (4, 12).

L. monocytogenes also utilizes deiminases to help maintain pH homeostasis during infection. The arginine deiminase system is comprised of ArcABCD, which encode for an arginine deiminase (ArcA), catabolic ornithine carbamoyltransferase (ArcB), carbamate kinase (ArcC), and arginine-ornithine antiporter (ArcD) (13). ArcA catabolizes arginine to citrulline and NH_3. Citrulline is subsequently converted to ornithine and carbamoyl-phosphate by ArcB. ArcC converts carbamoyl-phosphate to NH_3 and CO_2 while producing ATP in the process. The NH_3 produced during these enzymatic steps combines with H^+ ions to yield NH^{4+}, which in turn raises pH levels within the bacterium. The arginine-ornithine antiporter exports ornithine out of the cell while bringing in additional arginine to undergo further enzymatic reactions by ArcABC (13). The importance of the arginine deiminase system has been demonstrated using murine *Listeria* infection experiments which revealed a 10-fold reduction in the number of $\Delta arcA$ mutant bacteria in the spleen relative to the wild type strain (14). Furthermore, the $\Delta arcA$ mutant was found to be significantly more sensitive to acid exposure (pH 3.5) over 150 minutes relative to wild type *Listeria*, revealing the role this system plays in acid survival (14).

Urease is another well-characterized direct defense mechanism against acid stress. *H. pylori* predominantly utilizes cytoplasmic urease enzymes to survive the acidic conditions found within the stomach. The mechanism that *H. pylori* employs to maintain the neutral pH within the cytoplasm includes an H^+ gated urea channel, cytoplasmic urease, and a membrane-bound carbonic anhydrase (15). Urea is found in the gastric juices of the stomach and enters the cell via porins. Urea is then subsequently transported into the cytoplasmic space from the periplasm in an energy-independent manner by the H^+ gated urea channel, UreI (16). Once the urea is within the cytoplasm, a multisubunit complex urease enzyme (UreAB) hydrolyzes the urea into ammonia and carbamic acid. UreA and UreB form the structural subunits of the apoenzyme (17, 18) and further require the UreEFGH proteins to insert Ni^{2+} into the UreAB apoenzyme to form the active urease enzyme (19). The carbamic acid produced can subsequently react with H_2O to produce H_2CO_3 and NH_3. The H_2CO_3 that has been produced is then converted to CO_2 and H_2O by cytoplasmic carbonic anhydrase. Finally, the NH_3 and CO_2 gases produced diffuse back through the inner membrane to the periplasm, whereby the NH_3 consumes a proton (producing NH^{4+}), and a membrane-anchored carbonic anhydrase converts the CO_2 to HCO^{3-} and H^+. The proton produced can combine with available NH_3 while the HCO^{3-} acts as a buffer to maintain the pH of the periplasm to approximately 6.1 (20, 21). Acid survival by *H. pylori* using urea hydrolysis to maintain cell pH neutrality has been shown to be critical for bacterial colonization studies of the mouse stomach (22). Indeed, both $\Delta ureI$ and $\Delta ureB$ mutants are attenuated for gastric colonization of mice (22, 23).

Bacteria can also use F_1F_0 ATPase pumps to increase pH in response to acid exposure. The F_1F_0 ATPase pump generates ATP during oxidative phosphorylation under aerobic conditions. The F_1 subunit of the enzyme functions to generate ATP from ADP + Pi or can hydrolyze ATP. Proton translocation across the inner membrane is performed by the F_0 subunit. The generation of a proton gradient during oxidative phosphorylation drives ATP synthesis via proton translocation back into the cytoplasm via the F_1F_0 ATPase. However, the F_1F_0 ATPase can also function to expel H^+ from the cytoplasm during anaerobic growth conditions to generate a proton gradient which is coupled with ATP hydrolysis. The expulsion of H^+ ions from the cytoplasm by F_1F_0 ATPase pumps increases the internal pH of the cell as has been demonstrated in bacteria such as *L. monocytogenes* (24) and *Salmonella enterica* serovar Typhimurium (25).

Indirect Defenses Against Acid Stress

Interestingly, not all enteric pathogens utilize these well-characterized direct acid defense mechanisms and rely on alternative strategies to survive stressful acidic conditions. The human food-borne pathogen *Campylobacter jejuni* does not encode for any annotated urease or amino acid decarboxylase enzymes (26) and yet may remain within the stomach for up to 1 hour before passaging into the duodenum (27). *C. jejuni* infection is one of the leading causes of gastroenteritis in humans, with typical symptoms including mild to severe abdominal pain and diarrhea. With an infectious dose as low as 800 organisms, *C. jejuni* is clearly well equipped to survive acid stress encountered within the stomach (28). Indeed, *C. jejuni* can survive up to 30 minutes of exposure to pH 3.5 without any loss in cell viability (29).

To gain greater insight into the acid adaptation strategies of this bacteria, transcriptional profiling of *C. jejuni* exposed to pH stress under *in vitro* conditions (Mueller-Hinton broth buffered at pH 4.5) and *in vivo* conditions (piglet stomach contents) was performed to identify important mechanisms for acid stress survival (30). Transcriptional analysis of *C. jejuni* that was isolated from piglet stomach contents revealed significant upregulation of genes involved in heat shock response. These genes included the transcriptional regulator *hrcA* and protein chaperones involved in heat shock response (*groEL*, *groES*, *dnaK*, *grpE*, and *clpB*). Oxidative stress (*cft*) and nitrosative stress (*ctb*) responses were similarly upregulated. Genes that were significantly downregulated included those encoding for ribosomal proteins (*rplABEFLOPRVX*, *rpsBCEHNQ*, and *rpmC*), transcription (*rpoC* and *nusG*), and translation (*infC*, *prfA*, *fusA*, *trmD*, and *tilS*) (30).

Transcript changes in response to acid of *C. jejuni* cultured under *in vitro* conditions identified many of the genes found to be differentially expressed *in vivo*. Genes that were highly upregulated *in vitro* include flagellum biogenesis (*flgDEI*, *fliD*), glycosylation (*pseA*, *cj1321*, *cj1325*, *maf3*, and *neuA2*), oxidative stress defense (*ahpC*, *tpx*, *cj1064*, *katA*, *perR*, and *cft*), iron uptake (*cfbpABcj1658*, *cj1660*, and *cj1224*), and citric acid cycle genes (*icd*, *mdh*, *gltA*, *mfrABE*, and *sucCD*). In addition, several transcripts showed increasing induction with increased acid exposure times, including the acid stress resistance gene *cfa* (cyclopropane fatty acid synthase), the nitrosative stress defense gene (*cgb*), and the FeS cluster assembly gene (*nifU*). Genes that were downregulated included chemotaxis genes (*cetA/cetB* and *cj0262c*), protein glycosylation genes (*pglABC*), and fatty acid biosynthesis genes (*plsX*, *fabH*, and *ispA*) (30).

These studies suggest an important role for heat shock proteins in response to acid as well as induction of cross-protective stress defense mechanisms such as oxidative stress defense. Indeed, mutation of *clpB* (a cochaperone involved in refolding aggregated proteins along with DnaK-GrpE-DnaJ) resulted in increased acid sensitivity, demonstrating the importance of protein refolding for cell viability during pH stress in *C. jejuni* (30). Furthermore, ribosomal protein genes were downregulated, possibly indicating an effort by the cell to redirect energy toward acid-stress survival gene expression.

Cell surface proteins also play an important role in the *C. jejuni* acid-stress response. Transposon mutants into capsular polysaccharide genes *kpsS*, *hddC*, *cj1432c*, *cj1437c*, and *cj1442c* revealed growth defects when cultured under low pH conditions, suggesting that the capsule plays an important role in protecting the cell from potential H^+ influx (31). Flagellum biogenesis genes are also important in acid-stress survival. Both Le et al. and Reid et al. identified significant upregulation of flagellar biogenesis genes upon acid exposure (29, 30). It is thought that induction of flagellum biogenesis might be a general stress response by *C. jejuni* (similar responses are observed for expression of oxidative and nitrosative stress genes) (31). Alternatively, acid exposure may be used as a signal for *C. jejuni* to induce motility gene expression to prepare for intestinal colonization and invasion (29). Indeed, functional flagella have been shown to be an important factor for adherence and invasion of *C. jejuni* into INT407 cells (32, 33) and also for oxidative stress resistance (34). In support of this hypothesis, *C. jejuni* that was acid stressed at pH 5 displayed increased invasion of mouse intestinal crypt cells (m-ICc12) compared to nonstressed cells (pH 7) when grown using a transwell model (29). This result suggests that acid exposure helps prime the bacteria for colonization and invasion, potentially by upregulation of flagellum biogenesis genes (29).

OSMOTIC STRESS RESPONSE

Gastrointestinal pathogens are exposed to different levels of osmotic stress within the host as well as during transit between the environment and the host. Additionally, salting of foods as a method of preservation exposes food-borne pathogens to further osmotic stress, which must be overcome during the transmission phase from food to the host. Bacteria utilize numerous strategies to survive exposure to hyperosmotic or hypoosmotic environmental conditions. Two types of responses are involved during osmotic shock, consisting of immediate and long-term survival mechanisms. The immediate bacterial response involves sensing changes in the extracellular osmotic pressure due to the entry or exit of water from the cytoplasm, which results in changes in membrane tension, cell volume, turgor pressure, and intracellular ion concentrations (35). To combat these changes, bacteria selectively release or uptake ions and small molecules using specific enzymes and membrane channels to prevent the rupture or dehydration of cells (35). The long-term bacterial responses to osmotic stress involve the differential expression of transport systems as well as modifications to the composition of the cell membrane to survive hyper- or hypo-osmotic conditions (35). During hyperosmotic stress, *Escherichia coli* uptakes K^+ ions (immediate response) and organic osmolytes (trehalose, proline, glycine betaine) (long-term response) to prevent cellular dehydration (Fig. 1) (35). Cells can also synthesize these organic osmolytes as a response to changes in the osmotic environment. The organic osmolytes also serve a secondary role by maintaining protein stability and preventing degradation (36).

Immediate Bacterial Responses to Osmotic Shock

The two osmosensing K^+ ion uptake systems within *E. coli* are the Trk and Kdp systems. The Trk system is a multimeric ATP-dependent, low affinity K^+/H^+ symporter composed of TrkAEH(G) (Fig. 1A) (35). TrkA encodes for an essential peripheral cytoplasmic regulatory subunit that is thought to regulate K^+ conductance by potentially sensing the redox state of the cell (37). TrkE contains an ATP-binding cassette involved in import, and TrkH (or TrkG) encodes for the ion-conducting translocation subunit (35). The Trk transport system is constitutively expressed in *E. coli* and utilizes the proton motive force of the cell and ATP to provide the energy required for K^+ uptake (38).

E. coli expresses a second inducible high-affinity K^+ uptake system, KdpFABC. In contrast to the Trk system, the high K^+ affinity of the Kdp uptake system allows for cellular scavenging of K^+ ions during conditions of K^+ limitation or osmotic stress (39). The KdpA subunit is the K^+ ion translocation subunit, KdpB is an ATPase, KdpF plays a role in maintaining complex stability, and KdpC functions in assembly of the Kdp-ATPase complex (Fig. 1A) (35). The expression of this inducible K^+ ion transport system is controlled by the two-component response regulator KdpDE (40). KdpD is a histidine kinase that senses and responds to the ionic strength, K^+, and ATP concentrations within the cytoplasm (41). Under hyperosmotic stress, KdpD is autophosphorylated and subsequently phosphorylates the response regulator protein KdpE, leading to induction of *kdpFABC* (40, 42). The importance of the Trk and Kdp K^+ uptake systems in pathogenesis has been investigated in *Salmonella* using both mouse and chick virulence models (43). $\Delta trkA$ single and $\Delta kdpA\Delta trkA$ double deletion mutants were found to be significantly attenuated in virulence using a pathogenic mouse model. Furthermore, the $\Delta trkA$ and $\Delta kdpA\Delta trkA$ mutant strains were also attenuated for virulence using a chick survival assay. Indeed, inoculation of chicks with the mutant strains resulted in greater chick survival over a 2-week period relative to chicks that received the wild type strain. Clearly,

A) Immediate Response

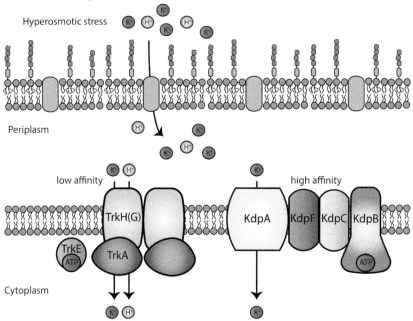

B) Long Term Response

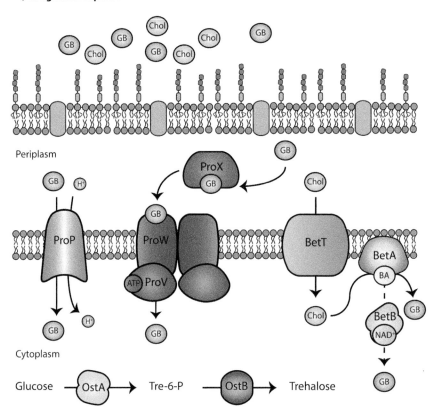

these K$^+$ acquisition systems are important for *Salmonella* host colonization and virulence (43).

Long-Term Bacterial Survival of Osmotic Shock

The Trk and Kdp ion transport systems are part of the immediate cellular responses to osmotic shock. However, bacteria, including *E. coli*, preferentially use alternative osmoprotectant molecules (trehalose, proline, glycine betaine) as part of their long-term survival mechanisms to hyperosmotic shock. *E. coli* cells show preferential uptake of proline and glycine betaine followed by trehalose synthesis after the initial K$^+$ ion intake (44). Indeed, it has been demonstrated that K$^+$ uptake is the initial transient response of the cells to osmotic shock. High intracellular levels of K$^+$ ions inhibit *E. coli* growth and thus necessitate the use of alternative organic osmolytes for sustained protection against hyperosmotic stress (44). Several uptake systems have been characterized for these organic osmolytes consisting of the ProP, ProU, and BetT transporters (Fig. 1B). ProP encodes for an H$^+$/osmoprotectant symporter which displays a high affinity for glycine betaine import as well as a lower affinity for uptake of a series of substances including proline, proline betaine, and ectoine (45). Import of these substances by ProP occurs in response to environmental osmolarity, as well as cytoplasmic levels of K$^+$ ions and osmolytes (46). The energy required for the uptake of osmoprotectant substances is provided by the proton motive force (46).

Deletion of Δ*proP* in uropathogenic *E. coli* results in a 100-fold decrease in bacteria recovered from the bladders of mice, suggesting the importance of osmoprotectant uptake by ProP for successful colonization and virulence (47).

ProU, like ProP, also has a broad range of substrates and has a high affinity for glycine betaine (48). The ATP-binding cassette transport system, ProU, is a multisubunit complex consisting of ProV, ProW, and ProX (Fig. 1B). The ProV subunit is a cytoplasmic, inner-membrane ATPase protein and has an important role in osmosensing (48, 49). ProW is an integral transmembrane protein (50), and ProX is a periplasmic binding protein which delivers specific substrates to the ProVW transport complex (48). In *E. coli*, ProU activity has been shown to be induced in response to increased osmotic stress (48). OpuC, an ortholog of ProU, was found to play an important role in the colonization and virulence of *L. monocytogenes* in a murine model of infection. Mutation of *opuC* resulted in a significant decrease in colonization of the mouse small intestine and decreased systemic infection of the spleen and liver (51).

Additional long-term adaptation responses to osmotic stress in *E. coli* include the uptake of choline by the BetT transporter followed by the synthesis of the osmoprotectant molecule glycine betaine (Fig. 1B). The Bet system is composed of an integral membrane, BetT, which utilizes the energy provided by the proton motive force to transport choline into the cytoplasm with high affinity (52). Once choline enters the cytoplasm, *betA* and *betB*, which encode for choline dehydrogenase

FIGURE 1 **The immediate and long-term osmotic shock responses of bacterial pathogens protect against changes in osmolarity during host colonization. (A) During initial exposure to hyperosmotic shock, pathogens transport K$^+$ ions from the external environment into the cytoplasm to prevent cellular dehydration. K$^+$ ion uptake can occur utilizing the low-affinity TrkAEH(G) or high-affinity KdpFABC acquisition systems. (B) Following initial K$^+$ uptake, uptake of glycine betaine and choline, and synthesis of trehalose are part of the long-term bacterial adaptations to osmotic stress. Uptake of glycine betaine is mediated by the ProP and ProVWX systems. Choline is transported by BetT into the cytoplasm and converted into betaine aldehyde and then glycine betaine by BetA. Alternatively, BetB can catalyze the conversion of betaine aldehyde into glycine betaine. Finally, trehalose can be synthesized from glucose by either BetA or BetB. Chol, choline; GB, glycine betaine; BA, betaine aldehyde.**

and betaine aldehyde dehydrogenase, respectively, convert choline into glycine betaine (52). BetA is membrane bound and catalyzes the oxidation of choline into betaine aldehyde and then into glycine betaine. BetB is a soluble, cytosolic enzyme which specifically converts betaine aldehyde into glycine betaine and requires a NAD^+ cofactor to function (53). High osmolarity was found to increase the enzymatic activity of these enzymes in E. coli (53).

Finally, E. coli also synthesizes trehalose to protect against the hyperosmotic stress conditions encountered by the cell. OstA and OstB catalyze the synthesis of trehalose from glucose (Fig. 1B). OstA is a trehalose 6-phosphate synthase and OstB is a trehalose 6-phosphate phosphatase (54). Induction of the ostAB genes occurs under conditions of both osmotic stress as well as during stationary phase growth (55).

Alternative Strategies for Osmotic Stress Survival in C. jejuni

In contrast to enteric pathogens such as E. coli, other bacteria such as C. jejuni are relatively sensitive to osmotic stress. C. jejuni will not grow under osmolarities of ~1 osmol/liter, in contrast to E. coli, which can grow in 1.7 to 2 osmol/liter and even survive for periods in solutions of 10 osmol/liter (56, 57). In support of this increased sensitivity, C. jejuni does not contain many of the primary defense systems against osmotic shock that are present in other bacteria, such as potassium transporters and the ability to produce compatible solutes (i.e., trehalose) (58). In addition to dealing with increases in osmolality, C. jejuni must also be able to adapt to sudden decreases in osmolality. For example, the osmolality of the human intestine is estimated to be 0.3 osmol/liter, compared to 0.9 osmol/liter in the chicken duodenum (59, 60). C. jejuni would also presumably be exposed to sudden downshifts in osmolarity when expelled from the host gastrointestinal tract into the environment.

Conditions of hypo-osmolarity occur when the bacterium is exposed to a low-solute-containing solution. This increases pressure on the bacterium as solvent rushes into the cell and threatens to expand the cell until it bursts. One of the primary defense mechanisms against this threat is mechanosensitive channels (MSCs). These channels are sensitive to external pressures on the cell membrane (61). Alterations in the membrane tension result in conformational changes that lead to a pore opening in the MSC. This pore allows for the passage of solvent/solute molecules that relieves the membrane tension (61). While E. coli has four types of MSC (large- conductance, small-conductance, mini-conductance, and potassium-dependent), C. jejuni contains only two versions of the small-conductance types (Cjj0263 and Cjj1025) (61, 62). Deletion mutants into these two channels revealed that the Δcjj0263 mutant was more sensitive to osmotic downshifts compared to the wild type, Δcjj1025, or the Δcjj0263Δcjj1025 double deletion mutant (62). When tested in chick colonization assays, only the Δcjj0263Δcjj1025 double deletion mutant was significantly affected in its ability to colonize the host. This suggests that when inoculated under experimental conditions (i.e., oral gavage), either cjj0263 or cjj1025 is dispensable. Interestingly, the recovered bacteria from the chick ceca (wild type, Δcjj0263, or Δcjj0263Δcjj1025) showed differing phenotypes to subsequent hypo-osmotic shock (62). The resuspended Δcjj0263 and Δcjj0263Δcjj1025 isolates were less able to survive the osmotic downshift induced by diluting the inoculum 10-fold in water. This suggests that while the MSC mutants may be able to colonize, they may be defective during environmental transit to new hosts (62).

Both Cjj0263 and Cjj1025 were found to contain potential N-linked glycosylation sites. When whole cell lysates from wild type and ΔpglB mutants were immunoblotted with anti-Cjj0263 and anti-Cjj1025, both channels showed a PglB-dependent shift in their molecular size (62). Testing the ΔpglB mutant for its sensitivity to hypo-osmolality revealed a slight decrease in its survivability (~2- to 3-fold reduction) compared to the wild type (62). This compares to the ~500-fold decrease seen in the Δ*cjj0263* mutant and suggests that N-linked glycosylation is not required for Cjj0263 function (62). Nonetheless, these results do indicate that the *C. jejuni* N-linked glycosylation system does play a role during osmotic shifts. The level of free oligosaccharides derived from the N-linked glycosylation pathway has been shown to be correlated with salt levels, with low free oligosaccharides under high salt conditions and correspondingly higher free oligosaccharides under low salt growth conditions (63). Indeed, mutants defective in various steps of the N-linked glycosylation pathway are sensitive to high salt levels (64). Recent work has also revealed that the *C. jejuni* Δ*kpsM* mutant that is defective in capsule biogenesis is also more sensitive to high salt conditions (58).

While *C. jejuni* may not contain the prototypical defense mechanisms against hyper-osmotic conditions, recent work has suggested the presence of a novel strategy to combat this stress. When *C. jejuni* is exposed to high salt conditions, it appears to form distinct sub-populations of cells that differ in their expression of key proteins such as AtpF (F_1F_0 ATP synthase) (58). Sampling of *C. jejuni* cultures grown under normal conditions revealed the presence of subpopulations of cells that were either more sensitive or resistant to hyper-osmotic conditions compared to the wild type (58). Moreover, *C. jejuni* appears to form a bistable population of differently sized colonies under high salt conditions. The authors speculate that this may be a form of "hedge-betting" by *C. jejuni* to ensure that there are always members of the population that are capable of overcoming future stresses such as osmolality shifts (58). Given that *C. jejuni* is missing many of the known DNA repair systems, these bistable populations could arise from phase variation in known/unidentified contingency regions or from point mutations during replication (58, 65).

OXIDATIVE STRESS RESPONSE

One of the major strategies used by host organisms to fight bacterial infections is by exposing invading pathogens to reactive oxygen species (ROS). The major host innate immune defenses against bacterial colonization and invasion include macrophages, neutrophils, and inflammatory monocytes. These phagosomes use a multisubunit plasma membrane–associated enzyme (NADPH oxidase) to initiate the oxidative burst by generating superoxide ($O_2^{\bullet-}$). The NADPH oxidase transports electrons into the phagosome which are then available for the reduction of molecular oxygen to produce $O_2^{\bullet-}$. Subsequent dismutation of $O_2^{\bullet-}$ produces a second ROS hydrogen peroxide, H_2O_2 (Fig. 2) (66). Neutrophils and monocytes (but not macrophages) also express myeloperoxidase, which produces bactericidal compounds by converting $O_2^{\bullet-}$ and H_2O_2 into hypochlorite, hypobromite, or hypoiodite (67). The pathogenic bacteria that are engulfed within these phagosomes are exposed to ROS, which can either inhibit growth or kill the bacteria by damaging important biological molecules such as DNA, proteins, and lipids (66). Furthermore, enteric pathogens can also be exposed to ROS from host microbiota, such as lactic acid bacteria, that produce and secrete H_2O_2 into the gastrointestinal tract (68). Consequently, pathogens encode for numerous direct oxidant detoxification enzymes to survive the harmful effects of oxidative stress encountered during host colonization and pathogenesis (Fig. 2). These enzymes include the intensely studied and well-characterized superoxide dismutase, catalase, and alkyl hydroperoxide reductase enzymes.

Direct Oxidative Stress Defenses

Bacterial pathogens typically encode for one or more superoxide dismutase enzymes which differ in their metal cofactors, cellular location, and regulation. Despite the diversity and number of these enzymes across

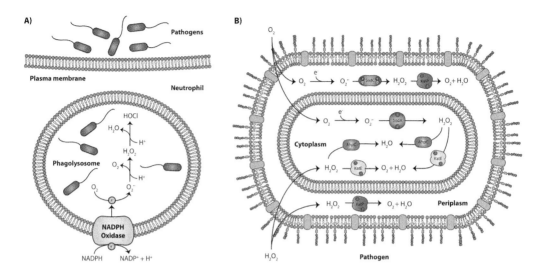

FIGURE 2 The oxidant detoxification mechanisms of bacterial pathogens provide defense against the oxidative burst encountered within the host neutrophil. (A) Invading pathogens are engulfed within the neutrophil phagolysosome and exposed reactive oxygen species and bactericidal compounds. Electrons supplied by NADPH oxidase reduce O_2 into $O_2^{\bullet-}$, which is subsequently converted into H_2O_2 and HOCl. (B) The oxidative stress defenses present pathogens (such as Shiga-toxin-producing *E. coli*) that contribute to bacterial survival against neutrophil oxidative burst. Uncharged O_2 and H_2O_2 freely diffuse across the bacterial membranes into the periplasmic and cytoplasmic spaces of the bacterial cell. O_2 can undergo one electron reduction to produce $O_2^{\bullet-}$. $O_2^{\bullet-}$ and H_2O_2 can be detoxified within the periplasm by SodC and KatP, respectively. Within the cytoplasm, $O_2^{\bullet-}$ and H_2O_2 are detoxified by SodA and KatE/AhpC, respectively. SodA and KatE are both induced under conditions of oxidative stress and are under the control of the transcriptional regulators SoxSR and OxyR.

bacterial species, the superoxide dismutase enzymes function by converting $O_2^{\bullet-}$ into H_2O_2 and O_2 (Fig. 2). Bacteria such as *C. jejuni* only encode for one iron cofactored superoxide dismutase, SodB (26, 69). Conversely, *E. coli* contains three superoxide dismutase enzymes (SodA, SodB, and SodC), which are cofactored with manganese, iron, and copper-zinc, respectively. SodA and SodB are cytoplasmic enzymes, in contrast to SodC, which is located within the periplasmic space (70, 71). Furthermore, the *sodA* and *sodB* genes are under regulatory control by different transcriptional regulators. *sodA* is induced by SoxSR (superoxide stress response) and is Fur (ferric uptake regulator) and AcrA (aerobic regulation control) repressed (72), whereas *sodB* is indirectly activated by Fur through the action of the non-coding RNA (ncRNA) RyhB (73).

S. Typhimurium expresses two periplasmic copper-zinc superoxide dismutases, SodCI and SodCII (74), in addition to cytosolic SodA and SodB. *sodCII* is encoded on the bacterial chromosome in all *S. enterica* strains, whereas *sodCI* is expressed from the Gifsy-2 bacteriophage located within the more virulent serovars of *S. enterica* (Typhimurium, Enteritidis, Dublin, Choleraesuis, Heidelberg, Gallinarum, Pullorum, Typhisuis, Haifa, Newport, Paratyphi B, and Saintpaul) (74). Studies involving the two periplasmic Sod enzymes revealed that SodCI has greater stability and catalytic activity than SodCII (75). *In vivo* experiments using a mouse virulence model have further demonstrated that SodCI plays a greater role in bacterial virulence compared to SodCII. Indeed, deletion of *sodCI* results in a significant decrease in mouse mortality relative to wild type

S. Typhimurium, whereas the $\Delta sodCII$ mutant showed only a modest (but not statistically significant) reduction. In addition, *sodCI* was also found to be significantly upregulated in *S.* Typhimurium recovered from macrophages (75).

The enzymatic reaction carried out by SOD enzymes produces a second ROS, H_2O_2. H_2O_2 detoxification can be carried out by numerous enzymes within bacteria, including catalase and alkyl hydroperoxide reductase (Fig. 2). Catalase enzymes dismutate H_2O_2 into H_2O and O_2. There are three classes of catalases: monofunctional catalases, bifunctional catalase-peroxidases, and nonheme-containing manganese catalases (76). The monofunctional catalases consist of two subgroups: large (>75 kDa) and small (>54 kDa) subunit catalases. Monofunctional catalases are typically tetrameric proteins consisting of four identical subunits. Each subunit has a heme prosthetic group which facilitates the two-step oxidation and reduction reaction required to catalyze H_2O_2 dismutation (equations 1 and 2).

$$\text{Enz}\,(\text{Por-Fe}^{III}) + H_2O_2 {\rightarrow} \text{Enz} \atop (\text{Por}^{\bullet +}\text{-Fe}^{IV} = O) + H_2O \tag{1}$$

$$\text{Enz}\,(\text{Por}^{\bullet +}\text{-Fe}^{IV} = O) + H_2O_2 {\rightarrow} \text{Enz} \atop (\text{Por-Fe}^{III}) + H_2O + O_2 \tag{2}$$

During the first reaction, the heme group is oxidized to a high valent, oxoferryl porphyrin cation radical intermediate by H_2O_2. During the second step, a second H_2O_2 molecule reduces the oxoferryl porphyrin cation radical back to its resting ferric state. Overall, this reaction consumes two molecules of H_2O_2 and yields two H_2O and one O_2 (77).

Bifunctional catalase-peroxidase enzymes are typically homodimers which display both catalase activity and peroxidase activity (78). In addition to the catalase reaction mechanism, the catalase-peroxidase enzyme can also use a peroxidase reaction mechanism to detoxify H_2O_2 and other organic compounds if a suitable electron donor is available within the cell. Following the oxidation of the heme iron (equation 1), the electron donor reduces the heme iron back to its resting state by two one-electron transfers (equations 3 and 4) or one two-electron transfer (equation 5) (78).

$$\text{Enz}\,(\text{Por}^{\bullet +}\text{-Fe}^{IV} = O) + AH {\rightarrow} \text{Enz} \atop (\text{Por} - \text{Fe}^{IV}\text{-OH}) + A^{\bullet +} \tag{3}$$

$$\text{Enz}\,(\text{Por-Fe}^{IV}\text{-OH}) + AH {\rightarrow} \text{Enz} \atop (\text{Por-Fe}^{III}) + H_2O + A^{\bullet +} \tag{4}$$

$$\text{Enz}\,(\text{Por}^{\bullet +}\text{-Fe}^{IV} = O) + X^- + H^+ {\rightarrow} \atop \textit{Enz}\,(\text{Por-Fe}^{III}) + H_2O + \text{HOX} \tag{5}$$

The third type of catalase is the nonheme manganese-containing catalase. The enzyme is hexameric in structure, with each subunit containing a di-manganese active center. Manganese catalases display lower specific enzyme activities compared to other catalase types, providing a possible explanation for why they are found in lower abundance across bacterial species (79). The reaction catalyzed by manganese catalases involves the di-manganese active site, which utilizes a distinct reaction mechanism compared to heme-containing catalases (equations 6 and 7).

$$H_2O_2 + \text{Mn}^{II}\text{-Mn}^{II} \atop (2\,H^+) {\rightarrow} \text{Mn}^{III}\text{-Mn}^{III} + 2\,H_2O \tag{6}$$

$$H_2O_2 + \text{Mn}^{III}\text{-Mn}^{III} {\rightarrow} \text{Mn}^{II}\text{-Mn}^{II} \atop (2\,H^+) + O_2 \tag{7}$$

Manganese catalases are able to detoxify H_2O_2 in either the 2^+ or 3^+ oxidation state. Therefore, either reaction 6 or 7 can occur depending on the oxidation state of the enzyme, with H_2O_2 acting as either an oxidant (Mn-Mn^{II} state) or reductant (Mn-Mn^{III} state). Furthermore, detoxification of

H_2O_2 only involves the transfer of electrons with the active center, unlike heme catalases, which require the formation of a reactive intermediate species (79).

Much like Sod enzymes, the types, cellular location, and regulation of catalases can differ vastly across different enteric pathogens. *H. pylori* and *C. jejuni* contain only one monofunctional catalase enzyme, KatA (26, 80). KatA from *H. pylori* has also been shown to localize within both the cytoplasmic and periplasmic cellular compartments. KatA is transported to the periplasm in a twin-arginine translocation–dependent manner using the KatA accessory protein, KapA (81). *E. coli* contains two catalases: one monofunctional large-subunit catalase (KatE) and one catalase peroxidase (KatG). The *katE* gene is upregulated under stationary phase and controlled by the stationary-phase-specific sigma factor, σs (82–84). *katG* expression is inducible upon exposure to H_2O_2 and is regulated by OxyR (66). The highly virulent O157:H7 Shiga-toxin-producing *E. coli* strain also expresses a third catalase peroxidase, periplasmic KatP (Fig. 2) (85). The *katP* gene is encoded within the pO157 plasmid, and it is predicted to be an important virulence factor (85, 86). *S.* Typhimurium encodes for three catalase enzymes: *katE*, *katG*, and *katN* (manganese catalase). *katN*, like *katE*, is regulated by the stationary-phase-specific sigma factor, σs (87). Interestingly, during stationary phase growth, a *katN* mutant did not display increased sensitivity toward H_2O_2 relative to the wild type strain, suggesting a relatively minor role for this enzyme within the cell (87).

Catalase enzymes have been extensively characterized in *in vivo* infectious models and play highly critical roles for successful bacterial colonization and pathogenesis. Deletion of *katA* in *C. jejuni* results in decreased fitness compared to the wild type strain in a pathogenic neonate piglet model of infection (88). Similarly, mutation of the *C. jejuni* KatA heme trafficking protein, Cj1386, also resulted in out-competition by the wild type

strain in piglets (88). Using a murine model of infection, both *katA* and *kapA H. pylori* mutants were attenuated for colonization of the gastric mucosa and were found to be required for long-term colonization (89). *In vivo* pathogenesis models involving KatA, Cj1386, and KapA highlight that catalase biogenesis and accessory proteins play an equally critical role during infection like KatA and provide potential novel therapeutic targets.

Hydrogen peroxide and organic peroxide detoxification is also performed within bacteria using alkyl hydroperoxide reductase (Ahp) enzymes (Fig. 2). Ahp consists of two subunits, AhpC and AhpF, where AhpC is a peroxidase and AhpF is an NADH-reducing flavoprotein. AhpCF detoxifies H_2O_2 by the transfer of electrons from NADH to H_2O_2 to produce two molecules of H_2O (90). In *E. coli*, AhpC scavenges low levels of cellular H_2O_2 (<20 μM) and helps maintain the concentration of H_2O_2 within the cell to approximately 20 nM (91). However, due to the requirement of using an NADH cofactor to regenerate the AhpC subunit, when extracellular levels of H_2O_2 exceed 20 μM, AhpC activity becomes saturated and catalase becomes the primary detoxifier of H_2O_2 (66). In *H. pylori*, Δ*ahpC* mutants failed to colonize the gastric mucosa of mice (92). Deletion of *ahpC* in *C. jejuni* also results in attenuated colonization in a chick colonization model (93).

In some bacterial species, catalase and alkyl hydroperoxide reductase enzymes have compensatory roles requiring tandem deletion of two or more H_2O_2 detoxification enzymes to observe an *in vivo* phenotype. Indeed, in *S.* Typhimurium, mutation of *katE*, *katG*, *katN*, *ahpC*, and *tsaA* (alkyl hydroperoxide reductase) is required to observe attenuation in virulence in a mouse model of infection (94). Similar findings have been observed in *Brucella abortus* in which a double deletion Δ*ahpCD*Δ*katE* mutant displayed a significant reduction in virulence in both C57BL/6 and BALB/c mice compared to the parental strain

(95). Attenuation in virulence, however, was not observed for the single $\Delta ahpCD$ and $\Delta katE$ mutants, suggesting functional redundancy between these two detoxification enzymes during host colonization and exposure to ROS (95).

Indirect Oxidative Stress Defenses

In addition to the major ROS detoxification enzymes which play significant roles in oxidative stress survival during host colonization and pathogenesis, indirect defenses have been identified that also contribute significantly to bacterial virulence. Repair mechanisms play crucial roles during colonization to reverse the damage inflicted on biological molecules as a result of oxidative stress. Oxidants can damage DNA, proteins, and lipids, which can disrupt important cellular processes leading to growth inhibition and cell death. Consequently, these molecules must be repaired to restore proper biological function. Methionine is one amino acid that is frequently damaged by oxidative stress due to its highly oxidizable sulphur atom (96). Oxidation of methionine produces two isomers: S and R methionine sulfoxide (MetO). S-MetO and R-MetO can be reduced by MsrA (methionine sulfoxide reductase) and MsrB/MsrC, respectively (97). Free S-MetO can also be reduced by biotin sulfoxide reductase, BisC. Additionally, BisC reduces biotin sulfoxide—an inactive molecule produced from the oxidation of biotin (98). Biotin is involved in many important cellular metabolic processes because it functions as a cofactor for a multitude of carboxylase enzymes (99). Thus, it has been found that biological repair mechanisms such as Msr and BisC are indirectly important for oxidative stress resistance and pathogenesis (97, 98). Deletion mutants of $\Delta msrA$ and $\Delta msrB\Delta msrC$ in S. Typhimurium were found to have increased sensitivity toward exogenous H_2O_2 (97). Additionally, the $\Delta msrA$ and $\Delta msrB\Delta msrC$ mutants displayed reduced growth in activated murine macrophages

and were attenuated for virulence in mice (97). Recently, BisC has also been shown to be important for H_2O_2 resistance as well as pathogenesis as assessed in a murine infectious model (98). Overall, these repair mechanisms play highly important roles in repairing cellular components damaged by oxidative stress and are essential for colonization and virulence.

Uptake of D-alanine by S. Typhimurium during infection has also been characterized as an indirect defense mechanism to protect the organism against oxidative stress (100, 101). Within the neutrophil phagosome, the flavin cofactored D-amino acid oxidase (DAAO) catalyzes the production of an α-ketoacid and NH^{4+} from the deamination of D-amino acids (i.e., D-alanine, D-serine). During the reaction, the reduced flavin cofactor is reoxidized by O_2 to yield H_2O_2 (102). Therefore, the production of H_2O_2 by DAAO represents part of the host innate defense mechanism against bacterial invasion. S. Typhimurium encodes for an ATP-binding cassette transporter for D-alanine acquisition, DalSTUV (100). The periplasmic binding protein of the transporter is encoded by dalS and specifically binds D-alanine. In vivo virulence experiments in C57BL/6 mice result in increased survival of mice orally inoculated with a $\Delta dalS$ mutant strain relative to the parental strain (100). Furthermore, the $\Delta dalS$ strain displayed decreased fitness relative to the wild type strain as determined from enumeration of the bacterial load within the spleen, liver, and cecum (100). The $\Delta dalS$ strain had decreased survival after 2 hours of exposure to purified DAAO in the presence of D-alanine (101). Reporter assays designed to determine intracellular S. Typhimurium H_2O_2 stress levels found a significant increase in DAAO-dependent H_2O_2 killing in the $\Delta dalS$ strain (101). In support of this finding, purified neutrophils were infected with wild type and the $\Delta dalS$ mutant strain and revealed decreased survival of the $\Delta dalS$ mutant strain (101). Inhibition of DAAO using 6-chloro-1,2-benzisoxazol-3(2H)-one (CBIO) rescued the survival defect of the $\Delta dalS$ mutant (101). Thus, uptake of D-alanine by *S.* Typhimurium likely decreases the available D-alanine that can be utilized by DAAO to produce H_2O_2 and other bactericidal compounds. Overall, these results demonstrate the importance of D-alanine import for bacterial survival within neutrophils by helping to evade DAAO-mediated bacterial killing.

NITROSATIVE STRESS RESPONSE

Basic Chemistry of Nitric Oxide (NO) and Reactive Nitrogen Species (RNS)

In addition to ROS stress, pathogenic bacteria must also contend with the presence of NO and various other RNS during colonization (collectively referred to as nitrosative stress [NS]). The full repertoire of targets and defenses against NS remains incomplete due to the complex chemistry of NO and related nitrogen species in the cell. This complexity is further enhanced by the fact that many of these RNS interact with each other, with ROS, and with reactive metal centers. What follows is a brief discussion of RNS to orient the reader to the essential elements of NS, and readers are encouraged to refer to several excellent reviews for a more thorough discussion of RNS chemistry (103–109).

NO is the base component for many RNS. Although uncharged, NO contains an unpaired electron and can thus be considered to be a "free radical" (103). In contrast to some other stereotypical free radicals (such as $O_2^{\cdot-}$ or $^{\cdot}OH$), NO is a weak oxidant and does not initiate oxidation pathways strongly by itself. NO rapidly reacts with existing free radicals. This contributes to the complex chemistry of RNS, because depending on the circumstances, NO can be considered a potent antioxidant by quenching oxidizing free radicals or NO can exacerbate oxidative reactions through its interaction with other relatively benign free radicals. For example, NO readily interacts with dioxygen to form nitrogen dioxide (NO_2) (both of which are uncharged free radicals) (equation 8).

$$2NO + O_2 \rightarrow 2NO_2 \qquad (8)$$

In contrast to NO, NO_2 (note that NO_2 is not equivalent to nitrite [NO^{2-}]) is an oxidant and oxidizes thiols, tyrosines, etc. (103). NO_2 also reacts with NO to form dinitrogen trioxide (N_2O_3) (equation 9).

$$NO_2 + NO \leftrightarrow N_2O_3 \qquad (9)$$

It is important to note that equations 8 and 9 are likely to be more biologically relevant in membrane environments. This is because two molecules of NO are required to initiate this cascade, and levels of both NO and O_2 tend to be higher in lipophilic environments than in the aqueous cytoplasm (110). N_2O_3 formed from NO_2 and NO subsequently either reacts with H_2O to generate two NO^{2-} (equation 10) or reacts with nitrosylated nucleophiles (Nuc-) to generate NO^{2-} (equation 11).

$$N_2O_3 + H_2O \leftrightarrow 2NO^{2-} + 2H^+ \qquad (10)$$

$$N_2O_3 + Nuc^- \rightarrow Nuc\text{-}OH + NO^{2-} \qquad (11)$$

NO also reacts with superoxide anions to form peroxynitrate ($ONOO^-$) (equation 12), which rapidly oxidizes a variety of biologically relevant substrates or eventually decomposes to nitrate and carbonic acid (equation 13) (103, 107–109).

$$NO + O_2^{\cdot-} \rightarrow ONOO^- \qquad (12)$$

$$ONOO^- + CO_2 \rightarrow ONOO\text{-}C(O)O^-$$
$$\rightarrow O_2NO\text{-}CO^{2-} + H_2O \rightarrow NO^{3-} \qquad (13)$$
$$+ HCO^{3-} + H^+$$

In addition, NO reacts with dioxygen bound to metals (i.e., oxymyoglobin, oxyhemoglobin) in a similar manner as superoxide due to the extensive electron donation of dioxygen to the metal center (equation 14).

$$[\text{Mb-Fe}^{\text{III}}] + O_2 \rightarrow [\text{Mb-Fe}^{\text{II}}\text{-}O_2 \leftrightarrow$$
$$\text{Mb-Fe}^{\text{III}}\text{-}O_{2-}] + NO \rightarrow \text{Mb-Fe}^{\text{III}} \quad (14)$$
$$+ NO^{3-}$$

In contrast to the analogous sequential reactions seen above (equations 12 and 13), this reaction does not appear to generate an intermediate peroxynitrite (111). Hemoproteins are also important biological targets of NO (104). When NO reacts with ferric heme it becomes slightly positively charged and can thus be attacked by an appropriate nucleophile (e.g., thiols, H_2O) which will become nitrosylated (equation 15) (103). The ferrous ion in the heme center must, of course, be reoxidized for the process to be catalytic.

$$[\text{Por-Fe}^{\text{III}}] + NO \rightarrow [\text{Por-Fe}^{\text{III}}\text{-}NO \leftrightarrow$$
$$\text{Por-Fe}^{\text{II}}\text{-}NO^+] + \text{Nuc-H} \rightarrow \text{Por-Fe}^{\text{II}} \quad (15)$$
$$+ \text{Nuc-NO} + H^+$$

Sources of NS in the Gastrointestinal Tract

The primary sources of NS in the gastrointestinal tract arise from the action of the host NO synthases (NOSs). There are three forms of NOS: endothelial (eNOS), neuronal (nNOS), and inducible (iNOS) (112). All three NOSs catalyze the formation of NO from the conversion of L-arginine to L-citrulline with the concomitant consumption of NADPH and O_2. eNOS and nNOS are constitutively expressed and are involved in cellular signaling, whereas iNOS is specifically induced upon exposure to cytokines (113). iNOS is also able to produce much more NO than either eNOS or nNOS. NO produced by iNOS is part of the oxidative burst generated by macrophages during an infection. However, NO production does not occur as rapidly as superoxide generation and is believed to commence ~8 hours postinfection (114).

NS can also arise from the presence of nitrate (NO^{3-}) and nitrite (NO^{2-}) in the gastrointestinal tract (106). These compounds originate from both ingested food and from the host itself. The primary dietary source of nitrate is from vegetables. Nitrate can also be produced by the host through the action of NOS (primarily eNOS), because the NO produced can react with oxidized hemoglobin to form nitrate (106, 115). Interestingly, saliva contains high levels of nitrate, with up to 25% of plasma nitrate actively secreted by the salivary glands (116). Oral microbiota reduce the nitrate present in saliva to nitrite (105, 117). When fasting, saliva normally contains 50 to 150 ×M nitrite (10 time greater than plasma levels) but can increase to concentrations of 1 to 2 mM upon ingestion of nitrate-rich food (116). Because humans ingest approximately 1 liter of saliva a day, this represents an important influx of nitrite into the gastrointestinal tract (106). Ingested nitrite is protonated in the acidic environment of the stomach, forming nitrous acid, which ultimately forms nitrogen trioxide and its downstream NS products (including NO) (equations 9–11) (105, 106). Indeed, the concentration of NO in the stomach can increase from a baseline level of 20 ppm (from fasting levels of nitrite present in saliva) to >400 ppm after the ingestion of a nitrate-rich meal (118). While the former concentration of NO is insufficient to kill enteric pathogens (i.e., *E. coli*, *Salmonella*, etc.), the latter kills most enteric pathogens in approximately 1 hour (119).

The gut microbiota is able to generate NO using nitrate or nitrite as a substrate. In particular, several commensal bacterial genera (i.e., *Bifidobacteria*, *Lactobacilli*) are capable of generating NO from nitrite (120). In contrast, typical pathogens such as *E. coli* and *Clostridium difficile* were not only unable to generate substantial NO, but they actively consumed NO instead (120). It should be noted, however, that some pathogens such as *Salmonella* species are capable of producing NO in a nitrate-dependent manner (121).

Certain bacteria also contain their own NOSs and can thus catalyze the formation of NO from L-arginine (122).

Bacterial Nitrosative Stress Defenses

Among the most important protein families involved in NS survival are bacterial globins (103, 123). These heme-containing proteins have been classified into three families: flavohemoglobins, single-domain globins, and truncated globins. Bacterial globins are induced under conditions of NS and detoxify NO. Currently, flavohemoglobins are the best-understood class. These proteins are composed of an N-terminal globin domain (which contains the heme cofactor) and a C-terminal reductase domain. Flavohemoglobins are not believed to be involved in the metabolism of oxygen. The C-terminal domain catalyzes the oxidation of NADH/NADPH, which results in the reduction of N-terminal heme via a flavin adenine dinucleotide cofactor (123). The flavohemoglobins' reduced heme subsequently converts NO and O_2 into nitrate. In contrast to the structure of flavohemoglobins, the single-domain globins are missing a C-terminal reductase domain. They are believed to function analogously to the flavohemoglobins with regard to their enzymatic activity but presumably require another protein to reduce their heme cofactors after each round of detoxification. Some single-domain globins may also have a role in oxygen metabolism (124). The last group of bacterial globins, the truncated globins, are the most recently discovered group and are thus the least characterized. Their direct function is somewhat unclear. Some appear to be involved in NO detoxification (125), while others appear to modulate the internal concentration of NO as a function of oxygen concentration (126). Like the single-domain globins, truncated globins do not have a reductase domain. However, it has been speculated that rather than being reduced by another protein, truncated globins may simply use reducing agents present in the cytoplasm (i.e., glutathione) (127–129).

Another defense mechanism that bacteria use to detoxify NO is through the use of NO reductases (103). NO reduction is performed through the concerted action of a flavorubredoxin (NorV) and associated flavoprotein (NorW) which reduce NO to the less toxic N_2O (130–132). In nitrifying bacteria N_2O undergoes fixation to N_2. Because the flavorubredoxin is sensitive to oxygen (132), NO reduction typically only occurs under microaerophilic or anaerobic conditions. Thus, numerous bacteria possess both bacterial globins and NO reductases to detoxify NO under both oxygen-rich and -limiting conditions (103).

Many bacteria can use nitrite as an electron acceptor under conditions of low oxygen availability (106). The periplasmic nitrite NrfA catalyzes the reduction of nitrate to ammonia with six electrons consumed in the process, and it has been proposed that NO is an intermediate in this reaction (103, 106). There is evidence that NrfA may also play a role in NO detoxification because it can also use NO as a direct substrate (133–135). Indeed, NrfA's location in the periplasm could also conceivably detoxify NO prior to entry into the cytoplasm (134).

The Effect of NS on Virulence: Inducible Host NS Generation

As discussed above, one of the primary sources of NS in the host is through the iNOS system. iNOS is highly expressed in specialized immune cells such as macrophages and is often targeted at engulfed pathogens present in phagosomes (112, 113). Macrophages that have iNOS function deleted or impaired through the use of inhibitors are defective in killing various pathogens in vitro (136, 137). The effect of NS in controlling pathogens in vivo is more complex. While ROS generators appear to be essential for short-term killing of bacterial pathogens (hour time spans), studies have indicated that iNOS-induced NS is primarily focused at controlling enteric pathogens over longer periods of time (days to weeks) (138–140). In fact, iNOS does not appear to be required for controlling *Salmonella* infection over the first week of infection but is instead required for long-term clearance (140). Recent work has suggested that the primary role of iNOS and its inducible NO response may be to eliminate pathogens that survived the initial oxidative burst generated by macrophages and to kill bacteria that have infected cells that are unable to mount a potent oxidative killing response (138).

Much of the biochemical work on bacterial resistance against NS has been done with *E. coli*, and thus its defenses against NS are particularly well characterized. *E. coli* encodes for both a flavohemoglobin (*hmp*) (141–143) and an NO reductase (*norVW*) (131) that are important for aerobic and anaerobic NO detoxification, respectively. Mutants in either system show impaired survival against NS (103, 141, 142, 144, 145). Interestingly, there are certain circumstances where the presence of NS appears to be beneficial for *E. coli* colonization or pathogenesis. In a mouse model of meningitis, iNOS$^{-/-}$ mice were more resistant to infection with *E. coli* K1 and showed reduced levels of inflammation compared to wild type controls (146). Treating wild type mice with an iNOS inhibitor also resulted in reduced damage and complete clearance of the bacteria (146). Recent work has also shown that commensal *E. coli* benefit from the production of host-derived nitrate in an inflamed gut and increase in numbers (147). This increased growth was not apparent in iNOS$^{-/-}$ mice. It is unclear whether pathogenic *E. coli* could also indirectly benefit from endogenously produced nitrate because this would appear to upend our current understanding of how NO production works to control pathogenic infections. It should be noted, however, that a recent paper has also identified a link between iNOS activity (and thus nitrate levels) and increased colonization potential of *E. coli* in streptomycin-treated mice (148).

Salmonella species have evolved numerous systems for dealing with NS generated by the host. *Salmonella* species encode a flavohemoglobin (*hmp*) that has been shown to be induced under NS and catalyze the detoxification of NO (141). A mutant in *hmp* was compromised in its ability to survive NO stress both *in vitro* (149) and *in vivo* (150). *Salmonella* also encodes for NO reductases (*norVW*) to allow for detoxification of NO under anoxic conditions (151). Moreover, *Salmonella* nitrate reductase also plays a role in NO detoxification under conditions of anaerobic respiration (151). Finally, *Salmonella* can directly inhibit the colocalization of iNOS with phagosomes via its SPI2 pathogenicity island and thus prevent the accumulation of NS and cellular injury (152).

In *C. jejuni* the single-domain hemoglobin Cgb is believed to be the primary inducible defense mechanism against RNS in *C. jejuni* (153, 154). Mutants in *cgb* showed increased sensitivity to various nitrosative stress agents. While Δ*cgb* mutants were unaffected in their adhesion to and invasion of Caco-2 cells, the Δ*cgb*-infected Caco-2 cells overproduced NO compared to cells infected with wild type *C. jejuni* (153). *C. jejuni* also contains a constitutively expressed defense mechanism against NO toxicity. The NrfA protein has been shown to be the sole nitrate reductase in *C. jejuni* (133). Deleting *nrfA* results in sensitivity to several different sources of RNS and reduced growth in the presence of nitrite. However, both the sensitivity and growth defect are less severe in the Δ*nrfA* mutant than in the Δ*cgb* mutant (133). Mutants in Δ*nrfA* were not affected in their ability to colonize the chick gastrointestinal tract, indicating that the constitutively expressed NO detoxification provided by NrfA is not required when colonizing this *C. jejuni* host (133). This result suggests that there is either minimal RNS present during commensal colonization (as one would expect) or that the inducible RNS defense systems (e.g., Cgb) are sufficient to overcome any RNS stresses present.

CONCLUSION

The host gastrointestinal tract exposes pathogens to a diverse range of physical and chemical stresses which must be detoxified or tolerated by the bacteria until more favorable conditions are encountered. Bacteria are able to maintain pH homeostasis during transit through the low pH of the stomach by several well-characterized direct H$^+$ consumption or expulsion mechanisms, such as those characterized in *Helicobacter*, *Listeria*, and *Salmonella* species. Interestingly, bacterial pathogens such as *Campylobacter* lack these well-defined direct detoxification mechanisms to resist pH fluctuations. Instead, *Campylobacter* relies on indirect defenses to survive acid exposure using its protective capsule and also induction of heat shock proteins. Resistance to changes in osmolarity have been found to consist of an immediate response followed by long-term responses which utilize proteins involved in K$^+$ influx and osmoprotectant molecules (trehalose, proline, glycine betaine), respectively. A novel strategy to survive osmotic shock has been characterized in *Campylobacter*, which was found to form distinct subpopulations that varied in expression of key genes upon exposure to increased salt concentrations. Furthermore, the presence of phase variability and the lack of characterized DNA repair mechanisms are thought to contribute to the observed heterogeneity in *Campylobacter*. The presence of bacteria with differing sensitivities to increased salt concentrations likely ensures that there are cells able to resist variations in environmental conditions.

Survival of bacterial pathogens against oxidative and nitrosative stresses has been well characterized over the years. Key enzymes against oxidative stress include catalases, alkyl hydroperoxide reductases, and superoxide dismutases, whereas globins are the primary detoxification enzymes against nitrosative stress. Defenses against these noxious compounds are highly critical for bacterial virulence during colonization. The innate immune system exposes bacteria to oxidative and nitrosative stress as a strategy to kill invading bacterial cells. Indeed, deletion of key bacterial oxidant and nitrosative defense enzymes results in significant attenuation in virulence in animal models and survival in macrophage models. These results highlight the critical role these enzymes have in resistance to host immune defenses. Overall, as our knowledge of bacterial virulence and adaptation mechanisms continues to expand, it is hoped that this key research will yield novel findings leading to new strategies to treat or prevent illness induced by bacterial pathogens.

ACKNOWLEDGMENTS

Research in Alain Stintzi's laboratory has been supported by CIHR (MOP#84224).

CITATION

Flint A, Butcher J, Stintzi A. 2016. Stress responses, adaptation, and virulence of bacterial pathogens during host gastrointestinal colonization. Microbiol Spectrum 4(2):VMBF-0007-2015.

REFERENCES

1. **Dressman JB, Berardi RR, Dermentzoglou LC, Russell TL, Schmaltz SP, Barnett JL, Jarvenpaa KM.** 1990. Upper gastrointestinal (GI) pH in young, healthy men and women. *Pharm Res* **7:**756–761.
2. **Rowbury RJ.** 1995. An assessment of environmental factors influencing acid tolerance and sensitivity in *Escherichia coli*, *Salmonella* spp. and other enterobacteria. *Lett Appl Microbiol* **20:**333–337.
3. **Raja N, Goodson M, Smith DG, Rowbury RJ.** 1991. Decreased DNA damage by acid and increased repair of acid-damaged DNA in acid-habituated *Escherichia coli*. *J Appl Bacteriol* **70:**507–511.
4. **Gahan CG, Hill C.** 2014. *Listeria monocytogenes*: survival and adaptation in the gastrointestinal tract. *Front Cell Infect Microbiol* **4:**9.

5. **Alvarez-Ordonez A, Begley M, Prieto M, Messens W, Lopez M, Bernardo A, Hill C.** 2011. *Salmonella* spp. survival strategies within the host gastrointestinal tract. *Microbiology* **157:**3268–3281.

6. **Fischer W, Prassl S, Haas R.** 2009. Virulence mechanisms and persistence strategies of the human gastric pathogen *Helicobacter pylori*. *Curr Top Microbiol Immunol* **337:**129–171.

7. **Kusters JG, van Vliet AH, Kuipers EJ.** 2006. Pathogenesis of *Helicobacter pylori* infection. *Clin Microbiol Rev* **19:**449–490.

8. **Kieboom J, Abee T.** 2006. Arginine-dependent acid resistance in *Salmonella enterica* serovar *Typhimurium*. *J Bacteriol* **188:**5650–5653.

9. **Heithoff DM, Conner CP, Hanna PC, Julio SM, Hentschel U, Mahan MJ.** 1997. Bacterial infection as assessed by *in vivo* gene expression. *Proc Natl Acad Sci USA* **94:**934–939.

10. **Eriksson S, Lucchini S, Thompson A, Rhen M, Hinton JC.** 2003. Unravelling the biology of macrophage infection by gene expression profiling of intracellular *Salmonella enterica*. *Mol Microbiol* **47:**103–118.

11. **Chen J, Fang C, Zheng T, Zhu N, Bei Y, Fang W.** 2012. Genomic presence of gadD1 glutamate decarboxylase correlates with the organization of ascB-dapE internalin cluster in *Listeria monocytogenes*. *Foodborne Pathog Dis* **9:**175–178.

12. **Archambaud C, Nahori MA, Soubigou G, Becavin C, Laval L, Lechat P, Smokvina T, Langella P, Lecuit M, Cossart P.** 2012. Impact of lactobacilli on orally acquired listeriosis. *Proc Natl Acad Sci USA* **109:**16684–16689.

13. **Ryan S, Hill C, Gahan CG.** 2008. Acid stress responses in *Listeria monocytogenes*. *Adv Appl Microbiol* **65:**67–91.

14. **Ryan S, Begley M, Gahan CG, Hill C.** 2009. Molecular characterization of the arginine deiminase system in *Listeria monocytogenes*: regulation and role in acid tolerance. *Environ Microbiol* **11:**432–445.

15. **Sachs G, Kraut JA, Wen Y, Feng J, Scott DR.** 2006. Urea transport in bacteria: acid acclimation by gastric *Helicobacter* spp. *J Membr Biol* **212:**71–82.

16. **Rektorschek M, Buhmann A, Weeks D, Schwan D, Bensch KW, Eskandari S, Scott D, Sachs G, Melchers K.** 2000. Acid resistance of *Helicobacter pylori* depends on the UreI membrane protein and an inner membrane proton barrier. *Mol Microbiol* **36:**141–152.

17. **Hu LT, Mobley HL.** 1990. Purification and N-terminal analysis of urease from *Helicobacter pylori*. *Infect Immun* **58:**992–998.

18. **Labigne A, Cussac V, Courcoux P.** 1991. Shuttle cloning and nucleotide sequences of *Helicobacter pylori* genes responsible for urease activity. *J Bacteriol* **173:**1920–1931.

19. **Cussac V, Ferrero RL, Labigne A.** 1992. Expression of *Helicobacter pylori* urease genes in *Escherichia coli* grown under nitrogen-limiting conditions. *J Bacteriol* **174:**2466–2473.

20. **Scott DR, Weeks D, Hong C, Postius S, Melchers K, Sachs G.** 1998. The role of internal urease in acid resistance of *Helicobacter pylori*. *Gastroenterology* **114:**58–70.

21. **Marcus EA, Moshfegh AP, Sachs G, Scott DR.** 2005. The periplasmic alpha-carbonic anhydrase activity of *Helicobacter pylori* is essential for acid acclimation. *J Bacteriol* **187:**729–738.

22. **Skouloubris S, Thiberge JM, Labigne A, De Reuse H.** 1998. The *Helicobacter pylori* UreI protein is not involved in urease activity but is essential for bacterial survival *in vivo*. *Infect Immun* **66:**4517–4521.

23. **Tsuda M, Karita M, Morshed MG, Okita K, Nakazawa T.** 1994. A urease-negative mutant of *Helicobacter pylori* constructed by allelic exchange mutagenesis lacks the ability to colonize the nude mouse stomach. *Infect Immun* **62:**3586–3589.

24. **Cotter PD, Gahan CG, Hill C.** 2000. Analysis of the role of the *Listeria monocytogenes* F0F1-AtPase operon in the acid tolerance response. *Int J Food Microbiol* **60:**137–146.

25. **Foster JW, Hall HK.** 1991. Inducible pH homeostasis and the acid tolerance response of *Salmonella typhimurium*. *J Bacteriol* **173:**5129–5135.

26. **Parkhill J, Wren BW, Mungall K, Ketley JM, Churcher C, Basham D, Chillingworth T, Davies RM, Feltwell T, Holroyd S, Jagels K, Karlyshev AV, Moule S, Pallen MJ, Penn CW, Quail MA, Rajandream MA, Rutherford KM, van Vliet AH, Whitehead S, Barrell BG.** 2000. The genome sequence of the food-borne pathogen *Campylobacter jejuni* reveals hypervariable sequences. *Nature* **403:**665–668.

27. **Siegel JA, Urbain JL, Adler LP, Charkes ND, Maurer AH, Krevsky B, Knight LC, Fisher RS, Malmud LS.** 1988. Biphasic nature of gastric emptying. *Gut* **29:**85–89.

28. **Black RE, Levine MM, Clements ML, Hughes TP, Blaser MJ.** 1988. Experimental *Campylobacter jejuni* infection in humans. *J Infect Dis* **157:**472–479.

29. **Le MT, Porcelli I, Weight CM, Gaskin DJ, Carding SR, van Vliet AH.** 2012. Acid-shock of *Campylobacter jejuni* induces flagellar gene expression and host cell invasion. *Eur J Microbiol Immunol* **2:**12–19.

30. **Reid AN, Pandey R, Palyada K, Naikare H, Stintzi A.** 2008. Identification of *Campylobacter jejuni* genes involved in the response to acidic pH and stomach transit. *Appl Environ Microbiol* **74:**1583–1597.

31. **Reid AN, Pandey R, Palyada K, Whitworth L, Doukhanine E, Stintzi A.** 2008. Identification of *Campylobacter jejuni* genes contributing to acid adaptation by transcriptional profiling and genome-wide mutagenesis. *Appl Environ Microbiol* **74:**1598–1612.

32. **Yao R, Burr DH, Doig P, Trust TJ, Niu H, Guerry P.** 1994. Isolation of motile and non-motile insertional mutants of *Campylobacter jejuni*: the role of motility in adherence and invasion of eukaryotic cells. *Mol Microbiol* **14:**883–893.

33. **Konkel ME, Klena JD, Rivera-Amill V, Monteville MR, Biswas D, Raphael B, Mickelson J.** 2004. Secretion of virulence proteins from *Campylobacter jejuni* is dependent on a functional flagellar export apparatus. *J Bacteriol* **186:**3296–3303.

34. **Flint A, Sun YQ, Butcher J, Stahl M, Huang H, Stintzi A.** 2014. Phenotypic screening of a targeted mutant library reveals *Campylobacter jejuni* defenses against oxidative stress. *Infect Immun* **82:**2266–2275.

35. **Wood JM.** 1999. Osmosensing by bacteria: signals and membrane-based sensors. *Microbiol Mol Biol Rev* **63:**230–262.

36. **Bolen DW.** 2001. Protein stabilization by naturally occurring osmolytes. *Methods Mol Biol* **168:**17–36.

37. **Corratge-Faillie C, Jabnoune M, Zimmermann S, Very AA, Fizames C, Sentenac H.** 2010. Potassium and sodium transport in non-animal cells: the Trk/Ktr/HKT transporter family. *Cell Mol Life Sci* **67:**2511–2532.

38. **Rhoads DB, Epstein W.** 1977. Energy coupling to net K$^+$ transport in *Escherichia coli* K-12. *J Biol Chem* **252:**1394–1401.

39. **Laimins LA, Rhoads DB, Epstein W.** 1981. Osmotic control of kdp operon expression in *Escherichia coli*. *Proc Natl Acad Sci USA* **78:**464–468.

40. **Altendorf K, Voelkner P, Puppe W.** 1994. The sensor kinase KdpD and the response regulator KdpE control expression of the kdpFABC operon in *Escherichia coli*. *Res Microbiol* **145:**374–381.

41. **Heermann R, Jung K.** 2010. The complexity of the 'simple' two-component system KdpD/KdpE in *Escherichia coli*. *FEMS Microbiol Lett* **304:**97–106.

42. **Voelkner P, Puppe W, Altendorf K.** 1993. Characterization of the KdpD protein, the sensor kinase of the K(+)-translocating Kdp system of *Escherichia coli*. *Eur J Biochem* **217:**1019–1026.

43. **Liu Y, Ho KK, Su J, Gong H, Chang AC, Lu S.** 2013. Potassium transport of *Salmonella* is important for type III secretion and pathogenesis. *Microbiology* **159:**1705–1719.

44. **Dinnbier U, Limpinsel E, Schmid R, Bakker EP.** 1988. Transient accumulation of potassium glutamate and its replacement by trehalose during adaptation of growing cells of *Escherichia coli* K-12 to elevated sodium chloride concentrations. *Arch Microbiol* **150:**348–357.

45. **MacMillan SV, Alexander DA, Culham DE, Kunte HJ, Marshall EV, Rochon D, Wood JM.** 1999. The ion coupling and organic substrate specificities of osmoregulatory transporter ProP in *Escherichia coli*. *Biochim Biophys Acta* **1420:**30–44.

46. **Culham DE, Henderson J, Crane RA, Wood JM.** 2003. Osmosensor ProP of *Escherichia coli* responds to the concentration, chemistry, and molecular size of osmolytes in the proteoliposome lumen. *Biochemistry* **42:**410–420.

47. **Culham DE, Dalgado C, Gyles CL, Mamelak D, MacLellan S, Wood JM.** 1998. Osmoregulatory transporter ProP influences colonization of the urinary tract by *Escherichia coli*. *Microbiology* **144**(Pt 1):91–102.

48. **May G, Faatz E, Villarejo M, Bremer E.** 1986. Binding protein dependent transport of glycine betaine and its osmotic regulation in *Escherichia coli* K12. *Mol Gen Genet* **205:**225–233.

49. **Gul N, Poolman B.** 2013. Functional reconstitution and osmoregulatory properties of the ProU ABC transporter from *Escherichia coli*. *Mol Membr Biol* **30:**138–148.

50. **Haardt M, Bremer E.** 1996. Use of phoA and lacZ fusions to study the membrane topology of ProW, a component of the osmoregulated ProU transport system of *Escherichia coli*. *J Bacteriol* **178:**5370–5381.

51. **Sleator RD, Wouters J, Gahan CG, Abee T, Hill C.** 2001. Analysis of the role of OpuC, an osmolyte transport system, in salt tolerance and virulence potential of *Listeria monocytogenes*. *Appl Environ Microbiol* **67:**2692–2698.

52. **Lamark T, Kaasen I, Eshoo MW, Falkenberg P, McDougall J, Strom AR.** 1991. DNA sequence and analysis of the bet genes encoding the osmoregulatory choline-glycine betaine pathway of *Escherichia coli*. *Mol Microbiol* **5:**1049–1064.

53. **Landfald B, Strom AR.** 1986. Choline-glycine betaine pathway confers a high level of osmotic tolerance in *Escherichia coli*. *J Bacteriol* **165:**849–855.

54. **Giaever HM, Styrvold OB, Kaasen I, Strom AR.** 1988. Biochemical and genetic characterization of osmoregulatory trehalose synthesis in *Escherichia coli*. *J Bacteriol* **170:**2841–2849.

55. **Kaasen I, McDougall J, Strom AR.** 1994. Analysis of the otsBA operon for osmoregulatory trehalose synthesis in *Escherichia coli* and homology of the OtsA and OtsB proteins to the yeast trehalose-6-phosphate synthase/phosphatase complex. *Gene* **145:**9–15.

56. **McLaggan D, Logan TM, Lynn DG, Epstein W.** 1990. Involvement of gamma-glutamyl peptides in osmoadaptation of *Escherichia coli*. *J Bacteriol* **172:**3631–3636.

57. **Doyle MP, Roman DJ.** 1982. Response of *Campylobacter jejuni* to sodium chloride. *Appl Environ Microbiol* **43:**561–565.

58. **Cameron A, Frirdich E, Huynh S, Parker CT, Gaynor EC.** 2012. Hyperosmotic stress response of *Campylobacter jejuni*. *J Bacteriol* **194:**6116–6130.

59. **Fordtran JS, Locklear TW.** 1966. Ionic constituents and osmolality of gastric and small-intestinal fluids after eating. *Am J Dig Dis* **11:**503–521.

60. **Klasing KC, Adler KL, Remus JC, Calvert CC.** 2002. Dietary betaine increases intraepithelial lymphocytes in the duodenum of coccidia-infected chicks and increases functional properties of phagocytes. *J Nutr* **132:**2274–2282.

61. **Haswell ES, Phillips R, Rees DC.** 2011. Mechanosensitive channels: what can they do and how do they do it? *Structure* **19:**1356–1369.

62. **Kakuda T, Koide Y, Sakamoto A, Takai S.** 2012. Characterization of two putative mechanosensitive channel proteins of *Campylobacter jejuni* involved in protection against osmotic downshock. *Vet Microbiol* **160:**53–60.

63. **Nothaft H, Liu X, McNally DJ, Li J, Szymanski CM.** 2009. Study of free oligosaccharides derived from the bacterial *N*-glycosylation pathway. *Proc Natl Acad Sci USA* **106:**15019–15024.

64. **Nothaft H, Liu X, Li J, Szymanski CM.** 2010. *Campylobacter jejuni* free oligosaccharides: function and fate. *Virulence* **1:**546–550.

65. **Gaasbeek EJ, van der Wal FJ, van Putten JP, de Boer P, van der Graaf-van Bloois L, de Boer AG, Vermaning BJ, Wagenaar JA.** 2009. Functional characterization of excision repair and RecA-dependent recombinational DNA repair in *Campylobacter jejuni*. *J Bacteriol* **191:**3785–3793.

66. **Imlay JA.** 2008. Cellular defenses against superoxide and hydrogen peroxide. *Annu Rev Biochem* **77:**755–776.

67. **Klebanoff SJ, Kettle AJ, Rosen H, Winterbourn CC, Nauseef WM.** 2013. Myeloperoxidase: a front-line defender against phagocytosed microorganisms. *J Leukoc Biol* **93:**185–198.

68. **Annuk H, Shchepetova J, Kullisaar T, Songisepp E, Zilmer M, Mikelsaar M.** 2003. Characterization of intestinal lactobacilli as putative probiotic candidates. *J Appl Microbiol* **94:**403–412.

69. **Purdy D, Park SF.** 1994. Cloning, nucleotide sequence and characterization of a gene encoding superoxide dismutase from *Campylobacter jejuni* and *Campylobacter coli*. *Microbiology* **140**(Pt 5)**:**1203–1208.

70. **Gort AS, Ferber DM, Imlay JA.** 1999. The regulation and role of the periplasmic copper, zinc superoxide dismutase of *Escherichia coli*. *Mol Microbiol* **32:**179–191.

71. **Carlioz A, Touati D.** 1986. Isolation of superoxide dismutase mutants in *Escherichia coli*: is superoxide dismutase necessary for aerobic life? *EMBO J* **5:**623–630.

72. **Compan I, Touati D.** 1993. Interaction of six global transcription regulators in expression of manganese superoxide dismutase in *Escherichia coli* K-12. *J Bacteriol* **175:**1687–1696.

73. **Dubrac S, Touati D.** 2000. Fur positive regulation of iron superoxide dismutase in *Escherichia coli*: functional analysis of the sodB promoter. *J Bacteriol* **182:**3802–3808.

74. **Fang FC, DeGroote MA, Foster JW, Baumler AJ, Ochsner U, Testerman T, Bearson S, Giard JC, Xu Y, Campbell G, Laessig T.** 1999. Virulent *Salmonella typhimurium* has two periplasmic Cu, Zn-superoxide dismutases. *Proc Natl Acad Sci USA* **96:**7502–7507.

75. **Ammendola S, Pasquali P, Pacello F, Rotilio G, Castor M, Libby SJ, Figueroa-Bossi N, Bossi L, Fang FC, Battistoni A.** 2008. Regulatory and structural differences in the Cu,Zn-superoxide dismutases of *Salmonella enterica* and their significance for virulence. *J Biol Chem* **283:**13688–13699.

76. **Zamocky M, Gasselhuber B, Furtmuller PG, Obinger C.** 2012. Molecular evolution of hydrogen peroxide degrading enzymes. *Arch Biochem Biophys* **525:**131–144.

77. **Alfonso-Prieto M, Biarnes X, Vidossich P, Rovira C.** 2009. The molecular mechanism of the catalase reaction. *J Am Chem Soc* **131:**11751–11761.

78. **Vlasits J, Jakopitsch C, Bernroitner M, Zamocky M, Furtmuller PG, Obinger C.** 2010. Mechanisms of catalase activity of heme peroxidases. *Arch Biochem Biophys* **500:**74–81.

79. **Chelikani P, Fita I, Loewen PC.** 2004. Diversity of structures and properties among catalases. *Cell Mol Life Sci* **61:**192–208.

80. **Odenbreit S, Wieland B, Haas R.** 1996. Cloning and genetic characterization of *Helicobacter pylori* catalase and construction of a catalase-deficient mutant strain. *J Bacteriol* **178:**6960–6967.

81. **Harris AG, Hazell SL.** 2003. Localisation of *Helicobacter pylori* catalase in both the periplasm and cytoplasm, and its dependence on the twin-arginine target protein, KapA, for activity. *FEMS Microbiol Lett* **229:**283–289.

82. **Mulvey MR, Switala J, Borys A, Loewen PC.** 1990. Regulation of transcription of katE and katF in *Escherichia coli*. *J Bacteriol* **172:**6713–6720.

83. **Schellhorn HE, Hassan HM.** 1988. Transcriptional regulation of katE in *Escherichia coli* K-12. *J Bacteriol* **170:**4286–4292.

84. **Von Ossowski I, Mulvey MR, Leco PA, Borys A, Loewen PC.** 1991. Nucleotide sequence of *Escherichia coli* katE, which encodes catalase HPII. *J Bacteriol* **173:**514–520.

85. **Brunder W, Schmidt H, Karch H.** 1996. KatP, a novel catalase-peroxidase encoded by the large plasmid of enterohaemorrhagic *Escherichia coli* O157:H7. *Microbiology* **142**(Pt 11):3305–3315.

86. **Varnado CL, Hertwig KM, Thomas R, Roberts JK, Goodwin DC.** 2004. Properties of a novel periplasmic catalase-peroxidase from *Escherichia coli* O157:H7. *Arch Biochem Biophys* **421:**166–174.

87. **Robbe-Saule V, Coynault C, Ibanez-Ruiz M, Hermant D, Norel F.** 2001. Identification of a non-haem catalase in *Salmonella* and its regulation by RpoS (sigmaS). *Mol Microbiol* **39:**1533–1545.

88. **Flint A, Sun YQ, Stintzi A.** 2012. Cj1386 is an ankyrin-containing protein involved in heme trafficking to catalase in *Campylobacter jejuni*. *J Bacteriol* **194:**334–345.

89. **Harris AG, Wilson JE, Danon SJ, Dixon MF, Donegan K, Hazell SL.** 2003. Catalase (KatA) and KatA-associated protein (KapA) are essential to persistent colonization in the *Helicobacter pylori* SS1 mouse model. *Microbiology* **149:**665–672.

90. **Imlay JA.** 2013. The molecular mechanisms and physiological consequences of oxidative stress: lessons from a model bacterium. *Nat Rev Microbiol* **11:**443–454.

91. **Seaver LC, Imlay JA.** 2001. Alkyl hydroperoxide reductase is the primary scavenger of endogenous hydrogen peroxide in *Escherichia coli*. *J Bacteriol* **183:**7173–7181.

92. **Olczak AA, Seyler RW Jr, Olson JW, Maier RJ.** 2003. Association of *Helicobacter pylori* antioxidant activities with host colonization proficiency. *Infect Immun* **71:**580–583.

93. **Palyada K, Sun YQ, Flint A, Butcher J, Naikare H, Stintzi A.** 2009. Characterization of the oxidative stress stimulon and PerR regulon of *Campylobacter jejuni*. *BMC Genomics* **10:**481.

94. **Hebrard M, Viala JP, Meresse S, Barras F, Aussel L.** 2009. Redundant hydrogen peroxide scavengers contribute to *Salmonella* virulence and oxidative stress resistance. *J Bacteriol* **191:**4605–4614.

95. **Steele KH, Baumgartner JE, Valderas MW, Roop RM 2nd.** 2010. Comparative study of the roles of AhpC and KatE as respiratory antioxidants in *Brucella abortus* 2308. *J Bacteriol* **192:**4912–4922.

96. **Moskovitz J.** 2005. Roles of methionine suldfoxide reductases in antioxidant defense, protein regulation and survival. *Curr Pharm Des* **11:**1451–1457.

97. **Denkel LA, Horst SA, Rouf SF, Kitowski V, Bohm OM, Rhen M, Jager T, Bange FC.** 2011. Methionine sulfoxide reductases are essential for virulence of *Salmonella typhimurium*. *PloS One* **6:**e26974. doi:10.1371/journal.pone.0026974.

98. **Denkel LA, Rhen M, Bange FC.** 2013. Biotin sulfoxide reductase contributes to oxidative stress tolerance and virulence in *Salmonella enterica* serovar *Typhimurium*. *Microbiology* **159:**1447–1458.

99. **Streit WR, Entcheva P.** 2003. Biotin in microbes, the genes involved in its biosynthesis, its biochemical role and perspectives for biotechnological production. *Appl Microbiol Biotechnol* **61:**21–31.

100. **Osborne SE, Tuinema BR, Mok MC, Lau PS, Bui NK, Tomljenovic-Berube AM, Vollmer W, Zhang K, Junop M, Coombes BK.** 2012. Characterization of DalS, an ATP-binding cassette transporter for D-alanine, and its role in pathogenesis in *Salmonella enterica*. *J Biol Chem* **287:**15242–15250.

101. **Tuinema BR, Reid-Yu SA, Coombes BK.** 2014. *Salmonella* evades d-amino acid oxidase to promote infection in neutrophils. *mBio* **5**(6): e01886-14. doi:10.1128/mBio.01886-14.

102. **Sacchi S.** 2013. D-Serine metabolism: new insights into the modulation of D-amino acid oxidase activity. *Biochem Soc Trans* **41:**1551–1556.

103. **Bowman LA, McLean S, Poole RK, Fukuto JM.** 2011. The diversity of microbial responses to nitric oxide and agents of nitrosative stress: close cousins but not identical twins. *Adv Microb Physiol* **59:**135–219.

104. **Ford PC.** 2010. Reactions of NO and nitrite with heme models and proteins. *Inorg Chem* **49:**6226–6239.

105. **Lundberg JO.** 2008. Nitric oxide in the gastrointestinal tract: role of bacteria. *Biosci Microflora* **27:**109–112.

106. **Lundberg JO, Weitzberg E, Cole JA, Benjamin N.** 2004. Nitrate, bacteria and human health. *Nat Rev Microbiol* **2:**593–602.

107. **Ferrer-Sueta G, Radi R.** 2009. Chemical biology of peroxynitrite: kinetics, diffusion, and radicals. *ACS Chem Biol* **4:**161–177.

108. **Beckman JS, Koppenol WH.** 1996. Nitric oxide, superoxide, and peroxynitrite: the good, the bad, and ugly. *Am J Physiol* **271:** C1424–C1437.

109. **Pryor WA, Squadrito GL.** 1995. The chemistry of peroxynitrite: a product from the reaction of nitric oxide with superoxide. *Am J Physiol* **268:** L699–L722.

110. **Liu X, Miller MJ, Joshi MS, Thomas DD, Lancaster JR, Jr.** 1998. Accelerated reaction of nitric oxide with O2 within the hydrophobic interior of biological membranes. *Proc Natl Acad Sci USA* **95:**2175–2179.

111. **Yukl ET, de Vries S, Moenne-Loccoz P.** 2009. The millisecond intermediate in the reaction of nitric oxide with oxymyoglobin is an iron(III)–nitrato complex, not a peroxynitrite. *J Am Chem Soc* **131:**7234–7235.

112. **Bogdan C.** 2001. Nitric oxide and the immune response. *Nat Immunol* **2:**907–916.

113. **Lowenstein CJ, Padalko E.** 2004. iNOS (NOS2) at a glance. *J Cell Sci* **117:**2865–2867.

114. **Eriksson S, Chambers BJ, Rhen M.** 2003. Nitric oxide produced by murine dendritic cells is cytotoxic for intracellular *Salmonella enterica* sv. *Typhimurium. Scand J Immunol* **58:**493–502.

115. **Doyle MP, Hoekstra JW.** 1981. Oxidation of nitrogen oxides by bound dioxygen in hemoproteins. *J Inorg Biochem* **14:**351–358.

116. **Spiegelhalder B, Eisenbrand G, Preussmann R.** 1976. Influence of dietary nitrate on nitrite content of human saliva: possible relevance to *in vivo* formation of N-nitroso compounds. *Food Cosmet Toxicol* **14:**545–548.

117. **Govoni M, Jansson EA, Weitzberg E, Lundberg JO.** 2008. The increase in plasma nitrite after a dietary nitrate load is markedly attenuated by an antibacterial mouthwash. *Nitric Oxide* **19:**333–337.

118. **McKnight GM, Smith LM, Drummond RS, Duncan CW, Golden M, Benjamin N.** 1997. Chemical synthesis of nitric oxide in the stomach from dietary nitrate in humans. *Gut* **40:**211–214.

119. **Dykhuizen RS, Frazer R, Duncan C, Smith CC, Golden M, Benjamin N, Leifert C.** 1996. Antimicrobial effect of acidified nitrite on gut pathogens: importance of dietary nitrate in host defense. *Antimicrob Agents Chemother* **40:**1422–1425.

120. **Sobko T, Huang L, Midtvedt T, Norin E, Gustafsson LE, Norman M, Jansson EÅ, Lundberg JO.** 2006. Generation of NO by probiotic bacteria in the gastrointestinal tract. *Free Radic Biol Med* **41:**985–991.

121. **Gilberthorpe NJ, Poole RK.** 2008. Nitric oxide homeostasis in *Salmonella typhimurium*: roles of respiratory nitrate reductase and flavohemoglobin. *J Biol Chem* **283:**11146–11154.

122. **Crane BR, Sudhamsu J, Patel BA.** 2010. Bacterial nitric oxide synthases. *Annu Rev Biochem* **79:**445–470.

123. **Poole RK, Hughes MN.** 2000. New functions for the ancient globin family: bacterial responses to nitric oxide and nitrosative stress. *Mol Microbiol* **36:**775–783.

124. **Frey AD, Shepherd M, Jokipii-Lukkari S, Haggman H, Kallio PT.** 2011. The single-domain globin of *Vitreoscilla*: augmentation of aerobic metabolism for biotechnological applications. *Adv Microb Physiol* **58:**81–139.

125. **Ouellet H, Ouellet Y, Richard C, Labarre M, Wittenberg B, Wittenberg J, Guertin M.** 2002. Truncated hemoglobin HbN protects *Mycobacterium bovis* from nitric oxide. *Proc Natl Acad Sci USA* **99:**5902–5907.

126. **Smith HK, Shepherd M, Monk C, Green J, Poole RK.** 2011. The NO-responsive hemoglobins of *Campylobacter jejuni*: concerted responses of two globins to NO and evidence *in vitro* for globin regulation by the transcription factor NssR. *Nitric Oxide* **25:**234–241.

127. **Gusarov I, Starodubtseva M, Wang ZQ, McQuade L, Lippard SJ, Stuehr DJ, Nudler E.** 2008. Bacterial nitric-oxide synthases operate without a dedicated redox partner. *J Biol Chem* **283:**13140–13147.

128. **Smagghe BJ, Trent JT 3rd, Hargrove MS.** 2008. NO dioxygenase activity in hemoglobins is ubiquitous *in vitro*, but limited by reduction *in vivo*. *PLoS One* **3:**e2039. doi:10.1371/journal.pone.0002039.

129. **Giuffre A, Moschetti T, Vallone B, Brunori M.** 2008. Neuroglobin: enzymatic reduction and oxygen affinity. *Biochem Biophys Res Commun* **367:**893–898.

130. **Gardner AM, Gardner PR.** 2002. Flavohemoglobin detoxifies nitric oxide in aerobic, but not anaerobic, *Escherichia coli*. Evidence for a novel inducible anaerobic nitric oxide-scavenging activity. *J Biol Chem* **277:**8166–8171.

131. **Gardner AM, Helmick RA, Gardner PR.** 2002. Flavorubredoxin, an inducible catalyst

for nitric oxide reduction and detoxification in *Escherichia coli*. *J Biol Chem* **277**:8172–8177.

132. **Gomes CM, Giuffre A, Forte E, Vicente JB, Saraiva LM, Brunori M, Teixeira M.** 2002. A novel type of nitric-oxide reductase. *Escherichia coli* flavorubredoxin. *J Biol Chem* **277**:25273–25276.

133. **Pittman MS, Elvers KT, Lee L, Jones MA, Poole RK, Park SF, Kelly DJ.** 2007. Growth of *Campylobacter jejuni* on nitrate and nitrite: electron transport to NapA and NrfA via NrfH and distinct roles for NrfA and the globin Cgb in protection against nitrosative stress. *Mol Microbiol* **63**:575–590.

134. **Mills PC, Richardson DJ, Hinton JC, Spiro S.** 2005. Detoxification of nitric oxide by the flavorubredoxin of *Salmonella enterica* serovar *Typhimurium*. *Biochem Soc Trans* **33**:198–199.

135. **Poock SR, Leach ER, Moir JW, Cole JA, Richardson DJ.** 2002. Respiratory detoxification of nitric oxide by the cytochrome c nitrite reductase of *Escherichia coli*. *J Biol Chem* **277**: 23664–23669.

136. **Vazquez-Torres A, Jones-Carson J, Mastroeni P, Ischiropoulos H, Fang FC.** 2000. Antimicrobial actions of the NADPH phagocyte oxidase and inducible nitric oxide synthase in experimental salmonellosis. I. Effects on microbial killing by activated peritoneal macrophages *in vitro*. *J Exp Med* **192**:227–236.

137. **Iovine NM, Pursnani S, Voldman A, Wasserman G, Blaser MJ, Weinrauch Y.** 2008. Reactive nitrogen species contribute to innate host defense against *Campylobacter jejuni*. *Infect Immun* **76**:986–993.

138. **Burton NA, Schurmann N, Casse O, Steeb AK, Claudi B, Zankl J, Schmidt A, Bumann D.** 2014. Disparate impact of oxidative host defenses determines the fate of *Salmonella* during systemic infection in mice. *Cell Host Microbe* **15**:72–83.

139. **White JK, Mastroeni P, Popoff JF, Evans CA, Blackwell JM.** 2005. *Slc11a1*-mediated resistance to *Salmonella enterica* serovar *Typhimurium* and *Leishmania donovani* infections does not require functional inducible nitric oxide synthase or phagocyte oxidase activity. *J Leukoc Biol* **77**:311–320.

140. **Mastroeni P, Vazquez-Torres A, Fang FC, Xu Y, Khan S, Hormaeche CE, Dougan G.** 2000. Antimicrobial actions of the NADPH phagocyte oxidase and inducible nitric oxide synthase in experimental salmonellosis. II. Effects on microbial proliferation and host survival *in vivo*. *J Exp Med* **192**:237–248.

141. **Membrillo-Hernandez J, Coopamah MD, Anjum MF, Stevanin TM, Kelly A, Hughes MN, Poole RK.** 1999. The flavohemoglobin of *Escherichia coli* confers resistance to a nitrosating agent, a "nitric oxide releaser," and paraquat and is essential for transcriptional responses to oxidative stress. *J Biol Chem* **274**:748–754.

142. **Poole RK, Anjum MF, Membrillo-Hernandez J, Kim SO, Hughes MN, Stewart V.** 1996. Nitric oxide, nitrite, and Fnr regulation of *hmp* (flavohemoglobin) gene expression in *Escherichia coli* K-12. *J Bacteriol* **178**:5487–5492.

143. **Gardner PR, Gardner AM, Martin LA, Salzman AL.** 1998. Nitric oxide dioxygenase: an enzymic function for flavohemoglobin. *Proc Natl Acad Sci USA* **95**:10378–10383.

144. **Stevanin TM, Read RC, Poole RK.** 2007. The *hmp* gene encoding the NO-inducible flavohaemoglobin in *Escherichia coli* confers a protective advantage in resisting killing within macrophages, but not *in vitro*: links with swarming motility. *Gene* **398**:62–68.

145. **Hutchings MI, Mandhana N, Spiro S.** 2002. The NorR protein of *Escherichia coli* activates expression of the flavorubredoxin gene *norV* in response to reactive nitrogen species. *J Bacteriol* **184**:4640–4643.

146. **Mittal R, Gonzalez-Gomez I, Goth KA, Prasadarao NV.** 2010. Inhibition of inducible nitric oxide controls pathogen load and brain damage by enhancing phagocytosis of *Escherichia coli* K1 in neonatal meningitis. *Am J Pathol* **176**:1292–1305.

147. **Winter SE, Winter MG, Xavier MN, Thiennimitr P, Poon V, Keestra AM, Laughlin RC, Gomez G, Wu J, Lawhon SD, Popova IE, Parikh SJ, Adams LG, Tsolis RM, Stewart VJ, Baumler AJ.** 2013. Host-derived nitrate boosts growth of *E. coli* in the inflamed gut. *Science* **339**:708–711.

148. **Spees AM, Wangdi T, Lopez CA, Kingsbury DD, Xavier MN, Winter SE, Tsolis RM, Baumler AJ.** 2013. Streptomycin-induced inflammation enhances *Escherichia coli* gut colonization through nitrate respiration. *mBio* **4** (4):e00430-13. doi:10.1128/mBio.00430-13.

149. **Stevanin TM, Poole RK, Demoncheaux EA, Read RC.** 2002. Flavohemoglobin Hmp protects *Salmonella enterica* serovar *Typhimurium* from nitric oxide-related killing by human macrophages. *Infect Immun* **70**:4399–4405.

150. **Bang IS, Liu L, Vazquez-Torres A, Crouch ML, Stamler JS, Fang FC.** 2006. Maintenance of nitric oxide and redox homeostasis by the *Salmonella* flavohemoglobin Hmp. *J Biol Chem* **281**:28039–28047.

151. **Mills PC, Rowley G, Spiro S, Hinton JC, Richardson DJ.** 2008. A combination of cytochrome c nitrite reductase (NrfA) and flavorubredoxin (NorV) protects *Salmonella enterica*

serovar *Typhimurium* against killing by NO in anoxic environments. *Microbiology* **154:**1218–1228.

152. **Chakravortty D, Hansen-Wester I, Hensel M.** 2002. *Salmonella* pathogenicity island 2 mediates protection of intracellular *Salmonella* from reactive nitrogen intermediates. *J Exp Med* **195:**1155–1166.

153. **Elvers KT, Wu G, Gilberthorpe NJ, Poole RK, Park SF.** 2004. Role of an inducible single-domain hemoglobin in mediating resistance to nitric oxide and nitrosative stress in *Campylobacter jejuni* and *Campylobacter coli. J Bacteriol* **186:**5332–5341.

154. **Pickford JL, Wainwright L, Wu G, Poole RK.** 2008. Expression and purification of Cgb and Ctb, the NO-inducible globins of the foodborne bacterial pathogen *C. jejuni. Methods Enzymol* **436:**289–302.

Bacterial Evasion of Host Antimicrobial Peptide Defenses

15

JASON N. COLE[1,2,3] and VICTOR NIZET[1,4,5]

INTRODUCTION

Antimicrobial peptides (AMPs) are small (<10 kDa) soluble host defense peptides that play an important role in the mammalian innate immune response, helping to prevent infection by inhibiting pathogen growth on skin and mucosal surfaces and subsequent dissemination to normally sterile sites. These natural antibiotics are produced by many cell types including epithelial cells, leukocytes (neutrophils, macrophages, dendritic cells, and mast cells), platelets, endothelial cells, and adipocytes in response to tissue damage or infectious stimuli and are found in body fluids and secretions including saliva, urine, sweat, and breast milk. To date, more than 2,000 AMPs have been identified from a wide variety of organisms including bacteria, insects, plants, amphibians, birds, reptiles, and mammals including humans (1, 2). Whereas prokaryotic AMPs are produced as a competitive strategy to facilitate the acquisition of nutrients and promote niche colonization (3), AMPs produced by higher organisms are generally conceived to carry out immune defense functions. In humans, the principal AMPs are hydrophobic molecules

[1]Department of Pediatrics, University of California San Diego, La Jolla, CA 92093; [2]School of Chemistry and Molecular Biosciences; [3]Australian Infectious Diseases Research Center, University of Queensland, St Lucia, Queensland 4072, Australia; [4]Skaggs School of Pharmacy and Pharmaceutical Sciences; [5]Center for Immunity, Infection & Inflammation, University of California San Diego, La Jolla, CA 92093.
Virulence Mechanisms of Bacterial Pathogens, 5th edition
Edited by Indira T. Kudva, Nancy A. Cornick, Paul J. Plummer, Qijing Zhang, Tracy L. Nicholson, John P. Bannantine, and Bryan H. Bellaire
© 2016 American Society for Microbiology, Washington, DC
doi:10.1128/microbiolspec.VMBF-0006-2015

composed of ~10 to 50 amino acid residues with a net positive charge, which exhibit varying degrees of broad-spectrum bioactivity against Gram-positive and Gram-negative bacteria, fungi, protozoan parasites, and certain enveloped viruses (4, 5). AMPs may be expressed constitutively or induced in response to infection (e.g., proinflammatory cytokines, toll-like receptor [TLR] signaling) (6) and are commonly produced as propeptides that undergo subsequent proteolytic processing to the mature bioactive peptide (7). AMPs with central roles in host defense are active at micromolar to nanomolar concentrations and facilitate microbial killing through perturbation of the cytoplasmic membrane (8). Several important human pathogens display significant resistance to AMPs, which appears to play a key role in their potential to produce serious invasive infections.

AMPs can be classified into four main groups according to their secondary structure: (i) α-helical peptides, (ii) β-sheet peptides, (iii) loop peptides, and (iv) extended peptides (1, 9). The two major AMP families in mammals are the cathelicidins and the defensins (Table 1). In their mature form, cathelicidins are often α-helical cationic AMPs that do not contain cysteine residues. LL-37 is the sole human cathelicidin (10). Defensins are β-sheet-stabilized peptides classified as either α- or β-defensins according to the pattern formed by three disulphide bridges. α-defensins are primarily produced by neutrophils and intestinal Paneth cells, while β-defensins are expressed by epithelial tissues in the respiratory, gastrointestinal, and urinary tracts (11, 12). Mammalian defensins produced by human epithelial and immune cells are cysteine-rich peptides ~30 to 40 amino acid residues in length (13). Humans produce six α-defensins: HNP 1 to HNP 4 are found in the azurophilic granules of neutrophil granulocytes (14), while human α-defensins HD-5 and HD-6 are expressed in Paneth cells located in the small intestine (15) and female urogenital tract (16) (Table 1). Six human β-defensins, HBD-1 through HBD-6, have

been identified and are expressed by epithelial cells, monocytes, macrophages and dendritic cells (11, 17). Cathelicidins are found in skin cells, gastrointestinal cells, neutrophils, and myeloid bone marrow cells (18) (Table 1). Activated platelets produce additional groups of cationic chemokine-related AMPs called thrombocidins and kinocidins (19–21).

These prototypical AMPs have a net positive charge to facilitate interaction with the net negative charge of bacterial surfaces (22). While cationic peptides comprise the largest class of AMPs, certain anionic peptides such as dermcidin, produced by eccrine sweat glands, also contribute to host epithelial defense (23). In addition to charge, other factors influencing the AMP spectrum and mechanism of action include size, amino acid composition, structural conformation, amphipathicity, and hydrophobicity (24). A primary mechanism of AMP action is through electrostatic interaction with the anionic phospholipid headgroups in the outer bacterial cytoplasmic membrane or cell wall components (22, 25). Upon penetration of the outer membrane or cell wall, AMP insertion into the cytoplasmic membrane causes membrane rupture and cell death (11).

Three general modes of AMP action have been proposed to explain the membrane disruption: (i) the "barrel-stave" mechanism where AMPs directly integrate into the target membrane forming membrane-spanning pores (26), (ii) the toroidal-pore mechanism where AMPs form membrane-spanning pores with intercalated lipids inducing a curvature in the membrane (27), and (iii) the "carpet" mechanism where AMPs at high concentration accumulate on the cell surface and dissolve the cell membrane in a detergent-like manner without forming membrane-spanning pores (28). In addition to cell membrane perturbation, some AMPs may exert downstream antimicrobial effects by inhibiting the bacterial DNA, RNA, or protein synthesis machinery or biosynthesis of cell wall components (29, 30). Nisin, an AMP commonly used in the food industry as a preservative, is a member of the bacteriocin or

TABLE 1 Human antimicrobial peptides and murine cathelicidin mCRAMP[a,b]

Class	Peptide	Gene	Species	Producing cells	References	Amino acid sequence[c]
α-defensins	HNP-1	DEFA1	Human	Azurophilic granules of neutrophil granulocytes	14	$AC_1YC_2RIPAC_3IAGERRYGTC_2IYQGRLWAFC_3C_1$
	HNP-2	DEFA1	Human			$C_1YC_2RIPAC_3IAGERRYGTC_2IYQGRLWAFC_3C_1$
	HNP-3	DEFA3	Human			$DC_1YC_2RIPAC_3IAGERRYGTC_2IYQGRLWAFC_3C_1$
	HNP-4	DEFA4	Human			$VC_1SC_2RLVFC_3RRTELRVGNC_2LIGGVSFTYC_3C_1TRV$
	HD-5	DEFA5	Human	Paneth cells in small intestine and female urogenital tract	15, 16	$ATC_1YC_2RTGRC_3ATRESLSGVC_2EISGRLYRLC_3C_1R$
	HD-6	DEFA6	Human			$AFTC_1HC_2RRSC_3YSTEYSYGTC_2TVMGINHRFC_3C_1L$
β-defensins	HBD-1	DEFB1	Human	Epithelial cells, monocytes, macrophages and dendritic cells	11, 17	$DHYNC_1VSSGGQC_2LYSAC_3PIFTKIQGTC_2YRGKAKC_1C_3K$
	HBD-2	DEFB4	Human			$GIGDPVTC_1LKSGAIC_2HPVFC_3PRRYKQIGTC_2GLPGTKC_1C_3KKP$
	HBD-3	DEFB103	Human			$GIINTLQKYYC_1RVRGGRC_2AVLSC_3LPKEEQIGKC_2STRGRKC_1C_3RRKK$
	HBD-4	DEFB104	Human			$ELDRIC_1GYGTARC_2RKKC_3RSQEYRIGRC_2PNTYAC_1C_3LRK$
Cathelicidins	LL-37	CAMP	Human	Skin cells, gastrointestinal cells, neutrophils, and myeloid bone marrow cells	18	LLGDFFRKSKEKIGKEFKRIVQRIKDFLRNLVPRTES
	mCRAMP	Cnlp	Murine			GLLRKGGEKIGEKLKKIGQKIKNFFQKLVPQPEQ
Others	C18G	n/a	Synthetic	n/a	253	ALYKKLLKLLKSAKKLG

[a] Abbreviations: HNP, human neutrophil defensin; HD, human α-defensin; HBD, human β-defensin; LL-37, human cathelicidin; mCRAMP, murine cathelicidin-related peptides; C18G, α-helical peptide derived from the carboxy terminus of platelet factor IV.
[b] Modified from Gruenheid and Moual (229).
[c] Numbers denote cysteine residues involved in disulfide bonds.

lantibiotic family of AMPs that inhibits the biosynthesis of teichoic acid (TA) and lipoteichoic acid (LTA) in Gram-positive bacteria (31). Another bacteriocin, mersacidin, inhibits cell wall peptidoglycan biosynthesis and is active against methicillin-resistant *Staphylococcus aureus* (32). Some eukaryotic defensins target the lipid II biosynthesis pathway, an essential component of peptidoglycan, to inhibit cell wall biosynthesis. Several AMPs inhibit nucleic acid biosynthesis including buforin II (33), indolicidin (34), and puroindoline (35). Human neutrophil peptide 1 (HNP-1), also known as human α-defensin 1, inhibits cell wall, DNA, and protein synthesis (36).

Genetic animal models have established an essential role for AMPs in the innate immune system. For example, mice deficient in the murine cathelicidin (mCRAMP) suffer more severe necrotic skin lesions than wild-type (WT) littermates following subcutaneous infection with *Streptococcus pyogenes* (group A *Streptococcus* [GAS]), a Gram-positive human pathogen (37, 38). GAS is killed less efficiently by whole blood and mast cells isolated from mCRAMP knockout mice (37, 38), and *Salmonella enterica* serovar Typhimurium (*S.* Typhimurium) proliferates better within macrophages of mCRAMP knockout mice (39). Cathelicidin-deficient mice are likewise more susceptible to *Escherichia coli* urinary tract infection (40), meningococcal septicemia (41), *Pseudomonas aeruginosa* keratitis (42), *Klebsiella pneumoniae* lung infection (43), and *Helicobacter pylori* gastritis, while mice deficient in β-defensin production show impaired defense against *P. aeruginosa* (44) or *Fusarium solani* keratitis (45). In gain-of-function analyses, transgenic mice overexpressing porcine cathelicidin were more resistant to bacterial skin infection (46), while transgenic expression of the human defensin-5 in mouse Paneth cells provided enhanced defense against *S.* Typhimurium enteritis (47).

Beyond their direct antimicrobial activities, AMPs including cathelicidins have also been reported to modulate cytokine produc-

tion, apoptosis, functional angiogenesis, or wound repair by stimulating keratinocyte migration and proliferation (48–50). Serving as an important link between the innate and adaptive immune system, AMPs may induce the expression of cytokines and chemokines (51, 52); exert direct chemotactic action on neutrophils, macrophages, immature dendritic cells, mast cells, monocytes, and T lymphocytes (53–55); and stimulate histamine release from mast cells to promote neutrophil migration to the site of infection (56).

The resistance mechanisms employed by commensals or microbial pathogens to combat AMPs have been intensively studied over the past two decades. This chapter highlights current information on the direct and indirect mechanisms of action used by human pathogenic bacteria to counteract AMPs, including surface charge alteration, external sequestration by secreted or surface-associated molecules, energy-dependent membrane efflux pumps, peptidase degradation, and the downregulation of AMP expression by host cells. Perturbation of these AMP resistance mechanisms may impair bacterial colonization capacity and reduce virulence in animal infection models. Understanding the molecular mechanisms of AMP resistance may identify novel targets for intervention in difficult to treat bacterial infections.

BACTERIAL AMP RESISTANCE MECHANISMS

Bacterial Surface Charge Modification Increases AMP Resistance

The cationic nature of human AMPs such as defensins and cathelicidin LL-37 provides an electrostatic affinity for bacterial cell surfaces, which are composed of negatively charged hydroxylated phospholipids including phosphatidylglycerol (PG), cardiolipin (also known as diphosphatidylglycerol), and phosphatidylserine (57). In contrast, mammalian and eukaryotic cell membranes contain neutral lipids (phosphatidylcholine, phosphatidylethanolamine, sphingomyelin) and sterols (cholesterol, ergosterol) and carry a net neutral charge that allows selectivity of AMPs for the mostly anionic bacterial cell membranes (3, 57). The amphipathic structure of AMPs resulting from the separation of charged or polar and hydrophobic moieties within the molecule enables their integration into the lipid bilayer of Gram-positive and Gram-negative bacteria, fungi, or viruses and the formation of destabilizing transmembrane pores that induce cell rupture and death (58, 59).

While Gram-positive bacteria lack an outer membrane, AMP access to the cytoplasmic membrane is inhibited by a thick peptidoglycan-containing cell wall cross-linked with polymers of TA or LTA. In Gram-negative bacteria, AMPs must traverse the outer membrane envelope composed of negatively charged lipopolysaccharide (LPS; up to 70% of the outer membrane) (60) and the periplasmic space beneath the outer membrane, which contains a thin peptidoglycan matrix. Surface-associated proteins and large capsular polysaccharides also hinder AMP access to the cytoplasmic membrane.

One common AMP-resistance strategy used by Gram-positive and Gram-negative bacteria is to increase their net positive surface charge through modification with cationic molecules, resulting in the electrostatic repulsion of cationic AMPs, thus preventing access to and disruption of the cytoplasmic membrane (Table 2). Several Gram-negative bacteria reduce the net negative charge of LPS lipid A through the addition of 4-amino-4-deoxy-L-arabinose (L-Ara4N), phosphoethanolamine (pEtN), or palmitoyl groups (61). Lipid A is negatively charged and consists of two glucosamine units with free phosphate groups linked to four or more acyl chains (62). Lipid A acylation coordinated by the PhoPQ regulatory system masks the negative surface charge in Gram-negative human pathogens such as *E. coli*, *Salmonella* spp., *Yersinia enterocolitica*, *Haemophilus influenzae*, *K. pneumoniae*, and

Legionella pneumophila (3, 63). Some Gram-positive pathogens alter their surface charge through the modification of TAs composed of linear anionic glycopolymers of polyglycerol phosphate and polyribitol phosphate linked by phosphodiester bonds. LTAs are noncovalently inserted into the cell membrane with a glycolipid anchor, while wall TAs are covalently attached to the peptidoglycan cell wall by a glycosidic bridge (64, 65). TAs play important roles in bacterial virulence, the adherence and invasion of host cells, biofilm formation (65), antimicrobial resistance (66–68), and activation of the immune response (69, 70). The D-alanylation of TAs by the *dlt* operon and integration of L-lysine into PG by membrane protein multipeptide resistance factor (MprF) are common strategies employed by Gram-positive bacteria to reduce the negative surface charge and enhance AMP resistance (65, 71–73). D-alanylation of TAs is only known to occur in the bacterial *Firmicutes* phylum (65).

D-Alanylation of Cell Wall TAs

S. aureus, a major Gram-positive human pathogen, is the etiologic agent of abscesses, cellulitis, osteomyelitis, septic arthritis, septicemia, and endocarditis. *S. aureus* resists killing by human AMPs through the D-alanylation of cell wall TA. Incorporation of D-alanyl esters into the cell wall by the action of four proteins encoded by the *dltABCD* operon exposes a positively charged amino group, reducing the net negative charge of TAs and diminishing the electrostatic attraction between cationic AMPs and the bacterial cell envelope (66–68, 72, 74, 75) (Fig. 1A). D-alanine is activated by D-alanyl carrier protein ligase (encoded by *dltA*) and delivered to D-alanine carrier protein (encoded by *dltC*) with assistance from chaperone protein DltD (encoded by *dltD*). The putative transmembrane protein DltB (encoded by *dltB*) is thought to facilitate transfer of the D-alanyl–D-alanine carrier protein complex across the cytoplasmic membrane (65). The D-alanylation of TA is also dependent upon environmental factors such as temperature, pH, and salt (e.g.,

TABLE 2 Bacterial antimicrobial peptide resistance mechanisms[a,b]

AMP resistance mechanism	AMP resistance phenotype	Genes	Target AMPs	Bacteria[c]	References
Cell surface alterations	D-alanylation of lipoteichoic acid and teichoic acid in bacterial cell wall	dlt operon, dltA	Cecropin B, colistin, gallidermin, HNP1-3, indolicidin, mCRAMP, magainin II, nisin, polymyxin B' protegrin 1, 3, and 5, tachyplesin 1 and 3, daptomycin, vancomycin	Staphylococcus aureus, Listeria monocytogenes, Group B Streptococcus, Group A Streptococcus, Streptococcus pneumoniae, Streptococcus suis, Enterococcus faecalis, Bacillus anthracis, Bacillus cereus, Clostridium difficile	66–68, 71, 72, 83, 254–259
	Addition of L-lysine or L-alanine to phosphatidylglycerol in cell membrane	mprF, lysC, lysX, PA0920	Arenicin-1, CAP18, gallidermin, HBD-3, HNP1-3, LL-37, lugworm beta-sheet peptide, lysozyme, magainin II, melittin, nisin, NK-2, polymyxin B, protamine, protegrin 3 and 5, tachyplesin 1, vancomycin	S. aureus, B. anthracis, L. monocytogenes, Mycobacterium tuberculosis, Pseudomonas aeruginosa	73, 81, 82, 85, 87, 91, 93–95
	Synthesis and extension of lipooligosaccharide	lpxA, lgtF, galT, cstII, waaF	Crp4, Fowl-1, HD-5, LL-37, polymyxin B	Neisseria meningitidis, Campylobacter jejuni	113–115
	Addition of ethanolamine (pEtN) to lipid A	lpxE_HP, cj0256, pmrC, lptA	LL-37, protegrin 1, polymyxin B	Helicobacter pylori, C. jejuni, S. Typhimurium, Neisseria gonorrhoeae, N. meningitidis	101, 108, 110, 111, 260
	Addition of aminoarabinose to lipid A in LPS	pmr genes	C18G, HBD-2, polymyxin B, protegrin 1, synthetic protegrin analogs	S. Typhimurium, Proteus mirabilis, Pseudomonas aeruginosa, Klebsiella pneumoniae	100, 103, 105, 106
	Acylation of lipid A in LPS	pagP, rcp, htrB msbB, lpxM	C18G, colistin, CP28, HBD-2, LL-37, magainin II, mCRAMP, protegrin 1, PGLa, polymyxin B and E	Salmonella spp., Legionella pneumophila, Haemophilus influenzae, Vibrio cholerae, K. pneumoniae	63, 117, 118, 120, 121
	Phosphorylcholine in LPS	licD	LL-37	H. influenzae	119

Category	Function	Gene	Target peptide(s)	Organism	Reference
	Synthesis of polysaccharide capsule	cps siaD sia operon ica genes cap hasABC	HBD-1 and 3, HNP-1 and 2, lactoferrin, polymyxin B, protamine, mCRAMP, CRAMP-18, LL-37, protegrin 1, polymyxin B, β-defensin-1, 2, and 3	K. pneumoniae N. meningitidis Staphylococcus epidermidis S. pneumoniae Group A Streptococcus	113, 139–143, 146
	PCN-binding protein PBP1a	ponA	HNP-1, LL-37, mCRAMP	Group B Streptococcus	96
	Mycolic acid synthesis	kasB	HNP-1, protamine, lysozyme	Mycobacterium marinum	99
	Production of carotenoids	crtOPQMN	HNP-1, thrombin-induced platelet microbicidal proteins, polymyxin B	S. aureus	261–263
Binding and inactivation	Staphylokinase	sak	HNP-1 and 2	S. aureus	122, 123
	M1 surface protein	emm1	LL-37	Group A Streptococcus	130
	SIC protein	sic	LL-37, α-defensins, lysozyme	Group A Streptococcus	124, 125
	Shedding of host proteoglycans	lasA	LL-37, HNP-1	P. aeruginosa E. faecalis Group A Streptococcus	136, 264
	PilB	pilB	LL-37, mCRAMP, polymyxin B	Group B Streptococcus	132
	LciA	lciA	Lactococcin A	Lactococcus lactis	265, 266
	Lanl lipoproteins	lanl	Lantibiotics	L. lactis Bacillus subtilis	267–269
Active efflux	ATP-dependent efflux system	mtr genes	LL-37, mCRAMP, PC-8, TP-1, protegrin-1 (PG1)	Neisseria gonorrhoeae N. meningitidis	111, 168, 170, 270
	K⁺-linked efflux pump	sap	Protamine	S. Typhimurium	167
	Plasmid-encoded efflux pump	qacA	Rabbit thrombin-induced platelet microbicidal protein	S. aureus	177
	VraFG ABC transporter	vraFG	Nisin, colistin, bacitracin, vancomycin, indolicidin, LL-37, hBD3	S. aureus S. epidermidis	155, 271–274
Proteolytic degradation	Elastase	lasB	LL-37	P. aeruginosa	181
	Gelatinase	gelE	LL-37	E. faecalis	181, 275
	Metalloproteinase	zapA aur degP	LL-37, lactoferricin	P. mirabilis S. aureus Escherichia coli	181, 183, 184, 192
	Cysteine protease	speB ideS	LL-37	Group A Streptococcus	181, 182
	Surface protease	pgtE	C18G	S. Typhimurium	188
	Gingipains (serine proteases)	rgpA/B	Cecropin B	Porphyromonas gingivalis	193

(Continued on next page)

TABLE 2 Bacterial antimicrobial peptide resistance mechanisms[a,b] *(Continued)*

AMP resistance mechanism	AMP resistance phenotype	Genes	Target AMPs	Bacteria[c]	References
	Aureolysin	*aur*	LL-37	*S. aureus*	183, 276
	V8 protease	*sspA*	LL-37	*S. aureus*	183
	SepA protease	*sepA*	Dermcidin	*S. epidermidis*	277, 278
Alteration of host processes	Downregulate AMP transcription	*mxiE*	LL-37, human beta-defensin-1, human beta-defensin HBD-3	*Shigella dysenteriae* *Shigella flexneri* *S.* Typhimurium *Neisseria gonorrhoeae*	225, 226, 279, 280
	Stimulation of host cysteine proteases and cathepsins	Unknown	HBD-2, HBD-3	*P. aeruginosa*	227, 281
Regulatory networks	Two-component regulator	*phoP/phoQ*	Defensins, protamine	*S.* Typhimurium *P. aeruginosa*	200, 205
	Two-component regulator	*pmrA/pmrB*	Defensins, polymyxin B	*S.* Typhimurium *P. aeruginosa*	100, 206
	Thermoregulated transcription factor	*prfA*	Defensins	*L. monocytogenes*	224

[a]Abbreviations: C18G, α-helical peptide derived from the carboxy terminus of platelet factor IV; CAP18, cationic LPS-binding protein 18 from rabbit; CP28, α-helical synthetic cationic peptide based on the cecropin-mellitin hybrid peptide CEME; mCRAMP and CRAMP-18, murine cathelicidin-related peptides; Crp4, murine homologous to human α-defensin-5; Fowl-1, heterophil-derived cathelicidin homolog fowlicidin-1; HBD, human β-defensin; HD-5, human α-defensin-5; HNP, human neutrophil defensin; LL-37, human cathelicidin, C-terminal part of the human cationic antimicrobial protein (hCAP-18); NK-2, α-helical fragment of mammalian NK-lysin; PGLa, peptide starting with a glycine and ending with a leucine amide from magainin peptide family.

[b]Modified from Anaya-Lopez et al. (3).

[c]Not all bacteria are resistant to the CAMP indicated; please see reference for specific resistance profile.

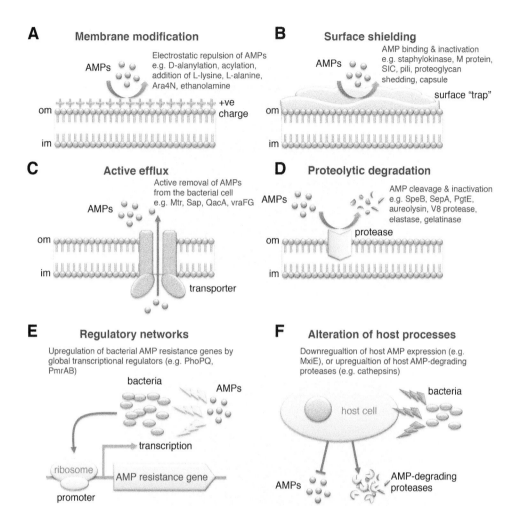

FIGURE 1 **Schematic representation of the multiple resistance mechanisms developed by bacteria to overcome host antimicrobial peptides. (A) Modification of the bacterial outer membrane. Bacterial resistance to cationic antimicrobial peptides is mediated by alterations in surface charge. Gram-positive bacteria: D-alanine modification of cell wall teichoic acid (*dlt*), L-lysine (*mprf*), or L-alanine modification of phosphatidylglycerol (*mprf*). Gram-negative bacteria: aminoarabinose or acylation modifications of lipid A in LPS (*pmr, pagP*), or addition of ethanolamine to lipid A (*pmrC, lptA*). The increased positive charge on bacterial surface repels cationic AMPs. (B) Shielding of the bacterial surface through the trapping and inactivation of AMPs in the extracellular milieu enhances resistance and pathogenicity. Surface-associated capsule traps AMP (e.g., *K. pneumoniae cps* operon), surface protein binds AMP (e.g., GAS M1 protein, GBS PilB pilus protein), secreted protein binds AMP (e.g., GAS SIC protein or *S. aureus* staphylokinase), or bacterial proteases release host proteoglycans to block AMP (e.g., *P. aeruginosa* LasA). (C) Membrane efflux pumps function by translocating the AMP out of the cell (e.g., *Neisseria* spp. Mtr, *S.* Typhimurium Sap, *S. aureus* QacA, and *Staphylococcus* spp. VraFG). (D) Degradation and inactivation of AMPs by bacterial proteases (e.g., GAS streptococcal pyrogenic exotoxin B protease, *S. epidermidis* SepA, *S.* Typhimurium PgtE, *S. aureus* aureolysin and V8 protease, *P. aeruginosa* elastase, and *E. faecalis* gelatinase). (E) Bacterial exposure to AMPs upregulates the expression of AMP-resistance genes through global gene regulatory networks (e.g., *S.* Typhimurium and *P. aeruginosa* PhoPQ and PmrAB). (F) Alteration of host processes by bacteria, including the downregulation of host AMP production (e.g., *Shigella* spp. transcriptional factor MxiE) or the upregulation and activation of host AMP-degrading proteases (e.g., *P. aeruginosa*). Abbreviations: om, bacterial outer membrane; im, bacterial inner membrane.**

NaCl) concentration (76, 77). Transcriptional regulators of TA D-alanylation have been identified for several species, including *Bacillus subtilis* (global transcriptional regulators AbrB and Spo0A) (78), group B *Streptococcus* (GBS) (two-component system DltRS) (79), and *S. aureus* (global regulators Agr and Rot, two-component system ArlRS) (20). In a recently proposed model, the increased density of the peptidoglycan sacculus resulting from cell wall D-alanylation may also sterically hinder AMP access to the cell membrane and contribute to AMP resistance (80). As a consequence, the cell wall of a GBS mutant lacking *dltA* was less compact and more permeable to AMPs than the WT parent strain (80). However, additional research is required to ascertain whether or not this mechanism applies to other Gram-positive species.

Compared to WT strains, *S. aureus dltA* null mutants and *dltA*, *dltB*, and *dltD* mutants of *Staphylococcus xylosus* are deficient in D-alanine esters of LTAs are hypersensitive to human α-defensins and cathelicidin due to an increase in negative surface charge and enhanced AMP binding (66, 72, 75). Furthermore, the overexpression of *dlt* in WT *S. aureus* enhances AMP resistance by increasing the cell surface positive charge (72). An *S. aureus dltA* mutant has reduced adherence to artificial surfaces, diminished biofilm formation, and reduced virulence in murine infection models (75, 81, 82). Several Gram-positive human pathogens have *dlt* operons, including GAS (71), GBS (66), *Streptococcus pneumoniae* (68), *Enterococcus faecalis* (67), *Listeria monocytogenes* (83), and *B. subtilis*. Inactivation of *dltA* in these and other Gram-positive species enhances sensitivity to human α-defensins and cathelicidin LL-37 (66, 71, 72, 83). Correspondingly, LTA D-alanylation is required for full virulence in mouse models of GAS (71), *L. monocytogenes* (83), and GBS infection (66). D-alanylation promotes GAS neutrophil intracellular survival as well as *L. monocytogenes in vivo* whole blood survival and *in vitro* adherence to macrophages, hepatocytes, and epithelial cells (83). In *Lactobacillus*, TA D-alanylation plays an important role in establishing gastrointestinal tract colonization (84).

Aminoacylation with L-Lysine or L-Alanine

The multiple peptide resistance factor MprF (also known as LysS), encoded by the *mprF* gene, is a highly conserved ~97-kDa integral membrane protein found in both Gram-positive and Gram-negative bacteria. MprF possesses a conserved C-terminal hydrophilic cytoplasmic domain and a large N-terminal flippase domain (85) that reduces the net negative surface charge of Gram-positive bacteria by incorporating L-lysine or L-alanine into cell wall PG (82, 85, 86). MprF is a lysine-substituted phosphatidylglycerol synthase that alters surface charge through the formation of a positively charged membrane phospholipid (82, 87) (Fig. 1A). Both the N- and C-terminal domains of MprF are necessary for AMP resistance in *S. aureus* (85), and *mprF* gene expression is controlled by the ApsRSX regulator (88). An *S. aureus* mutant strain lacking *mprF* has an increase in negative surface charge compared to WT, is more sensitive to killing by a broad range of bacterial and mammalian AMPs, including neutrophil defensins (82), and is less virulent in mouse infection models (75, 81, 82).

Aminoacylation of PG by MprF homologues increases AMP resistance in multiple bacterial species, including *Clostridium perfringens*, *E. faecalis*, *P. aeruginosa*, *Mycobacterium tuberculosis*, *Bacillus anthracis*, *B. subtilis*, *Enterococcus faecium*, and *L. monocytogenes* (89). *C. perfringens*, a Gram-positive spore-forming bacterium and common cause of foodborne illness, expresses two *mprF* genes designated *mprF1* and *mprF2*, which encode for alanyl phosphatidylglycerol synthase and lysylphosphatidylglycerol synthase, respectively (86, 90). In *M. tuberculosis*, the addition of positively charged amino acid L-lysine to PG is encoded by the *lysX* gene encoding for MprF homolog LysX and is essential for resistance to cationic antibiotics and AMPs (91, 92). Lysinylation of PG has also been described for *L. monocytogenes* (93), *P. aeruginosa* (94), and *B. anthracis* (95).

Additional cell wall modifications in Gram-positive bacteria have also been reported to influence AMP resistance. In GBS, the *ponA* gene encodes for penicillin-binding protein 1a and promotes resistance to human cathelicidin and defensins (96). The *pgm* gene, encoding a phosphoglucomutase, contributes to AMP resistance in porcine pathogen *Bordetella bronchiseptica* and the fish pathogen *Streptococcus iniae* (97, 98). In *Mycobacterium marinum*, mutation of the *kasB* gene, encoding beta-ketoacyl-acyl carrier protein synthase B, reduces growth in human macrophages and bacterial survival in the presence of human defensins (99).

Modification of LPS with L-Ara4N or pEtN

The outer membrane of Gram-negative bacteria is composed of lipid A, an anionic dimer of glucosamine linked to fatty acid chains and flanked by polar phosphate groups synthesized on the cytoplasmic surface of the inner membrane by highly conserved enzymes. The lipid A moiety has an attached core polysaccharide and species-specific side-chain "O" polysaccharides (62). Modification of this complex, known as LPS, with amine substituents L-Ara4N or pEtN reduces the net negative surface charge and AMP affinity, thereby promoting AMP resistance in Gram-negative bacteria such as *Salmonella* spp., important human pathogens and the causative agents of enteric/typhoid fever (Fig. 1A). In *S.* Typhimurium, two-component regulatory system PmrAB plays an important role in sensing extracellular cationic AMPs *in vivo*, and coordinates the expression of *pmrC* to decorate lipid A with ethanolamine and *pmrEHFIJKLM* for the attachment of positively charged L-Ara4N to the 4-phosphate group of the lipid A backbone, which together reduce the net negative charge of lipid A and enhance resistance to cationic AMPs (100, 101). All genes except for *pmrM* are required for the addition of L-Ara4N and increased resistance to cationic AMPs in

S. Typhimurium (100). *S.* Typhimurium lacking the LPS modifying enzyme PmrA are more sensitive to AMPs and have reduced virulence in a murine model of enteric infection (100, 102). L-Ara4N modification of LPS enhances AMP resistance of several Gram-negative species including *Proteus mirabilis*, responsible for urinary tract infections (103), *Yersinia pseudotuberculosis*, a causative agent of enterocolitis (104), *K. pneumoniae*, a human lung pathogen (105), and *P. aeruginosa* (106), associated with chronic airway infections in cystic fibrosis patients (107).

In the Gram-negative pathogen *H. pylori*, an etiologic agent of peptic ulcers and increased gastrointestinal cancer risk, the addition of pEtN to dephosphorylated lipid A of LPS increases AMP resistance and reduces TLR4-mediated activation of the innate immune system (108, 109). Mutation of the *H. pylori lpxEHP* genes disrupted direct attachment of pEtN to the disaccharide backbone of lipid A, increased the net negative charge of LPS, and concomitantly reduced the MIC of polymyxin B, a bacterial-derived AMP, by 25-fold compared to WT (108). In *Neisseria gonorrhoeae*, the *lptA* gene catalyzes addition of pEtN to lipid A and is necessary for polymyxin B resistance and survival in humans (110). Similarly, mutagenesis of *lptA* in *Neisseria meningitidis* decreased resistance to polymyxin B, protegrin-1, and LL-37 (111). Deletion of the *lpxA* gene encoding an enzyme in the lipid A biosynthesis pathway of *N. meningitidis* abolishes lipo-oligosaccharide (LOS) production and increases sensitivity to cationic AMPs (112, 113). Similarly, mutation of *waaF*, *cstII*, *galT*, or *lgtF* genes in *Campylobacter jejuni* results in LOS truncation and hypersensitivity to AMPs including polymyxin B, human α-defensin-5 (HD-5), and the murine HD-5 homologue Crp4 (114, 115).

Acylation and Phosphorylcholination of LPS

The *pagP* gene encoding acetyltransferase PagP in the outer membrane of *S.* Typhimurium acylates lipid A and increases AMP (C18G, pGLa, and protegrin-1) resistance by reducing outer membrane permeability (63, 116) (Fig. 1A). Inactivation of the *pagP* homologue *rcp* in the respiratory tract pathogen *L. pneumophila* reduces growth rate, AMP resistance, intracellular survival, and mouse lung colonization (117). LOS acylation by the *H. influenzae htrB* gene product is required for resistance to human AMP β-defensin 2 (HBD-2) (118). Addition of phosphorylcholine to the oligosaccharide portion of LPS promotes *H. influenzae* resistance to human cathelicidin LL-37 (119), conceivably through the cell surface exposure of the positively charged quaternary amine on choline to promote electrostatic repulsion (Fig. 1A). Inactivation of the *lpxM* gene in *K. pneumoniae*, which encodes an enzyme necessary for secondary acylation of immature lipid A, increases sensitivity to α-helical cationic AMPs through enhanced outer membrane permeability (120). In pathogenic *Vibrio cholerae* strain El Tor, the *msbB* gene is required for full acylation of the lipid A moiety and resistance to cationic AMPs (121).

Trapping of AMPs by Surface Molecules

Proteins and polysaccharides associated with the bacterial surface or secreted into the extracellular milieu may directly bind AMPs (Fig. 1B), thereby blocking access to the cytoplasmic membrane target of action and the formation of lytic pores. Another indirect AMP neutralization strategy employed by bacterial pathogens involves the release of the bound AMP from the bacterial surface (Table 2).

Surface-Associated Proteins, Secreted Proteins, and Polysaccharides

Plasminogen is the inactive form of plasmin, a host serine protease involved in the degradation of blood clots and tissue remodeling. *S. aureus* secretes a plasminogen-activating protein known as staphylokinase (SK). The accumulation of active plasmin activity on the *S. aureus* cell surface promotes host tis-

sue invasion and dissemination to normally sterile sites (122). SK binds and inactivates mCRAMP and α-defensins released from human neutrophils including HNP 1-3 (122, 123) (Fig. 1B), reducing AMP activity against *S. aureus* by more than 80%. Further, *S. aureus* strains expressing SK are more resistant to killing by α-defensins in a mouse model of arthritis, and the addition of purified SK to SK-deficient strains enhanced survival in the presence of α-defensin *in vitro* (123). The secreted hydrophilic GAS protein streptococcal inhibitor of complement (SIC) binds and inactivates human LL-37, α-defensin, and lysozyme to promote bacterial survival (Fig. 1B) (124–126). A *sic* knockout mutant in the highly invasive M1T1 GAS genetic background was more sensitive to killing by AMPs and shows diminished virulence in animal infection models (124, 125).

The M protein of GAS, encoded by the *emm* gene, is a major cell wall–anchored coiled-coil protein required for resistance to opsonophagocytosis, adherence to host cells, and full virulence in animal models of GAS infection (127). The C-terminal region of M protein is highly conserved and contains the canonical LPXTG cell wall anchor motif. GAS is classified into *emm* types according to the nucleotide sequence of the hypervariable N-terminal region. Currently, there are more than 200 known GAS serotypes, and the M1 GAS serotype is the most frequently isolated serotype from invasive GAS infections worldwide (128, 129). Mutation of the *emm1* gene, encoding M1 protein, significantly increased the sensitivity to LL-37 or mCRAMP compared to WT (130), while the heterologous expression of M1 protein in serotype M49 GAS or *Lactococcus lactis* enhanced LL-37 resistance. The trapping of LL-37 through the hypervariable extracellular N-terminal domain of M protein impedes LL-37 access to the cell membrane and promotes bacterial survival in LL-37-containing neutrophil extracellular traps (NETs) (Fig. 1B) (130). In GBS, surface-associated penicillin-binding protein-1a and the PilB surface pilus protein promotes adherence to host cells and resistance to cathelicidin AMPs through surface sequestration of LL-37 and mCRAMP *in vitro* (131, 132). Inactivation of *pilB* in GBS also reduces virulence in a mouse infection model (132).

Serological classification of streptococci in groups is based upon expression of unique carbohydrate antigens in the bacterial cell wall (133) known to play a structural role in cell wall biogenesis (134). Approximately 50% of the GAS cell wall by weight is made up of a single polysaccharide molecule termed the group A carbohydrate (GAC) antigen. All strains of GAS express GAC, which is composed of a polyrhamnose core with an immunodominant *N*-acetylglucosamine (GlcNAc) side chain (134). Inactivation of the *gacI* gene, encoding for a glycosyltransferase, abolished expression of the GlcNAc side chain in serotype M1 GAS. The *gacI* mutant was more susceptible to killing within NETs and to human cathelicidin LL-37, a component of neutrophil-specific granules important for intracellular killing and deployed within NETs (135). Similarly, the *gacI* mutant had reduced growth in human serum and was hypersensitive to killing by the antimicrobial releasate from thrombin-activated human platelets. Loss of the GlcNAc epitope on GAC attenuated GAS virulence in a rabbit model of pulmonary infection and a mouse model of systemic infection (135). In studies with purified WT and mutant GAC, the GlcNAc side chain was shown to impede LL-37 interaction with the underlying polyrhamnose core (135).

The active shedding of negatively charged surface exposed proteoglycans on host epithelial cells by proteases from bacterial pathogens is another resistance mechanism to trap and inactivate AMPs in tissues (Fig. 1B). Proteases secreted by GAS, *E. faecalis*, and *P. aeruginosa* degrade decorin and release dermatan sulfate, which can bind and inactivate human α defensin HNP-1 (136). Syndecan-1, a proteoglycan derived from the degradation of heparan sulfate, is released from the host

cell surface by *P. aeruginosa* virulence factor LasA to bind and impede AMP function (137). *S. epidermidis* synthesizes polysaccharide intercellular adhesin, a positively charged extracellular matrix polymer encoded by the *ica* gene locus (*icaADBC*) and the *cap* gene (138), to enhance electrostatic repulsion and resistance to cationic AMPs LL-37 and human β-defensin-3 (HBD-3) (139–141).

Capsular Polysaccharides

Several bacterial pathogens express surface capsules composed of high molecular mass polysaccharides that promote *in vivo* survival and trap cationic AMPs to impede interactions with the microbial cell surface (Fig. 1B). The hyaluronan capsule of GAS promotes survival in NETs through enhanced resistance to LL-37 (142). In *K. pneumoniae*, the *cps* capsule biosynthesis operon is transcriptionally upregulated in the presence of AMPs to enhance resistance to polymyxin B, protamine sulfate, defensin-1, β-defensin-1, and lactoferrin (143). The capsule of *K. pneumoniae* prevents engagement of TLR 2 and 4 and subsequent activation of the nuclear factor-κB and MAPK pathways to inhibit the expression of human β-defensins (144). Administration of capsular polysaccharide extracts from *S. pneumoniae* serotype 3 and *P. aeruginosa* enhanced the resistance of nonencapsulated *K. pneumoniae* to α-defensin HNP-1 and polymyxin B, suggesting that the release of capsule from the bacterial surface promotes the trapping of AMPs to prevent access to the site of action (145). Further, polymyxin B and HNP-1 also stimulate the release of capsule from the *S. pneumoniae* cell surface to sequester AMPs and increase AMP resistance (145). Studies of encapsulated WT and nonencapsulated serotype B mutant *N. meningitidis* demonstrate that capsule promotes resistance to protegrins, α- and β-defensins, polymyxin B, and cathelicidins LL-37 and mCRAMP (146). Moreover, the release of capsule from the surface of *N. meningitidis* is reported to promote resistance to LL-37 (113), and sublethal concentrations of AMP induce capsule biosynthesis (113, 146). Other bacterial species shield AMP targets with surface polymers. For example, LOS expression in *C. jejuni* increases LL-37, α-defensins, and polymyxin B resistance (114). *P. aeruginosa* biofilms produce alginate polysaccharide, a polymer of β-D-mannuronate and α-L-guluronate, to sequester and induce AMP conformational changes and peptide aggregation to prevent AMP access to the cell membrane (147).

Efflux Systems for AMP Resistance

Well studied for their prominent role in resistance to pharmaceutical antibiotics, certain adenosine triphosphate–binding cassette (ABC)–driven efflux pumps are used by human bacterial pathogens to resist AMPs through the extrusion of AMPs from the cell membrane site of action to the extracellular environment (148) (Fig. 1C). Three major classes of ABC transporter systems play a role in AMP resistance: (i) three-component ABC-transporters, (ii) two-component ABC-transporters, and (iii) single-protein multidrug-resistance transporters (149). Several three-component ABC transporters implicated in AMP resistance have been described in Gram-positive species, including NisFEG (*L. lactis*) (150), SpaFEG (*B. subtilis*) (151), and CprABC (*Clostridium difficile*) (152, 153) (Table 2). Common two-component systems involved in AMP resistance include the BceAB transporter system identified in *B. subtilis* (154), *S. aureus* (155), *L. lactis* (156), *S. pneumoniae* (157), and *L. monocytogenes* (158) and the BcrAB(C) transporter identified in some species of *Bacillus* (159), *Enterococcus* (160), *Clostridium* (161), and *Streptococcus* (162). The energy-driven efflux pumps RosA/RosB and AcrAB are required for polymyxin B resistance in *Y. enterocolitica* and *K. pneumoniae*, respectively (163, 164). In *Y. enterocolitica*, RosA and RosB upregulate the *ros* locus and are necessary and sufficient for resistance to cationic AMPs. In *K. pneumoniae*, AacrAB also enhances resistance to α- and β-defensins

(164). The MefE/Mel efflux pump contributes to LL-37 resistance in *S. pneumoniae* (165), while the TrkA and SapG potassium transport proteins in *Vibrio vulnificus* and *S.* Typhimurium, respectively, are essential for cationic AMP resistance (166, 167).

The energy-dependent MtrCDE efflux pump is a member of the resistance-nodulation-division efflux family. In the pathogens *N. gonorrhoeae* and *N. meningitidis*, MtrCDE is involved in actively transporting AMPs out of the bacterial cytoplasm and periplasmic space to promote resistance to LL-37, mCRAMP, PC-8, tachyplesin-1, and protegrin-1 (61, 111, 168). In addition, the Mtr efflux pump increases resistance to β-lactam and macrolide antibiotics and *in vivo* resistance to innate immune clearance (61, 168, 169). MtrCDE is necessary for *N. gonorrhoeae* colonization in a mouse model of genital tract infection (170), and inactivation of *mtrC* in *Haemophilus ducreyi* induces hypersensitivity to β-defensins and human LL-37 (171). The *sapABCDF* operon encoding ABC importer Sap (sensitive to antimicrobial peptides) in *S.* Typhimurium enhances resistance to protamine, bee-derived AMP melittin, and crude extracts from human neutrophil granule extracts (167, 172, 173). The Sap transporter also contributes to AMP resistance in other Gram-negative species, including *H. influenzae* (172) and *H. ducreyi* (174). Deletion of the *S.* Typhimurium *yejF* gene from the *yejABEF* operon encoding an ABC-type peptide import system, reduced resistance to polymyxin B, melittin, protamine, and human β-defensins 1 and 2 (175). In *S. aureus*, single-protein efflux pump QacA, encoded on naturally occurring plasmid pSK1, belongs to the major facilitator superfamily of transport proteins and uses proton motive force to extrude substrates (176). QacA promotes resistance to rabbit platelet AMP and host-derived thrombin-induced platelet microbicidal protein (177) and may also induce secondary changes in membrane fluidity to promote AMP resistance (178). Increased resistance to thrombin-induced platelet microbicidal protein in *S. aureus* is correlated with *in vivo* survival in animal infection models and endocarditis in humans (177, 179).

Inactivation of AMPs by Proteolytic Degradation

AMPs are relatively resistant to proteolytic degradation by surface-associated or secreted proteases produced by bacterial pathogens (180). However, some bacterial proteases with broad substrate specificity promote disease pathogenesis by efficiently cleaving and inactivating AMPs (Fig. 1D). The human AMP LL-37 is cleaved into nonfunctional breakdown products by proteases expressed by several human pathogens including *E. faecalis* (metallopeptidase gelatinase) (181), GAS (broad-spectrum cysteine protease streptococcal pyrogenic exotoxin B) (182), *S. aureus* (aureolysin) (183), and *P. mirabilis* (50-kDa metalloprotease) (184). Aureolysin inactivates LL-37 by cleaving the C-terminal peptide bonds between the Arg_{19}-Ile_{20}, Arg_{23}-Ile_{24}, and Leu_{31}-Val_{32} (183) and promotes survival within the LL-37-rich environment of macrophage phagolysosomes (185). The GAS protease inhibitor α2-macroglobulin binds broad-spectrum cysteine protease streptococcal pyrogenic exotoxin B (SpeB) to the cell surface with the help of surface-associated G-related α2-macroglobulin-binding protein to facilitate LL-37 cleavage and bacterial survival (186, 187). The metalloprotease ZapA, a major virulence factor of *P. mirabilis* that degrades antibodies, extracellular matrix molecules, and complement components C1q and C3, also contributes to AMP resistance by cleaving human β-defensin 1, LL-37, and protegrin-1 (184). The elastase of *P. aeruginosa* completely degrades and inactivates LL-37, promoting survival in an *ex vivo* wound fluid model (181). The *S.* Typhimurium *pgtE* gene that encodes for outer membrane protease PgtE, enhances resistance to LL-37 and C18G, an α-helical cationic AMP (188). Plasminogen-activating streptokinase secreted by GAS results in the accumulation of cell surface plasmin activity capable of degrading LL-37

(189). In *Burkholderia cenocepacia*, ZmpA and ZmpB zinc-dependent metalloproteases cleave and inactivate AMPs LL-37 and β-defensin 1, respectively (190). High-level expression of outer membrane protease OmpT of enterohemorrhagic *E. coli* promotes AMP resistance through the efficient degradation of LL-37 at dibasic sites (191). Proteases secreted by other pathogens also efficiently cleave and inactivate AMPs, including *B. anthracis* (LL-37), *Porphyromonas gingivalis* (α- and β-defensins, cecropin B), and *Prevotella* spp. (brevinin) (192–196) (Table 2).

Regulatory Networks and AMP Resistance

Bacterial pathogens use two-component regulatory systems to modulate gene expression in response to extracellular metal ion concentrations, metabolic requirements, growth phase or to subvert the host innate immune response mounted by neutrophils or macrophages within host tissue, resulting in the up- or downregulation of genes necessary for survival and disease progression. Several pathogens achieve maximal resistance to AMPs through the coordinated transcriptional upregulation of AMP resistance factors (Fig. 1E). PhoPQ is a well-studied two-component system in *S.* Typhimurium that responds to changes in magnesium ion (Mg^{2+}) concentration, pH, and the presence of cationic AMPs (20, 197) (Table 2). Sensor kinase PhoP directly or indirectly coordinates the expression of >100 genes in *S.* Typhimurium that encode for proteins involved in Mg^{2+} transport (MgtA and MgtCB), transcriptional regulators important for intracellular macrophage survival (SlyA), oxidative stress resistance (RpoS), LPS modification by amino arabinose (PmrAB), and lipid A acylation (PagP) to reduce the fluidity and permeability of the bacterial membrane and enhance AMP resistance (20, 188, 198). Consequently, PhoPQ plays a role in modifying LPS surface charge (63) and in enhancing macrophage resistance through the upregulation of the AMP-degrading outer membrane protease PgtE (188, 199–201) and is required for full virulence in a mouse model of gastrointestinal infection (167). Additional *S.* Typhimurium transcriptional factors associated with resistance to bacterially derived AMP polymyxin B include *virK*, *somA*, and *rcsC* (202). PhoPQ homologs have been identified in other Gram-negative pathogens, including *Yersinia pestis*, *Shigella flexneri*, and *P. aeruginosa* (203). Mutant strains of *Y. pestis* deficient in PhoPQ are more sensitive to AMPs and neutrophil intracellular killing (204). In *P. aeruginosa*, the presence of AMPs or divalent cations activates the PhoPQ and PmrAB systems to enhance resistance to cationic AMPs such as LL-37 and polymyxin B (205–207). The two-component system PmrAB in *P. aeruginosa* coordinates the incorporation of positively charged L-Ara4N subunits into LPS and promotes AMP resistance through electrostatic repulsion (106, 206).

Upon encountering bacteria at the site of infection, NETs are released to help trap and kill the bacteria. NETs are composed of DNA backbone and antimicrobial effectors such as histones, granule proteases and AMPs (in particular, cathelicidin) that promote microbe killing (208, 209). Degradation of the DNA scaffold by secreted bacterial DNases promotes NET escape and survival for several bacterial pathogens including GAS (210–212), *S. pneumoniae* (213), GBS (214), and *S. aureus* (215). Subinhibitory concentrations of exogenous DNA promote *P. aeruginosa* AMP resistance through the chelation of divalent cations and the resultant upregulation of AMP resistance genes (216). In *S.* Typhimurium, extracellular DNA also induces *pmr* expression and AMP resistance (217).

The D-alanylation of teichoic acid by the *dlt* operon is regulated by the *agr* locus in *S. aureus* and promotes AMP resistance (282). Exposure of *S. aureus* to AMPs activates the VraSR and VraDE operons involved in resistance to AMPs and cell wall-targeting antibiotics such as bacitracin (28). Human β-defensin (HBD-3) triggers the upregulation of the cell wall stress response pathway in *S. aureus* to counteract HBD-3-induced perturbation of peptidoglycan synthesis (13). Exposure of *S. aureus* to sublethal concentrations of magainin 2 and gramicidin D promotes resistance to these AMPs through the enhancement of membrane rigidity (218). Changes in membrane fluidity induced by incorporation of longer-chain unsaturated fatty acids into the lipid bilayer (resulting in increased membrane fluidity) or carotenoid staphyloxanthin pigment (resulting in increased membrane rigidity) promotes *S. aureus* resistance to platelet-derived AMPs (tPMPs) or polymyxin B and human neutrophil defensin 1, respectively (219, 220). While the precise resistance mechanism has yet to be determined, a significant increase or reduction in membrane fluidity may hinder AMP insertion into the cellular membrane (89, 221). In *L. monocytogenes*, an increase in the concentration of membrane saturated fatty acids and phosphatidylethanolamine, and a decrease in phosphatidylglycerol concentration, reduces the fluidity of the cell membrane to promote nisin resistance (222, 223). PrfA, a temperature-regulated transcription factor in *L. monocytogenes*, contributes to defensin resistance (224).

Modulation of Host AMP Production by Bacterial Pathogens

While low levels of AMPs are produced by epithelial and host immune cells at baseline, AMP expression is typically dramatically upregulated in response to bacterial infection. Some bacterial pathogens resist AMP-mediated innate immune clearance by interfering with, or suppressing, host AMP expression levels (Fig. 1F). *Shigella* spp. are Gram-negative rods capable of causing life-threatening invasive human infections such as bacillary dysentery. *Shigella dysenteriae* and *S. flexneri* downregulate the expression of LL-37 and β-defensin-1 in intestinal epithelial cells during early infection through a mechanism dependent on transcriptional factor MxiE and the type III secretion system to promote bacterial survival, colonization, and invasion of the gastrointestinal tract (225, 226) (Table 2). *P. aeruginosa*, a human pathogen commonly isolated from the lungs of cystic fibrosis patients, induces the expression of the host cysteine proteases cathepsins B, L, and S to cleave and inactivate β-defensins 2 and 3 and thwart AMP-mediated clearance of the bacteria in airway fluid (227). Enterotoxigenic *E. coli* and *V. cholerae* exotoxins reportedly repress the expression of host cell HBD-1 and LL-37 (228), while *N. gonorrhoeae* downregulates the expression of AMP genes (229). *Burkholderia* spp. are human pathogens associated with opportunistic infections in cystic fibrosis patients and chronic granulomatous disease (230). The high-level AMP resistance exhibited by this genus has been attributed to the constitutive incorporation of L-Ara4N into the LPS molecule (230, 231). Alternative sigma factor RpoE coordinates *Burkholderia* gene expression under stress conditions and contributes to AMP resistance in a temperature-dependent manner (230, 232).

CONCLUDING REMARKS AND FUTURE DIRECTIONS

AMPs are present in most organisms and are an ancient and diverse group of naturally occurring anti-infective molecules that play an integral part in the host innate immune defense against bacterial infection. Bacterial AMP resistance mechanisms have evolved as a result of selection pressures from direct competition among species (bacteriocins) and during host-pathogen interactions (innate defense AMPs). Human bacterial pathogens have evolved a broad diversity of intrinsic or inducible AMP-defense mechanisms to promote survival, colonization, and subsequent dissemination to normally sterile sites within the body to cause life-threatening invasive syndromes. Bacterial pathogens with intrinsic high-level resistance to AMPs, such as *S. aureus* and *Salmonella* spp. can bypass normally effective mucosal defenses and are consequently among the leading causes of deep tissue and systemic infections. AMP resistance is mediated by a variety of molecular mechanisms including net cell surface charge alteration, efflux, restricting AMP access to their targets, and proteolytic cleavage of AMPs. Bacterial mutants sensitive to AMPs in *in vitro* assays are attenuated for virulence in systemic animal infection models. An improved comprehension of AMP modes of action, resistance mechanisms and host pathogen interactions may inspire the development of alternative antibacterial therapeutics that target the cell wall, efflux pumps, or AMP-inactivating proteases, ultimately enhancing bacterial sensitivity to the AMPs of the host innate immune system. Understanding the interaction between conventional antibiotics and endogenous AMPs can also lead to improved therapeutic strategies for drug-resistant pathogens. The action of beta-lactam antibiotics to sensitize methicillin-resistant *S. aureus* and vancomycin-resistant *Enterococcus* spp. to killing by human cathelicidin LL-37 and cationic peptide antibiotic daptomycin has shown promise in synergy studies and small clinical series in patients with previously recalcitrant infections (233, 234).

The emergence of antibiotic-resistant microbes through the excessive and inappropriate use of conventional antibiotics is a critical public health threat responsible for high morbidity rates and significant socioeconomic costs worldwide. Moreover, the antibiotic development pipelines of the major pharmaceutical companies have steadily declined over the past 20 years. Consequently, there is considerable interest in alternative therapeutic approaches to facilitate the fight against multidrug-resistant pathogens, including the development of novel broad-spectrum AMPs against bacteria, fungi, protozoa, and enveloped viruses (30, 235). Importantly, the AMP mechanism of action is very rapid at concentrations close to the MIC, in comparison to conventional antibiotics (236). In recent years, intensive research has led to the establishment of several bioinformatics tools and databases (e.g., APD2, cathelicidin antimicrobial peptide, iAMP-2L) to identify and isolate new AMP classes and to elucidate their structure, function, and biological activity (237). However, prolonged *in vitro* exposure of bacteria to sublethal AMP concentrations (238), and preclinical trials with naturally occurring cationic AMPs have detected resistant strains, indicating that optimization of AMP composition and structures are required to enhance stability and efficacy (237). Cross-resistance to AMPs with disparate modes of action has also been reported. For example, *S. aureus* is resistant to pexiganan and cross-resistant to HNP-1 (239). *S. aureus* isolates resistant to daptomycin, a cyclic lipopeptide antibiotic that associates with Ca^{2+} to form a cationic complex (240), are also more resistant host defense AMPs with diverse mechanisms of action, including HNP-1, polymyxin B, and tPMPs (241). Human pathogens resistant to nisin, an AMP used as a food preservative (*L. monocytogenes*, *Streptococcus bovis*) (242, 243), and colistin, also known as polymyxin E (*Acinetobacter baumannii*, *P. aeruginosa*, *Brevundimonas diminuta*, *Ochrobactrum anthropi*, *K. pneumoniae*) (244, 245) have recently been reported.

The transfer of broad-spectrum resistance mechanisms between bacteria and the development of resistance against our own host defense peptides remain valid concerns moving forward with the development of AMPs for clinical use (246, 247). Systemic toxicity and decreased blood and/or serum activity of natural peptides have significantly hampered clinical AMP development and provided the impetus for *de novo*–designed peptide sequences (1). To this end, multiple new classes of AMPs have been reported (e.g., mimetic peptides, hybrid peptides, peptide congeners, stabilized AMPs, peptide conjugates, immobilized peptides) with potential applications in medicine, veterinary medicine, and agriculture (248). Rationally designed synthetic AMPs have recently been demonstrated to be active against antibiotic-resistant *A. baumannii* and *K. pneumoniae* (249). Synthetic peptides could also be designed to resist bacterial and host proteases through the incorporation of D-amino acids (229). While pathogenic bacteria have successfully evolved AMP-resistance mechanisms, resistance to a broad range of AMPs has not yet occurred. Enhanced microbicidal activity of phagocytic cells and enhanced resistance to bacterial infection *in vivo* has been achieved by genetic or pharmacological augmentation of transcriptional regulator hypoxia-inducible factor (250, 251), which regulates the expression of human and murine cathelicidin at the transcriptional level (250, 252). Combination therapy with AMPs and classical antibiotics that target more than one site of action, such as the inhibition of cell wall synthesis coupled with cell membrane disruption, may help to combat the increasing emergence of multidrug-resistant microbes associated with challenging and deadly microbial infections.

ACKNOWLEDGMENTS

The authors thank Anna Henningham, University of California San Diego School of Medicine, for the critical reading of this manuscript and many helpful suggestions.

This work was supported by the National Health and Medical Research Council of Australia (APP1033258 to J.N.C.) and the National Institutes of Health (AI093451, AR052728, AI077780, AI052453, and HD071600 to V.N.).

CITATION

Cole JN, Nizet V. 2016. Bacterial evasion of host antimicrobial peptide defenses. Microbiol Spectrum 4(1):VMBF-0006-2015.

REFERENCES

1. **Steckbeck JD, Deslouches B, Montelaro RC.** 2014. Antimicrobial peptides: new drugs for bad bugs? *Expert Opin Biol Ther* **14:**11–14.

2. **Di Francesco A, Favaroni A, Donati M.** 2013. Host defense peptides: general overview and an update on their activity against *Chlamydia* spp. *Expert Rev Anti Infect Ther* **11:**1215–1224.

3. **Anaya-Lopez JL, Lopez-Meza JE, Ochoa-Zarzosa A.** 2013. Bacterial resistance to cationic antimicrobial peptides. *Crit Rev Microbiol* **39:**180–195.

4. **Jenssen H, Hamill P, Hancock RE.** 2006. Peptide antimicrobial agents. *Clin Microbiol Rev* **19:**491–511.

5. **Nakatsuji T, Gallo RL.** 2012. Antimicrobial peptides: old molecules with new ideas. *J Invest Dermatol* **132:**887–895.

6. **Pinheiro da Silva F, Machado MC.** 2012. Antimicrobial peptides: clinical relevance and therapeutic implications. *Peptides* **36:** 308–314.

7. **Morrison G, Kilanowski F, Davidson D, Dorin J.** 2002. Characterization of the mouse beta defensin 1, Defb1, mutant mouse model. *Infect Immun* **70:**3053–3060.

8. **Guralp SA, Murgha YE, Rouillard JM, Gulari E.** 2013. From design to screening: a new antimicrobial peptide discovery pipeline. *PLoS One* **8:**e59305. doi:10.1371/journal.pone.0059305.

9. **Nguyen LT, Haney EF, Vogel HJ.** 2011. The expanding scope of antimicrobial peptide structures and their modes of action. *Trends Biotechnol* **29:**464–472.

10. **Lehrer RI, Ganz T.** 2002. Cathelicidins: a family of endogenous antimicrobial peptides. *Curr Opin Hematol* **9:**18–22.

11. **Ganz T.** 2003. Defensins: antimicrobial peptides of innate immunity. *Nat Rev Immunol* **3:** 710–720.

12. **Ayabe T, Satchell DP, Wilson CL, Parks WC, Selsted ME, Ouellette AJ.** 2000. Secretion of microbicidal alpha-defensins by intestinal Paneth cells in response to bacteria. *Nat Immunol* **1:**113–118.

13. **Yount NY, Yeaman MR.** 2013. Peptide antimicrobials: cell wall as a bacterial target. *Ann N Y Acad Sci* **1277:**127–138.

14. **Ganz T, Lehrer RI.** 1997. Antimicrobial peptides of leukocytes. *Curr Opin Hematol* **4:** 53–58.

15. **Jones DE, Bevins CL.** 1992. Paneth cells of the human small intestine express an antimicrobial peptide gene. *J Biol Chem* **267:**23216–23225.

16. **Quayle AJ, Porter EM, Nussbaum AA, Wang YM, Brabec C, Yip KP, Mok SC.** 1998. Gene expression, immunolocalization, and secretion of human defensin-5 in human female reproductive tract. *Am J Pathol* **152:**1247–1258.

17. **Duits LA, Ravensbergen B, Rademaker M, Hiemstra PS, Nibbering PH.** 2002. Expression of beta-defensin 1 and 2 mRNA by human monocytes, macrophages and dendritic cells. *Immunology* **106:**517–525.

18. **Kosciuczuk EM, Lisowski P, Jarczak J, Strzalkowska N, Jozwik A, Horbanczuk J, Krzyzewski J, Zwierzchowski L, Bagnicka E.** 2012. Cathelicidins: family of antimicrobial peptides. A review. *Mol Biol Rep* **39:**10957–10970.

19. **Yeaman MR.** 2010. Platelets in defense against bacterial pathogens. *Cell Mol Life Sci* **67:**525–544.

20. **Koprivnjak T, Peschel A.** 2011. Bacterial resistance mechanisms against host defense peptides. *Cell Mol Life Sci* **68:**2243–2254.

21. **Kwakman PH, Krijgsveld J, de Boer L, Nguyen LT, Boszhard L, Vreede J, Dekker HL, Speijer D, Drijfhout JW, te Velde AA, Crielaard W, Vogel HJ, Vandenbroucke-Grauls CM, Zaat SA.** 2011. Native thrombocidin-1 and unfolded thrombocidin-1 exert antimicrobial activity via distinct structural elements. *J Biol Chem* **286:** 43506–43514.

22. **Zasloff M.** 2002. Antimicrobial peptides of multicellular organisms. *Nature* **415:**389–395.

23. **Senyurek I, Paulmann M, Sinnberg T, Kalbacher H, Deeg M, Gutsmann T, Hermes M, Kohler T, Gotz F, Wolz C, Peschel A, Schittek B.** 2009. Dermcidin-derived peptides show a different mode of action than the cathelicidin LL-37 against *Staphylococcus aureus*. *Antimicrob Agents Chemother* **53:**2499–2509.

24. **Gennaro R, Zanetti M.** 2000. Structural features and biological activities of the cathelicidin-derived antimicrobial peptides. *Biopolymers* **55:** 31–49.

25. **Yeaman MR, Yount NY.** 2003. Mechanisms of antimicrobial peptide action and resistance. *Pharmacol Rev* **55:**27–55.

26. **Ehrenstein G, Lecar H.** 1977. Electrically gated ionic channels in lipid bilayers. *Q Rev Biophys* **10:**1–34.

27. **Matsuzaki K, Murase O, Fujii N, Miyajima K.** 1996. An antimicrobial peptide, magainin 2, induced rapid flip-flop of phospholipids coupled with pore formation and peptide translocation. *Biochemistry* **35:**11361–11368.

28. **Pietiainen M, Francois P, Hyyrylainen HL, Tangomo M, Sass V, Sahl HG, Schrenzel J, Kontinen VP.** 2009. Transcriptome analysis of the responses of *Staphylococcus aureus* to antimicrobial peptides and characterization of

the roles of *vraDE* and *vraSR* in antimicrobial resistance. *BMC Genomics* **10:**429.

29. **Straus SK, Hancock RE.** 2006. Mode of action of the new antibiotic for Gram-positive pathogens daptomycin: comparison with cationic antimicrobial peptides and lipopeptides. *Biochim Biophys Acta* **1758:**1215–1223.

30. **Brogden KA.** 2005. Antimicrobial peptides: pore formers or metabolic inhibitors in bacteria? *Nat Rev Microbiol* **3:**238–250.

31. **Muller A, Ulm H, Reder-Christ K, Sahl HG, Schneider T.** 2012. Interaction of type A lantibiotics with undecaprenol-bound cell envelope precursors. *Microb Drug Resist* **18:**261–270.

32. **Islam MR, Nagao J, Zendo T, Sonomoto K.** 2012. Antimicrobial mechanism of lantibiotics. *Biochem Soc Trans* **40:**1528–1533.

33. **Cho JH, Sung BH, Kim SC.** 2009. Buforins: histone H2A-derived antimicrobial peptides from toad stomach. *Biochim Biophys Acta* **1788:**1564–1569.

34. **Subbalakshmi C, Sitaram N.** 1998. Mechanism of antimicrobial action of indolicidin. *FEMS Microbiol Lett* **160:**91–96.

35. **Haney EF, Petersen AP, Lau CK, Jing W, Storey DG, Vogel HJ.** 2013. Mechanism of action of puroindoline derived tryptophanrich antimicrobial peptides. *Biochim Biophys Acta* **1828:**1802–1813.

36. **Lehrer RI, Barton A, Daher KA, Harwig SS, Ganz T, Selsted ME.** 1989. Interaction of human defensins with *Escherichia coli*. Mechanism of bactericidal activity. *J Clin Invest* **84:**553–561.

37. **Di Nardo A, Vitiello A, Gallo RL.** 2003. Cutting edge: mast cell antimicrobial activity is mediated by expression of cathelicidin antimicrobial peptide. *J Immunol* **170:**2274–2278.

38. **Nizet V, Ohtake T, Lauth X, Trowbridge J, Rudisill J, Dorschner RA, Pestonjamasp V, Piraino J, Huttner K, Gallo RL.** 2001. Innate antimicrobial peptide protects the skin from invasive bacterial infection. *Nature* **414:**454–457.

39. **Rosenberger CM, Gallo RL, Finlay BB.** 2004. Interplay between antibacterial effectors: a macrophage antimicrobial peptide impairs intracellular *Salmonella* replication. *Proc Natl Acad Sci USA* **101:**2422–2427.

40. **Chromek M, Slamova Z, Bergman P, Kovacs L, Podracka L, Ehren I, Hokfelt T, Gudmundsson GH, Gallo RL, Agerberth B, Brauner A.** 2006. The antimicrobial peptide cathelicidin protects the urinary tract against invasive bacterial infection. *Nat Med* **12:**636–641.

41. **Bergman P, Johansson L, Wan H, Jones A, Gallo RL, Gudmundsson GH, Hokfelt T, Jonsson AB, Agerberth B.** 2006. Induction of the antimicrobial peptide CRAMP in the blood-brain barrier and meninges after meningococcal infection. *Infect Immun* **74:**6982–6991.

42. **Kumar A, Gao N, Standiford TJ, Gallo RL, Yu FS.** 2010. Topical flagellin protects the injured corneas from *Pseudomonas aeruginosa* infection. *Microbes Infect* **12:**978–989.

43. **Kovach MA, Ballinger MN, Newstead MW, Zeng X, Bhan U, Yu FS, Moore BB, Gallo RL, Standiford TJ.** 2012. Cathelicidin-related antimicrobial peptide is required for effective lung mucosal immunity in Gram-negative bacterial pneumonia. *J Immunol* **189:**304–311.

44. **Augustin DK, Heimer SR, Tam C, Li WY, Le Due JM, Evans DJ, Fleiszig SM.** 2011. Role of defensins in corneal epithelial barrier function against *Pseudomonas aeruginosa* traversal. *Infect Immun* **79:**595–605.

45. **Kolar SS, Baidouri H, Hanlon S, McDermott AM.** 2013. Protective role of murine betadefensins 3 and 4 and cathelin-related antimicrobial peptide in *Fusarium solani* keratitis. *Infect Immun* **81:**2669–2677.

46. **Lee PH, Ohtake T, Zaiou M, Murakami M, Rudisill JA, Lin KH, Gallo RL.** 2005. Expression of an additional cathelicidin antimicrobial peptide protects against bacterial skin infection. *Proc Natl Acad Sci USA* **102:**3750–3755.

47. **Salzman NH, Ghosh D, Huttner KM, Paterson Y, Bevins CL.** 2003. Protection against enteric salmonellosis in transgenic mice expressing a human intestinal defensin. *Nature* **422:**522–526.

48. **Niyonsaba F, Ushio H, Nakano N, Ng W, Sayama K, Hashimoto K, Nagaoka I, Okumura K, Ogawa H.** 2007. Antimicrobial peptides human beta-defensins stimulate epidermal keratinocyte migration, proliferation and production of proinflammatory cytokines and chemokines. *J Invest Dermatol* **127:**594–604.

49. **Zanetti M.** 2004. Cathelicidins, multifunctional peptides of the innate immunity. *J Leukoc Biol* **75:**39–48.

50. **Koczulla R, von Degenfeld G, Kupatt C, Krotz F, Zahler S, Gloe T, Issbrucker K, Unterberger P, Zaiou M, Lebherz C, Karl A, Raake P, Pfosser A, Boekstegers P, Welsch U, Hiemstra PS, Vogelmeier C, Gallo RL, Clauss M, Bals R.** 2003. An angiogenic role for the human peptide antibiotic LL-37/hCAP-18. *J Clin Invest* **111:**1665–1672.

51. **Elssner A, Duncan M, Gavrilin M, Wewers MD.** 2004. A novel P2X7 receptor activator,

the human cathelicidin-derived peptide LL37, induces IL-1 beta processing and release. *J Immunol* **172**:4987–4994.

52. **Davidson DJ, Currie AJ, Reid GS, Bowdish DM, MacDonald KL, Ma RC, Hancock RE, Speert DP.** 2004. The cationic antimicrobial peptide LL-37 modulates dendritic cell differentiation and dendritic cell-induced T cell polarization. *J Immunol* **172**:1146–1156.

53. **Territo MC, Ganz T, Selsted ME, Lehrer R.** 1989. Monocyte-chemotactic activity of defensins from human neutrophils. *J Clin Invest* **84**:2017–2020.

54. **Kurosaka K, Chen Q, Yarovinsky F, Oppenheim JJ, Yang D.** 2005. Mouse cathelin-related antimicrobial peptide chemoattracts leukocytes using formyl peptide receptor-like 1/mouse formyl peptide receptor-like 2 as the receptor and acts as an immune adjuvant. *J Immunol* **174**:6257–6265.

55. **Niyonsaba F, Iwabuchi K, Someya A, Hirata M, Matsuda H, Ogawa H, Nagaoka I.** 2002. A cathelicidin family of human antibacterial peptide LL-37 induces mast cell chemotaxis. *Immunology* **106**:20–26.

56. **Niyonsaba F, Someya A, Hirata M, Ogawa H, Nagaoka I.** 2001. Evaluation of the effects of peptide antibiotics human beta-defensins-1/-2 and LL-37 on histamine release and prostaglandin D(2) production from mast cells. *Eur J Immunol* **31**:1066–1075.

57. **Lohner K.** 2009. New strategies for novel antibiotics: peptides targeting bacterial cell membranes. *Gen Physiol Biophys* **28**:105–116.

58. **Gutsmann T, Hagge SO, Larrick JW, Seydel U, Wiese A.** 2001. Interaction of CAP18-derived peptides with membranes made from endotoxins or phospholipids. *Biophys J* **80**:2935–2945.

59. **Oren Z, Lerman JC, Gudmundsson GH, Agerberth B, Shai Y.** 1999. Structure and organization of the human antimicrobial peptide LL-37 in phospholipid membranes: relevance to the molecular basis for its non-cell-selective activity. *Biochem J* **341**:501–513.

60. **Schmidtchen A, Pasupuleti M, Malmsten M.** 2014. Effect of hydrophobic modifications in antimicrobial peptides. *Adv Colloid Interface Sci* **205**:265–274.

61. **Guilhelmelli F, Vilela N, Albuquerque P, Derengowski L da S, Silva-Pereira I, Kyaw CM.** 2013. Antibiotic development challenges: the various mechanisms of action of antimicrobial peptides and of bacterial resistance. *Front Microbiol* **4**:353.

62. **Raetz CR, Reynolds CM, Trent MS, Bishop RE.** 2007. Lipid A modification systems in Gram-negative bacteria. *Annu Rev Biochem* **76**:295–329.

63. **Guo L, Lim KB, Poduje CM, Daniel M, Gunn JS, Hackett M, Miller SI.** 1998. Lipid A acylation and bacterial resistance against vertebrate antimicrobial peptides. *Cell* **95**:189–198.

64. **Brown S, Santa Maria JP Jr, Walker S.** 2013. Wall teichoic acids of Gram-positive bacteria. *Annu Rev Microbiol* **67**:313–336.

65. **Neuhaus FC, Baddiley J.** 2003. A continuum of anionic charge: structures and functions of D-alanyl-teichoic acids in Gram-positive bacteria. *Microbiol Mol Biol Rev* **67**:686–723.

66. **Poyart C, Pellegrini E, Marceau M, Baptista M, Jaubert F, Lamy MC, Trieu-Cuot P.** 2003. Attenuated virulence of *Streptococcus agalactiae* deficient in D-alanyl-lipoteichoic acid is due to an increased susceptibility to defensins and phagocytic cells. *Mol Microbiol* **49**:1615–1625.

67. **Fabretti F, Theilacker C, Baldassarri L, Kaczynski Z, Kropec A, Holst O, Huebner J.** 2006. Alanine esters of enterococcal lipoteichoic acid play a role in biofilm formation and resistance to antimicrobial peptides. *Infect Immun* **74**:4164–4171.

68. **Kovacs M, Halfmann A, Fedtke I, Heintz M, Peschel A, Vollmer W, Hakenbeck R, Bruckner R.** 2006. A functional *dlt* operon, encoding proteins required for incorporation of D-alanine in teichoic acids in Gram-positive bacteria, confers resistance to cationic antimicrobial peptides in *Streptococcus pneumoniae*. *J Bacteriol* **188**:5797–5805.

69. **Morath S, Geyer A, Hartung T.** 2001. Structure-function relationship of cytokine induction by lipoteichoic acid from *Staphylococcus aureus*. *J Exp Med* **193**:393–397.

70. **Grangette C, Nutten S, Palumbo E, Morath S, Hermann C, Dewulf J, Pot B, Hartung T, Hols P, Mercenier A.** 2005. Enhanced anti-inflammatory capacity of a *Lactobacillus plantarum* mutant synthesizing modified teichoic acids. *Proc Natl Acad Sci USA* **102**:10321–10326.

71. **Kristian SA, Datta V, Weidenmaier C, Kansal R, Fedtke I, Peschel A, Gallo RL, Nizet V.** 2005. D-alanylation of teichoic acids promotes group A *Streptococcus* antimicrobial peptide resistance, neutrophil survival, and epithelial cell invasion. *J Bacteriol* **187**:6719–6725.

72. **Peschel A, Otto M, Jack RW, Kalbacher H, Jung G, Gotz F.** 1999. Inactivation of the *dlt* operon in *Staphylococcus aureus* confers sensitivity to defensins, protegrins, and other antimicrobial peptides. *J Biol Chem* **274**:8405–8410.

73. Andra J, Goldmann T, Ernst CM, Peschel A, Gutsmann T. 2011. Multiple peptide resistance factor (MprF)-mediated resistance of *Staphylococcus aureus* against antimicrobial peptides coincides with a modulated peptide interaction with artificial membranes comprising lysyl-phosphatidylglycerol. *J Biol Chem* **286:**18692–18700.

74. Peschel A. 2002. How do bacteria resist human antimicrobial peptides? *Trends Microbiol* **10:**179–186.

75. Kristian SA, Lauth X, Nizet V, Goetz F, Neumeister B, Peschel A, Landmann R. 2003. Alanylation of teichoic acids protects *Staphylococcus aureus* against Toll-like receptor 2-dependent host defense in a mouse tissue cage infection model. *J Infect Dis* **188:**414–423.

76. Heptinstall S, Archibald AR, Baddiley J. 1970. Teichoic acids and membrane function in bacteria. *Nature* **225:**519–521.

77. MacArthur AE, Archibald AR. 1984. Effect of culture pH on the $_{pere}$-alanine ester content of lipoteichoic acid in *Staphylococcus aureus*. *J Bacteriol* **160:**792–793.

78. Perego M, Glaser P, Minutello A, Strauch MA, Leopold K, Fischer W. 1995. Incorporation of D-alanine into lipoteichoic acid and wall teichoic acid in *Bacillus subtilis*. Identification of genes and regulation. *J Biol Chem* **270:**15598–15606.

79. Poyart C, Lamy MC, Boumaila C, Fiedler F, Trieu-Cuot P. 2001. Regulation of D-alanyl-lipoteichoic acid biosynthesis in *Streptococcus agalactiae* involves a novel two-component regulatory system. *J Bacteriol* **183:**6324–6334.

80. Saar-Dover R, Bitler A, Nezer R, Shmuel-Galia L, Firon A, Shimoni E, Trieu-Cuot P, Shai Y. 2012. D-alanylation of lipoteichoic acids confers resistance to cationic peptides in group B *Streptococcus* by increasing the cell wall density. *PLoS Pathog* **8:**e1002891. doi:10.1371/journal. ppat.1002891.

81. Kristian SA, Durr M, Van Strijp JA, Neumeister B, Peschel A. 2003. MprF-mediated lysinylation of phospholipids in *Staphylococcus aureus* leads to protection against oxygen-independent neutrophil killing. *Infect Immun* **71:**546–549.

82. Peschel A, Jack RW, Otto M, Collins LV, Staubitz P, Nicholson G, Kalbacher H, Nieuwenhuizen WF, Jung G, Tarkowski A, van Kessel KP, van Strijp JA. 2001. *Staphylococcus aureus* resistance to human defensins and evasion of neutrophil killing via the novel virulence factor MprF is based on modification of membrane lipids with L-lysine. *J Exp Med* **193:**1067–1076.

83. Abachin E, Poyart C, Pellegrini E, Milohanic E, Fiedler F, Berche P, Trieu-Cuot P. 2002. Formation of D-alanyl-lipoteichoic acid is required for adhesion and virulence of *Listeria monocytogenes*. *Mol Microbiol* **43:**1–14.

84. Walter J, Loach DM, Alqumber M, Rockel C, Hermann C, Pfitzenmaier M, Tannock GW. 2007. D-alanyl ester depletion of teichoic acids in *Lactobacillus reuteri* 100-23 results in impaired colonization of the mouse gastrointestinal tract. *Environ Microbiol* **9:**1750–1760.

85. Ernst CM, Staubitz P, Mishra NN, Yang SJ, Hornig G, Kalbacher H, Bayer AS, Kraus D, Peschel A. 2009. The bacterial defensin resistance protein MprF consists of separable domains for lipid lysinylation and antimicrobial peptide repulsion. *PLoS Pathog* **5:**e1000660. doi:10.1371/journal.ppat.1000660.

86. Staubitz P, Neumann H, Schneider T, Wiedemann I, Peschel A. 2004. MprF-mediated biosynthesis of lysylphosphatidylglycerol, an important determinant in staphylococcal defensin resistance. *FEMS Microbiol Lett* **231:**67–71.

87. Nishi H, Komatsuzawa H, Fujiwara T, McCallum N, Sugai M. 2004. Reduced content of lysyl-phosphatidylglycerol in the cytoplasmic membrane affects susceptibility to moenomycin, as well as vancomycin, gentamicin, and antimicrobial peptides, in *Staphylococcus aureus*. *Antimicrob Agents Chemother* **48:**4800–4807.

88. Izadpanah A, Gallo RL. 2005. Antimicrobial peptides. *J Am Acad Dermatol* **52:**381–390; quiz 391–392.

89. Nawrocki KL, Crispell EK, McBride SM. 2014. Antimicrobial peptide resistance mechanisms of Gram-positive bacteria. *Antibiotics* **3:**461–492.

90. Roy H, Ibba M. 2008. RNA-dependent lipid remodeling by bacterial multiple peptide resistance factors. *Proc Natl Acad Sci USA* **105:**4667–4672.

91. Maloney E, Stankowska D, Zhang J, Fol M, Cheng QJ, Lun S, Bishai WR, Rajagopalan M, Chatterjee D, Madiraju MV. 2009. The two-domain LysX protein of *Mycobacterium tuberculosis* is required for production of lysinylated phosphatidylglycerol and resistance to cationic antimicrobial peptides. *PLoS Pathog* **5:**e1000534. doi:10.1371/journal.ppat.1000534.

92. Maloney E, Lun S, Stankowska D, Guo H, Rajagoapalan M, Bishai WR, Madiraju MV. 2011. Alterations in phospholipid catabolism in *Mycobacterium tuberculosis lysX* mutant. *Front Microbiol* **2:**19.

93. Thedieck K, Hain T, Mohamed W, Tindall BJ, Nimtz M, Chakraborty T, Wehland J,

Jansch L. 2006. The MprF protein is required for lysinylation of phospholipids in listerial membranes and confers resistance to cationic antimicrobial peptides (CAMPs) on *Listeria monocytogenes*. *Mol Microbiol* **62**:1325–1339.

94. **Klein S, Lorenzo C, Hoffmann S, Walther JM, Storbeck S, Piekarski T, Tindall BJ, Wray V, Nimtz M, Moser J.** 2009. Adaptation of *Pseudomonas aeruginosa* to various conditions includes tRNA-dependent formation of alanyl-phosphatidylglycerol. *Mol Microbiol* **71:** 551–565.

95. **Samant S, Hsu FF, Neyfakh AA, Lee H.** 2009. The *Bacillus anthracis* protein MprF is required for synthesis of lysylphosphatidylglycerols and for resistance to cationic antimicrobial peptides. *J Bacteriol* **191**:1311–1319.

96. **Hamilton A, Popham DL, Carl DJ, Lauth X, Nizet V, Jones AL.** 2006. Penicillin-binding protein 1a promotes resistance of group B *Streptococcus* to antimicrobial peptides. *Infect Immun* **74**:6179–6187.

97. **West NP, Jungnitz H, Fitter JT, McArthur JD, Guzman CA, Walker MJ.** 2000. Role of phosphoglucomutase of *Bordetella bronchiseptica* in lipopolysaccharide biosynthesis and virulence. *Infect Immun* **68**:4673–4680.

98. **Buchanan JT, Stannard JA, Lauth X, Ostland VE, Powell HC, Westerman ME, Nizet V.** 2005. *Streptococcus iniae* phosphoglucomutase is a virulence factor and a target for vaccine development. *Infect Immun* **73**:6935–6944.

99. **Gao LY, Laval F, Lawson EH, Groger RK, Woodruff A, Morisaki JH, Cox JS, Daffe M, Brown EJ.** 2003. Requirement for *kasB* in *Mycobacterium* mycolic acid biosynthesis, cell wall impermeability and intracellular survival: implications for therapy. *Mol Microbiol* **49:** 1547–1563.

100. **Gunn JS, Ryan SS, Van Velkinburgh JC, Ernst RK, Miller SI.** 2000. Genetic and functional analysis of a PmrA-PmrB-regulated locus necessary for lipopolysaccharide modification, antimicrobial peptide resistance, and oral virulence of *Salmonella enterica* serovar Typhimurium. *Infect Immun* **68**:6139–6146.

101. **Tamayo R, Choudhury B, Septer A, Merighi M, Carlson R, Gunn JS.** 2005. Identification of *cptA*, a PmrA-regulated locus required for phosphoethanolamine modification of the *Salmonella enterica* serovar Typhimurium lipopolysaccharide core. *J Bacteriol* **187**:3391–3399.

102. **Gunn JS.** 2001. Bacterial modification of LPS and resistance to antimicrobial peptides. *J Endotoxin Res* **7**:57–62.

103. **McCoy AJ, Liu H, Falla TJ, Gunn JS.** 2001. Identification of *Proteus mirabilis* mutants with increased sensitivity to antimicrobial peptides. *Antimicrob Agents Chemother* **45:** 2030–2037.

104. **Marceau M, Sebbane F, Collyn F, Simonet M.** 2003. Function and regulation of the *Salmonella*-like *pmrF* antimicrobial peptide resistance operon in *Yersinia pseudotuberculosis*. *Adv Exp Med Biol* **529**:253–256.

105. **Cheng HY, Chen YF, Peng HL.** 2010. Molecular characterization of the PhoPQ-PmrD-PmrAB mediated pathway regulating polymyxin B resistance in *Klebsiella pneumoniae* CG43. *J Biomed Sci* **17**:60.

106. **Moskowitz SM, Ernst RK, Miller SI.** 2004. PmrAB, a two-component regulatory system of *Pseudomonas aeruginosa* that modulates resistance to cationic antimicrobial peptides and addition of aminoarabinose to lipid A. *J Bacteriol* **186**:575–579.

107. **Ernst RK, Yi EC, Guo L, Lim KB, Burns JL, Hackett M, Miller SI.** 1999. Specific lipopolysaccharide found in cystic fibrosis airway *Pseudomonas aeruginosa*. *Science* **286**:1561–1565.

108. **Tran AX, Whittimore JD, Wyrick PB, McGrath SC, Cotter RJ, Trent MS.** 2006. The lipid A 1-phosphatase of *Helicobacter pylori* is required for resistance to the antimicrobial peptide polymyxin. *J Bacteriol* **188**:4531–4541.

109. **Cullen TW, Giles DK, Wolf LN, Ecobichon C, Boneca IG, Trent MS.** 2011. *Helicobacter pylori* versus the host: remodeling of the bacterial outer membrane is required for survival in the gastric mucosa. *PLoS Pathog* **7**:e1002454. doi:10.1371/journal.ppat.1002454.

110. **Lewis LA, Choudhury B, Balthazar JT, Martin LE, Ram S, Rice PA, Stephens DS, Carlson R, Shafer WM.** 2009. Phosphoethanolamine substitution of lipid A and resistance of *Neisseria gonorrhoeae* to cationic antimicrobial peptides and complement-mediated killing by normal human serum. *Infect Immun* **77**:1112–1120.

111. **Tzeng YL, Ambrose KD, Zughaier S, Zhou X, Miller YK, Shafer WM, Stephens DS.** 2005. Cationic antimicrobial peptide resistance in *Neisseria meningitidis*. *J Bacteriol* **187**:5387–5396.

112. **Albiger B, Johansson L, Jonsson AB.** 2003. Lipooligosaccharide-deficient *Neisseria meningitidis* shows altered pilus-associated characteristics. *Infect Immun* **71**:155–162.

113. **Jones A, Georg M, Maudsdotter L, Jonsson AB.** 2009. Endotoxin, capsule, and bacterial attachment contribute to *Neisseria meningitidis* resistance to the human antimicrobial peptide LL-37. *J Bacteriol* **191**:3861–3868.

114. **Keo T, Collins J, Kunwar P, Blaser MJ, Iovine NM.** 2011. *Campylobacter* capsule and

lipooligosaccharide confer resistance to serum and cationic antimicrobials. *Virulence* **2**:30–40.

115. **Naito M, Frirdich E, Fields JA, Pryjma M, Li J, Cameron A, Gilbert M, Thompson SA, Gaynor EC.** 2010. Effects of sequential *Campylobacter jejuni* 81-176 lipooligosaccharide core truncations on biofilm formation, stress survival, and pathogenesis. *J Bacteriol* **192**:2182–2192.

116. **Bishop RE, Gibbons HS, Guina T, Trent MS, Miller SI, Raetz CR.** 2000. Transfer of palmitate from phospholipids to lipid A in outer membranes of Gram-negative bacteria. *EMBO J* **19**:5071–5080.

117. **Robey M, O'Connell W, Cianciotto NP.** 2001. Identification of *Legionella pneumophilarcp*, a *pagP*-like gene that confers resistance to cationic antimicrobial peptides and promotes intracellular infection. *Infect Immun* **69**:4276–4286.

118. **Starner TD, Swords WE, Apicella MA, McCray PB Jr.** 2002. Susceptibility of nontypeable *Haemophilus influenzae* to human beta-defensins is influenced by lipooligosaccharide acylation. *Infect Immun* **70**:5287–5289.

119. **Lysenko ES, Gould J, Bals R, Wilson JM, Weiser JN.** 2000. Bacterial phosphorylcholine decreases susceptibility to the antimicrobial peptide LL-37/hCAP18 expressed in the upper respiratory tract. *Infect Immun* **68**:1664–1671.

120. **Clements A, Tull D, Jenney AW, Farn JL, Kim SH, Bishop RE, McPhee JB, Hancock RE, Hartland EL, Pearse MJ, Wijburg OL, Jackson DC, McConville MJ, Strugnell RA.** 2007. Secondary acylation of *Klebsiella pneumoniae* lipopolysaccharide contributes to sensitivity to antibacterial peptides. *J Biol Chem* **282**:15569–15577.

121. **Matson JS, Yoo HJ, Hakansson K, Dirita VJ.** 2010. Polymyxin B resistance in El Tor *Vibrio cholerae* requires lipid acylation catalyzed by MsbB. *J Bacteriol* **192**:2044–2052.

122. **Braff MH, Jones AL, Skerrett SJ, Rubens CE.** 2007. *Staphylococcus aureus* exploits cathelicidin antimicrobial peptides produced during early pneumonia to promote staphylokinase-dependent fibrinolysis. *J Infect Dis* **195**:1365–1372.

123. **Jin T, Bokarewa M, Foster T, Mitchell J, Higgins J, Tarkowski A.** 2004. *Staphylococcus aureus* resists human defensins by production of staphylokinase, a novel bacterial evasion mechanism. *J Immunol* **172**:1169–1176.

124. **Frick IM, Akesson P, Rasmussen M, Schmidtchen A, Bjorck L.** 2003. SIC, a secreted protein of *Streptococcus pyogenes* that inactivates antibacterial peptides. *J Biol Chem* **278**:16561–16566.

125. **Pence MA, Rooijakkers SH, Cogen AL, Cole JN, Hollands A, Gallo RL, Nizet V.** 2010. Streptococcal inhibitor of complement promotes innate immune resistance phenotypes of invasive M1T1 group A *Streptococcus. J Innate Immun* **2**:587–595.

126. **Fernie-King BA, Seilly DJ, Davies A, Lachmann PJ.** 2002. Streptococcal inhibitor of complement inhibits two additional components of the mucosal innate immune system: secretory leukocyte proteinase inhibitor and lysozyme. *Infect Immun* **70**:4908–4916.

127. **Walker MJ, Barnett TC, McArthur JD, Cole JN, Gillen CM, Henningham A, Sriprakash KS, Sanderson-Smith ML, Nizet V.** 2014. Disease manifestations and pathogenic mechanisms of group A *Streptococcus. Clin Microbiol Rev* **27**:264–301.

128. **Cole JN, Barnett TC, Nizet V, Walker MJ.** 2011. Molecular insight into invasive group A streptococcal disease. *Nat Rev Microbiol* **9**:724–736.

129. **Steer AC, Law I, Matatolu L, Beall BW, Carapetis JR.** 2009. Global *emm* type distribution of group A streptococci: systematic review and implications for vaccine development. *Lancet Infect Dis* **9**:611–616.

130. **Lauth X, von Kockritz-Blickwede M, McNamara CW, Myskowski S, Zinkernagel AS, Beall B, Ghosh P, Gallo RL, Nizet V.** 2009. M1 protein allows group A streptococcal survival in phagocyte extracellular traps through cathelicidin inhibition. *J Innate Immun* **1**:202–214.

131. **Jones AL, Mertz RH, Carl DJ, Rubens CE.** 2007. A streptococcal penicillin-binding protein is critical for resisting innate airway defenses in the neonatal lung. *J Immunol* **179**:3196–3202.

132. **Maisey HC, Quach D, Hensler ME, Liu GY, Gallo RL, Nizet V, Doran KS.** 2008. A group B streptococcal pilus protein promotes phagocyte resistance and systemic virulence. *FASEB J* **22**:1715–1724.

133. **Lancefield RC.** 1928. The antigenic complex of *Streptococcus haemolyticus*. I. Demonstration of a type-specific substance in extracts of *Streptococcus haemolyticus. J Exp Med* **47**:91–103.

134. **McCarty M.** 1952. The lysis of group A hemolytic streptococci by extracellular enzymes of *Streptomyces albus*. II. Nature of the cellular substrate attacked by the lytic enzymes. *J Exp Med* **96**:569–580.

135. **van Sorge NM, Cole JN, Kuipers K, Henningham A, Aziz RK, Kasirer-Friede A, Lin L, Berends ET, Davies MR, Dougan G, Zhang F, Dahesh S, Shaw L, Gin J, Cunningham M, Merriman JA, Hutter J, Lepenies B, Rooijakkers SH, Malley R, Walker**

MJ, Shattil SJ, Schlievert PM, Choudhury B, Nizet V. 2014. The classical lancefield antigen of group A *Streptococcus* is a virulence determinant with implications for vaccine design. *Cell Host Microbe* **15**:729–740.

136. Schmidtchen A, Frick IM, Bjorck L. 2001. Dermatan sulphate is released by proteinases of common pathogenic bacteria and inactivates antibacterial alpha-defensin. *Mol Microbiol* **39**:708–713.

137. Park PW, Pier GB, Preston MJ, Goldberger O, Fitzgerald ML, Bernfield M. 2000. Syndecan-1 shedding is enhanced by LasA, a secreted virulence factor of *Pseudomonas aeruginosa*. *J Biol Chem* **275**:3057–3064.

138. Heilmann C, Schweitzer O, Gerke C, Vanittanakom N, Mack D, Gotz F. 1996. Molecular basis of intercellular adhesion in the biofilm-forming *Staphylococcus epidermidis*. *Mol Microbiol* **20**:1083–1091.

139. Vuong C, Kocianova S, Voyich JM, Yao Y, Fischer ER, DeLeo FR, Otto M. 2004. A crucial role for exopolysaccharide modification in bacterial biofilm formation, immune evasion, and virulence. *J Biol Chem* **279**:54881–54886.

140. Vuong C, Voyich JM, Fischer ER, Braughton KR, Whitney AR, DeLeo FR, Otto M. 2004. Polysaccharide intercellular adhesin (PIA) protects *Staphylococcus epidermidis* against major components of the human innate immune system. *Cell Microbiol* **6**:269–275.

141. Kocianova S, Vuong C, Yao Y, Voyich JM, Fischer ER, DeLeo FR, Otto M. 2005. Key role of poly-gamma-DL-glutamic acid in immune evasion and virulence of *Staphylococcus epidermidis*. *J Clin Invest* **115**:688–694.

142. Cole JN, Pence MA, von Kockritz-Blickwede M, Hollands A, Gallo RL, Walker MJ, Nizet V. 2010. M protein and hyaluronic acid capsule are essential for *in vivo* selection of *covRS* mutations characteristic of invasive serotype M1T1 group A *Streptococcus*. *mBio* **1**:e00191-10. doi:10.1128/mBio.00191-10.

143. Campos MA, Vargas MA, Regueiro V, Llompart CM, Alberti S, Bengoechea JA. 2004. Capsule polysaccharide mediates bacterial resistance to antimicrobial peptides. *Infect Immun* **72**:7107–7114.

144. Moranta D, Regueiro V, March C, Llobet E, Margareto J, Larrarte E, Garmendia J, Bengoechea JA. 2010. *Klebsiella pneumoniae* capsule polysaccharide impedes the expression of beta-defensins by airway epithelial cells. *Infect Immun* **78**:1135–1146.

145. Llobet E, Tomas JM, Bengoechea JA. 2008. Capsule polysaccharide is a bacterial decoy for antimicrobial peptides. *Microbiology* **154**:3877–3886.

146. Spinosa MR, Progida C, Tala A, Cogli L, Alifano P, Bucci C. 2007. The *Neisseria meningitidis* capsule is important for intracellular survival in human cells. *Infect Immun* **75**:3594–3603.

147. Chan C, Burrows LL, Deber CM. 2004. Helix induction in antimicrobial peptides by alginate in biofilms. *J Biol Chem* **279**:38749–38754.

148. Piddock LJ. 2006. Multidrug-resistance efflux pumps: not just for resistance. *Nat Rev Microbiol* **4**:629–636.

149. Davidson AL, Dassa E, Orelle C, Chen J. 2008. Structure, function, and evolution of bacterial ATP-binding cassette systems. *Microbiol Mol Biol Rev* **72**:317–364.

150. Stein T, Heinzmann S, Solovieva I, Entian KD. 2003. Function of *Lactococcus lactis* nisin immunity genes *nisI* and *nisFEG* after coordinated expression in the surrogate host *Bacillus subtilis*. *J Biol Chem* **278**:89–94.

151. Stein T, Heinzmann S, Dusterhus S, Borchert S, Entian KD. 2005. Expression and functional analysis of the subtilin immunity genes *spaIFEG* in the subtilin-sensitive host *Bacillus subtilis* MO1099. *J Bacteriol* **187**:822–828.

152. Suarez JM, Edwards AN, McBride SM. 2013. The *Clostridium difficile cpr* locus is regulated by a noncontiguous two-component system in response to type A and B lantibiotics. *J Bacteriol* **195**:2621–2631.

153. McBride SM, Sonenshein AL. 2011. Identification of a genetic locus responsible for antimicrobial peptide resistance in *Clostridium difficile*. *Infect Immun* **79**:167–176.

154. Mascher T, Margulis NG, Wang T, Ye RW, Helmann JD. 2003. Cell wall stress responses in *Bacillus subtilis*: the regulatory network of the bacitracin stimulon. *Mol Microbiol* **50**:1591–1604.

155. Meehl M, Herbert S, Gotz F, Cheung A. 2007. Interaction of the GraRS two-component system with the VraFG ABC transporter to support vancomycin-intermediate resistance in *Staphylococcus aureus*. *Antimicrob Agents Chemother* **51**:2679–2689.

156. Kramer NE, van Hijum SA, Knol J, Kok J, Kuipers OP. 2006. Transcriptome analysis reveals mechanisms by which *Lactococcus lactis* acquires nisin resistance. *Antimicrob Agents Chemother* **50**:1753–1761.

157. Majchrzykiewicz JA, Kuipers OP, Bijlsma JJ. 2010. Generic and specific adaptive responses of *Streptococcus pneumoniae* to challenge with three distinct antimicrobial peptides, bacitracin, LL-37, and nisin. *Antimicrob Agents Chemother* **54**:440–451.

158. Mandin P, Fsihi H, Dussurget O, Vergassola M, Milohanic E, Toledo-Arana A, Lasa I, Johansson J, Cossart P. 2005. VirR, a response regulator critical for *Listeria monocytogenes* virulence. *Mol Microbiol* **57:**1367–1380.

159. Podlesek Z, Comino A, Herzog-Velikonja B, Zgur-Bertok D, Komel R, Grabnar M. 1995. *Bacillus licheniformis* bacitracin-resistance ABC transporter: relationship to mammalian multidrug resistance. *Mol Microbiol* **16:**969–976.

160. Manson JM, Keis S, Smith JM, Cook GM. 2004. Acquired bacitracin resistance in *Enterococcus faecalis* is mediated by an ABC transporter and a novel regulatory protein, BcrR. *Antimicrob Agents Chemother* **48:**3743–3748.

161. Charlebois A, Jalbert LA, Harel J, Masson L, Archambault M. 2012. Characterization of genes encoding for acquired bacitracin resistance in *Clostridium perfringens*. *PLoS One* **7:**e44449. doi:10.1371/journal.pone.0044449.

162. Tsuda H, Yamashita Y, Shibata Y, Nakano Y, Koga T. 2002. Genes involved in bacitracin resistance in *Streptococcus mutans*. *Antimicrob Agents Chemother* **46:**3756–3764.

163. Bengoechea JA, Skurnik M. 2000. Temperature-regulated efflux pump/potassium antiporter system mediates resistance to cationic antimicrobial peptides in *Yersinia*. *Mol Microbiol* **37:**67–80.

164. Padilla E, Llobet E, Domenech-Sanchez A, Martinez-Martinez L, Bengoechea JA, Alberti S. 2010. *Klebsiella pneumoniae* AcrAB efflux pump contributes to antimicrobial resistance and virulence. *Antimicrob Agents Chemother* **54:**177–183.

165. Zahner D, Zhou X, Chancey ST, Pohl J, Shafer WM, Stephens DS. 2010. Human antimicrobial peptide LL-37 induces MefE/Mel-mediated macrolide resistance in *Streptococcus pneumoniae*. *Antimicrob Agents Chemother* **54:**3516–3519.

166. Chen YC, Chuang YC, Chang CC, Jeang CL, Chang MC. 2004. A K$^+$ uptake protein, TrkA, is required for serum, protamine, and polymyxin B resistance in *Vibrio vulnificus*. *Infect Immun* **72:**629–636.

167. Parra-Lopez C, Lin R, Aspedon A, Groisman EA. 1994. A *Salmonella* protein that is required for resistance to antimicrobial peptides and transport of potassium. *EMBO J* **13:**3964–3972.

168. Shafer WM, Qu X, Waring AJ, Lehrer RI. 1998. Modulation of *Neisseria gonorrhoeae* susceptibility to vertebrate antibacterial peptides due to a member of the resistance/nodulation/division efflux pump family. *Proc Natl Acad Sci USA* **95:**1829–1833.

169. Veal WL, Nicholas RA, Shafer WM. 2002. Overexpression of the MtrC-MtrD-MtrE efflux pump due to an *mtrR* mutation is required for chromosomally mediated penicillin resistance in *Neisseria gonorrhoeae*. *J Bacteriol* **184:**5619–5624.

170. Jerse AE, Sharma ND, Simms AN, Crow ET, Snyder LA, Shafer WM. 2003. A gonococcal efflux pump system enhances bacterial survival in a female mouse model of genital tract infection. *Infect Immun* **71:**5576–5582.

171. Rinker SD, Trombley MP, Gu X, Fortney KR, Bauer ME. 2011. Deletion of *mtrC* in *Haemophilus ducreyi* increases sensitivity to human antimicrobial peptides and activates the CpxRA regulon. *Infect Immun* **79:**2324–2334.

172. Mason KM, Munson RS Jr, Bakaletz LO. 2005. A mutation in the *sap* operon attenuates survival of nontypeable *Haemophilus influenzae* in a chinchilla model of otitis media. *Infect Immun* **73:**599–608.

173. Parra-Lopez C, Baer MT, Groisman EA. 1993. Molecular genetic analysis of a locus required for resistance to antimicrobial peptides in *Salmonella typhimurium*. *EMBO J* **12:**4053–4062.

174. Mount KL, Townsend CA, Rinker SD, Gu X, Fortney KR, Zwickl BW, Janowicz DM, Spinola SM, Katz BP, Bauer ME. 2010. *Haemophilus ducreyi* SapA contributes to cathelicidin resistance and virulence in humans. *Infect Immun* **78:**1176–1184.

175. Eswarappa SM, Panguluri KK, Hensel M, Chakravortty D. 2008. The *yejABEF* operon of *Salmonella* confers resistance to antimicrobial peptides and contributes to its virulence. *Microbiology* **154:**666–678.

176. Saidijam M, Benedetti G, Ren Q, Xu Z, Hoyle CJ, Palmer SL, Ward A, Bettaney KE, Szakonyi G, Meuller J, Morrison S, Pos MK, Butaye P, Walravens K, Langton K, Herbert RB, Skurray RA, Paulsen IT, O'Reilly J, Rutherford NG, Brown MH, Bill RM, Henderson PJ. 2006. Microbial drug efflux proteins of the major facilitator superfamily. *Curr Drug Targets* **7:**793–811.

177. Kupferwasser LI, Skurray RA, Brown MH, Firth N, Yeaman MR, Bayer AS. 1999. Plasmid-mediated resistance to thrombin-induced platelet microbicidal protein in staphylococci: role of the *qacA* locus. *Antimicrob Agents Chemother* **43:**2395–2399.

178. Bayer AS, Kupferwasser LI, Brown MH, Skurray RA, Grkovic S, Jones T, Mukhopadhay K, Yeaman MR. 2006. Low-level resistance of *Staphylococcus aureus* to thrombin-induced platelet microbicidal protein 1 *in vitro* associated with *qacA* gene carriage is independent of

multidrug efflux pump activity. *Antimicrob Agents Chemother* **50:**2448–2454.

179. **Bayer AS, Cheng D, Yeaman MR, Corey GR, McClelland RS, Harrel LJ, Fowler VG Jr.** 1998. *In vitro* resistance to thrombin-induced platelet microbicidal protein among clinical bacteremic isolates of *Staphylococcus aureus* correlates with an endovascular infectious source. *Antimicrob Agents Chemother* **42:** 3169–3172.

180. **Shinnar AE, Butler KL, Park HJ.** 2003. Cathelicidin family of antimicrobial peptides: proteolytic processing and protease resistance. *Bioorg Chem* **31:**425–436.

181. **Schmidtchen A, Frick IM, Andersson E, Tapper H, Bjorck L.** 2002. Proteinases of common pathogenic bacteria degrade and inactivate the antibacterial peptide LL-37. *Mol Microbiol* **46:**157–168.

182. **Johansson L, Thulin P, Sendi P, Hertzen E, Linder A, Akesson P, Low DE, Agerberth B, Norrby-Teglund A.** 2008. Cathelicidin LL-37 in severe *Streptococcus pyogenes* soft tissue infections in humans. *Infect Immun* **76:**3399–3404.

183. **Sieprawska-Lupa M, Mydel P, Krawczyk K, Wojcik K, Puklo M, Lupa B, Suder P, Silberring J, Reed M, Pohl J, Shafer W, McAleese F, Foster T, Travis J, Potempa J.** 2004. Degradation of human antimicrobial peptide LL-37 by *Staphylococcus aureus*-derived proteinases. *Antimicrob Agents Chemother* **48:**4673–4679.

184. **Belas R, Manos J, Suvanasuthi R.** 2004. *Proteus mirabilis* ZapA metalloprotease degrades a broad spectrum of substrates, including antimicrobial peptides. *Infect Immun* **72:** 5159–5167.

185. **Kubica M, Guzik K, Koziel J, Zarebski M, Richter W, Gajkowska B, Golda A, Maciag-Gudowska A, Brix K, Shaw L, Foster T, Potempa J.** 2008. A potential new pathway for *Staphylococcus aureus* dissemination: the silent survival of *S. aureus* phagocytosed by human monocyte-derived macrophages. *PLoS One* **3:**e1409. doi:10.1371/journal.pone.0001409.

186. **Nyberg P, Rasmussen M, Bjorck L.** 2004. alpha2-Macroglobulin-proteinase complexes protect *Streptococcus pyogenes* from killing by the antimicrobial peptide LL-37. *J Biol Chem* **279:**52820–52823.

187. **Rasmussen M, Muller HP, Bjorck L.** 1999. Protein GRAB of *Streptococcus pyogenes* regulates proteolysis at the bacterial surface by binding alpha2-macroglobulin. *J Biol Chem* **274:**15336–15344.

188. **Guina T, Yi EC, Wang H, Hackett M, Miller SI.** 2000. A PhoP-regulated outer membrane protease of *Salmonella enterica* serovar Typhimurium promotes resistance to alpha-helical antimicrobial peptides. *J Bacteriol* **182:**4077–4086.

189. **Ly D, Taylor JM, Tsatsaronis JA, Monteleone MM, Skora AS, Donald CA, Maddocks T, Nizet V, West NP, Ranson M, Walker MJ, McArthur JD, Sanderson-Smith ML.** 2014. Plasmin(ogen) acquisition by group A *Streptococcus* protects against C3b-mediated neutrophil killing. *J Innate Immun* **6:**240–250.

190. **Kooi C, Sokol PA.** 2009. *Burkholderia cenocepacia* zinc metalloproteases influence resistance to antimicrobial peptides. *Microbiology* **155:**2818–2825.

191. **Thomassin JL, Brannon JR, Gibbs BF, Gruenheid S, Le Moual H.** 2012. OmpT outer membrane proteases of enterohemorrhagic and enteropathogenic *Escherichia coli* contribute differently to the degradation of human LL-37. *Infect Immun* **80:**483–492.

192. **Ulvatne H, Haukland HH, Samuelsen O, Kramer M, Vorland LH.** 2002. Proteases in *Escherichia coli* and *Staphylococcus aureus* confer reduced susceptibility to lactoferricin B. *J Antimicrob Chemother* **50:**461–467.

193. **Devine DA, Marsh PD, Percival RS, Rangarajan M, Curtis MA.** 1999. Modulation of antibacterial peptide activity by products of *Porphyromonas gingivalis* and *Prevotella* spp. *Microbiology* **145:**965–971.

194. **Carlisle MD, Srikantha RN, Brogden KA.** 2009. Degradation of human alpha- and beta-defensins by culture supernatants of *Porphyromonas gingivalis* strain 381. *J Innate Immun* **1:**118–122.

195. **Bachrach G, Altman H, Kolenbrander PE, Chalmers NI, Gabai-Gutner M, Mor A, Friedman M, Steinberg D.** 2008. Resistance of *Porphyromonas gingivalis* ATCC 33277 to direct killing by antimicrobial peptides is protease independent. *Antimicrob Agents Chemother* **52:**638–642.

196. **Thwaite JE, Hibbs S, Titball RW, Atkins TP.** 2006. Proteolytic degradation of human antimicrobial peptide LL-37 by *Bacillus anthracis* may contribute to virulence. *Antimicrob Agents Chemother* **50:**2316–2322.

197. **Chamnongpol S, Cromie M, Groisman EA.** 2003. Mg^{2+} sensing by the Mg^{2+} sensor PhoQ of *Salmonella enterica*. *J Mol Biol* **325:**795–807.

198. **Guo L, Lim KB, Gunn JS, Bainbridge B, Darveau RP, Hackett M, Miller SI.** 1997. Regulation of lipid A modifications by *Salmonella* Typhimurium virulence genes phoP-phoQ. *Science* **276:**250–253.

199. **Ernst RK, Guina T, Miller SI.** 1999. How intracellular bacteria survive: surface modifications that promote resistance to host innate immune responses. *J Infect Dis* **179**(Suppl 2): S326–S330.

200. **Ernst RK, Guina T, Miller SI.** 2001. *Salmonella* Typhimurium outer membrane remodeling: role in resistance to host innate immunity. *Microbes Infect* **3:**1327–1334.

201. **Garcia Vescovi E, Soncini FC, Groisman EA.** 1994. The role of the PhoP/PhoQ regulon in *Salmonella* virulence. *Res Microbiol* **145:**473–480.

202. **Detweiler CS, Monack DM, Brodsky IE, Mathew H, Falkow S.** 2003. *virK, somA* and *rcsC* are important for systemic *Salmonella enterica* serovar Typhimurium infection and cationic peptide resistance. *Mol Microbiol* **48:** 385–400.

203. **Prost LR, Daley ME, Bader MW, Klevit RE, Miller SI.** 2008. The PhoQ histidine kinases of *Salmonella* and *Pseudomonas* spp. are structurally and functionally different: evidence that pH and antimicrobial peptide sensing contribute to mammalian pathogenesis. *Mol Microbiol* **69:**503–519.

204. **O'Loughlin JL, Spinner JL, Minnich SA, Kobayashi SD.** 2010. *Yersinia pestis* two-component gene regulatory systems promote survival in human neutrophils. *Infect Immun* **78:**773–782.

205. **Macfarlane EL, Kwasnicka A, Hancock RE.** 2000. Role of *Pseudomonas aeruginosa* PhoP-phoQ in resistance to antimicrobial cationic peptides and aminoglycosides. *Microbiology* **146:**2543–2554.

206. **McPhee JB, Lewenza S, Hancock RE.** 2003. Cationic antimicrobial peptides activate a two-component regulatory system, PmrA-PmrB, that regulates resistance to polymyxin B and cationic antimicrobial peptides in *Pseudomonas aeruginosa*. *Mol Microbiol* **50:**205–217.

207. **McPhee JB, Bains M, Winsor G, Lewenza S, Kwasnicka A, Brazas MD, Brinkman FS, Hancock RE.** 2006. Contribution of the PhoP-PhoQ and PmrA-PmrB two-component regulatory systems to Mg^{2+}-induced gene regulation in *Pseudomonas aeruginosa*. *J Bacteriol* **188:**3995–4006.

208. **Amulic B, Cazalet C, Hayes GL, Metzler KD, Zychlinsky A.** 2012. Neutrophil function: from mechanisms to disease. *Annu Rev Immunol* **30:**459–489.

209. **von Kockritz-Blickwede M, Nizet V.** 2009. Innate immunity turned inside-out: antimicrobial defense by phagocyte extracellular traps. *J Mol Med* **87:**775–783.

210. **Buchanan JT, Simpson AJ, Aziz RK, Liu GY, Kristian SA, Kotb M, Feramisco J, Nizet V.** 2006. DNase expression allows the pathogen group A *Streptococcus* to escape killing in neutrophil extracellular traps. *Curr Biol* **16:** 396–400.

211. **Sumby P, Barbian KD, Gardner DJ, Whitney AR, Welty DM, Long RD, Bailey JR, Parnell MJ, Hoe NP, Adams GG, Deleo FR, Musser JM.** 2005. Extracellular deoxyribonuclease made by group A *Streptococcus* assists pathogenesis by enhancing evasion of the innate immune response. *Proc Natl Acad Sci USA* **102:** 1679–1684.

212. **Walker MJ, Hollands A, Sanderson-Smith ML, Cole JN, Kirk JK, Henningham A, McArthur JD, Dinkla K, Aziz RK, Kansal RG, Simpson AJ, Buchanan JT, Chhatwal GS, Kotb M, Nizet V.** 2007. DNase Sda1 provides selection pressure for a switch to invasive group A streptococcal infection. *Nat Med* **13:**981–985.

213. **Beiter K, Wartha F, Albiger B, Normark S, Zychlinsky A, Henriques-Normark B.** 2006. An endonuclease allows *Streptococcus pneumoniae* to escape from neutrophil extracellular traps. *Curr Biol* **16:**401–407.

214. **Derre-Bobillot A, Cortes-Perez NG, Yamamoto Y, Kharrat P, Couve E, Da Cunha V, Decker P, Boissier MC, Escartin F, Cesselin B, Langella P, Bermudez-Humaran LG, Gaudu P.** 2013. Nuclease A (Gbs0661), an extracellular nuclease of *Streptococcus agalactiae*, attacks the neutrophil extracellular traps and is needed for full virulence. *Mol Microbiol* **89:**518–531.

215. **Berends ET, Horswill AR, Haste NM, Monestier M, Nizet V, von Kockritz-Blickwede M.** 2010. Nuclease expression by *Staphylococcus aureus* facilitates escape from neutrophil extracellular traps. *J Innate Immun* **2:**576–586.

216. **Mulcahy H, Charron-Mazenod L, Lewenza S.** 2008. Extracellular DNA chelates cations and induces antibiotic resistance in *Pseudomonas aeruginosa* biofilms. *PLoS Pathog* **4:** e1000213. doi:10.1371/journal.ppat.1000213.

217. **Johnson L, Horsman SR, Charron-Mazenod L, Turnbull AL, Mulcahy H, Surette MG, Lewenza S.** 2013. Extracellular DNA-induced antimicrobial peptide resistance in *Salmonella enterica* serovar Typhimurium. *BMC Microbiol* **13:**115.

218. **Shireen T, Singh M, Das T, Mukhopadhyay K.** 2013. Differential adaptive responses of *Staphylococcus aureus* to *in vitro* selection with different antimicrobial peptides. *Antimicrob Agents Chemother* **57:**5134–5137.

219. **Bayer AS, Prasad R, Chandra J, Koul A, Smriti M, Varma A, Skurray RA, Firth N, Brown MH,**

Koo SP, Yeaman MR. 2000. *In vitro* resistance of *Staphylococcus aureus* to thrombin-induced platelet microbicidal protein is associated with alterations in cytoplasmic membrane fluidity. *Infect Immun* **68:**3548–3553.

220. **Mishra NN, Liu GY, Yeaman MR, Nast CC, Proctor RA, McKinnell J, Bayer AS.** 2011. Carotenoid-related alteration of cell membrane fluidity impacts *Staphylococcus aureus* susceptibility to host defense peptides. *Antimicrob Agents Chemother* **55:**526–531.

221. **Subczynski WK, Wisniewska A.** 2000. Physical properties of lipid bilayer membranes: relevance to membrane biological functions. *Acta Biochim Pol* **47:**613–625.

222. **Verheul A, Russell NJ, Van THR, Rombouts FM, Abee T.** 1997. Modifications of membrane phospholipid composition in nisin-resistant *Listeria monocytogenes* Scott A. *Appl Environ Microbiol* **63:**3451–3457.

223. **Crandall AD, Montville TJ.** 1998. Nisin resistance in *Listeria monocytogenes* ATCC 700302 is a complex phenotype. *Appl Environ Microbiol* **64:**231–237.

224. **Lopez-Solanilla E, Gonzalez-Zorn B, Novella S, Vazquez-Boland JA, Rodriguez-Palenzuela P.** 2003. Susceptibility of *Listeria monocytogenes* to antimicrobial peptides. *FEMS Microbiol Lett* **226:**101–105.

225. **Islam D, Bandholtz L, Nilsson J, Wigzell H, Christensson B, Agerberth B, Gudmundsson G.** 2001. Downregulation of bactericidal peptides in enteric infections: a novel immune escape mechanism with bacterial DNA as a potential regulator. *Nat Med* **7:**180–185.

226. **Sperandio B, Regnault B, Guo J, Zhang Z, Stanley SL Jr, Sansonetti PJ, Pedron T.** 2008. Virulent *Shigella flexneri* subverts the host innate immune response through manipulation of antimicrobial peptide gene expression. *J Exp Med* **205:**1121–1132.

227. **Taggart CC, Greene CM, Smith SG, Levine RL, McCray PB Jr, O'Neill S, McElvaney NG.** 2003. Inactivation of human beta-defensins 2 and 3 by elastolytic cathepsins. *J Immunol* **171:**931–937.

228. **Chakraborty K, Ghosh S, Koley H, Mukhopadhyay AK, Ramamurthy T, Saha DR, Mukhopadhyay D, Roychowdhury S, Hamabata T, Takeda Y, Das S.** 2008. Bacterial exotoxins downregulate cathelicidin (hCAP-18/LL-37) and human beta-defensin 1 (HBD-1) expression in the intestinal epithelial cells. *Cell Microbiol* **10:**2520–2537.

229. **Gruenheid S, Le Moual H.** 2012. Resistance to antimicrobial peptides in Gram-negative bacteria. *FEMS Microbiol Lett* **330:**81–89.

230. **Loutet SA, Valvano MA.** 2011. Extreme antimicrobial peptide and polymyxin B resistance in the genus *Burkholderia*. *Front Microbiol* **2:**159.

231. **Cox AD, Wilkinson SG.** 1991. Ionizing groups in lipopolysaccharides of *Pseudomonas cepacia* in relation to antibiotic resistance. *Mol Microbiol* **5:**641–646.

232. **Loutet SA, Mussen LE, Flannagan RS, Valvano MA.** 2011. A two-tier model of polymyxin B resistance in *Burkholderia cenocepacia*. *Environ Microbiol Rep* **3:**278–285.

233. **Dhand A, Bayer AS, Pogliano J, Yang SJ, Bolaris M, Nizet V, Wang G, Sakoulas G.** 2011. Use of antistaphylococcal beta-lactams to increase daptomycin activity in eradicating persistent bacteremia due to methicillin-resistant *Staphylococcus aureus*: role of enhanced daptomycin binding. *Clin Infect Dis* **53:**158–163.

234. **Sakoulas G, Bayer AS, Pogliano J, Tsuji BT, Yang SJ, Mishra NN, Nizet V, Yeaman MR, Moise PA.** 2012. Ampicillin enhances daptomycin- and cationic host defense peptide-mediated killing of ampicillin- and vancomycin-resistant *Enterococcus faecium*. *Antimicrob Agents Chemother* **56:**838–844.

235. **Hancock RE, Sahl HG.** 2006. Antimicrobial and host-defense peptides as new anti-infective therapeutic strategies. *Nat Biotechnol* **24:**1551–1557.

236. **Wiesner J, Vilcinskas A.** 2010. Antimicrobial peptides: the ancient arm of the human immune system. *Virulence* **1:**440–464.

237. **Tavares LS, Silva CS, de Souza VC, da Silva VL, Diniz CG, Santos MO.** 2013. Strategies and molecular tools to fight antimicrobial resistance: resistome, transcriptome, and antimicrobial peptides. *Front Microbiol* **4:**412.

238. **Peschel A, Sahl HG.** 2006. The co-evolution of host cationic antimicrobial peptides and microbial resistance. *Nat Rev Microbiol* **4:**529–536.

239. **Habets MG, Brockhurst MA.** 2012. Therapeutic antimicrobial peptides may compromise natural immunity. *Biol Lett* **8:**416–418.

240. **Jung D, Rozek A, Okon M, Hancock RE.** 2004. Structural transitions as determinants of the action of the calcium-dependent antibiotic daptomycin. *Chem Biol* **11:**949–957.

241. **Mishra NN, McKinnell J, Yeaman MR, Rubio A, Nast CC, Chen L, Kreiswirth BN, Bayer AS.** 2011. *In vitro* cross-resistance to daptomycin and host defense cationic antimicrobial peptides in clinical methicillin-resistant *Staphylococcus aureus* isolates. *Antimicrob Agents Chemother* **55:**4012–4018.

242. Gravesen A, Jydegaard Axelsen AM, Mendes da Silva J, Hansen TB, Knochel S. 2002. Frequency of bacteriocin resistance development and associated fitness costs in *Listeria monocytogenes*. *Appl Environ Microbiol* 68: 756–764.

243. Gravesen A, Ramnath M, Rechinger KB, Andersen N, Jansch L, Hechard Y, Hastings JW, Knochel S. 2002. High-level resistance to class IIa bacteriocins is associated with one general mechanism in *Listeria monocytogenes*. *Microbiology* 148:2361–2369.

244. Menuet M, Bittar F, Stremler N, Dubus JC, Sarles J, Raoult D, Rolain JM. 2008. First isolation of two colistin-resistant emerging pathogens, *Brevundimonas diminuta* and *Ochrobactrum anthropi*, in a woman with cystic fibrosis: a case report. *J Med Case Rep* 2:373.

245. Antoniadou A, Kontopidou F, Poulakou G, Koratzanis E, Galani I, Papadomichelakis E, Kopterides P, Souli M, Armaganidis A, Giamarellou H. 2007. Colistin-resistant isolates of *Klebsiella pneumoniae* emerging in intensive care unit patients: first report of a multiclonal cluster. *J Antimicrob Chemother* 59:786–790.

246. Huddleston JR. 2014. Horizontal gene transfer in the human gastrointestinal tract: potential spread of antibiotic resistance genes. *Infect Drug Resist* 7:167–176.

247. Napier BA, Band V, Burd EM, Weiss DS. 2014. Colistin heteroresistance in *Enterobacter cloacae* is associated with cross-resistance to the host antimicrobial lysozyme. *Antimicrob Agents Chemother* 58:5594–5597.

248. Costa F, Carvalho IF, Montelaro RC, Gomes P, Martins MC. 2011. Covalent immobilization of antimicrobial peptides (AMPs) onto biomaterial surfaces. *Acta Biomater* 7:1431–1440.

249. Deslouches B, Steckbeck JD, Craigo JK, Doi Y, Mietzner TA, Montelaro RC. 2013. Rational design of engineered cationic antimicrobial peptides consisting exclusively of arginine and tryptophan, and their activity against multidrug-resistant pathogens. *Antimicrob Agents Chemother* 57:2511–2521.

250. Peyssonnaux C, Datta V, Cramer T, Doedens A, Theodorakis EA, Gallo RL, Hurtado-Ziola N, Nizet V, Johnson RS. 2005. HIF-1alpha expression regulates the bactericidal capacity of phagocytes. *J Clin Invest* 115:1806–1815.

251. Okumura CY, Hollands A, Tran DN, Olson J, Dahesh S, von Kockritz-Blickwede M, Thienphrapa W, Corle C, Jeung SN, Kotsakis A, Shalwitz RA, Johnson RS, Nizet V. 2012. A new pharmacological agent (AKB-4924) stabilizes hypoxia inducible factor-1 (HIF-1) and increases skin innate defenses against bacterial infection. *J Mol Med* 90:1079–1089.

252. Nizet V, Johnson RS. 2009. Interdependence of hypoxic and innate immune responses. *Nat Rev Immunol* 9:609–617.

253. Darveau RP, Blake J, Seachord CL, Cosand WL, Cunningham MD, Cassiano-Clough L, Maloney G. 1992. Peptides related to the carboxyl terminus of human platelet factor IV with antibacterial activity. *J Clin Invest* 90:447–455.

254. Peschel A, Vuong C, Otto M, Gotz F. 2000. The D-alanine residues of *Staphylococcus aureus* teichoic acids alter the susceptibility to vancomycin and the activity of autolytic enzymes. *Antimicrob Agents Chemother* 44: 2845–2847.

255. Abi Khattar Z, Rejasse A, Destoumieux-Garzon D, Escoubas JM, Sanchis V, Lereclus D, Givaudan A, Kallassy M, Nielsen-Leroux C, Gaudriault S. 2009. The *dlt* operon of *Bacillus cereus* is required for resistance to cationic antimicrobial peptides and for virulence in insects. *J Bacteriol* 191:7063–7073.

256. Cox KH, Ruiz-Bustos E, Courtney HS, Dale JB, Pence MA, Nizet V, Aziz RK, Gerling I, Price SM, Hasty DL. 2009. Inactivation of DltA modulates virulence factor expression in *Streptococcus pyogenes*. *PLoS One* 4:e5366. doi:10.1371/journal.pone.0005366.

257. Fisher N, Shetron-Rama L, Herring-Palmer A, Heffernan B, Bergman N, Hanna P. 2006. The *dltABCD* operon of *Bacillus anthracis* sterne is required for virulence and resistance to peptide, enzymatic, and cellular mediators of innate immunity. *J Bacteriol* 188:1301–1309.

258. Fittipaldi N, Sekizaki T, Takamatsu D, Harel J, Dominguez-Punaro Mde L, Von Aulock S, Draing C, Marois C, Kobisch M, Gottschalk M. 2008. D-alanylation of lipoteichoic acid contributes to the virulence of *Streptococcus suis*. *Infect Immun* 76:3587–3594.

259. Collins LV, Kristian SA, Weidenmaier C, Faigle M, Van Kessel KP, Van Strijp JA, Gotz F, Neumeister B, Peschel A. 2002. *Staphylococcus aureus* strains lacking D-alanine modifications of teichoic acids are highly susceptible to human neutrophil killing and are virulence attenuated in mice. *J Infect Dis* 186:214–219.

260. Cullen TW, Trent MS. 2010. A link between the assembly of flagella and lipooligosaccharide of the Gram-negative bacterium *Campylobacter jejuni*. *Proc Natl Acad Sci USA* 107: 5160–5165.

261. Pelz A, Wieland KP, Putzbach K, Hentschel P, Albert K, Gotz F. 2005. Structure and

biosynthesis of staphyloxanthin from *Staphylococcus aureus*. *J Biol Chem* **280:**32493–32498.

262. **Clauditz A, Resch A, Wieland KP, Peschel A, Gotz F.** 2006. Staphyloxanthin plays a role in the fitness of *Staphylococcus aureus* and its ability to cope with oxidative stress. *Infect Immun* **74:**4950–4953.

263. **Liu GY, Essex A, Buchanan JT, Datta V, Hoffman HM, Bastian JF, Fierer J, Nizet V.** 2005. *Staphylococcus aureus* golden pigment impairs neutrophil killing and promotes virulence through its antioxidant activity. *J Exp Med* **202:**209–215.

264. **Park PW, Pier GB, Hinkes MT, Bernfield M.** 2001. Exploitation of syndecan-1 shedding by *Pseudomonas aeruginosa* enhances virulence. *Nature* **411:**98–102.

265. **Diep DB, Havarstein LS, Nes IF.** 1996. Characterization of the locus responsible for the bacteriocin production in *Lactobacillus plantarum* C11. *J Bacteriol* **178:**4472–4483.

266. **Diep DB, Skaugen M, Salehian Z, Holo H, Nes IF.** 2007. Common mechanisms of target cell recognition and immunity for class II bacteriocins. *Proc Natl Acad Sci USA* **104:**2384–2389.

267. **Klein C, Entian KD.** 1994. Genes involved in self-protection against the lantibiotic subtilin produced by *Bacillus subtilis* ATCC 6633. *Appl Environ Microbiol* **60:**2793–2801.

268. **Kuipers OP, Beerthuyzen MM, Siezen RJ, De Vos WM.** 1993. Characterization of the nisin gene cluster *nisABTCIPR* of *Lactococcus lactis*. Requirement of expression of the *nisA* and *nisI* genes for development of immunity. *Eur J Biochem* **216:**281–291.

269. **Saris PE, Immonen T, Reis M, Sahl HG.** 1996. Immunity to lantibiotics. *Antonie Van Leeuwenhoek* **69:**151–159.

270. **Warner DM, Shafer WM, Jerse AE.** 2008. Clinically relevant mutations that cause derepression of the *Neisseria gonorrhoeae* MtrC-MtrD-MtrE Efflux pump system confer different levels of antimicrobial resistance and *in vivo* fitness. *Mol Microbiol* **70:**462–478.

271. **Kawada-Matsuo M, Yoshida Y, Zendo T, Nagao J, Oogai Y, Nakamura Y, Sonomoto K, Nakamura N, Komatsuzawa H.** 2013. Three distinct two-component systems are involved in resistance to the class I bacteriocins, Nukacin ISK-1 and nisin A, in *Staphylococcus aureus*. *PLoS One* **8:**e69455. doi:10.1371/journal.pone.0069455.

272. **Li M, Cha DJ, Lai Y, Villaruz AE, Sturdevant DE, Otto M.** 2007. The antimicrobial peptide-sensing system *aps* of *Staphylococcus aureus*. *Mol Microbiol* **66:**1136–1147.

273. **Hiron A, Falord M, Valle J, Debarbouille M, Msadek T.** 2011. Bacitracin and nisin resistance in *Staphylococcus aureus*: a novel pathway involving the BraS/BraR two-component system (SA2417/SA2418) and both the BraD/BraE and VraD/VraE ABC transporters. *Mol Microbiol* **81:**602–622.

274. **Falord M, Karimova G, Hiron A, Msadek T.** 2012. GraXSR proteins interact with the VraFG ABC transporter to form a five-component system required for cationic antimicrobial peptide sensing and resistance in *Staphylococcus aureus*. *Antimicrob Agents Chemother* **56:**1047–1058.

275. **Thurlow LR, Thomas VC, Narayanan S, Olson S, Fleming SD, Hancock LE.** 2010. Gelatinase contributes to the pathogenesis of endocarditis caused by *Enterococcus faecalis*. *Infect Immun* **78:**4936–4943.

276. **Sabat A, Kosowska K, Poulsen K, Kasprowicz A, Sekowska A, van Den Burg B, Travis J, Potempa J.** 2000. Two allelic forms of the aureolysin gene (*aur*) within *Staphylococcus aureus*. *Infect Immun* **68:**973–976.

277. **Lai Y, Villaruz AE, Li M, Cha DJ, Sturdevant DE, Otto M.** 2007. The human anionic antimicrobial peptide dermcidin induces proteolytic defence mechanisms in staphylococci. *Mol Microbiol* **63:**497–506.

278. **Cheung GY, Rigby K, Wang R, Queck SY, Braughton KR, Whitney AR, Teintze M, DeLeo FR, Otto M.** 2010. *Staphylococcus epidermidis* strategies to avoid killing by human neutrophils. *PLoS Pathog* **6:**e1001133. doi:10.1371/journal.ppat.1001133.

279. **Bergman P, Johansson L, Asp V, Plant L, Gudmundsson GH, Jonsson AB, Agerberth B.** 2005. *Neisseria gonorrhoeae* downregulates expression of the human antimicrobial peptide LL-37. *Cell Microbiol* **7:**1009–1017.

280. **Salzman NH, Chou MM, de Jong H, Liu L, Porter EM, Paterson Y.** 2003. Enteric *Salmonella* infection inhibits Paneth cell antimicrobial peptide expression. *Infect Immun* **71:**1109–1115.

281. **Yanagi S, Ashitani J, Imai K, Kyoraku Y, Sano A, Matsumoto N, Nakazato M.** 2007. Significance of human beta-defensins in the epithelial lining fluid of patients with chronic lower respiratory tract infections. *Clin Microbiol Infect* **13:**63–69.

282. **Dunman PM, Murphy E, Haney S, Palacios D, Tucker-Kellogg G, Wu S, Brown EL, Zagursky RJ, Shlaes D, Projan SJ.** 2001. Transcription profiling-based identification of *Staphylococcus aureus* genes regulated by the agr and/or sarA loci. *J Bacteriol* **183:**7341–7353.

16

Antigenic Variation in Bacterial Pathogens

GUY H. PALMER,[1] TROY BANKHEAD,[1] and H. STEVEN SEIFERT[2]

OVERVIEW

Ross and Thompson's 1910 report of periodic spikes of *Trypanosoma gambiense* parasitemia (1), made possible by the relatively large size of the parasite, which allowed quantitation using light microscopy, was seminal in understanding how pathogens persist and led to later studies defining how trypanosomes and numerous other pathogens use antigenic variation to evade host immunity and clearance. Antigenic variation is a strategy used by a broad diversity of microbial pathogens to persist within mammalian hosts, from small RNA viruses, notably the human immunodeficiency virus (HIV), to large eukaryotic parasites with multiple chromosomes, illustrated by trypanosomal and malarial parasites (2, 3). Using a variety of genetic mechanisms to generate antigenic variants, immune evasion results in the infected host serving as a microbial reservoir for subsequent transmission. Unlike respiratory and gastrointestinal pathogens that have essentially continual opportunities for transmission, arthropod vector-borne and sexually transmitted pathogens have episodic transmission opportunities.

[1]Department of Veterinary Microbiology and Pathology, Paul G. Allen School for Global Animal Health, Washington State University, Pullman, WA 99164; [2]Department of Microbiology-Immunology, Feinberg School of Medicine, Northwestern University, Chicago, IL 60611.
Virulence Mechanisms of Bacterial Pathogens, 5th edition
Edited by Indira T. Kudva, Nancy A. Cornick, Paul J. Plummer, Qijing Zhang, Tracy L. Nicholson, John P. Bannantine, and Bryan H. Bellaire
© 2016 American Society for Microbiology, Washington, DC
doi:10.1128/microbiolspec.VMBF-0005-2015

Correspondingly, both vector-borne and sexually transmitted agents are overrepresented among antigenically variant pathogens (3, 4).

Pathogens use a breadth of genetic mechanisms to generate antigenic variants (3, 4). The large progeny size and minimal proofreading capacity allow viruses to use random mutation to generate variants. In contrast, antigenically variant bacteria have evolved mechanisms using a stable genome that safeguards progeny fitness. In this chapter, we focus on three well-characterized, highly antigenically variant bacterial pathogens: *Anaplasma*, *Borrelia*, and *Neisseria*. Collectively, these pathogens represent a diversity of bacterial genetic mechanisms used to create variation, structural and antigenic changes required for in-host persistence, and escape phenotypes. While the focus is on intrahost antigenic variation, as opposed to the evolution of new strain variants at the population level, the potential for the same mechanisms used to allow escape from immunity within the individual to allow escape at the population level is also presented.

ANAPLASMA

Introduction

In the same year that Ross and Thompson reported the aforementioned observation of recurrent, episodic spikes in trypanosome parasitemia, Arnold Theiler (later Sir Arnold Theiler) published a monograph in which he described the microscopically detectable appearance, disappearance, and then reappearance of organisms "resembling to a certain extent, the bacteria" in the blood of infected cattle (5). Although 75 years would pass before molecular techniques would define the cyclic waves of bacteremia, Theiler clearly understood that the pathogen, which he termed *Anaplasma* for its lack of eosinophilic cytoplasm as observed in other tick-borne agents (which

at that time were predominantly protozoa), persisted in the host and served as a reservoir for onward transmission (6). In the past decade the availability of complete genome sequences has driven the discovery of the genetic mechanisms used to generate *Anaplasma marginale*, and later *Anaplasma ovis* and *Anaplasma phagocytophilum*, antigenic variants that escape immune detection and allow persistence. Although the occurrence of outer membrane structural variation resulting in immune evasion is common to numerous bacterial pathogens, study of *A. marginale* has uncovered two broadly applicable findings that will be the focus here. The first is the mechanism of segmental gene conversion to exponentially expand the capacity of a small, stable bacterial genome to generate thousands of outer membrane protein (OMP) variants. The second is the relevance of gene conversion and its permissiveness for allelic duplication and generation of novel OMP-encoding alleles that permits strain superinfection—essentially immune evasion at the level of the host population rather than within an individual. Strikingly, both these findings also apply broadly to African trypanosomes, highlighting the principle of convergent evolution and unifying the original observations made by Ross and Theiler 75 years ago.

The genus *Anaplasma* includes *A. marginale*, the type species, *Anaplasma bovis*, *A. ovis*, *A. phagocytophilum*, and *Anaplasma platys* (7). *A. marginale* and *A. phagocytophilum* are well-described tick-borne pathogens, while the other three recognized species remain less studied and characterized, although there is evidence that all members of the genus persist in their respective reservoir hosts and are tick-transmitted. *A. marginale* infects both wild and domestic ruminants, while *A. phagocytophilum* infects multiple mammalian species (7). The severity of disease varies by host species and ranges from inapparent infection to severe acute febrile syndromes that progress to severe morbidity and mortality. *A. marginale* infections in most wild ruminants and *Bos indicus* breeds are asymptomatic or cause only mild disease. Acute infection of *Bos taurus* breeds commonly results in severe morbidity and can progress to fatal disease. *A. phagocytophilum* is also asymptomatic in many reservoir species but is responsible for human granulocytic anaplasmosis, canine and equine granulocytic anaplasmosis, and tick-borne fever in ruminants (7). Antigenic variation, immune evasion, persistence, and transmission have been most completely studied in *A. marginale* and are the focus here. However, detailed studies, including complete genome sequencing, of *A. phagocytophilum* have supported common genetic mechanisms underlying antigenic variation (8–10), as have more limited studies for *A. ovis* and *A. platys* (11–12).

A. marginale Persistence and Transmission

Following initial tick-borne transmission into an immunologically naïve host, *A. marginale* replicates to >10^8 organisms per ml of blood (reviewed in 13). In surviving animals, the immune response controls this acute-phase bacteremia but results not result in clearance, but rather, in persistence (Fig. 1). Bacteremia levels decrease concomitantly with the detection of IgG antibodies directed against *A. marginale* OMPs and resolve into a cyclical pattern composed of bacteremic waves ranging between 10^2 and 10^7 organisms/ml (14). Epidemiologically, persistence provides the reservoir for subsequent tick-borne transmission. As tick populations vary in presence, abundance, and activity seasonally and by macro- and micro-climatic variables, transmission opportunities are episodic rather than continuous. Consequently, persistence in the animal host is required for long-term survival of *A. marginale*, and achieving persistence is a primary evolutionary force shaping the organism's genome. Importantly, ticks that acquisition-feed on infected hosts

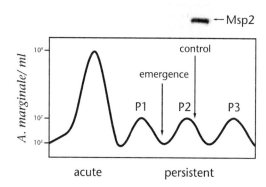

FIGURE 1 **Emergence of Msp2 antigenic variants during cyclic *Anaplasma marginale* bacteremia. *A. marginale* replicates to >10^8 organisms per ml during acute infection; the immune response does not completely clear the infection, which persists in a series of sequential bacteremia peaks. Organisms in each peak express an antigenically variant immunodominant surface protein, Msp2, which is not recognized by existing antibody at the time of emergence (as illustrated by the IgG immunoblot for the peak 2 variant). Immune recognition of the variant results in clearance followed by emergence of novel variants in peak 3. Original data from references 14 and 27.**

during the lower bacteremia levels associated with persistence still successfully acquire *A. marginale* (15–17). Subsequent replication within the tick salivary gland at the time of transmission-feeding to a new host makes up for the initially lower number of organisms ingested, and efficient onward transmission is achieved (17).

Cyclic Bacteremia and OMP Variation

A combination of bioinformatics, immunologic, and proteomic approaches has identified ~60 OMPs in *A. marginale* (18–22). Of these, two closely related proteins, major surface protein (Msp) 2 and Msp3, are both highly abundant and highly immunodominant (12, 22, 23). The two proteins are similar in structure, with a central surface-exposed region flanked by hydrophobic membrane domains (24, 25). Msp2 and Msp3 share a common C-terminus and likely were derived from a single ancestral gene. This is supported by the presence of only Msp2 in the closely related *A. phagocytophilum* but with an allelic repertoire that incorporates the complexity of the *A. marginale* Msp2/Msp3. In contrast to the other identified OMPs in *A. marginale*, which are encoded by single-copy genes and are invariant within a strain and during infection of the host, the surface-exposed domains of Msp2 and Msp3 are encoded by multiple chromosomal alleles, and recombination during infection generates structural and antigenic variants (18, 26). Studies by French et al. established that the variants expressed in sequential cyclic bacteremic peaks were both structurally and antigenically unique; variants were unrecognized by existing antibody at the time of their emergence and replicated to form a new bacteremic peak (Fig. 1) (27). Using quantitative analysis, Brayton et al., confirmed that both Msp2- and Msp3-specific variants emerged in sequential peaks with dramatic loss of the previously predominant variant (28).

Antibody responses are preferentially directed against the central surface-exposed domains, representing the structurally and antigenically unique regions of Msp2/3 and designated as the hypervariable region (HVR) (29, 30). Correspondingly, there is minimal antibody recognition of the conserved membrane domains (29, 30). The variant-specific IgG antibody responses are highly dynamic, with antibody against the HVR being remarkably short-lived compared to the responses against other conserved *A. marginale* OMPs (30). This short-lived response was unexpected given the richness of CD4$^+$ T cell epitopes in both variant-specific HVRs and the flanking conserved domains (29, 31); the latter would be predicted to provide abundant T cell help for HVR-directed B cell responses due to the principle of linked recognition. However, a series of studies conducted by Wendy Brown and colleagues demonstrated that Msp2-specific CD4$^+$ T cell responses, which can be strongly

induced by immunization, were suppressed during *A. marginale* bacteremia and only restored following antibiotic-mediated clearance of the organism (32–34). Although the mechanism of suppression remains incompletely defined, these findings suggest that the ability of Msp2 to evade immune recognition and clearance involves both the structural variation and immunologic modulation.

Genomic Structure and Mechanisms Underlying *A. marginale* Antigenic Variation

Although Msp2/3 antigenic variation had been identified prior to *A. marginale* genome sequencing, the completion of the first strain sequenced, the St. Maries strain, fully identified the allelic repertoire responsible for variation and allowed dissection of the mechanisms for long-term persistence (18). While only a single full-length Msp2/3 is expressed at one time, using a single operon-linked expression site, multiple alleles encoding unique HVRs are maintained within widely dispersed chromosomal loci (Fig. 2A). The nonexpression site alleles are each composed of a variable sequence encoding a unique HVR flanked by highly conserved 5' and 3' sequences that are identical to those of the single expression site copy (26). These alleles lack elements for transcription and translation and are silent in their loci: recombination into the expression site, mediated by the conserved flanking sequences, is required for expression of the unique HVR. Recombination, which occurs by gene conversion and retains the allelic donor unchanged, results in the expression site encoding a structurally and antigenically unique HVR, replacing the pre-existing Msp2/3 and allowing evasion of immune clearance and replication to form a new bacteremic peak. Detailed tracking of variant progression over time revealed that there is no set order in use of the potential donor alleles; each is capable of being recombined to the expression site and generating a replication-competent *A. marginale*

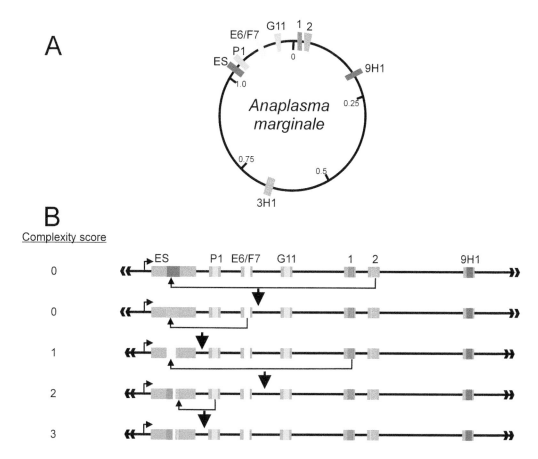

FIGURE 2 Generation of *Anaplasma marginale* Msp2 variants through gene conversion. (A) Genomic structure of the *A. marginale msp2* donor and expression site loci. The 1.2-Mb genome is a single circular chromosome and encodes a single Msp2 expression site (ES). Multiple *msp2* donor alleles, silent in their chromosomal loci, encode unique hypervariable regions (HVRs), which are expressed only when recombined into the expression site. The allelic repertoire shown is for the St. Maries strain; alleles encoding a unique HVR are shown in different colors; duplicated alleles (2, 3H1; 1, 9H1) are shown in the same color. The expression site *msp2* variant, in this example, corresponds to that encoded by the full 9H1 (or 1) allele. (B) Gene conversion generates unique *msp2* expression site variants. Sequential rounds of recombination result in replacement of the existing expression site copy by either a whole allelic donor sequence (as shown in the first gene conversion event in which allele 2 is the donor) or progressive modification of the existing expression site copy by segmental gene conversion. Over time, this process of segmental gene conversion generates complex expression site mosaics derived from multiple allelic donors and is reflected in a complexity score. The light blue regions flanking the expression site represent the conserved 5′ and 3′ domains; identical, truncated domains flank each donor allele and direct recombination. Figure and legend are from reference 41 with permission.

variant (35). The position of the locus itself relative to the expression site or origin of replication has no direct effect on variant progression; rather, the encoded HVR itself is deterministic, consistent with the importance of immune escape (36).

Notably, the *A. marginale* genome contains approximately 10 to 12 total unique *msp2* and *msp3* donor alleles (18, 37), too few to account for the number of bacteremic peaks observed and required for years of persistence. This paradox was resolved by a series of detailed studies that identified segmental gene conversion as a combinatorial mechanism to exponentially expand the potential repertoire (Fig. 2B) (35, 38, 39). Recombination of an oligonucleotide segment derived from the donor allele *hvr* into the existing expression site *hvr* generates a novel, mosaic expression site *msp2* not previously represented anywhere in the genome. Two further keys to understanding this mechanism were definition of how recombination was guided and how a mosaic could maintain minimal Msp2 structure. Futse et al. demonstrated an anchoring mechanism in which only either the 5′ or the 3′ conserved flanking sequence was required for recombination of a segment (35). The lack of a requirement for internal sequence identity allows tremendous expansion in the number of possible variants —assuming these would maintain a protein structure required for at least minimal fitness. Examination of several hundred mosaic HVRs identified stretches of 2 to 10 highly conserved amino acids, including conserved cysteines, which serve as structural "tethers" to maintain overall Msp2 structure (40). Thus, the HVR is itself composed of hypervariable microdomains that provide the diversity underlying antigenic variation with overall Msp2 structure maintained by the conserved tether elements. The resulting combinatorial diversity in the variant repertoire is estimated at 4^5 variants (four microdomains generated by segmental gene conversion using a minimum of five unique alleles per genome), consistent with continual antigenic variation.

Competing Selective Pressures for Immune Escape and Variant Fitness

Unlike the Msp2 variants generated from recombination of the intact *hvr* encoded by a donor allele, mosaic variants generated by segmental gene conversion exist only in the expression site and only transiently—due to the unidirectional recombination which results in the loss of the expression site

copy. As a consequence, mosaic variants are under long-term selection not for maximal structural fitness but only for short-term ability to evade immune recognition and clearance. In the absence of an adaptive immune response in the host, variants generated by recombination of the intact *hvr* from the chromosomal alleles (designated "simple variants") have a competitive advantage over mosaics generated by segmental gene conversion ("complex variants"). This is supported by two lines of evidence—both of which have relevance for pathogenesis and epidemiology. The first is that acute bacteremia in a newly infected host is composed of simple variants; over time as the repertoire of simple variants is expressed and sequentially cleared, mosaics generated by segmental gene conversion appear and predominate (35). As the infection continues to persist, variants become increasingly complex, with mosaics assembled with oligonucleotide segments derived from multiple alleles (Fig. 3A). This selection for complex variants occurs only under selective pressure of the adaptive immune response; direct inoculation into an immunologically naïve host results in acute bacteremia, again composed of simple variants (Fig. 3B) (41). The high-level bacteremia in acute infection reflects, at least in part, the core fitness of simple variants with a 10^2 to 10^3 reduction in fitness as complex variants emerge. The second supporting observation is that upon natural acquisition-feeding by ixodid ticks on a persistently infected host, ingested complex variants are rapidly lost from the *A. marginale* organism, and simple variants predominate in the tick midgut and, importantly, in the salivary gland upon onward transmission-feeding (Fig. 3C, D) (41–43). These findings underlie the paradox whereby a persistently infected host cannot clear its existing infection—due to sequential assembly of new mosaic variants by segmental gene conversion—but is immune to a new infection with the same strain, which expresses simple variants previously encountered. Importantly, this provides the

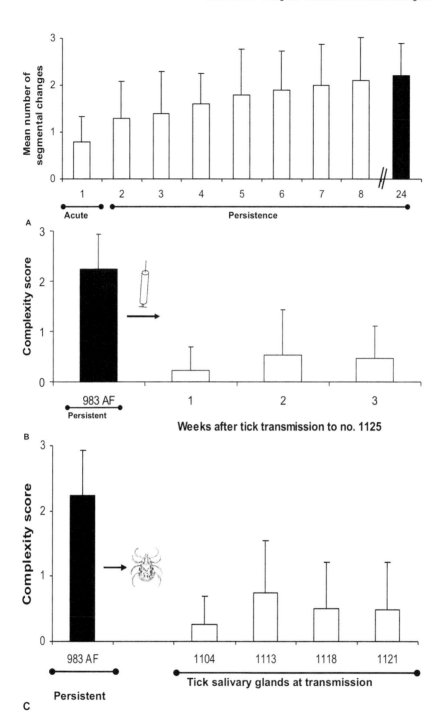

A

B

Weeks after tick transmission to no. 1125

Tick salivary glands at transmission

C

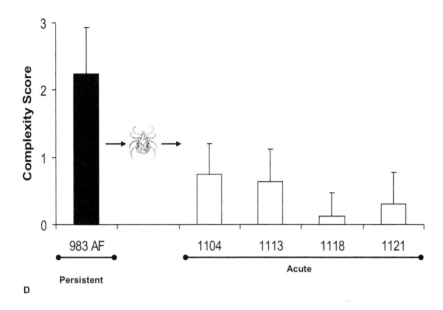

FIGURE 3 Complex variants are favored only under selection pressure of the adaptive immune response. (A) Development of complex Msp2 variants during persistent infection; complexity, measured by the number of expression site segments derived from different donor alleles (see Fig. 2B) is plotted on the *y* axis, and duration of infection (in months) is shown on the *x* axis. At 24 months of infection (solid bar), this animal was used as the source for direct transmission by intravenous inoculation of *Anaplasma marginale* into immunologically naïve animals (B) or for acquisition feeding of *Dermacentor andersoni* for tick transmission (C, D). (B) Expression of simple Msp2 variants following direct inoculation of complex variants into an immunologically naïve animal. Solid bar, complexity score of *A. marginale* variants in persistently infected calf 983. These were inoculated intravenously into immunologically naïve calf 1125. Open bars, complexity of the Msp2 variants emergent during the 3 weeks of acute bacteremia. (C) Expression of simple Msp2 variants in the tick salivary gland. Solid bar, complexity score of *A. marginale* Msp2 variants in persistently infected calf 983 during the acquisition feeding of ticks. Open bars, complexity of the variants in the salivary glands of ticks subsequently transmission-fed on each of four calves (calves 1104, 1113, 1118, and 1121). (D) Expression of simple Msp2 variants following tick transmission to immunologically naïve animals. Solid bar, complexity score of *A. marginale msp2* variants in persistently infected calf 983 during the acquisition-feeding of ticks. Open bars, complexity of the variants arising during acute infection following tick transmission to each of four immunologically naïve calves (1104, 1113, 1118, and 1121). Data, figure, and legend from reference 41 with permission.

framework for understanding antigenic variation at the level of the host population and how population immunity drives divergence in strain structure.

Population Immunity as a Driver of Strain Superinfection

Strain superinfection occurs when a second, genetically distinct pathogen strain infects a host that has already been infected with and mounted an immune response to a primary strain. Perhaps best understood in viruses, as illuminated by studies of HIV and hepatitis C virus (44, 45), the principles can be more broadly applied to more complex pathogens, including bacteria and protozoa. Following initial identification of *A. marginale* strain superinfection under conditions of natural transmission (46), Rodriguez et al. found that superinfecting strains differed in their *msp2* allelic repertoire (47), and Futse et al. demonstrated that even a single unique allele was sufficient to allow a second strain to superinfect and that strain superinfection required sole expression of the unique allele as an antigenically distinct Msp2 (48). This was in marked contrast to nonsuperinfecting strains that shared only identical alleles.

The complete *msp2* allelic repertoire was determined for multiple strains using a combination of targeted and whole-genome sequencing (48). Unlike the overall *A. marginale* genome, which is considered to be "closed core" with a high level of conservation in gene content and within individual genes (47), alleles encoding Msp2/3 differed as much between superinfecting strain pairs as they did within a strain (48)—the latter being the basis for continual antigenic variation within an individual infected host. This led to the hypothesis that immunity at the population level was selecting for strain divergence, specifically in the variant-encoding alleles, with the capacity to evade pre-existing immunity raised by a primary, existing strain. Three lines of evidence have supported this hypothesis. The first is that strain-specific variation in the primary structure of encoded simple variants is reflected in the lack of immune recognition—allowing evasion of immunity raised by the primary strain. Successful transmission of the secondary strain, which expresses simple variants in the tick vector, requires that one of the simple variants be sufficiently different to allow initial replication without immune recognition (48). Second, once established, superinfecting strains continue to generate, via segmental gene conversion, complex variants that reflect the greater level of overall antigenic diversity compared to single-strain primary infection (40). Third, the incidence of superinfection increases with the overall prevalence of *A. marginale* infection (40, 49). At low levels of infection prevalence and consequent population immunity, there is a large proportion of immunologically naïve hosts and therefore minimal selective pressure for divergence. However, as infection prevalence rises—especially toward saturation, as occurs in the tropics—the selective pressure markedly increases (40, 49). A "newly emergent" strain, defined as having at least one unique allele, whether derived *de novo* or exogenously introduced, has a clear selective advantage because the host population is immunologically naïve to the new strain (Fig. 4).

This duality of *A. marginale* antigenic variation for persistence both within the individual host and at the level of the host population role of interaction is consistent with propagation of self. Not surprisingly, this duality has also been recently observed in other highly antigenically variable bacterial pathogens, including but not limited to *Borrelia burgdorferi* (50), which is discussed in a subsequent section of this chapter.

Knowledge Gaps

Several significant knowledge gaps remain regarding mechanisms and selection determinants of *A. marginale* strain structure. How a new strain evolves from an existing one is not understood; both the rate of allelic change and mechanism(s) of change are unknown. One clue comes from the presence of exactly duplicated alleles in different loci within a strain (18, 37). This suggests that the duplicate allele could serve as a template for change, essentially experimentation to result in a sufficiently diverse allele to allow superinfection, without jeopardizing the existing complement of alleles that allow antigenic variation within the individual host. This is supported by identification of two unique alleles in a second strain that are in the identical loci occupied by duplicated alleles in the first strain (37). The mechanism by which a new sequence is introduced is also currently uncertain. Although 99% of variants map completely to one or more donor alleles, novel expression site variants characterized by mutation, insertions, and deletions at sites of segmental recombination have been identified (35). Gene conversion in reverse, resulting in an expression site sequence replacing a pre-existing allelic *hvr*,

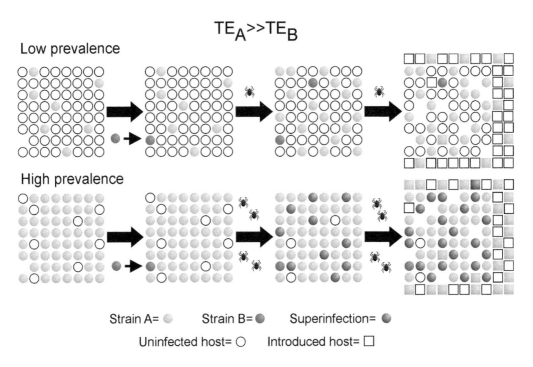

FIGURE 4 *Anaplasma marginale* strain superinfection is favored under the selective pressure of high population immunity. Circles indicate the existing animal population at T_o: white represents uninfected and immunologically naïve hosts; blue represents hosts carrying strain A; orange represents strain B; and purple represents hosts superinfected with strains A and B. Squares represent individual hosts introduced to the population by birth or immigration. The intrinsic transmission fitness is greater for strain A than strain B ($TE_A \gg TE_B$). Under conditions of low prevalence of infection (and hence low population immunity), strain A predominates. Following introduction of strain B, its transmission is at a strong disadvantage and there is minimal selective pressure for strain B superinfection. Consequently, strain A predominance is maintained over time. Under conditions of high prevalence of infection (and high population immunity), strain A is predominant, but there is strong selective pressure for strain B superinfection. Strain A transmission is favored for newly introduced naïve hosts and thus remains predominant but accompanied by prevalent superinfection. Figure and legend from reference 54 with permission.

could generate *de novo* allelic change with "successful" alleles being retained in the genome.

Finally, the trade-off between variant diversity that allows strain superinfection and maintaining minimal structure for bacterial fitness represents a clear knowledge gap with major epidemiological implications. Unchecked pressure only for allelic divergence would be expected to result in strain "chaos"—with dozens or more unique strains within a defined host population. However, study of naturally occurring infections identifies a much more limited strain structure, often defined by a predominant strain (40, 46, 51–53). The current hypothesis is that there is a dynamic balance between allelic divergence to allow superinfection and retention of minimal protein structure for bacterial fitness (54). Only under conditions of high population immunity do the lower fitness strains compete successfully and only within the structural limits of maintaining minimal function (Fig. 4). Addition of new hosts, by birth or exogenous introduction, favors the most fit strain, maintaining its predominance. Testing of this hypothesis under conditions of natural transmission is proposed as a needed and potentially illuminating set of experiments with broad relevance.

BORRELIA

Introduction

The genus *Borrelia* represents a genetically unique and highly separated lineage within the *Spirochaetes* branch of the bacterial kingdom (55, 56). These pathogenic spirochetes are obligated to a life cycle that requires transmission by hematophagous arthropods and long-term maintenance within a vertebrate host. All members of the *Borrelia* genus are defined by an unusual genome that consists of a linear chromosome and multiple linear plasmids containing covalently closed hairpin ends. *Borrelia hermsii* and *B. burgdorferi* are two well-studied members that exemplify relapsing fever and Lyme disease agents, respectively (55, 57, 58). A number of *Borrelia* species have been implicated in causing either the epidemic or endemic form of relapsing fever (56). *Borrelia recurrentis* is the only representative species responsible for causing epidemic relapsing fever, which is transmitted by the human body louse, *Pediculus humanus*. The remaining species are agents of the endemic form of relapsing fever and are primarily transmitted by soft-bodied ticks of the genus *Ornithodoros*. Both forms of the disease are characterized by recurrent spikes of high fever that correlate with periods of bacteremia that can reach levels as high as 10^8 spirochetes per milliliter of blood (59). Each febrile episode corresponds to spirochetes that produce a different form of the Vlp or Vsp lipoprotein through an antigenic variation system that is crucial to the success of relapsing fever borreliae as pathogens (60, 61). An effective host humoral response against Vlp/Vsp reduces the bacterial load in the blood, which brings about the resolution of fever in the host (62, 63). New *vlp/vsp*

variants arise in the host at a frequency of 10^{-3} to 10^{-4} per cell per generation (59) and in turn proliferate and seed the next wave of spirochetemia.

The multisystem disease known as Lyme disease (or Lyme borreliosis) is the most prevalent vector-borne infection affecting humans in both North America and Europe (64, 65). *B. burgdorferi*, *Borrelia garinii*, and *Borrelia afzelii* are the causative bacterial agents of the disease and are transmitted by hard-bodied ticks of the genus *Ixodes*. Infected ticks transmit Lyme disease borreliae to humans during feeding, which can result in a localized infection (erythema migrans) at the site of the tick bite. Disseminated and chronic stages of infection follow; these are characterized by neurological, cardiological, and arthritic manifestations of disease. Infection with Lyme disease borreliae can last from months to years due to avoidance of the host immune response, and key to its successful evasion tactics is recombination at the *vls* locus located at the telomeric end of a 28-kilobase linear plasmid (4, 66, 67). Gene conversion events within the *vls* locus result in sequence variations of the VlsE surface lipoprotein that in turn alter its antigenic properties and provide the spirochete with the ability to evade the host's antibody-mediated response (67–69). Although similarities and differences exist between the antigenic variation systems of relapsing fever and Lyme disease borreliae, this chapter will focus on the more well-studied *vls* system of the Lyme disease spirochete.

A schematic of the *vls* locus from the *B. burgdorferi* B31 strain is shown in Fig. 5. The locus consists of the *vlsE* expression site that encodes the 35-kDa lipoprotein, which is located 82 base pairs (bp) from the right telomere end of the linear plasmid, lp28-1 (66–68). The locus also includes a tandem array of 15 silent cassettes (*vls2-16*; each approximately 500 bp in length) that are oriented in the opposite direction of the *vlsE* gene. A short intergenic region (~160 bp) separates the *vlsE* locus and the silent

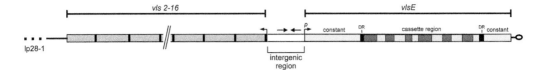

FIGURE 5 The *vls* locus of *Borrelia burgdorferi* B31. The illustration shows the arrangement of the *vls* expression site, *vlsE*, and the contiguous array of 15 silent cassettes comprising the *vls* locus on the right telomeric end of lp28-1. The six variable regions of the central *vlsE* cassette are colored light blue, while the six invariant regions are colored dark blue. The black bars flanking the *vlsE* cassette region and silent cassettes represent the 17-bp direct repeats. The silent cassettes (*vls2* to *vls16*) are not drawn to scale. Arrows positioned at the beginning of *vlsE* and silent cassettes indicate the respective orientations. The arrows located within the intergenic region denote the inverted DNA repeat. DR, 17-bp direct repeat; *p*, *vlsE* promoter. Figure adapted from reference 191 with permission.

cassettes, and this intergenic space contains a near-perfect inverted repeat of a 51-bp sequence capable of forming a highly stable DNA stem loop (70). In addition, a portion of the promoter sequence required for *vlsE* expression is located within this inverted repeat (70). The *vlsE* expression region is comprised of a central variable cassette (Fig. 5, blue region) that is flanked by constant regions (yellow). At the junction of the variable and constant regions are 17-bp direct repeats. With the exception of the final cassette, 17-bp direct repeat sequences are also found at either end of the silent cassettes. The *vlsE* cassette region exhibits roughly 90% sequence identity with each of the silent cassettes (67), and most of the sequence differences reside in six variable regions (Fig. 5, light blue) that are flanked by six highly conserved, or invariant, sequences (dark blue).

The *vls* Locus in Immune Evasion and Persistence

A number of experimental findings over the years have provided strong evidence implicating the importance of VlsE antigenic variation for *B. burgdorferi* persistence. The first studies involved determining the kinetics of gene conversion, and recombination events were observed as early as four days after infection of mice and continued to occur throughout infection (69).

However, assessing the exact rate of variation has proven difficult; this is because *vlsE* antigenic switching only occurs during mammalian infections (71), and *B. burgdorferi* is not readily sampled from the blood. VlsE variation occurs to such a degree that each clone examined from a single mouse skin biopsy can have a different *vlsE* sequence after only 28 days postinfection, and the sequence changes primarily occur within the six variable regions. Early work also demonstrated that antibodies specific for the variable regions of VlsE were produced during experimental infection of mice (72).

More evidence for the role of the *vls* system in immune evasion came from studies involving the *vls*-resident plasmid, lp28-1 (73, 74). Clones lacking lp28-1 were shown to exhibit an infectivity phenotype whereby these spirochetes were able to disseminate to tissue sites but were unable to persist in the murine host. Notably, these same clones are capable of long-term survival in severe-combined immunodeficient (SCID) mice that lack an effective antibody response (75, 76). Lp28-1-deficient isolates also grow normally in a dialysis membrane chamber implanted in the peritoneal cavity of rats, where exposure to either antibodies or immune cells is restricted (76). Finally, immunocompetent mice infected with an lp28-1 minus strain complemented with only the *vlsE* gene (*sans* the *vls* silent cassettes) are able to clear infection, demonstrating that it is not the mere presence of VlsE that provides the capacity for persistent infection, but rather the ability to undergo *vls* antigenic variation to produce VlsE variants (77). Although these studies provided a strong indication that lp28-1, and presumably the *vls* locus, are required for persistence only in the presence of an effective humoral immune response, definitive evidence for the role of VlsE antigenic variation in immune evasion remained elusive until the generation of a genetic deletion of the *vls* locus.

The construction of a *vls* knockout mutant in *B. burgdorferi* was made possible by taking advantage of the linear nature of lp28-1 (Fig. 6A). The method used involves integration of a plasmid containing a replicated telomere within a chosen linear plasmid of *B. burgdorferi* (78–80). The end result of the internal placement of the replicated telomere is deletion of DNA through the action of the *Borrelia* telomere resolvase, ResT (80, 81). Spirochetes that lost the *vls* locus due to telomere-mediated removal were completely cleared from immunocompetent C3H mice by day 21 postinfection (78), matching the phenotype observed with clones that lacked the lp28-1 plasmid. Consistent with the findings that lp28-1 is not required for persistent infection in the absence of an adaptive immune response (75–77), the *vls* deletion mutant exhibited long-term survival in SCID mice, thereby confirming the hypothesis that *vls* recombination functions to evade the humoral immune response in the mouse host (66, 67).

Targeted deletion was also utilized to obtain lp28-1 mutants containing mainly the *vls* locus and the necessary genes for autonomous replication of the plasmid (Fig. 6B). The only other potential genes retained on the lp28-1 mutant plasmid were eight very small open reading frames (*bbf19 to bbf22* and *bbf27 to bbf30*) predicted to potentially encode for proteins consisting of only 82 amino acids or less. Infectivity experiments showed that these *B. burgdorferi* clones are fully infectious and persistent in immunocompetent mice, providing further evidence that the silent *vls* cassettes and *vlsE* are involved in spirochete persistence (78). Moreover, these mutant clones carried out *vlsE* recombination in immunocompetent C3H mice, indicating that protein factors required for antigenic switching are likely not carried on lp28-1 but encoded elsewhere.

The remaining presence of the small ORF regions *bbf19* to *bbf22* and *bbf27* to *bbf30* left open the possibility that the loss of genes within these loci could have some role in the intermediate infectivity phenotype exhibited by the lp28-1-deficient clones and was not due solely to an absence of the *vls* locus. A study published by Embers et al. reported that expression of the immunodominant outer surface protein C (OspC) by an lp28-1-deficient *B. burgdorferi* clone was abnormally high *in vivo*, suggesting that downregulation of this protein is impaired (82). Previous studies have shown that OspC is downregulated in *B. burgdorferi* shortly after establishing infection in the animal host, and it has been suggested that this provides the spirochete with a mechanism to avoid clearance mediated by anti-OspC antibodies (83–85). The overall conclusion from the Embers et al. study was that failure of OspC repression by lp28-1-deficient spirochetes renders them susceptible to immune-mediated clearance, which could potentially be responsible in part for the intermediate infectivity phenotype associated with these *B. burgdorferi* clones. Thus, the possibility was raised that one or more genes involved in *ospC* repression may be present on the lp28-1 plasmid. However, recently generated mutants lacking either region *bbf19* to *bbf22* or *bbf27* to *bbf30* were found to be capable of persistent infection of immunocompetent C3H mice for up to 91 days (Hove and Bankhead, unpublished data). Together with previously published results involving additional lp28-1 deletion mutants, this raises the likelihood that the *vls* locus is the only lp28-1-resident genetic system responsible for

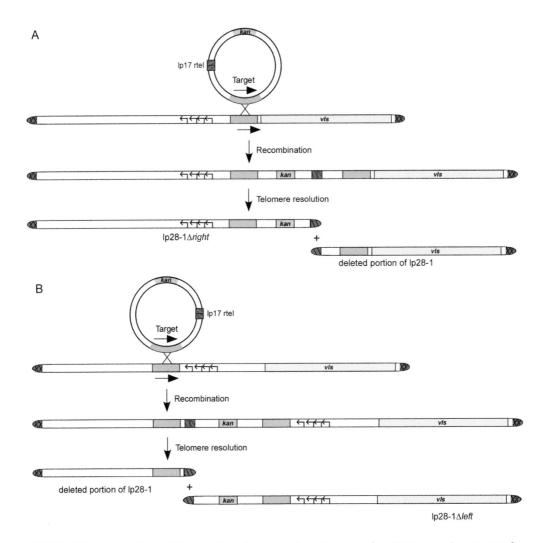

FIGURE 6 **Telomere-mediated deletion of the *vls* locus in *Borrelia burgdorferi*. (A) Construction strategy for the generation of the *vls* deletion mutant clone of *B. burgdorferi* B31. The target sequence for insertion (green) is chosen so that only the *vls* locus would be deleted from the lp28-1 plasmid. The genes encoding plasmid maintenance proteins that have been previously shown to allow autonomous replication are shown as black arrows. (B) Schematic of the construction strategy for the lp28-1Δ*left* plasmid. The target sequence for insertion (green) was chosen so that only the genes encoding proteins that allow autonomous replication of lp28-1 (shown as arrows arranged from left to right) and the right side of lp28-1 would remain. Hairpin telomeres are shown as red hatched regions. Figure adapted from reference 78 with permission.**

persistence during infection of the mammalian host.

Mechanism of Recombination

Although gene conversion has been implicated in *vlsE* antigenic variation, little is known about the exact mechanism of re-combination and the proteins involved in this process. Since the discovery of the *vls* system almost two decades ago, progress toward elucidating the mechanistic details of recombinational switching has been impeded by two factors. First, switching does not occur in either culture or the tick vector, but instead requires passage through a mammalian host (66), and second, the *vls* locus is genetically unstable when cloned in *E. coli* (67, 86).

The proposed model for *vlsE* antigenic switching involves a nonreciprocal gene conversion mechanism whereby segments within the *vlsE* central cassette region are replaced by sections of varied length and location from the silent cassettes (Fig. 7). Only the cassette region of *vlsE* displays sequence variation resulting from gene conversion; the sequence and organization of the silent cassettes remain unaltered (69). An elaborate study by Norris and colleagues examined 1,399 clones isolated from various tissue sites of mice infected from 4 to 365 days (87). Detailed analysis of the *vlsE* sequence changes found that the *vls* antigenic variation system promotes both short and long recombination events within each cassette region. Along with the gene conversion events, template-independent changes also

occur that lead to additional sequence variation of *vlsE*. The end result of these accumulated changes is a new *vlsE* sequence with a mosaic structure, and the total combined potential for sequence variation makes the *vlsE* switching process one of the most dynamic antigenic variation systems known.

Surprisingly, the RecA protein does not seem to be required for the generation of VlsE antigenic variants, despite being involved in DNA repair and homologous recombination in the spirochete (88). This is in sharp contrast to other well-studied antigenic variation systems that are RecA-dependent, such as the *pilE* locus of *Neisseria gonorrhoeae* (89). Similarly, disruption of a large number of genes involved in DNA recombination, repair, and replication ruled out the involvement of their respective encoded proteins in *vlsE* switching (90, 91). However, these same studies did find that the RuvAB complex of *B. burgdorferi* is required for *vls* antigenic variation, presumably by promoting branch migration of Holliday junctions during *vlsE* recombination (90, 91). Interestingly, while *B. burgdorferi* contains genes that encode the branch-migration complex RuvAB, these spirochetes are noticeably lacking the gene for the Holliday junction resolvase, RuvC. In fact, no recognizable ortholog exists in the *B. burgdorferi* genomic sequence, which suggests that a specialized Holliday junction resolvase may be expressed in the spirochete. This raises the question of how the Lyme disease pathogen promotes recombination at the *vls* locus with such a limited involvement of the usual collection of DNA recombination proteins.

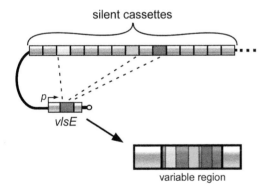

FIGURE 7 Overview of *vlsE* antigenic switching in *Borrelia burgdorferi*. Variant-specific segments act as a source of DNA for nonreciprocal recombination events with the *vlsE* expression locus. Through this process, segments of the variable region (blue) are replaced by sections of varied length and location from the donor sequences. In the example shown, three sequential gene conversion events (represented by dashed lines) occur within each expression site through recombination with the colored donor sections (yellow, green, or red) to generate a new expression site sequence with a mosaic structure. Figure adapted from reference 4 with permission.

One possible answer is that the *vlsE* antigenic switching process may involve the formation of G-quadruplex DNA structures. A study by Walia and Chaconas found that guanine quartet (G4) DNA could be formed by G-runs located in the 17-bp direct repeats of the *vlsE* gene (92). A G-quadruplex DNA structure has been shown to have a role in pilin antigenic variation in *N. gonorrhoeae* by acting as a signal for DNA strand nicking (93,

94). However, this process involves recombination proteins that are either known not to exist in *B. burgdorferi* or have been shown not to have a role in antigenic switching. Moreover, the G-runs found in the *vls* locus are not separated by short stretches of DNA similar to that typically found with G4 DNA. Thus, it remains unclear whether G-quadruplex formation has an actual role in *vlsE* recombination or if intermolecular interactions between the G-runs of the direct repeats promote gene conversion through an entirely different mechanism.

The VlsE Lipoprotein

The crystal structure of the recombinant-variant VlsE outer surface lipoprotein presents a three-dimensional protein fold that is substantially different from most other solved protein structures (95). Despite this unique configuration, analysis of the VlsE protein structure did reveal a resemblance to the variable surface protein of the relapsing fever agent, *B. hermsii*. The VlsE monomer is also quite similar to the overall protein fold of the OspC dimer structure, with both presenting membrane distal alpha-helical bundles to the host environment (95, 96). The overall primary structure of VlsE consists of N-terminal and C-terminal constant domains that flank the central cassette region. The loops containing the variable regions are localized at the distal surface of the protein, while the C terminus is positioned close to the N terminus that is attached to the bacterial lipid outer membrane. Gel filtration chromatography of VlsE showed that that the protein is primarily monomeric in solution, although the observed interface in the crystal structure raises the possibility that VlsE could exist as a dimer on the bacterial cell surface.

The observed position of the variable regions at the distal surface of VlsE confirms their accessibility to antibodies. In contrast to the variant regions, the invariant regions of VlsE have very limited surface exposure. Despite the apparent inaccessibility to antibodies, a strong humoral response is mounted against the conserved regions of VlsE (most notably invariant region 6). In fact, VlsE-based recombinant proteins or synthetic peptides are used for the immunodiagnosis of Lyme disease (97–101). The function of VlsE independent of its antigenic variation properties is not currently known. There have been previous indications that VlsE may be involved in tissue tropism, including reports that VlsE production is elevated during mammalian infection (102), with higher levels observed in spirochetes recovered from joint and skin tissues than from heart tissue (103). However, a recent study found no obvious differences in the amino acid sequence of VlsE variants recovered from different tissue sites, suggesting the absence of any VlsE role in tissue tropism (87).

Knowledge Gaps

Past research involving *B. burgdorferi* antigenic variation has focused on either analyzing *vlsE* sequence changes, the dynamics of those changes, or the role of *vlsE* switching in *B. burgdorferi* pathogenesis. However, studies that address the fundamental question of how antigenic variation occurs in *B. burgdorferi* have been seriously lacking. In addition, the use of molecular approaches to study *vls* recombination has been limited. Despite the widespread nature of this effective pathogenic strategy, few molecular details of the recombinational switching process have been reported for any organism.

A number of aspects regarding the molecular details of VlsE antigenic variation remain unknown and will likely be the focus of future experimental studies. For example, the subtelomeric positioning of the *vls* locus is a common feature associated with many antigenic variation systems found in both eubacterial and protozoal pathogens (104, 105).

The reasons behind this phenomenon are still unclear and could potentially be of great significance to the overall mechanism of antigenic variation. The importance of the 17-bp direct repeats that demarcate the *vlsE* variable region and flank the silent cassettes is also currently unknown. Although it was originally thought that these sequences might play a role in recombinational switching (67), sequence analysis showed that these repeats are not well conserved across *Borrelia* species and even within some species, casting doubt on a proposed role in recombination (106). However, the recent finding that G4 DNA can be formed at the guanine-rich 17-bp direct repeats may warrant further investigation into the potential mechanistic importance of these sequences for *vls* gene conversion. Nevertheless, any potential roles of these direct repeat elements for *vlsE* recombination during host infection have not been directly investigated. Also remaining to be determined is whether the *vlsE*–silent cassette intergenic region is required for *vls* antigenic variation. One intriguing idea is that the stem loop–forming potential of the intergenic region between *vlsE* and the silent cassette array delivers the cassette copies to *vlsE* during the gene conversion process. Finally, a study demonstrated that antigenic switching does not occur with a *trans* copy of *vlsE* during infection, suggesting a possible *cis* requirement for the *vls* recombination mechanism (77). However, the *trans* copy of *vlsE* was carried on a circular shuttle vector, as opposed to the linear lp28-1 plasmid in which *vlsE* normally resides, and whether this may have inhibited recombination between the shuttle plasmid and lp28-1 will require additional studies.

A role for the VlsE protein other than providing an antigenic disguise is not currently known, but it has been proposed that the protein might function in other forms of immune evasion (107, 108). An elegant study by Tilly, Bestor, and Rosa demonstrated that VlsE and OspC may share similar but distinct roles during host infection (109). Unfortunately, the exact function(s) of the OspC protein also remains undefined, and thus exactly what common role these two lipoproteins may share is still a mystery. Based on previous studies, it has been speculated that they may protect the pathogen from host defenses. Alternatively, they may aid in stabilizing the bacterial structure during host infection similar to the role recently demonstrated for OspA and OspB in lipid rafts on the spirochete membrane (110, 111). Though OspC was not found to be associated with these lipid rafts (111), high levels of either OspC or VlsE may still function in some fashion as an essential component for overall stability of the bacterial outer membrane.

Although a number of other surface proteins exist that are immunogenic, VlsE is the only known *B. burgdorferi* antigen that exhibits variation of its surface epitope. A daunting question regarding *B. burgdorferi* immune escape has been how such a feat is accomplished through sequence variation of this single lipoprotein, despite the presence of a substantial number of additional antigens residing on the bacterial surface. Many pathogens use their antigenically variable proteins in a number of ways as an evasion strategy, and several models have been suggested for how VlsE might become the primary target for the host immune response. In other pathogen systems, such as that found in *Trypanosoma brucei*, the variable surface protein hides other antigens by essentially coating the surface of the organism (112, 113).

It is possible that VlsE may act as a shield to obscure the epitopes of other surface antigens. In fact, crystallography data suggests that the binding of VlsE to other proteins on the membrane surface may block antibody binding to the lateral surface of VlsE (95). This in turn may protect other surface antigens that are tightly juxtaposed to VlsE from antibody recognition (Fig. 8A). A precedent for this type of interaction has

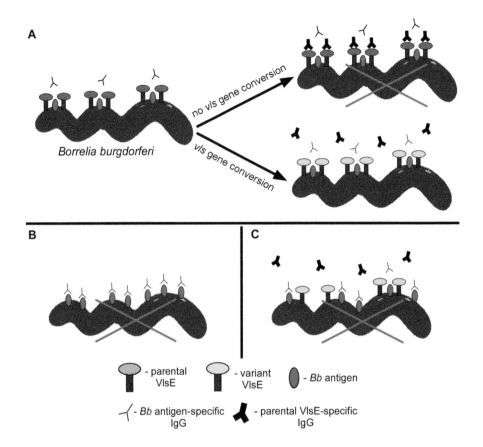

FIGURE 8 Model for VlsE-mediated protection of *Borrelia burgdorferi* surface antigens. **(A)** Shortly after host infection, upregulation of *vlsE* expression leads to surface localization of the encoded lipoprotein. Interaction of VlsE with other proteins results in a complex that functions to shield epitopes of these surface antigens. Continued *vls* gene conversion leading to production of VlsE variants is necessary to avoid killing by antibodies raised against the parental and subsequent VlsE variants, allowing for sustained epitope masking. Absence **(B)** or low expression **(C)** of VlsE allows binding of neutralizing antibodies to *B. burgdorferi* surface antigens that ultimately leads to spirochete death (denoted by a large red X). A legend indicating the identity of the various molecular cartoon depictions is provided at the bottom of the figure.

been demonstrated in studies with the *Borrelia* protein P66, in which the protein is protected from proteolytic cleavage in Lyme *Borrelia* expressing high levels of the outer surface protein OspA (114).

With respect to VlsE-mediated shielding, experiments using either *in vitro*–grown or host-adapted wild-type *B. burgdorferi* were conducted to determine whether VlsE expression could provide Lyme disease spirochetes with the capacity to reinfect mice (115). The levels of VlsE expression have been shown to be upregulated 32-fold during host

infection relative to those measured *in vitro* (102). Unlike the highly susceptible *in vitro*–grown spirochetes, *B. burgdorferi* that have adapted within the animal host have been demonstrated to be relatively invulnerable to the protective effects of immune sera (116, 117). The study showed that cultured (low VlsE–expressing) wild-type *B. burgdorferi* are unable to reinfect mice, while host-adapted (high VlsE-expressing) wild-type spirochetes are fully competent for host reinfection (115). Additional experiments involving wild-type and VlsE mutant clones found that only the wild type could reinfect mice initially infected and cleared of spirochetes devoid of VlsE. In other words, the immune response of these mice was sufficient to prevent reinfection by a VlsE-deficient clone but could not block reinfection by spirochetes capable of expressing variable VlsE (see Fig. 8B). It was also shown that SCID mice treated with immune sera generated to a VlsE-deficient mutant were resistant to infection by this same clone but could be successfully challenged by host-adapted wild-type B31 spirochetes expressing VlsE (115). The finding that passively transferred antibodies developed to non-VlsE surface antigens can provide immunity against the VlsE-deficient clone but were not borreliacidal to wild-type spirochetes, may hint at a possible VlsE-mediated shielding mechanism. Finally, VlsE expression is known to be highly reduced while in the tick environment, and in agreement with findings described above, mice fed with wild-type-infected ticks are immune to reinfection (Rogovskyy and Bankhead, unpublished report). Together, these data indicate that the adaptation state of infecting spirochetes, likely due to its respective effects on VlsE expression, can greatly influence *B. burgdorferi* evasion from the host antibody-mediated response (see Fig. 8C). Determining whether this VlsE-mediated immune avoidance system involves epitope shielding will require further investigation.

It has also been proposed that VlsE might be a T-cell-independent antigen that could directly stimulate certain B cell subsets (78, 108). The resulting humoral response generated by VlsE may override antibody production against other potential surface antigens. It has been observed that *vls* mutant *B. burgdorferi* clones complemented with a nonswitchable form of *vlsE* are cleared faster in immunocompetent mice relative to non VlsE-complemented mutants (78). It is conceivable that this outcome could be the result of direct stimulation of B cells by VlsE, and this modulating ability could result in more

effective clearance of these spirochetes due to the absence of VlsE antigenic variation in those clones. In support of this, a recent study found that sera derived from nude mice infected with wild-type *B. burgdorferi* contained anti-VlsE T-cell independent antibodies at sufficient levels to prevent infection by *in vitro*–grown wild-type *B. burgdorferi* but were at inadequate quantities to prevent infection by the VlsE-deficient mutant clone. This finding is suggestive that the T-cell independent antibody response is directed primarily to VlsE, with subdominant titers of these antibodies against non-VlsE surface antigens as demonstrated by their inability to prevent infection by the VlsE-deficient mutant clone.

Finally, because survival of the Lyme pathogen in nature is completely dependent on its enzootic life cycle, it would be interesting to assess whether the variant-generating capacity of the *vls* system is required for the Lyme pathogen to be efficiently and successfully perpetuated throughout its life cycle. Although never tested, the expected outcome would be that antigenic variation of VlsE is required for persistence in the natural reservoir host. Also unknown, and potentially more interesting, are the effects of *vls* mutation on the ability of *B. burgdorferi* to be acquired, persist, and be transmitted to naïve mice by *Ixodes* ticks. In all, continued efforts toward identifying the mechanism responsible for *B. burgdorferi* immune escape has important implications in the development of vaccines against the pathogen and other *Borrelia* species. If the protective effects of VlsE can be minimized using therapeutics, then an effective vaccine can be developed and used in conjunction to prevent infection or reinfection by the Lyme disease spirochete. Additionally, such knowledge could lead to the development of novel strategies for targeting Lyme disease *Borrelia* in the tick vector and/or reservoir host. Overall, such future studies will significantly advance our knowledge of immune evasion by *B. burgdorferi* and could in turn have broad implications for other animal and human pathogens.

NEISSERIA

Introduction

The genus *Neisseria* contains groups of Gram-negative, proteobacterial species, most of which colonize mucosal surfaces of mammals but are commensal organisms that do not normally elicit pathology or cause disease (118). Whether they have a mutualistic relationship with their hosts has not been established, but considering their long co-evolution with their host, it is likely. There are 11 species that colonize humans, and these species appear to be host-restricted since they are not known to inhabit any other natural ecological niche. It is unknown whether a progenitor of the human-restricted *Neisseria* colonized a human and the 11 species evolved from this one progenitor or whether a progenitor colonized one or more different hosts and then transferred and adapted to life exclusively within humans. While all of these organisms have the ability to colonize mucosal surfaces and grow, only two members of the genus are considered to be frank pathogens with serious sequelae of morbidity and mortality (118). The pathogenic *Neisseria* are *N. gonorrhoeae* (the gonococcus or Gc), the sole causative agent of gonorrhea, and *Neisseria meningitidis* (the meningococcus or Mc), the major cause of bacterial meningitis in teenagers and young adults. While these organisms are true pathogens that have the ability to cause disease in otherwise healthy people, they represent pathogens that have evolved from and share many of the colonization determinants with the commensal *Neisseria* and can behave either as nonpathogenic (commensal or asymptomatic) or pathogenic organisms when colonizing different individuals.

N. gonorrhoeae was the first member of the genus described and is a unique member of the genus since it mainly colonizes the human genital tract, and not the nasopharynx or oral cavity. A disease similar to gonorrhea has been described throughout human history (119). Gonorrhea is still prevalent worldwide today, and the rise in antibiotic resistance makes gonorrhea a major public health concern (120). Gonococcal infection usually results in symptomatic disease in men, with an obvious purulent exudate and painful urination; it is more linked to asymptomatic infections in women, with a less obvious exudate and little or no pain during uncomplicated infection (121, 122). However, there are no general population studies that measure the frequency of asymptomatic infection in either gender. In the developed world, a significant portion of infections are found within populations of men who have sex with men (123). Of the human-adapted *Neisseria*, Gc more often elicits inflammation than the other species. While the reasons for this are unknown, it is a reasonable hypothesis that inflammation increases sexual transmission.

N. meningitidis, like the commensal *Neisseria*, colonizes the nasopharynx and usually behaves similarly to the commensal *Neisseria* (124). However, in a small number of colonized people (<1%) the meningococcus can leave the nasopharynx and become systemic to cause meningococcemia or bacterial meningitis (125). Localized outbreaks of meningococcal disease occur when young adults from different geographical regions come in close contact with one another (e.g., dormitories or military barracks) or during the dry season in sub-Saharan Africa (126). These epidemiological correlations suggest that there are both immunological and environmental factors that can contribute to meningococcal disease. However, since many outbreaks are clonal in nature, it is postulated that there are hyperinvasive Mc clones that are more able to become systemic and/or cross the blood-brain barrier (124). While many genes or gene products have been correlated with hyperinvasive lineages, there is no single virulence factor that correlates with systemic disease (127–130). Although the frequency of invasive disease is low relative to commensal carriage, the high level of mortality associated with Mc meningitis makes this the most dangerous member of the genus.

Gc and Mc appear to have evolved from a common progenitor since they show greater than 90% identity in their core genomic sequences and are closely related (131). Not surprisingly, due to their different sites of colonization, transmission, and pathogenesis, each species has unique defining genetic determinants (e.g., the capsule of Mc), but the genetic similarities between these species are more impressive than their differences (132). One genetic characteristic that differentiates the pathogenic from the commensal *Neisseria* is the greater amount of phenotypic variation that is found in the pathogenic species. For reasons that are not well understood, the commensal *Neisseria* have low potential for variation; Mc has extensive variation but does not have the vast capacity that Gc encodes. One plausible hypothesis is that both Gc and Mc use variation for functional reasons not needed by the commensal *Neisseria*, while as an STI, Gc requires a greater amount of variation for immune evasion.

Phase and Antigenic Variation in the *Neisseria*

The pathogenic *Neisseria* are notable in the number of genes that can undergo stochastic variation of gene expression. The types of stochastic variation that have been described in the pathogenic *Neisseria* include on/off phase variation, which is the reversible expression or nonexpression of gene products, and antigenic variation, the expression of multiple antigenic forms of a gene product or structure. There are three major surface structures that all can undergo both phase and antigenic variation: the lipooligosaccharide (LOS) glycan struc-

ture that constitutes the outer layer of the outer membrane (133), the family of outer membrane adhesins called opacity proteins (134), and the type IV pilus (135). The properties and mechanism of variation of each of these important antigenically variable surface structures will be discussed in detail below.

There are also 50 to 100 genes in each pathogenic *Neisseria* strain that undergo simple on/off phase variation (136). Many of the phase-variable genes are involved in pathogenesis, but other functions are controlled by phase variation, and not all of the

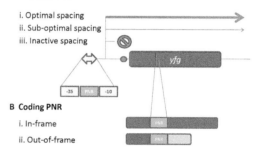

FIGURE 9 **Polynucleotide repeat (PNR)–based phase variation in *Neisseria*. (A) PNR within a promoter of your favorite gene (*yfg*). The yellow double-headed arrow represents the promoter with a -35 and -10 sequence and a PNR in between these promoter elements. The blue circle shows a ribosome binding site to initiate translation. (i) When the PNR repeat number is in the optimal spacing, the promoter initiates maximal transcription as long as other regulatory signals do not prevent expression. (ii) When the PNR changes ±1 nucleotide, the spacing between the -35 and -10 elements is not optimal, but there is still transcriptional initiation to produce a low level of gene expression. (iii) When the PNR number increases or decreases due to a spacing that does not allow RNA polymerase to effectively interact with the promoter, there is essentially no transcription. (B) PNR within a coding sequence. (i) The PNR length maintains the reading frame to translate the entire gene product. (ii) Change in the PNR length by ±1 or 2 changes the reading frame downstream of the PNR and usually terminates translation prematurely. It is possible that this change in reading frame could result in a different protein product.**

gene products have a known function. The phase-variable genes mostly alter expression through changes in polynucleotide repeats (PNR) located either in the promoter of the gene or within the coding sequence (Fig. 9). The number of nucleotides within the PNR can change ±1 during DNA replication through a process called slipped-strand mispairing (137). If the PNR is located within the promoter region of a gene, the size of the PNR therefore sets whether the -10 and -35 elements of the promoter are within an optimal distance of one another (high expression), a suboptimal distance (moderate expression), or a nonfunctional distance (no expression) (Fig. 9A). If the PNR is within a coding region, the change in repeat number can alter the translational reading frame and allows expression of the full-length gene product, or with a frame-shift that alters the reading frame this usually results in a premature stop codon (Fig. 9B). This large number of phase-variable genes with pathogenic *Neisseria* creates a situation where every population is a heterogeneous mix of phenotypic variants. This is one reason why genetic complementation is so critical in laboratory studies using mutants.

LOS Variation

As Gram-negative bacteria, members of the *Neisseria* genus have two phospholipid bilayer membranes. The outer membrane is an asymmetric bilayer, with the outer leaflet being comprised of LOS molecules. LOS is similar to the lipopolysaccharide expressed by many Gram-negative bacteria but does not have the long extended O-antigen polymeric sugars characteristic of lipopolysaccharide (133). The LOS has many functions for *Neisseria* including the barrier function of the outer membrane, immuno-stimulatory endotoxin activity, and providing complex glycosylation substrates that are recognized as being similar to host glycans and binding host lectins (138). LOS is a major component

of the outer membrane vesicles that are the basis of experimental vaccines (139) and an important immune-stimulatory component of the new Mc group B vaccine Bexsero (140).

In the pathogenic *Neisseria*, there are several invariant glycosyltransferases that help build the LOS glycan structure and a few phase-variable glycosyltransferases that each can be on or off in different cells (141–143). The glycan structure of the LOS is defined by the combination of the phase-variable glycosyltransferases that produce each enzyme. Phase variation of the LOS biosynthetic glycosyltransferase is mediated by changes in PNRs (polyG) found within the coding region of each variable gene, allowing for a simple on/off alteration in expression of the protein. The effect of these variable expression genes on the bacteria surface is amplified by the further modification of some but not all glycan structures by sialylation (141, 142, 144, 145) (Fig. 10A). LOS variation is a powerful way to use replication error to create multiple sugar structures to vary the bacterial surface. The reasons why Mc retains LOS variation despite having a distinct polysaccharide capsule covering the outer surface is not well-established, but the existence of acapsular strains and the ability of outer membrane proteins to engage host cell receptors suggests that the capsule is not a complete barrier to the bacterial surface (146).

Opa Variation

The pathogenic *Neisseria* can express a family of outer membrane proteins called opacity (Opa) proteins because some of these proteins cause change in colony opacity when cells are grown on agar plates (134, 147). Mc encodes 4 to 5 variable *opa* loci, Gc encodes 11 to 13 *opa* loci, and commensal *Neisseria* encode 1 to 2 *opa* loci. Opa proteins are beta-barrel outer membrane proteins that mainly act as adhesins. Different Opa variants bind to different members of the human carcinoembryonic antigen-related cell adhesion molecules (CEACAM) receptor family or to

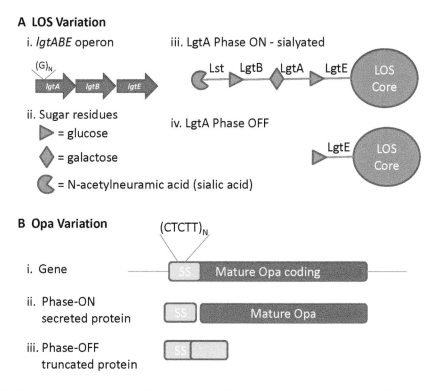

FIGURE 10 **Lipooligosaccharide (LOS) and opacity (Opa) protein phase variation. (A) LOS variation. Shown is one of the variable LOS biosynthetic gene clusters. (i) The *ltgA* glycosyltransferase gene has a guanine polynucleotide repeat (PNR) within the coding sequence that can change the repeat number ±1. (ii) Sugar residues added by each transglycosylase. (iii) When the *ltgA* PNR is in the correct reading frame, the glycosyltransferase is produced to add a galactose residue to the acceptor glucose. This galactose is then a substrate for the LgtB glycosyltransferase to add a glucose, which is then a substrate for the sialyltransferase (Lst). (iv) When the *lgtA* PNR changes number and causes a frame shift, this form of the LOS cannot be modified or sialylated. (B) Opa variation. (i) A representative *opa* gene showing the pentamer repeat within the signal sequence (SS). (ii) Phase-ON: when the pentamer repeat number encodes an in-frame protein, the full protein is translated and the signal sequence is cleaved during secretion. (iii) Phase-OFF: when the pentamer repeat number changes to be out of frame and an altered protein coding sequence is produced (blue), leading to a premature stop codon.**

heparin sulphate (148–150). It is possible that Opa protein variation is driven more by receptor specificity than by immune selection, but this has never been directly tested.

Each *opa* locus is independently transcribed, and each locus is under independent phase variation control. There is a pentamer nucleotide repeat (CTCTT) contained within the DNA segment that encodes the protein secretion signal sequence (134, 151). During DNA replication, this pentamer repeat adds or removes one repeat and puts the mature Opa protein coding sequence in or out of the reading frame of the initiating AUG (Fig. 10B). Therefore, each *Neisseria* cell can have any combination of Opa proteins expressed in a stochastic manner. The frequency of Opa phase variation is influenced by promoter strength, and the rate is larger when the repeat length is longer (152, 153).

Pilin Variation

Both the pathogenic and commensal *Neisseria* express a type IV pilus. The type

IV pilus is an important colonization factor that also plays many roles in the pathogenesis of disease. Pili help mediate adherence to host cells and tissues (154), twitching motility (155), resistance to polymorphonuclear leukocyte killing mechanisms (156), and genetic transfer (157). Only the pathogenic *Neisseria* have the ability to antigenically vary the pilus, with all Gc strains and most Mc strains having the ability; however, a small subset of Mc strains express a nonvariable pilus that is more similar to the commensal type IV pilus but still can cause invasive disease (158).

In the pathogenic *Neisseria*, pilus expression and antigenicity is modulated by many different mechanisms. There is transcriptional regulation of pilus expression in Mc (159), and if there is transcriptional regulation of pilus expression in Gc, it is by unknown mechanisms. There is stochastic phase variation of pilus expression that can result in three major levels of expression. Most clinical isolates of Gc are piliated, expressing many pili per cell (160, 161). Since Mc do not express the pilus-dependent colony morphology characteristic of Gc, it is less certain whether Mc piliation is also strongly selected for *in vivo*. It is likely that loss of full piliation occurs in both Gc and Mc infections, but this has not been extensively studied. Loss of piliation would allow individual bacterial cells to escape from bacterial communities (either microcolonies or biofilms) to move to different anatomical sites or to different hosts.

Both Gc and Mc can lose a majority of pilus expression through phase variation of the pilus-associated *pilC* genes (162). Both species have two independent *pilC* loci that each have a PNR in their coding sequences that allow them to vary on and off. Expression of either the *pilC1* or *pilC2* locus allows for full piliation (162), although in Mc there have been different reported phenotypes for the PilC1 and PilC2 pili, but this has been disputed (163). However, even when both *pilC* genes are phased off, there remains a low level of pilus expression, and pilus expression can be restored by inactivating the PilT traffic ATPase (164, 165). Low piliation variants can also result from pilin antigenic variation reactions that result in a full-length pilin protein, but one that is either inefficiently assembled into pili or cannot maintain an extended pilus conformation (166, 167). True off phase variation of pilus expression is only achieved when Gc incorporates a silent copy sequence encoding a nonsense codon (89, 166, 168), but not all Gc isolates have silent copies with stop codons, and silent copy-encoded stop codons have not been reported for Mc. Therefore, all of Mc pilus phase variation and a majority of Gc phase variation occurs between full piliation and poor piliation and not between on and off.

Most of the work on the mechanisms of pilin antigenic variation has been done using Gc, and while the central mechanisms are likely to be shared between Gc and Mc, this section will exclusively feature results from Gc, and the relationship to Mc is assumed but has not always been tested. Both Gc strains MS11 and FA1090 have been used to study pilin antigenic variation and have 15 and 19 silent copies, respectively, arranged in different loci both upstream and downstream of the expression locus (169, 170). The silent copies differ from the expression locus in that the silent copies are missing the conserved N-terminal coding sequences, the ribosome binding site, and the transcriptional promoter (Fig. 11A). Thus, although the silent copies do not produce a functional protein, they supply variant sequences to *pilE*. Transcription of the *pilE* gene is not required for pilin antigenic variation, disproving the hypothesis that transcription could differentiate the donor silent copies from the recipient *pilE* locus (171).

Pilin antigenic variation results from the nonreciprocal transfer of variant pilin coding sequences from one of the silent copies to the *pilE* locus (Fig. 11B); thus, the silent copies do not normally change during pilin

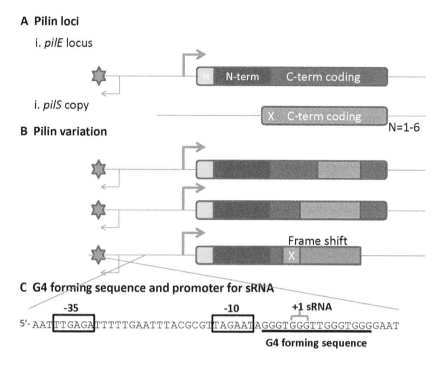

A Pilin loci

i. *pilE* locus

i. *pilS* copy

B Pilin variation

Frame shift

C G4 forming sequence and promoter for sRNA

-35   -10   +1 sRNA

5'- AATTTGAGATTTTTGAATTTACGCGTTAGAATAGGGTGGGTTGGGTGGGGAAT

G4 forming sequence

FIGURE 11 *Neisseria* pilin antigenic variation. **(A) The pilin loci. (i) The pilin expression locus (*pilE*) has a promoter sequence to initiate transcription; a seven-amino-acid signal sequence (SS, green), an absolutely conserved, N-terminal constant coding sequence (N-term, purple), and a variable carboxy-terminal coding sequence (C-term, red). The G4-forming sequence is represented by the blue star, and the sRNA transcript is represented by the thin arrow. (ii) A variant *pilS* gene copy that has variant pilin C-terminal coding sequences (C-term, orange) but cannot express a protein product. This *pilS* copy has a frame shift in the 5′-coding sequences (X). Each *pilS* locus can have one to six repeated *pilS* copies (*N* = 1 to 6). (B) Pilin variation. Nonreciprocal transfer of variant *pilS* copy sequences into the *pilE* locus produces pilin variants. The *pilS* sequences that are transferred can be from any part of the *pilS* copy that overlaps with the *pilE* sequence as long as there are regions of microhomology at the ends of the transferred sequence (not shown). Some (but not all) *pilS* copies encode a frame shift in their 5′ potential coding sequences that can result in an altered reading frame (blue), a premature stop codon, and a nonpiliated variant. (C) The G4-forming sequence and promoter for the *cis*-acting sRNA. The sequence shown is on the bottom strand of the cartoons in parts A and B. The sRNA promoter is indicated by the boxed -10 and -35 sequences. The sRNA required for pilin antigenic variation initiates (+1 sRNA) within the second set of guanines in the G4 forming sequence.**

antigenic variation. However, this may not be true for the silent copies that are located immediately upstream of the *pilE* gene (H.S. Seifert, unpublished observations). The segment of DNA that is transferred can be any part of the silent copy that aligns with the *pilE* sequence (168, 172), and the changes can be as small as one nucleotide or the replacement of the entire sequence by the donor *pilS* copy sequence (168, 172). Many *pilE* variants have sequence information from two silent donors, and some have

three or more. The transferred sequence is always bordered by regions of micro homology that can be as small as 3 bp (168, 172). The frequency of variants can be from 3 to 15% depending on the species and strain, and not all silent copies recombine at the same frequency (168, 173, 174). However, the rules that govern the frequency of each donor silent copy used have not been determined. The multiple donor silent copies located at positions on either side of the recipient *pilE* gene create an issue for modeling how gene conversion can occur within a bacterial chromosome. This led to the hypothesis that recombination might occur between sister chromosomes, and it was found that both Gc and Mc have two chromosomal copies, while the most closely related commensal that does not undergo pilin antigenic variation (*Neisseria lactamica*) has one chromosomal copy (175, 176). These pathogenic *Neisseria* are still genetically haploid since Gc cannot maintain different alleles at the same locus (176).

Pilin antigenic variation relies on the general recombination and repair systems common to most bacterial species. The process is absolutely dependent on having functional RecA, RecO, and RecR recombinases and shows reduced frequencies when RecQ, RecJ, Rep, RecX, RdgC, RuvABC, or RecG are inactivated by mutation (89, 177–182). The partial phenotypes of some of these factors may be due to redundancy (e.g., the helicases RecQ and Rep), an enhancing role on another factor (e.g., RecX on RecA), or the processing of different substrates that can lead to antigenic variation (not known). In addition, the Holliday junction–processing helicases RuvAB and RecG are both individually required for pilin antigenic variation, but a double mutant with *recG* and any one of the *ruvABC* genes produces synthetic lethality only when pilin antigenic variation can occur (183). Thus, cells that do not initiate pilin antigenic variation can survive, as do cells that have deleted the *pilE* locus (183). Inactivation of many of the recombinases required for pilin antigenic variation can also prevent the synthetic lethality (183; H.S. Seifert, unpublished data). Inactivation of mismatch correction increases the frequency of pilin antigenic variation (and also PilC phase variation) (184), and loss of mismatch correction also increases the level of synthetic lethality (192).

Several sequences are required for pilin antigenic variation. The first identified was called the Sma/Cla repeat since it often has sites for the *Sma* I and *Cla* I restriction endonucleases (185). This repeat is present at the 3′ end of all pilin loci, both *pilE* and each *pilS* locus, regardless of the number of *pilS* copies in that locus. It has been suggested that the Sma/Cla repeat binds an unknown recombinase (186), but it is likely that the Sma/Cla sequence provides an extended region of 3′-homology for recombination during pilin antigenic variation. The second site that has been suggested to be important for pilin antigenic variation is the *cys2* sequence within the *pilE* and *pilS* copies. This sequence encodes an invariant 10-amino-acid segment of the pilin protein that contains one of the two conserved cysteines. If the ~30-bp conserved *cys2* region is interrupted with an antibiotic resistance cassette or a 10-bp linker, normal pilin antigenic variation is disrupted, even though the same 10-bp linker inserted into the neighboring hypervariable loop sequences has no effect on the reactions (187). It has not been determined whether the *cys2* sequence is important to provide a stretch of homology during recombination or plays a more active role in the process.

The most important *cis*-acting sequence that has been described is the *pilE*-associated G4-forming sequence (93). The existence of this element was suggested by transposon insertions that totally inactivated pilin antigenic variation (171, 182). These transposons were located upstream of the *pilE* gene, were not within an open reading frame, and did not alter pilin expression (171, 182). Saturation mutagenesis of the region containing the transposon insertions showed that single point mutations in any one of 12 G-C bps disrupt pilin antigenic variation (93) (Fig. 11). Mutation of the four T-A bp within the region of G-C bp or sequences immediately adjacent to this GC-rich segment had no effect on pilin antigenic variation (93). The G-rich strand was predicted to form a G4 structure, and this prediction was confirmed by a series of *in vitro* assays (93). The structure of this G4 determined by nuclear magnetic resonance spectroscopy predicted that the G4 structure could bind to RecA, and this was confirmed experimentally (94). Interestingly, other G4-forming sequences precisely replacing the *pilE* G4 sequence could not mediate pilin antigenic variation and did not bind RecA (93, 94). Whether RecA binding to the *pilE* G4 structure is important for pilin antigenic variation has not been determined.

Activity of the G4-forming sequence was also found to depend on a promoter element that was located between the G4-forming sequence and the *pilE* that transcribes the G-rich strand the opposite direction from the *pilE* gene (188). The transcript produced initiates within the second set of guanines within the G4-forming sequence, but this transcript is of low abundance and does not appear to have a defined 3′-end (188). It is likely that this transcript allows the G4 structure to form by melting the DNA duplex and occluding the C-rich strand through the formation of an R-loop. What molecular steps follow these reactions are not known. Expression of the G4 structure and transcript at an ectopic locus does not rescue a promoter mutation, showing that this element must be present in *cis* (188). Moreover, the G4-forming sequence and associated transcript only work in the normal orientation at the normal location in the chromosome. If the direction is reversed or the G-rich and C-rich strand are exchanged, antigenic variation cannot proceed (188). One hypothesis that might explain the orientation is that the G4 structure is on the lagging strand, while the putative R-loop is on the leading strand and that these elements act by specifically interacting with the replication apparatus. A replication-interrupting structure may be a common mechanism of initiating recombination-based diversity generation since other G-rich sequences have been subsequently proposed to have roles in *Borrelia* (92) and *Treponema pallidum* antigenic variation (189). When replication stalls at the G-rich site, a programmed recombina-tion/repair process occurs to initiate each phenotypic variation process.

Knowledge Gaps

The three major variation systems expressed by the pathogenic *Neisseria* species strongly suggest that they are under strong selection for stochastically produced subpopulations. While we assume that this selection is immune-based, it is almost certain that the initial evolution of these diversity-generating systems was based on functional alterations (e.g., different Opa receptors) and not immune selection. Like many issues in biology, these diversity-generation systems are used for more than one function. Regardless of whether it is functional, immune selection, or both, the existence and conservation of these systems also suggest that the pathogenic *Neisseria* function as populations to allow subpopulations to be selected for rather than regulation that effects the entire population.

What is most notable about *Neisseria* antigenic variation is that these are mostly mucosal pathogens, while many of the other antigenically variable organisms are blood-borne and regularly exposed to antibody and phagocyte surveillance. It is possible that the ability to continually infect the high-risk, core group of the sexually active population is the driving selective force behind Gc variation. However, there are reports that Gc infection is immune-suppressive (190), which begs the question of why such a large amount of antigenic variation is necessary. The case for immune selection is less obvious for Mc, with its largely commensal lifestyle and smaller capacity for variation. With Mc it may be functional selection that remains the driving force for phenotypic variation, and whether phenotypic variation contributes to invasive disease remains unanswered.

While there have been many advances into understanding the mechanisms behind the gene conversion reactions that underlie pilin antigenic variation, there are many open questions remaining. Are the mechanisms used by Mc identical to those used by Gc? Does recombination occur between diploid chromosomes? Does the G4 sRNA play a direct role in the process? Is there a factor that facilitates G4 structure formation? Does G4 structure formation promote recombination through inhibiting replication, binding a recombinase, or both? What other sites are required to complete this high-frequency, gene conversion process? Is this a homologous recombination process using heteroduplex, an annealing process, or both? Answering these questions will increase our understanding of the possible mechanisms that allow all of the phenotypic variation in prokaryotes and eukaryotes that rely on recombination.

ACKNOWLEDGMENTS

This work was supported by National Institute of Allergy and Infectious Diseases (NIAID) grants R37 AI44005 (GHP); RO1 AI108704 and R21 AI101230 (TB); R37 AI033493 and RO1 AI044239 (HSS).

CITATION

Palmer GH, Bankhead T, Seifert HS. 2016. Antigenic variation in bacterial pathogens. Microbiol Spectrum 4(1):VMBF-0005-2015.

REFERENCES

1. **Ross T, Thomson D.** 1910. A case of sleeping sickness studied by precise enumerative methods: regular periodic increase of the parasites disclosed. *Ann Trop Med Parasitol* **4:**261–264.
2. **Holland J, Spindler K, Horodyski F, Grabau E, Nichol S, VandePol S.** 1982. Rapid evolution of RNA genomes. *Science* **215:**1577–1585.
3. **Deitsch KW, Lukehart SA, Stringer JR.** 2009. Common strategies for antigenic variation by bacterial, fungal and protozoan pathogens. *Nature Rev Microbiol* **7:**493–503.
4. **Palmer GH, Bankhead T, Lukehart SA.** 2009. Nothing is permanent but change: antigenic variation in persistent bacterial pathogens. *Cell Microbiol* **11:**1697–1705.
5. **Theiler A.** 1910. *Anaplasma marginale* (gen. spec. nov.). The marginal points in the blood of cattle suffering from a specific disease. Report of the government veterinary bacteriologist, 1908–1909. Transvaal, South Africa.
6. **Palmer GH.** 2009. Sir Arnold Theiler and the discovery of anaplasmosis: a centennial perspective. *Onderstepoort J Vet Res* **76:**75–79.
7. **Dumler JS, Barbet AF, Bekker CPJ, Dasch GA, Palmer GH, Ray SC, Rikihisa Y, Rurangirwa FR.** 2001. Reorganization of genera in the families *Rickettsiaceae* and *Anaplasmataceae* in the order *Rickettsiales*; unification of some species of *Ehrlichia* with *Anaplasma, Cowdria* with *Ehrlichia,* and *Ehrlichia* with *Neorickettsia*; descriptions of six new species combinations; and designation of *Ehrlichia equi* and "HGE agent" as subjective synonyms of *Ehrlichia phagocytophila. Int J Sys Evol Microbiol* **51:**2145–2165.
8. **Dunning Hotopp JC, Lin M, Madupu R, Crabtree J, Angiuoli SV, Eisen JA, Seshadri R, Ren Q, Wu M, Utterback TR, Smith S, Lewis M, Khouri H, Zhang C, Niu H, Lin Q, Ohashi N, Zhi N, Nelson W, Brinkac LM, Dodson RJ, Rosovitz MJ, Sundaram J, Daugherty SC, Davidsen T, Durkin AS, Gwinn M, Haft DH, Selengut JD, Sullivan SA, Zafar N, Zhou L, Benahmed F, Forberger H, Halpin R, Mulligan S, Robinson J, White O, Rikihisa Y, Tettelin H.** 2006. Comparative genomics of emerging human ehrlichiosis agents. *PLoS Genet* **2:**e21.
9. **Granquist EG, Stuen S, Crosby L, Lundgren AM, Alleman AR, Barbet AF.** 2010. Variant-specific and diminishing immune responses towards the highly variable MSP2(P44) outer membrane protein of *Anaplasma phagocytophilum* during persistent infection in lambs. *Vet Immunol Immunopathol* **133:**117–124.
10. **Rejmanek D, Foley P, Barbet A, Foley J.** 2012. Antigenic variability in *Anaplasma phagocytophilum* during chronic infection of a reservoir host. *Microbiol* **158:**2632–2641.
11. **Lai TH, Orellana NG, Yuasa Y, Rikihisa Y.** 2011. Cloning of the major outer membrane protein expression locus in *Anaplasma platys* and seroreactivity of a species-specific antigen. *J Bacteriol* **193:**2924–2930.
12. **Palmer GH, Abbott JR, French DM, McElwain TF.** 1998. Persistence of *Anaplasma ovis* infection and conservation of the *msp2* and *msp3* multigene families within the genus *Anaplasma. Infect Immun* **66:**6035–6039.
13. **Palmer GH, Brown WC, Rurangirwa FR.** 2000. Antigenic variation in the persistence and

transmission of the ehrlichia *Anaplasma marginale. Microb Infect* **2:**167–176.

14. **French DF, McElwain TF, McGuire TC, Palmer GH.** 1998. Expression of *Anaplasma marginale* major surface protein 2 variants during persistent cyclic rickettsemia. *Infect Immun* **66:**1200–1207.

15. **Eriks IS, Stiller D, Palmer GH.** 1993. Impact of persistent *Anaplasma marginale* rickettsemia on tick infection and transmission. *J Clin Microbiol* **31:**2091–2096.

16. **Scoles GA, Broce AB, Lysyk TJ, Palmer GH.** 2005. Relative efficiency of biological transmission of *Anaplasma marginale* (Rickettsiales: Anaplasmataceae) by *Dermacentor andersoni* Stiles (Acari: Ixodidae) compared to mechanical transmission by the stable fly, *Stomoxys calcitrans* (L.) (Diptera: Muscidae). *J Med Entomol* **42:**668–675.

17. **Ueti MW, Knowles DP, Davitt CM, Scoles GA, Baszler TV, Palmer GH.** 2009. Quantitative differences in salivary pathogen load during tick transmission underlie strain-specific variation in transmission efficiency of *Anaplasma marginale. Infect Immun* **77:**70–75.

18. **Brayton KA, Kappmeyer LS, Herndon DR, Dark MJ, Tibbals DL, Palmer GH, McGuire TC, Knowles DP.** 2005. Complete genome sequencing of *Anaplasma marginale* reveals that the surface is skewed to two superfamilies of outer membrane proteins. *Proc Natl Acad Sci USA* **102:**844–849.

19. **Noh SM, Brayton KA, Knowles DP, Agnes JT, Dark MJ, Brown WC, Baszler TV, Palmer GH.** 2006. Differential expression and sequence conservation of the *Anaplasma marginale msp2* gene superfamily outer membrane proteins. *Infect Immun* **74:**3471–3479.

20. **Noh SM, Brayton KA, Brown WC, Norimine J, Munske GR, Davitt CM, Palmer GH.** 2008. Composition of the surface proteome of *Anaplasma marginale* and its role in protective immunity induced by outer membrane immunization. *Infect Immun* **76:**2219–2226.

21. **Palmer GH, Brown WC, Noh SM, Brayton KA.** 2012. Genome-wide screening and identification of antigens for rickettsial vaccine development. *FEMS Immunol Med Microbiol* **64:**115–119.

22. **Palmer GH, Barbet AF, Kuttler KL, McGuire TC.** 1986. Detection of an *Anaplasma marginale* common surface protein present in all stages of infection. *J Clin Micro* **23:**1078–1083.

23. **McGuire TC, Davis WC, Brassfield AL, McElwain TF, Palmer GH.** 1991. Identification of *Anaplasma marginale* long-term carrier cattle by detection of serum antibody to isolated MSP-3. *J Clin Microbiol* **29:**788–793.

24. **Palmer GH, Eid G, Barbet AF, McGuire TC, McElwain TF.** 1994. The immunoprotective *Anaplasma marginale* major surface protein-2 (MSP-2) is encoded by a polymorphic multigene family. *Infect Immun* **62:**3808–3816.

25. **Meeus PFM, Brayton KA, Palmer GH, Barbet AF.** 2003. Conservation of a gene conversion mechanism in two distantly related paralogues of *Anaplasma marginale. Mol Microbiol* **47:**633–643.

26. **Brayton KA, Knowles DP, McGuire TC, Palmer GH.** 2001. Efficient use of small genome to generate antigenic diversity in tick-borne ehrlichial pathogens. *Proc Natl Acad Sci USA* **98:**4130–4135.

27. **French DM, Brown WC, Palmer GH.** 1999. Emergence of *Anaplasma marginale* antigenic variants during persistent rickettsemia. *Infect Immun* **67:**5834–5840.

28. **Brayton KA, Meeus PFM, Barbet AF, Palmer GH.** 2003. Simultaneous variation of the immunodominant outer membrane proteins MSP2 and MSP3 during *Anaplasma marginale* persistence *in vivo. Infect Immun* **71:**6627–6632.

29. **Abbott JR, Palmer GH, Howard CJ, Hope JC, Brown WC.** 2004. *Anaplasma marginale* major surface protein 2 CD4$^+$ T-cell epitopes are evenly distributed in conserved and hypervariable regions (HVR), whereas linear B-cell epitopes are predominantly located in the HVR. *Infect Immun* **72:**7360–7366.

30. **Zhuang Y, Futse JE, Brown WC, Brayton KA, Palmer GH.** 2007. Maintenance of antibody to pathogen epitopes generated by segmental gene conversion is highly dynamic during long-term persistent infection. *Infect Immun* **75:**5185–5190.

31. **Brown WC, Brayton KA, Styer CM, Palmer GH.** 2003. The hypervariable region of *Anaplasma marginale* major surface protein 2 (MSP2) contains multiple immunodominant CD4$^+$ T lymphocyte epitopes that elicit variant-specific proliferative and IFN-γ responses in MSP2 vaccinates. *J Immunol* **170:**3790–3798.

32. **Han S, Norimine J, Palmer GH, Mwangi W, Lahmers KK, Brown WC.** 2008. Rapid deletion of antigen-specific CD4+ T 1 cells following infection represents a strategy of immune evasion and persistence for *Anaplasma marginale. J Immunol* **181:**7759–7769.

33. **Han S, Norimine J, Brayton KA, Palmer GH, Scoles GA, Brown WC.** 2010. *Anaplasma marginale* infection with persistent high load

bacteremia induces a dysfunctional memory CD4+ T lymphocyte response but sustained high IgG titers. *Clin Vaccine Immunol* **17:**1881–1890.

34. **Turse JE, Scoles GA, Deringer JR, Fry LM, Brown WC.** 2014. Immunization-induced *Anaplasma marginale*-specific T-lymphocyte responses impaired by *A. marginale* infection are restored after eliminating infection with tetracycline. *Clin Vaccine Immunol* **21:**1369–1375.

35. **Futse JE, Brayton KA, Knowles DP, Palmer GH.** 2005. Structural basis for segmental gene conversion in generation of *Anaplasma marginale* outer membrane protein variants. *Mol Microbiol* **57:**212–221.

36. **Futse JE, Brayton KA, Nydam SD, Palmer GH.** 2009. Generation of antigenic variants by gene conversion: evidence for recombination fitness selection at the locus level in *Anaplasma marginale*. *Infect Immun* **71:**6627–6632.

37. **Dark MJ, Herndon D, Kappmeyer LS, Gonzales MP, Nordeen E, Palmer GH, Knowles DP, Brayton KA.** 2009. Conservation in the face of diversity: multistrain analysis of an intracellular bacterium. *BMC Genomics* **10:**16–28.

38. **Barbet AF, Lundgren A, Yi J, Rurangirwa FR, Palmer GH.** 2000. Antigenic variation of *Anaplasma marginale* by expression of MSP2 sequence mosaics. *Infect Immun* **68:**6133–6138.

39. **Brayton KA, Palmer GH, Lundgren A, Yi J, Barbet AF.** 2002. Antigenic variation of *Anaplasma marginale msp2* occurs by combinatorial gene conversion. *Mol Microbiol* **43:**1151–1159.

40. **Ueti MW, Tan Y, Broschat SL, Castañeda Ortiz EJ, Camacho-Nuez M, Mosqueda JJ, Scoles GA, Grimes M, Brayton KA, Palmer GH.** 2012. Expansion of variant diversity associated with high prevalence of pathogen strain superinfection under conditions of natural transmission. *Infect Immun* **80:**2354–2360.

41. **Palmer GH, Futse JE, Leverich CK, Knowles DP, Rurangirwa FR, Brayton KA.** 2007. Selection for simple Msp2 variants during *Anaplasma marginale* transmission to immunologically naïve animals. *Infect Immun* **75:**1502–1506.

42. **Löhr CV, Rurangirwa FR, McElwain TF, Stiller D, Palmer GH.** 2002. Specific expression of *Anaplasma marginale* major surface protein 2 salivary gland variants occurs in the midgut and is an early event during tick transmission. *Infect Immun* **70:**114–120.

43. **Rurangirwa FR, Stiller DS, French DM, Palmer GH.** 1999. Restriction of major surface protein 2 (MSP2) variants during tick transmission of the ehrlichiae *Anaplasma marginale*. *Proc Natl Acad Sci USA* **96:**3171–3176.

44. **Smith DM, Richman DD, Little SJ.** 2005. HIV superinfection. *J Infect Dis* **192:**438–444.

45. **Blackard JT.** 2012. HCV superinfection and reinfection. *Antivir Ther* **17:**1443–1448.

46. **Palmer GH, Knowles DP, Rodriguez JL, Gnad DP, Hollis LC, Marston T, Brayton KA.** 2004. Stochastic transmission of multiple genotypically distinct *Anaplasma marginale* strains within an endemic herd. *J Clin Microbiol* **42:**5381–5384.

47. **Rodriguez JL, Palmer GH, Knowles DP, Brayton KA.** 2005. Distinctly different *msp2* pseudogene repertoires in *Anaplasma marginale* strains that are capable of superinfection. *Gene* **361:**127–132.

48. **Futse JE, Brayton KA, Dark MJ, Knowles DP, Palmer GH.** 2008. Superinfection as a driver of genomic diversification in antigenically variant pathogens. *Proc Natl Acad Sci USA* **105:**2123–2127.

49. **Vallejo Esquerra E, Herndon DR, Alpirez Mendoza F, Mosqueda J, Palmer GH.** 2014. *Anaplasma marginale* superinfection attributable to pathogen strains with distinct genomic backgrounds. *Infect Immun* **82:**5286–5292.

50. **Rogovsky AS, Bankhead T.** 2014. Bacterial heterogeneity is a requirement for host superinfection by the Lyme disease spirochete. *Infect Immun* **82:**4542–4552.

51. **Palmer GH, Rurangirwa FR, McElwain TF.** 2001. Strain composition of the ehrlichia *Anaplasma marginale* within persistently infected cattle, a mammalian reservoir for tick-transmission. *J Clin Microbiol* **39:**631–635.

52. **De la Fuente J, Passos LM, Van Den Bussche RA, Ribeiro MF, Facury-Filho EJ, Kocan KM.** 2004. Genetic diversity and molecular phylogeny of *Anaplasma marginale* isolates from Minas Gerais, Brazil. *Vet Parasitol* **121:**307–316.

53. **Ruybal P, Moretta R, Perez A, Petrigh R, Zimmer P, Alcarez E, Echaide I, Torioni de Echaide S, Kocan KM, de la Fuente J, Farber M.** 2009. Genetic diversity of *Anaplasma marginale* in Argentina. *Vet Parasitol* **162:**176–180.

54. **Palmer GH, Brayton KA.** 2013. Antigenic variation and transmission fitness as drivers of bacterial strain structure. *Cell Microbiol* **15:**1969–1975.

55. **Paster BJ, Dewhirst FE, Weisburg WG, Tordoff LA, Fraser GJ, Hespell RB, Stanton TB, Zablen L, Mandelco L, Woese CR.** 1991. Phylogenetic analysis of the spirochetes. *J Bacteriol* **173:**6101–6109.

56. **Radolf JD, Samuels DS.** 2010. *Borrelia: Molecular Biology, Host Interaction, and Pathogenesis.* Caister Academic Press, Norfolk, UK.

57. **Ras NM, Lascola B, Postic D, Cutler SJ, Rodhain F, Baranton G, Raoult D.** 1996. Phylogenesis of relapsing fever *Borrelia* spp. *Int J Sys Bacteriol* **46:**859–865.

58. **Schwan TG, Raffel SJ, Schrumpf ME, Porcella SF.** 2007. Diversity and distribution of *Borrelia hermsii. Emerg Infect Dis* **13:**436–442.

59. **Stoenner HG, Dodd T, Larsen C.** 1982. Antigenic variation of *Borrelia hermsii. J Exp Med* **156:**1297–1311.

60. **Barbour AG, Restrepo BI.** 2000. Antigenic variation in vector-borne pathogens. *Emerg Infect Dis* **6:**449–457.

61. **Plasterk RH, Simon MI, Barbour AG.** 1985. Transposition of structural genes to an expression sequence on a linear plasmid causes antigenic variation in the bacterium *Borrelia hermsii. Nature* **318:**257–263.

62. **Barbour AG, Bundoc V.** 2001. *In vitro* and *in vivo* neutralization of the relapsing fever agent *Borrelia hermsii* with serotype-specific immunoglobulin M antibodies. *Infect Immun* **69:**1009–1015.

63. **Connolly SE, Benach JL.** 2001. Cutting edge: the spirochetemia of murine relapsing fever is cleared by complement-independent bactericidal antibodies. *J Immunol* **167:**3029–3032.

64. **Barbour AG.** 2001. *Borrelia*: a diverse and ubiquitous genus of tick-borne pathogens, p 153–173. *In* Scheld MW, Craig WA, Hughes JM (ed), *Emerging Infections 5.* ASM Press, Washington, DC.

65. **Steere AC, Coburn J, Glickstein L.** 2004. The emergence of Lyme disease. *J Clin Invest* **113:**1093–1101.

66. **Norris SJ.** 2006. Antigenic variation with a twist: the *Borrelia* story. *Mol Microbiol* **60:**1319–1322.

67. **Zhang JR, Hardham JM, Barbour AG, Norris SJ.** 1997. Antigenic variation in Lyme disease borreliae by promiscuous recombination of VMP-like sequence cassettes. *Cell* **89:**275–285.

68. **Zhang JR, Norris SJ.** 1998. Genetic variation of the *Borrelia burgdorferi* gene *vlsE* involves cassette-specific, segmental gene conversion. *Infect Immun* **66:**3698–3704.

69. **Zhang JR, Norris SJ.** 1998. Kinetics and *in vivo* induction of genetic variation of *vlsE* in *Borrelia burgdorferi. Infect Immun* **66:**3689–3697.

70. **Hudson CR, Frye JG, Quinn FD, Gherardini FC.** 2001. Increased expression of *Borrelia burgdorferi* vlsE in response to human endothelial cell membranes. *Mol Microbiol* **41:**229–239.

71. **Indest KJ, Howell JK, Jacobs MB, Scholl-Meeker D, Norris SJ, Philipp MT.** 2001. Analysis of *Borrelia burgdorferi* vlsE gene expression and recombination in the tick vector. *Infect Immun* **69:**7083–7090.

72. **McDowell JV, Sung SY, Hu LT, Marconi RT.** 2002. Evidence that the variable regions of the central domain of VlsE are antigenic during infection with Lyme disease spirochetes. *Infect Immun* **70:**4196–4203.

73. **Labandeira-Rey M, Skare JT.** 2001. Decreased infectivity in *Borrelia burgdorferi* strain B31 is associated with loss of linear plasmid 25 or 28-1. *Infect Immun* **69:**446–455.

74. **Purser JE, Norris SJ.** 2000. Correlation between plasmid content and infectivity in *Borrelia burgdorferi. Proc Natl Acad Sci USA* **97:**13865–13870.

75. **Labandeira-Rey M, Seshu J, Skare JT.** 2003. The absence of linear plasmid 25 or 28-1 of *Borrelia burgdorferi* dramatically alters the kinetics of experimental infection via distinct mechanisms. *Infect Immun* **71:**4608–4613.

76. **Purser JE, Lawrenz MB, Caimano MJ, Howell JK, Radolf JD, Norris SJ.** 2003. A plasmid-encoded nicotinamidase (PncA) is essential for infectivity of *Borrelia burgdorferi* in a mammalian host. *Mol Microbiol* **48:**753–764.

77. **Lawrenz MB, Wooten RM, Norris SJ.** 2004. Effects of *vlsE* complementation on the infectivity of *Borrelia burgdorferi* lacking the linear plasmid lp28-1. *Infect Immun* **72:**6577–6585.

78. **Bankhead T, Chaconas G.** 2007. The role of VlsE antigenic variation in the Lyme disease spirochete: persistence through a mechanism that differs from other pathogens. *Mol Microbiol* **65:**1547–1558.

79. **Beaurepaire C, Chaconas G.** 2005. Mapping of essential replication functions of the linear plasmid lp17 of *B. burgdorferi* by targeted deletion walking. *Mol Microbiol* **57:**132–142.

80. **Chaconas G.** 2005. Hairpin telomere and genome plasticity in *Borrelia*: all mixed up in the end. *Mol Microbiol* **58:**625–635.

81. **Kobryn K, Chaconas G.** 2002. ResT, a telomere resolvase encoded by the Lyme disease spirochete. *Mol Cell* **9:**195–201.

82. **Embers ME, Alvarez X, Ooms T, Philipp MT.** 2008. The failure of immune response evasion by linear plasmid 28-1-deficient *Borrelia burgdorferi* is attributable to persistent expression of an outer surface protein. *Infect Immun* **76:**3984–3991.

83. **Fung BP, McHugh GL, Leong JM, Steere AC.** 1994. Humoral immune response to outer

surface protein C of *Borrelia burgdorferi* in Lyme disease: role of the immunoglobulin M response in the serodiagnosis of early infection. *Infect Immun* **62:**3213–3221.

84. **Liang FT, Brown EL, Wang T, Iozzo RV, Fikrig E.** 2004. Protective niche for *Borrelia burgdorferi* to evade humoral immunity. *Am J Pathol* **165:**977–985.

85. **Xu Q, Seemanapalli SV, McShan K, Liang FT.** 2006. Constitutive expression of outer surface protein C diminishes the ability of *Borrelia burgdorferi* to evade specific humoral immunity. *Infect Immun* **74:**5177–5184.

86. **Casjens S, Palmer N, Van Vugt R, Huang WH, Stevenson B, Rosa P, Lathigra R, Sutton G, Peterson J, Dodson RJ, Haft D, Hickey E, Gwinn M, White O, Fraser CM.** 2000. A bacterial genome in flux: the twelve linear and nine circular extrachromosomal DNAs in an infectious isolate of the Lyme disease spirochete *Borrelia burgdorferi*. *Mol Microbiol* **35:**490–516.

87. **Coutte L, Botkin DJ, Gao L, Norris SJ.** 2009. Detailed analysis of sequence changes occurring during vlsE antigenic variation in the mouse model of *Borrelia burgdorferi* infection. *PLoS Pathog* **5:**e1000293. doi:10.1371/journal.ppat.1000293.

88. **Liveris D, Mulay V, Sandigursky S, Schwartz I.** 2008. *Borrelia burgdorferi* vlsE antigenic variation is not mediated by RecA. *Infect Immun* **76:**4009–4018.

89. **Koomey M, Gotschlich EC, Robbins K, Bergstrom S, Swanson J.** 1987. Effects of recA mutations on pilus antigenic variation and phase transitions in *Neisseria gonorrhoeae*. *Genetics* **117:**391–398.

90. **Dresser AR, Hardy PO, Chaconas G.** 2009. Investigation of the genes involved in antigenic switching at the vlsE locus in *Borrelia burgdorferi*: an essential role for the RuvAB branch migrase. *PLoS Pathog* **5:**e1000680. doi:10.1371/journal.ppat.1000680.

91. **Lin T, Gao L, Edmondson DG, Jacobs MB, Philipp MT, Norris SJ.** 2009. Central role of the Holliday junction helicase RuvAB in vlsE recombination and infectivity of *Borrelia burgdorferi*. *PLoS Pathog* **5:**e1000679. doi:10.1371/journal.ppat.1000679.

92. **Walia R, Chaconas G.** 2013. Suggested role for G4 DNA in recombinational switching at the antigenic variation locus of the Lyme disease spirochete. *PLoS One* **8:**e57792. doi:10.1371/journal.pone.0057792.

93. **Cahoon LA, Seifert HS.** 2009. An alternative DNA structure is necessary for pilin antigenic variation in *Neisseria gonorrhoeae*. *Science* **325:**764–767.

94. **Kuryavyi V, Cahoon LA, Seifert HS, Patel DJ.** 2012. RecA-binding pilE G4 sequence essential for pilin antigenic variation forms monomeric and 5′ end-stacked dimeric parallel G-quadruplexes. *Structure* **20:**2090–2102.

95. **Eicken C, Sharma V, Klabunde T, Lawrenz MB, Hardham JM, Norris SJ, Sacchettini JC.** 2002. Crystal structure of Lyme disease variable surface antigen VlsE of *Borrelia burgdorferi*. *J Biol Chem* **277:**21691–21696.

96. **Zuckert WR.** 2013. A call to order at the spirochaetal host-pathogen interface. *Mol Microbiol* **89:**207–211.

97. **Bacon RM, Biggerstaff BJ, Schriefer ME, Gilmore RD Jr, Philipp MT, Steere AC, Wormser GP, Marques AR, Johnson BJ.** 2003. Serodiagnosis of Lyme disease by kinetic enzyme-linked immunosorbent assay using recombinant VlsE1 or peptide antigens of *Borrelia burgdorferi* compared with 2-tiered testing using whole-cell lysates. *J Infect Dis* **187:**1187–1199.

98. **Embers ME, Jacobs MB, Johnson BJ, Philipp MT.** 2007. Dominant epitopes of the C6 diagnostic peptide of *Borrelia burgdorferi* are largely inaccessible to antibody on the parent VlsE molecule. *Clin Vaccine Immunol* **14:**931–936.

99. **Embers ME, Wormser GP, Schwartz I, Martin DS, Philipp MT.** 2007. *Borrelia burgdorferi* spirochetes that harbor only a portion of the lp28-1 plasmid elicit antibody responses detectable with the C6 test for Lyme disease. *Clin Vaccine Immunol* **14:**90–93.

100. **Liang FT, Steere AC, Marques AR, Johnson BJ, Miller JN, Philipp MT.** 1999. Sensitive and specific serodiagnosis of Lyme disease by enzyme-linked immunosorbent assay with a peptide based on an immunodominant conserved region of *Borrelia burgdorferi* vlsE. *J Clin Microbiol* **37:**3990–3996.

101. **Schulte-Spechtel U, Lehnert G, Liegl G, Fingerle V, Heimerl C, Johnson BJ, Wilske B.** 2003. Significant improvement of the recombinant *Borrelia*-specific immunoglobulin G immunoblot test by addition of VlsE and a DbpA homologue derived from *Borrelia garinii* for diagnosis of early neuroborreliosis. *J Clin Microbiol* **41:**1299–1303.

102. **Liang FT, Yan J, Mbow ML, Sviat SL, Gilmore RD, Mamula M, Fikrig E.** 2004. *Borrelia burgdorferi* changes its surface antigenic expression in response to host immune responses. *Infect Immun* **72:**5759–5767.

103. **Crother TR, Champion CI, Wu XY, Blanco DR, Miller JN, Lovett MA.** 2003. Antigenic composition of *Borrelia burgdorferi* during

infection of SCID mice. *Infect Immun* **71**:3419–3428.

104. **Barry JD, Ginger ML, Burton P, McCulloch R.** 2003. Why are parasite contingency genes often associated with telomeres? *Int J Parasitol* **33**:29–45.

105. **Kraemer SM, Smith JD.** 2006. A family affair: *var* genes, PfEMP1 binding, and malaria disease. *Curr Opin Microbiol* **9**:374–380.

106. **Wang D, Botkin DJ, Norris SJ.** 2003. Characterization of the *vls* antigenic variation loci of the Lyme disease spirochaetes *Borrelia garinii* Ip90 and *Borrelia afzelii* ACAI. *Mol Microbiol* **47**:1407–1417.

107. **Liang FT, Jacobs MB, Bowers LC, Philipp MT.** 2002. An immune evasion mechanism for spirochetal persistence in Lyme borreliosis. *J Exp Med* **195**:415–422.

108. **Philipp MT, Bowers LC, Fawcett PT, Jacobs MB, Liang FT, Marques AR, Mitchell PD, Purcell JE, Ratterree MS, Straubinger RK.** 2001. Antibody response to IR6, a conserved immunodominant region of the VlsE lipoprotein, wanes rapidly after antibiotic treatment of *Borrelia burgdorferi* infection in experimental animals and in humans. *J Infect Dis* **184**:870–878.

109. **Tilly K, Bestor A, Rosa PA.** 2013. Lipoprotein succession in *Borrelia burgdorferi*: similar but distinct roles for OspC and VlsE at different stages of mammalian infection. *Mol Microbiol* **89**:216–227.

110. **LaRocca TJ, Crowley JT, Cusack BJ, Pathak P, Benach J, London E, Garcia-Monco JC, Benach JL.** 2010. Cholesterol lipids of *Borrelia burgdorferi* form lipid rafts and are required for the bactericidal activity of a complement-independent antibody. *Cell Host Microbe* **8**:331–342.

111. **Toledo A, Crowley JT, Coleman JL, LaRocca TJ, Chiantia S, London E, Benach JL.** 2014. Selective association of outer surface lipoproteins with the lipid rafts of *Borrelia burgdorferi*. *mBio* **5**:e00899-00814. doi:10.1128/mBio.00899-14.

112. **Dzikowski R, Templeton TJ, Deitsch K.** 2006. Variant antigen gene expression in malaria. *Cell Microbiol* **8**:1371–1381.

113. **Taylor JE, Rudenko G.** 2006. Switching trypanosome coats: what's in the wardrobe? *Trends Genet* **22**:614–620.

114. **Bunikis J, Barbour AG.** 1999. Access of antibody or trypsin to an integral outer membrane protein (P66) of *Borrelia burgdorferi* is hindered by Osp lipoproteins. *Infect Immun* **67**:2874–2883.

115. **Rogovskyy AS, Bankhead T.** 2013. Variable VlsE is critical for host reinfection by the Lyme disease spirochete. *PLoS One* **8**:e61226. doi:10.1371/journal.pone.0061226.

116. **Barthold SW.** 1999. Specificity of infection-induced immunity among *Borrelia burgdorferi sensu lato* species. *Infect Immun* **67**:36–42.

117. **de Silva AM, Fikrig E, Hodzic E, Kantor FS, Telford SR 3rd, Barthold SW.** 1998. Immune evasion by tickborne and host-adapted *Borrelia burgdorferi*. *J Infect Dis* **177**:395–400.

118. **Virji M.** 2009. Pathogenic *Neisseriae*: surface modulation, pathogenesis and infection control. *Nat Rev Microbiol* **7**:274–286.

119. **Morton RS.** 1977. Gonorrhoea in earlier times, p 1–24. *In* Morton RS (ed), *Gonorrhoea*, vol. 9, W.B. Saunders, London, UK.

120. **Ndowa FJ, Ison CA, Cole MJ, Lusti-Narasimhan M.** 2013. Gonococcal antimicrobial resistance: challenges for public health control. *Sex Transm Infect* **89**(Suppl 4):iv3–4.

121. **Kellogg DS Jr, Thayer JD.** 1969. Virulence of gonococci. *Annu Rev Med* **20**:323–328.

122. **Morse SA.** 1978. The biology of the gonococcus. *CRC Crit Rev Microbiol* **7**:93–189.

123. **Lewis DA.** 2013. The role of core groups in the emergence and dissemination of antimicrobial-resistant *N gonorrhoeae*. *Sex Transm Infect* **89**(Suppl 4):iv47–51.

124. **Caugant DA, Maiden MC.** 2009. Meningococcal carriage and disease: population biology and evolution. *Vaccine* **27**(Suppl 2):B64–70.

125. **Pizza M, Rappuoli R.** 2014. *Neisseria meningitidis*: pathogenesis and immunity. *Curr Opin Microbiol* **23c**:68–72.

126. **Rouphael NG, Stephens DS.** 2012. *Neisseria meningitidis*: biology, microbiology, and epidemiology. *Methods Mol Biol* **799**:1–20.

127. **Callaghan MJ, Jolley KA, Maiden MC.** 2006. Opacity-associated adhesin repertoire in hyperinvasive *Neisseria meningitidis*. *Infect Immun* **74**:5085–5094.

128. **Urwin R, Russell JE, Thompson EA, Holmes EC, Feavers IM, Maiden MC.** 2004. Distribution of surface protein variants among hyperinvasive meningococci: implications for vaccine design. *Infect Immun* **72**:5955–5962.

129. **Bille E, Zahar JR, Perrin A, Morelle S, Kriz P, Jolley KA, Maiden MC, Dervin C, Nassif X, Tinsley CR.** 2005. A chromosomally integrated bacteriophage in invasive meningococci. *J Exp Med* **201**:1905–1913.

130. **Harrison OB, Maiden MC, Rokbi B.** 2008. Distribution of transferrin binding protein B gene (tbpB) variants among *Neisseria* species. *BMC Microbiol* **8**:66.

131. **Bennett JS, Jolley KA, Earle SG, Corton C, Bentley SD, Parkhill J, Maiden MC.** 2012. A genomic approach to bacterial taxonomy: an

examination and proposed reclassification of species within the genus *Neisseria*. *Microbiol* **158:**1570–1580.

132. **Snyder LA, Saunders NJ.** 2006. The majority of genes in the pathogenic *Neisseria* species are present in non-pathogenic *Neisseria lactamica*, including those designated as 'virulence genes.' *BMC Genomics* **7:**128.

133. **Zhang G, Meredith TC, Kahne D.** 2013. On the essentiality of lipopolysaccharide to Gram-negative bacteria. *Curr Opin Microbiol* **16:**779–785.

134. **Stern A, Brown M, Nickel P, Meyer TF.** 1986. Opacity genes in *Neisseria gonorrhoeae*: control of phase and antigenic variation. *Cell* **47:**61–71.

135. **Swanson J, Kraus SJ, Gotschlich EC.** 1971. Studies on gonococcus infection. I. Pili and zones of adhesion: their relation to gonococcal growth patterns. *J Exp Med* **134:**886–906.

136. **Snyder LA, Butcher SA, Saunders NJ.** 2001. Comparative whole-genome analyses reveal over 100 putative phase-variable genes in the pathogenic *Neisseria* spp. *Microbiol* **147:**2321–2332.

137. **Levinson G, Gutman GA.** 1987. Slipped-strand mispairing: a major mechanism for DNA sequence evolution. *Mol Biol Evol* **4:**203–221.

138. **Lo H, Tang CM, Exley RM.** 2009. Mechanisms of avoidance of host immunity by *Neisseria meningitidis* and its effect on vaccine development. *Lancet Infect Dis* **9:**418–427.

139. **Moran EE, Burden R, Labrie JE 3rd, Wen Z, Wang XM, Zollinger WD, Zhang L, Pinto VB.** 2012. Analysis of the bactericidal response to an experimental *Neisseria meningitidis* vesicle vaccine. *Clin Vaccine Immunol* **19:**659–665.

140. **Granoff DM.** 2010. Review of meningococcal group B vaccines. *Clin Infect Dis* **50:**S54–S65.

141. **Gotschlich EC.** 1994. Genetic locus for the biosynthesis of the variable portion of *Neisseria gonorrhoeae* lipooligosaccharide. *J Exp Med* **180:**2181–2190.

142. **Danaher RJ, Levin JC, Arking D, Burch CL, Sandlin R, Stein DC.** 1995. Genetic basis of *Neisseria gonorrhoeae* lipooligosaccharide antigenic variation. *J Bacteriol* **177:**7275–7279.

143. **Yang QL, Gotschlich EC.** 1996. Variation of gonococcal lipooligosaccharide structure is due to alterations in poly-G tracts in *lgt* genes encoding glycosyl transferases. *J Exp Med* **183:**323–327.

144. **Kahler CM, Stephens DS.** 1998. Genetic basis for biosynthesis, structure, and function of meningococcal lipooligosaccharide (endotoxin). *Crit Rev Microbiol* **24:**281–334.

145. **Burch CL, Danaher RJ, Stein DC.** 1997. Antigenic variation in *Neisseria gonorrhoeae*:

production of multiple lipooligosaccharides. *J Bacteriol* **179:**982–986.

146. **Johswich KO, Zhou J, Law DK, St Michael F, McCaw SE, Jamieson FB, Cox AD, Tsang RS, Gray-Owen SD.** 2012. Invasive potential of nonencapsulated disease isolates of *Neisseria meningitidis*. *Infect Immun* **80:**2346–2353.

147. **Bhat KS, Gibbs CP, Barrera O, Morrison SG, Jahnig F, Stern A, Kupsch EM, Meyer TF, Swanson J.** 1991. The opacity proteins of *Neisseria gonorrhoeae* strain MS11 are encoded by a family of 11 complete genes. *Mol Microbiol* **5:**1889–1901.

148. **Gray-Owen SD, Lorenzen DR, Haude A, Meyer TF, Dehio C.** 1997. Differential Opa specificities for CD66 receptors influence tissue interactions and cellular response to *Neisseria gonorrhoeae*. *Mol Microbiol* **26:**971–980.

149. **Dehio C, Gray-Owen SD, Meyer TF.** 1998. The role of neisserial Opa proteins in interactions with host cells. *Trends Microbiol* **6:**489–495.

150. **Sadarangani M, Pollard AJ, Gray-Owen SD.** 2011. Opa proteins and CEACAMs: pathways of immune engagement for pathogenic *Neisseria*. *FEMS Microbiol Rev* **35:**498–514.

151. **Murphy GL, Connell TD, Barritt DS, Koomey M, Cannon JG.** 1989. Phase variation of gonococcal protein II: regulation of gene expression by slipped-strand mispairing of a repetitive DNA sequence. *Cell* **56:**539–547.

152. **Belland RJ, Morrison SG, van der Ley P, Swanson J.** 1989. Expression and phase variation of gonococcal P.II genes in *Escherichia coli* involves ribosomal frameshifting and slipped-strand mispairing. *Mol Microbiol* **3:**777–786.

153. **Belland RJ, Morrison SG, Carlson JH, Hogan DM.** 1997. Promoter strength influences phase variation of neisserial opa genes. *Mol Microbiol* **23:**123–135.

154. **Virji M, Heckels JE.** 1984. The role of common and type-specific pilus antigenic domains in adhesion and virulence of gonococci for human epithelial cells. *J Gen Microbiol* **130:**1089–1095.

155. **Koomey M, Fox R, Brossay L, Hebe'rt J.** 1994. The gonococcal PilT protein plays an essential role in pilus-associated phenotypes of twitching motility and natural competence for transformation, p 64–65. *In* Evans JS, Yost SE, Maiden MCJ, Feavers IM (ed), *Proceedings of the 9th Pathogenic Neisseria Conference*, Winchester, UK.

156. **Stohl EA, Dale EM, Criss AK, Seifert HS.** 2013. *Neisseria gonorrhoeae* metalloprotease NGO1686 is required for full piliation, and piliation is required for resistance to H2O2- and

neutrophil-mediated killing. *mBio* **4:**e00399-13. doi:10.1128/mBio.00399-13.

157. **Biswas GD, Sox T, Blackman E, Sparling PF.** 1977. Factors affecting genetic transformation of *Neisseria gonorrhoeae*. *J Bacteriol* **129:**983–992.

158. **Wormann ME, Horien CL, Bennett JS, Jolley KA, Maiden MC, Tang CM, Aho EL, Exley RM.** 2014. Sequence, distribution and chromosomal context of class I and class II pilin genes of *Neisseria meningitidis* identified in whole genome sequences. *BMC Genomics* **15:**253.

159. **De Reuse H, Taha MK.** 1997. RegF, an SspA homologue, regulates the expression of the *Neisseria gonorrhoeae pilE* gene. *Res Microbiol* **148:**289–303.

160. **Kellogg DS Jr, Cohen IR, Norins LC, Schroeter AL, Reising G.** 1968. *Neisseria gonorrhoeae*. II. Colonial variation and pathogenicity during 35 months in vitro. *J Bacteriol* **96:**596–605.

161. **Kellogg DS, Jr, Peacock WL, Deacon WE, Brown L, Pirkle CI.** 1963. *Neisseria gonorrhoeae*. I. Virulence genetically linked to clonial variation. *J Bacteriol* **85:**1274–1279.

162. **Jonsson AB, Nyberg G, Normark S.** 1991. Phase variation of gonococcal pili by frameshift mutation in *pilC*, a novel gene for pilus assembly. *EMBO J* **10:**477–488.

163. **Morand PC, Drab M, Rajalingam K, Nassif X, Meyer TF.** 2009. *Neisseria meningitidis* differentially controls host cell motility through PilC1 and PilC2 components of type IV pili. *PLoS One* **4:**e6834. doi:10.1371/journal.pone.0006834.

164. **Rudel T, Boxberger HJ, Meyer TF.** 1995. Pilus biogenesis and epithelial cell adherence of *Neisseria gonorrhoeae* pilC double knockout mutants. *Mol Microbiol* **17:**1057–1071.

165. **Wolfgang M, Park HS, Hayes SF, van Putten JP, Koomey M.** 1998. Suppression of an absolute defect in type IV pilus biogenesis by loss-of-function mutations in *pilT*, a twitching motility gene in *Neisseria gonorrhoeae*. *Proc Natl Acad Sci USA* **95:**14973–14978.

166. **Swanson J, Bergstrom S, Robbins K, Barrera O, Corwin D, Koomey JM.** 1986. Gene conversion involving the pilin structural gene correlates with pilus+ in equilibrium with pilus- changes in *Neisseria gonorrhoeae*. *Cell* **47:**267–276.

167. **Long CD, Madraswala RN, Seifert HS.** 1998. Comparisons between colony phase variation of *Neisseria gonorrhoeae* FA1090 and pilus, pilin, and S-pilin expression. *Infect Immun* **66:**1918–1927.

168. **Criss AK, Kline KA, Seifert HS.** 2005. The frequency and rate of pilin antigenic variation in *Neisseria gonorrhoeae*. *Mol Microbiol* **58:**510–519.

169. **Meyer TF, Billyard E, Haas R, Storzbach S, So M.** 1984. Pilus genes of *Neisseria gonorrheae*: chromosomal organization and DNA sequence. *Proc Natl Acad Sci USA* **81:**6110–6114.

170. **Snodgrass TL, Dempsey JAF, Cannon JG.** 1994. The repertoire of silent pilin gene copies and their chromosomal location is similar but not identical in gonococcal strains FA1090 and MS11, p 113–115. *In* Evans JS, Yost SE, Maiden MCJ, Feavers IM (ed), *Proceedings of the Ninth International Pathogenic Neisseria Conference*, Winchester, UK.

171. **Kline KA, Criss AK, Wallace A, Seifert HS.** 2007. Transposon mutagenesis identifies sites upstream of the *Neisseria gonorrhoeae pilE* gene that modulate pilin antigenic variation. *J Bacteriol* **189:**3462–3470.

172. **Howell-Adams B, Seifert HS.** 2000. Molecular models accounting for the gene conversion reactions mediating gonococcal pilin antigenic variation. *Mol Microbiol* **37:**1146–1158.

173. **Rohrer MS, Lazio MP, Seifert HS.** 2005. A real-time semi-quantitative RT-PCR assay demonstrates that the pilE sequence dictates the frequency and characteristics of pilin antigenic variation in *Neisseria gonorrhoeae*. *Nucleic Acids Res* **33:**3363–3371.

174. **Helm RA, Seifert HS.** 2010. Frequency and rate of pilin antigenic variation of *Neisseria meningitidis*. *J Bacteriol* **192:**3822–3823.

175. **Tobiason DM, Seifert HS.** 2006. The obligate human pathogen, *Neisseria gonorrhoeae*, is polyploid. *PLoS Biol* **4:**e185. doi:10.1371/journal.pbio.0040185.

176. **Tobiason DM, Seifert HS.** 2010. Genomic content of *Neisseria* species. *J Bacteriol* **192:**2160–2168.

177. **Mehr IJ, Seifert HS.** 1998. Differential roles of homologous recombination pathways in *Neisseria gonorrhoeae* pilin antigenic variation, DNA transformation, and DNA repair. *Mol Microbiol* **30:**697–710.

178. **Mehr IJ, Long CD, Serkin CD, Seifert HS.** 2000. A homologue of the recombination-dependent growth gene, rdgC, is involved in gonococcal pilin antigenic variation. *Genetics* **154:**523–532.

179. **Stohl EA, Seifert HS.** 2001. The *recX* gene potentiates homologous recombination in *Neisseria gonorrhoeae*. *Mol Microbiol* **40:**1301–1310.

180. **Skaar EP, Lazio MP, Seifert HS.** 2002. Roles of the *recJ* and *recN* genes in homologous

recombination and DNA repair pathways of *Neisseria gonorrhoeae*. *J Bacteriol* **184:**919–927.

181. **Kline KA, Seifert HS.** 2005. Role of the Rep helicase gene in homologous recombination in *Neisseria gonorrhoeae*. *J Bacteriol* **187:**2903–2907.

182. **Sechman EV, Rohrer MS, Seifert HS.** 2005. A genetic screen identifies genes and sites involved in pilin antigenic variation in *Neisseria gonorrhoeae*. *Mol Microbiol* **57:**468–483.

183. **Sechman EV, Kline KA, Seifert HS.** 2006. Loss of both Holliday junction processing pathways is synthetically lethal in the presence of gonococcal pilin antigenic variation. *Mol Microbiol* **61:**185–193.

184. **Criss AK, Bonney KM, Chang RA, Duffin PM, LeCuyer BE, Seifert HS.** 2010. Mismatch correction modulates mutation frequency and pilus phase and antigenic variation in *Neisseria gonorrhoeae*. *J Bacteriol* **192:**316–325.

185. **Segal E, Hagblom P, Seifert HS, So M.** 1986. Antigenic variation of gonococcal pilus involves assembly of separated silent gene segments. *Proc Natl Acad Sci USA* **83:**2177–2181.

186. **Wainwright LA, Frangipane JV, Seifert HS.** 1997. Analysis of protein binding to the Sma/Cla DNA repeat in pathogenic *Neisseriae*. *Nucleic Acids Res* **25:**1362–1368.

187. **Howell-Adams B, Wainwright LA, Seifert HS.** 1996. The size and position of heterologous insertions in a silent locus differentially affect pilin recombination in *Neisseria gonorrhoeae*. *Mol Microbiol* **22:**509–522.

188. **Cahoon LA, Seifert HS.** 2013. Transcription of a cis-acting, noncoding, small RNA is required for pilin antigenic variation in *Neisseria gonorrhoeae*. *PLoS Pathog* **9:**e1003074. doi:10.1371/journal.ppat.1003074.

189. **Giacani L, Brandt SL, Puray-Chavez M, Reid TB, Godornes C, Molini BJ, Benzler M, Hartig JS, Lukehart SA, Centurion-Lara A.** 2012. Comparative investigation of the genomic regions involved in antigenic variation of the TprK antigen among treponemal species, subspecies, and strains. *J Bacteriol* **194:**4208–4225.

190. **Liu Y, Liu W, Russell MW.** 2014. Suppression of host adaptive immune responses by *Neisseria gonorrhoeae*: role of interleukin 10 and type 1 regulatory T cells. *Mucosal Immunol* **7:**165–176.

191. **Bankhead T.** 2012. Antigenic variation of VlsE in *Borrelia burgdorferi*, p 113–124. *In* Embers ME (ed), *The Pathogenic Spirochetes*, Springer, New York, NY.

192. **Rotman E, Seifert HS.** 2015. *Neisseria gonorrhoeae* MutS affects pilin antigenic variation through mismatch correction and not by pilE guanine quartet binding. *J Bacteriol* **197:**1828–1838.

Mechanisms of Antibiotic Resistance 17

JOSE M. MUNITA[1,2,4] and CESAR A. ARIAS[1,2,3]

INTRODUCTION

The discovery, commercialization, and routine administration of antimicrobial compounds to treat infections revolutionized modern medicine and changed the therapeutic paradigm. Indeed, antibiotics have become one of the most important medical interventions needed for the development of complex medical approaches such as cutting-edge surgical procedures, solid organ transplantation, and management of patients with cancer, among others. Unfortunately, the marked increase in antimicrobial resistance among common bacterial pathogens is now threatening this therapeutic accomplishment, jeopardizing the successful outcomes of critically ill patients. In fact, the World Health Organization has named antibiotic resistance as one of the three most important public health threats of the 21st century (1).

Infections caused by multidrug-resistant (MDR) organisms are associated with increased mortality compared to those caused by susceptible bacteria, and they carry an important economic burden, estimated at over 20 billion dollars per year in the United States alone (2–4). The Centers for Disease

[1]Department of Internal Medicine, Division of Infectious Diseases, University of Texas Medical School at Houston, Houston, TX 77030; [2]International Center for Microbial Genomics; [3]Molecular Genetics and Antimicrobial Resistance Unit, Universidad El Bosque, Bogota, Colombia; [4]Clinica Alemana de Santiago, Universidad del Desarrollo School of Medicine, Santiago, Chile.

Virulence Mechanisms of Bacterial Pathogens, 5th edition
Edited by Indira T. Kudva, Nancy A. Cornick, Paul J. Plummer, Qijing Zhang, Tracy L. Nicholson, John P. Bannantine, and Bryan H. Bellaire
© 2016 American Society for Microbiology, Washington, DC
doi:10.1128/microbiolspec.VMBF-0016-2015

Control and Prevention conservatively estimates that at least 23,000 people die annually in the United States as a result of an infection with an antibiotic-resistant organism (5). Moreover, according to a recent report, antibiotic resistance is estimated to cause around 300 million premature deaths by 2050, with a loss of up to $100 trillion to the global economy (6). This situation is worsened by a paucity of a robust antibiotic pipeline, resulting in the emergence of infections that are almost untreatable and leaving clinicians with no reliable alternatives to treat infected patients.

To understand the problem of antimicrobial resistance, it is useful to discuss some relevant concepts. First, antimicrobial resistance is ancient, and it is the expected result of the interaction of many organisms with their environment. Most antimicrobial compounds are naturally produced molecules, and as such, coresident bacteria have evolved mechanisms to overcome their action to survive. Thus, these organisms are often considered to be intrinsically resistant to one or more antimicrobials. However, when discussing the antimicrobial resistance conundrum, bacteria harboring intrinsic determinants of resistance are not the main focus of the problem. Rather, in clinical settings, we are typically referring to the expression of acquired resistance in a bacterial population that was originally susceptible to the antimicrobial compound. As will be discussed later in the chapter, the development of acquired resistance can be the result of mutations in chromosomal genes or be due to the acquisition of external genetic determinants of resistance, likely obtained from intrinsically resistant organisms present in the environment.

Second, it is important to recognize that the concept of antimicrobial resistance/ susceptibility in clinical practice is a relative phenomenon with many layers of complexity. The establishment of clinical susceptibility breakpoints (susceptible, intermediate, and resistant) mainly relies on the *in vitro* activity of an antibiotic against a sizeable bacterial sample, combined with some pharmacological parameters (e.g., blood and infection site concentrations of the antimicrobial, among others). Thus, when treating antibiotic-resistant bacteria, the interpretation of susceptibility patterns may vary according to the clinical scenario and the availability of treatment options. For instance, the concentration of gentamicin achieved in the urine may be sufficiently high to treat a lower urinary tract infection caused by an organism reported as gentamicin resistant. Similarly, different penicillin breakpoints have been established for *Streptococcus pneumoniae* depending on if the isolate is causing meningitis as opposed to other types of infections, taking into account the levels of the drug that actually reach the cerebrospinal fluid (7). In addition, the *in vivo* susceptibility of an organism to a particular antibiotic may vary according to the size of the bacterial inoculum, a situation that has been well documented in *Staphylococcus aureus* infections treated with some cephalosporins. Indeed, there is evidence to suggest that some cephalosporins (e.g., cefazolin) may fail in the setting of high-inocula, deep-seated infections caused by cephalosporin-susceptible *S. aureus* (8). Therefore, in the following sections, we will focus on the molecular and biochemical mechanisms of bacterial resistance, illustrating specific situations that are often encountered in clinical practice.

GENETIC BASIS OF ANTIMICROBIAL RESISTANCE

Bacteria have a remarkable genetic plasticity that allows them to respond to a wide array of environmental threats, including the presence of antibiotic molecules that may jeopardize their existence. Bacteria sharing the same ecological niche with antimicrobial-producing organisms have evolved ancient mechanisms to withstand the effect of the harmful antibiotic molecule and, consequently, their intrinsic resistance permits them to thrive in its presence. From an evolutionary perspective, bacteria use two major genetic strategies to adapt to the antibiotic "attack": (i) mutations in gene(s) often associated with the mechanism of action of the compound and (ii) acquisition of foreign DNA coding for resistance determinants through horizontal gene transfer (HGT).

Mutational Resistance

In this scenario, a subset of bacterial cells derived from a susceptible population develops mutations in genes that affect the activity of the drug, resulting in preserved cell survival in the presence of the antimicrobial molecule. Once a resistant mutant emerges, the antibiotic eliminates the susceptible population, and the resistant bacteria predominate. In many instances, mutational changes leading to resistance are costly to cell homeostasis (i.e., decreased fitness) and are only maintained if needed in the presence of the antibiotic. In general, mutations resulting in antimicrobial resistance alter the antibiotic action via one of the following mechanisms: (i) modifications of the antimicrobial target (decreasing the affinity for the drug; see below), (ii) a decrease in the drug uptake, (iii) activation of efflux mechanisms to extrude the harmful molecule, or (iv) global changes in important metabolic pathways via modulation of regulatory networks. Thus, resistance arising due to acquired mutational changes is diverse and varies in complexity. In this chapter, we will give several examples of antimicrobial resistance arising through mutational changes (see below).

HGT

Acquisition of foreign DNA material through HGT is one of the most important drivers of bacterial evolution, and it is frequently responsible for the development of antimicrobial resistance. Most antimicrobial agents used in clinical practice are (or derive from) products naturally found in the environment (mostly soil). Bacteria sharing the environment with these molecules harbor intrinsic genetic determinants of resistance, and there is robust evidence suggesting that such "environmental resistome" is a prolific source of the acquisition of antibiotic resistance genes in clinically relevant bacteria. Furthermore, this genetic exchange has been implicated in the dissemination of resistance to many frequently used antibiotics.

Classically, bacteria acquire external genetic material through three main strategies: (i) transformation (incorporation of naked DNA), (ii) transduction (phage mediated), and (iii) conjugation (bacterial "sex"). Transformation is perhaps the simplest type of HGT, but only a handful of clinically relevant bacterial species are able to naturally incorporate naked DNA to develop resistance. Emergence of resistance in the hospital environment often involves conjugation, a very efficient method of gene transfer that involves cell-to-cell contact and is likely to occur at high rates in the gastrointestinal tract of humans under antibiotic treatment. As a general rule, conjugation uses mobile genetic elements (MGEs) as vehicles to share valuable genetic information, although direct transfer from chromosome to chromosome has also been well characterized (9). The most important MGEs are plasmids and transposons, both of which play a crucial role in the development and dissemination of antimicrobial resistance among clinically relevant organisms.

Finally, one of the most efficient mechanisms for accumulating antimicrobial resistance genes is represented by integrons, which are site-specific recombination systems capable of recruiting open reading frames in the form of mobile gene cassettes. Integrons provide an efficient and rather simple mechanism for the addition of new genes into bacterial chromosomes, along with the necessary machinery to ensure their expression: a robust strategy of genetic interchange and one of the main drivers of bacterial evolution. For details on the mechanisms of HGT, readers are directed to a recent state-of-the-art review (10).

MECHANISTIC BASIS OF ANTIMICROBIAL RESISTANCE

Not surprisingly, bacteria have evolved sophisticated mechanisms of drug resistance to avoid killing by antimicrobial molecules, a process that has likely occurred over millions of years of evolution. Of note, resistance to one antimicrobial class can usually be achieved through multiple biochemical pathways, and one bacterial cell may be capable ofusing a cadre of mechanisms of resistance to survive the effect of an antibiotic. As an example, fluoroquinolone resistance can occur by three biochemical routes, all of which may coexist in the same bacteria at a given time (producing an additive effect and, often, increasing the levels of resistance): (i) mutations in genes encoding the target site of fluoroquinolones (DNA gyrase and topoisomerase IV), (ii) overexpression of efflux pumps that extrude the drug from the cell, and (iii) protection of the fluoroquinolone target site by a protein designated Qnr (see below for details on each of these mechanisms). However, bacterial species seem to have evolved a preference for some mechanisms of resistance over others. For example, the predominant mechanism of resistance to β-lactams in Gram-negative bacteria is the production of β-lactamases, whereas resistance to these compounds in Gram-positive organisms is mostly achieved by modifications of their target site, the penicillin-binding proteins (PBPs). It has been argued that this phenomenon is likely due to major differences in the cell envelope between Gram-negative and Gram-positive organisms. In the former, the presence of an outer membrane permits "control" of the entry of molecules to the periplasmic space. Indeed, most β-lactams require specific porins to reach the PBPs, which are located in the inner membrane. Therefore, the bacterial cell controls the access of these molecules to the periplasmic space, allowing the production of β-lactamases in sufficient concentrations to tip the kinetics in favor of the destruction of the antibiotic molecule. Conversely, this "compartmentalization" advantage is absent in Gram-positive organisms, although production of β-lactamases also seems to be successful in certain scenarios (e.g., staphylococcal penicillinase).

To provide a comprehensive classification of the antibiotic resistance mechanisms, we will categorize them according to the biochemical route involved in resistance, as follows: (i) modifications of the antimicrobial molecule, (ii) prevention of the compound reaching the antibiotic target (by decreasing penetration or actively extruding the antimicrobial compound), (iii) changes to and/or bypassing of target sites, and (iv) resistance due to global cell-adaptive processes. Each of these mechanistic strategies encompasses specific biochemical pathways that will be described in detail in the reminder of the chapter. Of note, we will focus the discussion on the most important mechanisms, giving examples that have relevant clinical impact.

Modifications of the Antibiotic Molecule

One of the most successful bacterial strategies to cope with the presence of antibiotics is to produce enzymes that inactivate the drug by adding specific chemical moieties to the compound or that destroy the molecule itself, rendering the antibiotic unable to interact with its target.

Chemical alterations of the antibiotic
The production of enzymes capable of introducing chemical changes to the antimicrobial molecule is a well-known mechanism of acquired antibiotic resistance in both Gram-negative and Gram-positive bacteria.

Interestingly, most of the antibiotics affected by these enzymatic modifications exert their mechanism of action by inhibiting protein synthesis at the ribosome level (11). Many types of modifying enzymes have been described, and the most frequent biochemical reactions they catalyze include (i) acetylation (aminoglycosides, chloramphenicol, streptogramins), (ii) phosphorylation (aminoglycosides, chloramphenicol), and (iii) adenylation (aminoglycosides, lincosamides). Regardless of the biochemical reaction, the resulting effect is often related to steric hindrance that decreases the avidity of the drug for its target, which in turn, is reflected in higher bacterial MICs.

One of the best examples of resistance via modification of the drug is the presence of aminoglycoside modifying enzymes (AMEs) that covalently modify the hydroxyl or amino groups of the aminoglycoside molecule. Multiple AMEs have been described to date, and they have become the predominant mechanism of aminoglycoside resistance worldwide. These enzymes are usually harbored in MGEs, but genes coding for AMEs have also been found as part of the chromosome in certain bacterial species, as seen with some aminoglycoside acetyltransferases in *Providencia stuartii*, *Enterococcus faecium* and *Serratia marcescens* (12). The nomenclature to classify the multiple AMEs considers their biochemical activity (acetyltransferase [ACC], adenyltransferase [ANT] or phosphotransferase [APH]), the site of the modification, which is depicted by a number from 1 to 6 corresponding to the particular carbon on the sugar ring, and a single or double prime symbol to symbolize that the reaction occurs in the first or second sugar moiety, respectively. In addition, whenever there is more than one enzyme catalyzing the exact same reaction, a roman numeral is used to differentiate them (Fig. 1).

There are important differences in the geographical distribution, the bacterial species in which these enzymes disseminate, and the specific aminoglycosides they affect. For instance, the APH(3) family is widely distributed in Gram-positive and Gram-negative bacteria and alters kanamycin and streptomycin but spares gentamicin and tobramycin. On the other hand, AAC(6′)-I is mainly found in Gram-negative clinical isolates including *Enterobacteriaceae*, *Pseudomonas*, and *Acinetobacter* and affects most aminoglycosides including amikacin and gentamicin (12). In addition, the activity and distribution of AMEs from the same family also varies. For instance, among the adenyltransferases, which classically affect both gentamicin and tobramycin, the genes encoding ANT(4′), ANT(6′), and ANT(9′) are usually harbored in MGEs of Gram-positive bacteria, and ANT(2″) and ANT(3″) are more prevalent in Gram-negative organisms (12).

Finally, it is worth mentioning that some of these enzymes have evolved more than a single biochemical activity. Indeed, AAC(6′) APH(2″), which is mainly found in Gram-positive organisms, is a bifunctional enzyme (with acetylation and phosphotransferase activities) that likely arose from the fusion of two AMEs encoding genes. This protein confers high-level resistance to all aminoglycosides except for streptomycin and is located on a Tn*4001*-like transposon that is widely distributed among enterococci and staphylococci. Furthermore, the presence of this bifunctional enzyme accounts for most of the high-level gentamicin resistance detected in enterococci (including in vancomycin-resistant strains) and methicillin-resistant *S. aureus* worldwide (13).

Another classical example of enzymatic alteration of an antibiotic involves the modification of chloramphenicol, an antibiotic that inhibits protein synthesis by interacting with the peptidyl-transfer center of the 50S ribosomal subunit. The chemical modification of chloramphenicol is mainly driven by the expression of acetyltransferases known as CATs (chloramphenicol acetyltransferases). Multiple *cat* genes have been described in both Gram-positive and Gram-negative organisms, and they have been classified into two

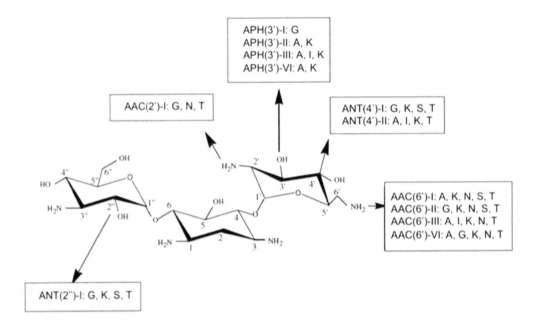

FIGURE 1 Representation of different types of aminoglycoside-modifying enzymes and their nomenclature. Each group of enzymes is identified by their biochemical activity as follows: acetyltransferase (AAC), adenyltransferase (ANT), and phosphotransferase (APH). Next in the enzyme name, an algebraic number in parentheses indicates the number of the carbon that is inactivated. The ring of the sugar in which the reaction takes place is symbolized by one (first sugar moiety) or two apostrophes (second sugar moiety). Roman numerals are used to differentiate distinct isoenzymes acting in the same site. Not all existing enzymes are shown. A, amikacin; G, gentamicin; I, isepamicin; K, kanamycin; N, netilmicin; S, sisomicin; T, tobramycin. Modified from reference 106.

main types: type A, which usually results in high-level resistance, and type B, which confers low-level chloramphenicol resistance (14). Although these determinants are usually harbored in MGEs such us plasmids and transposons, they have also been reported as being part of the core genome (chromosome) of certain bacteria.

Destruction of the antibiotic molecule

The main mechanism of β-lactam resistance relies on the destruction of these compounds by the action of β-lactamases. These enzymes destroy the amide bond of the β-lactam ring, rendering the antimicrobial ineffective. β-lactamases were first described in the early 1940s, one year before penicillin was introduced to the market, but there is evidence of their existence for millions of years (15, 16). Infections caused by penicillin-resistant

S. aureus became clinically relevant after penicillin became widely available and the mechanism of resistance was found to be a plasmid-encoded penicillinase that was readily transmitted between *S. aureus* strains, resulting in rapid dissemination of the resistance trait (17). To overcome this problem, new β-lactam compounds with a wider spectrum of activity and less susceptibility to penicillinases (such as ampicillin) were manufactured. However, during the 1960s a new plasmid-encoded β-lactamase capable of hydrolyzing ampicillin was found among Gram-negative organisms (termed TEM-1 after the name of the patient in which it was originally found [Temoneira]) (18). From then on, the development of newer generations of β-lactams has systematically been followed by the rapid appearance of enzymes capable of destroying any novel compound that reaches the market, in a process that is a prime example of antibiotic-driven adaptive bacterial evolution.

Genes encoding for β-lactamases are generally termed *bla*, followed by the name of the specific enzyme (e.g., *bla*$_{KPC}$), and they have been found in the chromosome or localized in MGEs as part of the accessory genome. These genes can also be found forming part of integrons, a situation that facilitates their dissemination. In terms of their expression, transcription of these genes can be constitutive, or it may require an external signal to induce their production.

To date, more than 1,000 β-lactamases have been described (www.lahey.org/studies), and many more are likely to continue to be reported as part of the normal process of bacterial evolution. Two main classification schemes have been proposed in an attempt to group this large number of enzymes. First, the Ambler classification relies on amino acid sequence identity and separates β-lactamases into four groups (A, B, C, and D). On the other hand, the Bush-Jacoby classification divides β-lactamases into four categories (each with several subgroups) according to their biochemical function, mainly based on substrate specificity (19, 20). A summary of the most important enzymes and their classification is presented in Fig 2.

It is important to note that both of these classification schemes have caveats and that they do not fully overlap. For instance, Ambler class A and D enzymes are all considered to be within group 2 in the Jacoby-Bush system. In addition, while the Ambler classification seems to be easier to follow, the lack of correlation with functional characteristics of the enzymes may lead to confusion. As an example, the Ambler class A group encompasses enzymes with a wide range of biochemical activities, from narrow-spectrum β-lactamases to enzymes capable of destroying almost all available β-lactams, including carbapenems. Moreover, enzymes originally classified within a group harboring a particular biochemical profile can evolve into novel

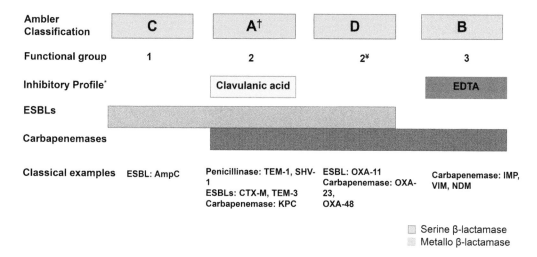

FIGURE 2 Schematic representation of β-lactamases. Molecular classification of β-lactamases follows the Ambler classification. Correlation with the main functional group of the Bush and Jacobi classification is also shown. Of note, the latter classification has several subgroups that are not shown. Representative examples of each group of enzymes are provided. [†]Class A enzymes are the most diverse and include penicillinases, ESBLs, and carbapenemases. [¥]Ambler class D enzymes belong to the functional group/subgroup 2d. [*]Class A enzymes belonging to the subgroup 2br are resistant to clavulanic acid inhibition. EDTA, ethylenediaminetetraacetic acid; ESBLs, extended-spectrum β-lactamases.

enzymes with different substrate specificities, usually due to mutations in the active site. A good example of this process is TEM-3, an enzyme that evolved from the original TEM-1 penicillinase after acquiring the ability to hydrolyze third-generation cephalosporins and aztreonam (a functional profile that defines it as an "extended spectrum β-lactamase" [ESBL]) due to the development of two amino acid substitutions that altered its function (18, 21).

Deciphering the role of the different types of enzymes and their characteristics is a complex task that requires understanding some of the terminology frequently used in the literature. As mentioned above, an ESBL enzyme has the ability to hydrolyze penicillins, third-generation cephalosporins (the hallmark characteristic), and monobactams, but it harbors modest (or no) activity against cephamycins and carbapenems. Most of the ESBLs belong to Ambler class A and, as such, they are generally inhibited by clavulanic acid or tazobactam. This property distinguishes them from AmpC enzymes, which are class C β-lactamases that also hydrolyze third-generation cephalosporins but are not inhibited by clavulanic acid or tazobactam. Of note, a subgroup of class D OXA enzymes capable of destroying third-generation cephalosporins is also considered within the ESBL group (see below and Fig. 2). Another clinically relevant group of enzymes is the carbapenemases, a diverse group of β-lactamases with the ability to hydrolyze carbapenems, the most potent β-lactams available in clinical practice. These enzymes can be divided into serine carbapenemases (Ambler class A or D) and metallo-carbapenemases (Ambler class B). In the rest of this section, we will provide examples of the different types of β-lactamases using the Ambler classification as the backbone for discussion.

Class A β-lactamases have a serine residue in the catalytic site, a property that they share with class C and D enzymes. Most class A enzymes are inhibited by clavulanic acid, and

their spectrum of activity includes monobactams but not cephamycins (cefoxitin and cefotetan). Class A enzymes include a wide range of proteins with very different catalytic activities, from penicillinases (TEM-1 and SHV-1, which only hydrolyze penicillin) to ESBLs (such as CTX-M) to carbapenemases such as KPC (*Klebsiella pneumoniae* carbapenemase), an enzyme that is currently prevalent in several Gram-negative species. We will discuss details of CTX-M (ESBL) and KPC carbapenemases, both class A enzymes with high clinical impact.

CTX-M is a plasmid-encoded ESBL commonly found in *K. pneumoniae*, *Escherichia coli*, and other *Enterobacteriaceae* around the world. In contrast to other Ambler class A ESBLs such as TEM-3, this enzyme did not derive from TEM or SHV; rather, the current evidence suggests that it was likely acquired from *Kluyvera* spp. (an environmental bacterium with no major human pathogenic significance) through HGT (22). Genes encoding CTX-M enzymes have been found in association with insertion sequences (IS*Ecp1*) and with transposable elements such as Tn*402*-like transposons. These mobile elements can be captured by a broad range of conjugative plasmids or phage-like sequences that can serve as vehicles for dissemination (23). Consequently, CTX-M enzymes have become the most prevalent ESBL worldwide and are responsible for a large proportion of cephalosporin resistance in *E. coli* and *K. pneumoniae*.

To date, five families of class A carbapenemases have been described, of which three are typically chromosomally encoded (IMI [imipenem-hydrolyzing enzyme], SME [*S. marcescens* enzyme], and NMC [not-metallo-enzyme carbapenemase]), and the remaining two (KPC and GES) are classically harbored in plasmids or other MGEs (24). As with other class A enzymes they are all inhibited by clavulanic acid and tazobactam, and they hydrolyze aztreonam but not cephamycins. KPC was first reported in 1996 from a *K. pneumoniae* strain recovered from a patient in North Carolina (25). Although these enzymes are predominantly found in *Klebsiella* spp. (thus its name, *K. pneumoniae* carbapenemase), they have been reported in several other Gram-negative organisms, including *Enterobacter* spp., *E. coli*, *Proteus mirabilis*, and *Salmonella* spp., among others. Furthermore, they have also been found in nonlactose fermenter organisms such as *Pseudomonas aeruginosa*. A total of 22 variants of the bla_{KPC} gene have been described to date, most of them located in plasmids harboring transposable elements (e.g., Tn*4401*) or in association with insertion sequences such as ISKpn6 and ISKpn7 (26).

Class B enzymes are also known as metallo-β-lactamases because they utilize a metal ion (usually zinc) as a cofactor (instead of a serine residue) for the nucleophilic attack of the β-lactam ring. They are inhibited by the presence of ion-chelating agents such as EDTA and, similar to class A carbapenemases, they are active against a wide range of β-lactams, including carbapenems. Metallo-β-lactamases are not inhibited by clavulanic acid or tazobactam, and while they efficiently hydrolyze cephamycins, aztreonam is typically a poor substrate. These enzymes were discovered over 50 years ago encoded by genes usually located in the chromosome of nonpathogenic bacteria. However, the situation dramatically changed during the 1990s, when enzymes such as IMP and VIM were increasingly reported in clinical strains of *Enterobacteriaceae*, *Pseudomonas* spp., and *Acinetobacter* spp. (24). Indeed, genes encoding these enzymes have been found as part of the accessory genome of pathogenic bacteria, which suggests HGT. There are about 10 types of metallo-carbapenemases, but most of the clinically important ones belong to 4 families: IMP, VIM, SPM, and NDM. Considering their high frequency and worldwide spread, we will briefly discuss IMP, VIM, and NDM.

The first IMP-type enzymes were described in Japan in the early 1990s in *S. marcescens*, and since then, more than 20 subtypes have been described worldwide in *Enterobacteriaceae*, *Pseudomonas* spp., and *Acinetobacter* spp., among other organisms. The bla_{IMP} genes have been found on large plasmids and forming part of class 1 integrons (27). The VIM-type enzymes were first described in the late 1990s in Verona, Italy (Verona integron-encoded metallo β-lactamase) and have since spread throughout the globe. These enzymes were initially found in *P. aeruginosa*, but their association with class 1 integrons, along with reports locating them in different types of MGEs, has likely contributed to their dissemination to many different bacterial species, making them a major concern around the globe. Among the many variants of VIM described to date, VIM-2 is the most widely distributed enzyme, with reports from Europe, Asia, Africa, and the Americas (28).

More recently (2008), a new carbapenemase was identified in a *K. pneumoniae* isolate recovered from a Swedish patient who had been previously admitted to a hospital in New Delhi, India. The enzyme was designated NDM-1, in reference to its origin (New Delhi metallo β-lactamase) (29). NDM-1 shares little amino acid identity with other members of the Ambler class B enzymes (e.g., 32% with VIM-1), but its hydrolytic profile is very similar to all of them. The bla_{NDM} gene has been found in several types of plasmids that are readily transferable among different species of Gram-negative organisms, and it has also been associated with the presence of insertion sequences such as the ISAba125. In contrast to other genes encoding metallo-enzymes, bla_{NDM} is not usually related to integron-like structures (30). Nevertheless, NDM-1 rapidly spread around the globe, becoming a prime example of how a resistance determinant can readily disseminate worldwide despite many efforts to avoid its transmission. Moreover, MGEs containing genes coding for NDM enzymes generally carry multiple other resistance determinants such as genes encoding other carbapenemases (e.g., VIM-type and OXA-type

enzymes), ESBL, AMEs, methylases conferring resistance to macrolides, the quinolone
resistance Qnr protein, enzymes that modify
rifampin, and proteins involved in resistance
to sulfamethoxazole, among others. Thus, the
presence of NDM-1 is frequently accompanied by an MDR phenotype.

The emergence of NDM-1 is particularly
concerning because the bla_{NDM} gene has
been shown to be readily transmissible
among different types of Gram-negative
organisms, spreading to many countries in
a short span of time and becoming one of
the most feared resistance determinants in
several parts of the world (28). In addition,
in the Indian subcontinent (i.e., India and
Pakistan), the bla_{NDM} gene is not only
extensively disseminated among nosocomial pathogens, but it is frequently found
in community-associated isolates. Furthermore, several reports have found NDM-1-
producing Gram-negative bacteria in soil
and in drinking water, suggesting that these
genes may be disseminating through the
human microbiota (31).

Class C β-lactamases confer resistance to
all penicillins and cephalosporins (although
cefepime is usually a poor substrate), including cephamycins. They do not reliably
hydrolyze aztreonam and are not inhibited
by clavulanic acid. The most clinically
relevant class C enzyme is AmpC, which is
a cephalosporinase that is generally encoded on the chromosome (although the
bla_{AMPc} gene has also been found in plasmids). Production of chromosomal AmpC is
a hallmark of *Enterobacter cloacae, Enterobacter aerogenes, Citrobacter freundii, S.
marcescens, Providencia* spp., *Morganella
morganii*, and *P. aeruginosa*, among others.
In contrast, *Proteus mirabilis, Proteus vul-
garis, Klebsiella* spp., and *Stenotrophomonas*
spp. are classical examples of species in
which the bla_{ampC} gene is absent from the
core genome (32).

The expression of *ampC* is generally
inducible and is under strict control of a
complex regulatory mechanism that has

been best studied in *Enterobacter* spp.
AmpR is a transcriptional regulator of the
LysR family that acts as a repressor of
the transcription of bla_{AMPc}. Under noninducing conditions (absence of β-lactams),
AmpR is bound to peptidoglycan precursors
(UDP-MurNAc pentapeptides), and interaction of AmpR with its cognate promoter does
not occur (resulting in absence of bla_{AMPc}
transcription). In contrast, in the presence
of β-lactams, the alterations in cell wall
homeostasis result in accumulation of peptidoglycan byproducts such as anhydro-
muropeptides that compete for the same
AmpR binding site with the UDP-MurNAc
pentapeptides. As a result of this competition,
AmpR is released and is able to interact with
the bla_{AMPc} promoter, activating transcription of the gene (33, 34).

Another mechanism by which *ampC* is
overexpressed is through AmpD, a cytosolic
amidase that recycles muropeptides. AmpD
effectively reduces the concentration of
anhydro-UDP-MurNAc tri-, tetra-, and pentapeptides, preventing displacement of UDP-
MurNAc pentapeptide from AmpR and, therefore, *ampC* overexpression. Mutations in
ampD are often seen in isolates that constitutively overproduce AmpC, affecting the clinical efficacy of cephalosporins. As mentioned,
cefepime is not a good substrate for AmpC
enzymes; however, high-level production of
AmpC may markedly increase cefepime MICs
(32, 35).

Class D β-lactamases include a wide range
of enzymes that were initially differentiated
from the class A penicillinases due to their
ability to hydrolyze oxacillin (hence their
name) and because they were poorly inhibited by clavulanic acid. Many OXA variants
have been described, including enzymes
with the ability to degrade third-generation
cephalosporins (ESBLs) (e.g., OXA-11 from
P. aeruginosa) and carbapenems (e.g., OXA-
23 from *Acinetobacter baumannii*). For example, OXA-48 is a widely disseminated class
D carbapenemase which was originally described in 2001 in Turkey from an MDR

isolate of *K. pneumoniae*. OXA-48 and its variants are now widely spread in clinical isolates of *K. pneumoniae* and other *Enterobacteriaceae* and have also been found in *A. baumannii* (36). Many other types of OXA enzymes have been described to date, possessing a variety of hydrolytic profiles and encoded by genes that are often found in a wide range of MGEs. In certain instances, the OXA-containing MGE inserts in the chromosome result in core-genome genes encoding OXA enzymes. This phenomenon has often been described in *Acinetobacter*, with both OXA-51 and OXA-69 encoded by genes located in the chromosome (36).

Although class D enzymes are particularly prevalent in *A. baumannii*, they have been reported in many other clinically relevant organisms, such as *E. coli*, *Enterobacter* spp., *K. pneumoniae*, and *P. aeruginosa*, among others. Furthermore, intra- and interspecies transmission of some of these genes has been particularly successful, with enzymes such as OXA-23 and OXA-58 currently being spread around the globe.

Decreased Antibiotic Penetration and Efflux

Decreased permeability

Many of the antibiotics used in clinical practice have intracellular bacterial targets or, in the case of Gram-negative bacteria, targets located in the cytoplasmic membrane (the inner membrane). Therefore, the compound must penetrate the outer and/or cytoplasmic membrane to exert its antimicrobial effect. Bacteria have developed mechanisms to prevent the antibiotic from reaching its intracellular or periplasmic target by decreasing the uptake of the antimicrobial molecule. This mechanism is particularly important in Gram-negative bacteria (for the reason specified above), limiting the influx of substances from the external milieu. In fact, the outer membrane acts as the first line of defense against the penetration of multiple toxic compounds, including

several antimicrobial agents. Hydrophilic molecules such as β-lactams, tetracyclines, and some fluoroquinolones are particularly affected by changes in permeability of the outer membrane since they often use water-filled diffusion channels known as porins to cross this barrier (37). The prime example of the efficiency of this natural barrier is the fact that vancomycin, a glycopeptide antibiotic, is not active against Gram-negative organisms due to the lack of penetration through the outer membrane. Likewise, the innate low susceptibility of *Pseudomonas* and *A. baumannii* to β-lactams (compared to *Enterobacteriaceae*) can be explained, at least in part, to a reduced number and/or differential expression of porins (38).

Several types of porins have been described, and they can be classified according to their structure (trimeric or monomeric), their selectivity, and the regulation of their expression. Among the best-characterized porins, the three major proteins produced by *E. coli* (known as OmpF, OmpC, and PhoE) and the *P. aeruginosa* OprD (also known as protein D2) are classical examples of porin-mediated antibiotic resistance. Alterations of porins can be achieved by three general processes: (i) a shift in the type of porins expressed, (ii) a change in the level of porin expression, and (iii) impairment of the porin function. Changes in permeability through any of these mechanisms frequently result in low-level resistance and are often associated with other mechanisms of resistance, such as increased expression of efflux pumps (see below) (39).

One classic example of porin-mediated resistance is the aberrant production of OprD in *P. aeruginosa*, which is normally used for the uptake of basic amino acids and antibiotics (i.e., imipenem, a potent antipseudomonal antibiotic from the carbapenem class). Mutations in the *oprD* gene have been shown to arise in clinical isolates of *P. aeruginosa* during therapy (40). Furthermore, clinical and *in vitro* studies have shown that these changes can produce resistance alone or in conjunction with overexpression of an efflux pump and/or the production of a carbapenem-hydrolyzing enzyme, resulting in high levels of resistance to carbapenems.

Another example relates to clinical isolates of *K. pneumoniae* recovered before and after antimicrobial therapy. The posttherapy isolates were found to exhibit a shift in porin expression from OmpK35 to OmpK36 (the latter possessing a smaller channel size). This alteration in the type of porin expressed correlated with a 4- to 8-fold decrease in susceptibility for a wide range of β-lactam antimicrobials (41, 42). Similar examples are found in other bacterial species of clinical importance such as *E. cloacae*, *Salmonella* spp., *Neisseria gonorrhoeae*, and *A. baumannii*.

Efflux pumps

The production of complex bacterial machineries capable of extruding a toxic compound out of the cell can also result in antimicrobial resistance. The description of an efflux system able to pump tetracycline out of the cytoplasm of *E. coli* dates from the early 1980s and was among the first to be described (43). Since then, many classes of efflux pumps have been characterized in both Gram-negative and Gram-positive pathogens. These systems may be substrate-specific (for a particular antibiotic such as *tet* determinants for tetracycline and *mef* genes for macrolides in pneumococci) or have broad substrate specificity, which is usually found in MDR bacteria (44). This mechanism of resistance affects a wide range of antimicrobial classes including protein synthesis inhibitors, fluoroquinolones, β-lactams, carbapenems, and polymyxins. The genes encoding efflux pumps can be located in MGEs (as initially described for the *tet* gene) or in the chromosome. Chromosomally encoded pumps can explain the inherent resistance of some bacterial species to a particular antibiotic (e.g., *Enterococcus faecalis* intrinsic resistance to streptogramin A; see below) (45).

There are five major families of efflux pumps: (i) the major facilitator superfamily, (ii) the small multidrug resistance family (SMR), (iii) the resistance-nodulation-cell-division family (RND), (iv) the ATP-binding cassette family, and (v) the multidrug and toxic compound extrusion family. These families differ in terms of structural conformation, energy source, range of substrates they are able to extrude, and the type of bacterial organisms in which they are distributed (46) (Fig. 3).

Tetracycline resistance is one of the classic examples of efflux-mediated resistance, where the Tet efflux pumps (belonging to the major facilitator superfamily family) extrude tetracyclines using proton exchange as the source of energy. Currently, more than 20 *tet* genes have been described, most of which are harbored in MGEs. The majority of these pumps are preferentially found in Gram-negative organisms, with Tet(K) and Tet(L) being among the few exceptions that predominate in Gram-positive organisms. Many of these pumps affect tetracycline and doxycycline but do not decrease minocycline or tigecycline susceptibility, because they are not able to use these compounds as substrates (44, 47). In addition to the tetracycline-specific transport systems, several MDR efflux pumps such as AcrAB-TolC in *Enterobacteriaceae* and MexAB-OprM in *P. aeruginosa* (both belonging to the RND family) are able to extrude tetracyclines (including tigecycline) as part of their contribution to multidrug resistance (48, 49).

Of note, MDR pumps belonging to the RND family are frequently found in the chromosome of clinically relevant Gram-negative bacteria and determine varying degrees of intrinsic resistance to several antimicrobials. Efflux pumps that belong to this family are organized as tripartite structures spanning the width of the Gram-negative cell envelope and selectively communicating the cytoplasm with the external environment. Among them, one of the best studied is the AcrAB-TolC system (classically found in *E. coli*), which is com-

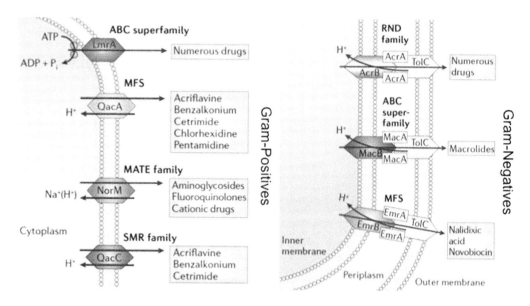

FIGURE 3 Representation of different types of efflux pumps in Gram-positive and Gram-negative bacteria. The five major families of efflux pumps are shown: ATP-binding cassette (ABC) superfamily, the major facilitator superfamily (MFS), the multidrug and toxic-compound extrusion (MATE) family, the small multidrug resistance (SMR) family, and the resistance nodulation division (RND) family. A diagrammatic comparison of all the families showing their source of energy and examples of drugs and compounds that serve as a substrate are shown. Modified from reference 107 with permission.

posed of a transporter protein located in the inner membrane (AcrB), a linker protein located in the periplasmic space (AcrA), and a protein channel located in the outer membrane (TolC) (108). RND pumps function as proton antiporters and are able to transport a wide array of substrates, conferring resistance to tetracyclines, chloramphenicol, some β-lactams, novobiocin, fusidic acid, and fluoroquinolones. In addition, they are capable of extruding several toxic compounds such as bile salts, cationic dyes, and disinfectants, among many others. Crystallographic studies have provided insight on the structure and function of these pumps, improving our understanding of how these systems operate. Indeed, they have shown that AcrB has two binding pockets with different substrate preferences and that compounds are moved out of the cell through a series of conformational changes in a functionally rotating mechanism that finishes with the substrate being extruded via TolC (a process that

requires an interaction with the periplasmic accessory protein AcrA) (109). Of note, recent investigations have described a small protein named ArcZ, which has been shown to modulate and enhance the affinity of AcrB for certain molecules such as chloramphenicol and tetracycline through a mechanism that is yet to be determined (110).

Another important phenotype of clinical relevance mediated by the efflux mechanism is that of resistance to macrolides. The best-characterized efflux pumps are encoded by the *mef* genes (*mefA* and *mefE*) that extrude the macrolide class of antibiotics (e.g., erythromycin). The Mef pumps are mainly found in *Streptococcus pyogenes* and *S. pneumoniae*, along with other streptococci and Gram-positive organisms. MefA is usually carried in a transposon (Tn*1207*) located in the chromosome, and MefE is harbored in the so called "MEGA-element," a fragment of DNA known as the macrolide efflux genetic assembly element that has been found inserted in different regions of the bacterial chromosome. Macrolide resistance due to these pumps does not result in cross-resistance to lincosamides and streptogramins (the so called MLS$_B$ group) (50).

Other efflux pumps resulting in macrolide resistance in Gram positive organisms include MsrA and MsrC, which belong to the ATP-binding cassette transporter family. MsrA is a plasmid-borne determinant that was initially described in *Staphylococcus epidermidis*. MsrC is a chromosomally encoded protein described in *E. faecalis* that produces low-level resistance to macrolides and streptogramin B. Finally, another predicted efflux pump is Lsa (encoded by the chromosomal gene *lsa*), which is responsible for the intrinsic resistance of *E. faecalis* to lincosamides and streptogramin A (LS$_A$ phenotype) (44, 45).

Changes in Target Sites

A common strategy for bacteria to develop antimicrobial resistance is to avoid the action of the antibiotic by interfering with their target site. To achieve this, bacteria have evolved different tactics, including protection of the target (preventing the antibiotic from reaching its binding site) and modifications of the target site that result in decreased affinity for the antibiotic molecule.

Target protection

Although some of the genetic determinants coding for proteins that mediate target protection have been found in the bacterial chromosome, most of the clinically relevant genes involved in this mechanism of resistance are carried by MGEs. Examples of drugs affected by this mechanism include tetracycline (Tet[M] and Tet[O]), fluoroquinolones (Qnr), and fusidic acid (FusB and FusC).

One of the classic and best-studied examples of the target protection mechanism

is the tetracycline resistance determinants Tet(M) and Tet(O). Tet(M) was initially described in *Streptococcus* spp. and Tet(O) in *Campylobacter jejuni*, but they are now both widely distributed among different bacterial species, likely because they have been found in several plasmids and in broad-range conjugative transposons (51). These proteins belong to the translation factor superfamily of GTPases and act as homologues of elongation factors (EF-G and EF-Tu) used in protein synthesis. TetO and TetM interact with the ribosome and dislodge the tetracycline from its binding site in a GTP-dependent manner. Dönhöfer et al. recently showed that TetM directly dislodges and releases tetracycline from the ribosome by an interaction between the domain IV of the 16S rRNA and the tetracycline binding site. Furthermore, this interaction alters the ribosomal conformation, preventing rebinding of the antibiotic (52). Similarly, TetO has also been shown to compete with tetracycline for the same ribosomal space and to alter the geometry of the binding site of the antibiotic, displacing the molecule from the ribosome and allowing protein synthesis to resume (53).

Another example of target protection is the quinolone resistance protein Qnr, which is a plasmid-mediated fluoroquinolone resistance determinant frequently found in clinical isolates. Initially described in a clinical isolate of *K. pneumoniae* in the mid-1990s (54), Qnr belongs to the pentapeptide repeat protein family, and it acts as a DNA homologue that competes for the DNA binding site of the DNA gyrase and topoisomerase IV. It is thought that this reduction in the DNA gyrase-DNA interaction decreases the opportunities of the quinolone molecule to form and stabilize the gyrase-cleaved DNA-quinolone complex that is lethal for the cell (55). Several different *qnr* alleles have been described to date, namely *qnrA*, *qnrB*, *qnrC*, *qnrD*, *qnrS*, and *qnrVC*, all of which have a similar mechanism of action. Notably, the presence of Qnr confers low-level quinolone resistance. However, harboring Qnr-encoding genes has been shown to promote the emergence of highly resistant isolates by facilitating the selection of mutants with point mutations in genes encoding the DNA gyrase and/or topoisomerase IV (56) (the predominant target of the fluoroquinolone class of antibiotics; see below).

Modification of the target site

Introducing modifications to the target site is one of the most common mechanisms of antibiotic resistance in bacterial pathogens affecting almost all families of antimicrobial compounds. These target changes may consist of (i) point mutations in the genes encoding the target site, (ii) enzymatic alterations of the binding site (e.g., addition of methyl groups), and/or (iii) replacement or bypass of the original target. As mentioned, regardless of the type of change, the final effect is always the same: a decrease in the affinity of the antibiotic for the target site. Classical examples of each of these strategies will be detailed below.

Mutations of the target site

One of the classical examples of mutational resistance is the development of rifampin resistance. Rifampin is a rifamycin that blocks bacterial transcription by inhibiting the DNA-dependent RNA polymerase, which is a complex enzyme with a $\alpha_2\beta\beta'\sigma$ subunit structure. The rifampin binding pocket is a highly conserved structure located in the β subunit of the RNA polymerase (encoded by *rpoB*), and after binding, the antibiotic molecule interrupts transcription by directly blocking the path of the nascent RNA (57). High-level rifampin resistance has been shown to occur by single-step point mutations resulting in amino acid substitutions in the *rpoB* gene, and many different genetic changes have been reported. Of note, while these mutations result in decreased affinity of the drug for its target, they usually spare the catalytic activity of the polymerase, permitting transcription to continue (58).

Another well-characterized example of mutational resistance involves the mechanism of fluoroquinolone resistance (as briefly mentioned above). Fluoroquinolones kill bacteria by altering DNA replication through the inhibition of two crucial enzymes, DNA gyrase and topoisomerase IV. Development of chromosomal mutations in the genes encoding subunits of the above-mentioned enzymes (*gyrA-gyrB* and *parC-parE* for DNA gyrase and topoisomerase IV, respectively) is the most frequent mechanism of acquired resistance to these compounds. Importantly, since fluoroquinolones interact with two enzymes (DNA gyrase and topoisomerase), and both of them are essential for bacterial survival, the level of resistance achieved by developing changes in one of the enzymes depends on the potency with which the antimicrobial inhibits the unaltered target. Thus, in contrast to rifampin, clinically relevant fluoroquinolone resistance frequently requires an accumulation of genetic changes over time, with the first mutation producing minor increases in the MIC (59).

Finally, another good example of antibiotic resistance arising due to mutational changes is resistance to oxazolidinones (linezolid and tedizolid). These drugs are synthetic bacteriostatic antibiotics with broad Gram-positive activity that exert their mechanism through an interaction with the A site of bacterial ribosomes. Such interaction inhibits protein synthesis by interfering with the positioning of the aminoacyl-tRNA. Linezolid is the most widely used antibiotic of this class, because tedizolid was only recently approved for clinical use. Although linezolid resistance remains an uncommon phenomenon, it has been well described in most clinically relevant Gram-positive organisms. The most commonly characterized mechanisms of linezolid resistance include mutations in genes encoding domain V of the 23S rRNA and/or the ribosomal proteins L3 and L4 (*rplC* and *rplD*, respectively), and methylation of A2503 (*E. coli* numbering) in the 23S rRNA mediated by the Cfr enzyme (see below) (Fig. 4) (60).

Mutations in genes encoding the central loop of domain V of the 23S rRNA in the 50S ribosomal subunit are the most frequent determinants of linezolid resistance. A number of mutations have been described to date, and the most frequent change found in clinical isolates appears to be the transition G2576T (*E. coli* numbering). Regardless of the position and type of genetic change, these mutations result in decreased affinity of the drug for its ribosomal target. Since bacteria carry multiple copies of the 23S rRNA genes, mutations need to accumulate in multiple alleles to yield a clinically relevant phenotype (gene-dose effect) (61). In addition, substitutions in the L3 and L4 ribosomal proteins have also been associated with development of linezolid resistance *in vivo* and *in vitro*, both alone and in

combination with other resistance determinants (60).

Enzymatic alteration of the target site

One of the best-characterized examples of resistance through enzymatic modification of the target site is the methylation of the ribosome catalyzed by an enzyme encoded by the *erm* genes (erythromycin ribosomal methylation), which results in macrolide resistance. These enzymes are capable of mono- or dimethylating an adenine residue in position A2058 of domain V of the 23rRNA of the 50S ribosomal subunit. Due to this biochemical change, the binding of the antimicrobial molecule to its target is impaired. Since macrolides, lincosamides, and streptogramin B antibiotics have overlapping binding sites in the 23S rRNA, expression of

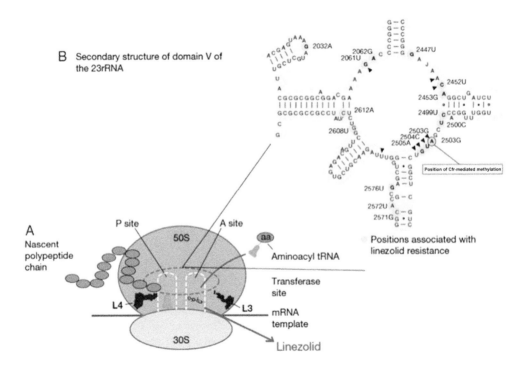

FIGURE 4 **Schematic representation of the mechanism of action and resistance to linezolid. (A) Linezolid interferes with the positioning of aminoacyl-tRNA by interactions with the peptidyl-transferase center (PTC). Ribosomal proteins L3 and L4 associated with resistance are shown. (B) Representation of domain V of 23S rRNA showing mutations associated with linezolid resistance. Position A2503, which is the target of Cfr methylation, is highlighted. Adapted from reference 92.**

the *erm* genes confers cross-resistance to all members of the MLS$_B$ group (62, 63). More than 30 *erm* genes have been described, many of them located in MGEs, which may account for their ample distribution among different genera, including aerobic and anaerobic Gram-positive and Gram-negative bacteria. In staphylococci, the most important *erm* genes are *erm*(A) (mostly distributed in a transposon in methicillin-susceptible *S. aureus* [MRSA]) and *erm*(C) (found in plasmids in MRSA). On the other hand, *erm*(B) has been more frequently reported in enterococci and pneumococci (where it was first described), located in plasmids and conjugative and nonconjugative transposons such as Tn*917* and Tn*551*. These genes are widely distributed and have now been found in over 30 bacterial genera (64).

Erm-mediated resistance carries an important bacterial fitness cost due to less efficient translation by the methylated ribosome. Hence, although the MLS$_B$ phenotype can be constitutively expressed, in most cases it is subject to strict control via complex posttranscriptional gene regulation. Through this mechanism, bacteria growing in the absence of antibiotics produce an inactive mRNA transcript that cannot be translated into the desired protein (in this case a methylase). Conversely, in the presence of antibiotic, the transcript becomes active and the system is primed to confer rapid resistance. This is best characterized by the inducible MLS$_B$ phenotype of the *erm*(C) operon in *S. aureus*, which is conformed by the *erm*(C) gene, an upstream gene encoding a leader peptide and an intergenic region (Fig. 5). In the absence of an inducer, transcription of the operon generates an mRNA with a secondary structure that conceals the ribosomal binding site upstream of *erm*. Translation proceeds through the leader peptide and then terminates, preventing the production of ErmC. In the presence erythromycin (but also other macrolides), the ribosome stalls due to inhibition by the antibiotic during translation of the leader

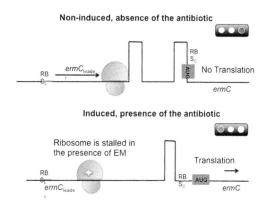

FIGURE 5 Schematic representation of the post-transcriptional control of the *ermC* gene. Under noninducing conditions, the ErmC leader peptide is produced and the *ermC* mRNA forms two hairpins, preventing the ribosome from recognizing the ribosomal binding site (RBS) of *ermC*. As a result, translation is inhibited. After exposure to erythromycin (EM, yellow star), the antibiotic interacts with the ribosome and binds tightly to the leader peptide, stalling progression of translation. This phenomenon releases the *ermC* RBS and permits translation. RBS$_L$, ribosomal binding site of the leader; RBS$_C$, ribosomal binding site of *ermC*; AUG, initiation codon. Ribosome represented in blue and erythromycin in yellow.

peptide, allowing a conformational change in the *ermC* mRNA that unmasks its ribosomal binding site, resulting in efficient translation of *erm*(C) (65). Thus, bacteria have evolved a sophisticated mRNA-based control mechanism to tightly regulate the expression of these methylases, ensuring a high efficiency of action in the presence of the antibiotic while minimizing the fitness costs for the bacterial population. The array of compounds capable of inducing the MLS$_B$ phenotype varies among different *erm* genes, but as a general rule the best inducer is erythromycin, while the inducing ability of other macrolides varies. Similarly, the system is usually not induced by lincosamides or streptogramins. However, the use of these agents against isolates carrying inducible *erm* genes may result in the selection of constitutive mutants *in vivo* (particularly in severe infections), leading to therapeutic failures.

Another relevant example of enzymatic alteration of the target is Cfr-mediated linezolid resistance. The *cfr* gene is a plasmid-borne determinant initially described in 2000 in a bovine isolate of *Staphylococcus sciuri* and first reported in humans in 2005 in an *S. aureus* strain isolated from a patient in Colombia (66). Since then, it has been found in several species of human pathogens, including *S. aureus, E. faecalis, E. faecium,* and some Gram-negative bacteria. This gene encodes the Cfr enzyme, which is a member of the S-adenosyl-L-methionine (SAM) methylase family, which also confers resistance to phenicols, lincosamides, pleuromutilins, and streptogramin A. Moreover, *cfr* has been associated with various MGEs, suggesting that it has an enhanced potential to spread and to cause transferable linezolid resistance in the future. Carriage of *cfr* does not appear to confer resistance to the recently FDA-approved oxazolidinone tedizolid (67).

Complete replacement or bypass of the target site

Using this strategy, bacteria are capable of evolving new targets that accomplish similar biochemical functions of the original target but are not inhibited by the antimicrobial molecule. The most relevant clinical examples include methicillin resistance in *S. aureus* due to the acquisition of an exogenous PBP (PBP2a) and vancomycin resistance in enterococci through modifications of the peptidoglycan structure mediated by the *van* gene clusters. Finally, another route to avoid the antimicrobial action is to "bypass" the metabolic pathway that the antibiotic inhibits by overproducing the antibiotic target. A relevant example of this mechanism is resistance to trimethoprim-sulfamethoxazole (TMP-SMX). In the remainder of this section we will provide further details of the examples mentioned above.

The antibacterial activity of β-lactams relies on their ability to disrupt cell wall synthesis through inhibition of PBPs, which are important enzymes responsible for the transpeptidation and transglycosylation of peptidoglycan units emerging from the cytoplasm. Resistance to methicillin (a semisynthetic penicillin that is stable against the staphylococcal penicillinase) in *S. aureus* results from the acquisition of a foreign gene (likely from *S. sciuri*) designated *mecA* that is often located in a large DNA fragment designated staphylococcal chromosomal cassette *mec* (SCC*mec*). The *mecA* gene encodes PBP2a, a PBP that has low affinity for all β-lactams, including penicillins, cephalosporins (except for last-generation compounds), and carbapenems. Acquisition of *mecA* renders most β-lactams useless against MRSA, and alternative therapies need to be used in serious infections. Of note, PBP2a carries a transpeptidase domain, but it does not function as a transglycosylase (class B PBP), so it requires the activity of other native PBPs to perform the latter function and fully cross-link peptidoglycan. Specifically, the penicillin-insensitive transglycosylase domain of PBP2 (a class A PBP) is particularly important to achieve transglycosylation of peptidoglycan in the presence of β-lactams in *mecA*-carrying MRSA isolates.

The *mecA* gene is usually found as part of a gene cassette inserted into a larger MGE (SCC*mec*), whose basic components include *mecA, mecR1* (encoding the signal transducer protein MecR1), *mecI* (encoding the repressor protein MecI), and *ccr* (encoding a recombinase: cassette chromosome recombinase). To date, 11 SCC*mec* allotypes have been described with varying degrees of genetic homology and different sizes, insertion sequences, and accompanying resistance genes (68, 69). SCC*mec* types seem to differ among different MRSA clones. Indeed, community-associated MRSA strains appear to harbor shorter SCC*mec* cassettes (e.g., SCC*mec* type IV) and carry fewer antibiotic resistance determinants, whereas hospital-associated isolates possess longer elements (e.g., SCC*mec* type II) and are usually MDR (70).

A two-component regulatory system that includes the repressor protein MecI and the signal transducer MecR1 regulates the expression of *mecA*. Once MecR1 senses the presence of β-lactams in the environment, it triggers a signal transduction cascade that removes the MecI repressor from its DNA binding site, resulting in transcription of *mecA* and its regulatory genes. These events culminate with the production of PBP2a, which is the hallmark of methicillin resistance in *S. aureus* (70, 71).

Another important example of the replacement and bypass strategy to achieve resistance is related to vancomycin resistance. Similar to β-lactams, glycopeptides (i.e., vancomycin and teicoplanin) kill bacteria by inhibiting cell wall synthesis. However, unlike β-lactams, glycopeptides do not directly interact with PBPs. Instead, they bind to the terminal D-alanine-D-alanine (D-Ala-D-Ala) of the pentapeptide moiety of the nascent peptidoglycan precursors (lipid II), preventing PBP-mediated cross-linking and resulting in inhibition of cell wall synthesis. It has been postulated that the main effect of the binding of vancomycin to D-Ala-D-Ala-ending precursors emerging from the cytoplasm is alteration of transglycosylation (presumably due to steric hindrance) preventing further processing of the cell wall and leading to bacterial death (72).

Vancomycin resistance is especially relevant in enterococci (particularly *E. faecium*), and it is usually accompanied by the presence of other resistance determinants, making the treatment of infections caused by these organisms an important clinical challenge (73). Vancomycin resistance in enterococci involves the acquisition of a group of genes (designated *van* gene clusters) that code for a biochemical machinery that remodels the synthesis of peptidoglycan by (i) changing the last D-Ala for either D-lactate (high-level resistance) or D-serine (low-level resistance) and (ii) destroying the "normal" D-Ala-D-Ala-ending precursors to prevent vancomycin from binding to the cell wall precursors. The change of D-Ala for D-lactate removes a single hydrogen bond between the vancomycin molecule and its target (D-Ala-D-Ala moiety), decreasing the antibiotic affinity for the precursor about 1,000-fold. Although the change of D-Ala for D-Ser does not remove any of the five hydrogen bonds between vancomycin and its target, the presence of the hydroxyl group of serine affects the interaction of the antibiotic with the precursors, reducing its affinity, albeit less markedly than with the D-Lac replacement (74).

The origin of the *van* genes has been a topic of intense investigation. Genes nearly identical to those of the *vanA* gene cluster (the most prevalent in clinical enterococcal strains) have been found in soil organisms such as *Paenibacillus thiaminolyticus* and *Paenibacillus apiarius* (75). To date, nine distinct enterococcal *van* clusters have been described (*vanA, vanB, vanC, vanD, vanE, vanG, vanL, vanM,* and *vanN*). The *vanADLM* clusters synthesize precursors ending in D-Lac, whereas the *vanCEGN* produce D-Ser-ending peptidoglycan. Most clinical vancomycin-resistant enterococci (VRE) isolates carry the *vanA* or *vanB* gene clusters, which are usually found in MGEs either associated with plasmids or inserted in the chromosome. We will provide further details of the biochemical mechanism of VanA-mediated resistance (involving both vancomycin and teicoplanin). The reader is referred to other comprehensive reviews for additional details on glycopeptide resistance (13, 74, 76).

The *vanA* gene cluster is usually located on a Tn3-family transposon designated Tn*1546*, which has been found on both conjugative and nonconjugative plasmids. This gene cluster consists of seven genes coding for three groups of proteins: (i) a classical two-component regulatory system that regulates the expression of resistance (VanS is the histidine kinase and VanR the response regulator of the system), (ii) enzymes necessary for the synthesis of new peptidoglycan precursors, namely a dehydrogenase (VanH) and an amino acid ligase with altered substrate specificity (VanA) capable of producing D-Ala-D-Lac, and (iii) enzymes that destroy the normal D-Ala-D-Ala-ending precursors (VanX and VanY). Of note, an additional gene, *vanZ*, is present in Tn*1546*, but its function remains unknown.

Induction of the *vanA* gene cluster appears to involve initial sensing by VanS of the accumulation of substrates resulting from inhibition of glycosyltransferase activity (77). This initial step results in an ATP-dependent phosphorylation of the response regulator VanR, which subsequently binds to two promoters, one of them located upstream of its own gene (*vanR*) and the other upstream of *vanH* in Tn*1546* (78). The *vanH* gene encodes a dehydrogenase enzyme necessary for the production of D-lactate using pyruvate as the substrate. D-Lac is then bound to a molecule of D-Ala by the VanA ligase, and the D-Ala-D-Lac dipeptide is subsequently added to the nascent tripeptide (MurNAc-L-Ala^1-γ-D-Glu^2-L-Lys^3) to form the altered peptidoglycan unit (UDP-MurNAc-pentadepsipeptide; Mur-NAc-L-Ala^1-γ-D-Glu^2-L-Lys^3-D-Ala^4-D-Lac^5) (Fig. 6).

The other genes of Tn*1546* code for enzymes that destroy D-Ala-ending precursors. The *vanX* gene encodes a D,D-dipeptidase that hydrolyzes any D-Ala-D-Ala produced in the "normal" peptidoglycan synthesis pathway, and *vanY* codes for a membrane-bound D,D-carboxypeptidase that removes the last D-Ala of normal ending precursors, ensuring that no D-Ala-D-Ala-ending pentapeptides (which could potentially bind vancomycin) are exposed on the cell surface. Finally, Tn*1546* harbors another gene (designated *vanZ*) that appears to be involved in teicoplanin resistance (but not vancomycin) and whose function is unknown (76).

Development of high-level vancomycin resistance in *S. aureus* (vancomycin-resistant *S. aureus*) was first described in 2002 and was the result of acquisition by an MRSA strain of the *vanA* gene cluster from a VRE

(*E. faecalis*) isolate (79). However, occurrence of this phenomenon continues to be rare. Although transfer of an enterococcal plasmid containing the *vanA* gene cluster in Tn*1546* to *S. aureus* has been shown to occur *in vitro*, the efficiency of this mechanism is low since replication of enterococcal plasmids in staphylococci is frequently suboptimal. However, a potentially more worrisome scenario is the acquisition of the *vanA* gene cluster by community-associated strains using native staphylococcal plasmids. Indeed, a recent report described such a phenomenon where the *vanA* gene cluster was harbored in a highly transferable staphylococcal plasmid originally identified in community-associated *S. aureus* isolates. The isolate was found in a bloodstream isolate of MRSA recovered from a Brazilian patient (80), and transfer to a methicillin-susceptible isolate within the same patient was also documented.

The *vanB* gene cluster harbors genes similar to those carried by the *vanA* cluster, with the difference that the VanS$_B$ sensor kinase does not appear to be activated by the presence of teicoplanin. Thus, isolates harboring the *vanB* cluster remain susceptible to this glycopeptide. The *vanB* gene cluster is also carried by mobile elements in Tn*1547* or related conjugative transposons and has been identified in pheromone-responsive plasmids. In addition, the *vanB* cluster lacks the *vanZ* gene and carries an additional gene (designated *vanW*) whose function remains to be established.

The prototypical gene cluster responsible for low-level vancomycin resistance and the production of D-Ala-D-Ser peptidoglycan precursors is *vanC*. Of note, enterococci carrying the *vanEGLN* clusters also produce D-Ala-D-Ser, exhibit a low level of vancomycin resistance, and carry genes similar to those described in *vanC*. The main differences in terms of gene content and biochemical activities of VanC-type mediated resistance compared with VanA and VanB are that (i) they encode a unique racemase (VanT)

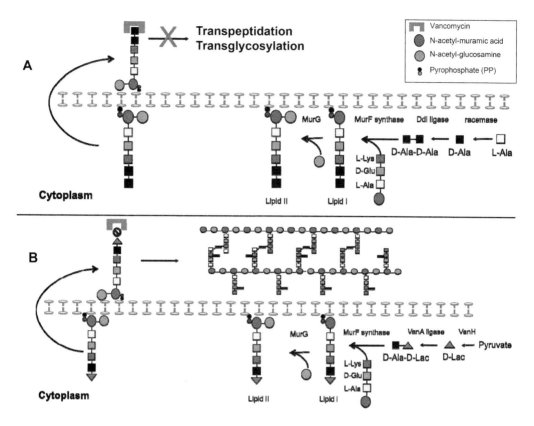

FIGURE 6 Schematic representation of peptidoglycan biosynthesis and mechanisms of vancomycin action (A) and resistance (B). (A) Normal peptidoglycan production. Binding of the antibiotic to the terminal D-Ala-D-Ala of the peptidoglycan precursors prevents transpeptidation and transglycosylation, interrupting cell wall synthesis and resulting in bacterial death. (B) The change in peptidoglycan synthesis produced by the expression of the *vanA* gene cluster. Change of the terminal dipeptide from D-Ala-D-Ala to D-Ala-D-Lac markedly reduces the binding of vancomycin to the peptidoglycan target permitting cell wall synthesis to continue.

capable of producing D-serine using L-serine as a substrate, (ii) they possess a ligase (*vanCEGLN*) with the ability to synthesize D-Ala-D-Ser dipeptides, and (iii) they often harbor a single gene (*vanXY*) encoding both D-Ala-D-Ala dipeptidase and carboxypeptidase activities that are normally coded for two distinct genes in the other clusters (*vanX* and *vanY*; see above).

On rare occasions, VRE strains can develop null mutations in the native D-Ala-D-Ala ligase (*ddl*) that abolish the normal production of D-Ala-D-Ala for peptidoglycan synthesis. Thus, strains harboring such mutations rely on the production of altered peptidoglycan

precursors for cell wall synthesis by the inducible *van* clusters (e.g., *vanA*). Therefore, cell survival depends on the permanent presence of the antibiotic to induce the system (hence, these isolates are designated vancomycin-dependent enterococci). This phenotype seems to be unstable since mutations in the VanS sensor or promoter regions frequently revert the phenotype (81).

As mentioned above, another well-described strategy of "target bypass" is to increase the production of the antimicrobial target with the objective of overwhelming the antibiotic by increasing the amount of targets available. One of the best examples of this mechanism is the development of resistance to TMP-SMX. This drug impairs bacterial synthesis of purines and some important amino acids by altering the production of folate, exploiting the fact that most bacteria are unable to incorporate folate from external sources. Therefore, bacteria rely on their own biochemical machinery for folate synthesis. The synthetic pathway of folate involves two major enzymes: (i) dihydropteroic acid synthase (DHPS), which forms dihydrofolate from para-aminobenzoic acid (inhibited by SMX), and (ii) dihydrofolate reductase (DHFR), which catalyzes the formation of tetrahydrofolate from dihydrofolate (inhibited by TMP).

Although development of resistance to TMP-SMX can be achieved through several strategies including amino acid changes in the above enzymes (decreasing their affinity for the antibiotic molecules, target modification) and acquisition of external genes encoding DHPS or DHFR that are less sensitive to inhibition by TMP-SMX (target bypass), a clever bypass strategy is the overproduction of DHFR or DHPS through mutations in the promoter region of the DNA encoding these enzymes. These mutations result in the production of increased quantities of the above enzymes, overwhelming the ability of TMP-SMX to inhibit folate production and permitting bacterial survival (82, 83). Interestingly, enterococci use another bypass strategy by incorporating exogenous tetrahydrofolic acid and folinic acid when added to the media. This ability to use folate from different sources is correlated with an up to 25-fold increase in the MICs of TMP-SMX and is thought to impair the antimicrobial activity *in vivo* (84, 85).

Resistance Due to Global Cell Adaptations

Through years of evolution, bacteria have developed sophisticated mechanisms to cope with environmental stressors and pressures in order to survive in the most hostile environments, including the human body. Bacteria need to compete for nutrients and avoid the attack of molecules produced by rival organisms to gain the "upper hand." Inside a particular host, bacterial organisms are constantly attacked by the host's immune system, and to establish themselves in particular biological niches, it is crucial that they adapt and cope with these stressful situations. Thus, bacterial pathogens have devised very complex mechanisms to avoid the disruption of pivotal cellular processes such as cell wall synthesis and membrane homeostasis. Development of resistance to daptomycin (DAP) and vancomycin (low-level in *S. aureus*) are the most clinically relevant examples of resistance phenotypes that are the result of a global cell-adaptive response to the antibacterial attack.

DAP is a lipopeptide antibiotic related to cationic antimicrobial peptides produced by the innate immune system that exerts its bactericidal effect by altering cell envelope homeostasis. The bactericidal activity of DAP requires four important steps (Fig. 7). First, DAP is complexed with calcium (rendering the molecule positively charged) and, subsequently, is directed to the cell membrane (CM) target by electrostatic interactions with the usually negatively charged CM. Of note, recent evidence suggests that DAP mainly targets the CM at the level of the division septum (86). Second, once the antibiotic molecules reach the CM, they initially oligomerize at the outer leaflet of the CM and, subsequently, these DAP oligomers reach the inner CM leaflet. DAP's oligomerization at the outer leaflet of the CM appears to be dependent on the presence of the phospholipid phosphatidylglycerol (PG) (87). Additionally, another phospholipid (cardiolipin), seems to play an important role in the translocation of DAP oligomers from the outer to the inner leaflet, but its contribution is not completely understood. In fact, there is evidence to suggest that the presence of cardiolipin in high concentrations may

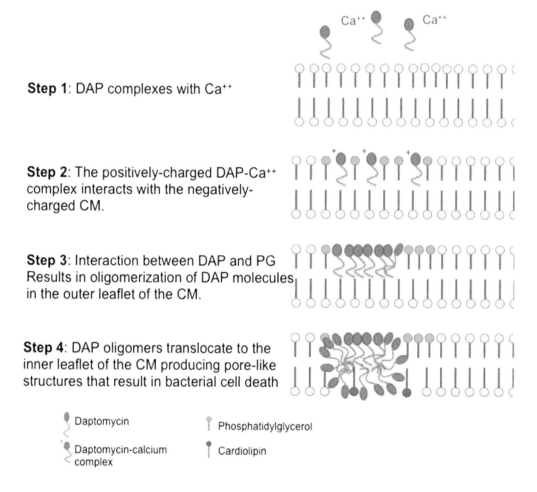

Step 1: DAP complexes with Ca⁺⁺

Step 2: The positively-charged DAP-Ca⁺⁺ complex interacts with the negatively-charged CM.

Step 3: Interaction between DAP and PG Results in oligomerization of DAP molecules in the outer leaflet of the CM.

Step 4: DAP oligomers translocate to the inner leaflet of the CM producing pore-like structures that result in bacterial cell death

Daptomycin

Daptomycin-calcium complex

Phosphatidylglycerol

Cardiolipin

FIGURE 7 **Diagrammatic representation of the mechanism of action of daptomycin. DAP, daptomycin; PG, phosphatidylglycerol; CM, cell membrane.**

prevent translocation of DAP oligomers into the inner leaflet of the phospholipid bilayer (87). Third, once the DAP oligomers reach the inner leaflet of the CM, they organize and form transmembrane pore-like structures that are likely to alter the physicochemical properties of the CM and promote leakage of ions (e.g., potassium) from the cytoplasm, causing important electrochemical alterations. Finally, these structural and functional CM alterations lead to bacterial death in the absence of cell lysis by mechanisms that are not fully understood.

Bacteria have developed ancient systems of defense to withstand cAMP action and possess a cadre of regulatory systems that are involved in protecting the cell envelope when under attack by cationic antimicrobial peptides. In enterococci, work using whole-genome sequencing of a clinical strain-pair of *E. faecalis* that developed DAP resistance (DAP-R) over the course of therapy revealed that changes in a three-component regulatory system designated LiaFSR (which orchestrates the cell-envelope stress response in Gram-positive organisms) are paramount in the development of DAP-R (88). In *Bacillus subtilis*, where the system was first characterized, and other Gram-positive bacteria, LiaFSR (and the homolog system VraTSR in

S. aureus) is composed of three proteins: (i) LiaF (VraT), a transmembrane protein that appears to negatively regulate the system, (ii) LiaS (VraS), a classical sensor-histidine kinase protein that phosphorylates the response regulator, and (iii) LiaR (VraR), the response regulator of the system. Indeed, a single deletion of an isoleucine at position 177 of LiaF increased the DAP MIC from 1 to 4 µg/ml (established clinical breakpoint is 4 µg/ml) and, more importantly, was sufficient to abolish the bactericidal activity of DAP (89). Moreover, in recent genomic analyses of 19 DAP-nonsusceptible *E. faecium* (DAP MICs from 3 to 48 µg/ml; clinical breakpoint is 4 µg/ml), the most frequently identified mutations were in *liaFSR*, supporting the hypothesis that changes in this system are a pivotal step toward DAP-R in enterococci (90). Furthermore, the majority (75%) of DAP-susceptible *E. faecium* isolates recovered from bacteremic patients whose MIC was in the higher range of susceptibility (i.e., between 3 and 4 µg/ml) harbored mutations in LiaFSR. Conversely, none of the isolates of the same collection with DAP MIC ≤ 2 µg/ml exhibited changes in this system (91). More importantly, these changes were sufficient to abolish the *in vitro* bactericidal activity of DAP and were associated with a clinical failure in a neutropenic patient with VRE bacteremia (92).

The mechanism by which LiaFSR results in DAP-R is not fully understood. Furthermore, the specific mechanism through which this system orchestrates the cell-envelope response to stress is still a matter of active research. In *B. subtilis*, the *lia* locus consists of six genes, *liaIH-liaGFSR*, of which *liaGFSR* are constitutively expressed at a low basal level due to the presence of a weak constitutive promoter upstream of *liaG*. In contrast, expression of *liaIH* is completely LiaR-dependent. Although LiaR regulates other genes, Wolf et al. provided evidence indicating that *liaIH* is the only relevant target of LiaR-dependent gene expression in wild-type cells. The physiological role of LiaI and LiaH

are not completely understood. LiaI is a small hydrophobic protein of unknown function with two putative transmembrane helices, and LiaH is a member of the phage-shock protein family that forms large oligomeric ring-like structures (resembling what has been reported with PspA in *E. coli*). The LiaFSR system constitutes a cell envelope stress-sensing/response system that is highly conserved in *Firmicutes* bacteria (93).

In enterococci, recent evidence suggests that LiaR mediates a reorganization of anionic phospholipids (i.e., cardiolipin) in the CM associated with DAP-R. In a clinical strain of DAP-R, development of resistance was clearly associated with redistribution of cardiolipin microdomains from the septum to other CM areas (94). This mislocalization seems to divert DAP from its principle CM septal target, resulting in bacterial survival of the DAP attack. Furthermore, deletion of LiaR completely reverted DAP susceptibility and restored the organization of cardiolipin domains (95).

Other regulatory systems involved in cell envelope homeostasis have also been associated with DAP-R. For example, YycFG (WalKR), an essential two-component regulatory system that has been implicated in cell-wall synthesis and homeostasis, has been found to be important to DAP-R in both enterococci and *S. aureus* (96, 97). Although the exact mechanism mediating this phenomenon has not been fully elucidated, it appears to involve alteration in cell wall metabolism that results in changes in surface-charge-producing electrostatic repulsion of the positively charged calcium-DAP complex from the cell envelope.

A second group of genes that have been shown to contribute to the development of DAP-R correspond to enzymes involved in the metabolism of CM phospholipids. For example, two enzymes, a glycerol-phosphodiester phosphodiesterase (GdpD) and cardiolipin synthase (Cls), were found to enhance the DAP-R phenotype in the background of *liaFSR* mutations in *E. faecalis* (88).

These changes seem to alter the CM phospholipid composition mainly by decreasing the amount of PG. Other enzymes such as MprF, PG synthase (PgsA), cyclic fatty acid synthase (Cfa), and geranyltransferase (98) involved in CM phospholipid homeostasis have also been linked to DAP-R. In *S. aureus*, MprF (a lysyl-PG synthase) has been one of the most studied enzymes, and inactivation of this protein reversed DAP-R. This enzyme harbors two domains: (i) a lysyl-transferase domain that transfers the positively charged amino acid lysine from its tRNA carrier to PG (lysyl-PG) in the inner leaflet of the CM and (ii) a flipase domain, through which newly synthesized lysyl-PG is translocated from the inner to the outer leaflet of the CM (99). Mutations in *mprF* appear to produce a gain of function of the enzyme and, as a result, the cell surface becomes more positively charged, repelling the DAP-calcium complex (also with positive charge). Of interest, a homolog of LiaFSR (VraTSR) seems also to contribute to the DAP-R phenotype mediated by changes in MprF in *S. aureus* (97).

The development of high-level vancomycin resistance mediated by the acquisition of the *van* gene cluster is a rare event in *S. aureus*. However, a much more common problem is the finding of *S. aureus* isolates with intermediate susceptibility to vancomycin (known as VISA isolates), exhibiting MICs between 4 to 8 μg/ml. This phenomenon was first reported in Japan in 1997 and led to therapeutic failure (100). The isolate, designated Mu50, was derived from a vancomycin-susceptible strain known as Mu3 (≤2 μg/ml). Population analyses of Mu3 later confirmed that this strain contained a subpopulation of bacterial cells capable of surviving at concentrations of vancomycin above 2 μg/ml (clinical breakpoint for susceptibility), a phenomenon that has now been designated the heterogenous-VISA (hVISA) phenotype. Because the resistant subpopulation is difficult to identify, detection of hVISA becomes very challenging, and some *S. aureus* strains reported as

susceptible to vancomycin by standard susceptibility testing may still exhibit this phenotype (101). Indeed, *S. aureus* within the range of susceptibility, with vancomycin MICs >1 and ≤2 μg/ml have been more frequently associated with the hVISA phenotype. Due to the difficulties in detecting these strains, vancomycin failures have been increasingly reported in deep-seated infections. Published studies estimate that the overall prevalence of MRSA strains with an hVISA/VISA profile range between 0 and 8.24%, but it can be as high as 30% in selected populations (e.g., patients with MRSA infective endocarditis) (102, 103).

The hVISA/VISA isolates usually emerge *in vivo* in patients with a history of an MRSA infection that failed to respond to a prolonged course of vancomycin therapy. From a mechanistic point of view, the development of the hVISA/VISA does not occur by the acquisition of foreign DNA material (as seen in vancomycin-resistant *S. aureus*); rather, the phenotype appears to be the result of sequential and ordered genetic changes that usually involve genes forming part of regulatory systems controlling cell envelope homeostasis (similar to that described above for DAP). The specific mechanisms that lead to the hVISA/VISA phenotype remain to be completely understood. However, the available evidence shows that the regulatory systems most consistently implicated in this mechanism of resistance are YycFG (WalKR), VraSR (homolog of LiaFSR), and GraRS (104). Interestingly, these two- and three-component regulatory systems are involved in cell wall homeostasis, supporting the notion that selection of the hVISA/VISA phenotype involves important remodeling of the cell wall to survive the antimicrobial attack.

Apart from the above regulatory systems, another change that has been frequently associated with the VISA phenotype is mutations in *rpoB* (encoding the B subunit of the RNA polymerase). Indeed, Watanabe et al. analyzed 38 VISA isolates from

10 countries and demonstrated that mutations in the *rpoB* gene were present in the majority (71%) of the isolates (105). However, the mechanisms by which mutation of *rpoB* led to reduced vancomycin and DAP susceptibility are unclear.

Phenotypically, hVISA/VISA strains exhibit distinct metabolic characteristics that may include (i) increased fructose utilization, (ii) increased fatty acid metabolism, (iii) impaired acetate metabolism and tricarboxylic acid cycle, (iv) decreased glutamate availability, and (iv) increased expression of cell wall synthesis genes. These global homeostatic changes appear to lead to a reduced autolytic activity with a thickened cell wall and an increased amount of free D-Ala-D-Ala dipeptides, with less peptidoglycan cross-linking (101, 104). In addition, VISA strains bind vancomycin more avidly than their non-VISA counterparts, but diffusion of the antibiotic molecule into the inner part of the cell wall appears to be impaired. Hence, it has been postulated that these changes result in trapping of vancomycin in the outer layers of the peptidoglycan, preventing the antibiotic molecule from reaching its target of precursors emerging from the cytoplasmic membrane. As a result, cell wall synthesis and peptidoglycan cross-linking continue to be uninterrupted.

Finally, a striking feature of many hVISA/VISA strains is their ability to revert from one phenotype to another (or even to a fully vancomycin-susceptible phenotype) in the absence of vancomycin exposure. Therefore, there seems to be a price to pay for developing resistance, and this is yet another example of the ability of bacteria to adapt to the environment by means of their remarkable genetic plasticity.

CONCLUDING REMARKS

The use of antimicrobials in clinical practice is a recent development compared to the emergence of bacterial organisms on our planet. Therefore, the development of antibiotic resistance should be viewed as a normal adaptive response and a clear manifestation of Darwin's principles of evolution. Arguably, the implementation of antimicrobial therapy in clinical practice has been one of the most successful advances of modern medicine, paving the way for complex and highly sophisticated medical interventions that have allowed us to significantly prolong the life span of the population around the globe. To survive, bacteria, in a process likely pressed by the increased use of antimicrobials in clinical practice, have developed complex and creative strategies to circumvent the antibiotic attack. Antibiotic resistance has rapidly evolved in the past few decades to become one of the greatest public health threats of the 21st century. Indeed, infections that are untreatable due to multidrug resistance of the infecting organism have become more common in clinical settings. This dire scenario has been worsened by a shortage of research and development on antibiotics. The "golden" pipeline of antibiotic discovery (1960s and 1970s) rapidly dried up as the identification of new compounds became more challenging. Big pharma concentrated their efforts on other more profitable and rewarding areas, leaving the wave of resistance to grow unabated.

If we are to tackle this problem, efforts in research and development need to be heavily increased and supported. A complete understanding of the mechanisms by which bacteria become resistant to antibiotics is of paramount importance to designing novel strategies to counter the resistance threat. We are in need of developing antibiotics, with the understanding that the microorganism will respond to them and resistance will develop (an evolutionary fact). Therefore, efforts to develop antibiotics and study mechanisms of resistance should be continuous, resilient, and steady. This is likely to be a long haul "war" against living entities with a major ability to adapt and survive.

ACKNOWLEDGMENTS

This work was funded by NIH-NIAID grant RO1 AI093749.

CITATION

Munita JM, Arias CA. 2016. Mechanisms of antibiotic resistance. Microbiol Spectrum 4(2):VMBF-0016-2015.

REFERENCES

1. **World Health Organization.** 2014. *Antimicrobial Resistance: Global Report on Surveillance 2014.* WHO, Geneva Switzerland. http://www.who.int/drugresistance/documents/surveillancereport/en/.

2. **Cosgrove SE.** 2006. The relationship between antimicrobial resistance and patient outcomes: mortality, length of hospital stay, and health care costs. *Clin Infect Dis* **42**(Suppl 2):S82–S89.

3. **DiazGranados CA, Zimmer SM, Klein M, Jernigan JA.** 2005. Comparison of mortality associated with vancomycin-resistant and vancomycin-susceptible enterococcal bloodstream infections: a meta-analysis. *Clin Infect Dis* **41**:327–333.

4. **Sydnor ER, Perl TM.** 2011. Hospital epidemiology and infection control in acute-care settings. *Clin Microbiol Rev* **24**:141–173.

5. **Centers for Disease Control and Prevention.** 2013. *Antibiotic Resistance Threats in the United States.* Centers for Disease Control and Prevention, 2013. CDC, Atlanta, GA. http://www.cdc.gov/drugresistance/threat-report-2013/index.html.

6. **The Review on Antimicrobial Resistance.** 2014. *Antimicrobial Resistance: Tackling a Crisis for the Future Health and Wealth of Nations.* http://amr-review.org.

7. **Clinical and Laboratory Standards Institute.** 2014. *Performance Standards for Antimicrobial Susceptibility Testing; 24th informational supplement.* CLSI document M100-S24. CLSI, Wayne, PA.

8. **Nannini EC, Singh KV, Arias CA, Murray BE.** 2013. *In vivo* effect of cefazolin, daptomycin, and nafcillin in experimental endocarditis with a methicillin-susceptible *Staphylococcus aureus* strain showing an inoculum effect against cefazolin. *Antimicrob Agents Chemother* **57:** 4276–4281.

9. **Manson JM, Hancock LE, Gilmore MS.** 2010. Mechanism of chromosomal transfer of *Enterococcus faecalis* pathogenicity island, capsule, antimicrobial resistance, and other traits. *Proc Natl Acad Sci USA* **107:**12269–12274.

10. **Thomas CM, Nielsen KM.** 2005. Mechanisms of, and barriers to, horizontal gene transfer between bacteria. *Nat Rev Microbiol* **3:**711–721.

11. **Wilson DN.** 2014. Ribosome-targeting antibiotics and mechanisms of bacterial resistance. *Nat Rev Microbiol* **12:**35–48.

12. **Ramirez MS, Tolmasky ME.** 2010. Aminoglycoside modifying enzymes. *Drug Resist Updat* **13:**151–171.

13. **Hollenbeck BL, Rice LB.** 2012. Intrinsic and acquired resistance mechanisms in enterococcus. *Virulence* **3:**421–433.

14. **Schwarz S, Kehrenberg C, Doublet B, Cloeckaert A.** 2004. Molecular basis of bacterial resistance to chloramphenicol and florfenicol. *FEMS Microbiol Rev* **28:**519–542.

15. **Abraham EP, Chain E.** 1940. An enzyme from bacteria able to destroy penicillin. *Nature* **146:**837.

16. **D'Costa VM, King CE, Kalan L, Morar M, Sung WW, Schwarz C, Froese D, Zazula G, Calmels F, Debruyne R, Golding GB, Poinar HN, Wright GD.** 2011. Antibiotic resistance is ancient. *Nature* **477:**457–461.

17. **Bush K.** 2013. Proliferation and significance of clinically relevant β-lactamases. *Ann N Y Acad Sci* **1277:**84–90.

18. **Paterson DL, Bonomo RA.** 2005. Extended-spectrum beta-lactamases: a clinical update. *Clin Microbiol Rev* **18:**657–686.

19. **Bush K.** 2013. The ABCD's of β-lactamase nomenclature. *J Infect Chemother* **19:**549–559.

20. **Bush K, Jacoby GA.** 2010. Updated functional classification of β-lactamases. *Antimicrob Agents Chemother* **54:**969–976.

21. **Sirot D, Sirot J, Labia R, Morand A, Courvalin P, Darfeuille-Michaud A, Perroux R, Cluzel R.** 1987. Transferable resistance to third-generation cephalosporins in clinical isolates of *Klebsiella pneumoniae*: identification of CTX-1, a novel beta-lactamase. *J Antimicrob Chemother* **20:** 323–334.

22. **Bonnet R.** 2004. Growing group of extended-spectrum beta lactamases: the CTX-M enzymes. *Antimicrob Agents Chemother* **48:**1–14.

23. **Poirel L, Lartigue M-F, Decousser J-W, Nordmann P.** 2005. ISEcp1B-mediated transposition of $bla_{\mathrm{CTX-M}}$ in *Escherichia coli*. *Antimicrob Agents Chemother* **49:**447–450.

24. **Queenan AM, Bush K.** 2007. Carbapenemases: the versatile beta-lactamases. *Clin Microbiol Rev* **20:**440–458.

25. **Yigit H, Queenan AM, Anderson GJ, Domenech-Sanchez A, Biddle JW, Steward**

CD, Alberti S, Bush K, Tenover FC. 2001. Novel carbapenem-hydrolyzing beta-lactamase, KPC-1, from a carbapenem-resistant strain of *Klebsiella pneumoniae*. *Antimicrob Agents Chemother* **45:**1151–1161.

26. Nordmann P, Cuzon G, Naas T. 2009. The real threat of *Klebsiella pneumoniae* carbapenemase-producing bacteria. *Lancet Infect Dis* **9:**228–236.

27. Poirel L, Pitout JD, Nordmann P. 2007. Carbapenemases: molecular diversity and clinical consequences. *Future Microbiol* **2:** 501–512.

28. Cornaglia G, Giamarellou H, Rossolini GM. 2011. Metallo-β-lactamases: a last frontier for β-lactams? *Lancet Infect Dis* **11:**381–393.

29. Kumarasamy KK, Toleman MA, Walsh TR, Bagaria J, Butt F, Balakrishnan R, Chaudhary U, Doumith M, Giske CG, Irfan S, Krishnan P, Kumar AV, Maharjan S, Mushtaq S, Noorie T, Paterson DL, Pearson A, Perry C, Pike R, Rao B, Ray U, Sarma JB, Sharma M, Sheridan E, Thirunarayan MA, Turton J, Upadhyay S, Warner M, Welfare W, Livermore DM, Woodford N. 2010. Emergence of a new antibiotic resistance mechanism in India, Pakistan, and the UK: a molecular, biological, and epidemiological study. *Lancet Infect Dis* **10:**597–602.

30. Nordmann P, Poirel L, Walsh TR, Livermore DM. 2011. The emerging NDM carbapenemases. *Trends Microbiol* **19:**588–595.

31. Walsh TR, Weeks J, Livermore DM, Toleman MA. 2011. Dissemination of NDM-1 positive bacteria in the New Delhi environment and its implications for human health: an environmental point prevalence study. *Lancet Infect Dis* **11:**355–362.

32. Jacoby GA. 2009. AmpC beta-lactamases. *Clin Microbiol Rev* **22:**161–182.

33. Jacobs C, Frère JM, Normark S. 1997. Cytosolic intermediates for cell wall biosynthesis and degradation control inducible beta-lactam resistance in Gram-negative bacteria. *Cell* **88:**823–832.

34. Johnson JW, Fisher JF, Mobashery S. 2013. Bacterial cell wall recycling. *Ann N Y Acad Sci* **1277:**54–75.

35. Schmidtke AJ, Hanson ND. 2006. Model system to evaluate the effect of ampD mutations on AmpC-mediated beta-lactam resistance. *Antimicrob Agents Chemother* **50:**2030–2037.

36. Evans BA, Amyes SG. 2014. OXA β-lactamases. *Clin Microbiol Rev* **27:**241–263.

37. Pagès JM, James CE, Winterhalter M. 2008. The porin and the permeating antibiotic: a selective diffusion barrier in Gram-negative bacteria. *Nat Rev Microbiol* **6:**893–903.

38. Hancock RE, Brinkman FS. 2002. Function of pseudomonas porins in uptake and efflux. *Annu Rev Microbiol* **56:**17–38.

39. Nikaido H. 2003. Molecular basis of bacterial outer membrane permeability revisited. *Microbiol Mol Biol Rev* **67:**593–656.

40. Quinn JP, Dudek EJ, DiVincenzo CA, Lucks DA, Lerner SA. 1986. Emergence of resistance to imipenem during therapy for *Pseudomonas aeruginosa* infections. *J Infect Dis* **154:**289–294.

41. Hasdemir UO, Chevalier J, Nordmann P, Pagès J-M. 2004. Detection and prevalence of active drug efflux mechanism in various multidrug resistant *Klebsiella pneumoniae* strains from Turkey. *J Clin Microbiol* **42:**2701–2706.

42. Doménech-Sánchez A, Martínez-Martínez L, Hernández-Allés S, del Carmen Conejo M, Pascual A, Tomás JM, Albertí S, Benedí VJ. 2003. Role of *Klebsiella pneumoniae* OmpK35 porin in antimicrobial resistance. *Antimicrob Agents Chemother* **47:**3332–3335.

43. McMurry LM, Petrucci RE Jr, Levy SB. 1980. Active efflux of tetracycline encoded by four genetically different tetracycline resistance determinants in *Escherichia coli*. *Proc Natl Acad Sci USA* **77:**3974–3977.

44. Poole K. 2005. Efflux-mediated antimicrobial resistance. *J Antimicrob Chemother* **56:** 20–51.

45. Singh KV, Weinstock GM, Murray BE. 2002. An *Enterococcus faecalis* ABC homologue (Lsa) is required for the resistance of this species to clindamycin and quinupristin–dalfopristin. *Antimicrob Agents Chemother* **46:**1845–18450.

46. Piddock LJ. 2006. Clinically relevant chromosomally encoded multidrug resistance efflux pumps in bacteria. *Clin Microbiol Rev* **19:** 382–402.

47. Roberts MC. 2005. Update on acquired tetracycline resistance genes. *FEMS Microbiol Lett* **245:**195–203.

48. Visalli MA, Murphy E, Projan SJ, Bradford PA. 2003. AcrAB multidrug efflux pump is associated with reduced levels of susceptibility to tigecycline (GAR-936) in *Proteus mirabilis*. *Antimicrob Agents Chemother* **47:**665–669.

49. Dean CR, Visalli MA, Projan SJ, Sum PE, Bradford PA. 2003. Efflux-mediated resistance to tigecycline (GAR-936) in *Pseudomonas aeruginosa* PAO1. *Antimicrob Agents Chemother* **47:**972–978.

50. Ross JI, Eady EA, Cove JH, Cunliffe WJ, Baumberg S, Wootton JC. 1990. Inducible erythromycin resistance in staphylococci is encoded by a member of the ATP-binding transport super-gene family. *Mol Microbiol* **4:**1207–1214.

51. **Connell SR, Tracz DM, Nierhaus KH, Taylor DE.** 2003. Ribosomal protection proteins and their mechanism of tetracycline resistance. *Antimicrob Agents Chemother* **47:** 3675–3681.

52. **Dönhöfer A, Franckenberg S, Wickles S, Berninghausen O, Beckmann R, Wilson DN.** 2012. Structural basis for TetM-mediated tetracycline resistance. *Proc Natl Acad Sci USA* **109:**16900–16905.

53. **Li W, Atkinson GC, Thakor NS, Allas U, Lu CC, Chan KY, Tenson T, Schulten K, Wilson KS, Hauryliuk V, Frank J.** 2013. Mechanism of tetracycline resistance by ribosomal protection protein Tet(O). *Nat Commun* **4:**1477.

54. **Martinez-Martinez L, Pascual A, Jacoby GA.** 1998. Quinolone resistance from a transferable plasmid. *Lancet* **351:**797–799.

55. **Rodríguez-Martínez JM, Cano ME, Velasco C, Martínez-Martínez L, Pascual A.** 2011. Plasmid-mediated quinolone resistance: an update. *J Infect Chemother* **17:**149–12.

56. **Aldred KJ, Kerns RJ, Osheroff N.** 2014. Mechanism of quinolone action and resistance. *Biochemistry* **53:**1565–1574.

57. **Campbell EA, Korzheva N, Mustaev A, Murakami K, Nair S, Goldfarb A, Darst SA.** 2001. Structural mechanism for rifampicin inhibition of bacterial RNA polymerase. *Cell* **104:**901–912.

58. **Floss HG, Yu TW.** 2005. Rifamycin: mode of action, resistance, and biosynthesis. *Chem Rev* **105:**621–632.

59. **Hooper DC.** 2002. Fluoroquinolone resistance among Gram-positive cocci. *Lancet Infect Dis* **2:**530–538.

60. **Mendes RE, Deshpande LM, Jones RN.** 2014. Linezolid update: stable *in vitro* activity following more than a decade of clinical use and summary of associated resistance mechanisms. *Drug Resist Updat* **17:**1–12.

61. **Marshall SH, Donskey CJ, Hutton-Thomas R, Salata RA, Rice LB.** 2002. Gene dosage and linezolid resistance in *Enterococcus faecium* and *Enterococcus faecalis*. *Antimicrob Agents Chemother* **46:**3334–3336.

62. **Leclercq R.** 2002. Mechanisms of resistance to macrolides and lincosamides: nature of the resistance elements and their clinical implications. *Clin Infect Dis* **34:**482–492.

63. **Weisblum B.** 1995. Erythromycin resistance by ribosome modification. *Antimicrob Agents Chemother* **39:**577–585.

64. **Roberts MC.** 2008. Update on macrolide-lincosamide-streptogramin, ketolide, and oxazolidinone resistance genes. *FEMS Microbiol Lett* **282:**147–159.

65. **Katz L, Ashley GW.** 2005. Translation and protein synthesis: macrolides. *Chem Rev* **105:** 499–528.

66. **Toh SM, Xiong L, Arias CA, Villegas MV, Lolans K, Quinn J, Mankin AS.** 2007. Acquisition of a natural resistance gene renders a clinical strain of methicillin-resistant *Staphylococcus aureus* resistant to the synthetic antibiotic linezolid. *Mol Microbiol* **64:**1506–1514.

67. **Locke JB, Zurenko GE, Shaw KJ, Bartizal K.** 2014. Tedizolid for the management of human infections: *in vitro* characteristics. *Clin Infect Dis* **58**(Suppl 1):S35–S42.

68. **Hiramatsu K, Ito T, Tsubakishita S, Sasaki T, Takeuchi F, Morimoto Y, Katayama Y, Matsuo M, Kuwahara-Arai K, Hishinuma T, Baba T.** 2013. Genomic basis for methicillin resistance in *Staphylococcus aureus*. *Infect Chemother* **45:**117.

69. **Moellering RC.** 2012. MRSA: the first half century. *J Antimicrob Chemother* **67:**4–11.

70. **Chambers HF, Deleo FR.** 2009. Waves of resistance: *Staphylococcus aureus* in the antibiotic era. *Nat Rev Microbiol* **7:**629–641.

71. **Chambers HF.** 1997. Methicillin resistance in staphylococci: molecular and biochemical basis and clinical implications. *Clin Microbiol Rev* **10:**781–791.

72. **Reynolds PE.** 1989. Structure, biochemistry and mechanism of action of glycopeptide antibiotics. *Eur J Clin Microbiol Infect Dis* **8:**943–950.

73. **Arias CA, Murray BE.** 2012. The rise of the *Enterococcus*: beyond vancomycin resistance. *Nat Rev Microbiol* **10:**266–278.

74. **Miller WR, Munita JM, Arias CA.** 2014. Mechanisms of antibiotic resistance in enterococci. *Expert Rev Anti Infect Ther* **12:**1221–1236.

75. **Guardabassi L, Agersø Y.** 2006. Genes homologous to glycopeptide resistance vanA are widespread in soil microbial communities. *FEMS Microbiol Lett* **259:**221–225.

76. **Courvalin P.** 2006. Vancomycin resistance in Gram-positive cocci. *Clin Infect Dis* **42:**S25–S34.

77. **Arthur M.** 2010. Antibiotics: vancomycin sensing. *Nat Chem Biol* **6:**313–315.

78. **Arthur M, Molinas C, Courvalin P.** 1992. The VanS-VanR two-component regulatory system controls synthesis of depsipeptide peptidoglycan precursors in *Enterococcus faecium* BM4147. *J Bacteriol* **174:**2582–2591.

79. **Sievert DM, Rudrik JT, Patel JB, McDonald LC, Wilkins MJ, Hageman JC.** Vancomycin-resistant *Staphylococcus aureus* in the United States, 2002-2006. *Clin Infect Dis* **46:**668–674.

80. **Rossi F, Diaz L, Wollam A, Panesso D, Zhou Y, Rincon S, Narechania A, Xing G, Di Gioia TS, Doi A, Tran TT, Reyes J, Munita JM, Carvajal LP, Hernandez-Roldan A, Brandão D, van der Heijden IM, Murray BE, Planet PJ, Weinstock GM, Arias CA.** 2014. Transferable vancomycin resistance in a community-associated MRSA lineage. *N Engl J Med* **370:**1524–1531.

81. **Van Bambeke F, Chauvel M, Reynolds PE, Fraimow HS, Courvalin P.** 1999. Vancomycin-dependent *Enterococcus faecalis* clinical isolates and revertant mutants. *Antimicrob Agents Chemother* **43:**41–47.

82. **Flensburg J, Sköld O.** 1987. Massive overproduction of dihydrofolate reductase in bacteria as a response to the use of trimethoprim. *Eur J Biochem* **162:**473–476.

83. **Huovinen P.** 2001. Resistance to trimethoprim sulfamethoxazole. *Clin Infect Dis* **32:**1608–1614.

84. **Hamilton-Miller JM.** 1988. Reversal of activity of trimethoprim against Gram-positive cocci by thymidine, thymine and 'folates.' *J Antimicrob Chemother* **22:**35–39.

85. **Zervos MJ, Schaberg DR.** 1985. Reversal of the *in vitro* susceptibility of enterococci to trimethoprim–sulfamethoxazole by folinic acid. *Antimicrob Agents Chemother* **28:**446–448.

86. **Pogliano J, Pogliano N, Silverman JA.** 2012. Daptomycin-mediated reorganization of membrane architecture causes mislocalization of essential cell division proteins. *J Bacteriol* **194:**4494–4504.

87. **Zhang T, Muraih JK, Tishbi N, Herskowitz J, Victor RL, Silverman J, Uwumarenogie S, Taylor SD, Palmer M, Mintzer E.** 2014. Cardiolipin prevents membrane translocation and permeabilization by daptomycin. *J Biol Chem* **289:**11584–11591.

88. **Arias CA, Panesso D, McGrath DM, Qin X, Mojica MF, Miller C, Diaz L, Tran TT, Rincon S, Barbu EM, Reyes J, Roh JH, Lobos E, Sodergren E, Pasqualini R, Arap W, Quinn JP, Shamoo Y, Murray BE, Weinstock GM.** 2011. Genetic basis for *in vivo* daptomycin resistance in enterococci. *N Engl J Med* **365:**892–900.

89. **Munita JM, Tran TT, Diaz L, Panesso D, Reyes J, Murray BE, Arias CA.** 2013. A liaF codon deletion abolishes daptomycin bactericidal activity against vancomycin-resistant *Enterococcus faecalis. Antimicrob Agents Chemother* **57:**2831–2833.

90. **Diaz L, Tran TT, Munita JM, Miller WR, Rincon S, Carvajal LP, Wollam A, Reyes J, Panesso D, Rojas NL, Shamoo Y, Murray BE, Weinstock GM, Arias CA.** 2014. Whole-genome analyses of *Enterococcus faecium* isolates with diverse daptomycin MICs. *Antimicrob Agents Chemother* **58:**4527–4534.

91. **Munita JM, Panesso D, Diaz L, Tran TT, Reyes J, Wanger A, Murray BE, Arias CA.** 2012. Correlation between mutations in liaFSR of *Enterococcus faecium* and MIC of daptomycin: revisiting daptomycin breakpoints. *Antimicrob Agents Chemother* **56:**4354–4359.

92. **Munita JM, Mishra NN, Alvarez D, Tran TT, Diaz L, Panesso D, Reyes J, Murray BE, Adachi JA, Bayer AS, Arias CA.** 2014. Failure of high-dose daptomycin for bacteremia caused by daptomycin-susceptible *Enterococcus faecium* harboring LiaSR substitutions. *Clin Infect Dis* **59:**1277–1280.

93. **Wolf D, Kalamorz F, Wecke T, Juszczak A, Mäder U, Homuth G, Jordan S, Kirstein J, Hoppert M, Voigt B, Hecker M, Mascher T.** 2010. In-depth profiling of the LiaR response of *Bacillus subtilis. J Bacteriol* **192:**4680–4693.

94. **Tran TT, Panesso D, Mishra NN, Mileykovskaya E, Guan Z, Munita JM, Reyes J, Diaz L, Weinstock GM, Murray BE, Shamoo Y, Dowhan W, Bayer AS, Arias CA.** 2013. Daptomycin-resistant *Enterococcus faecalis* diverts the antibiotic molecule from the division septum and remodels cell membrane phospholipids. *MBio* **4**(4):e00281-13. doi:10.1128/mBio.00281-13.

95. **Reyes J, Panesso D, Tran TT, Mishra NN, Cruz MR, Munita JM, Singh KV, Yeaman MR, Murray BE, Shamoo Y, Garsin D, Bayer AS, Arias CA.** 2014. A liaR deletion restores susceptibility to daptomycin and antimicrobial peptides in multidrug-resistant *Enterococcus faecalis. J Infect Dis.* [Epub ahead of print.] doi:10.1093/infdis/jiu602.

96. **Tran TT, Panesso D, Gao H, Roh JH, Munita JM, Reyes J, Diaz L, Lobos EA, Shamoo Y, Mishra NN, Bayer AS, Murray BE, Weinstock GM, Arias CA.** 2013. Whole-genome analysis of a daptomycin-susceptible *Enterococcus faecium* strain and its daptomycin-resistant variant arising during therapy. *Antimicrob Agents Chemother* **57:**261–268.

97. **Bayer AS, Schneider T, Sahl HG.** 2013. Mechanisms of daptomycin resistance in *Staphylococcus aureus*: role of the cell membrane and cell wall. *Ann N Y Acad Sci* **1277:**139–158.

98. **Krute CN, Carroll RK, Rivera FE, Weiss A, Young RM, Shilling A, Botlani M, Varma S, Baker BJ, Shaw LN.** 2015. The disruption of prenylation leads to pleiotropic rearrangements in cellular behavior in *Staphylococcus aureus. Mol Microbiol* **95:**819–832.

99. **Ernst CM, Kuhn S, Slavetinsky CJ, Krismer B, Heilbronner S, Gekeler C, Kraus D, Wagner S, Peschel A.** 2015. The lipid-modifying multiple peptide resistance factor is an oligomer consisting of distinct interacting synthase and flippase subunits. *MBio* **6**(1):e02340-14. doi:10.1128/mBio.02340-14.

100. **Hiramatsu K, Hanaki H, Ino T, Yabuta K, Oguri T, Tenover FC.** Methicillin-resistant *Staphylococcus aureus* clinical strain with reduced vancomycin susceptibility. *J Antimicrob Chemother* **40:**135–136.

101. **Howden BP, Davies JK, Johnson PD, Stinear TP, Grayson ML.** 2010. Reduced vancomycin susceptibility in *Staphylococcus aureus*, including vancomycin-intermediate and heterogeneous vancomycin-intermediate strains: resistance mechanisms, laboratory detection, and clinical implications. *Clin Microbiol Rev* **23:**99–139.

102. **Stryjewski ME, Corey GR.** 2014. Methicillin-resistant *Staphylococcus aureus*: an evolving pathogen. *Clin Infect Dis* **58**(Suppl 1):S10–S19.

103. **Bae IG, Federspiel JJ, Miró JM, Woods CW, Park L, Rybak MJ, Rude TH, Bradley S, Bukovski S, de la Maria CG, Kanj SS, Korman TM, Marco F, Murdoch DR, Plesiat P, Rodriguez-Creixems M, Reinbott P, Steed L, Tattevin P, Tripodi MF, Newton KL, Corey GR, Fowler VG Jr, International Collaboration on Endocarditis-Microbiology Investigator.** 2009. Heterogeneous vancomycin-intermediate susceptibility phenotype in bloodstream methicillin-resistant *Staphylococcus aureus* isolates from an international cohort of patients with infective endocarditis: prevalence, genotype, and clinical significance. *J Infect Dis* **200:**1355–1366.

104. **Gardete S, Tomasz A.** 2014. Mechanisms of vancomycin resistance in *Staphylococcus aureus*. *J Clin Invest* **124:**2836–2840.

105. **Watanabe Y, Cui L, Katayama Y, Kozue K, Hiramatsu K.** 2011. Impact of rpoB mutations on reduced vancomycin susceptibility in *Staphylococcus aureus*. *J Clin Microbiol* **49:**2680–2684.

106. **Jana S, Debb JK.** 2006. Molecular understanding of aminoglycoside action and resistance. *Appl Microbiol Biotechnol* **70:**140–150.

107. **Piddock LJ.** 2006. Multidrug-resistance efflux pumps: not just for resistance. *Nat Rev Microbiol* **4:**629–636.

108. **Du D, van Veen HW, Luisi BF.** 2015. Assembly and operation of bacterial tripartite multidrug efflux pumps. *Trends Microbiol* **23:**311–319.

109. **Du D, Wang Z, James NR, Voss JE, Klimont E, Ohene-Agyei T, Venter H, Chiu W, Luisi BF.** 2014. Structure of the AcrAB-TolC multidrug efflux pump. *Nature* **509:**512–515.

110. **Hobbs EC, Yin X, Paul BJ, Astarita JL, Storz G.** 2014. Conserved small protein associates with the multidrug efflux pump AcrB and differentially affects antibiotic resistance. *Proc Natl Acad Sci USA* **109:**16696–16701.

BACTERIAL PERSISTENCE: WITHIN AND BETWEEN HOSTS

18

Chronic Bacterial Pathogens: Mechanisms of Persistence

MARIANA X. BYNDLOSS[1] and RENEE M. TSOLIS[1]

INTRODUCTION

Persistent bacterial infections such as brucellosis and typhoid fever are characterized by a long incubation period that leads to chronic, sometimes lifelong, debilitating disease with serious clinical manifestations (1). Therefore, chronic bacterial diseases have a significant impact on public health, due to the utilization of resources for long-term treatment of patients (2). Additionally, chronic infections affect the ability of the ill to provide for their families, resulting in a significant socioeconomic burden in affected countries (3).

Brucellosis, caused by intracellular Gram-negative coccobacilli of the *Brucella* spp., is considered one of the most relevant bacterial zoonoses worldwide, with more than 500,000 new human cases reported each year (4). The disease targets organs of the mononuclear phagocyte system, resulting in a chronic debilitating infection with serious clinical manifestations such as fever, arthritis, hepatomegaly, and splenomegaly (3, 5).

Typhoid fever, caused by the human-adapted *Salmonella enterica* serovar Typhi (*S.* Typhi) affects between 10 and 20 million people each year (6, 7), causing an estimated 190,000 deaths (8). Similar to *Brucella*, *S.* Typhi

[1]Department of Medical Microbiology and Immunology, School of Medicine, University of California at Davis, Sacramento, CA 95817.

Virulence Mechanisms of Bacterial Pathogens, 5th edition
Edited by Indira T. Kudva, Nancy A. Cornick, Paul J. Plummer, Qijing Zhang, Tracy L. Nicholson, John P. Bannantine, and Bryan H. Bellaire
© 2016 American Society for Microbiology, Washington, DC
doi:10.1128/microbiolspec.VMBF-0020-2015

causes a systemic infection, which targets the mononuclear phagocyte system, and has the ability to persist inside host tissues for long periods, causing a chronic debilitating disease (9, 10). Interestingly, one study of brucellosis patients noted that over half had initially been misdiagnosed as having typhoid fever, which highlights the similar clinical presentation of these very different infections (11).

In the host, one of the preferential target cells for both *Salmonella* and *Brucella* spp. are macrophages (3, 12), in which the bacterium can persist and replicate (3, 12, 13). A hallmark of these chronic bacterial infections is the formation of granulomas, which contain epithelioid macrophages and are known to be a site of bacterial persistence during infection (Fig. 1) (3). The granulomatous response is viewed as an attempt by the host to isolate bacteria that have been taken up but not killed by macrophages (14) and is the result of an inefficient and/or insufficient immune response to these pathogens.

Intracellular *Brucella* survival involves a temporary fusion of the *Brucella*-containing vacuole with the lysosome and subsequent exclusion of the lysosomal proteins (15).

Interestingly enough, after this process, the *Brucella*-containing vacuole becomes associated with the rough endoplasmic reticulum, creating the compartment in which intracellular replication of *Brucella* occurs (16–18). Once inside the endoplasmic reticulum–associated compartment, *Brucella* spp. become practically invisible to the immune system (13), as demonstrated by a low production of cytokines and antibodies during the chronic phase of infection (19, 20). Therefore, the initial immune response becomes a key factor for the control of *Brucella* spp. infection.

Salmonella enters the host through the gastrointestinal tract, mainly through epithelial barrier translocation via microfold (M) cell invasion or via phagocytosis by CD-18+ antigen presenting cells (21). Like *Brucella*, after bypassing the intestinal barrier, *Salmonella* is able to survive within macrophages residing in systemic tissues (12). Intracellularly, *Salmonella* can avoid complete fusion with the lysosome through translocation of effector proteins that direct maturation of a *Salmonella*-containing vacuole (reviewed in reference 22). Once inside the *Salmonella*-containing vacuole, *Salmonella* is able to

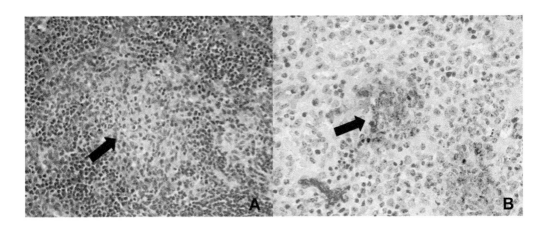

FIGURE 1 Microgranuloma formation in spleen of *Brucella*-infected mice. (A) Fully developed microgranuloma (black arrow) at 30 days postinfection. Granuloma is composed of epithelioid macrophages surrounded by lymphocytes. Hematoxylin and eosin stain, 400x magnification. (B) Immunolabeling of *Brucella abortus* within microgranulomas in spleen at 30 days postinfection. Note the presence of bacteria inside macrophages (black arrow). Immunohistochemistry, 400x magnification.

manipulate host cell functions, leading to replication and persistence.

Although *Brucella abortus*, and *S.* Typhi have the common goal to avoid elimination by the host, these pathogens use different strategies to persist. In this article we will discuss the different mechanisms used by these chronic bacterial pathogens to evade the initial host immune defense and colonize the host. Moreover, we will discuss the recent concept that bacterial pathogens have evolved to take advantage of the host cell metabolism and nutrient availability to survive and replicate inside target cells.

TRICKING THE HOST IMMUNE SYSTEM

Entry into the Host: the Role of Secretion Systems

In spite of their well-established immuno-evasive character, *Brucella* spp. do rely on an important virulence factor for intracellular survival: the type IV secretion system (T4SS) encoded by the genes *virB1* to *virB12* (13, 23–25). The critical role of the *Brucella* T4SS is demonstrated by the inability of T4SS-deficient mutants to persist *in vivo*, as demonstrated in the murine (25–27) and caprine infection models (28). This phenotype could be attributed to the essential role of the T4SS in establishing the endoplasmic reticulum–associated niche for *Brucella* replication (18), since *virB* mutants remain inside macrophage lysosomes and are degraded (3).

Interestingly, it has been demonstrated that the T4SS is required not only for establishment of long-term infection, but also for the induction of Th1 immune response in infected mice (29). This function was confirmed by the fact that a functional T4SS is necessary for B cell maturation, for activation of CD4+ T cells, and for initial secretion of interleukin-12 (IL-12) and interferon-γ (IFN-γ) (30, 31). Moreover, *B. abortus* detection by Nod-like

receptors, leading to apoptotic speck-like protein with a caspase recruitment domain–inflammasome–mediated production of IL-1β and IL-18, was also shown to be dependent on the T4SS (32).

S. Typhi enters the host through the gastrointestinal tract and uses different strategies to reach systemic sites where it can persist for long periods (33). *Salmonella* serovars encode two type III secretion systems, T3SS-1 and T3SS-2. Studies in the murine typhoid model using *Salmonella enterica* serovar Typhimurium have demonstrated that the T3SS-1 is essential for the initial contact of the pathogen with intestinal epithelial cells and invasion of the ileal and colonic mucosa (34). Subsequently, the T3SS-2 is activated to mediate *Salmonella* survival inside macrophages and persistence in systemic sites (35). While few studies have addressed directly whether findings from the mouse typhoid model hold true for human typhoid, a screen for *S.* Typhi genes involved in infection of humanized mice identified mutants in either structural genes or regulators of both T3SS-1 and T3SS-2, suggesting that both of these virulence factors are involved in the bacteremic phase of typhoid (36).

Innate Immune System Evasion

The innate immune system is considered the first line of host defense against invading pathogens. Therefore, the host has evolved mechanisms to detect the presence of bacteria in tissue through an innate immune surveillance system, which is able to recognize conserved pathogen-associated molecular patterns. These pathogen recognition receptors, present in cell membranes (Toll-like receptors [TLRs]) or in the cytosol (nucleotide oligomerization domain (NOD)–like receptors) are able to detect products considered unique to bacteria, such as lipopolysaccharides (LPS), lipoteichoic acids, lipoproteins, and flagellin (37), leading to induction of the initial proinflammatory response. However, chronic pathogens have evolved passive and active mechanisms to evade detection by both TLRs and NOD-like receptors of the innate immune system (Table 1).

The Stealthy Nature of *Brucella* Species

The LPS of *Brucella* spp. has several features that contribute to its near invisibility to the innate immune system. *Brucella* spp. can avoid detection by TLR4 via modification of the lipid A moiety of its LPS. While most bacterial pathogens such as *Enterobacteriaceae* have a lipid A moiety containing short fatty acid residues (C_{12} to C_{16}), *Brucella* lipid A contains a much longer one (C_{28}), resulting in its greatly reduced TLR4 agonist and endotoxic properties (38). TLR4 agonist activity is further reduced by glycosylation of the LPS core, which reduces its affinity for the TLR4 coreceptor MD-2 (39). Another LPS component, the O-antigen moiety, is recognized by complement (40). Therefore, an additional anti-inflammatory feature of *Brucella* LPS is its resistance to deposition of complement component C3 (41, 42), avoiding the generation of the anaphylatoxins C3a and C5a, which synergize with TLRs in the induction of proinflammatory cytokines (43, 44).

Recently, an additional role for *B. abortus* LPS in evasion of innate immunity has been described, namely, inhibition of neutrophil function. Once *B. abortus* has been phagocytosed by neutrophils, release of LPS within the pathogen vacuole appears to trigger a novel form of noninflammatory cell death, thereby preventing killing of the engulfed bacteria (45). It is not yet known whether *B. abortus* LPS can be recognized by caspase-11 (or its human orthologs caspase-4 and caspase-5); the lack of pyroptotic cell death observed during infection of macrophages suggests that either LPS is not released to the cytosol, where it can be accessed by these sensor caspases, or that it does not activate them in the same manner as described for other bacterial pathogens (46).

While *Brucella* spp. are nonmotile, their genomes encode the structural components of an unconventional flagellum of unknown function, which is sheathed by LPS (47, 48). Interestingly, *Brucella* flagellin is able to avoid TLR5 detection, because it lacks a domain that is essential for its recognition by this receptor (49). However, recent work has demonstrated that the cytosolic receptor NLCR4 is able to detect *Brucella* flagellin and is important for pathogen control in the mouse model of infection (50).

TABLE 1 Strategies for persistence[a]

Bacterial pathogen	TLR evasion	Complement evasion	Secretion systems
Brucella spp.	Modified lipid A moiety LPS (TLR4) Flagellin lacks TLR5 recognition moiety (TLR5) Btp1/TcpB protein degrades MyD88 adaptor-like (TLR2, TLR4)	O-antigen portion of LPS modification avoids C3 binding and release of anaphylatoxins C3a C5a	T4SS-mediated lysosome evasion and trafficking to endoplasmic reticulum
Salmonella enterica serovar Typhi	Expression of Vi-capsule (TLR4) TviA- mediated downregulation of flagellin (TLR5) TviA-mediated downregulation of T3SS1 (surface TLR2, TLR4)	Expression of Vi-capsule inhibits C3 binding and release of anaphylatoxins C3a C5a Vi-capsule inhibition of C3b binding and complement-mediated phagocytosis by neutrophils Vi-capsule inhibition of C5a-dependent neutrophils chemotaxis	T3SS1: downregulated during systemic infection T3SS2: mediates lysosome evasion and intracellular survival

[a]Abbreviations: LPS, lipopolysaccharides; TLR, Toll-like receptor; T4SS, type IV secretion system

In addition to TLR4, TLR2 and TLR9 have also been implicated in sensing *Brucella* infection (2, 51, 52). Therefore, as another strategy to avoid immune recognition, the *Brucella* genome encodes a protein that contains a Toll-interleukin-1 receptor domain, named Btp1/BtpA in *B. abortus* and TcpB in *Brucella melitensis* (53, 54). Btp1/TcpB acts by degrading the MyD88 adaptor-like, which is required for both TLR2 and TLR4 signaling, but not for TLR9 (53, 55). As a consequence, Btp1/TcpB is able to inhibit dendritic cell maturation and production of proinflammatory cytokines, contributing to long-term *Brucella* persistence. Recently, a second *Brucella* Toll-interleukin-1 receptor–containing effector protein has been described, named BtpB (56). BtpB is also believed to interfere with TLR signaling in a MyD88-dependent manner, although its role in modulating *Brucella*-induced inflammatory responses and bacterial persistence remains to be determined.

The *viaB* Locus: the "Cloaking Device" of *S.* Typhi

In contrast to *Brucella*, it has been demonstrated that the lipid A moiety of purified *S.* Typhi LPS is a potent TLR4 agonist (57), that *S.* Typhi flagellin is recognized by TLR5 (58), and that the O-antigen of purified *S.* Typhi LPS activates complement (59). Therefore, to persist, *S.* Typhi has evolved different strategies to avoid recognition by pathogen recognition receptors.

Whole-genome sequencing revealed the presence of an *S.* Typhi–specific pathogenicity island, named *Salmonella* pathogenicity island 7 (60), that contains the *viaB* locus that encodes for the production and export of the Vi capsular polysaccharide antigen, also known as Vi-antigen (61). Initial studies demonstrated that the expression of Vi-antigen was linked to reduced flagellin secretion and lower *Salmonella* invasiveness. Moreover, the expression of the Vi capsule was tightly regulated by osmolarity conditions, since high-osmolarity conditions suppressed Vi-antigen expression and led to increased *Salmonella* invasiveness and flagellin secretion (62, 63). Further studies demonstrated that the first gene in the *viaB* locus, named *tviA*, encoded the regulatory protein TviA, which is responsible for these osmolarity-dependent phenotypic changes (64).

Interestingly, regulation of *tviA* expression is directly linked to conditions encountered by *S.* Typhi in the intestinal lumen (65) and is key for this pathogen's ability to bypass the intestinal barrier. It turns out that TviA is responsible not only for regulation of the Vi-antigen, but also for the suppression of flagella production and regulation of T3SS-1 gene expression (64, 66). Therefore, the high-osmolarity environment encountered in the lumen leads to inhibition of *tviA* expression, which allows *S.* Typhi to be motile and invasive as it approaches the mucosal epithelium (66). In contrast, once *S.* Typhi reaches the intestinal lamina propria, it encounters an environment characterized by low osmolarity, which leads to rapid *tviA* expression (65). As a result, several *S.* Typhi pathogen-associated molecular patterns and pathogen-induced processes can no longer be detected by the host's immune system.

As described above, TviA-mediated repression of flagellin expression prevents detection of *S.* Typhi by host TLR5 and the consequent induction of the TLR5-dependent production of the proinflammatory cytokine IL-8 by colonocytes (67). Additionally, it has been demonstrated that *S.* Typhi is able to evade TLR4 recognition in a Vi-antigen dependent manner (reviewed in reference 66). Recent studies suggest that this TLR4 evasion could result indirectly from the ability of the Vi antigen to prevent complement activation (43), and consequent generation of the anaphylatoxins C3a and C5a, which are two known enhancers of the TLR4-mediated induction of proinflammatory cytokines in response to lipid A recognition (44). The Vi-dependent inhibition of complement activation also prevents deposition of C3b in the bacterial surface, which in turn inhibits phagocytosis of *S.* Typhi by neutrophils, a cell type crucial for avoiding *Salmonella* dissemination (43, 66). Moreover, the *S.* Typhi Vi-capsule is also able to inhibit bacteria-guided neutrophil chemotaxis in a C5a-dependent manner (68). Taken together, these mechanisms help explain the lack of neutrophils in intestinal infiltrates from *S.* Typhi–infected individuals (69, 70), which greatly contribute to this pathogen's ability to evade host immune defenses and leads to an invasive persistent infection.

Both *Brucella* and *S.* Typhi are able to conceal two crucial molecular signatures that would otherwise allow the host's immune system to identify them as Gram-negative bacteria. The host's inability to detect these molecular patterns through TLR receptors as well as the complement system prevents the induction of an appropriate initial antibacterial host response. As a consequence, the pathogen clearance and infection control is significantly impaired (3, 71).

Induction of Anti-Inflammatory Cytokines by *Brucella*

Interleukin 10 (IL-10) is considered an immunoregulatory cytokine that can be produced by different cell types, including B cells, T cells, macrophages, and keratinocytes (72). The main cell type responsible for IL-10 production in defined situations is dependent on the kind of stimulus, type of affected tissue, and time point in an immune process (73). Therefore, IL-10 is able to function at different stages of an immune response, affirming its crucial role as a regulator of both Th1 and Th2 cell responses (72, 74).

Therefore, a plausible strategy for a persistent pathogen would be the induction of a cytokine that is able to modulate the host proinflammatory response. Indeed, in addition to an early proinflammatory Th1 response, *B. abortus* also induces the anti-inflammatory cytokine IL-10 (1, 2, 75). Interestingly, anti-*Brucella* effector functions of IFNγ-activated macrophages such as bactericidal capacity and production of proinflammatory cytokines were dampened by IL-10 during *in vitro* infection (75, 76). *In vivo* experiments demonstrated that production of IL-10 by CD4+CD25+ T cells was key for modulation of macrophage function during early *Brucella* infection, since mice lacking IL-10 production by T cells or lacking the presence of the IL-10R in macrophages presented decreased bacterial survival in spleen and liver, as well as increased production of proinflammatory cytokines and pathology in affected organs (1). Moreover, a *B. abortus* proline racemase PrpA was shown to both stimulate mitogenic activity on B cells and induce IL-10 secretion by splenocytes, suggesting that it may be one of the factors involved in induction of IL-10 during infection (77). Taken together, these data suggest an important role of IL-10 in modulating the initial immune response to *Brucella* infection through regulation of macrophage function, resulting in increased pathogen survival and long-term persistence.

TAKING ADVANTAGE OF HOST CELL METABOLISM

The interactions of persistent bacterial pathogens with the host immune system have been extensively studied and contribute greatly to the ability of such pathogens to cause chronic infection. However, evasion of the immune response is not the sole mechanism for pathogen persistence, since studies have shown that factors required for establishment of chronic disease *in vivo* may not be necessarily dependent on the induction of an immune response. Interestingly, a variety of genes required for *Brucella* persistence, for example, are related to changes in bacterial metabolism and to the ability of the pathogen to use a specific nutrient (26). This fact gives rise to the possibility that chronic bacterial pathogens may have adapted not only to the different immune environment present during persistent infection, but also to differences in nutrient availability in target cells during this period.

Macrophage Subsets and Their Different Metabolism

Macrophage activation by IFNγ and TLRs leads to upregulation of the inducible form of nitric oxide synthase (78) and production of reactive oxygen species (79). Therefore, reactive oxygen species and nitric oxide production are key functional features of the inflammatory and bactericidal classical-ly activated macrophage (CAM) (Fig. 2), and the metabolic alterations that occur are integral to this process (80). Interestingly, nitric oxide competes with oxygen to inhibit cytochrome *c* oxidase, the terminal electron acceptor of the respiratory chain. This fact prevents the reoxidation of NADH, which in turn limits flux through the tricarboxylic acid cycle. Moreover, increased generation of reactive oxygen species by mitochondria also contributes to reduced macrophage reliance on the tricarboxylic acid cycle and the respiratory chain for energy and ATP production. However, CAMs still need to maintain ATP levels for biosynthesis, as well as to maintain mitochondrial membrane

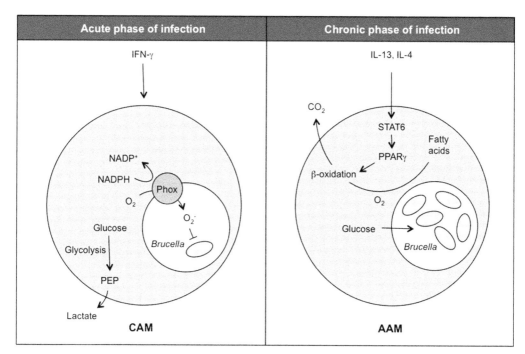

FIGURE 2 Macrophage metabolism during *Brucella* infection. During the acute phase of *Brucella abortus* infection (left), interferon-γ (IFN-γ) is transiently produced, resulting in a predominance of classically activated macrophages (CAMs). In these cells, oxygen is consumed by NADPH oxidase (Phox) to generate superoxide radicals, and energy is produced by anaerobic glycolysis. Since anaerobic glycolysis yields only 2ATP, the cell has to consume more glucose to meet its energy needs. In contrast, during the chronic infection phase (right), IFN-γ is absent, but interleukin-4 (IL-4) and IL-13 signal via STAT6 to induce the alternatively activated macrophage (AAM) phenotype. Activation of STAT6 increases the expression and activation of peroxisome proliferator-activated receptor gamma (PPARγ), which in turn upregulates genes controlling β-oxidation, thereby shifting cellular physiology toward oxidative pathways. As a result, less glucose is consumed for cellular metabolism, and the intracellular glucose concentration increases. This glucose can be utilized by *B. abortus* for growth within infected macrophages.

potential and to prevent apoptosis (80). Therefore, decreased tricarboxylic acid flux in CAMs leads to ATP production through anaerobic glycolysis and lactate production. Consequently, these cells show elevated expression of the glucose transporter GLUT1 as well as a marked switch from expression of the liver isoform of the enzyme 6-phosphofructo-2-kinase (encoded by *PFKFB1*) to the PFKFB3 isoform (81). This leads to increased glucose uptake and consumption, as well as to accumulation of fructose-2,6-bisphosphate, which in turn, increases glycolytic flux (80).

The opposite is true when macrophages are activated by IL-4 and IL-13, which promote development of alternatively activated macrophages (AAMs) (Fig. 2). This macrophage subpopulation exhibits a profound increase in the entire program of fatty-acid metabolism, including uptake and oxidation of fatty acids and mitochondrial biogenesis, as well as much lower rates of glycolysis (81, 82). Consequently, while CAMs preferentially utilize glucose, the alternative program of macrophage activation switches over to fatty acid oxidation for energy homeostasis (82). Since AAMs are involved in chronic processes and tissue repair, it is possible that the more energy-efficient oxidative metabolism is better suited to long-term roles of this subpopulation (80).

Interestingly, the control of the genetic program for long-term activation is dependent on STAT6 phosphorylation (80, 83). As a consequence, phosphorylated STAT6 dimerizes and translocates to the nucleus, where it induces expression of its target genes, including markers (*Arg1, Yml, Fizz1, Cd301*) and regulators of macrophage metabolism and alternative activation (i.e., *Pparγ, Pparδ*, and *PGC-1β*) (84).

Macrophage Metabolism and *Brucella* Persistence

It is well established that macrophages represent the main target cell for *Brucella* persistence in many tissue types (13, 85–89). Therefore, interactions between *Brucella* and the different macrophage subpopulations are key to understanding bacterial survival and disease progression. Interestingly, during infection of C57BL/6 mice the macrophage subpopulations differ significantly between acute and chronic stages of *Brucella* infection. During the acute and more proinflammatory stage of infection, there is a significant increase in the numbers of bactericidal CAMs, and this correlates well with higher IFNγ levels as well as the decrease in *B. abortus* survival in spleen of infected mice (88). Conversely, during chronic infection, there is a shift in the macrophage subpopulation, with predominance of the wound-healing AAM subtypes leading to persistent *Brucella* survival over time. Indeed, AAMs were shown to be more permissive for *B. abortus* survival and replication *in vitro*. Furthermore, during chronic infection of mice, two lines of evidence show persistence of *B. abortus* in AAMs: first, viable *B. abortus* was cultured primarily from the CD11b+ fraction, which consists predominantly of AAMs during chronic infection, and second, bacteria were localized by flow cytometry to splenic cells expressing markers of the AAM phenotype, $CD301^+CD11b^+$. The presence of *B. abortus*–infected AAMs was shown to be dependent on the activation of the intracellular receptor peroxisome proliferator-activated receptor gamma (PPARγ).

PPARγ is a nuclear receptor activated by fatty acids, which has recently been linked to the polarization of macrophage phenotype (90). Therefore, even though PPARγ is best known for its influence in adipocyte development and insulin resistance (84), it can also have a widespread influence on macrophage biology (91, 92). Interestingly, studies using PPARγ-deficient cells have demonstrated that, in the absence of PPARγ signaling, macrophages neither appropriately suppress inflammatory cytokine production nor acquire an oxidative metabolic program that is associated with the AAM phenotype (84, 90).

As previously discussed, one consequence of macrophage polarization is the shift in their cellular metabolism, which means that CAMs and AAMs utilize different sources of carbon and energy (93). This fact raises the possibility that different nutrients are available intracellularly in different macrophage subpopulations. Indeed, CAMs rely on glycolysis for energy production and, therefore, consume most intracellular glucose. Conversely, AAMs obtain their ATP via degradation of fatty acids via the β-oxidation pathway in a PPAR-dependent manner. As a consequence, there is an accumulation of glucose inside the cell, shown by higher intracellular glucose levels in AAMs compared to CAMs (88, 94). Interestingly, *Brucella* uses this nutrient availability for long-term persistence, since a *gluP* mutant, which lacks the ability to take up intracellular glucose, is no longer able to persist inside AAMs in the mouse model. Moreover, this phenotype was dependent on PPARγ expression by macrophages (26, 88).

Macrophage Metabolism and *Salmonella* Persistence

While *S*. Typhi is a strictly human-adapted pathogen, work done modeling *S*. Typhi infection by studying chronic infection of *S. enterica* serovar Typhimurium in mice has provided significant insights into mechanisms underlying persistence at systemic sites.

Recent work with mice has shown that there is a shift in the immune environment during *Salmonella* infection, characterized by predominance of a proinflammatory Th1 response during acute infection and the presence of Th2 cytokines such as IL-4 during chronic infection. As a result, there is an increase in the percentage of AAM during the persistence phase of the disease, and this cell type was shown to harbor the majority of the *Salmonella* population in infected organs (94). The increased susceptibility of this particular cell type was dependent on its metabolic program, rather than on its immunological status.

Interestingly, survival of *Salmonella* was dependent on the activation of one of the PPAR receptors, named PPARδ. As previously described for PPARγ, PPARδ regulates the host cell energy metabolism, mainly fatty acid β-oxidation (95). Indeed, *Salmonella* infection actively upregulated the expression of *Ppard*, which in turn led to a shift in the metabolism of infected cells to the oxidation of fatty acids. Consequently, infected AAMs presented increased intracellular levels of glucose, the carbon source used by macrophages when β-oxidation is downregulated (81, 94). This fact raised the possibility that *Salmonella* was taking advantage of this new available energy source to persist and proliferate inside AAMs. The inability of glucose uptake–deficient *Salmonella* mutants to survive inside AAMs confirmed that intracellular glucose utilization was key to *Salmonella* long-term persistence in AAMs and consequent establishment of chronic infection.

Although AAM-polarized cells of the human-derived monocytic cell line THP1 were shown to support higher levels of intracellular *S*. Typhi replication, it will be interesting to see if *S*. Typhi uses increased glucose availability to persist in the host, as was shown for *S*. Typhimurium, and whether PPARδ expression is linked with intracellular persistence of *S*. Typhi in human macrophages (94).

CONCLUSION

Recent work in both the *Brucella* and *Salmonella* fields of research has revealed shared strategies utilized by chronic bacterial pathogens to persist in the host. It is becoming more evident that both immune evasion and interactions with the host-cell metabolism play key roles during establishment of chronic infection. Therefore, the picture emerging from these studies is that persistence is determined not only by the pathogen's ability to evade the host immune response, but also by its ability to develop mechanisms to exploit the nutrients available during the chronic stages of infection. Since both preventive and therapeutic interventions remain difficult and costly, a better understanding of the new mechanisms responsible for bacterial pathogen persistence will be crucial for the proper control and treatment of such infections.

ACKNOWLEDGMENTS

This work was funded by NIH grants from the National Institute of Allergy and Infectious Diseases (NIAID): AI112258 and AI109799.

CITATION

Byndloss MX, Tsolis RM. 2016. Chronic bacterial pathogens: mechanisms of persistence. Microbiol Spectrum 4(2):VMBF-0020-2015.

REFERENCES

1. **Xavier MN, Winter MG, Spees AM, Nguyen K, Atluri VL, Silva TM, Baumler AJ, Muller W, Santos RL, Tsolis RM.** 2013. CD4+ T cell-derived IL-10 promotes *Brucella abortus* persistence via modulation of macrophage function. *PLoS Pathog* 9:e1003454. doi:10.1371/journal. ppat.1003454.
2. **Svetic A, Jian YC, Lu P, Finkelman FD, Gause WC.** 1993. *Brucella abortus* induces a novel cytokine gene expression pattern characterized by elevated IL-10 and IFN-γ in CD4+ T cells. *Int Immunol* 5:877–883.
3. **Atluri VL, Xavier MN, de Jong MF, den Hartigh AB, Tsolis RM.** 2011. Interactions of the human pathogenic *Brucella* species with their hosts. *Annu Rev Microbiol* 65:523–541.
4. **Pappas G, Papadimitriou P, Akritidis N, Christou L, Tsianos EV.** 2006. The new global map of human brucellosis. *Lancet Infect Dis* 6:91–99.
5. **Corbel MJ.** 1997. Brucellosis: an overview. *Emerg Infect Dis* 3:213–221.
6. **Crump JA, Luby SP, Mintz ED.** 2004. The global burden of typhoid fever. *Bull World Health Organ* 82:346–353.
7. **Keestra-Gounder AM, Tsolis RM, Baumler AJ.** 2015. Now you see me, now you don't: the interaction of *Salmonella* with innate immune receptors. *Nat Rev Microbiol* 13:206–216.
8. **Lozano R, Naghavi M, Foreman K, Lim S, Shibuya K, Aboyans V, Abraham J, Adair T, Aggarwal R.** 2012. Global and regional mortality from 235 causes of death for 20 age groups in 1990 and 2010: a systematic analysis for the Global Burden of Disease Study 2010. *Lancet* 380:2095–2128.
9. **House D, Bishop A, Parry C, Dougan G, Wain J.** 2001. Typhoid fever: pathogenesis and disease. *Curr Opin Infect Dis* 14:573–578.
10. **DelVecchio VG, Kapatral V, Elzer P, Patra G, Mujer CV.** 2002. The genome of *Brucella melitensis*. *Vet Microbiol* 90:587–592.
11. **Jennings GJ, Hajjeh RA, Girgis FY, Fadeel MA, Maksoud MA, Wasfy MO, El-Sayed N, Srikantiah P, Luby SP, Earhart K, Mahoney FJ.** 2007. Brucellosis as a cause of acute febrile illness in Egypt. *Trans R Soc Trop Med Hyg* 101:707–713.
12. **Monack DM, Bouley DM, Falkow S.** 2004. *Salmonella typhimurium* persists within macrophages in the mesenteric lymph nodes of chronically infected Nramp1+/+ mice and can be reactivated by IFNγ neutralization. *J Exp Med* 199:231–241.
13. **Xavier MN, Paxão TA, den Hartigh AB, Tsolis RM, Santos RL.** 2010. Pathogenesis of *Brucella* spp. *Open Vet Sci J* 4:109–118.
14. **Adams DO.** 1976. The granulomatous inflammatory response. A review. *Am J Pathol* 84:164–192.
15. **Starr T, Ng TW, Wehrly TD, Knodler LA, Celli J.** 2008. *Brucella* intracellular replication requires trafficking through the late endosomal/lysosomal compartment. *Traffic* 9:678–694.
16. **Anderson TD, Cheville NF.** 1986. Ultrastructural morphometric analysis of *Brucella abortus*-infected trophoblasts in experimental placentitis. Bacterial replication occurs in rough endoplasmic reticulum. *Am J Pathol* 124:226–237.
17. **Pizarro-Cerda J, Meresse S, Parton RG, van der Goot G, Sola-Landa A, Lopez-Goni I, Moreno E, Gorvel JP.** 1998. *Brucella abortus* transits through the autophagic pathway and replicates in the endoplasmic reticulum of nonprofessional phagocytes. *Infect Immun* 66:5711–5724.
18. **Celli J, de Chastellier C, Franchini DM, Pizarro-Cerda J, Moreno E, Gorvel JP.** 2003. *Brucella* evades macrophage killing via VirB-dependent sustained interactions with the endoplasmic reticulum. *J Exp Med* 198:545–556.
19. **Rodriguez-Zapata M, Matias MJ, Prieto A, Jonde MA, Monserrat J, Sanchez L, Reyes E,**

De la Hera A, Alvarez-Mon M. 2010. Human brucellosis is characterized by an intense Th1 profile associated with a defective monocyte function. *Infect Immun* **78:**3272–3279.

20. **Martirosyan A, Moreno E, Gorvel J-P.** 2011. An evolutionary strategy for a stealthy intracellular *Brucella* pathogen. *Immunol Rev* **240:** 211–234.

21. **Haraga A, Ohlson MB, Miller SI.** 2008. *Salmonellae* interplay with host cells. *Nat Rev Microbiol* **6:**53–66.

22. **Bakowski MA, Braun V, Brumell JH.** 2008. *Salmonella*-containing vacuoles: directing traffic and nesting to grow. *Traffic* **9:**2022–2031.

23. **O'Callaghan D, Cazevieille C, Allardet-Servent A, Boschiroli ML, Bourg G, Foulongne V, Frutos P, Kulakov Y, Ramuz M.** 1999. A homologue of the *Agrobacterium tumefaciens* VirB and *Bordetella pertussis* Ptl type IV secretion systems is essential for intracellular survival of *Brucella suis. Mol Microbiol* **33:**1210–1220.

24. **Delrue RM, Martinez-Lorenzo M, Lestrate P, Danese I, Bielarz V, Mertens P, De Bolle X, Tibor A, Gorvel JP, Letesson JJ.** 2001. Identification of *Brucella* spp. genes involved in intracellular trafficking. *Cell Microbiol* **3:** 487–497.

25. **den Hartigh AB, Rolan HG, de Jong MF, Tsolis RM.** 2008. VirB3-VirB6 and VirB8-VirB11, but not VirB7, are essential for mediating persistence of *Brucella* in the reticuloendothelial system. *J Bacteriol* **190:**4427–4436.

26. **Hong PC, Tsolis RM, Ficht TA.** 2000. Identification of genes required for chronic persistence of *Brucella abortus* in mice. *Infect Immun* **68:**4102–4107.

27. **den Hartigh AB, Sun YH, Sondervan D, Heuvelmans N, Reinders MO, Ficht TA, Tsolis RM.** 2004. Differential requirements for VirB1 and VirB2 during *Brucella abortus* infection. *Infect Immun* **72:**5143–5149.

28. **Zygmunt MS, Hagius SD, Walker JV, Elzer PH.** 2006. Identification of *Brucella melitensis* 16M genes required for bacterial survival in the caprine host. *Microbes Infect* **8:**2849–2854.

29. **Roux CM, Rolan HG, Santos RL, Beremand PD, Thomas TL, Adams LG, Tsolis RM.** 2007. *Brucella* requires a functional type IV secretion system to elicit innate immune responses in mice. *Cell Microbiol* **9:**1851–1869.

30. **Rolan HG, Tsolis RM.** 2007. Mice lacking components of adaptive immunity show increased *Brucella abortus virB* mutant colonization. *Infect Immun* **75:**2965–2973.

31. **Rolán HG, Tsolis RM.** 2008. Inactivation of the type IV secretion system reduces the Th1 polarization of the immune response to *Brucella abortus* infection. *Infection and Immunity* **76:**3207–3213.

32. **Gomes MT, Campos PC, Oliveira FS, Corsetti PP, Bortoluci KR, Cunha LD, Zamboni DS, Oliveira SC.** 2013. Critical role of ASC inflammasomes and bacterial type IV secretion system in caspase-1 activation and host innate resistance to *Brucella abortus* infection. *J Immunol* **190:**3629–3638.

33. **Monack DM.** 2012. *Salmonella* persistence and transmission strategies. *Curr Opin Microbiol* **15:**100–107.

34. **Galan JE, Curtiss R 3rd.** 1989. Cloning and molecular characterization of genes whose products allow *Salmonella typhimurium* to penetrate tissue culture cells. *Proc Natl Acad Sci USA* **86:**6383–6387.

35. **Khoramian-Falsafi T, Harayama S, Kutsukake K, Pechere JC.** 1990. Effect of motility and chemotaxis on the invasion of *Salmonella typhimurium* into HeLa cells. *Microb Pathog* **9:**47–53.

36. **Libby SJ, Brehm MA, Greiner DL, Shultz LD, McClelland M, Smith KD, Cookson BT, Karlinsey JE, Kinkel TL, Porwollik S, Canals R, Cummings LA, Fang FC.** 2010. Humanized nonobese diabetic-scid IL2rγnull mice are susceptible to lethal *Salmonella* Typhi infection. *Proc Natl Acad Sci USA* **107:**15589–15594.

37. **Hoebe K, Janssen E, Beutler B.** 2004. The interface between innate and adaptive immunity. *Nat Immunol* **5:**971–974.

38. **Lapaque N, Takeuchi O, Corrales F, Akira S, Moriyon I, Howard JC, Gorvel JP.** 2006. Differential inductions of TNF-alpha and IGTP, IIGP by structurally diverse classic and non-classic lipopolysaccharides. *Cell Microbiol* **8:**401–413.

39. **Conde-Alvarez R, Arce-Gorvel V, Iriarte M, Mancek-Keber M, Barquero-Calvo E, Palacios-Chaves L, Chacon-Diaz C, Chaves-Olarte E, Martirosyan A, von Bargen K, Grillo MJ, Jerala R, Brandenburg K, Llobet E, Bengoechea JA, Moreno E, Moriyon I, Gorvel JP.** 2012. The lipopolysaccharide core of *Brucella abortus* acts as a shield against innate immunity recognition. *PLoS Pathog* **8:** e1002675. doi:10.1371/journal.ppat.1002675.

40. **Joiner KA, Puentes SM, Warren KA, Scales RA, Judd RC.** 1989. Complement binding on serum-sensitive and serum-resistant transformants of *Neisseria gonorrhoeae*: effect of presensitization with a non-bactericidal monoclonal antibody. *Microb Pathog* **6:**343–350.

41. **Barquero-Calvo E, Chaves-Olarte E, Weiss DS, Guzman-Verri C, Chacon-Diaz C, Rucavado A,**

Moriyon I, Moreno E. 2007. *Brucella abortus* uses a stealthy strategy to avoid activation of the innate immune system during the onset of infection. *PLoS One* 2:e631. doi:10.1371/journal.pone.0000631.

42. **Hoffmann EM, Houle JJ.** 1983. Failure of *Brucella abortus* lipopolysaccharide (LPS) to activate the alternative pathway of complement. *Vet Immunol Immunopathol* 5:65–76.

43. **Wilson RP, Winter SE, Spees AM, Winter MG, Nishimori JH, Sanchez JF, Nuccio SP, Crawford RW, Tukel C, Baumler AJ.** 2011. The Vi capsular polysaccharide prevents complement receptor 3-mediated clearance of *Salmonella enterica* serotype Typhi. *Infect Immun* 79:830–837.

44. **Zhang X, Kimura Y, Fang C, Zhou L, Sfyroera G, Lambris JD, Wetsel RA, Miwa T, Song WC.** 2007. Regulation of Toll-like receptor-mediated inflammatory response by complement *in vivo*. *Blood* 110:228–236.

45. **Barquero-Calvo E, Mora-Cartin R, Arce-Gorvel V, de Diego JL, Chacon-Diaz C, Chaves-Olarte E, Guzman-Verri C, Buret AG, Gorvel JP, Moreno E.** 2015. *Brucella abortus* induces the premature death of human neutrophils through the action of its lipopolysaccharide. *PLoS Pathog* 11:e1004853. doi:10.1371/journal.ppat.1004853.

46. **Yang J, Zhao Y, Shao F.** 2015. Non-canonical activation of inflammatory caspases by cytosolic LPS in innate immunity. *Curr Opin Immunol* 32:78–83.

47. **Ferooz J, Letesson JJ.** 2010. Morphological analysis of the sheathed flagellum of *Brucella melitensis*. *BMC Res Notes* 3:333.

48. **Fretin D, Fauconnier A, Kohler S, Halling S, Leonard S, Nijskens C, Ferooz J, Lestrate P, Delrue RM, Danese I, Vandenhaute J, Tibor A, DeBolle X, Letesson JJ.** 2005. The sheathed flagellum of *Brucella melitensis* is involved in persistence in a murine model of infection. *Cell Microbiol* 7:687–698.

49. **Andersen-Nissen E, Smith KD, Strobe KL, Barrett SL, Cookson BT, Logan SM, Aderem A.** 2005. Evasion of Toll-like receptor 5 by flagellated bacteria. *Proc Natl Acad Sci USA* 102:9247–9252.

50. **Terwagne M, Ferooz J, Rolan HG, Sun YH, Atluri V, Xavier MN, Franchi L, Nunez G, Legrand T, Flavell RA, De Bolle X, Letesson JJ, Tsolis RM.** 2013. Innate immune recognition of flagellin limits systemic persistence of *Brucella*. *Cell Microbiol* 15:942–960.

51. **Macedo GC, Magnani DM, Carvalho NB, Bruna-Romero O, Gazzinelli RT, Oliveira SC.** 2008. Central role of MyD88-dependent dendritic cell maturation and proinflammatory cytokine production to control *Brucella abortus* infection. *J Immunol* 180:1080–1087.

52. **Copin R, De Baetselier P, Carlier Y, Letesson JJ, Muraille E.** 2007. MyD88-dependent activation of B220-CD11b+LY-6C+ dendritic cells during *Brucella melitensis* infection. *J Immunol* 178:5182–5191.

53. **Salcedo SP, Marchesini MI, Lelouard H, Fugier E, Jolly G, Balor S, Muller A, Lapaque N, Demaria O, Alexopoulou L, Comerci DJ, Ugalde RA, Pierre P, Gorvel JP.** 2008. *Brucella* control of dendritic cell maturation is dependent on the TIR-containing protein Btp1. *PLoS Pathog* 4:e21. doi:10.1371/journal.ppat.0040021.

54. **Cirl C, Wieser A, Yadav M, Duerr S, Schubert S, Fischer H, Stappert D, Wantia N, Rodriguez N, Wagner H, Svanborg C, Miethke T.** 2008. Subversion of Toll-like receptor signaling by a unique family of bacterial Toll/interleukin-1 receptor domain-containing proteins. *Nat Med* 14:399–406.

55. **Sengupta D, Koblansky A, Gaines J, Brown T, West AP, Zhang D, Nishikawa T, Park SG, Roop RM 2nd,Ghosh S.** 2010. Subversion of innate immune responses by *Brucella* through the targeted degradation of the TLR signaling adapter, MAL. *J Immunol* 184:956–964.

56. **Salcedo SP, Marchesini MI, Degos C, Terwagne M, Von Bargen K, Lepidi H, Herrmann CK, Santos Lacerda TL, Imbert PR, Pierre P, Alexopoulou L, Letesson JJ, Comerci DJ, Gorvel JP.** 2013. BtpB, a novel *Brucella* TIR-containing effector protein with immune modulatory functions. *Front Cell Infect Microbiol* 3:28.

57. **Bignold LP, Rogers SD, Siaw TM, Bahnisch J.** 1991. Inhibition of chemotaxis of neutrophil leukocytes to interleukin-8 by endotoxins of various bacteria. *Infect Immun* 59:4255–4258.

58. **Wyant TL, Tanner MK, Sztein MB.** 1999. *Salmonella typhi* flagella are potent inducers of proinflammatory cytokine secretion by human monocytes. *Infect Immun* 67:3619–3624.

59. **Gewurz H, Mergenhagen SE, Nowotny A, Phillips JK.** 1968. Interactions of the complement system with native and chemically modified endotoxinss. *J Bacteriol* 95:397–405.

60. **Baker S, Dougan G.** 2007. The genome of *Salmonella enterica* serovar Typhi. *Clin Infect Dis* 45(Suppl 1):S29–S33.

61. **Tischler AD, McKinney JD.** 2010. Contrasting persistence strategies in *Salmonella* and *Mycobacterium*. *Curr Opin Microbiol* 13:93–99.

62. **Arricau N, Hermant D, Waxin H, Ecobichon C, Duffey PS, Popoff MY.** 1998. The RcsB-RcsC regulatory system of *Salmonella typhi* differentially modulates the expression of invasion proteins, flagellin and Vi antigen in response to osmolarity. *Mol Microbiol* **29:**835–850.

63. **Zhao L, Ezak T, Li ZY, Kawamura Y, Hirose K, Watanabe H.** 2001. Vi-suppressed wild strain *Salmonella typhi* cultured in high osmolarity is hyperinvasive toward epithelial cells and destructive of Peyer's patches. *Microbiol Immunol* **45:**149–158.

64. **Winter SE, Winter MG, Thiennimitr P, Gerriets VA, Nuccio SP, Russmann H, Baumler AJ.** 2009. The TviA auxiliary protein renders the *Salmonella enterica* serotype Typhi RcsB regulon responsive to changes in osmolarity. *Mol Microbiol* **74:**175–193.

65. **Winter SE, Winter MG, Godinez I, Yang HJ, Russmann H, Andrews-Polymenis HL, Baumler AJ.** 2010. A rapid change in virulence gene expression during the transition from the intestinal lumen into tissue promotes systemic dissemination of *Salmonella*. *PLoS Pathog* **6:** e1001060. doi:10.1371/journal.ppat.1001060.

66. **Wangdi T, Winter SE, Baumler AJ.** 2012. Typhoid fever: "you can't hit what you can't see". *Gut Microbes* **3:**88–92.

67. **Winter SE, Raffatellu M, Wilson RP, Russmann H, Baumler AJ.** 2008. The *Salmonella enterica* serotype Typhi regulator TviA reduces interleukin-8 production in intestinal epithelial cells by repressing flagellin secretion. *Cell Microbiol* **10:**247–261.

68. **Wangdi T, Lee CY, Spees AM, Yu C, Kingsbury DD, Winter SE, Hastey CJ, Wilson RP, Heinrich V, Baumler AJ.** 2014. The Vi capsular polysaccharide enables *Salmonella enterica* serovar Typhi to evade microbe-guided neutrophil chemotaxis. *PLoS Pathog* **10:**e1004306. doi:10.1371/journal. ppat.1004306.

69. **Kraus MD, Amatya B, Kimula Y.** 1999. Histopathology of typhoid enteritis: morphologic and immunophenotypic findings. *Mod Pathol* **12:**949–955.

70. **Mukawi TJ.** 1978. Histopathological study of typhoid perforation of the small intestines. *Southeast Asian J Trop Med Public Health* **9:**252–255.

71. **Tsolis RM, Young GM, Solnick JV, Baumler AJ.** 2008. From bench to bedside: stealth of enteroinvasive pathogens. *Nat Rev Microbiol* **6:**883–892.

72. **Saraiva M, O'Garra A.** 2010. The regulation of IL-10 production by immune cells. *Nat Rev Immunol* **10:**170–181.

73. **Couper KN, Blount DG, Riley EM.** 2008. IL-10: the master regulator of immunity to infection. *J Immunol* **180:**5771–5777.

74. **Moore KW, de Waal Malefyt R, Coffman RL, O'Garra A.** 2001. Interleukin-10 and the interleukin-10 receptor. *Annu Rev Immunol* **19:**683–765.

75. **Fernandes DM, Baldwin CL.** 1995. Interleukin-10 downregulates protective immunity to *Brucella abortus*. *Infect Immun* **63:**1130–1133.

76. **Fernandes DM, Jiang X, Jung JH, Baldwin CL.** 1996. Comparison of T cell cytokines in resistant and susceptible mice infected with virulent *Brucella abortus* strain 2308. *FEMS Immunol Med Microbiol* **16:**193–203.

77. **Spera JM, Ugalde JE, Mucci J, Comerci DJ, Ugalde RA.** 2006. A B lymphocyte mitogen is a *Brucella abortus* virulence factor required for persistent infection. *Proc Natl Acad Sci USA* **103:**16514–16519.

78. **Everts B, Amiel E, van der Windt GJ, Freitas TC, Chott R, Yarasheski KE, Pearce EL, Pearce EJ.** 2012. Commitment to glycolysis sustains survival of NO-producing inflammatory dendritic cells. *Blood* **120:**1422–1431.

79. **West AP, Brodsky IE, Rahner C, Woo DK, Erdjument-Bromage H, Tempst P, Walsh MC, Choi Y, Shadel GS, Ghosh S.** 2011. TLR signalling augments macrophage bactericidal activity through mitochondrial ROS. *Nature* **472:**476–480.

80. **O'Neill LAJ, Hardie DG.** 2013. Metabolism of inflammation limited by AMPK and pseudo-starvation. *Nature* **493:**346–355.

81. **Rodriguez-Prados JC, Traves PG, Cuenca J, Rico D, Aragones J, Martin-Sanz P, Cascante M, Bosca L.** 2010. Substrate fate in activated macrophages: a comparison between innate, classic, and alternative activation. *J Immunol* **185:**605–614.

82. **Vats D, Mukundan L, Odegaard JI, Zhang L, Smith KL, Morel CR, Wagner RA, Greaves DR, Murray PJ, Chawla A.** 2006. Oxidative metabolism and PGC-1β attenuate macrophage-mediated inflammation. *Cell Metab* **4:**13–24.

83. **Martinez FO, Sica A, Mantovani A, Locati M.** 2008. Macrophage activation and polarization. *Front Biosci* **13:**453–461.

84. **Bensinger SJ, Tontonoz P.** 2008. Integration of metabolism and inflammation by lipid-activated nuclear receptors. *Nature* **454:**470–477.

85. **Ilhan F, Yener Z.** 2008. Immunohistochemical detection of *Brucella melitensis* antigens in cases of naturally occurring abortions in sheep. *J Vet Diagn Invest* **20:**803–806.

86. **Magnani DM, Lyons ET, Forde TS, Shekhani MT, Adarichev VA, Splitter GA.** 2013.

Osteoarticular tissue infection and development of skeletal pathology in murine brucellosis. *Dis Model Mech* **6:**811–818.

87. **Xavier MN, Paixao TA, Poester FP, Lage AP, Santos RL.** 2009. Pathological, immunohistochemical and bacteriological study of tissues and milk of cows and fetuses experimentally infected with *Brucella abortus*. *J Comp Pathol* **140:**149–157.

88. **Xavier MN, Winter MG, Spees AM, den Hartigh AB, Nguyen K, Roux CM, Silva TM, Atluri VL, Kerrinnes T, Keestra AM, Monack DM, Luciw PA, Eigenheer RA, Baumler AJ, Santos RL, Tsolis RM.** 2013. PPARγ -mediated increase in glucose availability sustains chronic Brucella abortus infection in alternatively activated macrophages. *Cell Host Microbe* **14:**159–170.

89. **Meador VP, Deyoe BL, Cheville NF.** 1989. Pathogenesis of *Brucella abortus* infection of the mammary gland and supramammary lymph node of the goat. *Vet Pathol* **26:**357–368.

90. **Odegaard JI, Ricardo-Gonzalez RR, Goforth MH, Morel CR, Subramanian V, Mukundan L, Red Eagle A, Vats D, Brombacher F,** Ferrante AW, Chawla A. 2007. Macrophage-specific PPARγ controls alternative activation and improves insulin resistance. *Nature* **447:**1116–1120.

91. **Tontonoz P, Spiegelman BM.** 2008. Fat and beyond: the diverse biology of PPARγ. *Annu Rev Biochem* **77:**289–312.

92. **Zhang L, Chawla A.** 2004. Role of PPARγ in macrophage biology and atherosclerosis. *Trends Endocrinol Metab* **15:**500–505.

93. **Roop RM 2nd, Caswell CC.** 2013. Bacterial persistence: finding the "sweet spot". *Cell Host Microbe* **14:**119–120.

94. **Eisele NA, Ruby T, Jacobson A, Manzanillo PS, Cox JS, Lam L, Mukundan L, Chawla A, Monack DM.** 2013. *Salmonella* require the fatty acid regulator PPARδ for the establishment of a metabolic environment essential for long-term persistence. *Cell Host Microbe* **14:** 171–182.

95. **Barak Y, Liao D, He W, Ong ES, Nelson MC, Olefsky JM, Boland R, Evans RM.** 2002. Effects of peroxisome proliferator-activated receptor δ on placentation, adiposity, and colorectal cancer. *Proc Natl Acad Sci USA* **99:**303–308.

The Staphylococcal Biofilm: Adhesins, Regulation, and Host Response

19

ALEXANDRA E. PAHARIK[1] and ALEXANDER R. HORSWILL[1]

INTRODUCTION

The *Staphylococcus* genus includes a diverse group of commensals that colonize mammals on the skin or mucous membranes. Some of the best-known members of this genus, such as *Staphylococcus aureus* and *Staphylococcus epidermidis*, are also opportunistic pathogens and are responsible for a tremendous burden on the health care system (1, 2). One of the reasons staphylococci are problematic is their well-known ability to attach to surfaces and develop into recalcitrant community structures, often referred to as "biofilms." Generally, biofilms are defined as communities of cells encased within an exopolymeric matrix and attached to a surface, and they are recognized as being resistant to antimicrobial therapy and host defenses (3).

The biofilm state was initially observed in studies of marine environments, in which adherent communities of bacteria were found in natural as well as industrial aquatic environments (4). Biofilm development was subsequently found to be important in many types of infections and is now a widely accepted bacterial mode of growth. According to the NIH, as many as 80% of human infections are biofilm-based (5). Biofilm infections present a clinical challenge, because they are highly resistant to antimicrobial therapies and often occur

[1]Department of Microbiology, Roy J. and Lucille A. Carver College of Medicine, University of Iowa, Iowa City, IA 52242.

Virulence Mechanisms of Bacterial Pathogens, 5th edition
Edited by Indira T. Kudva, Nancy A. Cornick, Paul J. Plummer, Qijing Zhang, Tracy L. Nicholson, John P. Bannantine, and Bryan H. Bellaire
© 2016 American Society for Microbiology, Washington, DC
doi:10.1128/microbiolspec.VMBF-0022-2015

in areas of the body that are not easily accessible for treatment (6, 7). Staphylococci, in particular, represent a large portion of biofilm-based infections. *S. aureus* and the coagulase-negative staphylococci are the number 1 and number 3 most common etiological agents of hospital-acquired infections in the United States, respectively, including infections of medical devices and surgical wounds (8). Biofilm infections clearly are a significant burden on the health care system today, and the *in vivo* biofilm state is an important area of study.

Definition of a Biofilm

The growth of staphylococci in a biofilm has been linked to many types of infections, but one of the ongoing challenges in the field is the lack of a consensus description of the biofilm state. There is no universal agreement on what constitutes a "staphylococcal biofilm" in terms of morphology, depth, surface coverage, regulatory state, antibiotic resistance level, or whether surface attachment is even necessary. In the field, a biofilm is defined mostly by subjective observations, as well as high antibiotic resistance relative to planktonic bacteria. There have been attempts to identify biomarkers of staphylococcal biofilm formation to provide a better definition. In one promising study, Secor et al. determined that the nonribosomally generated peptide aureusimine (phevalin) was produced in higher levels by biofilm-grown *S. aureus* (9), suggesting that this natural product could be a biofilm biomarker. While this finding is encouraging, there is not yet enough follow-up work on aureusimine or other potential biomarkers to reach a consensus.

The other ongoing challenge in defining biofilms is the enormity of growth states that have been linked to this term. Staphylococcal biofilm growth has been linked to foreign bodies (10), endocarditis (11), osteomyelitis (12), skin infection (13), colonization (14), cystic fibrosis (15), urinary tract infection (UTI) (16), and abscess communities (17). Under such a large umbrella of different growth conditions in the host, each requiring a unique suite of bacterial factors and regulatory machinery, it is impossible to obtain a universal definition of a staphylococcal biofilm that will be agreed upon in the field. Not surprisingly, the staphylococcal requirements to develop infective endocarditis or a skin abscess, such as specific toxins and superantigens (18, 19), are not the same as those needed for an indwelling catheter infection that can be caused by many types of staphylococci. Further, a much lower bacterial load (estimated at 10,000-fold lower) is needed to colonize a foreign body than to cause a skin abscess (20). The reason for this is likely the lack of vascularization at the site and, presumably, a reduced presence of innate immunity factors (10). Considering this point, it seems logical that the virulence factor profile of the invading bacterial pathogen will be different to survive these varied host environments. As one example, *S. aureus* strains deficient in the *agr* quorum-sensing system are unable to properly initiate infective endocarditis or osteomyelitis (21, 22), while the same regulatory system is not essential to initiate a staphylococcal foreign body infection (23); in fact, the *agr* system seems to inhibit colonization of the foreign body (24). Thus, it is increasingly important to consider the context of infection when comparing and contrasting results with other studies.

The Biofilm Life Cycle

The biofilm life cycle is thought to consist of at least three stages (see Fig. 1): initial attachment to an abiotic or biotic surface, maturation of the biofilm, and dispersal. Some consider "microcolony formation" to be an intermediate step between attachment and maturation, but the precise differences between a microcolony and a mature biofilm are not clearly defined. Attachment involves bacterial adhesins that can stick to the surface,

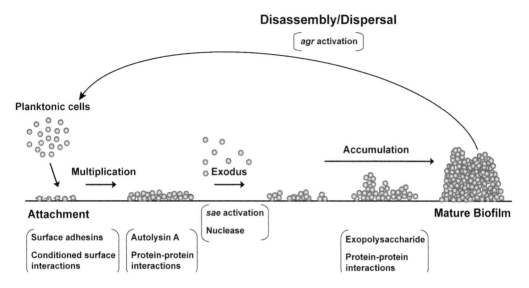

FIGURE 1 The biofilm life cycle. Recent studies have identified steps present in early stages of biofilm formation. After attachment, bacteria form a lawn of growth, which undergoes an exodus period that leaves several small foci of cells. The exodus phase is mediated by the SaeRS system via nuclease enzyme activity. The foci of cells then develop into a mature biofilm containing tower structures. Final dispersal is mediated by the *agr* system via secreted enzymes and phenol-soluble modulins.

while maturation is mediated by cell-cell adhesion, although some adhesins possess both properties. Dispersal or disassembly is mediated by enzymes that degrade the biofilm matrix (25–27). These enzymes may be produced by the bacteria itself or be present in the environment.

A recent paper provided new insights into the stages of early biofilm development using a microtiter flow-based biofilm system (28). This study found that in an *S. aureus* biofilm, attachment and early accumulation were followed by dispersal of a portion of the cells, leaving behind small foci of biofilm growth. These foci then matured into a biofilm with tower structures. Interestingly, the early dispersal phase, termed "exodus," was independent of the *agr* system but required the *sae* system and was specifically modulated by the *sae*-regulated nuclease. These findings provide novel insight into *S. aureus* biofilm development and the independent roles of staphylococcal regulatory systems in the biofilm life cycle.

Biofilm Matrix

The staphylococcal biofilm matrix has been a topic of interest in a number of reports, and various findings have demonstrated its heterogeneity and variability (29). The biofilm matrix contains extracellular DNA (eDNA), both from lysed bacteria and potentially from host neutrophil cell death, and is susceptible to dispersal by DNAses (30, 31). Proteinaceous adhesins have also been identified in the staphylococcal biofilm matrix. These may be directly associated with bacteria in the biofilm or be free in the biofilm matrix (32). A number of cytoplasmic proteins have been identified that appear to moonlight as matrix components and undoubtedly have an important function (33). Finally, the extracellular polysaccharide intercellular adhesin (PIA) has also been identified as a major component of the staphylococcal biofilm, especially in certain strains of *S. epidermidis* (34). Proteinaceous and polysaccharide-based biofilms are susceptible to disassembly by proteases and polysaccharide-degrading agents (26, 27). Teichoic acids have also been implicated in the biofilm matrix (35), although their relative role in biofilm mechanisms has not received as much attention. Presumably, other cellular components are also present and awaiting further investigation.

Coverage of this Review

This review will cover recent advances in staphylococcal biofilm studies. We will discuss the mechanism of biofilm formation by staphylococcal adhesins and regulatory systems, as well as the interaction of biofilms with the host immune system, with a focus on *S. aureus* and *S. epidermidis* as the model pathogens of the genus. Finally, we will discuss the current knowledge of biofilm formation and virulence in other species of staphylococci.

STAPHYLOCOCCAL ADHESINS

Staphylococci possess a number of surface-associated adhesins that mediate initial attachment of biofilm cells as well as intercellular adhesion during biofilm maturation (32, 36). The *S. aureus* genome encodes more than 20 adhesins (32, 36, 37), while coagulase-negative staphylococci have significantly fewer (38, 39). Staphylococcal adhesion and biofilm accumulation are mediated by covalently anchored cell wall proteins, noncovalently associated proteins, and nonprotein factors. The general properties of these adhesins are presented in this section, and their functions within biofilm development are included where information is available.

Covalently Linked Cell Wall–Anchored (CWA) Proteins

Staphylococcal CWA proteins are secreted by the Sec system and share a C-terminal cell wall anchoring motif, hydrophobic domain, and positively charged domain (40). In the majority of CWA proteins, cell wall anchoring is mediated by sortase A, which cleaves the LPXTG cell wall anchoring motif at the threonine-glycine junction and catalyzes the covalent linkage of the CWA protein to peptidoglycan (41). Some Isd proteins in the NEAT (near iron transporter) family are instead anchored by sortase B at the NPQT/PN/S motif (40). The staphylococcal CWA proteins were recently discussed in a review by Foster et al., who proposed classifying them into four groups (see Table 1 and Fig. 2) based on structural motifs (40). These are the MSCRAMMs (microbial surface component recognizing adhesive matrix molecules), the NEAT motif family, the three-helical bundle family, and the G5-E repeat family. All of these types of CWA proteins are involved in biofilm formation in the staphylococci.

MSCRAMMs were originally defined as a broad category of proteins that are cell surface–associated and able to interact with the host extracellular matrix (42). The recent definition proposed by Foster et al. limits the term MSCRAMM to adhesins that contain at least two IgG-like folds and employ a ligand-binding mechanism called "dock, lock, and latch" (40). The staphylococcal MSCRAMMs are the Clf-Sdr family proteins, including Bbp (bone sialoprotein-binding protein), the FnBPs (fibronectin-binding proteins), and CNA (collagen adhesion). Exposure of *S. aureus* to human plasma *in vitro* enhances both MSCRAMM expression and biofilm formation, suggesting the importance of their role in *in vivo* biofilm infections (43).

The Clf-Sdr family consists of clumping factor A (ClfA), clumping factor B (ClfB), and the Sdr proteins. In addition to the IgG-like folds, their structure contains a serine-aspartate repeat domain called the SD region (40). ClfA and ClfB are fibrinogen-binding proteins in *S. aureus* (40, 44), and both are upregulated in biofilm growth relative to planktonic growth (45). Rot and *agr* affect bacterial binding to fibrinogen by regulating *clfB* but not *clfA* (46) (see regulation section).

TABLE 1 **Categorized cell wall-anchored adhesins**

Family	Subfamily	Adhesin	Species	Ligand(s)	References
MSCRAMMs					
	Clf-Sdr				
		ClfA	*Staphylococcus aureus*	Fibrinogen γ-chain	45–56
		SdrG/Fbe	*Staphylococcus epidermidis*	Fibrinogen β-chain	57–64
		Fbl	*Staphylococcus lugdunensis*	Fibrinogen γ-chain	65–69
		ClfB	*S. aureus*	Fibrinogen α-chain, cytokeratin 10, cytokeratin 8, loricrin	45–48, 56, 70–79
		SdrC	*S. aureus*	β-neurexins, self-association	80–82
		SdrD	*S. aureus*	Nasal epithelial cells	80, 83, 84
		SdrE	*S. aureus*	Factor H, C4b-binding protein	80, 85–87
		Bbp	*S. epidermidis*	Bone sialoprotein, C4b-binding protein	87, 97–102
		SdrF	*S. epidermidis*	Type I collagen, Dacron	88–90
		SdrG	*S. epidermidis*	Unknown	91
		SdrH	*S. epidermidis*	Unknown	91
		SdrX	*Staphylococcus capitis*	Type VI collagen	92
		SdrI	*Staphylococcus saprophyticus*	Collagen, fibronectin	93–96
	FnBPs				
		FnBPA	*S. aureus*	Fibrinogen, elastin, fibronectin	103–113
		FnBPB	*S. aureus*	Fibrinogen, elastin, fibronectin	103–113
		CNA	*S. aureus*	Collagen	114–120
NEAT motif					
		IsdA	*S. aureus*	Heme, fibrinogen, fibronectin	122–125
Three helical bundle					
		SpA	*S. aureus*	Fc region of IgG	37, 128–132
G5-E					
		SasG	*S. aureus*	Nasal epithelial cells, self-association	133, 137, 138
		Aap	*S. epidermidis*	Corneocytes, self-association	133–136, 138–140

ClfA is present on the cell wall throughout the growth cycle (47) and promotes bacterial clumping in solution with fibrinogen as well as bacterial attachment to immobilized fibrinogen (48, 49). The ClfA IgG-like fold domains N2 and N3 bind at the C-terminal region of the γ-chain of fibrinogen, a region that also contains platelet binding sites (50, 51). ClfA has been shown to inhibit fibrinogen binding to platelets and fibrinogen-dependent platelet aggregation, indicating that its binding site occludes the platelet binding site (50, 52, 53). In a murine model of *S. aureus* septicemia, mice lacking the ClfA-binding motif of fibrinogen had better survival, suggesting that ClfA-fibrinogen interactions in the blood contribute to virulence (54). A *clfA* mutant in *S. aureus* had a decreased ability to cause vegetations in a rat endocarditis model (55) and reduced bacterial load in a murine abscess model (56).

The *S. epidermidis* MSCRAMM SdrG (also called Fbe) is homologous to *S. aureus* ClfA, although it binds to the β-chain of fibrinogen

MSCRAMMS

Clf-Sdr Family

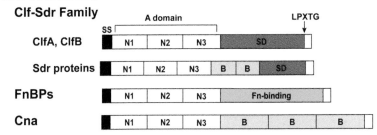

NEAT motif proteins

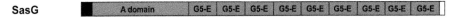

Three helical bundle

G5/E repeat proteins

FIGURE 2 Cell wall–anchored adhesins. All the cell wall–anchored adhesins contain an N-terminal signal sequence (SS) and a C-terminal portion that is cleaved by sortase A at the LPXTG sequence. MSCRAMMs contain three IgG-like folds (N1, N2, and N3) followed by specific ligand-binding domains. In the Sdr protein subfamily, a variable number of B repeats is found between the IgG-like folds and the SD repeat region. SdrC is shown, which contains two of these B repeats. Similarly, the Isd proteins contain one, two, or three NEAT motifs. IsdA is shown, which has one. In SpA, there are four or five IgG-binding domains, sometimes referred to as domains E, D, A, C, and B. There follows a region containing a variable number of tandem repeats.

rather than the γ-chain (57, 58). SdrG is the archetypal example of the dock, lock, and latch mechanism of binding using its IgG-like folds. The dock, lock, and latch model was proposed based on the crystal structure of the SdrG-fibrinogen interaction (59, 60). SdrG mediates adherence to fibrinogen-coated surfaces *in vitro* (61, 62) and is required for fibrinogen-dependent platelet aggregation (63). In a rat model of central venous catheter infection, wild type *S. epidermidis* was more likely to cause infection and formed a more robust biofilm on the catheter *in vivo* than an *sdrG* mutant, indicating its importance in the *in vivo* biofilm formation of *S. epidermidis* (64).

The coagulase-negative species *Staphylococcus lugdunensis* also has a ClfA homolog called Fbl (65, 66). Fbl promotes both adherence to immobilized fibrinogen and cell clumping in fibrinogen-rich solution (66). Fbl and ClfA have similar binding affinities to fibrinogen, and both interact with the C-terminus of the γ-chain (67). Fbl also is used as a species-specific detection method for *S. lugdunensis* (68, 69).

Like ClfA, the *S. aureus* ClfB IgG-like fold region binds to fibrinogen; however, it interacts with the α-chain of fibrinogen rather than the γ-chain (48, 70). ClfB promotes adherence to immobilized fibrinogen as well as *S. aureus* clumping in fibrinogen-rich solution (48, 70). In contrast to ClfA, ClfB becomes depleted from the cell wall beginning in the late exponential phase, suggesting that it is susceptible to proteolytic degradation (48). Further studies revealed that the metalloprotease aureolysin cleaves ClfB at two sites, resulting in the loss of fibrinogen binding (71, 72). ClfB promotes biofilm formation *in vitro*, and aureolysin treatment disrupts ClfB-mediated biofilms, suggesting that aureolysin might facilitate biofilm dispersal by processing ClfB (73). *In vivo*, ClfB is required for full virulence in a rat endocarditis model of infection, although the phenotype of the *clfB* mutant in this model was slight (74). A *clfB* mutant also had decreased bacterial load in a murine abscess model (56).

In addition to fibrinogen, ClfB also binds to the human epithelial proteins cytokeratin 10, cytokeratin 8, and loricrin. ClfB bound to the C-terminal tail region of purified cytokeratin 10, as well as cytokeratin 10 that was natively expressed in desquamated nasal epithelial cells (70, 75, 76). The ClfB IgG-like folds bind cytokeratin 10 by the dock, lock, and latch mechanism (70). Similarly, ClfB bound immobilized cytokeratin 8 and endogenous cytokeratin 8 from lysates of the HaCaT keratinocyte cell line (77). ClfB also binds loricrin, the primary protein in the cornified envelope of the stratum corneum, which is present in the anterior nares. In a murine model of nasal colonization, *clfB* mutant *S. aureus* was defective for colonization compared to wild type. Colonization by both wild type and *clfB* mutant *S. aureus* was also decreased in loricrin-deficient mice, suggesting that loricrin is a critical ligand for *S. aureus* nasal colonization (78). In an experimental model of human nasal colonization, *clfB* mutant *S. aureus* was eliminated significantly more quickly from the nares than its wild type parent, and ClfB was required for long-term colonization (79). These results demonstrate ClfB's versatility in ligand binding and its importance for *S. aureus* colonization.

S. aureus Sdr proteins SdrC, SdrD, and SdrE are encoded in a single locus and have striking similarity in sequence and structural arrangement with the Clf proteins (80). SdrC can bind a host ligand as well as self-associate to promote biofilm formation. A study using a phage display peptide library found that SdrC binds to human β-neurexins, which are expressed on neuronal cells (81). Although the effect of this has not been tested *in vivo*, *S. aureus* endocarditis and sepsis are associated with polyneuropathy, meaning that SdrC interactions with neurexins could contribute to *S. aureus* pathogenesis. A later study showed that SdrC self-associates at the N2 domain and promotes biofilm formation, a process that is inhibited by Mn^{2+} (82). In contrast to SdrC, the structural stability of SdrD appears to require binding to divalent cations, specifically Ca^{2+} (83). Like SdrC, SdrD mediates adherence to human desquamated nasal epithelial cells (84). SdrE in *S. aureus* (80) induces platelet aggregation (85). SdrE also inhibits complement activation by two mechanisms. It binds the complement regulatory protein factor H, which inhibits activation of the alternative complement pathway (86). SdrE also inhibits classical complement pathway-mediated opsonization and phagocytosis by binding to the classical complement regulator C4b-binding protein (87).

SdrF in *S. epidermidis* binds type I collagen, mediated by its B domain repeats (88). Interestingly, SdrF was also found to bind with high affinity to Dacron, the polymeric surface of drivelines that are used in ventricular assist devices (VAD) for end-stage congestive heart failure. Since *S. epidermidis* is a common etiological agent of medical device infections, including VAD infections, this finding is relevant to its pathogenesis. Anti-SdrF antibodies decreased infection in a murine model of *S. epidermidis* VAD driveline infection, suggesting possible therapeutic interventions for these infections (89). SdrF also was found to bind other plastic materials based on ionic interactions (90). These results suggest that inhibition of SdrF binding to prosthetic devices may be a promising avenue for treatment of *S. epidermidis* infections.

S. epidermidis also has SdrG and SdrH, whose sequences are similar to typical SD proteins but are not present in cell wall preparations of *S. epidermidis*, indicating that they may be improperly sorted to the cell wall. However, antisera from patients following infection with *S. epidermidis* were reactive to the A domains of SdrG and SdrH, suggesting that they are expressed during infection (91).

Other coagulase-negative staphylococci possess Sdr family proteins that have been characterized in limited detail. *Staphylococcus capitis* SdrX has an SD repeat region, although the N-terminal domain is not strongly similar to *S. aureus* Sdr proteins. SdrX was reported to bind type VI collagen and mediate bacterial adherence to a type VI collagen-coated surface (92). *Staphylococcus saprophyticus* has the Clf-Sdr family protein SdrI, which binds collagen (93) and fibronectin (94), the latter of which is a unique property among the Sdr proteins. SdrI was also found to contribute to the hydrophobicity of the *S. saprophyticus* surface, a property that is known to enable bacterial adherence to host epithelia (95). In a murine model of UTI, SdrI was critical for persistence but not initial colonization (96).

Bbp (bone sialoprotein-binding protein) is an Sdr-family protein in *S. aureus* that is considered to be an allelic variant of SdrE (87). *S. aureus* isolates from osteomyelitis infections were observed to bind bone sialoprotein by an unknown adhesin (97), which was eventually identified to be Bbp (98, 99). Like SdrE, Bbp binds the classical complement regulator C4b-binding protein, inhibiting classical-pathway-mediated opsonization and phagocytosis (87). Bbp appears to be associated with invasive osteomyelitis infections in particular. In 60 patients with deep *S. aureus* infections following orthopedic surgery, 95% of the isolates were positive for the *bbp* gene (100), while of 53 *S. aureus* isolates from bloodstream infections, 47% were positive for *bbp* (101). The presence of antibodies to Bbp was also shown to be effective in distinguishing osteomyelitis from soft tissue infections in patients with diabetic foot ulcers (102).

FnBPs

S. aureus has two fibronectin-binding proteins, FnBPA and FnBPB, which are encoded by *fnbA* and *fnbB*, respectively (103). Like the Clf-Sdr family proteins, the FnBPs contain an N-terminal region that forms IgG-like folds; these domains bind fibrinogen and elastin (104, 105). In place of the SD repeat region, the FNBPs have a region of 10 to 11 tandem repeats that recognize fibronectin (106). FnBP binding to fibronectin induces bacterial invasion into epithelial cells, endothelial cells, and keratinocytes (107–109). The FnBPs have been found to affect biofilm formation and virulence. In *S. aureus*, a double knockout of *fnbA* and *fnbB* lost the ability to bind fibronectin and to form biofilms on microtiter plates and under shear flow conditions. Complementation of either *fnbA* or *fnbB* alone on a plasmid restored these phenotypes, as well as the ability of *S. aureus* to agglutinate (110). The FnBPs are thought to promote biofilm formation by a self-association mechanism that is distinct from ligand binding, making them multifunctional in the *S. aureus* biofilm life cycle (111, 112). The FnBPs also were shown to enhance virulence in an experimental model of endocarditis (113).

The collagen-binding adhesin CNA was initially reported to be necessary and sufficient for *S. aureus* binding to the collagen-rich substrate cartilage (114). CNA consists of an A domain with several collagen-binding sites and a domain containing B repeats (114, 115). Crystal structure characterization of the CNA-collagen interaction suggested a "collagen hug" model, a variation of the dock, lock, and latch ligand-binding scheme (115). CNA blocks activation of the classical complement pathway (116) and contributes to virulence of *S. aureus* keratitis (117), osteomyelitis (118), septic arthritis (119), and endocarditis (120).

S. epidermidis also has a collagen-binding protein, the GehD lipase. GehD is not LPXTG-anchored, although it is cell wall–associated, and its structure does not resemble CNA of *S. aureus*. However, purified GehD binds to immobilized collagen and mediates *S. epider-*

midis binding to collagen and therefore may contribute to colonization or pathogenesis (121).

The NEAT motif family consists of the Isd (iron–regulated surface determinant) proteins. These CWA proteins bind heme or hemoglobin, facilitating its transport into the bacterial cell, and they are upregulated in iron limiting conditions (122). *S. aureus* IsdA and IsdC bind heme via their NEAT motifs (Fig. 2) (123). These proteins also play a role in survival against host immune defense. *S. aureus* IsdA is the most abundant CWA protein in iron starvation conditions and also decreases surface hydrophobicity, which makes *S. aureus* more resistant to bactericidal fatty acids and peptides in human skin (124). IsdA also is able to bind human fibrinogen and fibronectin (125). In a murine model of systemic infection, *S. aureus isdB* expression varied among organs to which bacteria localized in the host, and IsdB was required for colonization of the heart (126). This suggests that *isd* expression depends upon iron availability in each host niche of infection. In *S. lugdunensis*, IsdC was found to induce biofilm formation under iron-limiting conditions and to induce attachment to polystyrene as well as self-associate to promote intercellular adhesion (127).

The sole three-helical bundle cell wall–anchored protein is staphylococcal protein A (SpA), which is present in all strains of *S. aureus* and whose sequence variation is used for strain typing (128). SpA binds the conserved Fc region of immunoglobulin IgG, which allows immune evasion (129, 130) and has also been found in the biofilm matrix *in vitro* (131). SpA is also released from the cell wall, and released SpA has been shown to promote bacterial survival in human blood, suggesting that free SpA contributes to disruption of the host immune response (37, 132). Presumably, free SpA could also provide adhesion in the biofilm matrix.

G5-E Repeat Family: Aap/SasG

G5-E repeats are found in cell wall–anchored adhesins in Gram-positive organisms, and are so named because of the five conserved glycine residues in each repeat. G5 domains consist of 78 residues and form 6 beta strands, with E domain spacers that are of similar sequence to G5, but only 50 residues (133). The *S. aureus* G5-E repeat protein SasG and its *S. epidermidis* homolog Aap have similar structures and are thought to function similarly in adhesion and biofilm formation. SasG and Aap each have an N-terminal A domain that mediates attachment to abiotic and host surfaces via unknown ligands. In *S. epidermidis* Aap, the A domain alone promotes attachment to polystyrene (134, 135) as well as to human corneocytes (136). *S. aureus* SasG promotes attachment to human desquamated nasal epithelial cells via its A domain (137). Multiple studies have shown that the G5-E repeats of SasG and Aap are able to dimerize by binding to Zn^{2+}, forming a "twisted rope" structure (133, 138). This property is thought to enable intercellular adhesion when adjacent SasG or Aap proteins dimerize via their G5-E domains. In *S. epidermidis*, Aap has been shown to induce biofilm formation following proteolytic removal of its A domain by exogenous proteases, although the *S. epidermidis* proteases that may process Aap are not identified (139). Aap has also been shown to be required for full *in vitro* biofilm formation in *S. epidermidis*, as well as for virulence in a rat catheter model of infection (134). Recently, a small 18-kDa scaffolding protein, called small basic protein, or Sbp, was found in the *S. epidermidis* biofilm matrix and affects both PIA-dependent and Aap-dependent biofilm formation. In Aap-mediated biofilm formation, Sbp was found to interact with the B domain of Aap in the biofilm matrix, suggesting its role as a structural component of the biofilm (140).

Uncategorized CWA Proteins

The remaining uncategorized cell wall–anchored proteins are Bap and several Sas proteins, including SasA/SraP. Bap is an

S. aureus cell wall–anchored protein that was identified in a transposon screen for mutants defective in biofilm formation (141). It has a unique structure consisting of three major domains, each with sequence homology to different cell wall–anchored proteins in other bacterial genera. Bap was found to mediate attachment to an abiotic surface as well as intercellular adhesion, making it a potent enhancer of biofilm formation. In a murine model of catheter infection, the *bap* mutant had decreased bacterial load. Bap is also present in several coagulase-negative staphylococci, and a mutant of the *bap* homolog in *S. epidermidis* had decreased biofilm formation relative to wild type (142). A later study demonstrated that Bap promoted adherence, but inhibited invasion, of epithelial cells *in vitro* by binding the Gp96 receptor (143). The authors propose that this property of Bap enhances virulence of biofilm-based infections by resisting bacterial engulfment into host cells, although this has yet to be directly tested.

S. aureus SasA/SraP (serine-rich adhesin for platelets) is a member of the serine-rich repeat family of cell wall–bound proteins found in several Gram-positive pathogens, primarily oral streptococci (144, 145). Homologs of SraP have also been identified in the coagulase-negative staphylococcal species *S. epidermidis* and *Staphylococcus haemolyticus* (146, 147). SraP is a sortase-anchored, cell wall–bound adhesin that binds platelets, and it also possesses a ligand-binding domain that is thought to promote intercellular adhesion and biofilm formation. A *sraP* mutant was reported to have decreased biofilm formation, and SraP bound to *S. aureus* whole cell lysates, suggesting that SraP may self-associate or bind other targets on neighboring *S. aureus* cells to promote biofilm development (148). The ligand-binding domain was recently structurally characterized and found to contain a lectin-like module that binds N-acetylneuraminic acid (149), an abundant sugar on host glycosylated proteins. The *S. haemolyticus* serine-rich repeat protein UafB mediates binding to fibronectin, fibrinogen, and human uroepithelial cells (150).

SasX is another cell wall–anchored adhesin that has been shown to play an important role in virulence. SasX was linked to the spread of a methicillin-resistant *S. aureus* (MRSA) epidemic in China, because its prevalence in MRSA clones increased via horizontal transfer, suggesting its importance in the pathogenic success of MRSA. SasX was also shown to be crucial for a murine model of nasal colonization, murine MRSA skin infection, and bacterial aggregation *in vitro* (151). SasX has recently been shown to be a promising vaccine candidate for *S. aureus* infection. Active or passive immunization to SasX decreased *S. aureus* virulence in murine models of skin infection, lung infection, and nasal colonization (152).

There are also several *S. aureus* Sas proteins that are poorly characterized. SasC is an LPXTG-anchored protein that contains a FIVAR domain and a domain of unknown function consisting of repeats. SasC, specifically its FIVAR domain, induced cell aggregation, binding to polystyrene, and biofilm formation (153). Genome sequence analysis of *S. aureus* revealed the putative cell wall–anchored adhesins SasB, SasD, SasF, SasJ, SasK, and SasL, but their structure and function have not been studied further (154).

Surface-Associated Proteinaceous Adhesins

The autolysins AtlA and AtlE are found in *S. aureus* and *S. epidermidis*, respectively. Atl and AtlE share a similar amino acid sequence and structure, with bacteriolytic amidase and glucosoaminidase domains (155). They are known to be involved in cell wall turnover, cell division, and cell lysis (156, 157). Autolysins have two properties that could promote biofilm formation: the ability to attach to extracellular matrix materials and to augment the biofilm matrix with eDNA by inducing cell lysis. Adhesin activity was first identified in a transposon mutant of *S. epidermidis atlE* that had decreased ability to adhere to polystyrene and vitronectin (155). In an *S. epidermidis* biofilm grown on medical device biomaterials *in vitro*, *atlE* expression decreased during the first 12 hours of biofilm growth relative to planktonic culture, but by 48 hours, expression was up-regulated 10-fold (158). This may indicate that *atlE* is more important later in the bio-film life cycle, when autolysis is induced and eDNA is released.

Nonproteinaceous Surface-Associated Adhesins

Wall teichoic acids and lipoteichoic acids have been shown to play a role in adhesion, colonization of host cells, and biofilm forma-tion. Wall teichoic acids are covalently linked to the peptidoglycan and consist of alternat-ing phosphate and ribitol, while lipoteichoic acids attach to the outer leaflet of the cell membrane and have alternating phosphate and glycerol (36). Teichoic acids are highly charged, a property that was found to be critical for *S. aureus* colonization of abiotic surfaces. A mutant lacking D-alanine in its wall teichoic acid lost the ability to form a biofilm *in vitro*. This was due to its greater net negative charge, which decreased its adher-ence to plastic surfaces (159). In *S. epider-midis*, wall teichoic acids induced adherence to immobilized fibronectin (160). Teichoic acids have been identified in the biofilm matrices of *S. epidermidis* and *S. aureus* (35, 161, 162).

PIA is a secreted polysaccharide that is synthesized by the *ica* operon and has been thoroughly studied in the context of biofilm formation, immune evasion, and pathogene-sis. Several reports state that PIA is required for *S. epidermidis* biofilm formation and vir-ulence (163–165), and it is considered to be the most important intercellular adhesin of the staphylococci (34). The role of PIA in staphylococcal biofilm formation has been reviewed by O'Gara (166) and by Rohde et al.

(167), and the regulation of the *ica* locus in the staphylococci is reviewed in reference 168.

SECRETED PROTEINS IN THE BIOFILM MATRIX

A number of secreted staphylococcal proteins have been implicated in biofilm formation, the most prominent being AtlA/AtlE (dis-cussed above as surface associated), proteases, nucleases, and phenol-soluble modulins (PSMs). The exo-enzymes and PSMs will be discussed in more detail in the regulation section below, because their role in biofilm development relates more to dispersal than accumulation. Other secreted proteins that have been linked to biofilm formation are covered here.

Alpha-toxin (Hla) is a potent cytolysin secreted by *S. aureus* that also affects inflam-mation and contributes to pathogenesis by multiple mechanisms. Many studies have shown that alpha-toxin mutants are attenu-ated in virulence (169). However, the contri-bution of this toxin to biofilm formation is less clear. In a study of *in vitro* biofilm for-mation on polystyrene, an *S. aureus hla* mutant had dramatically reduced biofilm in a standard microtiter plate assay and under flow conditions. Its initial attachment to the surface was also decreased, indicating that an inability to bind to the surface contributes to decreased mature biofilm (170), although the exact mechanism of this phenotype remains unclear.

S. aureus beta-toxin (Hlb) is a secreted sphingomyelinase that has hemolytic and lymphocytic activities (171, 172). Beta-toxin also has a sphingomyelinase-independent "biofilm ligase" activity, which refers to its ability to cross-link strands of DNA in the biofilm matrix. Mutants in *hlb* were deficient in *in vitro* attachment, flow-cell biofilm formation, and vegetation formation in a rabbit endocarditis model (173). Hlb is the first staphylococcal protein identified that binds eDNA in the biofilm matrix, providing more evidence of the importance of this matrix component.

S. aureus secretes multiple proteins that have been called secreted expanded repertoire adhesive molecules (SERAM) (174). Two of the SERAMs, the extracellular adherence protein (Eap; also called the MHC class II analog protein or Map) and the extracellular matrix-binding protein (Emp) have a demonstrated connection to biofilm formation (175, 176). Eap is a secreted adhesin that enhances S. aureus adherence to the extracellular matrix, and it has been shown to bind fibrinogen, fibronectin, vitronectin, and thrombospondin-1 with varying affinities (177–180). Eap can also self-associate to induce aggregation of S. aureus (177). Due to its ability to bind several matrix proteins, Eap is required for biofilm formation in the presence of serum (175). Regulation of the eap gene is dependent on the SaeRS two-component system (181, 182), and the gene is upregulated under low-iron conditions (176). The eap mutant biofilm phenotype is dependent on these iron-limiting conditions (176). The Eap protein has a number of known immunomodulating properties that have been summarized elsewhere (174). Less is known about Emp, but this protein can also bind matrix proteins such as fibrinogen (174), and it is also SaeRS and iron regulated (176, 182). Similar to Eap, Emp is required for biofilm formation in iron limiting conditions (176).

REGULATION OF BIOFILM FORMATION

Global changes in gene regulation occur throughout the course of the staphylococcal biofilm life cycle. Microarray studies have shown that the biofilm lifestyle requires a gene expression profile to allow tolerance of the low pH within a biofilm, as well as a metabolic quiescence that includes down-regulation of transcription, translation, and aerobic processes (183, 184). Several global regulators, such as the agr quorum sensing system, sigma factor B, and SarA, have strong connections to staphylococcal biofilm formation in vitro and during infection and will be summarized further below. These regulators have also been examined in more acute pathogenesis mechanisms, and the focus here will be on the biofilm-like infections. The majority of these studies have been performed with S. aureus, but some studies of S. epidermidis are also included. It should be noted that a number of other regulators have also been linked to biofilm formation, including MgrA (185) and ArlRS (186), but these are beyond the scope of this review.

agr Quorum-Sensing System

The agr (accessory gene regulator) system is a peptide quorum-sensing system present in all the staphylococci and is a dominant regulator of pathogenesis and biofilm development in S. aureus. Its molecular characteristics and importance in pathogenesis have been thoroughly studied and reviewed in detail (187, 188). The agr system functions by sensing extracellular levels of an auto-inducing peptide (AIP) that is produced by staphylococci during growth. The chemical nature of this AIP signal is variable depending on the species and can even have multiple types within a species. Briefly, the AIP is released outside the cell, where it accumulates, and at a particular concentration (usually in the low nM range), the AIP binds to the surface-exposed AgrC histidine kinase, activating a two-component response. This results in phosphorylation of the response regulator AgrA, which in turn induces expression of the primary output of the system, the regulatory transcript RNAIII (189). In parallel, AgrA activates transcription of the PSMα and PSMβ transcripts (190) and autoinduces the quorum-sensing machinery. RNAIII is the main effector of the system and directly regulates production of virulence factors; it also regulates the translation of the repressor of toxins (Rot) (191). In the staphylococcal strains in which global changes in *agr*-dependent gene expression have been assessed (192, 193), the general dogma is that induction of the *agr* system leads to upregulation of secreted enzymes and toxins while simultaneously downregulating adhesins.

Understanding and interpreting the literature on the *agr* system is a challenging task, in part due to the depth of the literature but also due to the complexities of the system. Focusing on *S. aureus*, one of the most overlooked issues is that the dynamic range of the *agr* system is tremendously variable across strains (187), meaning some strains barely produce RNAIII, whereas others, such as the USA300 strains, produce very high levels (194). In recent years, the molecular nature of this variability has begun to be examined (195), providing preliminary explanations for why some *S. aureus* strains have muted *agr* function, resulting in reduced RNAIII levels. The challenge becomes interpreting the results of *agr* mutant studies, where in a USA300 strain the mutation has a dramatic impact on many phenotypes (196–198), but in others, such as some clonal complex 30 strains (195), it has little impact. Further complicating this issue, some older lab strains, such as 8325-4, have known mutations that lead to dysregulation of *agr* function (199). Thus, care must be taken in interpreting results of studies, especially in animal studies of infections, and unfortunately, the *agr* function of strains used for some of these studies is not known.

Several studies have investigated the role of quorum sensing in the biofilm life cycle. The current model is that biofilm initiation and maturation require low *agr* expression, while subsequent *agr* activation within the biofilm induces dispersion to the planktonic state. Indeed, multiple studies of *S. aureus* and *S. epidermidis* have shown that isogenic *agr* mutants display increased biofilm formation *in vitro* (24, 199–201). As the biofilm develops, small populations experience *agr* reactivation and disperse from the biofilm (27, 187, 202). An established *S. aureus* biofilm can be fully dispersed by the addition of AIP to induce *agr* activation (179, 203), and the dispersion process is mediated by *agr*-regulated proteases, most prominently the staphopain enzymes (204). The *agr* regulation of the proteases is via Rot, whose transcriptional repression of the proteases is relieved when *agr* is induced (205, 206). A model for this regulatory pathway is shown in Fig. 3. Currently, the major missing piece of this model is the specific biofilm matrix proteins that are targeted by the staphopain enzymes, and this is a topic of ongoing investigation. The other prominent *agr*-regulated factors linked to biofilm dispersion are the PSMs (23). These peptides have surfactant activity that is antibiofilm in nature. On the whole, these results support the model that under *agr*-repressive conditions or with *agr* null mutants, *S. aureus* cells have increased biofilm capacity *in vitro* due to the absence of secreted dispersal factors. However, in a biofilm infection, the importance of the *agr* system for initiation depends on the type of infection (see below), presumably because in some tissue sites *S. aureus* must secrete *agr*-regulated immunomodulating factors to survive. Once the biofilm has been established, both *in vitro* and *in vivo* studies indicate that activation of the *agr* system can lead to dispersal of the cells and dissemination to new sites.

Environmental conditions are a critical factor in controlling *agr* function. *S. aureus* can metabolize many sugars (207), and the low pH generated from excretion of short-chain fatty acids can repress *agr* activity (208). For development of an *in vitro S. aureus* biofilm, excess sugar (e.g., glucose) must be provided to trigger the pH decline and promote biofilm formation (179). The expression of *agr*-regulated factors, such as the staphopains, must be repressed for *S. aureus* cells to attach and initiate biofilm development. For other staphylococcal species, this low pH requirement is less clear. In *S. epidermidis*, the addition of excess glucose was not essential for promoting biofilm formation (134), but

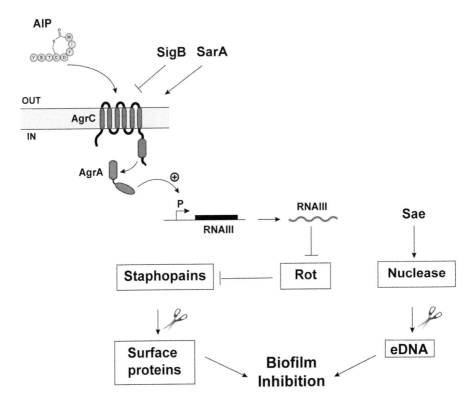

FIGURE 3 Regulatory networks in biofilm formation. The *agr* quorum-sensing system induces expression of secreted staphopain proteases by inhibiting translation of Rot (repressor of toxins), a negative regulator of the proteases. These proteases then degrade proteins on the staphylococcal surface and in the biofilm matrix. The SaeRS system induces production of the nuclease enzyme that cleaves eDNA in the matrix. Sigma factor B (SigB) inhibits *agr* expression, while SarA has been shown to directly enhance it.

whether this is related to *agr* function is not known. The control of *agr* function is also beginning to be appreciated in the host environment. Proteins found in human serum are known to repress *S. aureus agr* activity (209), including apolipoprotein B (210, 211). Hemoglobin is another abundant host protein with known *agr*-inhibitory properties (212). Environmental contaminants that accumulate in the body, such as triclosan, have also been linked to enhanced biofilm formation (213). Altered environmental conditions can impact biofilm structure as well, as recently demonstrated with the conversion of PSMs into protease-resistant amyloid fibers (214).

The role of *agr* during infection is complex and has been the focus of many studies. The contribution of *agr* to acute pathogenesis has been reviewed previously (187), and we will focus on chronic infections with biofilm-like properties. One of the most common models of biofilm infection is a catheter placed subcutaneously in the flank of a mouse. Staphylococci are inoculated into the lumen of the catheter and allowed to develop into a biofilm over an extended time (215). The inoculum dose can be varied, because it is known that foreign bodies greatly reduce the bacterial load required to colonize (10). Using this model, *S. aureus agr* mutants have no defect in their ability to colonize the catheter and develop a biofilm (C. Ibberson, C. Parlet, and A.R. Horswill, unpublished observations). However, these mutants are less able to disseminate into other tissues (23), consistent with the concept that the *agr* system is a dispersing mechanism. Using a similar rabbit model of indwelling medical device infection, an *S. epidermidis agr* mutant had an increased ability to colonize the device (24). For both *S. aureus* and *S. epidermidis*, it has been demonstrated that PSMs are important for dispersing from a foreign-body biofilm (23, 216). It seems likely that the many exo-enzymes secreted by these pathogens are also important for dissemination through the host, and our preliminary studies confirm this hypothesis (C. Ibberson, C. Parlet, and A.R. Horswill, unpublished observations).

For chronic infections involving host tissue, the function of the *agr* system has also been assessed. *S. aureus* is one of the leading causes of osteomyelitis, a chronic infection of the bone that has known biofilm-like properties (12). *S. aureus agr* mutants are attenuated in their ability to establish osteomyelitis (22). *S. aureus* is also the leading cause of infective endocarditis (217), another chronic infection, where bacteria attach to the heart valve and develop into a vegetation composed of matrix proteins, platelets, and immune cells. Similar to osteomyelitis, *S. aureus agr* mutants show a defect in their ability to establish infection (21). Interestingly, the *agr* system showed progressive activation within the endocarditis vegetations (218), which is in contrast to what is observed in biofilms under *in vitro* conditions (179). As an added complication of endocarditis, septic emboli can dislodge and enter the bloodstream, and these emboli have biofilm characteristics that make them more resistant to antibiotics than planktonic bacteria and are potentially life-threatening for the patient (219–222).

It is generally accepted that low levels of *agr* expression are observed in chronic infections (223–225), suggesting that the loss or decreased activity of *agr* is an adaptation to allow persistence in the host environment. However, this is somewhat misleading, since the comparison for these claims is usually *in vitro* broth culture, in which *agr* function and RNAIII levels are extremely high. The more informative experiment is tracking *agr* function over time within the infection, which was performed with infective endocarditis (218) but has not been attempted more systemically in other infection types. Some of the studies on low *agr* expression are based on *S. aureus* isolates from the cystic fibrosis lung. Growth of bacterial pathogens, such as *Pseudomonas aeruginosa*, in cystic fibrosis are known to be in a biofilm state, but there is limited information on *S. aureus*, although a link to biofilms has been suggested (15). What is clear is that *agr*-negative mutants do frequently appear during biofilm growth *in vitro* (226) and during biofilm infections (225, 227). In part, this could be due to the increased fitness cost of expressing the *agr* system in the presence of antibiotic pressure (228). When *S. aureus* reenters a normal state, the maintenance requirement of the *agr* system is restored (229).

As a global regulator, the *agr* quorum-sensing system has widespread effects on gene expression that can strongly impact the staphylococcal biofilm life cycle. However, the complexity of the system and the factors that alter its expression can result in varied effects of the *agr* system *in vivo*. When studying the role of the *agr* system during infection, the *agr* expression level of the staphylococcal strain must be considered, as well as the infection niche and the relevant host factors that may modify the importance of *agr*. Since inhibition of *agr* has begun to be investigated as a possible treatment for *S. aureus* infections (230–232), further work needs to be done to clarify the types of *in vivo* conditions and infections that would benefit from this.

AI-2

AI-2, or autoinducer-2, is another quorum-sensing molecule that is present in both Gram-positive and Gram-negative organisms, and it is thought to be a bacterial interspecies signaling molecule (233, 234). AI-2 has been shown to inhibit biofilm formation and virulence in both *S. aureus* and *S. epidermidis*. In *S. epidermidis*, a mutant that does not produce AI-2 had greatly increased biofilm formation *in vitro* and increased virulence in a rat central venous catheter infection model (235). This mutant also had increased expression of the secreted polysaccharide synthesis operon *ica* and increased polysaccharide production, which is thought to be the mechanism for its biofilm phenotype. Yu et al. reported similar findings, in which an AI-2 mutant had increased biofilm formation *in vitro* and in a murine catheter infection model. AI-2 was also shown to positively regulate expression of the *ica* operon repressor *icaR*, leading to increased production of extracellular polysaccharide in the AI-2 mutant (236). An *S. aureus* AI-2 mutant also displayed increased survival in human blood and macrophages (237). Yu et al. also investigated the relationship between AI-2 and *agr* regulation in *S. epidermidis* biofilm formation. The two were found to have an additive effect, in which a double mutant had higher biofilm formation than either single mutant (236).

SigB

Sigma B (SigB) is an alternative sigma factor of RNA polymerase that is activated in stress response and leads to global changes in promoter specificity and, thus, gene expression (238). Strains lacking SigB have tremendous changes in regulatory profiles that alter biofilm formation and virulence. *S. aureus* mutants in the global regulator *sigB* are unable to form a biofilm *in vitro* (199). This phenotype is mediated both by increased protease activity (239, 240) and increased nuclease activity (241). Part of the reason for increased protease activity has been linked to hyper-activation of the *agr* system in SigB-defective strains (199). In *S. epidermidis*, a *sigB* mutant also was reported to have decreased biofilm formation and increased

expression of *icaR*, which represses production of the extracellular polysaccharide PIA (242, 243).

SigB also plays an important role in the response of staphylococci to the *in vivo* environment. In a murine intravenous infection model with *S. aureus*, the SigB cascade was reported to be highly transcriptionally active, although a *sigB* mutant had no difference in disease outcome in the mice (244). However, an *S. epidermidis sigB* mutant did have a defect in colonization in a rat model of foreign body infection (245). Expression of *S. aureus* SigB is also activated by human pulmonary surfactant and after internalization by human bronchial epithelial cells (246, 247).

Spontaneous *sigB* mutants arise *in vitro* in biofilm formation and in chronic staphylococcal infections (248, 249). These mutants are small colony variants, which have elevated extracellular protease activity and decreased biofilm formation. They also have increased intracellular persistence and are thought to contribute to virulence of *S. aureus* infections (249). These results suggest that biofilm populations and infecting bacteria are heterogeneous in gene sequence as well as expression level of key virulence factors.

SarA

The *sar* (staphylococcal accessory regulator) locus was discovered in a transposon mutagenesis screen for fibrinogen-binding-negative mutants (250). In addition to decreased fibrinogen binding, the *sar* mutant had an altered exoprotein profile, with increased protease, lipase, and α-hemolysin. The *sar* locus produces three transcripts from three separate promoters, all of which contain the ORF for the DNA-binding protein SarA (251, 252). Early studies showed that a *sar* mutant had decreased levels of the *agr* transcripts RNAII and RNAIII (253–255). EMSA (electrophoretic mobility shift assay) studies have shown that purified SarA directly binds to three sites within a region spanning the P2 and P3 promoters of the *agr* locus (252). SarA regulatory activity therefore occurs partially via its effects on *agr*.

SarA also directly regulates several genes that affect biofilm formation. A putative SarA binding site has been identified upstream of several SarA-regulated genes, providing a mechanism for direct regulation by DNA binding (256). SarA represses transcription of *cna* even in the absence of *agr* and directly binds to the *cna* promoter region (257, 258). A microarray revealed that in addition to positively regulating *fnbA* and *fnbB*, SarA negatively regulates *isaB* and *spa*, and all of these gene promoters contain a putative SarA binding site (193). SarA also positively regulates *bap*, a cell wall adhesin found in bovine isolates of *S. aureus*, via direct binding to its promoter (259). Secreted proteases and nuclease are upregulated in *sarA* mutants (193, 260, 261). Since the opposite phenotypes are observed in *agr* mutants, it is apparent that this effect occurs via an *agr*-independent pathway.

Multiple studies have reported that in *S. aureus*, SarA is required for biofilm formation, both *in vitro* and *in vivo* (175, 262–264). Various mechanisms for this phenotype have been proposed. The first study to report the *S. aureus sarA* mutant biofilm defect also showed that this mutant had decreased *ica* transcription and PIA production and suggested that this could partially account for the biofilm phenotype (263). However, a later study showed that while an *S. aureus sarA* mutant did not produce a biofilm, an *ica* operon knockout had no decrease in biofilm formation (183). These studies were performed *in vitro* as well as *in vivo* using a murine model of catheter-associated biofilm infection. The results indicate that *ica* regulation is not the sole factor behind the *sarA* knockout biofilm phenotype and that PIA production may not be critical under certain biofilm conditions.

Biofilm formation in *sarA* mutants is also thought to be inhibited by their increased protease and nuclease activity. Although one study found that protease inhibitor treatment did not alter the phenotype of a *sarA* mutant, only the initial attachment was tested, rather than the endpoint of biofilm growth (263). A later report found that treatment with a cocktail of protease inhibitors for all the secreted proteases resulted in increased biofilm formation of an *S. aureus sarA* mutant in the clinical isolate UAMS-1 (265). This suggests that increased protease activity contributes to the *sarA* biofilm phenotype. The same study showed that a *sarA nuc* double mutant had improved biofilm formation relative to a single *sarA* mutant, demonstrating that the effect of SarA is also partially mediated by nuclease production. In a group of three *S. aureus* clinical isolates, *sarA* mutants had decreased biofilm formation regardless of their various levels of *agr* expression (266). This study also found that protease inhibitor treatment improved biofilm formation in *sarA* mutants of each clinical isolate, confirming the impact of secreted proteases on biofilm formation. On the whole, these results suggest that SarA-mediated effects on biofilm formation are mediated by secreted enzymes more than PIA and are at least partially independent of *agr*.

There are conflicting reports of the effect of *sarA* mutation on *S. epidermidis*. In two *S. epidermidis* clinical isolates, *sarA* mutation was found to drastically decrease biofilm formation (267). In the same study, *S. epidermidis* SarA was also found to positively regulate transcription of the *ica* operon and bind to the *icaA* promoter, indicating that SarA induces biofilm formation via PIA production. In contrast, Christner et al. showed that SarA represses biofilm formation in an *S. epidermidis* clinical isolate by two mechanisms (268). Mutation of *sarA* dramatically increased biofilm formation in the *aap*-negative, *ica*-negative *S. epidermidis* clinical isolate 1585 as well as in an *S. epidermidis* 1457 *icaA* mutant. The first mechanism of biofilm enhancement in the *sarA* mutant was increased expression of the cell wall adhesin *embp* (extracellular matrix binding protein). A double *sarA embp* mutant had decreased biofilm formation relative to the *sarA* mutant, indicating that the *sarA* phenotype was partially dependent on Embp. The second mechanism of biofilm enhancement was found to be increased protease expression in the *sarA* mutant, although this is contrary to previous findings in *S. aureus*. *S. epidermidis sarA* mutants have increased production of the metalloprotease SepA (269), which was shown by Christner et al. to induce processing of the autolysin AtlE, leading to increased lysis and eDNA release (268). This study shows that SarA is a positive regulator of the eDNA- and Embp-dependent biofilm.

EVASION OF THE HOST IMMUNE SYSTEM

Staphylococcal biofilms are noted for their resistance to host immune clearing, and there have been significant efforts to characterize the mechanisms that contribute to this resistance (270–272). Studies have investigated the effects of staphylococcal biofilms on immune cell function, the host antibody response to chronic staphylococcal infection, and the staphylococcal transcriptional response to host innate immune cells.

In the innate immune system, polymorphonuclear leukocytes (PMNs) and macrophages are the first responders to staphylococcal infection (17, 273–275). Although one study reported minimal PMN influx in a murine model of catheter-associated *S. aureus* biofilm growth (272), others have demonstrated that activated PMNs are prevalent at the site of infection in human patients with orthopedic device-associated staphylococcal biofilm infections (276, 277). Multiple studies have reported that human PMNs in *in vitro* coculture with *S. aureus* localize to the biofilm and can phagocytose bacteria (278, 279). In an *S. epidermidis* biofilm grown *in vitro*, PMNs were able to attach to the biofilm, release granule components from both primary and secondary granules, and phagocytose biofilm

bacteria (280). These effects were observed with or without opsonization, which suggests they are mediated at least in part by bacterial components that interact with the PMNs.

PMNs can attack staphylococcal biofilms by phagocytosis, release of toxic granule components, and production of neutrophil extracellular traps (NETs), although there is evidence that these effects are dampened relative to planktonic bacteria (281). *S. epidermidis* is more resistant to *in vitro* killing by human PMNs when grown in a biofilm than grown planktonically (282). The *S. epidermidis* extracellular polysaccharide PIA is thought to play a role in evading PMN killing, because it has been shown that an *S. epidermidis ica* mutant exhibits increased susceptibility to phagocytosis and killing by human PMNs *in vitro* (283). Similarly, the *S. aureus* capsular polysaccharide inhibits opsonophagocytosis of planktonic bacteria by PMNs *in vitro* and is required for full virulence in a murine model of septic arthritis (284, 285). Although these studies did not directly test phagocytosis of biofilm bacteria, the results suggest that PIA and capsule in a staphylococcal biofilm may shield the bacteria from the host immune response. The *agr* system may also allow the staphylococcal biofilm to resist PMN killing. In *S. aureus*, an *agr* mutant biofilm was less cytotoxic to PMNs in coculture than its wild type counterpart, suggesting that biofilm cells expressing *agr* could kill PMNs and therefore evade phagocytosis and killing by PMNs (278). This corroborates an earlier study testing interactions of planktonic wild type and *agr* mutant *S. aureus* with PMNs, which also found that the *agr* mutant induced decreased PMN lysis (198).

NETs were first described by Brinkmann et al., who showed that activated PMNs produce thread-like projections composed of DNA and granule components (286). NETs bind to microbes *in vitro* and degrade bacterial extracellular virulence factors as well as kill the bacteria. NET formation is thought to occur via a regulated cell death pathway termed NETosis that is distinct from necrosis and apoptosis (287). *S. aureus* extracellular nuclease has been shown to degrade NETs, thereby allowing the bacteria to resist NET-mediated killing (288, 289). Since the secreted nuclease is unique and not found in all staphylococci, species that lack it may be more susceptible to NETs, although an additional surface-attached nuclease (Nuc2) is more conserved among the staphylococci (290).

The interactions between staphylococcal biofilms and host macrophages have also been investigated. These studies have led to a model (see Fig. 4) in which staphylococci promote an anti-inflammatory, profibrotic environment via alternative macrophage activation (270, 272). Macrophages can undergo at least two varieties of activation, including classical and alternative (291). Classically activated (M1) macrophages are characterized by their ability to present antigen and degrade intracellular pathogens, while alternatively activated macrophages

are inefficient at both of these. Alternatively activated (M2) macrophages have high arginase (Arg–1) activity, which decreases their ability to destroy intracellular pathogens (292) and promotes collagen formation, extracellular matrix proliferation, and wound healing (293). Planktonic staphylococci have been shown to induce classical activation of macrophages and are readily phagocytosed (294). However, in an *S. aureus* biofilm coculture with macrophages, Scherr et al. observed little macrophage phagocytosis of *S. aureus* cells and few macrophages in close proximity to the biofilm (278). A coculture study of *S. aureus* biofilms and macrophages reported that macrophages that interacted closely with the biofilm performed little phagocytosis and exhibited gene expression patterns consistent with M2 activation. Further, the same study showed that macrophage death was induced in cells that were close to the biofilm (294). Another group has reported that *clfA* expression prevents macrophage phagocytosis by a mechanism that is independent of binding to fibrinogen (295). These results suggest that biofilms can promote a macrophage phenotype that favors the progression of infection and produce factors that are cytotoxic to macrophages.

Multiple studies have performed microarrays on *S. aureus* following coculture with innate immune cells to determine global regulatory changes that facilitate staphylococcal survival. A microarray study of *S. aureus* following interactions with PMNs and macrophages revealed more extensive changes in regulation after exposure to macrophages. Although various *S. aureus* genes were differentially regulated in response to PMNs, a striking global downregulation was observed following coculture with macrophages. In both an immature and a mature biofilm, downregulation of hundreds of genes was observed, corresponding to a global decrease in metabolic processes (278). Another report demonstrated that following coculture with phagocytic PMNs, *S. aureus* experienced widespread changes in regulation. Stress

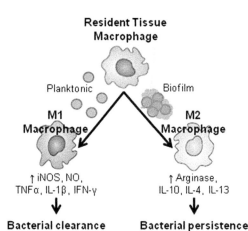

FIGURE 4 Macrophage activation pathways. Biofilm growth of *Staphylococci* has been shown to favor the M2 phenotype in macrophages, which is characterized by increased arginase and profibrotic activity, as well as decreased antimicrobial clearance. These changes are thought to contribute to the persistence of staphylococci in biofilm infections. This figure is reproduced from reference 272.

response proteins such as catalase were upregulated, as well as virulence factors such as hemolysins and fibrinogen-binding proteins. There was also a shift in the metabolic profile relative to broth culture, and changes in global regulators occurred. Of note, the Sae system, which positively regulates several secreted toxins and other virulence-associated proteins (196, 296–298), was upregulated several fold after exposure to PMNs (299). The Sae system was later shown to differentially regulate its various targets in response to specific neutrophil stimuli (300), and *sae* mutants have decreased survival in *in vitro* PMN phagocytosis assays (298). These results demonstrate that *S. aureus* has an arsenal of tools to survive PMN and innate immune assault and that the Sae system in particular is a crucial element.

Several studies have characterized the *S. aureus* proteins that are targeted by the host antibody response following infection or colonization (301–303). This group of antigens is referred to as the immune proteome, and it identifies proteins that are expressed *in vivo* and may be important to virulence. These findings also may suggest targets for the development of a vaccine for *S. aureus*, which has been an area of interest in recent years.

OTHER STAPHYLOCOCCAL SPECIES

The study of staphylococcal biofilm formation has largely focused on *S. aureus* and *S. epidermidis*. However, other staphylococcal species are also pathogenic biofilm-formers. Staphylococci are classified based on their production of the blood-clotting enzyme coagulase, a secreted protein that induces the conversion of fibrinogen to fibrin (304, 305). The genus *Staphylococcus* comprises 47 species: 8 are coagulase-positive or coagulase-variable, 38 are coagulase-negative, and 1, *Staphylococcus schleiferi*, has both a coagulase-negative and a coagulase-positive subspecies. Of the coagulase-positive staphy-

lococci, *S. aureus* is the sole species that is primarily associated with human disease (1). However, there have been reports of other coagulase-positive staphylococci colonizing or causing disease in human hosts who have significant contact with animals (306, 307). One example is *Staphylococcus pseudintermedius*, a commensal of dogs that is implicated in canine opportunistic infection (308). Bioinformatic and proteomic analyses have been employed to study the cell wall adhesins of *S. pseudintermedius*, leading to further study of two proteins (SpsD and SpsL) to which canines have antibodies, indicating their expression *in vivo* (309, 310).

The coagulase-negative staphylococci are the third most common cause of human health care–associated infections (8) and the number 1 cause of bovine intramammary infections (311–313). They have been reviewed thoroughly in references 1 and 44. Within the coagulase-negative staphylococci, *S. epidermidis* is the most frequent cause of medical device–related infections and is able to infect virtually any medical implant including catheters, central lines, ventilators, prosthetic joints, and pacemakers (8, 314–316). One reason for its high rate of infection may be its prevalence in the normal skin flora and ability to colonize many surfaces of the human body, including the anterior nares, axillae, and inguinal and perineal areas (1, 317). Other coagulase-negative staphylococci species inhabit various niches of the human body. *S. lugdunensis* is found particularly in the lower extremities of the body in the perineal and groin areas, as well as in the axillae (318, 319). *S. haemolyticus* is preferentially isolated from axillae and pubic areas (317, 320), and *S. saprophyticus*, from the gastrointestinal tract, rectum, and urogenital tract, typically in younger individuals (1, 321, 322).

Of the coagulase-negative staphylococci, *S. lugdunensis* is considered to be the most similar to coagulase-positive staphylococci (1). It is a skin commensal and opportunistic pathogen, responsible for 0.8 to 7.8% of infectious endocarditis cases in non–drug users (323), with mortality rates ranging from 38 to 42% (323, 324). These high mortality rates are similar to those of *S. aureus* endocarditis and are suggestive of aggressive infection. *S. lugdunensis* is also implicated in infections of medical devices, such as catheters and prosthetic joints (325–327). Recent studies have also demonstrated that *S. lugdunensis* is a significant cause of skin and soft-tissue infections, with up to 53 per 100,000 per year (328).

For mechanisms of pathogenesis, *S. lugdunensis* possesses several virulence factors, including surface adhesins, which are reviewed in reference 329. A mutant in the cell wall–anchoring enzyme sortase A was attenuated in an experimental endocarditis model, confirming that like in *S. aureus*, adhesins contribute to *S. lugdunensis*–mediated endocarditis (330). *S. lugdunensis* also has an *ica* locus for PIA synthesis, although its role in biofilm formation is not clear, since *S. lugdunensis* biofilms *in vitro* were not sensitive to degradation by either of the PIA-targeting factors Na-metaperiodate or dispersin B (331). Biofilm formation may be a significant factor in infection, because *S. lugdunensis* clinical isolates from prosthetic implant infections have been shown to be strong biofilm formers *in vitro* (332). In addition to its biofilm-forming activity, *S. lugdunensis* has several putative cytolysins, including the SLUSH (*S. lugdunensis* synergistic hemolytic) peptides, which are similar to *S. aureus* delta-toxin Hld, and another Hld-like protein (329, 333). However, the activity and virulence role of these SLUSH proteins is not known.

S. haemolyticus has been implicated in a range of opportunistic infections in humans, including prosthetic device infections (334) and postoperative endophthalmitis (335). In a study of *S. haemolyticus* isolated from bloodstream infections, 66% of the isolates formed robust biofilms *in vitro*, but the same strains were all negative for PCR of the *ica* operon for PIA synthesis (336). This suggests that *S. haemolyticus* has other means of biofilm formation. The Bap adhesin was present in several biofilm-positive *S. haemolyticus* nosocomial infection isolates, identifying at least one PIA-independent mechanism that may contribute to *S. haemolyticus* biofilm formation and infection (337).

Since *S. saprophyticus* colonizes the rectum and urogenital tract, it is unsurprising that it is a common cause of UTIs. *S. saprophyticus* is the second most frequent cause of UTI in young, sexually active women, although it also causes UTIs in populations of all ages (338, 339). *S. saprophyticus* has several adhesins that contribute to virulence, including SdrI and the serine-rich repeat protein UafB (see adhesins section). It also secretes urease, an enzyme that hydrolyzes urea to carbon dioxide and ammonia, which raises the pH of the urinary tract and can result in calculi formation. Urease was shown to be a virulence factor in a rat model of *S. saprophyticus* UTI (340). Chemical inhibition of urease was able to prevent the pH change caused by *S. saprophyticus* growth in an artificial urine medium, although the effectiveness of this as a treatment has yet to be tested *in vivo* (341).

CONCLUSIONS AND FUTURE PERSPECTIVES

The goal of this review on staphylococcal biofilms is to summarize the latest literature on the function of adhesins, regulatory cascades, and the host response to these biofilms, with a focus on the noted pathogens *S. aureus* and *S. epidermidis*, and also coverage on other coagulase-negative staphylococci biofilms. The significant body of work available indicates that there are numerous mechanisms to assemble a mature staphylococcal biofilm, and these structures vary depending on the substratum, the adhesins particular staphylococci express, and the matrix materials available. Within a biofilm infection, the host niche clearly also has an important role in biofilm matrix composition and impacting the regulatory pathways controlling expression of staphylococcal biofilm factors.

A number of recent studies provide convincing evidence that the staphylococcal biofilm cells are equipped to thwart the host immune response, making them more resistant to the host immune system than planktonic cells. Recent findings have also shown that staphylococcal biofilms contain heterogeneous populations, with a subset of cells contributing to the development of antibiotic resistance. In several bacteria, the phenomenon of persister cells has been observed, which are a small portion of a bacterial population that remains following antibiotic treatment (342, 343). *S. aureus* persisters were first observed in a murine model of deep wound infection. Treatment with vancomycin killed 99% of *S. aureus* cells, while the remaining 1% continued to be unaffected by vancomycin even after another day of treatment, suggesting a persister population (344). Other studies have demonstrated that the appearance of heterogeneous populations can develop within an *S. aureus* biofilm (226), and further studies have shown that these subpopulations can interact to promote vancomycin-intermediate resistance phenotypes (345). Clearly, biofilms are a diverse population with varying phenotypic properties that can contribute to the progress of an infection in complex ways.

Despite all the advancements, much remains to be elucidated regarding the defined nature of the *in vivo* biofilm state. Although the term "biofilm" is broadly applied to various growth states ranging from benign skin colonization to endocarditis, the universal qualities of these that specifically define biofilm characteristics are not clear, making it challenging at times to compare results across studies. There have been efforts to identify universal biomarkers of a staphylococcal biofilm (9), as well as to clarify the roles of virulence determinants that are unique to certain biofilm infection types, but there is still a pressing need for more studies in this direction to standardize the field. In part, researchers themselves have created this dilemma by trying to link every staphylococcal growth state to a biofilm without considering the limitations of such a diverse umbrella. Attempts have been made to rein in the enthusiasm by trying to keep certain growth states separate and uniquely defined, such as colonization (346), but the popularity of "biofilms" keeps this terminology at the forefront of any literature on staphylococcal communities. Further, with the growing literature on other community states, such as synovial aggregates (347), polysaccharide aggregates (348), and fibrinogen-based clumping (349), there is a growing need for investigations to compare and contrast properties of these states with classical biofilm features.

The study of staphylococcal biofilm development has advanced greatly over the past decade, and we have endeavored in this review to cover many of the recent advances. In the future, biofilm studies will need to be extended to more host-relevant conditions to properly model and understand the *in vivo* biofilm state. Too often, *in vitro* studies leave out host factors that can impact biofilm maturation in many ways, and these conditions need to be considered when modeling biofilm development *in vitro* or *in vivo*. We need to properly understand all these complexities to best position therapeutic development for treating biofilm infections.

ACKNOWLEDGMENTS

A.E.P was funded by an American Heart Association predoctoral fellowship (14PRE19910005). Studies in the laboratory of A.R.H are supported by grant AI083211 (Project 3) from the National Institute of Allergy and Infectious Diseases.

CITATION

Paharik AE, Horswill AR. 2016. The staphylococcal biofilm: adhesins, regulation, and host response. Microbiol Spectrum 4(2): VMBF-0022-2015.

REFERENCES

1. **Becker K, Heilmann C, Peters G.** 2014. Coagulase-negative staphylococci. *Clin Microbiol Rev* **27**:870–926.
2. **Lowy FD.** 1998. *Staphylococcus aureus* infections. *N Engl J Med* **339**:520–532.
3. **Kiedrowski MR, Horswill AR.** 2011. New approaches for treating staphylococcal biofilm infections. *Ann N Y Acad Sci* **1241**:104–121.
4. **Costerton JW, Cheng KJ, Geesey GG, Ladd TI, Nickel JC, Dasgupta M, Marrie TJ.** 1987. Bacterial biofilms in nature and disease. *Annu Rev Microbiol* **41**:435–464.
5. **Davies D.** 2003. Understanding biofilm resistance to antibacterial agents. *Nat Rev Drug Discov* **2**:114–122.
6. **del Pozo JL, Patel R.** 2007. The challenge of treating biofilm-associated bacterial infections. *Clin Pharmacol Ther* **82**:204–209.
7. **Jacqueline C, Caillon J.** 2014. Impact of bacterial biofilm on the treatment of prosthetic joint infections. *J Antimicrob Chemother* **69** (Suppl 1):i37–i40.
8. **Sievert DM, Ricks P, Edwards JR, Schneider A, Patel J, Srinivasan A, Kallen A, Limbago B, Fridkin S.** 2013. Antimicrobial-resistant pathogens associated with healthcare-associated infections: summary of data reported to the National Healthcare Safety Network at the Centers for Disease Control and Prevention, 2009-2010. *Infect Control Hosp Epidemiol* **34**:1–14.
9. **Secor PR, Jennings LK, James GA, Kirker KR, Pulcini ED, McInnerney K, Gerlach R, Livinghouse T, Hilmer JK, Bothner B, Fleckman P, Olerud JE, Stewart PS.** 2012. Phevalin (aureusimine B) production by *Staphylococcus aureus* biofilm and impacts on human keratinocyte gene expression. *PloS One* **7**:e40973. doi:10.1371/journal.pone.0040973.
10. **Zimmerli W, Trampuz A, Ochsner PE.** 2004. Prosthetic-joint infections. *N Engl J Med* **351**:1645–1654.
11. **Parsek MR, Singh PK.** 2003. Bacterial biofilms: an emerging link to disease pathogenesis. *Annu Rev Microbiol* **57**:677–701.
12. **Brady RA, Leid JG, Calhoun JH, Costerton JW, Shirtliff ME.** 2008. Osteomyelitis and the role of biofilms in chronic infection. *FEMS Immunol Med Microbiol* **52**:13–22.
13. **Percival SL, Emanuel C, Cutting KF, Williams DW.** 2012. Microbiology of the skin and the role of biofilms in infection. *Int Wound J* **9**:14–32.
14. **Iwase T, Uehara Y, Shinji H, Tajima A, Seo H, Takada K, Agata T, Mizunoe Y.** 2010. *Staphylococcus epidermidis* Esp inhibits *Staphylococcus aureus* biofilm formation and nasal colonization. *Nature* **465**:346–349.
15. **Goss CH, Muhlebach MS.** 2011. Review: *Staphylococcus aureus* and MRSA in cystic fibrosis. *J Cystic Fibrosis* **10**:298–306.
16. **Trautner BW, Darouiche RO.** 2004. Role of biofilm in catheter-associated urinary tract infection. *Am J Infect Control* **32**:177–183.
17. **Cheng AG, DeDent AC, Schneewind O, Missiakas D.** 2011. A play in four acts: *Staphylococcus aureus* abscess formation. *Trends Microbiol* **19**:225–232.
18. **Kobayashi SD, Malachowa N, Whitney AR, Braughton KR, Gardner DJ, Long D, Bubeck Wardenburg J, Schneewind O, Otto M, Deleo FR.** 2011. Comparative analysis of USA300 virulence determinants in a rabbit model of skin and soft tissue infection. *J Infect Dis* **204**:937–941.
19. **Salgado-Pabon W, Breshears L, Spaulding AR, Merriman JA, Stach CS, Horswill AR, Peterson ML, Schlievert PM.** 2013. Superantigens are critical for *Staphylococcus aureus* infective endocarditis, sepsis, and acute kidney injury. *mBio* **4**:e00494-13. doi:10.1128/mBio.00494-13.
20. **Nowakowska J, Landmann R, Khanna N.** 2014. Foreign body infection models to study host-pathogen response and antimicrobial tolerance of bacterial biofilm. *Antibiotics* **3**:378–397.
21. **Cheung AL, Eberhardt KJ, Chung E, Yeaman MR, Sullam PM, Ramos M, Bayer AS.** 1994. Diminished virulence of a sar-/agr- mutant of *Staphylococcus aureus* in the rabbit model of endocarditis. *J Clin Invest* **94**:1815–1822.
22. **Gillaspy AF, Hickmon SG, Skinner RA, Thomas JR, Nelson CL, Smeltzer MS.** 1995. Role of the accessory gene regulator (agr) in pathogenesis of staphylococcal osteomyelitis. *Infect Immuny* **63**:3373–3380.
23. **Periasamy S, Joo HS, Duong AC, Bach TH, Tan VY, Chatterjee SS, Cheung GY, Otto M.** 2012. How *Staphylococcus aureus* biofilms develop their characteristic structure. *Proc Natl Acad Sci USA* **109**:1281–1286.
24. **Vuong C, Kocianova S, Yao Y, Carmody AB, Otto M.** 2004. Increased colonization of indwelling medical devices by quorum-sensing mutants of *Staphylococcus epidermidis in vivo*. *J Infect Dis* **190**:1498–1505.
25. **Lister JL, Horswill AR.** 2014. *Staphylococcus aureus* biofilms: recent developments in biofilm dispersal. *Front Cell Infect Microbiol* **4**:178.
26. **Kaplan JB.** 2010. Biofilm dispersal: mechanisms, clinical implications, and potential therapeutic uses. *J Dent Res* **89**:205–218.

27. **Boles BR, Horswill AR.** 2011. Staphylococcal biofilm disassembly. *Trends Microbiol* **19:**449–455.

28. **Moormeier DE, Bose JL, Horswill AR, Bayles KW.** 2014. Temporal and stochastic control of *Staphylococcus aureus* biofilm development. *mBio* **5:**e01341-14. doi:10.1128/mBio.01341-14.

29. **Hobley L, Harkins C, MacPhee CE, Stanley-Wall NR.** 2015. Giving structure to the biofilm matrix: an overview of individual strategies and emerging common themes. *FEMS Microbiol Rev* **39:**649–669.

30. **Montanaro L, Poggi A, Visai L, Ravaioli S, Campoccia D, Speziale P, Arciola CR.** 2011. Extracellular DNA in biofilms. *Int J Artif Organs* **34:**824–831.

31. **Mann EE, Rice KC, Boles BR, Endres JL, Ranjit D, Chandramohan L, Tsang LH, Smeltzer MS, Horswill AR, Bayles KW.** 2009. Modulation of eDNA release and degradation affects *Staphylococcus aureus* biofilm maturation. *PloS One* **4:**e5822. doi:10.1371/journal.pone.0005822.

32. **Speziale P, Pietrocola G, Foster TJ, Geoghegan JA.** 2014. Protein-based biofilm matrices in staphylococci. *Front Cell Infect Microbiol* **4:**171.

33. **Foulston L, Elsholz AK, DeFrancesco AS, Losick R.** 2014. The extracellular matrix of *Staphylococcus aureus* biofilms comprises cytoplasmic proteins that associate with the cell surface in response to decreasing pH. *mBio* **5:**e01667-14. doi:10.1128/mBio.01667-14.

34. **Otto M.** 2013. Staphylococcal infections: mechanisms of biofilm maturation and detachment as critical determinants of pathogenicity. *Annu Rev Med* **64:**175–188.

35. **Jabbouri S, Sadovskaya I.** 2010. Characteristics of the biofilm matrix and its role as a possible target for the detection and eradication of *Staphylococcus epidermidis* associated with medical implant infections. *FEMS Immunol Med Microbiol* **59:**280–291.

36. **Heilmann C.** 2011. Adhesion mechanisms of staphylococci. *Adv Exp Med Biol* **715:**105–123.

37. **Becker S, Frankel MB, Schneewind O, Missiakas D.** 2014. Release of protein A from the cell wall of *Staphylococcus aureus*. *Proc Natl Acad Sci USA* **111:**1574–1579.

38. **Bowden MG, Chen W, Singvall J, Xu Y, Peacock SJ, Valtulina V, Speziale P, Hook M.** 2005. Identification and preliminary characterization of cell-wall-anchored proteins of *Staphylococcus epidermidis*. *Microbiology* **151:**1453–1464.

39. **Heilbronner S, Holden MT, van Tonder A, Geoghegan JA, Foster TJ, Parkhill J, Bentley SD.** 2011. Genome sequence of *Staphylococcus lugdunensis* N920143 allows identification of putative colonization and virulence factors. *FEMS Microbiol Lett* **322:**60–67.

40. **Foster TJ, Geoghegan JA, Ganesh VK, Hook M.** 2014. Adhesion, invasion and evasion: the many functions of the surface proteins of *Staphylococcus aureus*. *Nat Rev Microbiol* **12:**49–62.

41. **Mazmanian SK, Liu G, Ton-That H, Schneewind O.** 1999. *Staphylococcus aureus* sortase, an enzyme that anchors surface proteins to the cell wall. *Science* **285:**760–763.

42. **Patti JM, Allen BL, McGavin MJ, Hook M.** 1994. MSCRAMM-mediated adherence of microorganisms to host tissues. *Annu Rev Microbiol* **48:**585–617.

43. **Cardile AP, Sanchez CJ Jr, Samberg ME, Romano DR, Hardy SK, Wenke JC, Murray CK, Akers KS.** 2014. Human plasma enhances the expression of staphylococcal microbial surface components recognizing adhesive matrix molecules promoting biofilm formation and increases antimicrobial tolerance *in vitro*. *BMC Res Notes* **7:**457.

44. **Otto M.** 2004. Virulence factors of the coagulase-negative staphylococci. *Front Biosci* **9:**841–863.

45. **Resch A, Rosenstein R, Nerz C, Gotz F.** 2005. Differential gene expression profiling of *Staphylococcus aureus* cultivated under biofilm and planktonic conditions. *Appl Environ Microbiol* **71:**2663–2676.

46. **Xue T, You Y, Shang F, Sun B.** 2012. Rot and Agr system modulate fibrinogen-binding ability mainly by regulating clfB expression in *Staphylococcus aureus* NCTC8325. *Med Microbiol Immunol* **201:**81–92.

47. **Hartford O, Francois P, Vaudaux P, Foster TJ.** 1997. The dipeptide repeat region of the fibrinogen-binding protein (clumping factor) is required for functional expression of the fibrinogen-binding domain on the *Staphylococcus aureus* cell surface. *Mol Microbiol* **25:**1065–1076.

48. **Ni Eidhin D, Perkins S, Francois P, Vaudaux P, Hook M, Foster TJ.** 1998. Clumping factor B (ClfB), a new surface-located fibrinogen-binding adhesin of *Staphylococcus aureus*. *Mol Microbiol* **30:**245–257.

49. **McDevitt D, Francois P, Vaudaux P, Foster TJ.** 1994. Molecular characterization of the clumping factor (fibrinogen receptor) of *Staphylococcus aureus*. *Mol Microbiol* **11:**237–248.

50. **McDevitt D, Nanavaty T, House-Pompeo K, Bell E, Turner N, McIntire L, Foster T, Hook**

M. 1997. Characterization of the interaction between the *Staphylococcus aureus* clumping factor (ClfA) and fibrinogen. *Eur J Biochem* **247**:416–424.

51. **Ganesh VK, Rivera JJ, Smeds E, Ko YP, Bowden MG, Wann ER, Gurusiddappa S, Fitzgerald JR, Hook M.** 2008. A structural model of the *Staphylococcus aureus* ClfA-fibrinogen interaction opens new avenues for the design of anti-staphylococcal therapeutics. *PLoS Pathog* **4**:e1000226. doi:10.1586/erd. 11.36.

52. **Liu CZ, Shih MH, Tsai PJ.** 2005. ClfA(221-550), a fibrinogen-binding segment of *Staphylococcus aureus* clumping factor A, disrupts fibrinogen function. *Thromb Haemost* **94**:286–294.

53. **Liu CZ, Huang TF, Tsai PJ, Tsai PJ, Chang LY, Chang MC.** 2007. A segment of *Staphylococcus aureus* clumping factor A with fibrinogen-binding activity (ClfA221-550) inhibits platelet-plug formation in mice. *Thromb Res* **121**:183–191.

54. **Flick MJ, Du X, Prasad JM, Raghu H, Palumbo JS, Smeds E, Hook M, Degen JL.** 2013. Genetic elimination of the binding motif on fibrinogen for the *S. aureus* virulence factor ClfA improves host survival in septicemia. *Blood* **121**:1783–1794.

55. **Moreillon P, Entenza JM, Francioli P, McDevitt D, Foster TJ, Francois P, Vaudaux P.** 1995. Role of *Staphylococcus aureus* coagulase and clumping factor in pathogenesis of experimental endocarditis. *Infect Immun* **63**:4738–4743.

56. **Cheng AG, Kim HK, Burts ML, Krausz T, Schneewind O, Missiakas DM.** 2009. Genetic requirements for *Staphylococcus aureus* abscess formation and persistence in host tissues. *FASEB J* **23**:3393–3404.

57. **Nilsson M, Frykberg L, Flock JI, Pei L, Lindberg M, Guss B.** 1998. A fibrinogen-binding protein of *Staphylococcus epidermidis*. *Infect Immun* **66**:2666–2673.

58. **Pei L, Palma M, Nilsson M, Guss B, Flock JI.** 1999. Functional studies of a fibrinogen binding protein from *Staphylococcus epidermidis*. *Infect Immun* **67**:4525–4530.

59. **Ponnuraj K, Bowden MG, Davis S, Gurusiddappa S, Moore D, Choe D, Xu Y, Hook M, Narayana SV.** 2003. A "dock, lock, and latch" structural model for a staphylococcal adhesin binding to fibrinogen. *Cell* **115**:217–228.

60. **Bowden MG, Heuck AP, Ponnuraj K, Kolosova E, Choe D, Gurusiddappa S, Narayana SV, Johnson AE, Hook M.** 2008. Evidence for the "dock, lock, and latch" ligand

binding mechanism of the staphylococcal microbial surface component recognizing adhesive matrix molecules (MSCRAMM) SdrG. *J Biol Chem* **283**:638–647.

61. **Pei L, Flock JI.** 2001. Lack of *fbe*, the gene for a fibrinogen-binding protein from *Staphylococcus epidermidis*, reduces its adherence to fibrinogen coated surfaces. *Microb Pathog* **31**:185–193.

62. **Hartford O, O'Brien L, Schofield K, Wells J, Foster TJ.** 2001. The Fbe (SdrG) protein of *Staphylococcus epidermidis* HB promotes bacterial adherence to fibrinogen. *Microbiology* **147**:2545–2552.

63. **Brennan MP, Loughman A, Devocelle M, Arasu S, Chubb AJ, Foster TJ, Cox D.** 2009. Elucidating the role of *Staphylococcus epidermidis* serine-aspartate repeat protein G in platelet activation. *J Thromb Haemost* **7**:1364–1372.

64. **Guo B, Zhao X, Shi Y, Zhu D, Zhang Y.** 2007. Pathogenic implication of a fibrinogen-binding protein of *Staphylococcus epidermidis* in a rat model of intravascular-catheter-associated infection. *Infect Immun* **75**:2991–2995.

65. **Nilsson M, Bjerketorp J, Guss B, Frykberg L.** 2004. A fibrinogen-binding protein of *Staphylococcus lugdunensis*. *FEMS Microbiol Lett* **241**:87–93.

66. **Mitchell J, Tristan A, Foster TJ.** 2004. Characterization of the fibrinogen-binding surface protein Fbl of *Staphylococcus lugdunensis*. *Microbiology* **150**:3831–3841.

67. **Geoghegan JA, Ganesh VK, Smeds E, Liang X, Hook M, Foster TJ.** 2010. Molecular characterization of the interaction of staphylococcal microbial surface components recognizing adhesive matrix molecules (MSCRAMM) ClfA and Fbl with fibrinogen. *J Biol Chem* **285**: 6208–6216.

68. **Pereira EM, Oliveira FL, Schuenck RP, Zoletti GO, Dos Santos KR.** 2010. Detection of *Staphylococcus lugdunensis* by a new species-specific PCR based on the *fbl* gene. *FEMS Immunol Med Microbiol* **58**:295–298.

69. **Chatzigeorgiou KS, Siafakas N, Petinaki E, Zerva L.** 2010. *fbl* gene as a species-specific target for *Staphylococcus lugdunensis* identification. *J Clin Lab Anal* **24**:119–122.

70. **Ganesh VK, Barbu EM, Deivanayagam CC, Le B, Anderson AS, Matsuka YV, Lin SL, Foster TJ, Narayana SV, Hook M.** 2011. Structural and biochemical characterization of *Staphylococcus aureus* clumping factor B/ligand interactions. *J Biol Chem* **286**:25963–25972.

71. **McAleese FM, Walsh EJ, Sieprawska M, Potempa J, Foster TJ.** 2001. Loss of clumping

factor B fibrinogen binding activity by *Staphylococcus aureus* involves cessation of transcription, shedding and cleavage by metalloprotease. *J Biol Chem* **276**:29969–29978.

72. **Perkins S, Walsh EJ, Deivanayagam CC, Narayana SV, Foster TJ, Hook M.** 2001. Structural organization of the fibrinogen-binding region of the clumping factor B MSCRAMM of *Staphylococcus aureus*. *J Biol Chem* **276**:44721–44728.

73. **Abraham NM, Jefferson KK.** 2012. *Staphylococcus aureus* clumping factor B mediates biofilm formation in the absence of calcium. *Microbiology* **158**:1504–1512.

74. **Entenza JM, Foster TJ, Ni Eidhin D, Vaudaux P, Francioli P, Moreillon P.** 2000. Contribution of clumping factor B to pathogenesis of experimental endocarditis due to *Staphylococcus aureus*. *Infect Immun* **68**:5443–5446.

75. **O'Brien LM, Walsh EJ, Massey RC, Peacock SJ, Foster TJ.** 2002. *Staphylococcus aureus* clumping factor B (ClfB) promotes adherence to human type I cytokeratin 10: implications for nasal colonization. *Cell Microbiol* **4**:759–770.

76. **Walsh EJ, O'Brien LM, Liang X, Hook M, Foster TJ.** 2004. Clumping factor B, a fibrinogen-binding MSCRAMM (microbial surface components recognizing adhesive matrix molecules) adhesin of *Staphylococcus aureus*, also binds to the tail region of type I cytokeratin 10. *J Biol Chem* **279**:50691–50699.

77. **Haim M, Trost A, Maier CJ, Achatz G, Feichtner S, Hintner H, Bauer JW, Onder K.** 2010. Cytokeratin 8 interacts with clumping factor B: a new possible virulence factor target. *Microbiology* **156**:3710–3721.

78. **Mulcahy ME, Geoghegan JA, Monk IR, O'Keeffe KM, Walsh EJ, Foster TJ, McLoughlin RM.** 2012. Nasal colonisation by *Staphylococcus aureus* depends upon clumping factor B binding to the squamous epithelial cell envelope protein loricrin. *PLoS Pathog* **8**:e1003092. doi:10.1371/journal.ppat.1003092.

79. **Wertheim HF, Walsh E, Choudhurry R, Melles DC, Boelens HA, Miajlovic H, Verbrugh HA, Foster T, van Belkum A.** 2008. Key role for clumping factor B in *Staphylococcus aureus* nasal colonization of humans. *PLoS Med* **5**:e17.

80. **Josefsson E, McCrea KW, Ni Eidhin D, O'Connell D, Cox J, Hook M, Foster TJ.** 1998. Three new members of the serine-aspartate repeat protein multigene family of *Staphylococcus aureus*. *Microbiology* **144**:3387–3395.

81. **Barbu EM, Ganesh VK, Gurusiddappa S, Mackenzie RC, Foster TJ, Sudhof TC,**

Hook M. 2010. beta-Neurexin is a ligand for the *Staphylococcus aureus* MSCRAMM SdrC. *PLoS Pathog* **6**:e1000726. doi:10.1371/journal. ppat.1000726.

82. **Barbu EM, Mackenzie C, Foster TJ, Hook M.** 2014. SdrC induces staphylococcal biofilm formation through a homophilic interaction. *Mol Microbiol* **94**:172–185.

83. **Josefsson E, O'Connell D, Foster TJ, Durussel I, Cox JA.** 1998. The binding of calcium to the B-repeat segment of SdrD, a cell surface protein of *Staphylococcus aureus*. *J Biol Chem* **273**:31145–31152.

84. **Corrigan RM, Miajlovic H, Foster TJ.** 2009. Surface proteins that promote adherence of *Staphylococcus aureus* to human desquamated nasal epithelial cells. *BMC Microbiol* **9**:22.

85. **O'Brien L, Kerrigan SW, Kaw G, Hogan M, Penades J, Litt D, Fitzgerald DJ, Foster TJ, Cox D.** 2002. Multiple mechanisms for the activation of human platelet aggregation by *Staphylococcus aureus*: roles for the clumping factors ClfA and ClfB, the serine-aspartate repeat protein SdrE and protein A. *Mol Microbiol* **44**:1033–1044.

86. **Sharp JA, Echague CG, Hair PS, Ward MD, Nyalwidhe JO, Geoghegan JA, Foster TJ, Cunnion KM.** 2012. *Staphylococcus aureus* surface protein SdrE binds complement regulator factor H as an immune evasion tactic. *PLoS One* **7**:e38407. doi:10.1371/journal.pone. 0038407.

87. **Hair PS, Foley CK, Krishna NK, Nyalwidhe JO, Geoghegan JA, Foster TJ, Cunnion KM.** 2013. Complement regulator C4BP binds to *Staphylococcus aureus* surface proteins SdrE and Bbp inhibiting bacterial opsonization and killing. *Results Immunol* **3**:114–121.

88. **Arrecubieta C, Lee MH, Macey A, Foster TJ, Lowy FD.** 2007. SdrF, a *Staphylococcus epidermidis* surface protein, binds type I collagen. *J Biol Chem* **282**:18767–18776.

89. **Arrecubieta C, Toba FA, von Bayern M, Akashi H, Deng MC, Naka Y, Lowy FD.** 2009. SdrF, a *Staphylococcus epidermidis* surface protein, contributes to the initiation of ventricular assist device driveline-related infections. *PLoS Pathog* **5**:e1000411. doi:10.1371/journal.ppat.1000411.

90. **Toba FA, Visai L, Trivedi S, Lowy FD.** 2013. The role of ionic interactions in the adherence of the *Staphylococcus epidermidis* adhesin SdrF to prosthetic material. *FEMS Microbiol Lett* **338**:24–30.

91. **McCrea KW, Hartford O, Davis S, Eidhin DN, Lina G, Speziale P, Foster TJ, Hook M.** 2000. The serine-aspartate repeat (Sdr) protein

family in *Staphylococcus epidermidis*. *Microbiology* **146:**1535–1546.

92. **Liu Y, Ames B, Gorovits E, Prater BD, Syribeys P, Vernachio JH, Patti JM.** 2004. SdrX, a serine-aspartate repeat protein expressed by *Staphylococcus capitis* with collagen VI binding activity. *Infect Immun* **72:**6237–6244.

93. **Sakinc T, Kleine B, Gatermann SG.** 2006. SdrI, a serine-aspartate repeat protein identified in *Staphylococcus saprophyticus* strain 7108, is a collagen-binding protein. *Infect Immun* **74:**4615–4623.

94. **Sakinc T, Kleine B, Michalski N, Kaase M, Gatermann SG.** 2009. SdrI of *Staphylococcus saprophyticus* is a multifunctional protein: localization of the fibronectin-binding site. *FEMS Microbiol Lett* **301:**28–34.

95. **Kleine B, Ali L, Wobser D, Sakiotanc T.** 2015. The N-terminal repeat and the ligand binding domain A of SdrI protein is involved in hydrophobicity of *S. saprophyticus*. *Microbiol Res* **172:**88–94.

96. **Kline KA, Ingersoll MA, Nielsen HV, Sakinc T, Henriques-Normark B, Gatermann S, Caparon MG, Hultgren SJ.** 2010. Characterization of a novel murine model of *Staphylococcus saprophyticus* urinary tract infection reveals roles for Ssp and SdrI in virulence. *Infect Immun* **78:**1943–1951.

97. **Ryden C, Yacoub AI, Maxe I, Heinegard D, Oldberg A, Franzen A, Ljungh A, Rubin K.** 1989. Specific binding of bone sialoprotein to *Staphylococcus aureus* isolated from patients with osteomyelitis. *Eur J Biochem* **184:**331–336.

98. **Yacoub A, Lindahl P, Rubin K, Wendel M, Heinegard D, Ryden C.** 1994. Purification of a bone sialoprotein-binding protein from *Staphylococcus aureus*. *Eur J Biochem* **222:**919–925.

99. **Tung H, Guss B, Hellman U, Persson L, Rubin K, Ryden C.** 2000. A bone sialoprotein-binding protein from *Staphylococcus aureus*: a member of the staphylococcal Sdr family. *Biochem J* **345:**611–619.

100. **Aamot HV, Blomfeldt A, Skramm I, Muller F, Monecke S.** 2012. Molecular characterisation of methicillin-sensitive *Staphylococcus aureus* from deep surgical site infections in orthopaedic patients. *Eur J Clin Microbiol Infect Dis* **31:**1999–2004.

101. **Wisniewska K, Piorkowska A, Kasprzyk J, Bronk M, Swiec K.** 2014. Clonal distribution of bone sialoprotein-binding protein gene among *Staphylococcus aureus* isolates associated with bloodstream infections. *Folia Microbiol (Praha)* **59:**465–471.

102. **Persson L, Johansson C, Ryden C.** 2009. Antibodies to *Staphylococcus aureus* bone sialoprotein-binding protein indicate infectious osteomyelitis. *Clin Vaccine Immunol* **16:**949–952.

103. **Jonsson K, Signas C, Muller HP, Lindberg M.** 1991. Two different genes encode fibronectin binding proteins in *Staphylococcus aureus*. The complete nucleotide sequence and characterization of the second gene. *Eur J Biochem* **202:**1041–1048.

104. **Roche FM, Downer R, Keane F, Speziale P, Park PW, Foster TJ.** 2004. The N-terminal A domain of fibronectin-binding proteins A and B promotes adhesion of *Staphylococcus aureus* to elastin. *J Biol Chem* **279:**38433–38440.

105. **Keane FM, Loughman A, Valtulina V, Brennan M, Speziale P, Foster TJ.** 2007. Fibrinogen and elastin bind to the same region within the A domain of fibronectin binding protein A, an MSCRAMM of *Staphylococcus aureus*. *Mol Microbiol* **63:**711–723.

106. **Schwarz-Linek U, Werner JM, Pickford AR, Gurusiddappa S, Kim JH, Pilka ES, Briggs JA, Gough TS, Hook M, Campbell ID, Potts JR.** 2003. Pathogenic bacteria attach to human fibronectin through a tandem beta-zipper. *Nature* **423:**177–181.

107. **Peacock SJ, Foster TJ, Cameron BJ, Berendt AR.** 1999. Bacterial fibronectin-binding proteins and endothelial cell surface fibronectin mediate adherence of *Staphylococcus aureus* to resting human endothelial cells. *Microbiology* **145:**3477–3486.

108. **Sinha B, Francois PP, Nusse O, Foti M, Hartford OM, Vaudaux P, Foster TJ, Lew DP, Herrmann M, Krause KH.** 1999. Fibronectin-binding protein acts as *Staphylococcus aureus* invasin via fibronectin bridging to integrin alpha5beta1. *Cell Microbiol* **1:**101–117.

109. **Edwards AM, Potter U, Meenan NA, Potts JR, Massey RC.** 2011. *Staphylococcus aureus* keratinocyte invasion is dependent upon multiple high-affinity fibronectin-binding repeats within FnBPA. *PLoS One* **6:**e18899. doi:10.1371/journal.pone.0018899.

110. **McCourt J, O'Halloran DP, McCarthy H, O'Gara JP, Geoghegan JA.** 2014. Fibronectin-binding proteins are required for biofilm formation by community-associated methicillin-resistant *Staphylococcus aureus* strain LAC. *FEMS Microbiol Lett* **353:**157–164.

111. **Geoghegan JA, Monk IR, O'Gara JP, Foster TJ.** 2013. Subdomains N2N3 of fibronectin binding protein A mediate *Staphylococcus aureus* biofilm formation and adherence to fibrinogen using distinct mechanisms. *J Bacteriol* **195:**2675–2683.

112. Herman-Bausier P, El-Kirat-Chatel S, Foster TJ, Geoghegan JA, Dufrene YF. 2015. *Staphylococcus aureus* fibronectin-binding protein A mediates cell-cell adhesion through low-affinity homophilic bonds. *mBio* **6**:e00413-15. doi:10.1128/mBio.00413-15.

113. Menzies BE. 2003. The role of fibronectin binding proteins in the pathogenesis of *Staphylococcus aureus* infections. *Curr Opin Infect Dis* **16**:225–229.

114. Patti JM, Boles JO, Hook M. 1993. Identification and biochemical characterization of the ligand binding domain of the collagen adhesin from *Staphylococcus aureus*. *Biochemistry* **32**:11428–11435.

115. Zong Y, Xu Y, Liang X, Keene DR, Hook A, Gurusiddappa S, Hook M, Narayana SV. 2005. A 'collagen hug' model for *Staphylococcus aureus* CNA binding to collagen. *EMBO J* **24**:4224–4236.

116. Kang M, Ko YP, Liang X, Ross CL, Liu Q, Murray BE, Hook M. 2013. Collagen-binding microbial surface components recognizing adhesive matrix molecule (MSCRAMM) of Gram-positive bacteria inhibit complement activation via the classical pathway. *J Biol Chem* **288**: 20520–20531.

117. Rhem MN, Lech EM, Patti JM, McDevitt D, Hook M, Jones DB, Wilhelmus KR. 2000. The collagen-binding adhesin is a virulence factor in *Staphylococcus aureus* keratitis. *Infect Immun* **68**:3776–3779.

118. Elasri MO, Thomas JR, Skinner RA, Blevins JS, Beenken KE, Nelson CL, Smeltzer MS. 2002. *Staphylococcus aureus* collagen adhesin contributes to the pathogenesis of osteomyelitis. *Bone* **30**:275–280.

119. Xu Y, Rivas JM, Brown EL, Liang X, Hook M. 2004. Virulence potential of the staphylococcal adhesin CNA in experimental arthritis is determined by its affinity for collagen. *J Infect Dis* **189**:2323–2333.

120. Hienz SA, Schennings T, Heimdahl A, Flock JI. 1996. Collagen binding of *Staphylococcus aureus* is a virulence factor in experimental endocarditis. *J Infect Dis* **174**:83–88.

121. Bowden MG, Visai L, Longshaw CM, Holland KT, Speziale P, Hook M. 2002. Is the GehD lipase from *Staphylococcus epidermidis* a collagen binding adhesin? *J Biol Chem* **277**:43017–43023.

122. Hammer ND, Skaar EP. 2011. Molecular mechanisms of *Staphylococcus aureus* iron acquisition. *Annu Rev Microbiol* **65**:129–147.

123. Pluym M, Muryoi N, Heinrichs DE, Stillman MJ. 2008. Heme binding in the NEAT domains of IsdA and IsdC of *Staphylococcus aureus*. *J Inorg Biochem* **102**:480–488.

124. Clarke SR, Mohamed R, Bian L, Routh AF, Kokai-Kun JF, Mond JJ, Tarkowski A, Foster SJ. 2007. The *Staphylococcus aureus* surface protein IsdA mediates resistance to innate defenses of human skin. *Cell Host Microbe* **1**:199–212.

125. Clarke SR, Wiltshire MD, Foster SJ. 2004. IsdA of *Staphylococcus aureus* is a broad spectrum, iron-regulated adhesin. *Mol Microbiol* **51**:1509–1519.

126. Pishchany G, Dickey SE, Skaar EP. 2009. Subcellular localization of the *Staphylococcus aureus* heme iron transport components IsdA and IsdB. *Infect Immun* **77**:2624–2634.

127. Missineo A, Di Poto A, Geoghegan JA, Rindi S, Heilbronner S, Gianotti V, Arciola CR, Foster TJ, Speziale P, Pietrocola G. 2014. IsdC from *Staphylococcus lugdunensis* induces biofilm formation under low-iron growth conditions. *Infect Immun* **82**:2448–2459.

128. Shopsin B, Gomez M, Montgomery SO, Smith DH, Waddington M, Dodge DE, Bost DA, Riehman M, Naidich S, Kreiswirth BN. 1999. Evaluation of protein A gene polymorphic region DNA sequencing for typing of *Staphylococcus aureus* strains. *J Clin Microbiol* **37**:3556–3563.

129. Moks T, Abrahmsen L, Nilsson B, Hellman U, Sjoquist J, Uhlen M. 1986. Staphylococcal protein A consists of five IgG-binding domains. *Eur J Biochem* **156**:637–643.

130. Falugi F, Kim HK, Missiakas DM, Schneewind O. 2013. Role of protein A in the evasion of host adaptive immune responses by *Staphylococcus aureus*. *mBio* **4**:e00575-13. doi:10.1128/mBio.00575-13.

131. Merino N, Toledo-Arana A, Vergara-Irigaray M, Valle J, Solano C, Calvo E, Lopez JA, Foster TJ, Penades JR, Lasa I. 2009. Protein A-mediated multicellular behavior in *Staphylococcus aureus*. *J Bacteriol* **191**:832–843.

132. O'Halloran DP, Wynne K, Geoghegan JA. 2015. Protein A is released into the *Staphylococcus aureus* culture supernatant with an unprocessed sorting signal. *Infect Immun* **83**:1598–1609.

133. Conrady DG, Wilson JJ, Herr AB. 2013. Structural basis for Zn2+-dependent intercellular adhesion in staphylococcal biofilms. *Proc Natl Acad Sci USA* **110**:E202–E211.

134. Schaeffer CR, Woods KM, Longo GM, Kiedrowski MR, Paharik AE, Buttner H, Christner M, Boissy RJ, Horswill AR, Rohde H, Fey PD. 2015. Accumulation-associated protein enhances *Staphylococcus epidermidis* biofilm formation under dynamic conditions and is required for infection in a rat catheter model. *Infect Immun* **83**:214–226.

135. **Conlon BP, Geoghegan JA, Waters EM, McCarthy H, Rowe SE, Davies JR, Schaeffer CR, Foster TJ, Fey PD, O'Gara JP.** 2014. Role for the A domain of unprocessed accumulation-associated protein (Aap) in the attachment phase of the *Staphylococcus epidermidis* biofilm phenotype. *J Bacteriol* **196:**4268–4275.

136. **Macintosh RL, Brittan JL, Bhattacharya R, Jenkinson HF, Derrick J, Upton M, Handley PS.** 2009. The terminal A domain of the fibrillar accumulation-associated protein (Aap) of *Staphylococcus epidermidis* mediates adhesion to human corneocytes. *J Bacteriol* **191:**7007–7016.

137. **Roche FM, Meehan M, Foster TJ.** 2003. The *Staphylococcus aureus* surface protein SasG and its homologues promote bacterial adherence to human desquamated nasal epithelial cells. *Microbiology* **149:**2759–2767.

138. **Conrady DG, Brescia CC, Horii K, Weiss AA, Hassett DJ, Herr AB.** 2008. A zinc-dependent adhesion module is responsible for intercellular adhesion in staphylococcal biofilms. *Proc Natl Acad Sci USA* **105:**19456–19461.

139. **Rohde H, Burdelski C, Bartscht K, Hussain M, Buck F, Horstkotte MA, Knobloch JK, Heilmann C, Herrmann M, Mack D.** 2005. Induction of *Staphylococcus epidermidis* biofilm formation via proteolytic processing of the accumulation-associated protein by staphylococcal and host proteases. *Mol Microbiol* **55:**1883–1895.

140. **Decker R, Burdelski C, Zobiak M, Buttner H, Franke G, Christner M, Sass K, Zobiak B, Henke HA, Horswill AR, Bischoff M, Bur S, Hartmann T, Schaeffer CR, Fey PD, Rohde H.** 2015. An 18 kDa scaffold protein is critical for *Staphylococcus epidermidis* biofilm formation. *PLoS Pathog* **11:**e1004735. doi:10.1371/journal.ppat.1004735.

141. **Cucarella C, Solano C, Valle J, Amorena B, Lasa I, Penades JR.** 2001. Bap, a *Staphylococcus aureus* surface protein involved in biofilm formation. *J Bacteriol* **183:**2888–2896.

142. **Tormo MA, Knecht E, Gotz F, Lasa I, Penades JR.** 2005. Bap-dependent biofilm formation by pathogenic species of *Staphylococcus*: evidence of horizontal gene transfer? *Microbiology* **151:**2465–2475.

143. **Valle J, Latasa C, Gil C, Toledo-Arana A, Solano C, Penades JR, Lasa I.** 2012. Bap, a biofilm matrix protein of *Staphylococcus aureus* prevents cellular internalization through binding to GP96 host receptor. *PLoS Pathog* **8:** e1002843. doi:10.1371/journal.ppat.1002843.

144. **Bensing BA, Sullam PM.** 2002. An accessory sec locus of *Streptococcus gordonii* is required for export of the surface protein GspB and for normal levels of binding to human platelets. *Mol Microbiol* **44:**1081–1094.

145. **Lizcano A, Sanchez CJ, Orihuela CJ.** 2012. A role for glycosylated serine-rich repeat proteins in Gram-positive bacterial pathogenesis. *Mol Oral Microbiol* **27:**257–269.

146. **Zhang YQ, Ren SX, Li HL, Wang YX, Fu G, Yang J, Qin ZQ, Miao YG, Wang WY, Chen RS, Shen Y, Chen Z, Yuan ZH, Zhao GP, Qu D, Danchin A, Wen YM.** 2003. Genome-based analysis of virulence genes in a non-biofilm-forming *Staphylococcus epidermidis* strain (ATCC 12228). *Mol Microbiol* **49:**1577–1593.

147. **Takeuchi F, Watanabe S, Baba T, Yuzawa H, Ito T, Morimoto Y, Kuroda M, Cui L, Takahashi M, Ankai A, Baba S, Fukui S, Lee JC, Hiramatsu K.** 2005. Whole-genome sequencing of *Staphylococcus haemolyticus* uncovers the extreme plasticity of its genome and the evolution of human-colonizing staphylococcal species. *J Bacteriol* **187:**7292–7308.

148. **Sanchez CJ, Shivshankar P, Stol K, Trakhtenbroit S, Sullam PM, Sauer K, Hermans PW, Orihuela CJ.** 2010. The pneumococcal serine-rich repeat protein is an intra-species bacterial adhesin that promotes bacterial aggregation *in vivo* and in biofilms. *PLoS Pathog* **6:**e1001044. doi:10.1371/journal.ppat.1001044.

149. **Yang YH, Jiang YL, Zhang J, Wang L, Bai XH, Zhang SJ, Ren YM, Li N, Zhang YH, Zhang Z, Gong Q, Mei Y, Xue T, Zhang JR, Chen Y, Zhou CZ.** 2014. Structural insights into SraP-mediated *Staphylococcus aureus* adhesion to host cells. *PLoS Pathog* **10:**e1004169. doi:10.1371/journal.ppat.1004169.

150. **King NP, Beatson SA, Totsika M, Ulett GC, Alm RA, Manning PA, Schembri MA.** 2011. UafB is a serine-rich repeat adhesin of *Staphylococcus saprophyticus* that mediates binding to fibronectin, fibrinogen and human uroepithelial cells. *Microbiology* **157:**1161–1175.

151. **Li M, Du X, Villaruz AE, Diep BA, Wang D, Song Y, Tian Y, Hu J, Yu F, Lu Y, Otto M.** 2012. MRSA epidemic linked to a quickly spreading colonization and virulence determinant. *Nat Med* **18:**816–819.

152. **Liu Q, Du X, Hong X, Li T, Zheng B, He L, Wang Y, Otto M, Li M.** 2015. Targeting surface protein SasX by active and passive vaccination to reduce *Staphylococcus aureus* colonization and infection. *Infect Immun* **83:**2168–2174.

153. **Schroeder K, Jularic M, Horsburgh SM, Hirschhausen N, Neumann C, Bertling A, Schulte A, Foster S, Kehrel BE, Peters G, Heilmann C.** 2009. Molecular characterization

of a novel *Staphylococcus aureus* surface protein (SasC) involved in cell aggregation and biofilm accumulation. *PloS One* **4**:e7567. doi:10.1371/journal.pone.0007567.

154. **Roche FM, Massey R, Peacock SJ, Day NP, Visai L, Speziale P, Lam A, Pallen M, Foster TJ.** 2003. Characterization of novel LPXTG-containing proteins of *Staphylococcus aureus* identified from genome sequences. *Microbiology* **149**:643–654.

155. **Heilmann C, Hussain M, Peters G, Gotz F.** 1997. Evidence for autolysin-mediated primary attachment of *Staphylococcus epidermidis* to a polystyrene surface. *Mol Microbiol* **24**:1013–1024.

156. **Takahashi J, Komatsuzawa H, Yamada S, Nishida T, Labischinski H, Fujiwara T, Ohara M, Yamagishi J, Sugai M.** 2002. Molecular characterization of an atl null mutant of *Staphylococcus aureus*. *Microbiol Immunol* **46**:601–612.

157. **Biswas R, Voggu L, Simon UK, Hentschel P, Thumm G, Gotz F.** 2006. Activity of the major staphylococcal autolysin Atl. *FEMS Microbiol Lett* **259**:260–268.

158. **Patel JD, Colton E, Ebert M, Anderson JM.** 2012. Gene expression during *S. epidermidis* biofilm formation on biomaterials. *J Biomed Mater Res A* **100**:2863–2869.

159. **Gross M, Cramton SE, Gotz F, Peschel A.** 2001. Key role of teichoic acid net charge in *Staphylococcus aureus* colonization of artificial surfaces. *Infect Immun* **69**:3423–3426.

160. **Hussain M, Heilmann C, Peters G, Herrmann M.** 2001. Teichoic acid enhances adhesion of *Staphylococcus epidermidis* to immobilized fibronectin. *Microb Pathog* **31**:261–270.

161. **Sadovskaya I, Vinogradov E, Flahaut S, Kogan G, Jabbouri S.** 2005. Extracellular carbohydrate-containing polymers of a model biofilm-producing strain, *Staphylococcus epidermidis* RP62A. *Infect Immun* **73**:3007–3017.

162. **Vinogradov E, Sadovskaya I, Li J, Jabbouri S.** 2006. Structural elucidation of the extracellular and cell-wall teichoic acids of *Staphylococcus aureus* MN8m, a biofilm forming strain. *Carbohydr Res* **341**:738–743.

163. **Rupp ME, Ulphani JS, Fey PD, Bartscht K, Mack D.** 1999. Characterization of the importance of polysaccharide intercellular adhesin/hemagglutinin of *Staphylococcus epidermidis* in the pathogenesis of biomaterial-based infection in a mouse foreign body infection model. *Infect Immun* **67**:2627–2632.

164. **Vuong C, Kocianova S, Voyich JM, Yao Y, Fischer ER, DeLeo FR, Otto M.** 2004. A crucial role for exopolysaccharide modification in bacterial biofilm formation, immune evasion, and virulence. *J Biol Chem* **279**:54881–54886.

165. **Heilmann C, Schweitzer O, Gerke C, Vanittanakom N, Mack D, Gotz F.** 1996. Molecular basis of intercellular adhesion in the biofilm-forming *Staphylococcus epidermidis*. *Mol Microbiol* **20**:1083–1091.

166. **O'Gara JP.** 2007. ica and beyond: biofilm mechanisms and regulation in *Staphylococcus epidermidis* and *Staphylococcus aureus*. *FEMS Microbiol Lett* **270**:179–188.

167. **Rohde H, Frankenberger S, Zahringer U, Mack D.** 2010. Structure, function and contribution of polysaccharide intercellular adhesin (PIA) to *Staphylococcus epidermidis* biofilm formation and pathogenesis of biomaterial-associated infections. *Eur J Cell Biol* **89**:103–111.

168. **Cue D, Lei MG, Lee CY.** 2012. Genetic regulation of the intercellular adhesion locus in staphylococci. *Front Cell Infect Microbiol* **2**:38.

169. **Berube BJ, Bubeck Wardenburg J.** 2013. *Staphylococcus aureus* alpha-toxin: nearly a century of intrigue. *Toxins* **5**:1140–1166.

170. **Caiazza NC, O'Toole GA.** 2003. Alpha-toxin is required for biofilm formation by *Staphylococcus aureus*. *J Bacteriol* **185**:3214–3217.

171. **Marshall MJ, Bohach GA, Boehm DF.** 2000. Characterization of *Staphylococcus aureus* beta-toxin induced leukotoxicity. *J Nat Toxins* **9**:125–138.

172. **Huseby M, Shi K, Brown CK, Digre J, Mengistu F, Seo KS, Bohach GA, Schlievert PM, Ohlendorf DH, Earhart CA.** 2007. Structure and biological activities of beta toxin from *Staphylococcus aureus*. *J Bacteriol* **189**:8719–8726.

173. **Huseby MJ, Kruse AC, Digre J, Kohler PL, Vocke JA, Mann EE, Bayles KW, Bohach GA, Schlievert PM, Ohlendorf DH, Earhart CA.** 2010. Beta toxin catalyzes formation of nucleoprotein matrix in staphylococcal biofilms. *Proc Natl Acad Sci USA* **107**:14407–14412.

174. **Chavakis T, Wiechmann K, Preissner KT, Herrmann M.** 2005. *Staphylococcus aureus* interactions with the endothelium: the role of bacterial "secretable expanded repertoire adhesive molecules" (SERAM) in disturbing host defense systems. *Thromb Haemost* **94**:278–285.

175. **Zielinska AK, Beenken KE, Mrak LN, Spencer HJ, Post GR, Skinner RA, Tackett AJ, Horswill AR, Smeltzer MS.** 2012. sarA-mediated repression of protease production plays a key role in the pathogenesis of *Staphylococcus aureus* USA300 isolates. *Mol Microbiol* **86**:1183–1196.

176. Johnson M, Cockayne A, Morrissey JA. 2008. Iron-regulated biofilm formation in *Staphylococcus aureus* Newman requires ica and the secreted protein Emp. *Infect Immun* **76:**1756–1765.

177. Malone CL, Boles BR, Horswill AR. 2007. Biosynthesis of *Staphylococcus aureus* auto-inducing peptides by using the synechocystis DnaB mini-intein. *Appl Environ Microbiol* **73:**6036–6044.

178. Hammel M, Nemecek D, Keightley JA, Thomas GJ Jr, Geisbrecht BV. 2007. The *Staphylococcus aureus* extracellular adherence protein (Eap) adopts an elongated but structured conformation in solution. *Protein Sci* **16:**2605–2617.

179. Boles BR, Horswill AR. 2008. Agr-mediated dispersal of *Staphylococcus aureus* biofilms. *PLoS Pathog* **4:**e1000052. doi:10.1371/journal.ppat.1000052.

180. Harraghy N, Hussain M, Haggar A, Chavakis T, Sinha B, Herrmann M, Flock JI. 2003. The adhesive and immunomodulating properties of the multifunctional *Staphylococcus aureus* protein Eap. *Microbiology* **149:**2701–2707.

181. Harraghy N, Homerova D, Herrmann M, Kormanec J. 2008. Mapping the transcription start points of the *Staphylococcus aureus* eap, emp, and vwb promoters reveals a conserved octanucleotide sequence that is essential for expression of these genes. *J Bacteriol* **190:**447–451.

182. Harraghy N, Kormanec J, Wolz C, Homerova D, Goerke C, Ohlsen K, Qazi S, Hill P, and Herrmann M. 2005. sae is essential for expression of the staphylococcal adhesins Eap and Emp. *Microbiology* **151:**1789–1800.

183. Beenken KE, Dunman PM, McAleese F, Macapagal D, Murphy E, Projan SJ, Blevins JS, Smeltzer MS. 2004. Global gene expression in *Staphylococcus aureus* biofilms. *J Bacteriol* **186:**4665–4684.

184. Yao Y, Sturdevant DE, Otto M. 2005. Genome-wide analysis of gene expression in *Staphylococcus epidermidis* biofilms: insights into the pathophysiology of *S. epidermidis* biofilms and the role of phenol-soluble modulins in formation of biofilms. *J Infect Dis* **191:**289–298.

185. Trotonda MP, Tamber S, Memmi G, Cheung AL. 2008. MgrA represses biofilm formation in *Staphylococcus aureus*. *Infect Immun* **76:**5645–5654.

186. Toledo-Arana A, Merino N, Vergara-Irigaray M, Debarbouille M, Penades JR, Lasa I. 2005. *Staphylococcus aureus* develops an alternative, ica-independent biofilm in the absence of the arlRS two-component system. *J Bacteriol* **187:**5318–5329.

187. Thoendel M, Kavanaugh JS, Flack CE, Horswill AR. 2011. Peptide signaling in the staphylococci. *Chem Rev* **111:**117–151.

188. Novick RP, Geisinger E. 2008. Quorum sensing in staphylococci. *Annu Rev Genet* **42:**541–564.

189. Koenig RL, Ray JL, Maleki SJ, Smeltzer MS, Hurlburt BK. 2004. *Staphylococcus aureus* AgrA binding to the RNAIII-agr regulatory region. *J Bacteriol* **186:**7549–7555.

190. Queck SY, Jameson-Lee M, Villaruz AE, Bach TH, Khan BA, Sturdevant DE, Ricklefs SM, Li M, Otto M. 2008. RNAIII-independent target gene control by the agr quorum-sensing system: insight into the evolution of virulence regulation in *Staphylococcus aureus*. *Mol Cell* **32:**150–158.

191. Geisinger E, Adhikari RP, Jin R, Ross HF, Novick RP. 2006. Inhibition of rot translation by RNAIII, a key feature of agr function. *Mol Microbiol* **61:**1038–1048.

192. Olson ME, Todd DA, Schaeffer CR, Paharik AE, Van Dyke MJ, Buttner H, Dunman PM, Rohde H, Cech NB, Fey PD, Horswill AR. 2014. *Staphylococcus epidermidis* agr quorum-sensing system: signal identification, cross talk, and importance in colonization. *J Bacteriol* **196:**3482–3493.

193. Dunman PM, Murphy E, Haney S, Palacios D, Tucker-Kellogg G, Wu S, Brown EL, Zagursky RJ, Shlaes D, Projan SJ. 2001. Transcription profiling-based identification of *Staphylococcus aureus* genes regulated by the agr and/or sarA loci. *J Bacteriol* **183:**7341–7353.

194. Li M, Diep BA, Villaruz AE, Braughton KR, Jiang X, DeLeo FR, Chambers HF, Lu Y, Otto M. 2009. Evolution of virulence in epidemic community-associated methicillin-resistant *Staphylococcus aureus*. *Proc Natl Acad Sci USA* **106:**5883–5888.

195. DeLeo FR, Kennedy AD, Chen L, Bubeck Wardenburg J, Kobayashi SD, Mathema B, Braughton KR, Whitney AR, Villaruz AE, Martens CA, Porcella SF, McGavin MJ, Otto M, Musser JM, Kreiswirth BN. 2011. Molecular differentiation of historic phage-type 80/81 and contemporary epidemic *Staphylococcus aureus*. *Proc Natl Acad Sci USA* **108:**18091–18096.

196. Montgomery CP, Boyle-Vavra S, Daum RS. 2010. Importance of the global regulators Agr and SaeRS in the pathogenesis of CA-MRSA USA300 infection. *PLoS One* **5:**e15177. doi:10.1371/journal.pone.0015177.

197. Lauderdale KJ, Malone CL, Boles BR, Morcuende J, Horswill AR. 2010. Biofilm dispersal of community-associated methicillin-resistant *Staphylococcus aureus* on orthopedic implant material. *J Orthop Res* **28:**55–61.

198. **Pang YY, Schwartz J, Thoendel M, Ackermann LW, Horswill AR, Nauseef WM.** 2010. agr-Dependent interactions of *Staphylococcus aureus* USA300 with human polymorphonuclear neutrophils. *J Innate Immun* **2:**546–559.

199. **Lauderdale KJ, Boles BR, Cheung AL, Horswill AR.** 2009. Interconnections between Sigma B, agr, and proteolytic activity in *Staphylococcus aureus* biofilm maturation. *Infect Immun* **77:**1623–1635.

200. **Vuong C, Gerke C, Somerville GA, Fischer ER, Otto M.** 2003. Quorum-sensing control of biofilm factors in *Staphylococcus epidermidis*. *J Infect Dis* **188:**706–718.

201. **Batzilla CF, Rachid S, Engelmann S, Hecker M, Hacker J, Ziebuhr W.** 2006. Impact of the accessory gene regulatory system (Agr) on extracellular proteins, codY expression and amino acid metabolism in *Staphylococcus epidermidis*. *Proteomics* **6:**3602–3613.

202. **Yarwood JM, Bartels DJ, Volper EM, Greenberg EP.** 2004. Quorum sensing in *Staphylococcus aureus* biofilms. *J Bacteriol* **186:**1838–1850.

203. **Lauderdale KJ, Malone CL, Boles BR, Morcuende J, Horswill AR.** 2010. Biofilm dispersal of community-associated methicillin-resistant *Staphylococcus aureus* on orthopedic implant material. *J Orthop Res* **28:**55–61.

204. **Mootz JM, Malone CL, Shaw LN, Horswill AR.** 2013. Staphopains modulate *Staphylococcus aureus* biofilm integrity. *Infect Immun* **81:**3227–3238.

205. **Mootz JM, Benson MA, Heim CE, Crosby HA, Kavanaugh JS, Dunman PM, Kielian T, Torres VJ, Horswill AR.** 2015. Rot is a key regulator of *Staphylococcus aureus* biofilm formation. *Mol Microbiol* **96:**388–404.

206. **Hsieh HY, Tseng CW, Stewart GC.** 2008. Regulation of Rot expression in *Staphylococcus aureus*. *J Bacteriol* **190:**546–554.

207. **Olson ME, King JM, Yahr TL, Horswill AR.** 2013. Sialic acid catabolism in *Staphylococcus aureus*. *J Bacteriol* **195:**1779–1788.

208. **Regassa LB, Novick RP, Betley MJ.** 1992. Glucose and nonmaintained pH decrease expression of the accessory gene regulator (agr) in *Staphylococcus aureus*. *Infect Immun* **60:**3381–3388.

209. **Yarwood JM, McCormick JK, Paustian ML, Kapur V, Schlievert PM.** 2002. Repression of the *Staphylococcus aureus* accessory gene regulator in serum and *in vivo*. *J Bacteriol* **184:**1095–1101.

210. **Hall PR, Elmore BO, Spang CH, Alexander SM, Manifold-Wheeler BC, Castleman MJ, Daly SM, Peterson MM, Sully EK, Femling JK, Otto M, Horswill AR, Timmins GS, Gresham HD.** 2013. Nox2 modification of LDL is essential for optimal apolipoprotein B-mediated control of agr type III *Staphylococcus aureus* quorum-sensing. *PLoS Pathog* **9:**e1003166. doi:10.1371/journal.ppat.1003166.

211. **Peterson MM, Mack JL, Hall PR, Alsup AA, Alexander SM, Sully EK, Sawires YS, Cheung AL, Otto M, Gresham HD.** 2008. Apolipoprotein B Is an innate barrier against invasive *Staphylococcus aureus* infection. *Cell Host Microbe* **4:**555–566.

212. **Pynnonen M, Stephenson RE, Schwartz K, Hernandez M, Boles BR.** 2011. Hemoglobin promotes *Staphylococcus aureus* nasal colonization. *PLoS Pathog* **7:**e1002104. doi:10.1371/journal.ppat.1002104.

213. **Syed AK, Ghosh S, Love NG, Boles BR.** 2014. Triclosan promotes *Staphylococcus aureus* nasal colonization. *mBio* **5:**e01015. doi:10.1128/mBio.01015-13.

214. **Schwartz K, Syed AK, Stephenson RE, Rickard AH, Boles BR.** 2012. Functional amyloids composed of phenol soluble modulins stabilize *Staphylococcus aureus* biofilms. *PLoS Pathog* **8:**e1002744. doi:10.1371/journal.ppat.1002744.

215. **Cassat JE, Lee CY, Smeltzer MS.** 2007. Investigation of biofilm formation in clinical isolates of *Staphylococcus aureus*. *Methods Mol Biol* **391:**127–144.

216. **Wang R, Khan BA, Cheung GY, Bach TH, Jameson-Lee M, Kong KF, Queck SY, Otto M.** 2011. *Staphylococcus epidermidis* surfactant peptides promote biofilm maturation and dissemination of biofilm-associated infection in mice. *J Clin Invest* **121:**238–248.

217. **Fowler VG Jr, Miro JM, Hoen B, Cabell CH, Abrutyn E, Rubinstein E, Corey GR, Spelman D, Bradley SF, Barsic B, Pappas PA, Anstrom KJ, Wray D, Fortes CQ, Anguera I, Athan E, Jones P, van der Meer JT, Elliott TS, Levine DP, Bayer AS.** 2005. *Staphylococcus aureus* endocarditis: a consequence of medical progress. *JAMA* **293:**3012–3021.

218. **Xiong YQ, Van Wamel W, Nast CC, Yeaman MR, Cheung AL, Bayer AS.** 2002. Activation and transcriptional interaction between agr RNAII and RNAIII in *Staphylococcus aureus in vitro* and in an experimental endocarditis model. *J Infect Dis* **186:**668–677.

219. **Fux CA, Wilson S, Stoodley P.** 2004. Detachment characteristics and oxacillin resistance of *Staphyloccocus aureus* biofilm emboli in an *in vitro* catheter infection model. *J Bacteriol* **186:**4486–4491.

220. **Koh TW, Brecker SJ, Layton CA.** 1996. Successful treatment of *Staphylococcus lugdunensis*

endocarditis complicated by multiple emboli: a case report and review of the literature. *Int J Cardiol* **55:**193–197.

221. **Ye R, Zhao L, Wang C, Wu X, Yan H.** 2014. Clinical characteristics of septic pulmonary embolism in adults: a systematic review. *Respir Med* **108:**1–8.

222. **Plicht B, Janosi RA, Buck T, Erbel R.** 2010. Infective endocarditis as cardiovascular emergency. *Internist (Berl)* **51:**987–994. [In German.]

223. **Goerke C, Campana S, Bayer MG, Doring G, Botzenhart K, Wolz C.** 2000. Direct quantitative transcript analysis of the agr regulon of *Staphylococcus aureus* during human infection in comparison to the expression profile *in vitro*. *Infect Immun* **68:**1304–1311.

224. **Goerke C, Wolz C.** 2004. Regulatory and genomic plasticity of *Staphylococcus aureus* during persistent colonization and infection. *Int J Med Microbiol* **294:**195–202.

225. **Goerke C, Wolz C.** 2010. Adaptation of *Staphylococcus aureus* to the cystic fibrosis lung. *Int J Med Microbiol* **300:**520–525.

226. **Yarwood JM, Paquette KM, Tikh IB, Volper EM, Greenberg EP.** 2007. Generation of virulence factor variants in *Staphylococcus aureus* biofilms. *J Bacteriol* **189:**7961–6967.

227. **Traber KE, Lee E, Benson S, Corrigan R, Cantera M, Shopsin B, Novick RP.** 2008. agr function in clinical *Staphylococcus aureus* isolates. *Microbiology* **154:**2265–2274.

228. **Paulander W, Nissen Varming A, Baek KT, Haaber J, Frees D, Ingmer H.** 2013. Antibiotic-mediated selection of quorum-sensing-negative *Staphylococcus aureus*. *mBio* **3:**e00459-12. doi:10.1128/mBio.00459-12.

229. **Shopsin B, Eaton C, Wasserman GA, Mathema B, Adhikari RP, Agolory S, Altman DR, Holzman RS, Kreiswirth BN, Novick RP.** 2010. Mutations in agr do not persist in natural populations of methicillin-resistant *Staphylococcus aureus*. *J Infect Dis* **202:**1593–1599.

230. **Daly SM, Elmore BO, Kavanaugh JS, Triplett KD, Figueroa M, Raja HA, El-Elimat T, Crosby HA, Femling JK, Cech NB, Horswill AR, Oberlies NH, Hall PR.** 2015. omega-hydroxyemodin limits *Staphylococcus aureus* quorum sensing-mediated pathogenesis and inflammation. *Antimicrob Agents Chemother* **59:**2223–2235.

231. **Sully EK, Malachowa N, Elmore BO, Alexander SM, Femling JK, Gray BM, DeLeo FR, Otto M, Cheung AL, Edwards BS, Sklar LA, Horswill AR, Hall PR, Gresham HD.** 2014. Selective chemical inhibition of agr quorum sensing in *Staphylococcus aureus* promotes host defense with minimal impact on resistance.

PLoS Pathog **10:**e1004174. doi:10.1371/journal.ppat.1004174.

232. **Cech NB, Horswill AR.** 2013. Small-molecule quorum quenchers to prevent *Staphylococcus aureus* infection. *Future Microbiol* **8:**1511–1514.

233. **Schauder S, Shokat K, Surette MG, Bassler BL.** 2001. The LuxS family of bacterial autoinducers: biosynthesis of a novel quorum-sensing signal molecule. *Mol Microbiol* **41:**463–476.

234. **Li M, Villaruz AE, Vadyvaloo V, Sturdevant DE, Otto M.** 2008. AI-2-dependent gene regulation in *Staphylococcus epidermidis*. *BMC Microbiol* **8:**4.

235. **Xu L, Li H, Vuong C, Vadyvaloo V, Wang J, Yao Y, Otto M, Gao Q.** 2006. Role of the luxS quorum-sensing system in biofilm formation and virulence of *Staphylococcus epidermidis*. *Infect Immun* **74:**488–496.

236. **Yu D, Zhao L, Xue T, Sun B.** 2012. *Staphylococcus aureus* autoinducer-2 quorum sensing decreases biofilm formation in an icaR-dependent manner. *BMC Microbiol* **12:**288.

237. **Zhao L, Xue T, Shang F, Sun H, Sun B.** 2010. *Staphylococcus aureus* AI-2 quorum sensing associates with the KdpDE two-component system to regulate capsular polysaccharide synthesis and virulence. *Infect Immun* **78:**3506–3515.

238. **Kullik II, Giachino P.** 1997. The alternative sigma factor sigmaB in *Staphylococcus aureus*: regulation of the sigB operon in response to growth phase and heat shock. *Arch Microbiol* **167:**151–159.

239. **Mootz JM, Malone CL, Shaw LN, Horswill AR.** 2013. Staphopains modulate *Staphylococcus aureus* biofilm integrity. *Infect Immun* **81:**3227–3238.

240. **Marti M, Trotonda MP, Tormo-Mas MA, Vergara-Irigaray M, Cheung AL, Lasa I, Penades JR.** 2010. Extracellular proteases inhibit protein-dependent biofilm formation in *Staphylococcus aureus*. *Microbes Infect* **12:**55–64.

241. **Kiedrowski MR, Kavanaugh JS, Malone CL, Mootz JM, Voyich JM, Smeltzer MS, Bayles KW, Horswill AR.** 2011. Nuclease modulates biofilm formation in community-associated methicillin-resistant *Staphylococcus aureus*. *PLoS One* **6:**e26714. doi:10.1371/journal.pone.0026714.

242. **Knobloch JK, Jager S, Horstkotte MA, Rohde H, Mack D.** 2004. RsbU-dependent regulation of *Staphylococcus epidermidis* biofilm formation is mediated via the alternative sigma factor sigmaB by repression of the negative regulator gene icaR. *Infect Immun* **72:**3838–3848.

243. **Jager S, Jonas B, Pfanzelt D, Horstkotte MA, Rohde H, Mack D, Knobloch JK.** 2009. Regulation of biofilm formation by sigma B is a common mechanism in *Staphylococcus epidermidis* and is not mediated by transcriptional regulation of sarA. *Int J Artif Organs* **32:**584–591.

244. **Depke M, Burian M, Schafer T, Broker BM, Ohlsen K, Volker U.** 2012. The alternative sigma factor B modulates virulence gene expression in a murine *Staphylococcus aureus* infection model but does not influence kidney gene expression pattern of the host. *Int J Med Microbiol* **302:**33–39.

245. **Pintens V, Massonet C, Merckx R, Vandecasteele S, Peetermans WE, Knobloch JK, Van Eldere J.** 2008. The role of sigmaB in persistence of *Staphylococcus epidermidis* foreign body infection. *Microbiology* **154:**2827–2836.

246. **Ishii K, Adachi T, Yasukawa J, Suzuki Y, Hamamoto H, Sekimizu K.** 2014. Induction of virulence gene expression in *Staphylococcus aureus* by pulmonary surfactant. *Infect Immun* **82:**1500–1510.

247. **Pfortner H, Burian MS, Michalik S, Depke M, Hildebrandt P, Dhople VM, Pane-Farre J, Hecker M, Schmidt F, Volker U.** 2014. Activation of the alternative sigma factor SigB of *Staphylococcus aureus* following internalization by epithelial cells: an *in vivo* proteomics perspective. *Int J Med Microbiol* **304:**177–187.

248. **Savage VJ, Chopra I, O'Neill AJ.** 2013. Population diversification in *Staphylococcus aureus* biofilms may promote dissemination and persistence. *PloS One* **8:**e62513. doi:10.1371/journal.pone.0062513.

249. **Mitchell G, Fugere A, Pepin Gaudreau K, Brouillette E, Frost EH, Cantin AM, Malouin F.** 2013. SigB is a dominant regulator of virulence in *Staphylococcus aureus* small-colony variants. *PloS One* **8:**e65018. doi:10.1371/journal.pone.0065018.

250. **Cheung AL, Koomey JM, Butler CA, Projan SJ, Fischetti VA.** 1992. Regulation of exoprotein expression in *Staphylococcus aureus* by a locus (sar) distinct from agr. *Proc Natl Acad Sci USA* **89:**6462–6466.

251. **Bayer MG, Heinrichs JH, Cheung AL.** 1996. The molecular architecture of the sar locus in *Staphylococcus aureus*. *J Bacteriol* **178:**4563–4570.

252. **Rechtin TM, Gillaspy AF, Schumacher MA, Brennan RG, Smeltzer MS, Hurlburt BK.** 1999. Characterization of the SarA virulence gene regulator of *Staphylococcus aureus*. *Mol Microbiol* **33:**307–316.

253. **Cheung AL, Projan SJ.** 1994. Cloning and sequencing of sarA of *Staphylococcus aureus*, a gene required for the expression of agr. *J Bacteriol* **176:**4168–4172.

254. **Heinrichs JH, Bayer MG, Cheung AL.** 1996. Characterization of the sar locus and its interaction with agr in *Staphylococcus aureus*. *J Bacteriol* **178:**418–423.

255. **Cheung AL, Bayer MG, Heinrichs JH.** 1997. sar genetic determinants necessary for transcription of RNAII and RNAIII in the agr locus of *Staphylococcus aureus*. *J Bacteriol* **179:**3963–3971.

256. **Chien Y, Manna AC, Projan SJ, Cheung AL.** 1999. SarA, a global regulator of virulence determinants in *Staphylococcus aureus*, binds to a conserved motif essential for sar-dependent gene regulation. *J Biol Chem* **274:**37169–37176.

257. **Gillaspy AF, Lee CY, Sau S, Cheung AL, Smeltzer MS.** 1998. Factors affecting the collagen binding capacity of *Staphylococcus aureus*. *Infect Immun* **66:**3170–3178.

258. **Blevins JS, Gillaspy AF, Rechtin TM, Hurlburt BK, Smeltzer MS.** 1999. The staphylococcal accessory regulator (sar) represses transcription of the *Staphylococcus aureus* collagen adhesin gene (cna) in an agr-independent manner. *Mol Microbiol* **33:**317–326.

259. **Trotonda MP, Manna AC, Cheung AL, Lasa I, Penades JR.** 2005. SarA positively controls bap-dependent biofilm formation in *Staphylococcus aureus*. *J Bacteriol* **187:**5790–5798.

260. **Blevins JS, Beenken KE, Elasri MO, Hurlburt BK, Smeltzer MS.** 2002. Strain-dependent differences in the regulatory roles of sarA and agr in *Staphylococcus aureus*. *Infect Immun* **70:**470–480.

261. **Cassat J, Dunman PM, Murphy E, Projan SJ, Beenken KE, Palm KJ, Yang SJ, Rice KC, Bayles KW, Smeltzer MS.** 2006. Transcriptional profiling of a *Staphylococcus aureus* clinical isolate and its isogenic agr and sarA mutants reveals global differences in comparison to the laboratory strain RN6390. *Microbiology* **152:**3075–3090.

262. **Beenken KE, Blevins JS, Smeltzer MS.** 2003. Mutation of sarA in *Staphylococcus aureus* limits biofilm formation. *Infect Immun* **71:**4206–4211.

263. **Valle J, Toledo-Arana A, Berasain C, Ghigo JM, Amorena B, Penades JR, Lasa I.** 2003. SarA and not sigmaB is essential for biofilm development by *Staphylococcus aureus*. *Mol Microbiol* **48:**1075–1087.

264. **Snowden JN, Beaver M, Beenken K, Smeltzer M, Horswill AR, Kielian T.** 2013. *Staphylococcus aureus* sarA regulates inflammation and colonization during central nervous system biofilm formation. *PloS One* **8:**e84089. doi:10.1371/journal.pone.0084089.

265. **Tsang LH, Cassat JE, Shaw LN, Beenken KE, Smeltzer MS.** 2008. Factors contributing to the biofilm-deficient phenotype of *Staphylococcus aureus* sarA mutants. *PloS One* **3**:e3361. doi:10.1371/journal.pone.0003361.

266. **Beenken KE, Mrak LN, Griffin LM, Zielinska AK, Shaw LN, Rice KC, Horswill AR, Bayles KW, Smeltzer MS.** 2010. Epistatic relationships between sarA and agr in *Staphylococcus aureus* biofilm formation. *PloS One* **5**:e10790. doi:10.1371/journal.pone.0010790.

267. **Tormo MA, Marti M, Valle J, Manna AC, Cheung AL, Lasa I, Penades JR.** 2005. SarA is an essential positive regulator of *Staphylococcus epidermidis* biofilm development. *J Bacteriol* **187**:2348–2356.

268. **Christner M, Heinze C, Busch M, Franke G, Hentschke M, Bayard Duhring S, Buttner H, Kotasinska M, Wischnewski V, Kroll G, Buck F, Molin S, Otto M, Rohde H.** 2012. sarA negatively regulates *Staphylococcus epidermidis* biofilm formation by modulating expression of 1 MDa extracellular matrix binding protein and autolysis-dependent release of eDNA. *Mol Microbiol* **86**:394–410.

269. **Lai Y, Villaruz AE, Li M, Cha DJ, Sturdevant DE, Otto M.** 2007. The human anionic antimicrobial peptide dermcidin induces proteolytic defence mechanisms in staphylococci. *Mol Microbiol* **63**:497–506.

270. **Scherr TD, Heim CE, Morrison JM, Kielian T.** 2014. Hiding in plain sight: interplay between staphylococcal biofilms and host immunity. *Front Immunol* **5**:37.

271. **Costerton JW, Stewart PS, Greenberg EP.** 1999. Bacterial biofilms: a common cause of persistent infections. *Science* **284**:1318–1322.

272. **Hanke ML, Kielian T.** 2012. Deciphering mechanisms of staphylococcal biofilm evasion of host immunity. *Front Cell Infect Microbiol* **2**:62.

273. **Verdrengh M, Tarkowski A.** 1997. Role of neutrophils in experimental septicemia and septic arthritis induced by *Staphylococcus aureus*. *Infect Immun* **65**:2517–2521.

274. **Verdrengh M, Tarkowski A.** 2000. Role of macrophages in *Staphylococcus aureus*-induced arthritis and sepsis. *Arthritis Rheum* **43**:2276–2282.

275. **Rigby KM, DeLeo FR.** 2012. Neutrophils in innate host defense against *Staphylococcus aureus* infections. *Semin Immunopathol* **34**:237–259.

276. **Wagner C, Kondella K, Bernschneider T, Heppert V, Wentzensen A, Hansch GM.** 2003. Post-traumatic osteomyelitis: analysis of inflammatory cells recruited into the site of infection. *Shock* **20**:503–510.

277. **Wagner C, Kaksa A, Muller W, Denefleh B, Heppert V, Wentzensen A, Hansch GM.** 2004. Polymorphonuclear neutrophils in posttraumatic osteomyelitis: cells recovered from the inflamed site lack chemotactic activity but generate superoxides. *Shock* **22**:108–115.

278. **Scherr TD, Roux CM, Hanke ML, Angle A, Dunman PM, Kielian T.** 2013. Global transcriptome analysis of *Staphylococcus aureus* biofilms in response to innate immune cells. *Infect Immun* **81**:4363–4376.

279. **Leid JG, Shirtliff ME, Costerton JW, Stoodley P.** 2002. Human leukocytes adhere to, penetrate, and respond to *Staphylococcus aureus* biofilms. *Infect Immun* **70**:6339–6345.

280. **Meyle E, Brenner-Weiss G, Obst U, Prior B, Hansch GM.** 2012. Immune defense against *S. epidermidis* biofilms: components of the extracellular polymeric substance activate distinct bactericidal mechanisms of phagocytic cells. *Int J Artif Organs* **35**:700–712.

281. **Meyle E, Stroh P, Gunther F, Hoppy-Tichy T, Wagner C, Hansch GM.** 2010. Destruction of bacterial biofilms by polymorphonuclear neutrophils: relative contribution of phagocytosis, DNA release, and degranulation. *Int J Artif Organs* **33**:608–620.

282. **Kristian SA, Birkenstock TA, Sauder U, Mack D, Gotz F, Landmann R.** 2008. Biofilm formation induces C3a release and protects *Staphylococcus epidermidis* from IgG and complement deposition and from neutrophil-dependent killing. *J Infect Dis* **197**:1028–1035.

283. **Vuong C, Voyich JM, Fischer ER, Braughton KR, Whitney AR, DeLeo FR, Otto M.** 2004. Polysaccharide intercellular adhesin (PIA) protects *Staphylococcus epidermidis* against major components of the human innate immune system. *Cell Microbiol* **6**:269–275.

284. **Nilsson IM, Lee JC, Bremell T, Ryden C, Tarkowski A.** 1997. The role of staphylococcal polysaccharide microcapsule expression in septicemia and septic arthritis. *Infect Immun* **65**:4216–4221.

285. **Thakker M, Park JS, Carey V, Lee JC.** 1998. *Staphylococcus aureus* serotype 5 capsular polysaccharide is antiphagocytic and enhances bacterial virulence in a murine bacteremia model. *Infect Immun* **66**:5183–5189.

286. **Brinkmann V, Reichard U, Goosmann C, Fauler B, Uhlemann Y, Weiss DS, Weinrauch Y, Zychlinsky A.** 2004. Neutrophil extracellular traps kill bacteria. *Science* **303**:1532–1535.

287. **Fuchs TA, Abed U, Goosmann C, Hurwitz R, Schulze I, Wahn V, Weinrauch Y, Brinkmann V, Zychlinsky A.** 2007. Novel cell death program

leads to neutrophil extracellular traps. *J Cell Biol* **176**:231–241.

288. **Berends ET, Horswill AR, Haste NM, Monestier M, Nizet V, von Kockritz-Blickwede M.** 2010. Nuclease expression by *Staphylococcus aureus* facilitates escape from neutrophil extracellular traps. *J Innate Immun* **2**:576–586.

289. **Thammavongsa V, Missiakas DM, Schneewind O.** 2013. *Staphylococcus aureus* degrades neutrophil extracellular traps to promote immune cell death. *Science* **342**:863–866.

290. **Kiedrowski MR, Crosby HA, Hernandez FJ, Malone CL, McNamara JO 2nd, Horswill AR.** 2014. *Staphylococcus aureus* Nuc2 is a functional, surface-attached extracellular nuclease. *PLoS One* **9**:e95574. doi:10.1371/journal.pone.0095574.

291. **Mosser DM.** 2003. The many faces of macrophage activation. *J Leukoc Biol* **73**:209–212.

292. **Hesse M, Modolell M, La Flamme AC, Schito M, Fuentes JM, Cheever AW, Pearce EJ, Wynn TA.** 2001. Differential regulation of nitric oxide synthase-2 and arginase-1 by type 1/type 2 cytokines *in vivo*: granulomatous pathology is shaped by the pattern of L-arginine metabolism. *J Immunol* **167**:6533–6544.

293. **Song E, Ouyang N, Horbelt M, Antus B, Wang M, Exton MS.** 2000. Influence of alternatively and classically activated macrophages on fibrogenic activities of human fibroblasts. *Cell Immunol* **204**:19–28.

294. **Thurlow LR, Hanke ML, Fritz T, Angle A, Aldrich A, Williams SH, Engebretsen IL, Bayles KW, Horswill AR, Kielian T.** 2011. *Staphylococcus aureus* biofilms prevent macrophage phagocytosis and attenuate inflammation *in vivo*. *J Immunol* **186**:6585–6596.

295. **Palmqvist N, Patti JM, Tarkowski A, Josefsson E.** 2004. Expression of staphylococcal clumping factor A impedes macrophage phagocytosis. *Microbe Infect* **6**:188–195.

296. **Olson ME, Nygaard TK, Ackermann L, Watkins RL, Zurek OW, Pallister KB, Griffith S, Kiedrowski MR, Flack CE, Kavanaugh JS, Kreiswirth BN, Horswill AR, Voyich JM.** 2013. *Staphylococcus aureus* nuclease is an SaeRS-dependent virulence factor. *Infect Immun* **81**:1316–1324.

297. **Nygaard TK, Pallister KB, Ruzevich P, Griffith S, Vuong C, Voyich JM.** 2010. SaeR binds a consensus sequence within virulence gene promoters to advance USA300 pathogenesis. *J Infect Dis* **201**:241–254.

298. **Voyich JM, Vuong C, DeWald M, Nygaard TK, Kocianova S, Griffith S, Jones J, Iverson C, Sturdevant DE, Braughton KR, Whitney AR, Otto M, DeLeo FR.** 2009. The SaeR/S gene regulatory system is essential for innate immune evasion by *Staphylococcus aureus*. *J Infect Dis* **199**:1698–1706.

299. **Zurek OW, Nygaard TK, Watkins RL, Pallister KB, Torres VJ, Horswill AR, Voyich JM.** 2014. The role of innate immunity in promoting SaeR/S-mediated virulence in *Staphylococcus aureus*. *J Innate Immun* **6**:21–30.

300. **Malone CL, Boles BR, Lauderdale KJ, Thoendel M, Kavanaugh JS, Horswill AR.** 2009. Fluorescent reporters for *Staphylococcus aureus*. *J Microbiol Methods* **77**:251–260.

301. **Holtfreter S, Nguyen TT, Wertheim H, Steil L, Kusch H, Truong QP, Engelmann S, Hecker M, Volker U, van Belkum A, Broker BM.** 2009. Human immune proteome in experimental colonization with *Staphylococcus aureus*. *Clin Vaccine Immunol* **16**:1607–1614.

302. **Holtfreter S, Kolata J, Broker BM.** 2010. Towards the immune proteome of *Staphylococcus aureus*: the anti-*S. aureus* antibody response. *Int J Med Microbiol* **300**:176–192.

303. **Broker BM, van Belkum A.** 2011. Immune proteomics of *Staphylococcus aureus*. *Proteomics* **11**:3221–3231.

304. **Fairbrother RW.** 1940. Coagulase production as a criterion for the classification of the staphylococci. *J Pathol* **50**:5.

305. **Tager M.** 1956. Studies on the nature and the purification of the coagulase-reacting factor and its relation to prothrombin. *J Exp Med* **104**:675–686.

306. **Vandenesch F, Celard M, Arpin D, Bes M, Greenland T, Etienne J.** 1995. Catheter-related bacteremia associated with coagulase-positive *Staphylococcus intermedius*. *J Clin Microbiol* **33**:2508–2510.

307. **Hanselman BA, Kruth SA, Rousseau J, Weese JS.** 2009. Coagulase positive staphylococcal colonization of humans and their household pets. *Can Vet J* **50**:954–958.

308. **Bannoehr J, Guardabassi L.** 2012. *Staphylococcus pseudintermedius* in the dog: taxonomy, diagnostics, ecology, epidemiology and pathogenicity. *Vet Dermatol* **23**:253–266.

309. **Bannoehr J, Ben Zakour NL, Reglinski M, Inglis NF, Prabhakaran S, Fossum E, Smith DG, Wilson GJ, Cartwright RA, Haas J, Hook M, van den Broek AHM, Thoday KL, Fitzgerald JR.** 2011. Genomic and surface proteomic analysis of the canine pathogen *Staphylococcus pseudintermedius* reveals proteins that mediate adherence to the extracellular matrix. *Infect Immun* **79**:3074–3086.

310. **Pietrocola G, Geoghegan JA, Rindi S, Di Poto A, Missineo A, Consalvi V, Foster TJ, Speziale P.** 2013. Molecular characterization of the

multiple interactions of SpsD, a surface protein from *Staphylococcus pseudintermedius*, with host extracellular matrix proteins. *PloS One* **8**:e66901. doi:10.1371/journal.pone.0066901.

311. **Bergonier D, de Cremoux R, Rupp R, Lagriffoul G, Berthelot X.** 2003. Mastitis of dairy small ruminants. *Vet Res* **34**:689–716.

312. **Piessens V, De Vliegher S, Verbist B, Braem G, Van Nuffel A, De Vuyst L, Heyndrickx M, Van Coillie E.** 2012. Intra-species diversity and epidemiology varies among coagulase-negative *Staphylococcus* species causing bovine intramammary infections. *Vet Microbiol* **155**:62–71.

313. **Unal N, Cinar OD.** 2012. Detection of stapylococcal enterotoxin, methicillin-resistant and Panton-Valentine leukocidin genes in coagulase-negative staphylococci isolated from cows and ewes with subclinical mastitis. *Trop Anim Health Prod* **44**:369–375.

314. **Otto M.** 2009. *Staphylococcus epidermidis*: the 'accidental' pathogen. *Nat Rev Microbiol* **7**:555–567.

315. **Otto M.** 2012. Molecular basis of *Staphylococcus epidermidis* infections. *Semin Immunopathol* **34**:201–214.

316. **Mack D, Davies AP, Harris LG, Jeeves R, Pascoe B, Knobloch JK, Rohde H, Wilkinson TS.** 2013. *Staphylococcus epidermidis* in biomaterial-associated infections, p 25–56. *In* Moriarty F, Zaat SAJ, Busscher H (ed), *Biomaterials Associated Infection: Immunological Aspects and Antimicrobial Strategies.* Springer, New York.

317. **Schleifer KH.** 1975. Isolation and characterization of staphylococci from human skin. *Int J Syst Bacteriol* **25**:17.

318. **van der Mee-Marquet N, Achard A, Mereghetti L, Danton A, Minier M, Quentin R.** 2003. *Staphylococcus lugdunensis* infections: high frequency of inguinal area carriage. *J Clin Microbiol* **41**:1404–1409.

319. **Bieber L, Kahlmeter G.** 2010. *Staphylococcus lugdunensis* in several niches of the normal skin flora. *Clin Microbiol Infect* **16**:385–388.

320. **Kloos WE, Musselwhite MS.** 1975. Distribution and persistence of *Staphylococcus* and *Micrococcus* species and other aerobic bacteria on human skin. *Appl Microbiol* **30**:381–385.

321. **Rupp ME, Soper DE, Archer GL.** 1992. Colonization of the female genital tract with *Staphylococcus saprophyticus*. *J Clin Microbiol* **30**:2975–2979.

322. **Schneider PF, Riley TV.** 1996. *Staphylococcus saprophyticus* urinary tract infections: epidemiological data from Western Australia. *Eur J Epidemiol* **12**:51–54.

323. **Anguera I, Del Rio A, Miro JM, Matinez-Lacasa X, Marco F, Guma JR, Quaglio G, Claramonte X, Moreno A, Mestres CA, Mauri E, Azqueta M, Benito N, Garcia-de la Maria C, Almela M, Jimenez-Exposito MJ, Sued O, De Lazzari E, Gatell JM.** 2005. *Staphylococcus lugdunensis* infective endocarditis: description of 10 cases and analysis of native valve, prosthetic valve, and pacemaker lead endocarditis clinical profiles. *Heart* **91**:e10.

324. **Liu PY, Huang YF, Tang CW, Chen YY, Hsieh KS, Ger LP, Chen YS, Liu YC.** 2010. *Staphylococcus lugdunensis* infective endocarditis: a literature review and analysis of risk factors. *J Microbiol Immunol Infect* **43**:478–484.

325. **Tee WS, Soh SY, Lin R, Loo LH.** 2003. *Staphylococcus lugdunensis* carrying the *mecA* gene causes catheter-associated bloodstream infection in premature neonate. *J Clin Microbiol* **41**:519–520.

326. **Choi SH, Chung JW, Lee EJ, Kim TH, Lee MS, Kang JM, Song EH, Jun JB, Kim MN, Kim YS, Woo JH, Choi SH.** 2010. Incidence, characteristics, and outcomes of *Staphylococcus lugdunensis* bacteremia. *J Clin Microbiol* **48**:3346–3349.

327. **Sampathkumar P, Osmon DR, Cockerill FR 3rd.** 2000. Prosthetic joint infection due to *Staphylococcus lugdunensis*. *Mayo Clin Proc* **75**:511–512.

328. **Bocher S, Tonning B, Skov RL, Prag J.** 2009. *Staphylococcus lugdunensis*, a common cause of skin and soft tissue infections in the community. *J Clin Microbiol* **47**:946–950.

329. **Ravaioli S, Selan L, Visai L, Pirini V, Campoccia D, Maso A, Speziale P, Montanaro L, Arciola CR.** 2012. *Staphylococcus lugdunensis*, an aggressive coagulase-negative pathogen not to be underestimated. *Int J Artif Organs* **35**:742–753.

330. **Heilbronner S, Hanses F, Monk IR, Speziale P, Foster TJ.** 2013. Sortase A promotes virulence in experimental *Staphylococcus lugdunensis* endocarditis. *Microbiology* **159**:2141–2152.

331. **Frank KL, Patel R.** 2007. Poly-N-acetylglucosamine is not a major component of the extracellular matrix in biofilms formed by icaADBC-positive *Staphylococcus lugdunensis* isolates. *Infect Immun* **75**:4728–4742.

332. **Giormezis N, Kolonitsiou F, Makri A, Vogiatzi A, Christofidou M, Anastassiou ED, Spiliopoulou I.** 2015. Virulence factors among *Staphylococcus lugdunensis* are associated with infection sites and clonal spread. *Eur J Clin Microbiol Infect Dis* **34**:773–778.

333. **Donvito B, Etienne J, Denoroy L, Greenland T, Benito Y, Vandenesch F.** 1997. Synergistic

hemolytic activity of *Staphylococcus lugdunensis* is mediated by three peptides encoded by a non-agr genetic locus. *Infect Immun* **65**:95–100.

334. **Loverix L, Timmermans P, Benit E.** 2013. Successful non-surgical treatment of endocarditis caused by *Staphylococcus haemolyticus* following transcatheter aortic valve implantation (TAVI). *Acta Clin Belg* **68**:376–379.

335. **Wong RW, Rhodes KM.** 2015. Endophthalmitis caused by *Staphylococcus hominis* and two different colonies of *Staphylococcus haemolyticus* after cataract surgery. *Retin Cases Brief Rep* **9**:181–184.

336. **Silva PV, Cruz RS, Keim LS, Paula GR, Carvalho BT, Coelho LR, Carvalho MC, Rosa JM, Figueiredo AM, Teixeira LA.** 2013. The antimicrobial susceptibility, biofilm formation and genotypic profiles of *Staphylococcus haemolyticus* from bloodstream infections. *Mem Inst Oswaldo Cruz* **108**:812–813.

337. **Potter A, Ceotto H, Giambiagi-Demarval M, dos Santos KR, Nes IF, Bastos Mdo C.** 2009. The gene *bap*, involved in biofilm production, is present in *Staphylococcus* spp. strains from nosocomial infections. *J Microbiol* **47**:319–326.

338. **Latham RH, Running K, Stamm WE.** 1983. Urinary tract infections in young adult women caused by *Staphylococcus saprophyticus*. *JAMA* **250**:3063–3066.

339. **Hovelius B, Mardh PA.** 1984. *Staphylococcus saprophyticus* as a common cause of urinary tract infections. *Rev Infect Dis* **6**:328–337.

340. **Gatermann S, John J, Marre R.** 1989. *Staphylococcus saprophyticus* urease: characterization and contribution to uropathogenicity in unobstructed urinary tract infection of rats. *Infect Immun* **57**:110–116.

341. **Loes AN, Ruyle L, Arvizu M, Gresko KE, Wilson AL, Deutch CE.** 2014. Inhibition of urease activity in the urinary tract pathogen *Staphylococcus saprophyticus*. *Lett Appl Microbiol* **58**:31–41.

342. **Keren I, Kaldalu N, Spoering A, Wang Y, Lewis K.** 2004. Persister cells and tolerance to antimicrobials. *FEMS Microbiol Lett* **230**:13–18.

343. **Lewis K.** 2001. Riddle of biofilm resistance. *Antimicrob Agents Chemother* **45**:999–1007.

344. **Conlon BP.** 2014. *Staphylococcus aureus* chronic and relapsing infections: evidence of a role for persister cells: an investigation of persister cells, their formation and their role in *S. aureus* disease. *BioEssays* **36**:991–996.

345. **Koch G, Yepes A, Forstner KU, Wermser C, Stengel ST, Modamio J, Ohlsen K, Foster KR, Lopez D.** 2014. Evolution of resistance to a last-resort antibiotic in *Staphylococcus aureus* via bacterial competition. *Cell* **158**:1060–1071.

346. **Krismer B, Peschel A.** 2011. Does *Staphylococcus aureus* nasal colonization involve biofilm formation? *Future Microbiol* **6**:489–493.

347. **Dastgheyb S, Parvizi J, Shapiro IM, Hickok NJ, Otto M.** 2015. Effect of biofilms on recalcitrance of staphylococcal joint infection to antibiotic treatment. *J Infect Dis* **211**:641–650.

348. **Haaber J, Cohn MT, Frees D, Andersen TJ, Ingmer H.** 2012. Planktonic aggregates of *Staphylococcus aureus* protect against common antibiotics. *PloS One* **7**:e41075. doi:10.1371/journal.pone.0041075.

349. **Walker JN, Crosby HA, Spaulding AR, Salgado-Pabon W, Malone CL, Rosenthal CB, Schlievert PM, Boyd JM, Horswill AR.** 2013. The *Staphylococcus aureus* ArlRS two-component system is a novel regulator of agglutination and pathogenesis. *PLoS Pathog* **9**:e1003819. doi:10.1371/journal.ppat.1003819.

Surviving Between Hosts: Sporulation and Transmission

20

MICHELLE C. SWICK,[1] THERESA M. KOEHLER,[1] and ADAM DRIKS[2]

SPORE-FORMING BACTERIAL PATHOGENS

Bacillus anthracis and Other Pathogenic Bacillus Species

The *Bacillus* species are Gram-positive, spore-forming, facultative aerobes that are commonly found in the soil, sometimes associated with plants and nematodes. The *Bacillus cereus sensu lato* clade of this well-studied genus contains pathogens and nonpathogens, with a complex taxonomy that in recent years has been continuously modified to reflect DNA sequence data. In addition to DNA sequence similarities and gene synteny, horizontal transfer of closely related plasmids is apparent among these ubiquitous soil bacteria (1). Member species of the *B. cereus sensu lato* group include *B. cereus sensu stricto*, *B. anthracis*, *Bacillus thuringiensis*, *Bacillus mycoides*, *Bacillus pseudomycoides*, *Bacillus weihenstephanensis*, and *Bacillus cytotoxicus* (2–10). Of these, the best-studied species are *B. anthracis*, *B. cereus sensu stricto*, and *B. thuringiensis*. *B. anthracis* is the causative agent of anthrax in mammals, an often lethal disease. Human disease is generally acquired accidentally during outbreaks of anthrax in domestic livestock and wildlife, but has also been associated with bioterrorism (11). Certain strains of

[1]University of Texas Medical School at Houston, Houston, TX 77030; [2]Loyola University Chicago, Stritch School of Medicine, Maywood, IL 60153.

Virulence Mechanisms of Bacterial Pathogens, 5th edition
Edited by Indira T. Kudva, Nancy A. Cornick, Paul J. Plummer, Qijing Zhang, Tracy L. Nicholson, John P. Bannantine, and Bryan H. Bellaire
© 2016 American Society for Microbiology, Washington, DC
doi:10.1128/microbiolspec.VMBF-0029-2015

B. cereus can cause food poisoning in humans, while some strains of *B. thuringiensis* are lethal for invertebrates and are used as insecticides (12, 13). Other species of the *B. cereus sensu lato* group are only occasionally cited as disease-causing in mammals, but their potential virulence factors are not known.

B. anthracis and anthrax

B. anthracis infection can manifest as a cutaneous or systemic disease. Entry of spores via a preexisting lesion in the skin can result in cutaneous anthrax. This disease is distinguished by the presence of a characteristic black eschar on the skin and typically remains a localized infection. Systemic anthrax can take several forms. One of these, gastrointestinal anthrax, is the result of ingesting spores, which may occur in grass-fed mammals that consume the spores in the soil or in humans through the consumption of contaminated food products. The other systemic form, inhalational anthrax, is the most deadly form, in part because of its ambiguous set of symptoms and rapid onset. Spores are inhaled and deposited into the lung tissue, where they proceed to germinate and spread through lymph nodes, rapidly causing systemic disease, massive tissue damage, shock, and death (14). Recently, a fourth form, injectional anthrax, has been recognized in heroin addicts whose drug supply was likely contaminated by contact with infected animal material (15, 16).

Virulent *B. anthracis* carries two virulence plasmids. The anthrax toxin genes are located on virulence plasmid pXO1, and the capsule biosynthetic operon is located on pXO2 (17). Anthrax toxin is composed of three proteins: lethal factor, edema factor, and protective antigen. Lethal factor is a zinc-dependent metalloprotease that targets the mitogen-activated kinase kinases (MAPKKs, or Meks). Lethal factor cleaves the N-terminus of these proteins, disrupting the ERK1/2, JNK/SAPK, and p38 signaling pathways in host cells. These pathways are critical to proper cell cycle regulation, cellular proliferation, and defense against cellular stresses. Edema factor is a calmodulin-dependent adenylate cyclase, which, as the name implies, causes the intense edema observed with the disease. This enzyme influences many cellular signaling pathways in the host cell by increasing cyclic AMP (cAMP) levels. Protective antigen is required for the delivery of both lethal factor and edema factor to host cells. Protective antigen is cleaved into a fragment that can multimerize, forming a heptameric structure that binds to receptors on the host cell (TEM8 and CMG2), forms a pore within the membrane, and delivers lethal factor and edema factor to the host cell cytosol (18, 19). The capsule of *B. anthracis* is unique among capsule-forming bacteria in that it is composed of poly-D-glutamic acid instead of the more common polysaccharide or hyaluronic acid capsules seen in other pathogens. As is true for other bacterial capsules, the *B. anthracis* capsule has antiphagocytic and antiopsinogenic roles in infection. Recent reports have expanded the role of capsule, indicating that it can also act as an adhesin and suppress dendritic cell function. It, may also serve as a TLR2 agonist (20–22).

B. thuringiensis: the insect pathogen

B. thuringiensis is used extensively as a biological control agent for insect pests. During sporulation, certain *B. thuringiensis* strains produce parasporal crystals comprised of Cry proteins (also known as delta-endotoxins). These toxins are lethal for many invertebrates, including members of the orders *Lepidoptera*, *Diptera*, and *Coleoptera*; some nematodes; mites; and protozoa (12, 13). The Cry toxins vary in degree of toxicity, but generally disrupt host cell membranes, including those of epithelial cells in the insect gut (23). Cry-mediated formation of pores in cell membranes causes an osmotic imbalance, and/or the opening of ion channels, activating cell death (24). *B. thuringiensis* infection in insects includes three successive steps—virulence, necrotrophism, and sporulation—which are controlled by quorum sensing systems and multiple regulators. In addition to the Cry toxins, multiple other factors, including degradative enzymes, play roles in these different stages of infection (25).

B. thuringiensis is generally considered nonpathogenic to humans and other animals. However, there are some reports of association of the bacterium with human diseases including food-poisoning-associated diarrheas, periodontitis, and bacteremia. There are also rare instances of *B. thuringiensis*-associated ocular, burn, and wound infections (26, 27). Multiple secreted proteins of *B. thuringiensis*, including phospholipases, hemolysins, and enterotoxins, have been shown to contribute to disease in animal models of infection (28).

B. cereus and food poisoning

Some *B. cereus sensu stricto* strains are opportunistic human pathogens, and infection and intoxication can result from consumption of contaminated foods. Cereulide toxin–producing strains are responsible for an enteric syndrome that is acquired by eating contaminated rice or pasta. Diarrheal disease, linked with contaminated dairy products and vegetables, is caused by *B. cereus sensu stricto* strains producing three toxins: cytotoxin K and the heat-labile protein complexes hemolysin BL and nonhemolytic enterotoxin (29, 30).

Pathogenic *Clostridium* Species

Many members of the *Clostridiales*, like many *Bacillales*, are Gram-positive sporulating soil bacteria. Yet unlike the *Bacillales* species that form spores, the known spore-forming *Clostridiales* species are obligate anaerobes and are exquisitely sensitive to oxygen. The major pathogenic *Clostridiales* species are a genetically diverse group that includes *Clostridium difficile*, *Clostridium perfringens*, *Clostridium botulinum*, *Clostridium tetani*, and *Clostridium sordellii*. (We note that *C. difficile* is properly referred to as *Peptoclostridium difficile* [31]. However, for the purpose of this review, we will use the former and still very widespread nomenclature). *C. perfringens* is the second-most-common bacterial source of foodborne illness in the United States (32) and the most common *Clostridium* species associated with gas gangrene. *C. difficile* has emerged over the past 10 years as a causative agent of antibiotic-associated diarrhea (33). Other pathogenic *Clostridium* species include *C. tetani*, the agent of tetanus, *Clostridium botulinum*, which causes botulism, and *C. sordellii*, which has been associated with rare postabortion infections (34).

Hospital-acquired *C. difficile* infections

C. difficile is the leading cause of nosocomial diarrhea worldwide, and the bacterium can cause life-threatening infections in patients undergoing antibiotic treatment. Spores are transmitted via the fecal-oral route and are very easily spread by health care workers. *C. difficile* is a toxin-producing extracellular pathogen. Typically, the treatment of a patient with antibiotics for an unrelated infection negatively affects the normal flora within the gut. These commensals provide colonization resistance or the ability to prevent invasion by pathogens simply by colonizing the niche first. In the absence of these protective commensals, *C. difficile* spores can germinate, replicate, and produce toxins. Unlike other infections, *C. difficile*-infected patients have a high relapse rate, further complicating the treatment of the disease. This relapse rate may be due to the ability of *C. difficile* to sporulate and regerminate within the host environment, thereby persisting within the host. The ability of *C. difficile* to complete its life cycle within the host is one significant difference between *C. difficile* and *B. anthracis*, for which sporulation within the host has not been observed (35, 36).

The primary virulence factors of *C. difficile* are two enterotoxins: toxin A (TcdA) and toxin B (TcdB). These toxins are required for the development of clinical symptoms. They act by glycosylating members of the Rho family of host proteins, which causes remodeling of the host cell cytoskeleton and leads to massive damage to the epithelium and induction of a strong inflammatory response (37, 38). The results of these events are intestinal tissue injury and acute inflammation, leading to the diarrheal symptoms observed clinically. The ability to produce toxins A and/or B is essential for virulence; highly toxinogenic strains are capable of causing severe disease, while non-toxin-producing strains do not cause symptomatic disease (38). While the relative contributions of toxins A and B to disease are still an important area of investigation (39, 40), recent data suggest that toxin B is the primary contributor to disease (41). *C. difficile* produces a third toxin, called CDT (also known as binary toxin). This toxin is an ADP-ribosyltransferase, much like the diphtheria, cholera, and pertussis toxins. The role of this toxin in the causation of disease is unclear, because many pathogenic strains do not possess the gene to encode it. However, one hypothesis is that CDT augments the activity of TcdA and TcdB. Interestingly, one study has implicated CDT as a significant predictor of recurrent disease (42).

C. perfringens infections

C. perfringens can cause human clostridial myonecrosis and food poisoning as well as several enterotoxemic and enteritis diseases of animals. Clostridial myonecrosis, also known as gas gangrene, arises when spores from contaminated soil enter muscle tissue, often the result of traumatic injury (43). Spontaneous myonecrosis can also occur but is usually associated with *Clostridium septicum* or other related species (44). Clostridial myonecrosis in humans and other mammals spreads rapidly via tissue necrosis, often leading to systemic toxemia and shock with high mortality rates. *C. perfringens* gastroenteritis can be acquired from contaminated meat, including poultry. Spores, and vegetative cells from food stored in conditions that permit germination and multiplication, survive passage through the stomach and reach the intestine, where they can multiply and produce toxin (32). Pathogenesis of *C. perfringens* is mediated by multiple secreted toxins, many of which are plasmid-encoded (45). Strains are distinguished by the combinations of toxins that they produce. Toxigenic types A, B, C, D, and E, are based on distinct combinations of four toxins (alpha-, beta-, epsilon-, and iota-toxins). Some strains can produce additional toxins, including the beta 2 enterotoxin and *C. perfringens* enterotoxin (32, 46, 47).

THE SPORE AS AN INFECTIOUS PARTICLE

Spores of *Bacillus* and *Clostridium* represent a distinctive cell type that is made when vegetative cells experience a specific alteration in the environment that is usually associated with starvation (Fig. 1). Spores are distinguished from the vast majority of other cell types by their minimal metabolic activity and high resistance to environmental stressors (48). As a result, spores can survive in the environment for extended periods of time (49). In most cases where disease is initiated by a spore, the spore must germinate before the virulence factors that cause disease (such as toxins) are expressed (for an important exception, see discussion of *C. perfringens*, below). This is because the spore itself appears to be generally nontoxic to the host; rather, toxicity arises from factors produced after germination, when vegetative cell growth resumes.

Spore Structure and Function

All spores produced by species in the *Bacillales* and *Clostridiales* have a common architectural plan; they are spherical or roughly ovoid cells composed of a series of concentric shells (Fig. 1).

The inner membrane and its contents
The innermost structure is always a membrane-bound compartment harboring the spore's

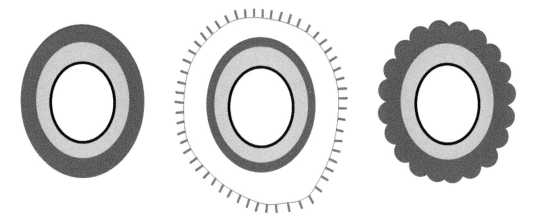

FIGURE 1 Schematic representation of spores of *B. subtilis* (left), *B. anthracis* (middle), and *C. difficile* (right) illustrating the major spore structures. The innermost compartment (housing the spore DNA), the core, is white. The inner membrane (the location of the germinant receptors in *B. subtilis* and *B. anthracis*, but not *C. difficile*) is the black oval surrounding the core. The gray region is the spore peptidoglycan and, surrounding that, the dark blue is the coat. Although an outer membrane is present during spore formation, it is most likely not present in the mature spore (72) and, therefore, is not shown here. For simplicity, the sublayers of the coat are not indicated. *B. anthracis* (but not the other two species) (65) possesses an additional outer layer, the exosporium, indicated by a red line (the exosporium basal layer) and protrusions extending from the basal layer surface (the hair-like projections, or nap). The region between the coat and the exosporium is the interspace. The *C. difficile* coat has a scalloped appearance in cross-section, as indicated in the figure.

DNA, which is tightly associated with small peptides called small acid-soluble proteins, or SASPs (50). This compartment also contains cations and pyridine-2,6-dicarboxylic acid (or dipicolinic acid [DPA]) in a 1:1 chelate with divalent calcium ions (Ca^{2+}DPA), which maintain the spore's dormant state and resistance to certain DNA-damaging agents. The membrane of this compartment retards the diffusion of water (51, 52).

An additional important function of the inner membrane, at least in many species, is to house the germinant receptors, which initiate a signal transduction pathway ultimately leading to the resumption of metabolism (51, 53). The receptors bind to specific small-molecule "germinants," which can be a subset of sugars, amino acids, and ribonucleosides, as well as other small molecules, depending on the spore species (53). Not all germinant receptors are located in the inner membrane; the *C. difficile* germinant receptor CspC is likely associated with either the coat

and/or cortex (54). CspC is distinct from the "canonical" germinant receptors, best studied in *Bacillus subtilis* and present in a variety of *Bacillaceae* and *C. perfringens* (55). In particular, unlike the typical germinant receptors, CspC does not contain membrane-spanning sequences. As will be discussed later, this difference between CspC and the other known germinant receptors suggests that germinant receptors in other spore-forming bacteria may vary from the examples studied so far. As a result, searches for novel germinant receptors should not be based solely on bioinformatics-driven analyses.

All known germinant receptors are located in deeper layers of the spore, suggesting that germinants must reach the receptors via diffusion. Therefore, it can be inferred that all the layers that encase the inner membrane (discussed below) are porous to molecules at least as large as the corresponding germinants. The porosity of the coat to small molecules has been demonstrated experimentally for a few *Bacillus* species and can be inferred for many others where data are available; these species possess sequences for canonical germinant receptors. The porosity of the cortex is a reasonable inference based on the known structure and composition of peptidoglycan layers.

Cortex and germ cell wall

Surrounding the forespore membrane is another spore layer that is common to all species examined: a shell of peptidoglycan containing two sublayers: the cortex and the germ cell wall. The germ cell wall is destined to become the nascent cell wall of the vegetative cell when outgrowth begins. The cortex encases the germ cell wall. In transmission electron micrographs, the cortex appears distinct from vegetative cell peptidoglycan and, at least in *B. anthracis* and *B. subtilis*, the cortex differs biochemically as well. A major role of the cortex is to retain the relatively dry state of the core. The cortex does this by constricting the core's volume. In the absence of this girdle-like effect of the cortex (if, for example, the integrity of the cortex is compromised by first extracting the coat and then treating with lysozyme [56]), the core will immediately begin to expand and rehydrate.

The spore coat

The next layer of the spore, the coat, is a protein shell that is universally present but varies significantly in composition and morphology among species (57–63). In many species, including *B. subtilis* and *C. difficile*, but not *B. anthracis* and its close relatives, the coat is the external layer of the spore (Fig. 1) (64, 65). The coat is biochemically complex, comprising approximately 70 protein species organized into several layers (60, 66–69). The spore coat of *B. anthracis* is relatively thin; in contrast, it is much thicker in *C. difficile* (65). The coat has a larger surface area than the cortex on which it sits. As a result, while much of the inner surface of the coat associates with the outer cortex surface, the mismatch in surface areas results in folds or buckles in the coat (70–72). In fact, the coat is relatively flexible and can fold and unfold in response to changes in the spore's degree of hydration. Such changes are evident in spores where cortex volume changes in response to alterations in ambient humidity (72–75).

As already mentioned, the coat acts as a sieve, restricting passage of large molecules. An important consequence of this constraint is that structures within the spore are protected from degradative enzymes such as mammalian lysozyme, which readily lyses the cortex, and other destructive enzymes common in the soil environment (57, 59). The coat also has roles in resistance to several types of small reactive chemicals (48). The mechanism(s) responsible for this type of resistance is (are) not yet known. The coat also provides resistance to digestion by eukaryotic microbes and nematodes (76, 77). Possibly, resistance to these organisms is due to exclusion of microbial degradative enzymes by sieving. It is reasonable to speculate that the evolution of resistance to degradative enzymes in the environment gave rise to the ability to exclude host-generated degradative enzymes during infection. In this view, the diversity in coat structures among pathogenic spores evolved prior to the appearance of pathogenic life styles in these lineages. As might be expected from its biochemical complexity, the coat probably has other functions, although these are still poorly understood (66). However, in *B. subtilis*, for which some information on these functions is available, it has been shown that the coat plays complex roles in germination. Because germination is central to pathogenesis in many if not all cases where the spore is the infectious particle (see below), a deeper understanding of the role of the coat in germination in pathogenic species would likely provide mechanistic insights into how these species cause disease and new therapeutics to target them.

Studies of spore structure and function have been limited to a small number of species, and the diversity in coat structure across the much larger number of known species remains poorly explored. Given that some species (such as the nonpathogenic species *Bacillus clausii*) possess long spike-like appendages, and others (such as *Clostridium taeniosporum*) harbor intriguing propeller-like ribbons extending from one end, no doubt more exotic structural variations remain to be discovered (63, 78, 79). It is unlikely that we will be able to understand fully the roles of the coat in natural environments until we have a better understanding of how coat architecture and composition varies among spore formers. One future challenge involves elucidating the environmental selective pressures that drive the diversity in coat morphology across species (80).

The exosporium
The outermost structure of many spores (and some, but not all, pathogens) is a structurally distinct layer called the exosporium. The exosporium is defined by its location and morphology: it is separated from the coat by a gap (referred to as the interspace) and, importantly, the interspace thickness varies around the circumference of the spore (58, 60, 64). As a result, the contours of the exosporium do not follow the folds of the coat. While it is reasonable to infer that some material must connect the exosporium to the coat (and, specifically, guide exosporium deposition during spore assembly [60]), the identity of this material and that of the interspace contents remains unknown. Regardless of which specific molecules compose the interspace, their organization almost certainly must be different than that of molecules in the coat, given that variation in interspace width is so prevalent among exosporium-bearing spores (63).

Like the coat, the exosporium has been studied in only a few species, primarily *B. anthracis* and *B. cereus* (60, 81–96). Structural studies provide strong support for the view that, like the coat, the exosporium serves as a sieve that excludes large molecules (84). There is also evidence that the *B. cereus* exosporium provides resistance to specific chemicals including ethanol, toluene, chloroform, phenol and, in the context of a macrophage, nitric oxide (86, 97). Spores from which the exosporium has been removed, due to mutations in genes encoding exosporium proteins or other proteins involved in assembly, are able to germinate, but at levels that are altered relative to wild type spores (83, 98, 99).

Characterizing the roles for the coat and/or the exosporium in pathogenesis is an important ongoing area of work. Clearly, the presence or absence of an exosporium is not an indication of a pathogenic lifestyle, given that many exosporium-bearing species are not virulent and that some spores without an exosporium cause disease. It is also notable that *B. anthracis*, a pathogen with an exosporium, can cause disease in several animal models when the exosporium has been removed mechanically or by mutation (60, 81, 100). Importantly, this ability to cause disease when the exosporium is absent does not necessarily imply that the *B. anthracis* exosporium has no role in natural infection. In fact, the *B. anthracis* exosporium surface protein BclA has been shown to bind to macrophage receptors and to mediate interactions with epithelial cells and extracellular matrix proteins (100–103).

An additional reasonable inference from the lack of an essential role for the exosporium in disease is the view that the coat provides significant protection against host defenses. This view is supported by the well characterized roles of the *B. subtilis* coat in resistance to diverse chemical and environmental stresses and the presence of spores of *B. subtilis*, *C. difficile*, and other species without exosporia in the mammalian gastrointestinal tract (59, 65, 104). Other roles for the *B. anthracis* exosporium have been identified which, while not directly connected with pathogenesis, could nonetheless plausibly facilitate infection. For example, the exosporium modulates germination, as already mentioned. It seems plausible that the exosporium could participate in a variety of other functions, including acting as a sieve to prevent entry of large molecules (and especially degradative enzymes) to the spore interior and providing appropriate surface chemistry for optimal interactions with surfaces in the environment (105). Of course, in the cases of the spores harboring exosporia produced by the many nonpathogenic species, these other roles will also be important, albeit to a nonpathogenic lifestyle.

The Decision to Sporulate

For maximal efficiency of infection, *B. anthracis* and *C. difficile*, and most likely other spore-forming bacterial pathogens, usually enter the body as spores rather than vegetative cells. The spores themselves, however, are not the direct cause of disease; rather, symptoms initiate only after the spores germinate and produce vegetative cells that, in turn, produce the toxins and other virulence factors that are direct causes of disease (bearing in mind the important exception of *C. perfringens*, already mentioned). Nonetheless, spore formation in the nonhost environment, in the case of *Bacillus*, and sporulation in the context of the host, in the case of *Clostridium*, leads to further dissemination of disease.

Complex regulation of *Bacillus* sporulation

The precise identities of the factors triggering sporulation are not known; even in the best-studied model, *B. subtilis*, these factors remain obscure. Nonetheless, it is known that sporulation is usually stimulated by depletion of nutrients and other molecules associated with growth. This environmental change is detected by a set of sensor kinases, which in turn, activate a phosphorylation cascade. This cascade appears to be a major part of a regulatory circuit responsible for pushing the cell toward one or another behavior, depending on the severity of the nutrient depletion and other environmental and cell-

internal factors (106–108). Sporulation is one such choice. The specific circuitry that couples activation of the sensor kinases with the decision to sporulate is likely to vary significantly among species, because each species will have evolved to sporulate in a manner that is adaptive in its specific niche. For example, *B. anthracis* does not sporulate during infection; spores appear only after an animal that has died of anthrax is scavenged and, as a result, the vegetative cells that have accumulated in the blood are exposed to the environment (109). By remaining vegetative, the bacterial load and toxin production in the host are maximized. By restricting the initiation of sporulation to a point when the bacterial titer is highest, the number of spores that can ultimately disseminate the infection is also maximized. There is strong evidence that this is achieved by the specific configuration of the phosphorylation cascade in *B. anthracis*, a cascade that has likely evolved to limit sporulation initiation during infection (110–113).

In *C. difficile*, the situation is different; spores are produced in the host during active infection, when the bacterium has colonized the gastrointestinal tract (36). It is not yet known how *C. difficile* initiates sporulation in the host. However, the genetic control of sporulation in this organism is being elucidated. An important lesson from these early studies is that the mechanism differs in important ways from what is known in *B. subtilis* (114, 115). As for the case of *B. anthracis*, it is likely that, in *C. difficile*, the control of sporulation initiation has adapted to support pathogenesis.

Spore development and toxin synthesis

Two distinct examples of how sporulation can participate in the initiation of disease are provided by the gastrointestinal disease caused by the *C. perfringens* enterotoxin and the insecticidal effect of *B. thuringiensis* (and several other members of the *Bacillaceae*, including *Lysinibacillus sphaericus*). In both organisms, a toxin produced concomitantly with the spore induces disease. In the case of *C. perfringens*, vegetative cells enter the body orally, often due to consumption of spoiled food that is stored anaerobically (such as when canned). The cells then sporulate in the gastrointestinal tract, resulting in the synthesis of toxin, an event that is governed by the sporulation developmental program. The result is the appearance of toxin in the mother cell compartment and the liberation of toxin into the gastrointestinal tract upon mother cell envelope lysis. The diarrhea that results from the toxin facilitates spore dissemination and the next round of infection.

B. thuringiensis produces an insecticidal crystal toxin during sporulation and under the control of the sporulation transcription factors that direct mother cell gene expression (σ^E and/or σ^K) (116). The crystal is typically in close association with the spore and can be underneath or outside of the exosporium (117–119). Unlike what usually results from the disease caused by the *C. perfringens* enterotoxin, *B. thuringiensis* kills its insect host and then replicates in the cadaver. A subset of these replicating cells goes on to sporulate (25, 120).

In both *C. perfringens* and *B. thuringiensis*, the association of a toxin with the spore facilitates disease and dissemination of spores after infection, although the resulting pathology and the mechanisms of dissemination differ. It is intriguing to consider that such similar mechanisms of toxin production and delivery arose in such phylogenetically different species.

Germination Dynamics and Signals

Germination is a multistep process in which spores transition from dormancy to metabolically active, dividing cells. Germination is broken down into stages: commitment, stage I, stage II, and cortex hydrolysis leading to outgrowth. Commitment is the time between germinant interaction and Stage I, which is characterized by a series of biophysical events that lead to a rapid influx of water

into the spore. Stage II is marked by completion of water influx and the degradation of the peptidoglycan cortex. Once the cortex is hydrolyzed and outgrowth is complete, the cells resume full metabolic activity.

Germination can be triggered in one of two ways: (i) nutrient-triggered germination or (ii) non-nutrient-triggered germination. In nutrient-triggered germination, the response is initiated by the sensing of environmental signals/nutrients; this pathway is more likely followed by spores that germinate in the host. Non-nutrient-triggered germination occurs in response to damage or degradation of the spore coat/cortex/inner membrane (121). This method is considered an attempt at vegetative growth when the spore is damaged. The process of germination is characterized by distinct and temporal structural and biochemical changes in spores. Because individual cells proceed asynchronously through these changes, and with varying rates and timing, germination in a spore population is understood to be heterogeneous. The stages of germination differ between *B. anthracis* and *C. difficile*. The process is best understood in *B. subtilis* and is thought to be similar in *B. anthracis*, given the conservation in germination proteins between the two species. In cases where pathogenic *Bacillus* species have been studied, results are comparable to those in *B. subtilis*.

Germinants

Germination is activated when the spore senses the appropriate external signals or molecules, termed germinants, to initiate the germination pathway. Germinants interact with their corresponding germinant receptors to initiate the germination cascade. The germinants for *B. anthracis* and *C. difficile* are distinct, and each pathogen germinates with different dynamics. Studies of *B. anthracis* germination *in vitro* have revealed major germinants for initiation of the process and functions of key spore proteins associated with development of the vegetative cell. The major germinants for

B. anthracis are alanine or purine ribonucleotides. One or more additional amino acids are required to act as cogerminants. *In vitro*, *B. anthracis* requires a minimum of two germinants, but the number of germinants affects the required concentration of each germinant. In other words, the more germinants that are present, the less of each is necessary to trigger germination initiation. In *B. anthracis*, six distinct germination pathways have been described (122–126). These pathways require different combinations of amino acids, sugars, and ions to initiate germination. Interestingly, D-amino acids are unable to trigger germination, while L-amino acids can (127).

Germinant receptors

The germinant receptors (GRs) are encoded by *ger* genes in *Bacillus*, located on the inner membrane, and composed of three or four subunits (GerA, GerB, GerC, and GerD). In general, GRs are thought to be present at very low protein levels (few copies per cell) (51, 128). GRs are clustered in one spot on the inner membrane. The cluster of GRs is termed the germinosome. GerD is important to the formation of the germinosome (cluster). Spores lacking GerD have GRs dispersed throughout the inner membrane. (129). Because GRs are located on the inner membrane, germinants must travel through the spore's outer layers to initiate germination. However, spores germinate within minutes after contact with germinants, so it is reasonable to hypothesize that germinant penetration of the outer layers is somehow selective or specific. The *gerP* operon (where "P" denotes permeation) may be involved in this process. First discovered in *B. cereus* (130), *gerP$_{ABCDEF}$* is regulated by σ^K, suggesting that it is expressed in the mother cell during sporulation (130, 131). This operon in *B. anthracis* is 99% similar by sequence similarity and 97% protein identity (132). Disruption of the GerP operon leads to a germination defect, but the functions of the genes in the operon are unknown. They are

not predicted to resemble any known enzymes. Mutations in *gerP* result in a normal, stable spore, suggesting that this operon does not affect the structure of the spore. GerP might function to enable the Ca^{2+} dipicolinic acid (CaPDA) release (133).

To date, there have been no *in vitro* studies showing the direct binding of a germinant receptor to a germinant. Thus, there is no definitive proof of the function of GRs. However, there is other strong evidence to support their function as receptors for germinants. Genetic studies involving point mutants of GRs result in altered response to germinants, most frequently demonstrated by changes in the concentration of germinant needed to trigger germination. These studies strongly suggest that GRs and germinants do interact (134, 135).

gerX, a tricistronic operon found on the pXO1 plasmid, is expressed exclusively in the developing spore. Deletion of the *gerX* locus altered germination *in vivo* (136, 137). However, no *in vitro* phenotype was uncovered. Many other *ger* genes have been discovered through whole-genome sequencing and annotation. These GRs are chromosomally encoded; *gerX* remains the only identified germinant receptor locus that is found on a virulence plasmid in *B. anthracis*.

Although the primary means of germination seems to be through response to germinants via GRs, germination can also occur in response to peptidoglycan fragments released by nearby bacteria (138). This response seems to be completely independent of the nutrient pathway, because no GRs are used to initiate germination. Instead of GRs, PrkC, a membrane-associated Ser/Thr kinase, binds directly to peptidoglycan fragments shed by neighboring vegetative cells. This phenomenon was shown in *B. subtilis* and *B. anthracis*. Although the role of PrkC in this germination pathway was well demonstrated, the signal transduction thereafter is not yet understood. It is reasonable to hypothesize that spores might use the presence of actively growing bacteria in the environment as a signal of favorable growth conditions; however, it is unclear whether this pathway has a role in anthrax pathogenesis.

Computationally, orthologs of the GerA family of GRs found in *B. anthracis* cannot be predicted in the *C. difficile* genome. Furthermore, even within *Clostridium* species, the conserved pathways are differentially regulated. Of the five pathogenic species of *Clostridium*, *C. perfringens* is the best studied with respect to germination. However, some recent research has shed light on the unique properties of germination in *C. difficile*. In contrast to *B. subtilis* and *C. perfringens*, which sense nucleosides, sugars, amino acids, and ions, *C. difficile* germinates in response to bile salts and derivatives, including cholate taurocholate, glycocholate, and deoxycholate (139, 140). In addition to bile salts, the amino acids L-glycine or L-histidine serve as cogerminants (139, 141, 142). Germination in *C. difficile* is inhibited by chenodeoxycholic acid derivatives (139, 143), including muricholic acids (54).

Commitment to germination

Commitment to germination can be defined as the point at which the dissociation of a nutrient germinant by a strong competitive inhibitor or acidification to a pH of ~4.5 no longer blocks completion of germination. It is hypothesized that germinant receptor–nutrient binding results in commitment (126). Commitment is characterized by major changes in the permeability and structure of the inner membrane. As a result, the spore releases monovalent cations, including Na^+, K^+, and H^+. Once this reaction has occurred, the spore is committed to germinate even if the germinant is displaced from the receptor (126, 144–146). Recently, Wang et al. measured germination in individual spores and found that a spore commits to germination at or very near the time at which the spore's inner membrane permeability changes (147).

The period between the moment germinants are mixed with spores and the initiation of germination is termed the lag period. The lag period ranges in length from a few minutes to more than 24 hours. Spores that have extremely long lag periods are termed superdormant. Superdormant spores represent only a small fraction of the total spore population. While superdormancy is not well understood, it appears to be due to very low levels of GRs present in the inner membrane (148–150). This variation may be epistatic in nature. Regardless of the length of the lag period, very little is known about what happens during this time in either species (151, 152).

Within the *Bacillales* spore core, water makes up only 25 to 50% of the total weight. Meanwhile, Ca^{2+}DPA makes up 10% of the dry weight of the spore. These biochemical properties change drastically in stage I. Stage I is characterized by a series of biophysical events that involve rapid release of Ca^{2+}DPA and the rapid influx of water molecules into the spore. These events are triggered by the interaction of the GRs with germinants. Stage II encompasses the events from Ca^{2+}DPA release to expansion of the core, until the cell contains similar amounts of water equivalent to growing cells (80%). During stage II, spore-cortex lytic enzymes, or SCLEs, degrade the peptidoglycan (PG) cortex. The increase in water enables metabolism to resume.

The dynamics of germination in *C. difficile* are distinct from those of the *Bacillales*. Francis et al. (123) compared the biochemical dynamics of germination in *C. difficile* to those in *B. subtilis*. They found that in *B. subtilis*, Ca^{2+}DPA release occurs first, followed by release of cortex fragments. These findings were similar to those reported previously. However, in *C. difficile*, the opposite is true; cortex fragments can be detected in the medium before Ca^{2+}DPA. Additionally, deletion of hydrolase genes from *B. subtilis* prevented cortex fragment release but not Ca^{2+}DPA release (123).

SCLEs recognize the muramic-δ-lactam molecule, which is found exclusively in cortex PG. This is one reason why SCLEs can degrade the cortex PG, but not the spore's cell wall PG, which is chemically identical to cell wall in vegetative cells (152).

In *B. subtilis*, two SCLEs, SleB and CwlJ, serve partially redundant roles in cortex hydrolysis and spore germination (153). SleB is a lytic transglycosylase that recognizes and hydrolyzes the modified bond between *N*-acetyl muramic acid and *N*-acetyl glucosamine (154). While the activity of CwlJ seems to be activated by the $Ca^{2+}DPA$ signal, the mechanism of activation is not yet known. CwlJ has not been shown to have specific enzymatic activity, but it bears one catalytic domain with homology to SleB (53), is located in the spore coat, and is necessary for spore germination by exogenous $Ca^{2+}DPA$ treatment (155).

In *B. subtilis* and *B. anthracis*, the *sleB* gene is located within a bicistronic operon with *ypeB*. YpeB is essential for the proper assembly of SleB during sporulation (154, 156). One hypothesis is that YpeB serves as an inhibitory molecule to SleB during sporulation, and proteolysis of YpeB during germination allows SleB proteolytic activity to resume (157). Similarly, in both organisms, *cwlJ* is located in an operon with *gerQ*, which is required for CwlJ activity (158). The *B. anthracis* genome, in contrast with those of *B. subtilis* and *B. cereus*, contains a second copy of *gerQ* (*gerQ*-like) and *cwlJ* (*cwlJ2*). SleB and CwlJ are required for full virulence in a murine model for inhalation anthrax, but deletion of *cwlJ2* alone does not affect virulence significantly (159). Deletion of *cwlJ2* along with *sleB* and *cwlJ* reduces virulence synergistically.

As mentioned above, the proteins involved in germination of *Clostridium* strains are distinctly different from those found in *Bacillus*, so much so that computational analysis could not predict the genes in *Clostridium* species based upon those known in *Bacillus* (37). In *C. perfringens*, the Csp family of subtilin-like serine proteases—CspA, CspB, and CspC—act to degrade the core. One protein of the Csp family cleaves SleC, the spore-cortex lytic enzyme (SleB in *B. anthracis*), which in turn degrades the core. In *C. difficile*, CspC and CspA are predicted to be catalytically dead because two of the three residues of the catalytic triad are mutated in each protein (160). Instead, CspC acts as a germinant receptor for bile salt (54). This interaction between germinant and germinant receptor is thought to be important for virulence, because a *cspC* mutant is attenuated in a Syrian hamster model of *C. difficile* infection (59). Furthermore, mutation of CspC (G457R) altered the specificity of this receptor for bile salt (54). Lastly, *cspC*-null *C. difficile* spores were able to germinate in the presence of chenodeoxycholate, which normally inhibits taurocholate-mediated germination (a competitive inhibitor).

CspB is the only Csp protease with an intact catalytic triad. One hypothesis is that, in response to bile salts, CspC activates CspB, which processes SleB to activate it for cortex degradation. Unlike the SleC-CwlJ system in *Bacillus*, CspC and SleB are not activated by $Ca^{2+}DPA$. In fact, the signals that activate the system in *C. difficile* are unknown (37).

Germination in the host

For *Bacillus* and *Clostridium* species, it is likely that successful pathogenesis depends on restricting germination to a specific point during infection; otherwise, the spore could become susceptible to host defenses before reaching a location in the host where survival in the vegetative form is feasible. Therefore, in considering the evolution of pathogenesis in spore-forming species, it is very important to analyze adaptations of the germination system to the host.

Although *B. anthracis* can exist outside of the mammalian host as spores or vegetative cells, spores are more highly infectious than cells by most routes of infection. Vegetative cells have been shown to cause anthrax disease only when inoculated directly into the bloodstream (161, 162). In contrast, spores were pathogenic by every infection route tested. Entry of spores by the inhalation route is most deadly, and therefore most studied. A landmark study by Ross (163) demonstrated that spores are phagocytosed quickly by phagocytes, which detach from the lung and migrate to the lymph nodes. This work was done in an inhalation anthrax model using guinea pigs as the host. Ross was able to document a large number of spore-containing phagocytes and some germinated bacterial cells within the host cells en route to the lymph node. *B. anthracis* cells can also be phagocytosed by dendritic cells, which are also able to capture spores and deliver them to lymph nodes (164). However, differences have been observed between strains. While the Sterne strain tends to germinate quickly (165), the Ames strain has been shown to remain in the lung in an ungerminated state for 96 hours (166). These differences are not fully understood, but they suggest that the timing of germination is not dependent solely upon the presence of germinants. Phagocytes can bind and phagocytose *B. anthracis* efficiently, but neither event is necessary for germination: spores can germinate in cell-free, macrophage conditioned media (125), suggesting that host cells add small-molecule germinants to the medium.

Despite these reports that capture snapshots in the establishment phase of infection, no conclusive study shows whether spores germinate before or after phagocytosis. Both scenarios have been demonstrated *in vitro*. However, there is evidence for the presence of at least one bottleneck during infection. From an inoculum containing equal numbers of three *B. anthracis* strains, each expressing a different fluorescent protein, only one fluorescent protein was detected in distal organs following aerosol infection (167). Another study proposed two bottlenecks dependent on the infection route. Infections of the nasal mucosa–associated lymphoid tissue resulted in a bottleneck at the cervical lymph node, whereas lung-based infections revealed a bottleneck in a focal region of growth within the lung (168).

For *C. difficile*, germination in the host depends heavily on the gut microbial metabolism (169, 170). The gut microbiota is responsible for the conversion of bile acids into secondary bile acids, which inhibit germination of *C. difficile*. Antibiotic treatment alters the structure of the gut microbiome and thereby alters the ability of these bacteria to synthesize secondary bile acids. Without such inhibitory molecules, *C. difficile* can germinate, grow, produce toxin, and cause *C. difficile* infection, known as CDI. Use of fecal transplants to regenerate the natural flora of the gut has proved successful for treatment of resistant and recurrent CDI (171).

TRANSMISSION AND LIFESTYLES OUTSIDE OF THE HUMAN HOST

For *Bacillus* and *Clostridium* species, the infectious form of the bacterium is the dormant spore. Thus, pathogenesis depends upon survival of spores in the nonhost environment prior to entry into susceptible hosts. Yet a fundamental difference between pathogenic *Clostridium* and *Bacillus* species is the state of the bacterium upon exit from a mammalian host. *C. difficile* and *C. perfringens* sporulate within the mammalian gut during infection, and bacteria are released from the colonic tract to the nonhost environment as dormant spores. As an obligate anaerobe, vegetative cells of *Clostridium* cannot survive for more than a few hours outside of the anaerobic host environment (172, 173). Thus, fecal-oral transmission of *Clostridium* species from person to person requires persistence of the bacterium in the dormant spore form in the nonhost environment. By contrast, *B. anthracis* is not released from mammalian hosts until death of the infected host, at which time vegetative cells of the bacterium are found in blood and other body tissues. Reasons for lack of sporulation in dead or dying hosts are not clear. It has been suggested that once nutrients are depleted, the oxygen tension is too low for sporulation

(174). Sporulation *in vivo* may also be repressed by the virulence gene regulator AtxA (175). Blood from dead *B. anthracis*–infected animals does not clot and can drain from orifices into the nonhost environment. In the wild, vegetative cells from infected tissues can also be released through damage imposed by scavenging carnivores. Sporulation of *B. anthracis* is initiated when vegetative cells are exposed to the air (176).

Transition from Host to Nonhost Environments

The developmental state of spore-forming bacteria is dependent upon the ability to sense niche-specific signals. Transition from the host to nonhost environment presents a major change in nutrient availability, temperature, and moisture. In the metabolically inactive spore state, the pathogens can withstand these challenges and others, including significant changes in pressure, pH, and ultraviolet light (177, 178). In the case of *C. difficile*, spores are intrinsically resistant to antibiotics and the host immune system (179). Upon shedding from the host, spores persist because they are resistant to inactivation by nonbleach disinfectants that are used commonly in hospital settings (180). Resistance of *B. anthracis* spores to the challenges of the nonhost environment is also considered essential for persistence, yet some studies suggest that the *B. anthracis* sporulation–germination cycle outside of the host plays a role in transmission.

Pathogenic *Bacillus* Lifestyles Outside of the Host

B. cereus group species exist in soil and water but can also be isolated from a diverse array of mammals, birds, reptiles, and invertebrates. The bacteria can be found in the intestinal tracts of poultry and turtles and on the udders of cows (9, 181–185). Multiple strains of *B. cereus* group species have been reported to exist as commensal inhabitants of invertebrate intestines, including the guts of termites, millipedes, sow bugs, and cockroaches (186, 187). The species may also associate with amoeba (188). It is not clear to what degree the pathogenic *Bacillus* species persist upon release from these organisms, as opposed to potential commensal lifestyles within complex ecosystems of these varied hosts. The epidemiology of human anthrax has livestock, wildlife, soil, and water components. Blood from *B. anthracis*-infected mammals can contain as much as 10^9 vegetative cells per milliliter (189). Processed animal products, such as leather and wool, can carry large numbers of spores, and human cases of anthrax generally result from direct contact with contaminated animal products. A few anthrax cases have been reported to result from insect bites, which are presumed to be due to feeding of insects on infected animals or carcasses (190, 191). In the soil, spores can remain viable for decades, especially when deposited 15 centimeters below the upper soil levels (176). Herbivores are most likely to be exposed to spores during grazing, and infection may occur via inhalation or ingestion.

B. cereus strains have been reported in multiple foods and are most often associated with rice and dairy products (184, 192). It is likely that the spores survive pasteurization and heating. They are also somewhat resistant to gamma-ray irradiation, which is used to reduce food pathogens. Spore hydrophobicity is thought to contribute to adherence to surfaces. In addition, biofilms of *B. cereus* are a recurrent problem in milk tanks at dairies (193–195).

B. anthracis germination in the nonhost environment

The lifestyle of *B. anthracis* in the nonhost environment is complex and somewhat controversial. Anthrax ecology is influenced by climate, but it is difficult to draw firm conclusions from various reports because of large variations in the timing and severity of outbreaks even within single ecosystems (109, 196, 197). Some studies suggest that spore germination in the soil can be triggered by alkaline pH, high organic content, moisture, and temperatures in excess of 15° C (177). Germination may also occur in response to components of exudates from grass plants. *B. anthracis*, *B. cereus*, and *B. thuringiensis* have been reported to germinate in the plant rhizosphere (198, 199). Cycles of germination, proliferation, and sporulation would ultimately result in amplification of the bacterium outside of its host. Yet it has been suggested that replication of *B. anthracis* vegetative cells in nonhost environments reduces virulence, possibly via loss of the virulence plasmid pXO2 that encodes the *B. anthracis* capsule. This plasmid, unlike the toxin-encoding plasmid pXO1, is unstable during growth in the absence of selection for the antiphagocytic property of the capsule (200). Moreover, it is likely, but has not been clearly demonstrated, that vegetative cells fall prey to other microbial species and protozoans in the soil (177).

B. anthracis and other *B. cereus* group species have been reported to germinate and replicate in response to factors excreted by the amoeba (188). The bacteria can colonize the surface of amoeba as microcolonies, resisting phagocytosis. At high amoeba densities, the bacteria form long filaments that cannot be ingested due to size exclusion. It has been proposed that these different cell morphologies may be significant not only outside of the host, but also during infection in the context of immune evasion (188).

Interestingly, genomic analyses indicate that *B. cereus* group species cannot efficiently utilize complex plant carbohydrates (201). Thus, in contrast to the common soil-borne nonpathogenic species *B. subtilis*, the *B. cereus* species appear to be adapted for use of animal-derived material. While the concept of *B. anthracis* germination in the soil is controversial, this difference in catabolism suggests that even in the event of germination in the nonhost environment, these species may proliferate to a lesser extent than the nonpathogenic *Bacillus* species.

Clostridium Species in the Nonhost Environment

A number of reports suggest that *Clostridium* species are ubiquitous in multiple nonhost environments, including soil and water close to urban areas (202). *C. perfringens* has been reported in wastewater treatment systems and can be isolated from animal intestinal tracts (5, 203). *C. botulinum* spores are found in animal carcasses and even algal mats, where accumulation of botulinum toxin is central to human disease occurrence (204). Multiple strains of *C. difficile*, including those associated with disease and those less commonly found in patients, have been isolated from water and sediments. The genetic diversity of *C. difficile* isolates found in close proximity and the complex network of their prophages have been suggested to contribute to the emergence of new strains in clinics (205).

The relative abundance of *C. difficile* spores in clinical settings is due in part to infected patients entering a "super-shedder" state in which high quantities of spores are released in feces. The spores can persist in these settings for extended periods (206). Therefore, measures to control and prevent *C. difficile* infection include enhanced compliance with cleaning and disinfection procedures. Decontamination protocols for patient rooms often include use of dilute hypochlorite solutions and other sporicidal products. Recently, ultraviolet light and hydrogen peroxide vapor systems have been introduced as "hands off" methods of disinfection (33). Nevertheless, there are few reports assessing the impact of these methods on *C. difficile* transmission.

IMPLICATIONS AND QUESTIONS

Sporulation as an Enabler of Pathogen Transmission

The ability of spores to resist diverse environmental stresses and to remain viable for extended periods in the absence of nutrients makes spores highly suited to the dissemination of disease. It is important to emphasize, however, that only a small number of spore-forming species are known to cause disease in humans or other animals. Most likely, the ability to form a spore was a relatively early event in the evolution of the *Firmicutes* (the phylum containing the *Bacillales* and *Clostridiales*), and only after their appearance did pathogenic lifestyles emerge for a subset of the spore-forming species. In those cases where survival in a host was beneficial, the resistance characteristics of spores may have provided the opportunity for rapid evolution of pathogenesis by, for example, acquisition of toxin genes. It is plausible that for a spore-forming species to acquire the ability to cause disease initially, the spore itself does not necessarily have to evolve, given its impressive resistance properties in most if not all species. Nonetheless, specific adaptations of spore structures that facilitate pathogenesis are possible, and their study remains an important open area of investigation. Regardless of whether the spore itself has adapted to facilitate disease, specific spore resistance properties and, therefore, specific spore structures must be considered in understanding the mechanistic basis of dissemination and infection by spores.

Spore–Vegetative Cell Interactions

Spore-forming bacteria are found in almost every environment where they have been sought. Given that the resistance properties of the spore are likely to have had a significant impact on survival in diverse niches, it is tempting to propose that spore formation is specifically an adaptation to the stresses of these environments. However, an important possible prediction of this view, that only spores, and not vegetative cells, would be found in the soil, is not borne out. The view that spores and vegetative cells coexist in the environment is suggested by analyses of biofilms in the pathogen *C. difficile* and the model spore-forming (and nonpathogenic) species *B. subtilis* (207, 208). In both species, spores are formed from vegetative cells as the biofilm matures, and both cell types are present in the biofilm for a significant period during biofilm development. Therefore, it is plausible that during an infection, both spores and vegetative cells are present in the host and that, in fact, the presence of both cell types contributes to survival in the host even when only the vegetative cell produces essential virulence factors such as toxins.

Gaps in Knowledge of the Ecology of Spore Formers

For pathogenic spore formers, increased understanding of the mechanisms for sporulation, germination, and interaction with non-host environments will facilitate development of strategies for more effective disease prevention and treatment. In particular, our poor understanding of the signals and pressures of the nonhost environment is directly related to the difficulty of establishing laboratory assays that authentically mimic natural environments. Further, the bio-complexity of the nonhost environment is likely to affect spore/cell viability and the developmental cycle. The nature of the mixed microbial communities and the threat of predation is another largely unknown area related to the lifestyles of spore formers outside of their host organisms. Development of a comprehensive understanding of the natural ecology of spore formers will enhance our understanding of these diverse developmental pathogens.

ACKNOWLEDGMENTS

This work was funded by NIH National Institute of Allergy and Infectious Diseases (NIAID) grants RO1 AI033537, RO1 AI093493, and R21 AI1097934.

CITATION

Swick MC, Koehler TM, Driks A. 2016. Surviving between hosts: sporulation and transmission. Microbiol Spectrum 4(2): VMBF-0029-2015.

REFERENCES

1. **Cardazzo B, Negrisolo E, Carraro L, Alberghini L, Patarnello T, Giaccone V.** 2008. Multiple-locus sequence typing and analysis of toxin genes in *Bacillus cereus* food-borne isolates. *Appl Environ Microbiol* **74**:850–860.

2. **Ash C, Farrow JA, Dorsch M, Stackebrandt E, Collins MD.** 1991. Comparative analysis of *Bacillus anthracis, Bacillus cereus*, and related species on the basis of reverse transcriptase sequencing of 16S rRNA. *Int J Syst Bacteriol* **41**:343–346.

3. **Helgason E, Caugant DA, Olsen I, Kolsto AB.** 2000. Genetic structure of population of *Bacillus cereus* and *B. thuringiensis* isolates associated with periodontitis and other human infections. *J Clin Microbiol* **38**:1615–1622.

4. **Helgason E, Tourasse NJ, Meisal R, Caugant DA, Kolsto AB.** 2004. Multilocus sequence typing scheme for bacteria of the *Bacillus cereus* group. *Appl Environ Microbiol* **70**:191–201.

5. **Drean P, McAuley CM, Moore SC, Fegan N, Fox EM.** 2015. Characterization of the spore-forming *Bacillus cereus* sensu lato group and *Clostridium perfringens* bacteria isolated from the Australian dairy farm environment. *BMC Microbiol* **15**:38.

6. **Guinebretiere MH, Auger S, Galleron N, Contzen M, De Sarrau B, De Buyser ML, Lamberet G, Fagerlund A, Granum PE, Lereclus D, De Vos P, Nguyen-The C, Sorokin A.** 2013. *Bacillus cytotoxicus* sp. nov. is a novel thermotolerant species of the *Bacillus cereus* group occasionally associated with food poisoning. *Int J Syst Evol Microbiol* **63**:31–40.

7. **Guinebretiere MH, Velge P, Couvert O, Carlin F, Debuyser ML, Nguyen-The C.** 2010. Ability of *Bacillus cereus* group strains to cause food poisoning varies according to phylogenetic affiliation (groups I to VII) rather than species affiliation. *J Clin Microbiol* **48**:3388–3391.

8. **Soufiane B, Cote JC.** 2009. Discrimination among *Bacillus thuringiensis* H serotypes, serovars and strains based on 16S rRNA, gyrB and aroE gene sequence analyses. *Antonie van Leeuwenhoek* **95**:33–45.

9. **Jensen GB, Hansen BM, Eilenberg J, Mahillon J.** 2003. The hidden lifestyles of *Bacillus cereus* and relatives. *Environ Microbiol* **5**:631–640.

10. **Tourasse NJ, Helgason E, Okstad OA, Hegna IK, Kolsto AB.** 2006. The *Bacillus cereus* group: novel aspects of population structure and genome dynamics. *J Appl Microbiol* **101**:579–593.

11. **Bengis RG, Frean J.** 2014. Anthrax as an example of the One Health concept. *Rev Sci Tech* **33**:593–604.

12. **Schnepf E, Crickmore N, Van Rie J, Lereclus D, Baum J, Feitelson J, Zeigler DR, Dean DH.** 1998. *Bacillus thuringiensis* and its pesticidal crystal proteins. *Microbiol Mol Biol Rev* **62**:775–806.

13. **van Frankenhuyzen K, Liu Y, Tonon A.** 2010. Interactions between *Bacillus thuringiensis* subsp. *kurstaki* HD-1 and midgut bacteria in larvae of gypsy moth and spruce budworm. *J Invertebr Pathol* **103**:124–131.

14. **Moayeri M, Leppla SH, Vrentas C, Pomerantsev AP, Liu S.** 2015. Anthrax pathogenesis. *Annu Rev Microbiol* **69**:185–208.

15. **Grunow R, Klee SR, Beyer W, George M, Grunow D, Barduhn A, Klar S, Jacob D, Elschner M, Sandven P, Kjerulf A, Jensen JS, Cai W, Zimmermann R, Schaade L.** 2013. Anthrax among heroin users in Europe possibly caused by same *Bacillus anthracis* strain since 2000. *Euro Surveill* **18**(13):pii=20437. http://www.eurosurveillance.org/ViewArticle.aspx?ArticleId=20437.

16. **Ringertz SH, Hoiby EA, Jensenius M, Maehlen J, Caugant DA, Myklebust A, Fossum K.** 2000. Injectional anthrax in a heroin skin-popper. *Lancet* **356**:1574–1575.

17. **Keim P, Gruendike JM, Klevytska AM, Schupp JM, Challacombe J, Okinaka R.** 2009. The genome and variation of *Bacillus anthracis*. *Mol Aspects Med* **30**:397–405.

18. **Liu S, Moayeri M, Leppla SH.** 2014. Anthrax lethal and edema toxins in anthrax pathogenesis. *Trends Microbiol* **22**:317–325.

19. **Lowe DE, Glomski IJ.** 2012. Cellular and physiological effects of anthrax exotoxin and its relevance to disease. *Front Cell Infect Microbiol* **2**:76.

20. **Jelacic TM, Chabot DJ, Bozue JA, Tobery SA, West MW, Moody K, Yang D, Oppenheim JJ, Friedlander AM.** 2014. Exposure to *Bacillus anthracis* capsule results in suppression of human monocyte-derived dendritic cells. *Infect Immun* **82**:3405–3416.

21. **Jeon JH, Lee HR, Cho MH, Park OK, Park J, Rhie GE.** 2015. The poly-gamma-d-glutamic acid capsule surrogate of the *Bacillus anthracis* capsule is a novel Toll-like receptor 2 agonist. *Infect Immun* **83**:3847–3856.

22. **Piris-Gimenez A, Corre JP, Jouvion G, Candela T, Khun H, Goossens PL.** 2009. Encapsulated *Bacillus anthracis* interacts closely with liver endothelium. *J Infect Dis* **200**:1381–1389.

23. **Soberon M, Gill SS, Bravo A.** 2009. Signaling versus punching hole: how do *Bacillus thuringiensis* toxins kill insect midgut cells? *Cell Mol Life Sci* **66:**1337–1349.

24. **Melo AL, Soccol VT, Soccol CR.** 2015. *Bacillus thuringiensis*: mechanism of action, resistance, and new applications: a review. *Crit Rev Biotechnol* **36:**317–326.

25. **Verplaetse E, Slamti L, Gohar M, Lereclus D.** 2015. Cell differentiation in a *Bacillus thuringiensis* population during planktonic growth, biofilm formation, and host infection. *MBio* **6:** e00138-15. doi:10.1128/mBio.00138-15.

26. **Hernandez E, Ramisse F, Ducoureau JP, Cruel T, Cavallo JD.** 1998. *Bacillus thuringiensis* subsp. *konkukian* (serotype H34) superinfection: case report and experimental evidence of pathogenicity in immunosuppressed mice. *J Clin Microbiol* **36:**2138–2139.

27. **Samples JR, Buettner H.** 1983. Corneal ulcer caused by a biologic insecticide (*Bacillus thuringiensis*). *Am J Ophthalmol* **95:**258–260.

28. **Celandroni F, Salvetti S, Senesi S, Ghelardi E.** 2014. *Bacillus thuringiensis* membrane-damaging toxins acting on mammalian cells. *FEMS Microbiol Lett* **361:**95–103.

29. **Arslan S, Eyi A, Kucuksari R.** 2014. Toxigenic genes, spoilage potential, and antimicrobial resistance of *Bacillus cereus* group strains from ice cream. *Anaerobe* **25:**42–46.

30. **Ehling-Schulz M, Fricker M, Scherer S.** 2004. *Bacillus cereus*, the causative agent of an emetic type of food-borne illness. *Mol Nutr Food Res* **48:**479–487.

31. **Yutin N, Galperin MY.** 2013. A genomic update on clostridial phylogeny: Gram-negative spore formers and other misplaced clostridia. *Environ Microbiol* **15:**2631–2641.

32. **Grass JE, Gould LH, Mahon BE.** 2013. Epidemiology of foodborne disease outbreaks caused by *Clostridium perfringens*, United States, 1998-2010. *Foodborne Pathog Dis* **10:**131–136.

33. **Barbut F.** 2015. How to eradicate *Clostridium difficile* from the environment. *J Hosp Infect* **89:**287–295.

34. **Aronoff DM.** 2013. *Clostridium novyi, sordellii*, and *tetani*: mechanisms of disease. *Anaerobe* **24:**98–101.

35. **Kelly CP, LaMont JT.** 2008. *Clostridium difficile*: more difficult than ever. *N Engl J Med* **359:** 1932–1940.

36. **Rupnik M, Wilcox MH, Gerding DN.** 2009. *Clostridium difficile* infection: new developments in epidemiology and pathogenesis. *Nat Rev Microbiol* **7:**526–536.

37. **Paredes-Sabja D, Shen A, Sorg JA.** 2014. *Clostridium difficile* spore biology: sporulation, germination, and spore structural proteins. *Trends Microbiol* **22:**406–416.

38. **Shields K, Araujo-Castillo RV, Theethira TG, Alonso CD, Kelly CP.** 2015. Recurrent *Clostridium difficile* infection: from colonization to cure. *Anaerobe* **34:**59–73.

39. **Kuehne SA, Cartman ST, Heap JT, Kelly ML, Cockayne A, Minton NP.** 2010. The role of toxin A and toxin B in *Clostridium difficile* infection. *Nature* **467:**711–713.

40. **Kuehne SA, Collery MM, Kelly ML, Cartman ST, Cockayne A, Minton NP.** 2014. Importance of toxin A, toxin B, and CDT in virulence of an epidemic *Clostridium difficile* strain. *J Infect Dis* **209:**83–86.

41. **Carter GP, Chakravorty A, Pham Nguyen TA, Mileto S, Schreiber F, Li L, Howarth P, Clare S, Cunningham B, Sambol SP, Cheknis A, Figueroa I, Johnson S, Gerding D, Rood JI, Dougan G, Lawley TD, Lyras D.** 2015. Defining the roles of TcdA and TcdB in localized gastrointestinal disease, systemic organ damage, and the host response during *Clostridium difficile* infections. *MBio* **6:**e00551-15. doi:10.1128/ mBio.00551-15.

42. **Stewart DB, Berg A, Hegarty J.** 2013. Predicting recurrence of *C. difficile* colitis using bacterial virulence factors: binary toxin is the key. *J Gastrointest Surg* **17:**118–124, discussion 124–115.

43. **Stevens DL, Aldape MJ, Bryant AE.** 2012. Life-threatening clostridial infections. *Anaerobe* **18:**254–259.

44. **Bryant AE, Stevens DL.** 2010. Clostridial myonecrosis: new insights in pathogenesis and management. *Curr Infect Dis Rep* **12:**383–391.

45. **Uzal FA, Freedman JC, Shrestha A, Theoret JR, Garcia J, Awad MM, Adams V, Moore RJ, Rood JI, McClane BA.** 2014. Towards an understanding of the role of *Clostridium perfringens* toxins in human and animal disease. *Future Microbiol* **9:**361–377.

46. **Fisher DJ, Fernandez-Miyakawa ME, Sayeed S, Poon R, Adams V, Rood JI, Uzal FA, McClane BA.** 2006. Dissecting the contributions of *Clostridium perfringens* type C toxins to lethality in the mouse intravenous injection model. *Infect Immun* **74:**5200–5210.

47. **Li J, Adams V, Bannam TL, Miyamoto K, Garcia JP, Uzal FA, Rood JI, McClane BA.** 2013. Toxin plasmids of *Clostridium perfringens*. *Microbiol Mol Biol Rev* **77:**208–233.

48. **Setlow P.** 2006. Spores of *Bacillus subtilis*: their resistance to and killing by radiation, heat and chemicals. *J Appl Microbiol* **101:**514–525.

49. **Nicholson WL, Munakata N, Horneck G, Melosh HJ, Setlow P.** 2000. Resistance of *Bacillus* endospores to extreme terrestrial and

extraterrestrial environments. *Microbiol Mol Biol Rev* **64:**548–572.

50. **Driks A.** 2002. Proteins of the spore core and coat, p 527–536. *In* Sonenshein AL, Hoch JA, Losick R (ed), *Bacillus subtilis and Its Closest Relatives.* ASM Press, Washington, DC.

51. **Setlow P.** 2003. Spore germination. *Curr Opin Microbiol* **6:**550–556.

52. **Knudsen SM, Cermak N, Feijo Delgado F, Setlow B, Setlow P, Manalis SR.** 2015. Water and small molecule permeation of dormant *Bacillus subtilis* spores. *J Bacteriol* **198:**168–177.

53. **Moir A.** 2006. How do spores germinate? *J Appl Microbiol* **101:**526–530.

54. **Francis MB, Allen CA, Shrestha R, Sorg JA.** 2013. Bile acid recognition by the *Clostridium difficile* germinant receptor, CspC, is important for establishing infection. *PLoS Pathog* **9:** e1003356. doi:10.1371/journal.ppat.1003356.

55. **Ross C, Abel-Santos E.** 2010. The Ger receptor family from sporulating bacteria. *Curr Issues Mol Biol* **12:**147–158.

56. **Cutting SM, Vander Horn PB.** 1990. *Molecular Biological Methods for Bacillus.* John Wiley & Sons, Chichester, United Kingdom.

57. **Aronson AI, Fitz-James P.** 1976. Structure and morphogenesis of the bacterial spore coat. *Bacteriol Rev* **40:**360–402.

58. **Holt SC, Leadbetter ER.** 1969. Comparative ultrastructure of selected aerobic spore-forming bacteria: a freeze-etching study. *Bacteriol Rev* **33:**346–378.

59. **Driks A.** 1999. The *Bacillus subtilis* spore coat. *Microbiol Mol Biol Rev* **63:**1–20.

60. **Giorno R, Bozue J, Cote C, Wenzel T, Moody K-S, Ryan M, Wang R, Zielke R, Maddock JM, Friedlander A, Welkos S, Driks A.** 2007. Morphogenesis of the *Bacillus anthracis* spore. *J Bacteriol* **189:**691–705.

61. **Henriques AO, Moran CP Jr.** 2000. Structure and assembly of the bacterial endospore coat. *Methods* **20:**95–110.

62. **Henriques AO, Costa TV, Martins LO, Zilhao R.** 2004. The functional architecture and assembly of the coat, p 65–86. *In* Ricca RE, Henriques AO, Cutting SM (ed), *Bacterial Spore Formers: Probiotics and Emerging Applications.* Horizon Biosciences, Norfolk, United Kingdom.

63. **Traag BA, Driks A, Stragier P, Bitter W, Broussard G, Hatfull G, Chu F, Adams KN, Ramakrishnan L, Losick R.** 2010. Do mycobacteria produce endospores? *Proc Natl Acad Sci USA* **107:**878–881.

64. **Driks A.** 2002. Maximum shields: the armor plating of the bacterial spore. *Trends Microbiol* **10:**251–254.

65. **Semenyuk EG, Laning ML, Foley J, Johnston PF, Knight KL, Gerding D, Driks A.** 2014. Spore formation and toxin production in *Clostridium difficile* biofilms. *PLoS One* **9:** e87757. doi:10.1371/journal.pone.0087757.

66. **McKenney PT, Driks A, Eichenberger P.** 2013. The *Bacillus subtilis* endospore: assembly and functions of the multilayered coat. *Nat Rev Microbiol* **11:**33–44.

67. **Kim H, Hahn M, Grabowski P, McPherson DC, Wang R, Ferguson C, Eichenberger P, Driks A.** 2006. The *Bacillus subtilis* spore coat protein interaction network. *Mol Microbiol* **59:**487–502.

68. **McKenney PT, Driks A, Eskandarian HA, Grabowski P, Guberman J, Wang KH, Gitai Z, Eichenberger P.** 2010. A distance-weighted interaction map reveals a previously uncharacterized layer of the *B. subtilis* spore coat. *Curr Biol* **29:**934–938.

69. **Henriques AO, Moran CP.** 2007. Structure, assembly and function of the spore surface layers. *Annu Rev Microbiol* **61:**555–588.

70. **Driks A.** 2003. The dynamic spore. *Proc Natl Acad Sci USA* **100:**3007–3009.

71. **Chada VG, Sanstad EA, Wang R, Driks A.** 2003. Morphogenesis of *Bacillus* spore surfaces. *J Bacteriol* **185:**6255–6261.

72. **Sahin O, Yong E-H, Driks A, Mahadevan L.** 2012. Physical basis for the adaptive flexibility of *Bacillus* spore coats. *J R Soc Interface* **9:**3156–3160.

73. **Westphal AJ, Price PB, Leighton TJ, Wheeler KE.** 2003. Kinetics of size changes of individual *Bacillus thuringiensis* spores in response to changes in relative humidity. *Proc Natl Acad Sci USA* **100:**3461–3466.

74. **Chen X, Goodnight D, Gao Z, Cavusoglu AH, Sabharwal N, DeLay M, Driks A, Sahin O.** 2015. Scaling up nanoscale water-driven energy conversion into evaporation-driven engines and generators. *Nat Commun* **6:**7346.

75. **Chen X, Mahadevan L, Driks A, Sahin O.** 2014. *Bacillus* spores as building blocks for stimuli-responsive materials and nanogenerators. *Nat Nanotechnol* **9:**137–141.

76. **Laaberki MH, Dworkin J.** 2008. Role of spore coat proteins in the resistance of *Bacillus subtilis* spores to *Caenorhabditis elegans* predation. *J Bacteriol* **190:**6197–6203.

77. **Klobutcher LA, Ragkousi K, Setlow P.** 2006. The *Bacillus subtilis* spore coat provides "eat resistance" during phagocytic predation by the protozoan *Tetrahymena thermophila. Proc Natl Acad Sci USA* **103:**165–170.

78. **Walker JR, Gnanam AJ, Blinkova AL, Hermandson MJ, Karymov MA, Lyubchenko**

YL, Graves PR, Haystead TA, Linse KD. 2007. *Clostridium taeniosporum* spore ribbon-like appendage structure, composition and genes. *Mol Microbiol* **63**:629–643.

79. **Driks A.** 2007. Surface appendages of bacterial spores. *Mol Microbiol* **63**:623–625.

80. **Qin H, Driks A.** 2013. Contrasting evolutionary patterns of spore coat proteins in two *Bacillus* species groups are linked to a difference in cellular structure. *BMC Evol Biol* **13**:261.

81. **Giorno R, Bozue J, Mallozzi M, Moody K-S, Slack A, Wang R, Friedlander A, Welkos S, Driks A.** 2009. Characterization of a *Bacillus anthracis* spore protein with roles in exosporium morphology. *Microbiology* **155**:1133–1145.

82. **Todd SJ, Moir AJ, Johnson MJ, Moir A.** 2003. Genes of *Bacillus cereus* and *Bacillus anthracis* encoding proteins of the exosporium. *J Bacteriol* **185**:3373–3378.

83. **Severson KM, Mallozzi M, Bozue J, Welkos SL, Cote CK, Knight KL, Driks A.** 2009. Roles of the *Bacillus anthracis* spore protein ExsK in exosporium maturation and germination. *J Bacteriol* **191**:7587–7596.

84. **Ball DA, Taylor R, Todd SJ, Redmond C, Couture-Tosi E, Sylvestre P, Moir A, Bullough PA.** 2008. Structure of the exosporium and sublayers of spores of the *Bacillus cereus* family revealed by electron crystallography. *Mol Microbiol* **68**:947–958.

85. **Kailas L, Terry C, Abbott N, Taylor R, Mullin N, Tzokov SB, Todd SJ, Wallace BA, Hobbs JK, Moir A, Bullough PA.** 2011. Surface architecture of endospores of the *Bacillus cereus/anthracis/thuringiensis* family at the sub-nanometer scale. *Proc Natl Acad Sci USA* **108**:16014–16019.

86. **Johnson MJ, Todd SJ, Ball DA, Shepherd AM, Sylvestre P, Moir A.** 2006. ExsY and CotY are required for the correct assembly of the exosporium and spore coat of *Bacillus cereus*. *J Bacteriol* **188**:7905–7913.

87. **Redmond C, Baille L, Hibbs S, Moir A, Charlton S.** 2001. Characterization of the exosporium of *Bacillus anthracis*. Abstract, 4th International Confernece on Anthrax, Annapolis, MD.

88. **Redmond C, Baillie LW, Hibbs S, Moir AJ, Moir A.** 2004. Identification of proteins in the exosporium of *Bacillus anthracis*. *Microbiology* **150**:355–563.

89. **Charlton S, Moir AJ, Baillie L, Moir A.** 1999. Characterization of the exosporium of *Bacillus cereus*. *J Appl Microbiol* **87**:241–245.

90. **Rodenburg CM, McPherson SA, Turnbough CL Jr, Dokland T.** 2014. Cryo-EM analysis of the organization of BclA and BxpB in the *Bacillus anthracis* exosporium. *J Struct Biol* **186**:181–187.

91. **Tan L, Turnbough CL Jr.** 2010. Sequence motifs and proteolytic cleavage of the collagen-like glycoprotein BclA required for its attachment to the exosporium of *Bacillus anthracis*. *J Bacteriol* **192**:1259–1268.

92. **Steichen C, Chen P, Kearney JF, Turnbough CL Jr.** 2003. Identification of the immunodominant protein and other proteins of the *Bacillus anthracis* exosporium. *J Bacteriol* **185**:1903–1910.

93. **Steichen CT, Kearney JF, Turnbough CL Jr.** 2005. Characterization of the exosporium basal layer protein BxpB of *Bacillus anthracis*. *J Bacteriol* **187**:5868–5876.

94. **Steichen CT, Kearney JF, Turnbough CL Jr.** 2007. Non-uniform assembly of the *Bacillus anthracis* exosporium and a bottle cap model for spore germination and outgrowth. *Mol Microbiol* **64**:359–367.

95. **Boydston JA, Chen P, Steichen CT, Turnbough CL Jr.** 2005. Orientation within the exosporium and structural stability of the collagen-like glycoprotein BclA of *Bacillus anthracis*. *J Bacteriol* **187**:5310–5317.

96. **Boydston JA, Yue L, Kearney JF, Turnbough CL Jr.** 2006. The ExsY protein is required for complete formation of the exosporium of *Bacillus anthracis*. *J Bacteriol* **188**:7440–7448.

97. **Weaver J, Kang TJ, Raines KW, Cao GL, Hibbs S, Tsai P, Baillie L, Rosen GM, Cross AS.** 2007. Protective role of *Bacillus anthracis* exosporium in macrophage-mediated killing by nitric oxide. *Infect Immun* **75**:3894–3901.

98. **Liang L, He X, Liu G, Tan H.** 2008. The role of a purine-specific nucleoside hydrolase in spore germination of *Bacillus thuringiensis*. *Microbiology* **154**:1333–1340.

99. **Chesnokova ON, McPherson SA, Steichen CT, Turnbough CL Jr.** 2009. The spore-specific alanine racemase of *Bacillus anthracis* and its role in suppressing germination during spore development. *J Bacteriol* **191**:1303–1310.

100. **Brahmbhatt TN, Janes BK, Stibitz ES, Darnell SC, Sanz P, Rasmussen SB, O'Brien AD.** 2007. *Bacillus anthracis* exosporium protein BclA affects spore germination, interaction with extracellular matrix proteins, and hydrophobicity. *Infect Immun* **75**:5233–5239.

101. **Bozue J, Moody KL, Cote CK, Stiles BG, Friedlander AM, Welkos SL, Hale ML.** 2007. *Bacillus anthracis* spores of the *bclA* mutant exhibit increased adherence to epithelial cells, fibroblasts, and endothelial cells but not to macrophages. *Infect Immun* **75**:4498–4505.

102. **Oliva C, Turnbough CL Jr, Kearney JF.** 2009. CD14-Mac-1 interactions in *Bacillus*

anthracis spore internalization by macrophages. *Proc Natl Acad Sci USA* **106**:13957–13962.

103. **Oliva CR, Swiecki MK, Griguer CE, Lisanby MW, Bullard DC, Turnbough CL Jr, Kearney JF.** 2008. The integrin Mac-1 (CR3) mediates internalization and directs *Bacillus anthracis* spores into professional phagocytes. *Proc Natl Acad Sci USA* **105**:1261–1266.

104. **Hong HA, Khaneja R, Tam NM, Cazzato A, Tan S, Urdaci M, Brisson A, Gasbarrini A, Barnes I, Cutting SM.** 2009. *Bacillus subtilis* isolated from the human gastrointestinal tract. *Res Microbiol* **160**:134–143.

105. **Chen G, Driks A, Tawfiq K, Mallozzi M, Patil S.** 2010. *Bacillus anthracis* and *Bacillus subtilis* spore surface properties as analyzed by transport analysis. *Colloids Surf B Biointerfaces* **76**:512–518.

106. **Grossman AD.** 1995. Genetic networks controlling the initiation of sporulation and the development of genetic competence in *Bacillus subtilis*. *Annu Rev Genet* **29**:477–508.

107. **Hoch JA.** 1993. Regulation of the phosphorelay and the initiation of sporulation in *Bacillus subtilis*. *Annu Rev Microbiol* **47**:441–465.

108. **van Gestel J, Vlamakis H, Kolter R.** 2015. Division of labor in biofilms: the ecology of cell differentiation. *Microbiol Spectr* **3**:MB-0002-2014. doi:10.1128/microbiolspec.MB-0002-2014.

109. **Hugh-Jones M, Blackburn J.** 2009. The ecology of *Bacillus anthracis*. *Mol Aspects Med* **30**:356–367.

110. **Perego M, Hoch JA.** 2008. Commingling regulatory systems following acquisition of virulence plasmids by *Bacillus anthracis*. *Trends Microbiol* **16**:215–221.

111. **Brunsing RL, La Clair C, Tang S, Chiang C, Hancock LE, Perego M, Hoch JA.** 2005. Characterization of sporulation histidine kinases of *Bacillus anthracis*. *J Bacteriol* **187**:6972–6981.

112. **Bongiorni C, Stoessel R, Shoemaker D, Perego M.** 2006. Rap phosphatase of virulence plasmid pXO1 inhibits *Bacillus anthracis* sporulation. *J Bacteriol* **188**:487–498.

113. **White AK, Hoch JA, Grynberg M, Godzik A, Perego M.** 2006. Sensor domains encoded in *Bacillus anthracis* virulence plasmids prevent sporulation by hijacking a sporulation sensor histidine kinase. *J Bacteriol* **188**:6354–6360.

114. **Edwards AN, McBride SM.** 2014. Initiation of sporulation in *Clostridium difficile*: a twist on the classic model. *FEMS Microbiol Lett* **358**:110–118.

115. **Edwards AN, Nawrocki KL, McBride SM.** 2014. Conserved oligopeptide permeases modulate sporulation initiation in *Clostridium difficile*. *Infect Immun* **82**:4276–4291.

116. **Aronson A.** 2002. Sporulation and delta-endotoxin synthesis by *Bacillus thuringiensis*. *Cell Mol Life Sci* **59**:417–425.

117. **Debro L, Fitz-James PC, Aronson A.** 1986. Two different parasporal inclusions are produced by *Bacillus thuringiensis* subsp. finitimus. *J Bacteriol* **165**:258–268.

118. **Ammons DR, Reyna A, Granados JC, Ventura-Suarez A, Rojas-Avelizapa LI, Short JD, Rampersad JN.** 2013. A novel *Bacillus thuringiensis* Cry-like protein from a rare filamentous strain promotes crystal localization within the exosporium. *Appl Environ Microbiol* **79**:5774–5776.

119. **Chai PF, Rathinam X, Solayappan M, Ahmad Ghazali AH, Subramaniam S.** 2014. Microscopic analysis of a native *Bacillus thuringiensis* strain from Malaysia that produces exosporium-enclosed parasporal inclusion. *Microscopy (Oxf)* **63**:371–375.

120. **Dubois T, Faegri K, Perchat S, Lemy C, Buisson C, Nielsen-LeRoux C, Gohar M, Jacques P, Ramarao N, Kolsto AB, Lereclus D.** 2012. Necrotrophism is a quorum-sensing-regulated lifestyle in *Bacillus thuringiensis*. *PLoS Pathog* **8**:e1002629. doi:10.1371/journal.ppat.1002629.

121. **Fisher N, Carr KA, Giebel JD, Hanna PC.** 2011. *Anthrax Spore Germination*. John Wiley & Sons, Hoboken, NJ.

122. **Fisher N, Hanna P.** 2005. Characterization of *Bacillus anthracis* germinant receptors *in vitro*. *J Bacteriol* **187**:8055–8062.

123. **Francis MB, Allen CA, Sorg JA.** 2015. Spore cortex hydrolysis precedes dipicolinic acid release during *Clostridium difficile* spore germination. *J Bacteriol* **197**:2276–2283.

124. **Ireland JA, Hanna PC.** 2002. Amino acid- and purine ribonucleoside-induced germination of *Bacillus anthracis* DeltaSterne endospores: gerS mediates responses to aromatic ring structures. *J Bacteriol* **184**:1296–1303.

125. **Weiner MA, Hanna PC.** 2003. Macrophage-mediated germination of *Bacillus anthracis* endospores requires the gerH operon. *Infect Immun* **71**:3954–3959.

126. **Yi X, Setlow P.** 2010. Studies of the commitment step in the germination of spores of *Bacillus* species. *J Bacteriol* **192**:3424–3433.

127. **Atluri S, Ragkousi K, Cortezzo DE, Setlow P.** 2006. Cooperativity between different nutrient receptors in germination of spores of *Bacillus subtilis* and reduction of this cooperativity by alterations in the GerB receptor. *J Bacteriol* **188**:28–36.

128. **Bergman NH, Anderson EC, Swenson EE, Niemeyer MM, Miyoshi AD, Hanna PC.**

2006. Transcriptional profiling of the *Bacillus anthracis* life cycle *in vitro* and an implied model for regulation of spore formation. *J Bacteriol* **188:**6092–6100.

129. **Griffiths KK, Zhang J, Cowan AE, Yu J, Setlow P.** 2011. Germination proteins in the inner membrane of dormant *Bacillus subtilis* spores colocalize in a discrete cluster. *Mol Microbiol* **81:**1061–1077.

130. **Behravan J, Chirakkal H, Masson A, Moir A.** 2000. Mutations in the gerP locus of *Bacillus subtilis* and *Bacillus cereus* affect access of germinants to their targets in spores. *J Bacteriol* **182:**1987–1994.

131. **Kroos L, Kunkel B, Losick R.** 1989. Switch protein alters specificity of RNA polymerase containing a compartment-specific sigma factor. *Science* **243:**526–529.

132. **Read TD, Peterson SN, Tourasse N, Baillie LW, Paulsen IT, Nelson KE, Tettelin H, Fouts DE, Eisen JA, Gill SR, Holtzapple EK, Okstad OA, Helgason E, Rilstone J, Wu M, Kolonay JF, Beanan MJ, Dodson RJ, Brinkac LM, Gwinn M, DeBoy RT, Madpu R, Daugherty SC, Durkin AS, Haft DH, Nelson WC, Peterson JD, Pop M, Khouri HM, Radune D, Benton JL, Mahamoud Y, Jiang L, Hance IR, Weidman JF, Berry KJ, Plaut RD, Wolf AM, Watkins KL, Nierman WC, Hazen A, Cline R, Redmond C, Thwaite JE, White O, Salzberg SL, Thomason B, Friedlander AM, Koehler TM, Hanna PC, Kolstø AB, Fraser CM.** 2003. The genome sequence of *Bacillus anthracis* Ames and comparison to closely related bacteria. *Nature* **423:**81–86.

133. **Paidhungat M, Ragkousi K, Setlow P.** 2001. Genetic requirements for induction of germination of spores of *Bacillus subtilis* by Ca(2+)-dipicolinate. *J Bacteriol* **183:**4886–4893.

134. **Christie G, Gotzke H, Lowe CR.** 2010. Identification of a receptor subunit and putative ligand-binding residues involved in the *Bacillus megaterium* QM B1551 spore germination response to glucose. *J Bacteriol* **192:**4317–4326.

135. **Mongkolthanaruk W, Cooper GR, Mawer JS, Allan RN, Moir A.** 2011. Effect of amino acid substitutions in the GerAA protein on the function of the alanine-responsive germinant receptor of *Bacillus subtilis* spores. *J Bacteriol* **193:**2268–2275.

136. **Guidi-Rontani C, Pereira Y, Ruffie S, Sirard JC, Weber-Levy M, Mock M.** 1999. Identification and characterization of a germination operon on the virulence plasmid pXO1 of *Bacillus anthracis*. *Mol Microbiol* **33:**407–414.

137. **McKevitt MT, Bryant KM, Shakir SM, Larabee JL, Blanke SR, Lovchik J, Lyons CR, Ballard JD.** 2007. Effects of endogenous

D-alanine synthesis and autoinhibition of *Bacillus anthracis* germination on *in vitro* and *in vivo* infections. *Infect Immun* **75:**5726–5734.

138. **Shah IM, Laaberki MH, Popham DL, Dworkin J.** 2008. A eukaryotic-like Ser/Thr kinase signals bacteria to exit dormancy in response to peptidoglycan fragments. *Cell* **135:**486–496.

139. **Sorg JA, Sonenshein AL.** 2008. Bile salts and glycine as cogerminants for *Clostridium difficile* spores. *J Bacteriol* **190:**2505–2512.

140. **Ridlon JM, Kang DJ, Hylemon PB.** 2006. Bile salt biotransformations by human intestinal bacteria. *J Lipid Res* **47:**241–259.

141. **Howerton A, Ramirez N, Abel-Santos E.** 2011. Mapping interactions between germinants and *Clostridium difficile* spores. *J Bacteriol* **193:**274–282.

142. **Wheeldon LJ, Worthington T, Lambert PA.** 2011. Histidine acts as a co-germinant with glycine and taurocholate for *Clostridium difficile* spores. *J Appl Microbiol* **110:**987–994.

143. **Sorg JA, Sonenshein AL.** 2009. Chenodeoxycholate is an inhibitor of *Clostridium difficile* spore germination. *J Bacteriol* **191:**1115–1117.

144. **Foster SJ, Johnstone K.** 1986. The use of inhibitors to identify early events during *Bacillus megaterium* KM spore germination. *Biochem J* **237:**865–870.

145. **Stewart GS, Johnstone K, Hagelberg E, Ellar DJ.** 1981. Commitment of bacterial spores to germinate. A measure of the trigger reaction. *Biochem J* **198:**101–106.

146. **Venkatasubramanian P, Johnstone K.** 1989. Biochemical analysis of the *Bacillus subtilis* 1604 spore germination response. *J Gen Microbiol* **135:**2723–2733.

147. **Wang S, Shen A, Setlow P, Li YQ.** 2015. Characterization of the dynamic germination of individual *Clostridium difficile* spores using Raman spectroscopy and differential interference contrast microscopy. *J Bacteriol* **197:**2361–2373.

148. **Ghosh S, Setlow P.** 2009. Isolation and characterization of superdormant spores of *Bacillus* species. *J Bacteriol* **191:**1787–1797.

149. **Yi X, Liu J, Faeder JR, Setlow P.** 2011. Synergism between different germinant receptors in the germination of *Bacillus subtilis* spores. *J Bacteriol* **193:**4664–4671.

150. **Chen Y, Ray WK, Helm RF, Melville SB, Popham DL.** 2014. Levels of germination proteins in *Bacillus subtilis* dormant, superdormant, and germinating spores. *PLoS One* **9:**e95781. doi:10.1371/journal.pone.0095781.

151. **Setlow P.** 2013. When the sleepers wake: the germination of spores of *Bacillus* species. *J Appl Microbiol* **115:**1251–1268.

152. **Setlow P.** 2014. Germination of spores of *Bacillus* species: what we know and do not know. *J Bacteriol* **196**:1297–1305.

153. **Heffron JD, Orsburn B, Popham DL.** 2009. Roles of germination-specific lytic enzymes CwlJ and SleB in *Bacillus anthracis. J Bacteriol* **191**:2237–2247.

154. **Boland FM, Atrih A, Chirakkal H, Foster SJ, Moir A.** 2000. Complete spore-cortex hydrolysis during germination of *Bacillus subtilis* 168 requires SleB and YpeB. *Microbiology* **146**(Pt 1):57–64.

155. **Bagyan I, Setlow P.** 2002. Localization of the cortex lytic enzyme CwlJ in spores of *Bacillus subtilis. J Bacteriol* **184**:1219–1224.

156. **Chirakkal H, O'Rourke M, Atrih A, Foster SJ, Moir A.** 2002. Analysis of spore cortex lytic enzymes and related proteins in *Bacillus subtilis* endospore germination. *Microbiology* **148**:2383–2392.

157. **Li Y, Butzin XY, Davis A, Setlow B, Korza G, Ustok FI, Christie G, Setlow P, Hao B.** 2013. Activity and regulation of various forms of CwlJ, SleB, and YpeB proteins in degrading cortex peptidoglycan of spores of *Bacillus* species *in vitro* and during spore germination. *J Bacteriol* **195**:2530–2540.

158. **Ragkousi K, Eichenberger P, van Ooij C, Setlow P.** 2003. Identification of a new gene essential for germination of Bacillus subtilis spores with Ca2+-dipicolinate. *J Bacteriol* **185**:2315–2329.

159. **Giebel JD, Carr KA, Anderson EC, Hanna PC.** 2009. The germination-specific lytic enzymes SleB, CwlJ1, and CwlJ2 each contribute to *Bacillus anthracis* spore germination and virulence. *J Bacteriol* **191**:5569–5576.

160. **Adams CM, Eckenroth BE, Putnam EE, Doublie S, Shen A.** 2013. Structural and functional analysis of the CspB protease required for *Clostridium* spore germination. *PLoS Pathog* **9**: e1003165. doi:10.1371/journal.ppat.1003165.

161. **Koch R.** 1881. *On the Etiology of Anthrax.* Greenwood Press, New York, New York.

162. **Koch R.** 1881. Mitt. *Kaisserliche Gesundheitsamte* **1**:174–206.

163. **Ross J.** 1957. The pathogenesis of anthrax following the administration of spores by the respiratory route. *J Pathol Bacteriol* **73**:485–494.

164. **Cleret A, Quesnel-Hellmann A, Vallon-Eberhard A, Verrier B, Jung S, Vidal D, Mathieu J, Tournier JN.** 2007. Lung dendritic cells rapidly mediate anthrax spore entry through the pulmonary route. *J Immunol* **178**:7994–8001.

165. **Sanz P, Teel LD, Alem F, Carvalho HM, Darnell SC, O'Brien AD.** 2008. Detection of *Bacillus anthracis* spore germination *in vivo* by bioluminescence imaging. *Infect Immun* **76**:1036–1047.

166. **Cote CK, Van Rooijen N, Welkos SL.** 2006. Roles of macrophages and neutrophils in the early host response to *Bacillus anthracis* spores in a mouse model of infection. *Infect Immun* **74**:469–480.

167. **Plaut RD, Kelly VK, Lee GM, Stibitz S, Merkel TJ.** 2012. Dissemination bottleneck in a murine model of inhalational anthrax. *Infect Immun* **80**:3189–3193.

168. **Lowe DE, Ernst SM, Zito C, Ya J, Glomski IJ.** 2013. *Bacillus anthracis* has two independent bottlenecks that are dependent on the portal of entry in an intranasal model of inhalational infection. *Infect Immun* **81**:4408–4420.

169. **Theriot CM, Koenigsknecht MJ, Carlson PE Jr, Hatton GE, Nelson AM, Li B, Huffnagle GB, Li JZ, Young VB.** 2014. Antibiotic-induced shifts in the mouse gut microbiome and metabolome increase susceptibility to *Clostridium difficile* infection. *Nat Commun* **5**:3114.

170. **Theriot CM, Young VB.** 2015. Interactions between the gastrointestinal microbiome and *Clostridium difficile. Annu Rev Microbiol* **69**:445–461.

171. **Bowman KA, Broussard EK, Surawicz CM.** 2015. Fecal microbiota transplantation: current clinical efficacy and future prospects. *Clin Exp Gastroenterol* **8**:285–291.

172. **Deakin LJ, Clare S, Fagan RP, Dawson LF, Pickard DJ, West MR, Wren BW, Fairweather NF, Dougan G, Lawley TD.** 2012. The *Clostridium difficile* spo0A gene is a persistence and transmission factor. *Infect Immun* **80**:2704–2711.

173. **Jump RL, Pultz MJ, Donskey CJ.** 2007. Vegetative *Clostridium difficile* survives in room air on moist surfaces and in gastric contents with reduced acidity: a potential mechanism to explain the association between proton pump inhibitors and *C. difficile*-associated diarrhea? *Antimicrob Agents Chemother* **51**:2883–2887.

174. **Roth NG, Livery DH, Hodge HM.** 1955. Influence of oxygen uptake and age of culture on sporulation of *Bacillus anthracis* and *Bacillus globigii. J Bacteriol* **69**:455–459.

175. **Mignot T, Mock M, Robichon D, Landier A, Lereclus D, Fouet A.** 2001. The incompatibility between the PlcR- and AtxA-controlled regulons may have selected a nonsense mutation in *Bacillus anthracis. Mol Microbiol* **42**:1189–1198.

176. **Goel AK.** 2015. Anthrax: a disease of biowarfare and public health importance. *World J Clin Cases* **3**:20–33.

177. **Dragon DC, Rennie RP.** 1995. The ecology of anthrax spores: tough but not invincible. *Can Vet J* **36:**295–301.

178. **Dutz W, Kohout-Dutz E.** 1981. Anthrax. *Int J Dermatol* **20:**203–206.

179. **Baines SD, O'Connor R, Saxton K, Freeman J, Wilcox MH.** 2009. Activity of vancomycin against epidemic *Clostridium difficile* strains in a human gut model. *J Antimicrob Chemother* **63:**520–525.

180. **Ali S, Moore G, Wilson AP.** 2011. Spread and persistence of *Clostridium difficile* spores during and after cleaning with sporicidal disinfectants. *J Hosp Infect* **79:**97–98.

181. **Andersson A, Ronner U, Granum PE.** 1995. What problems does the food industry have with the spore-forming pathogens *Bacillus cereus* and *Clostridium perfringens*? *Int J Food Microbiol* **28:**145–155.

182. **Barbosa TM, Serra CR, La Ragione RM, Woodward MJ, Henriques AO.** 2005. Screening for *Bacillus* isolates in the broiler gastrointestinal tract. *Appl Environ Microbiol* **71:**968–978.

183. **Jones TO, Turnbull PC.** 1981. Bovine mastitis caused by *Bacillus cereus*. *Vet Record* **108:**271–274.

184. **McAuley CM, McMillan K, Moore SC, Fegan N, Fox EM.** 2014. Prevalence and characterization of foodborne pathogens from Australian dairy farm environments. *J Dairy Sci* **97:**7402–7412.

185. **Nfor NN, Lapin CN, McLaughlin RW.** 2015. Isolation of *Bacillus cereus* group from the fecal material of endangered wood turtles. *Curr Microbiol* **71:**524–527.

186. **Feinberg L, Jorgensen J, Haselton A, Pitt A, Rudner R, Margulis L.** 1999. Arthromitus (*Bacillus cereus*) symbionts in the cockroach *Blaberus giganteus*: dietary influences on bacterial development and population density. *Symbiosis* **27:**109–123.

187. **Margulis L, Jorgensen JZ, Dolan S, Kolchinsky R, Rainey FA, Lo SC.** 1998. The *Arthromitus* stage of *Bacillus cereus*: intestinal symbionts of animals. *Proc Natl Acad Sci USA* **95:**1236–1241.

188. **Beeton ML, Atkinson DJ, Waterfield NR.** 2013. An amoeba phagocytosis model reveals a novel developmental switch in the insect pathogen *Bacillus thuringiensis*. *J Insect Physiol* **59:**223–231.

189. **Turnbull PC.** 2002. Introduction: anthrax history, disease and ecology. *Curr Topics Microbiol Immunol* **271:**1–19.

190. **Bradaric N, Punda-Polic V.** 1992. Cutaneous anthrax due to penicillin-resistant *Bacillus anthracis* transmitted by an insect bite. *Lancet* **340:**306–307.

191. **Turell MJ, Knudson GB.** 1987. Mechanical transmission of *Bacillus anthracis* by stable flies (*Stomoxys calcitrans*) and mosquitoes (*Aedes aegypti* and *Aedes taeniorhynchus*). *Infect Immun* **55:**1859–1861.

192. **Martinez-Blanch JF, Sanchez G, Garay E, Aznar R.** 2009. Development of a real-time PCR assay for detection and quantification of enterotoxigenic members of *Bacillus cereus* group in food samples. *Int J Food Microbiol* **135:**15–21.

193. **Christiansson A, Bertilsson J, Svensson B.** 1999. *Bacillus cereus* spores in raw milk: factors affecting the contamination of milk during the grazing period. *J Dairy Sci* **82:**305–314.

194. **Vissers MM, Te Giffel MC, Driehuis F, De Jong P, Lankveld JM.** 2007. Minimizing the level of *Bacillus cereus* spores in farm tank milk. *J Dairy Sci* **90:**3286–3293.

195. **Zottola EA, Sasahara KC.** 1994. Microbial biofilms in the food processing industry: should they be a concern? *Int J Food Microbiol* **23:**125–148.

196. **Blackburn JK, McNyset KM, Curtis A, Hugh-Jones ME.** 2007. Modeling the geographic distribution of *Bacillus anthracis*, the causative agent of anthrax disease, for the contiguous United States using predictive ecological [corrected] niche modeling. *Am J Trop Med Hyg* **77:**1103–1110.

197. **Hampson K, Lembo T, Bessell P, Auty H, Packer C, Halliday J, Beesley CA, Fyumagwa R, Hoare R, Ernest E, Mentzel C, Metzger KL, Mlengeya T, Stamey K, Roberts K, Wilkins PP, Cleaveland S.** 2011. Predictability of anthrax infection in the Serengeti, Tanzania. *J Appl Ecol* **48:**1333–1344.

198. **Halverson LJ, Clayton MK, Handelsman J.** 1993. Variable stability of antibiotic-resistance markers in *Bacillus cereus* UW85 in the soybean rhizosphere in the field. *Mol Ecol* **2:**65–78.

199. **Saile E, Koehler TM.** 2006. *Bacillus anthracis* multiplication, persistence, and genetic exchange in the rhizosphere of grass plants. *Appl Environ Microbiol* **72:**3168–3174.

200. **Green BD, Battisti L, Koehler TM, Thorne CB, Ivins BE.** 1985. Demonstration of a capsule plasmid in *Bacillus anthracis*. *Infect Immun* **49:**291–297.

201. **Ivanova N, Sorokin A, Anderson I, Galleron N, Candelon B, Kapatral V, Bhattacharyya A, Reznik G, Mikhailova N, Lapidus A, Chu L, Mazur M, Goltsman E, Larsen N, D'Souza M, Walunas T, Grechkin Y, Pusch G, Haselkorn R, Fonstein M, Ehrlich SD, Overbeek R, Kyrpides N.** 2003. Genome sequence of *Bacillus cereus* and comparative analysis with *Bacillus anthracis*. *Nature* **423:**87–91.

202. **Marcheggiani S, D'Ugo E, Puccinelli C, Giuseppetti R, D'Angelo AM, Gualerzi CO, Spurio R, Medlin LK, Guillebault D, Weigel W, Helmi K, Mancini L.** 2015. Detection of emerging and re-emerging pathogens in surface waters close to an urban area. *Int J Environ Res Public Health* **12:**5505–5527.

203. **Schneeberger CL, O'Driscoll M, Humphrey C, Henry K, Deal N, Seiber K, Hill VR, Zarate-Bermudez M.** 2015. Fate and transport of enteric microbes from septic systems in a coastal watershed. *J Environ Health* **77:**22–30.

204. **Espelund M, Klaveness D.** 2014. Botulism outbreaks in natural environments: an update. *Front Microbiol* **5:**287.

205. **Hargreaves KR, Clokie MR.** 2015. A taxonomic review of *Clostridium difficile* phages and proposal of a novel genus, "Phimmp04likevirus". *Viruses* **7:**2534–2541.

206. **Gerding DN, Muto CA, Owens RC Jr.** 2008. Measures to control and prevent *Clostridium difficile* infection. *Clin Infect Dis* **46**(Suppl 1): S43–S49.

207. **Cairns LS, Hobley L, Stanley-Wall NR.** 2014. Biofilm formation by *Bacillus subtilis*: new insights into regulatory strategies and assembly mechanisms. *Mol Microbiol* **93:**587–598.

208. **Pantaleon V, Bouttier S, Soavelomandroso AP, Janoir C, Candela T.** 2014. Biofilms of *Clostridium* species. *Anaerobe* **30:**193–198.

Staying Alive: *Vibrio cholerae's* Cycle of Environmental Survival, Transmission, and Dissemination

21

JENNA G. CONNER,[1] JENNIFER K. TESCHLER,[1] CHRISTOPHER J. JONES,[1] and FITNAT H. YILDIZ[1]

INTRODUCTION

Vibrio cholerae causes 3 to 5 million cases of cholera annually, resulting in 100,000 to 120,000 deaths (1, 2). Infection occurs through the ingestion of contaminated water or food, primarily impacting regions that lack adequate sanitation and clean drinking water (3, 4). The disease is characterized by watery diarrhea and rapid dehydration, which, if untreated, can lead to hypotonic shock and death within 12 hours of the first symptoms (3, 4). Large outbreaks of the disease have occurred throughout the past two centuries, including several recent epidemics in Haiti, Vietnam, and Zimbabwe (5–7). Annual seasonal outbreaks also occur in many areas of the world where cholera is endemic, including countries in Asia, Africa, and the Americas, due to the ability of toxigenic *V. cholerae* to survive in the aquatic environment year-round (8, 9). The timing and severity of seasonal outbreaks vary depending on a number of environmental factors, including rainfall, salinity, temperature, and plankton blooms (10).

Transmission between individuals within the same household is common, and the spread of cholera during outbreaks is often exacerbated in highly

[1]Microbiology and Environmental Toxicology, University of California Santa Cruz, Santa Cruz, CA 95064.
Virulence Mechanisms of Bacterial Pathogens, 5th edition
Edited by Indira T. Kudva, Nancy A. Cornick, Paul J. Plummer, Qijing Zhang, Tracy L. Nicholson, John P. Bannantine, and Bryan H. Bellaire
© 2016 American Society for Microbiology, Washington, DC
doi:10.1128/microbiolspec.VMBF-0015-2015

populated areas with poor infrastructure (11). High bacterial loads of *V. cholerae* are shed in the stool of infected patients and exhibit a hyperinfective phenotype that can contribute to the aggressive nature of an epidemic (12). Intriguingly, not all individuals infected with pathogenic *V. cholerae* exhibit symptoms of cholera, and several host factors appear to impact immunity to cholera. Both retinol deficiency and blood type O have been associated with an increased susceptibility to infection (13–18). Independent of blood type, higher transmission rates of cholera are observed between first-degree relatives than between less closely related contacts living in the same household, indicating that additional genetic factors play a role in the susceptibility to cholera (14). Additionally, while cholera infections can occur across all age groups, there are disproportionately high incidences and mortalities in children under the age of 5 (2). Continued study of both the ecological and human dynamics influencing *V. cholerae* outbreaks and infectivity is essential to our understanding of cholera dissemination and transmission.

V. cholerae strains are classified into serogroups based on the structure of their cell surface lipopolysaccharides. Of the over 200 known serogroups of *V. cholerae*, only the O1 and O139 serotypes can produce the cholera toxin and cause pandemic cholera (3). The O1 serotype is further classified into the classical and El Tor biotypes based on a number of phenotypic differences, including their susceptibility to polymyxin B and phage infection (3, 9). Since 1817 there have been seven recorded cholera pandemics, the first six of which were most likely caused by the classical biotype. The El Tor biotype displaced the classical biotype as the predominant epidemic strain in 1961 and is responsible for the longest and most severe seventh pandemic, which continues today (19). After its initial appearance in 1992, the O139 serogroup temporarily displaced the El Tor biotype in India and Bangladesh before it was displaced by a new El Tor strain in 1994

(20). This serogroup switching occurred several times over the past decade in cholera-endemic regions, suggesting that acquired immunity plays an important role in the emergence of specific serogroups. It additionally suggests that rapid evolution and genetic rearrangement of O1 and O139 strains contribute to the persistence and reemergence of this disease (19, 21). New pathogenic variants of *V. cholerae* that have emerged in recent years have characteristics of both the classical and El Tor strains. These are termed altered or atypical El Tor and include the Matlab variants from Bangladesh, the Mozambique variants, the recent Haitian variants, as well as a number of additional atypical El Tor variants from around the world (22).

Historically, the El Tor strains are credited with having greater environmental fitness than the classical strains, while the classical strains are considered to induce a more severe form of cholera than the El Tor strains (3, 9). Genetic analysis of *V. cholerae* El Tor variants revealed the conservation of a predominately El Tor genomic backbone containing multiple genomic islands that match the classical strain, confirming that they are genetic hybrids (23). El Tor variants appear to combine the environmental fitness of El Tor strains and the higher infectivity of classical strains and are associated with increased ecological persistence, infectivity, disease severity, and dispersion worldwide (19, 23–26). As *V. cholerae* strains continue to adapt and evolve, understanding the underlying factors that contribute to enhanced environmental persistence and increased transmission will be essential to our ability to predict outbreaks and establish preventative measures.

V. cholerae is an ideal model environmental pathogen for understanding the cycle of environmental survival, transmission, and dissemination of bacterial pathogens between hosts. In this chapter, we describe *V. cholerae* strategies that impact environmental survival, as well as the environmental conditions that contribute to the initiation of an outbreak. We then describe the molecular and physiological responses *V. cholerae* undergoes during its initial transmission into the human host and during late-stage infection in preparation for dissemination. The ability of *V. cholerae* to transition between the human host and the aquatic environment is essential for the explosive waterborne spread of cholera during outbreaks, as well as the persistence of *V. cholerae* in endemic areas during nonepidemic periods.

MECHANISMS OF ENVIRONMENTAL SURVIVAL AND FACTORS INFLUENCING OUTBREAKS

V. cholerae is considered an environmental pathogen, because it spends much of its life cycle outside of the human host in estuarine and coastal environments. This pathogen's residence in the aquatic environment year round requires it to respond to a number of fluctuating conditions, including temperature shifts, osmotic stress, nutrient limitation, and predation. To survive these challenges, *V. cholerae* employs a number of strategies including formation of biofilms on abiotic and biotic surfaces, transition to a metabolically quiescent state, acquisition and storage of nutrients, and initiation of protective responses to specific physiological and biological stressors. In this section we detail major factors contributing to *V. cholerae* growth and persistence in the aquatic environment, as well as known drivers of seasonal outbreaks.

Biofilm Formation in the Aquatic Environment

In the aquatic environment *V. cholerae* is frequently found in microbial communities known as biofilms (8). These communities are often associated with surfaces and are composed of cell aggregates encased by a self-produced or acquired extracellular matrix. Biofilms contribute to the environmental persistence of *V. cholerae* and provide protection from a number of environmental stresses, including nutrient limitation and predation by protozoa and bacteriophages (27–29). While *V. cholerae* can form biofilms on many biotic and abiotic surfaces, it is predominately found in association with zooplankton, phytoplankton, and oceanic chitin rain (30).

Transmission may be enhanced by the ingestion of biofilms, which allow for the delivery of high numbers of bacteria to human hosts (31). The removal of particles larger than 20 µm via simple filtration resulted in a reduction of reported cholera cases, suggesting that manual removal of biofilms and zooplankton-associated biofilms from the environment impedes transmission (32, 33). Additionally, biofilm-like aggregates have been observed in patient stool and are known to exhibit a hyperinfectious phenotype, suggesting that biofilms play a role not only in transmission from the environment to the host, but also in the spread of cholera from host to host (34, 35). Given the importance of biofilms in *V. cholerae*'s environmental survival and subsequent transmission to the human host, we discuss the development, structure, and regulation of *V. cholerae* biofilms, as well as the impact of environmental signals on biofilm formation (Fig. 1).

Molecular basis of *V. cholerae* biofilm formation

V. cholerae biofilm formation is a multistep process that begins with surface scanning and initial attachment, followed by the production of extracellular matrix components and the formation of microcolonies, and finally the development of highly organized, three-dimensional structures (36–38). A single polar flagellum powered by a Na^+ motor drives *V. cholerae* motility; when *V. cholerae* cells swim near surfaces, hydrodynamic forces act on the flagellum and induce torque on the cell body, which deflects the swimming direction of cells into curved clockwise paths (38, 39, 40). A recent study

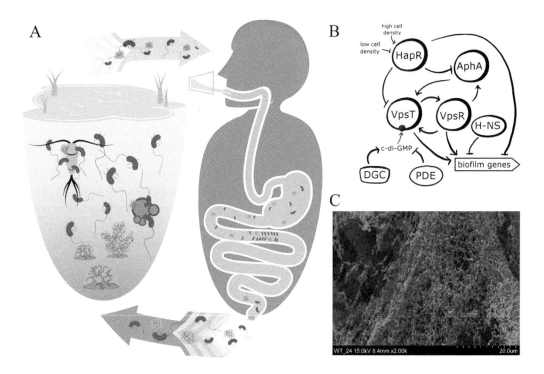

FIGURE 1 Role of biofilms in *V. cholerae* survival, transmission, and dissemination. (A) Biofilms play an important role in *V. cholerae* environmental protection, transmission into the human host, and dissemination to new hosts and back into environmental reservoirs. *V. cholerae* can be readily found growing in biofilms in the aquatic environment, often in association with zooplankton, phytoplankton, detritus, sediment, or oceanic chitin rain. This growth mode provides protection from a number of environmental stressors, including nutrient limitation and predation, and allows *V. cholerae* to survive in the aquatic environment year-round. The manual removal of biofilms and plankton-associated biofilms from the environment has been shown to decrease transmission during seasonal outbreaks. Additionally, the ingestion of *V. cholerae* grown in biofilms allows for the delivery of both higher numbers of bacteria and hyperinfectious cells. Though the role of biofilms during host infection is still being studied, biofilm-like aggregates have been observed in patient stool and also exhibit a hyperinfectious phenotype, suggesting that biofilms play a role not only in transmission from the environment to the host, but also in the spread of cholera from host to host. (B) VpsR and VpsT are the master positive regulators of biofilm genes and positively regulate one another's expression and genes involved in biofilm formation. VpsR additionally activates the expression of a master virulence regulator, AphA, which in turn activates VpsT expression. VpsT activity is dependent on its interaction with the small signaling molecule, c-di-GMP, which is synthesized by diguanylate cyclases (DGCs) and degraded by phosphodiesterases (PDEs). The quorum sensing regulator, HapR, represses expression of VpsR, VpsT, and AphA in response to high cell density. At low cell density, HapR is inactivated and biofilm formation is upregulated. H-NS (histone-like nucleoid structuring protein) is an additional negative regulator of biofilm formation. Its repressive function is silenced by VpsT. (C) An electron scanning microscopy image of a *V. cholerae* biofilm shows cells encased in biofilm matrix.

revealed that *V. cholerae* exhibits two distinct, clockwise motility modes when approaching a glass surface, known as "roaming" and "orbiting." The roaming mode involves weak interactions between the surface and *V. cholerae*'s mannose-sensitive hemagglutinin pili (MSHA), while orbiting results from stronger interactions between the surface and MSHA. Orbiting cells exhibit a distribution of intermittent pauses prior to attaching to the surface, while roaming cells pass over surface regions without attaching. Pausing and attachment were ablated in orbiting cells when MSHA attachment was interrupted, indicating that MSHA pili binding to the surface is mechanochemical in nature and likely plays an important role in *V. cholerae*'s transition from motile to sessile. Furthermore, sites of initial surface attachment in *V. cholerae* biofilm formation strongly correlate with the location of eventual microcolonies, which indicates that surface-associated motility does not occur following cell attachment and does not contribute to microcolony formation (37).

After *V. cholerae* attaches to a surface, it produces an extracellular matrix composed of polysaccharides, proteins, and nucleic acids (41, 42). Key components of the *V. cholerae* biofilm matrix include *Vibrio* polysaccharide (VPS); the biofilm matrix proteins RbmA, RbmC, and Bap1; and extracellular DNA (eDNA) (38, 41, 43–45). Each component plays a unique role in the formation and structure of the biofilm. The *V. cholerae* biofilm-matrix cluster (VcBMC) encodes the genes involved in the production of VPS and the RbmA and RbmC matrix proteins in a functional genetic module composed of the *vps-I*, *rbmA-E*, and *vps-II* gene clusters (38, 43, 44, 46). The gene encoding Bap1 is encoded elsewhere on the chromosome (44).

VPS is secreted shortly after attachment and is essential for the development of three-dimensional biofilm structures (Fig. 1C) (38, 42, 46). Two types of VPS were identified in the biofilm: the repeating unit of the major variant of the polysaccharide portion of VPS is [→4(-α-L-Gul*p*NAcAGly3OAc-(1→4)-β-D-Glc*p*-(1→4)-α-D-Glc*p*-(1→4)-α-D-Gal*p*-)1→]$_n$, while the minor variant (~20%) replaces the α-D-Glc with α-D-GlcNAc (47). Interaction of VPS with biofilm matrix proteins is critical for biofilm formation. Deletion mutants that cannot produce VPS are unable to retain RbmA, RbmC, and Bap1 at a solid-liquid interface, and RmbC was found to be critical for incorporation of VPS throughout the biofilm (42). During biofilm formation, RbmA, Bap1, and RbmC are secreted by the type II secretion system and maintain spatial and temporal patterns during this process (48). After initial attachment and VPS production, RbmA accumulates on the cell surface, where it facilitates cell-cell interaction, followed by Bap1 secretion at the cell-attachment surface interface. RbmC is then secreted at discrete sites on the cell surface. As the biofilm matures, RbmC and Bap1 form flexible envelopes that can grow as cells divide. Continued secretion of biofilm components results in a fully formed biofilm composed of organized clusters composed of cells, VPS, RbmA, Bap1, and RbmC (42). *V. cholerae* phenotypic variants with enhanced ability to form biofilms, termed rugose, arise and get selected during biofilm formation. Rugose variants are associated with higher production of VPS and have increased resistance to environmental stress (38).

There is limited information on dispersal of *V. cholerae* biofilms. Two extracellular nucleases, Dns and Xds, contribute to biofilm dispersal, presumably via their degradation of eDNA, though the exact role of Dns, Xds, and eDNA in dispersal is still unclear (45). Deletion of Dns and Xds also resulted in impaired *in vivo* colonization, suggesting that dispersal from the biofilm may be necessary for colonization of the host and effective transmission (45). Additionally, a putative polysaccharide lyase encoded by *rbmB* has been hypothesized to play a role in VPS degradation, and *rbmB* mutants exhibit enhanced biofilm formation (44). The negative regulation of biofilm matrix production likely plays a role in dispersal; however, genes involved in degradation of VPS and biofilm proteins have yet to be identified. Further study of this important step in the biofilm cycle is essential for a full understanding of the role biofilms play in survival, dissemination, and transmission.

A complex network of regulators govern *V. cholerae* biofilm formation

Various regulators participate in regulation of biofilm formation, including the transcriptional activators: VpsR, VpsT, and AphA;

repressors: HapR and H-NS; alternative sigma factors; small regulatory RNAs; and a multitude of signaling molecules (Fig. 1B). VpsR is the master regulator of biofilm formation, activating *vps* genes, matrix protein genes, and genes that encode part of the type II secretion system required for secretion of matrix proteins. Deletion of *vpsR* abolishes formation of biofilms (49–51). VpsT also upregulates biofilm formation and must bind to the small signaling molecule cyclic dimeric guanosine monophosphate (c-di-GMP) to activate its transcriptional regulation of VcBMC genes (52). While the VpsR and VpsT regulons extensively overlap, likely due to their ability to positively control each other's expression, VpsR has a greater impact on biofilm formation (49, 51). VpsR and VpsT can directly bind to the upstream regulatory region of the *vps*-II cluster; VpsR and VpsT binding sites have also been identified in the upstream regulatory regions of the *vps*-I cluster, the *rbmA* gene, and the *vpsT* gene (53). VpsR also upregulates a master virulence regulator, AphA, which was shown to enhance biofilm formation via its transcriptional control of *vpsT* (54). AphA provides a link between the expression of virulence genes and biofilm genes, potentially playing a role in *in vivo* biofilm formation and likely contributing to the hyperinfectivity of cells grown in biofilms (54).

HapR is the main repressor of biofilm formation; it is activated through a quorum sensing (QS) pathway that responds to cell density (55, 56). At low cell density, quorum-regulated small RNAs (sRNAs), Qrr1–4, work in conjunction with the sRNA chaperone Hfq to prevent the translation of *hapR* mRNA. This translational interference relieves HapR repression of biofilm genes. At high cell densities, production of Qrr1–4 diminishes and HapR levels rise, allowing HapR to repress biofilm formation by directly binding to the regulatory regions of *vpsT* and the *vps*-II operon (57). Though not detailed here, several additional regulators can influence the expression of *hapR* in response to signals

that are presently unknown (58–62). This indicates that, in addition to population dynamics, a number of other factors can influence the timing of HapR expression, which in turn modulates the formation of mature biofilms and subsequent dispersal from biofilms (55, 63). In addition to its role in modulating nucleoid topology, a histone-like protein, H-NS, also acts as a major negative regulator of biofilm and virulence genes and directly binds to the *vps-I*, *vps-II*, and *vpsT* promoter regions (64, 65).

Biofilm formation is also influenced by small nucleotide signaling, including c-di-GMP, cyclic adenosine-monophosphate (cAMP), and guanosine 3′-diphosphate 5′-triphosphate and guanosine 3′,5′-bis (diphosphate) (p)ppGpp signaling. C-di-GMP is a second messenger signaling molecule that is important in regulating *V. cholerae*'s transition from a motile to a sessile state; high cellular c-di-GMP levels enhance transcription of key genes involved in biofilm formation (66). C-di-GMP is synthesized by diguanylate cyclases (DGCs), which contain GGDEF domains, and is degraded by phosphodiesterases (PDEs), which contain EAL or HD-GYP domains. The *V. cholerae* genome encodes 62 predicted DGCs and PDEs, though only a fraction have been shown to impact c-di-GMP levels, and it is likely that many of these proteins are activated in response to specific environmental signals (49, 57, 67–70). In *V. cholerae*, c-di-GMP is sensed by receptor proteins, including PilZ, VpsT, and FlrA, or c-di-GMP riboswitches, which are activated by binding c-di-GMP (52, 71–73). In contrast to c-di-GMP, the second messenger cAMP acts as a repressor of *V. cholerae* biofilm formation (74). cAMP binds its cAMP receptor protein (CRP), forming the cAMP-CRP complex, which downregulates expression of *rbmA*, *rbmC*, *bap1*, *vpsR*, and other *vps* genes (61, 74, 75). cAMP-CRP also upregulates HapR and the biosynthesis of the QS autoinducer CAI-I, which allows *V. cholerae* to sense increases in cell density and further upregulates HapR (61, 75).

Finally, biofilm formation is promoted by the stringent response, which is triggered by nutritional stress and results in the synthesis of (p)ppGpp by RelA, SpoT, and RelV (76–78). Overexpression of (p)ppGpp was shown to increase biofilm formation. All three (p)ppGpp synthases are necessary for *vpsR* transcription, but only RelA is necessary for *vpsT* transcription, indicating that the synthases may also have a direct role in regulating biofilm genes (78). The c-di-GMP, cAMP, and (p)ppGpp pathways play key roles in regulating biofilm formation, allowing *V. cholerae* to quickly respond to various environmental inputs by modulating internal levels of these small nucleotide signals.

Regulation of biofilm formation in response to changing environmental conditions in the aquatic environment and the human host

Estuaries, which act as environmental reservoirs for *V. cholerae*, undergo significant nutrient, temperature, salinity, and osmolarity fluctuations that can impact biofilm formation and *vps* expression (79–81). Additionally, signals encountered during passage through a human host can impact biofilm formation, including bile and the organic compound indole (82, 83). Nutritional status appears to play a key role in biofilm formation, and the highly conserved bacterial phosphoenolpyruvate phosphotransferase system (PTS) was recently linked to the regulation of *V. cholerae* biofilm formation. Four independent PTS pathways have been identified in activation or repression of *V. cholerae* biofilm formation and are mainly responsible for the positive regulation of biofilm in response to PTS sugars (84, 85). In contrast, the parallel nitrogen-specific PTS pathway appears to repress biofilm formation in LB, but not in minimal media (84). The involvement of PTS in biofilm formation suggests that the PTS may play a role in determining environmental suitability for biofilm growth and provides a clear link

between *V. cholerae*'s nutrition status and ability to form biofilms.

In addition to PTS substrates, a number of other environmental signals can influence *V. cholerae* biofilm formation. Small organic cations known as polyamines are produced by both eukaryotic and bacterial cells and are known to influence biofilm formation in *V. cholerae* (86–88). Increased environmental concentrations of the polyamine norspermidine increases biofilm formation and leads to NspS-mediated activation of *vpsL* transcription (88). Spermidine, which has a similar structure to norspermidine, represses biofilm formation, and it has been hypothesized that excess exogenous spermidine may inhibit NspS interaction with norspermidine (87). Calcium (Ca^{+2}) levels can vary in the aquatic environment, and extracellular Ca^{+2} has been demonstrated to inhibit *vps* transcription and lead to the dissolution of biofilms (89, 90). Indole, which is produced by bacteria found in the human gut, is thought to activate expression of *vps* genes (82). Additional signals and their impacts on biofilm formation are discussed in the subsequent sections. Though the mechanisms by which many of these signals are sensed have yet to be determined, elucidation of signal sensing and response is essential to our understanding of *V. cholerae* survival and could lead to the development of targeted treatments that interrupt these pathways.

Nutrient Acquisition in the Aquatic Environment

V. cholerae is prototrophic and must acquire nutrients from its environment. Procuring essential nutrients can be challenging in the aquatic environment, where seasonally variable conditions and inter- and intraspecies competition limit access and availability. *V. cholerae* employs a number of tightly regulated nutrient acquisition strategies to enable its survival and persistence in the aquatic environment; some of these strategies are also utilized when similar conditions are met in the host.

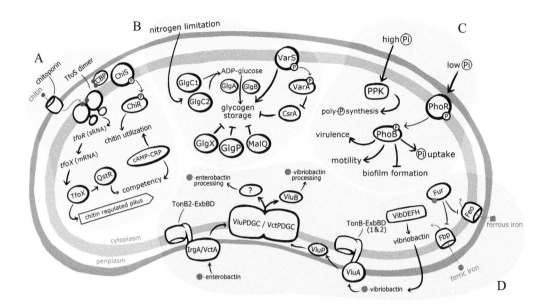

FIGURE 2 *V. cholerae* regulation of nutrient acquisition. *V. cholerae* utilizes various uptake systems to acquire nutrients from the external environment. (A) During chitin utilization, chitin oligomers enter the periplasm through chitoporins in the outer membrane. Once in the periplasm, chitin oligomers bind to the chitin binding protein (CBP), allowing it to release from and relive repression of the histidine kinase, ChiS, which is part of a two-component system (TCS). Once active, ChiS activates an as yet unidentified response regulator, ChiR, which upregulates genes involved in chitin catabolism and utilization. While ChiS is thought also to play a role in TfoS activation, the mechanism has not been identified. However, it is known that TfoS binds to chitin oligomers in the periplasm and dimerizes to become active. Once in its active conformation, TfoS upregulates the expression of the small RNA (sRNA), *tfor*, which in turn, activates translation of *tfox* mRNA. TfoX goes on to upregulate genes involved in competency, including the chitin regulated pilus and QstR. The activation of both the chitin catabolism and competency pathways are also dependent on the cAMP-CRP complex and in the absence of this complex are repressed. (B) Glycogen storage is activated in response to nitrogen limitation. The first reaction in glycogen synthesis is catalyzed by the ADP-glucose pyrophosphorylase enzymes GlgC1 and GlgC2, which generate ADP-glucose from ATP and glucose-1-phosphate. Subsequently, the enzymes GlgA and GlgB build glycogen by forming α-1,4 and α-1,6 linkages, respectively, between ADP-glucose monomers. Glycogen breakdown is initiated by three enzymes: the glycogen debranching GlgX, the maltodextrin phosphorylase GlgP, and the 4-α-glucanotransferase MalQ. Additionally, in response to unknown environmental stimuli, the TCS VarSA is activated and has been shown to enhance glycogen storage and posttranscriptionally repress the global transcriptional regulator, CsrA. (C) Environmental inorganic phosphate (Pi) levels regulate a number of cell processes in *V. cholerae*. When Pi is high, *V. cholerae* initiates the biosynthesis of large amounts of inorganic polyphosphate (poly-P), composed of long chains of linked Pi, via the polyphosphate kinase, PPK. When Pi is limited, the TCS PhoBR is activated and regulates a number of cellular processes, including virulence, motility, biofilm formation, and Pi uptake. (D) *V. cholerae* uses a number of mechanisms to facilitate iron acquisition. Iron uptake is regulated by the iron-dependent regulator, Fur. When iron levels are high, Fur complexes with ferrous iron (Fur-Fe^{2+}) and directly binds to conserved regions on the genome, called Fur boxes, to regulate the transcription of target genes. The Fur-Fe^{2+} complex upregulates genes involved in iron storage, metabolism, and antioxidant defense and represses iron uptake genes, including the genes encoding the Feo and Fbp transport systems, which facilitate uptake of ferrous and ferric iron, respectively. Under iron-limited conditions, *V. cholerae* produces and secretes the siderophore vibriobactin via the VibBDEFH system. Ferric vibriobactin is imported back into the cell via the outer membrane protein ViuA and both of *V. cholerae*'s TonB-ExbBD complexes. Ferric vibriobactin is then transported through the periplasm to the inner membrane by the periplasmic binding protein, ViuP, and then across the inner membrane by two transport systems, ViuPDGC and VctPDGC. The cytoplasmic esterase, ViuB, processes ferric vibriobactin

Chitin utilization

Chitin, an abundant insoluble polymer found in the exoskeleton of zooplankton and other marine crustaceans, provides a significant source of carbon and nitrogen for *V. cholerae* in the aquatic environment (30, 91–93). Composed of β-1,4-linked *N*-acetylglucosamine (GlcNAc) residues, chitin not only serves as a nutrient source, but also acts as a signaling molecule, a substrate for biofilm growth, and a mode of dissemination for *V. cholerae* (93). *V. cholerae* utilizes chemotaxis to swim toward chitin subunits, followed by attachment to chitin via a mechanism involving the MSHA pilus and the chitin-binding protein GbpA (93, 94). In response to chitin attachment, *V. cholerae* initiates a chitin catabolic response, which allows cells to degrade and catabolize chitin residues, and simultaneously induces natural competency, which allows cells to acquire new genetic material (Fig. 2) (95). Competent bacteria and eDNA are in close proximity in biofilms, so the bacteria can readily take up DNA and expand the genome to better cope with the stresses of the environmental lifestyle. Additionally, biofilm formation on chitinous zooplankton allows *V. cholerae* to disseminate to new waterways via passive locomotion or by mechanical transfer (96–98). Thus, *V. cholerae* growth on chitin supports survival, evolution, and transmission.

Two extracellular chitinases, ChiA-1 and ChiA-2, are activated during growth on chitin and degrade insoluble chitin polymers into shorter GlcNAc oligomers, which are then transported into the cell via an ATP-binding cassette (ABC) transporter (93, 99). The *V. cholerae* response to chitin is mediated by a two-component signal transduction system. In a typical two-component system (TCS) signal transduction cascade, the membrane-bound histidine kinase senses an environmental signal and autophosphorylates. The phosphate is then transferred to its cognate response regulator, which alters the conformation of its output domain and initiates changes in gene expression or enzymatic activities. The sensor kinase ChiS initiates the chitin signaling cascade, though it does not appear to utilize the canonical TCS signaling described above. Instead, a high-affinity chitin binding protein (CBP) interacts with ChiS in the periplasm to keep it in the inactive state. In the presence of chitin, chitin subunits enter the periplasm through chitoporins and bind to CBP. The binding of chitin subunits to CBP allows it to dissociate from ChiS and activates the ChiS signaling cascade; it is unknown if this activation is initiated by autophosphorylation or an alternative mechanism (99). ChiS regulates the expression of 41 chitin-induced genes, including the GlcNAc catabolic operon, two extracellular chitinases, a chitoporin, and a type IV pilus involved in natural competency (93, 100).

Recent work suggests that ChiS likely has two independent targets: a catabolic regulon and a competence regulon. ChiS activation of the catabolic regulon is mediated by a hypothetical canonical response regulator, ChiR, which remains to be identified and is required for transcription of the chitin catabolic genes in the *chb* operon (93, 100). Active ChiS also activates the transmembrane regulator, TfoS, which is responsible for regulating natural competency. TfoS subsequently promotes the transcription of the competence-inducing sRNA, *tfoR* (100, 101). Transcription of *tfoR* is essential for the translation of *tfoX* mRNA, a positive regula-

---

and removes the iron from the siderophore so that it may be used within the cell. *V. cholerae* can import siderophores produced by other bacteria, including enterobactin, which is recognized by two enterobactin receptors, IrgA and VctA, and then transported across the outer membrane with energy supplied by the TonB2-ExbBD complex, followed by shuttling across the inner membrane by the transport systems ViuPDGC and VctPDGC. The enzyme responsible for processing ferric enterobactin in *V. cholerae* has not been identified.

tor of natural competence and chitin metabolism genes in *V. cholerae* (102). TfoX and HapR activate expression of the regulator QstR, which is required for the expression of a subset of competence genes (103). Both activation of catabolism and competence appear to be independent of the ChiS conserved phosphorelay residues, indicating that ChiS activates chitin catabolism and natural competency through an atypical and, as yet, unidentified mechanism.

Provision of competing carbon sources can downregulate the chitin utilization program via carbon catabolite repression (96). Carbon catabolite repression allows *V. cholerae* to preferentially utilize easily metabolized carbon sources by repressing less desirable pathways, and glucose and other PTS sugars were shown to repress chitin utilization and natural competency. The PTS interferes with the accumulation of cAMP, which is required to work with its binding partner CRP, to initiate efficient colonization of the chitin surface, chitin degradation and utilization, and the induction of natural competency. Thus, PTS sugars inhibit the chitin utilization program via its repression of cAMP synthesis (96). Intriguingly, cAMP-CRP has been shown to repress biofilm formation, a phenotype associated with growth on chitin. This highlights the intricate and complex regulatory network that governs these phenotypes, and further investigation is needed to understand how biofilm formation evades repression via cAMP-CRP when growing on chitin.

The chitin utilization program alleviates starvation due to the lack of nutrients in the water column, promotes the formation of biofilms, and initiates natural competency in *V. cholerae*. Additionally, components of this system may play roles in survival and pathogenesis during infection. Similarities between chitin and intestinal mucins allow the *N*-acetylglucosamine binding protein (GbpA) to aid in both attachment to chitin and in intestinal colonization of the host (104, 105). The extracellular chitinase ChiA2 was re-

cently found to promote survival and pathogenesis in the host by allowing *V. cholerae* to utilize mucin as a nutrient source. ChiA2 was shown to deglycosylate mucin, resulting in the release of GlcNAc and its oligomers, which can then be utilized for growth and survival in the host (106). This link between environmental and host nutrient acquisition is important in the evolution of *V. cholerae* to become a successful environmental pathogen, allowing it readily to navigate two different systems using similar tools.

Nutrient storage granules

In addition to chitin utilization, *V. cholerae* copes with carbon limitation in the environment by using intracellular glycogen stores that are synthesized and accumulated when carbon sources are highly available. Glycogen, a polysaccharide made of glucose monomers with α-1,4 linkages and α-1,6 branches, serves as a common form of energy storage for many organisms. *V. cholerae* glycogen accumulation is regulated by nitrogen and carbon availability (Fig. 2). When nitrogen is in excess, glycogen is continually synthesized and degraded at basal levels. When nitrogen is limited, enzymes involved in glycogen synthesis are upregulated and glycogen accumulation within the cell is stimulated (107). During the first step of glycogen synthesis in *V. cholerae*, the ADP-glucose pyrophosphorylase enzymes GlgC1 and GlgC2 generate ADP-glucose from ATP and glucose-1-phosphate. Subsequently, the enzymes GlgA and GlgB build glycogen by forming α-1,4 and α-1,6 linkages, respectively, between ADP-glucose monomers (107). Depending on nitrogen and carbon availability, *V. cholerae* initiates glycogen breakdown via three enzymes: the glycogen debranching protein GlgX, the maltodextrin phosphorylase GlgP, and the 4-α-glucanotransferase MalQ (107, 108). The global transcriptional regulator CsrA (for carbon storage regulator) has been shown to negatively control the *glg* genes in *Escherichia coli* and is thought to play a similar role in *V. cholerae* (108, 109). In

V. cholerae, CsrA is posttranscriptionally regulated by the TCS VarSA, which represses CsrA translation via the activation of three sRNAs in response to an unknown environmental signal. A mutant lacking the histidine kinase gene *varS* had significantly less glycogen storage than wild type, indicating that this system and CsrA are involved in glycogen storage in *V. cholerae* (58, 108). Activation of VarSA and repression of CsrA are also known to inhibit biofilm formation via activation of HapR and may link carbon storage and nutritional status to QS and biofilm formation (58).

Glycogen storage and utilization promote *V. cholerae* dissemination and environmental survival in multiple ways. It is known that *V. cholerae* cells in rice water stool contain glycogen storage granules, indicating that the organism stores glycogen in preparation for dissemination from the nutrient-rich host into nutrient-poor environments such as stool or pond water (107). These glycogen stores have been shown to prolong *V. cholerae* survival in rice water stool, pond water, and the infant rabbit host (107, 108). Interestingly, a mutant unable to degrade glycogen survived as long as wild type in two of three rice water stool samples, while mutants defective in glycogen storage had reduced survival compared to wild type in all samples. This demonstrated that the presence of glycogen plays a protective role against environmental stresses, regardless of its ability to be metabolized, and can prolong survival after *V. cholerae* is shed in stool. However, in carbon-poor environments, the ability to degrade and utilize glycogen stores appears to be essential for survival, because mutants unable to degrade glycogen were dramatically attenuated in survival when compared to wild type under these conditions (107).

Glycogen-rich *V. cholerae* was also shown to be more virulent in an infant mouse model of transmission. Mutants lacking the ability to synthesize or degrade glycogen were attenuated for transmission in infant mice following incubation in pond water, indicating that the abilities to store and use glycogen are critical for *V. cholerae* to infect new hosts. Passage through pond water prior to infection was intended to mimic the environment *V. cholerae* encounters when it is shed in stool before it encounters a new host. This passage was necessary to observe the attenuated phenotype and supports the hypothesis that glycogen storage is important for transmission from host to host (107). Glycogen storage and metabolism appear to play significant roles in *V. cholerae* transmission, dissemination, and environmental survival.

Inorganic phosphate availability

V. cholerae must cope with the limited availability of inorganic phosphate (Pi), an essential nutrient, during its residence in the aquatic environment. In *V. cholerae*, PhoBR activates the Pho regulon, which includes genes involved in phosphate homeostasis, biofilm formation, motility, and virulence (Fig. 2) (110, 111). PhoBR is composed of the histidine kinase, PhoR, which phosphorylates its response regulator, PhoB, in response to low extracellular Pi levels. Once phosphorylated, PhoB regulates the expression of the genes that make up the Pho regulon through direct binding to DNA sequences known as Pho boxes. When Pi levels are sufficient, the phosphate-specific transport system (Pst) is inactive and represses activation of PhoBR through an unknown mechanism; this repression is lifted when Pi levels are low and the Pst becomes activated. Induction of PhoBR activity results in significant production of PstS, the periplasmic component of the Pst (112). Phosphorylated PhoB (P~PhoB) stimulates production of the alkaline phosphatase PhoA, which provides the cell with exogenous Pi, and two PhoH-family ATPases, which have unknown roles in mediating Pi limitation. P~PhoB also inhibits production of the outer membrane pore-forming proteins OmpU and OmpT, while stimulating production of the phosphate-specific porin, PhoE (112, 113). Pi limitation induces genes that are part of the general stress regulon, which is controlled by the alternative sigma factor RpoS, and likely contributes to the ability of *V. cholerae* to survive low Pi conditions (112).

PhoBR also plays a role during infection and dissemination, suggesting that *V. cholerae* may experience Pi limitation in the host. *phoB* mutants had diminished survival in low-phosphate medium and infant mouse and rabbit intestines, as well as in pond water after passage through a host (110, 113). The response regulator PhoB is also required for *V. cholerae* survival in pond water following dissemination from the host (110). *In vivo* Pi supplementation only partially restored the colonization defect of a *phoB* mutant, indicating that this response regulator may respond to other signals in the small intestine. Additionally, PhoBR is a negative regulator of the major virulence activator *tcpP* and appears to play a temporal role in infection, because both strains lacking PhoBR and strains with constitutively activated PhoBR resulted in attenuated colonization in an infant mouse model (110). During late-stage infection, PhoB is known to regulate genes involved in c-di-GMP metabolism that positively regulate motility, supporting a model in which phosphate limitation in the host prepares *V. cholerae* for dissemination by activating PhoB and motility (111). Together, these studies indicate that PhoBR is important for *V. cholerae* during much of its life cycle.

V. cholerae synthesizes large amounts of inorganic polyphosphate (poly-P), composed of long chains of linked Pi, in response to surplus extracellular phosphate (Fig. 2). Loss of *ppk*, which encodes for the polyphosphate kinase required for poly-P synthesis, did not impact *V. cholerae* motility, biofilm formation, starvation survival, virulence, or colonization of the suckling mouse intestine. However, sensitivity to other environmental stressors was enhanced, including sensitivity to acid stress, osmotic stress, and oxidative stress in a Pi-limited medium (114). Molecular mechanisms by which *ppk* provides

protection from these stresses are yet to be determined.

Iron availability

Iron is an essential nutrient needed for a variety of cellular processes, including energy metabolism, yet it is limited in aquatic environments due to poor solubility. To survive in iron-limited environments, *V. cholerae* has evolved a wide variety of mechanisms for acquiring iron and coping with iron starvation (Fig. 2). As is the case with many other bacterial species, iron uptake is controlled by the iron-dependent regulator Fur, which regulates the expression of genes involved in iron uptake, storage, and metabolism in response to intracellular iron levels. When iron levels are high, Fur complexes with ferrous iron (Fur-Fe^{2+}) and represses the transcription of target genes by directly binding to conserved regions in their promoters, called Fur boxes (115). The Fur-Fe^{2+} complex represses iron uptake genes, including the genes encoding the Feo and Fbp transport systems, which facilitate uptake of ferrous and ferric iron, respectively, and upregulates genes involved in iron storage, metabolism, and antioxidant defense (115–117). When iron is limited, uncomplexed Fur represses genes encoding nonessential iron-containing proteins and activates the expression of alternative proteins, such as manganese-containing superoxide dismutase (115). Independent of iron levels, Fur also appears to play a role in virulence by upregulating genes located in the *V. cholerae* pathogenicity island. Though the exact role of Fur during host infection is unknown, a *fur* deletion mutant displayed reduced colonization compared to wild type in the infant mouse model (115).

When iron is limited, *V. cholerae* utilizes small iron chelating compounds known as siderophores, which scavenge iron with extremely high efficiency. *V. cholerae* produces a unique catechol siderophore called vibriobactin from dihydroxybenzoate, threonine, and norspermidine via the VibBDEFH system (118–120). Ferric vibriobactin is recognized by the outer membrane protein ViuA, and its movement across the outer membrane is facilitated by both of *V. cholerae*'s TonB-ExbBD complexes, which harness the proton motive force to power the import of substrates (121, 122). Upon entering the periplasm, ferric vibriobactin is transported to the inner membrane by the periplasmic binding protein ViuP, followed by movement through the inner membrane by two ABC transport systems, ViuPDGC and VctPDGC (120, 123, 124). The cytoplasmic esterase ViuB is required for ferric vibriobactin processing or removal of iron from the siderophore (125). After being freed from vibriobactin, the ferric iron can be used in various cellular processes. Loss of the ability to synthesize vibriobactin had no effect on *V. cholerae* virulence in the infant mouse, indicating that use of this siderophore is not a critical iron acquisition mechanism in the host (126).

V. cholerae can also take advantage of siderophores produced by other Gram-negative bacteria, including the catechol siderophore enterobactin, thus maximizing iron uptake without the energetic costs of synthesizing vibriobactin (123). Uptake of ferric enterobactin is facilitated by two enterobactin receptors, IrgA and VctA, which recognize the compound on the outer membrane (124). The iron-enterobactin complex is then transported across the outer membrane with energy supplied by the TonB2-ExbBD complex, followed by shuttling across the inner membrane by the transport systems ViuPDGC and VctPDGC (123, 124, 127). The genes required for removal of iron from enterobactin are unknown. ViuB, the esterase that processes vibriobactin, is different in sequence and structure from Fes, the enterobactin-processing protein from *E. coli*, and is not expected to cleave iron from enterobactin (125). While it is not known whether *V. cholerae* encounters enterobactin at significant levels in the host, sewage-contaminated waters likely contain enterobactin-producers, and thus, the pathogen's coexistence with such bacteria in the environment may facilitate its survival and transmission to new hosts.

When iron is limited, *V. cholerae* maximizes cellular function without iron. Genes that encode nonessential iron-dependent proteins are repressed, and *V. cholerae* replaces proteins that require iron cofactors with alternative forms. For example, during iron limitation *V. cholerae* represses the gene for iron-dependent superoxide dismutase SodB while manganese-dependent SodA is upregulated, thus ensuring that the cell can resist oxidative damage despite the lack of iron (115). FumC, the alternative, non-iron-containing form of fumarate hydratase, is also produced, ensuring that the cells can perform the tricarboxylic acid cycle in the absence of iron (115). Iron limitation also activates the TCS CpxAR, which regulates cell envelope stress responses. Activation of the Cpx pathway results in elevated transcription of genes involved in iron acquisition and homeostasis and is required for adaption to iron-limited conditions (128). The wide variety of mechanisms used by *V. cholerae* to acquire iron and adapt to iron limitation further highlights the importance of this metal for the organism's survival in the environment and the host.

During infection, iron is sequestered within host cells and is relatively inaccessible to extracellular pathogens; however, *V. cholerae* is capable of using alternative iron acquisition mechanisms in the host. Iron limitation positively regulates the production of hemolysin, which lyses mammalian cells and frees heme and hemoglobin for *V. cholerae* to utilize (129). The TonB-dependent receptor proteins HutA, HutR, and HasR recognize heme and hemoglobin on the outer membrane (130, 131). Mutation of all three of these receptor genes renders *V. cholerae* completely unable to utilize heme or hemoglobin yet do not impact its ability to colonize an infant mouse, indicating that the pathogen possesses additional mechanisms for iron acquisition *in vivo* (131).

Response to Physiological and Biological Stressors in the Aquatic Environment

Physiological conditions such as salinity and temperature can change drastically in *V. cholerae*'s aquatic habitats and can alter the growth patterns and population dynamics of the organism. Biological stressors can also impact *V. cholerae* survival and abundance, including inter- and intraspecies competition and predation by protozoa and bacteriophages. *V. cholerae* has evolved mechanisms for adapting to these physiological and biological stressors, which allows it to survive in aquatic reservoirs when conditions are unfavorable.

Adaptations to changes in salinity

In the coastal and estuarine habitats of *V. cholerae*, fluctuations in salinity and osmolarity are common and vary seasonally. Additionally, *V. cholerae* must adapt to salinity shifts upon host entry and exit. While the optimal salinity for *V. cholerae* growth is equivalent to 200 mM NaCl, a concentration commonly observed in estuarine habitats, it has adapted to tolerate a wide range of salinities and osmolarities. In response to osmotic stress, *V. cholerae* synthesizes ectoine and imports glycine betaine; these molecules are compatible solutes or small, highly soluble molecules that balance extracellular osmotic pressure. Ectoine is synthesized via gene products from a four-gene operon composed of a putative aspartokinase gene and *ectABC* (132). Expression of *ectABC* genes is regulated by osmolarity (80). Because *V. cholerae* lacks the genes needed for glycine betaine synthesis, it imports glycine betaine produced by other organisms via the transporter OpuD (79).

V. cholerae also responds to changes in osmolarity by regulating biofilm formation. Biofilm formation is highest in media with osmolarity equal to that of 100 mM NaCl, which falls within the range typically found in estuaries, and it lessens with increased or decreased osmolarity (80). Low osmolarity induces expression of the transcriptional regulator gene *oscR*, which represses biofilm genes (80). In contrast, the transcriptional regulator CosR activates biofilm genes and represses motility genes in response to high ionic strength. Additionally, CosR represses compatible solute biosynthesis and transporter genes at optimal ionic strength (~200 mM), independently of its function as a regulator of biofilm formation (81). These regulators link changes in external conditions with the production of biofilms, demonstrating both the significance of this growth mode in environmental survival and the complex regulatory networks that govern it.

Adaptations to changes in temperature

Temperature fluctuations due to seasonal changes are known to correlate with other factors that influence *V. cholerae* growth and survival, including shifts in plankton concentration, nutrient availability, and salinity, making it a suitable marker for indirect detection of *V. cholerae* occurrence via remote sensing (133). Ecological studies have demonstrated that high water temperature, typically above 15°C, is a good predictor for the presence of *V. cholerae* (134–136). Temperature can also act as a signal for the transition between environment and host. When shifted to low temperatures relative to the host temperature of 37°C, *V. cholerae* has been shown to initiate biofilm formation via the activation of six DGCs that collectively increase c-di-GMP levels. Increased biofilm formation was observed at 15°C and 25°C when compared to growth at 37°C, with the greatest biofilm formation observed at the lowest temperature of 15°C (70). This indicates that biofilm formation may be initiated once *V. cholerae* transitions from the human host into the aquatic environment and may be upregulated when seasonal downshifts in temperature occur. In contrast, high water temperature has been shown to promote attachment to chitin by upregulating the production of the adhesins MSHA and

GpbA, potentially playing a role in increasing vector transmission to the host (137). Additionally, translation of a major *V. cholerae* virulence regulator, ToxT, appears to be activated via an RNA thermometer when the organism is shifted to 37°C, the internal temperature of its human host (138).

V. cholerae utilizes several survival mechanisms in response to suboptimal temperatures. Two cold shock proteins, CspA and CspV, are induced when *V. cholerae* experiences low temperatures, and appear to play roles in cold adaptation. However, the mechanism of adaptation and regulons of these cold shock proteins have not been extensively explored (139). CspA and CspV are hypothesized to play roles in induction of a nonculturable state in response to 4°C temperatures. The nonculturable state, which is induced in response to cold stress or nutritional starvation, allows *V. cholerae* to survive unfavorable environmental conditions and is described in greater detail at the end of this section (140). This process indicates that *V. cholerae* can respond to the broad range of temperatures it encounters during its life cycle and initiate the appropriate responses, either activating protective measures to improve environmental survival during seasonal temperature drops or inducing virulence factors that enhance intestinal colonization once it transitions from the aquatic environment into the human host.

Generation of metabolically dormant cells

In response to environmental stress, *V. cholerae* has been observed to reduce its metabolic activity, convert from its characteristic comma shape to a round, coccoid shape, and become nonculturable under traditional laboratory conditions (141). This state has been referred to as viable but nonculturable (VBNC), conditionally viable, environmental *V. cholerae* (CVEC), and persister cells, depending on the conditions under which they were observed, though it appears that these states are highly similar and can be induced by common cues (142–145). Nutrient

deprivation is one of the most commonly observed signals shown to induce this state and diminishes the lipid, carbohydrate, RNA, and protein content of the cell (146). The reduced needs of these cells appear to contribute significantly to environmental survival when conditions are unfavorable. Both QS and passage through a mammalian host return these cells to their active state, indicating that recovery from this state plays a significant role in transmission and the start of outbreaks (147–150).

Type VI secretion system

V. cholerae utilizes the type VI secretion system (T6SS) to translocate effector proteins into a diverse group of target cells, including other bacteria, phagocytic amoebas, and human macrophages. This secretion system contributes to environmental survival and persistence by providing a defense against other bacteria and eukaryotic predators and appears to play a role in host survival by interrupting host phagocytosis (151–154). The T6SS is ubiquitous among Gram-negative bacteria and is composed of a dynamic, contractile phage tail-like structure anchored to a membrane associated, cell-envelope-spanning assembly. T6SS delivers effector proteins in a contact-dependent manner, which occurs via assembly of the phage tail-like structure, composed of a base plate, tube, and sheath, onto the membrane complex. This is followed by the contraction of the sheath-like structure, resulting in the propulsion of the inner tube toward the target cell and the delivery the effector protein. The contracted sheath is then disassembled, and sheath components are recycled (155).

The T6SS delivery tube is composed of repeating units of the hemolysin coregulated protein, and a trimeric tip is composed of the valine–glycine repeat proteins G (VgrG1-3). Some VgrGs carry C-terminal extensions that are enzymatically active and can impact the target cell, including *V. cholerae*'s VgrG-1, which cross-links actin in eukaryotic cells, and VgrG-3, which carries a C-terminal domain with peptidoglycan-degrading activity that kills other bacterial cells (153, 156). The T6SS can be used to deliver VgrG-associated effectors or independent effectors, such as the *V. cholerae* T6SS toxins VasX and TseL, which disrupt both prokaryotic and eukaryotic cell membranes (157–159). Most T6SS effectors have corresponding antagonistic immunity proteins that inactivate the effector and prevent self-killing (159). Three main *V. cholerae* effectors, VgrG-3, VasX, and TseL, are known to be inactivated by the immunity genes *tsiV3*, *tsiV2*, and *tsiV1*, respectively, which are encoded directly downstream of their corresponding effectors (158, 160).

The T6SS plays an important role in inter- and intraspecies competition (152, 154). Strains of *V. cholerae* that constitutively express the T6SS are not only highly virulent toward other bacteria, but they are also more virulent against other *V. cholerae* strains that constitutively express the T6SS (154, 161). While all *V. cholerae* strains sequenced to date harbor T6SS genes, the effectors and immunity proteins within these conserved genes exhibit diversity between strains. Compatible strains do not kill one another because they harbor the same immunity proteins, but incompatible strains that carry different effector modules are subject to intraspecies killing (160). Some strains that do not constitutively express the T6SS carry the immunity proteins necessary for protection against the strains that constitutively express the T6SS; however, different strains that constitutively express the T6SS were shown to enhance killing of one another, likely due to heterologous effector-immunity sets (161).

Three genomic loci encode for the *V. cholerae* T6SS. The major, or large, cluster encodes for the structural components of the T6SS, while two auxiliary clusters encode hemolysin coregulated proteins (152). All three clusters harbor effector and immunity proteins (160). Though our understanding of the regulation of these genes is incomplete,

several regulators of the T6SS have been identified, including VasH, RpoN, HapR, LuxO, cAMP-CRP, FliA, TsrA, TfoX, QstR, and OscR (Fig. 3) (152, 162–168). VasH is an RpoN-dependent transcriptional regulator encoded within the T6SS large cluster that upregulates the expression of the *hcp* and *vasX* genes by binding to the promoter regions of the large T6SS cluster and the satellite cluster starting with *hcp-1* (152, 157). VasH is predicted to activate the alternative sigma factor RpoN, which positively regulates the *hcp* operons and *vgrG3*, but has no effect on the main T6SS cluster (163, 165, 169). QS also plays a role in T6SS regulation. T6SS genes are positively regulated by HapR and negatively regulated by phosphorylated LuxO and QS sRNAs, which inhibit HapR translation and base pair to the large T6SS to inhibit transcription (164–166). The regulatory complex cAMP-CRP, which is required for the biosynthesis of the cholera autoinducer (CAI-1) to activate QS, positively controls expression of *hcp*, and elimination of cAMP-CRP was shown to ablate production of hemolysin coregulated protein (165). Additional negative regulators of T6SS genes have been identified. Deletion of flagellar regulatory genes results in the upregulation of T6SS genes, including the alternative sigma factor responsible for activating late-stage flagellin genes, FliA (168, 170). The global transcriptional regulator TsrA has some structural similarity to H-NS and appears to play a similar silencing role to repress T6SS genes (164).

Environmental signals stimulating expression of T6SS genes have been identified. A recent study revealed that expression of the T6SS is positively controlled by two major regulators of competency, TfoX and QstR, which are activated in response to growth on chitin (167). Growth on chitin supports the formation of biofilms and allows predatory cells close access to neighboring bacteria within the densely packed microbial community. Upregulation of the T6SS by natural competency regulatory circuitry results in the killing of nonimmune neighboring cells

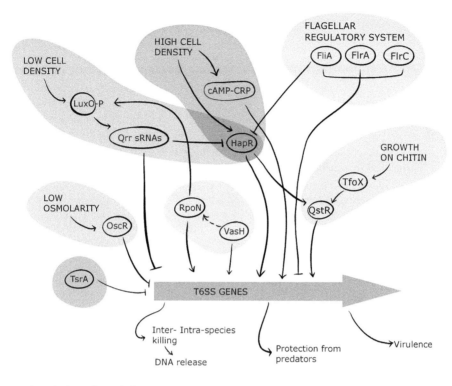

FIGURE 3 Regulation of *V. cholerae* type VI secretion system (T6SS). The *V. cholerae* T6SS plays an important role in the life cycle of this pathogen, enhancing inter- and intraspecies competition, protection from predators, and virulence. In strains where this system is not constitutively active, the T6SS is regulated in response to a number of environmental signals. Though it is unknown what signal TsrA responds to, this regulator represses the T6SS and the master virulence regulator ToxT, while activating HapA expression, which is involved in mucin degradation. Low osmolarity results in activation of the osmoregulator, OscR, which represses the T6SS. Quorum sensing also regulates the T6SS in response. At low cell density, LuxO is phosphorylated and activates the expression of quorum regulatory small RNAs (Qrr sRNAs), which repress the T6SS both through direct binding to the promoter regions of T6SS genes and through their inhibition of the positive regulator of T6SS, HapR. At high cell density, both HapR and the cAMP-CRP complex activate T6SS. HapR also actives QstR, which upregulates T6SS in response to growth on chitin. Flagellar regulatory genes are known to repress the T6SS through an unknown mechanism. Additionally, VasH, which is encoded by the T6SS pathogenicity island, is known to activate T6SS genes, potentially through its interaction with the alternative sigma factor RpoN, which appears to coregulate T6SS genes in a cAMP-CRP-dependent manner. Intriguingly, RpoN is also known to activate Qrr sRNAs, which repress the T6SS.

during growth on chitin. DNA is released from the lysed target cell, which is then taken up by the predatory cell via the competency machinery. This study demonstrated that in addition to its role in competition, the T6SS can enhance DNA uptake, potentially leading to increased evolution via horizontal gene transfer when the new DNA is incorporated into the genome (167).

T6SS expression was shown to be greatly enhanced under high osmolarity and low temperature conditions, which mimic estuarine conditions, suggesting that this system may be important in defense against predation and intraspecies competition in the aquatic environment. Genetic evidence suggests that the osmoregulator, OscR, represses the T6SS under low osmolarity at 37°C, though the mechanism of regulation has not been determined (171). It is hypothesized that expression of the T6SS in O1 strains is regulated in a pathoadaptive manner by osmolarity and temperature shifts; however, the T6SS also appears to play a role in the human host and likely responds to additional signals. The immunity gene *tsiV3* was shown to contribute to colonization of infant rabbit intestines when cocolonized with bacterial cells carrying a functional T6SS, indicating that *in vivo* species competition may contribute to virulence (172). Additionally, the effector VgrR-1 is known to increase inflammation and colonization in an infant mouse model (173). Thus, the T6SS contributes to both environmental and host survival, though further characterization of this important system is needed to fully determine its role in *V. cholerae* ecology.

Protozoan grazing

In aquatic environments, *V. cholerae* is preyed upon by a variety of bacterivorous predators, including ciliated and flagellated protozoa. In response to this biological stress, the bacterium has evolved mechanisms to shield itself from grazing and to actively kill predators. The T6SS described in the previous section can be mobilized to kill predatory protozoa and was, in fact, initially discovered for its ability to attack and kill the model host amoeba *Dictyostelium discoideum* (152). This defense mechanism requires direct contact with predator cells, because the T6SS structure must puncture the cell membrane to deliver the VasX and TseL toxins (157, 159).

Predator grazing also stimulates VPS production, leading to enhanced biofilm formation and a switch from smooth to rugose morphology associated with higher VPS production. VPS provides a physical barrier that partially protects *V. cholerae* from grazing (174). Additionally, *V. cholerae* biofilms grown on chitin appear to have higher antiprotozoal activity than those grown on abiotic surfaces and were shown to significantly reduce numbers of the surface-feeding flagellate *Rhynchomonas nasuta*, which is sensitive to ammonium produced by *V. cholerae* as a byproduct of chitin metabolism. The loss of QS in biofilms grown on chitin results in lower ammonium production and reduced toxicity to *R. nasuta* (175). Nonchitin biofilms have also been demonstrated to reduce predatory numbers at higher rates than planktonic cultures and promote predator killing via the production of QS-dependent antiprotozoal factors (29). While these antiprotozoal factors have not yet been identified, the HapR-regulated secreted protease PrtV is thought to be a candidate and was shown to be responsible for *V. cholerae* killing of *Cafeteria roenbergensis* and *Tetrahymena pyriformis* (176). The fact that both VPS and HapR contribute to grazing resistance is intriguing, because HapR downregulates *vps* expression. The role of HapR/QS in grazing resistance appears to be greater than that of VPS, because *hapR* mutants are less resistant to grazing than *vps* mutants (174). However, *hapR* mutants exhibit some grazing resistance in field and microcosm experiments, likely due to the increased biofilm formation phenotypes associated with *hapR* mutations. This physical protection from predators likely accounts for the enhanced grazing resistance of *hapR* mutants compared to wild type and demonstrates that *V. cholerae* uses multiple, independent mechanisms for evading predation (51, 177, 178).

Vibriophages

Bacterial viruses, known as bacteriophages or phages, play a critical role in the duration and severity of cholera outbreaks. Vibriophages specific for the serogroup dominating a particular outbreak can target and kill members of that serogroup in aquatic reservoirs or in infected hosts, thus promoting the decline of outbreaks by reducing transmission of infective *V. cholerae* (143, 179–181). An inverse correlation between the presence of environmental phages and the occurrence of viable *V. cholerae* in the aquatic environment, as well as the number of locally reported cholera cases, was observed over a 3-year study (180). This study suggests that epidemics are likely to begin when phage levels are diluted or diminished in the environment. In addition to influencing the timing of outbreaks and environmental competition of strains, lytic phages contribute to the self-limiting nature of seasonal cholera outbreaks. At the height of an epidemic, high levels of *V. cholerae* are observed in patient stool and in the environment, followed by high levels of lytic phages specific for the serogroup dominating the given epidemic, which contribute to the epidemic's decline. High levels of environmental phages correspond to high levels of phages observed in patient stool, suggesting that host-mediated phage amplification and subsequent dispersal into the environment is an important contributor to the self-limiting nature of seasonal outbreaks (143, 179). Additionally, studies that analyzed the impact of lytic phages naturally found in rice water stool on *V. cholerae* survival and infectious doses after coincubation in pond water revealed that high levels of lytic phages reduced infectivity and prevented transmission of *V. cholerae* to new hosts (181, 182). These findings suggest that phages modulate the infectious dose of *V. cholerae* and contribute to the collapse of cholera epidemics.

Evasion or adaptation to phage attack can also influence *V. cholerae* evolution. Often the O antigen is used as a major target of phages, and *V. cholerae* may modify its O antigen in an attempt to evade phage attack, resulting in new *V. cholerae* clones (183). Environmental phages displayed genetic and phenotypic diversity and, while many were specific to either O1 or O139 strains, some were able to use multiple *V. cholerae* strains as hosts, behaving as lysogenic phages in some strains and lytic phages in others. High phage concentrations may result in selective pressure for strains to become phage resistant or lysogenic for prevalent phages, and phage-related territorialism might be exploited to modulate epidemics and the rise of specific serogroups (180).

Phages not only play an essential role in the control of cholera outbreaks, but also contribute to the evolution of *V. cholerae* via horizontal gene transfer, genomic rearrangements, and vibriocidal selection. One of *V. cholerae*'s main virulence factors, cholera toxin, was introduced to *V. cholerae* via horizontal gene transfer. The cholera toxin genetic element (CTX), which encodes the genes necessary for the production of cholera toxin, is encoded by a lysogenic bacteriophage (CTXΦ) that uses the toxin coregulated pilus (TCP) as its receptor (184). Phage-bacteria interactions have a large influence on epidemic and evolutionary dynamics, playing dual roles in the rise of pathogenic *V. cholerae* and subsequent control of *V. cholerae* outbreaks.

ENTRY INTO THE HOST

V. cholerae undergoes a significant shift in environmental conditions as it is transmitted from the aquatic environment into the human host, and it continues to be exposed to diverse and changing signals throughout its infection cycle. This section outlines the challenges that *V. cholerae* experiences as it passes through the stomach and colonizes the small intestine, including stomach acid, nitric oxide (NO), bile, bicarbonate, antimicrobial peptides (AMPs), and mucin, and describes the molecular and physiological changes it undergoes to allow for efficient survival and transmission. Additionally, the induction of the virulence cascade in response to host signals is described, and we end this section by detailing how *V. cholerae* contacts host epithelial cells and initiates the production of the two major *V. cholerae* virulence factors, the TCP and cholera toxin. *In vitro* systems, human cholera patients, and various model organisms, including infant and adult mice, infant rabbits, and rabbit ligated ileal loops, were used to determine *V. cholerae*'s molecular and physiological responses to the host environment.

Responses to Challenges Encountered in the Stomach

When *V. cholerae* is ingested by the host, it enters the stomach and must respond to extreme physiological stresses, including exposure to acid and DNA-damaging agents. Adaptation to these damaging agents is essential for passage on to the small intestine, where the pathogen targets epithelial cells and induces virulence. In this section we describe the main challenges encountered by *V. cholerae* in the stomach and detail known survival responses and their impact on transmission and infection.

Adaptation to low pH

After ingestion, *V. cholerae* cells experience extreme acidity as they pass through the stomach, where the pH typically ranges from 1 to 3. *V. cholerae* grows best at neutral pH and has been shown to have a relatively low tolerance for acidic conditions, yet it survives prolonged acid exposure in the stomach, where average dwell times range from 20 to 60 minutes (185, 186). Growth in biofilm was shown to enhance the pathogen's acid tolerance by providing physical protection against acid shock, and ingestion of biofilms has been hypothesized to increase survival of *V. cholerae* in the host (56).

Exposure to acidic pH before infection greatly enhances colonization in the infant mouse due to *V. cholerae*'s ability to mount a robust acid tolerance response (ATR) (Fig. 4) (12). Many of the genes induced in response to low pH are heat shock proteins and chaperones, presumably to protect proteins from acid hydrolysis (187). *cadA*, which encodes a lysine decarboxylase, is critical for *V. cholerae*'s ATR, and disruption of *cadA* rendered the pathogen unable to survive acid shock after acid adaptation (188). Lysine decarboxylases consume H+ ions to produce cadaverine and carbon dioxide, and therefore

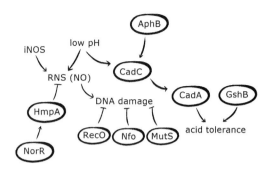

FIGURE 4 *V. cholerae* adaptation to low pH and radical nitrogen species (RNS). After ingestion, *V. cholerae* must adapt to low pH and RNS encountered in the stomach and small intestine. CadC, a ToxR-like transcriptional regulator, mediates the acid tolerance response and is known to be activated in response to low pH and by the LysR-type regulator AphB. CadC activates the expression of a lysine decarboxylase, CadA, which is thought to pump H+ ions out of the cell, thus raising internal pH. The glutathione synthetase, GshB, is also known to increase acid tolerance, likely through its regulation of the Kef system, which is responsible for potassium ion transport and plays a role in pH homeostasis. Low pH also contributes to the production of RNS, because acidified nitrite generated in response to low pH can be reduced to RNS. Inducible NO synthase (iNOS) produced by epithelial cells is also used to generate RNS. *V. cholerae* exposure to RNS can result in DNA damage that may be counteracted through the expression of RecO, a protein involved in daughter strand gap repair, Nfo, an endonuclease involved in base excision repair, and MutS, a DNA mismatch repair protein. Additionally, activation of HmpA, an enzyme responsible for destroying nitric oxide (NO), via the transcriptional regulator NorR contributes to *V. cholerae* resistance to RNS stress.

CadA likely protects *V. cholerae* from acid stress by pumping H+ ions out of the cell and raising internal pH. *cadA* expression is induced during infection of infant mice and adult rabbit ileal loops but not during growth in LB (188). Expression of *cadA* was also induced by other conditions potentially encountered during host infection, including oxygen limitation, sucrose or glucose exposure, and low pH in the presence of lysine (189). *cadA* is encoded in the *cadBA* operon, which is activated by the ToxR-like transcriptional regulator CadC. Expression of *cadC* is activated by the LysR-type regulator AphB, which also controls the virulence regulatory cascade in conjunction with the QS-regulated transcriptional activator, AphA. AphB and CadC are important for the *V. cholerae* ATR due to their regulation of *cadA*, and AphB's role in the ATR establishes a link between acid stress and virulence in *V. cholerae* (189).

Furthermore, the *V. cholerae* ATR likely involves *gshB*, which encodes glutathione synthetase, the enzyme that catalyzes the final step of glutathione synthesis. Disruption of *gshB* resulted in a 1,000-fold decrease in colonization of the infant mouse compared to wild-type *V. cholerae* (190). Glutathione regulates the Kef system, which is required for potassium ion transport, and pH homeostasis is believed to involve Na^+ and K^+ transport. Thus, the inability to produce glutathione and regulate K^+ transport likely renders bacteria unable to cope with pH stress.

Interestingly, acid-adaptation does not appear to increase *V. cholerae* survival during passage through the infant mouse stomach (191). Instead, it has been proposed that acid-adapted cells have enhanced colonization because they begin multiplying earlier and/or have a faster multiplication rate compared to unadapted cells. Although pretreating *V. cholerae* with acid does not aid in passage through the stomach, ATR genes are induced during infection and bolster colonization of the small intestine, indicating that the response to acid stress is critical for host infection and the transmission cycle of *V. cholerae*.

Adaptation to reactive nitrogen species (RNS)

In addition to acid shock, *V. cholerae* must cope with DNA damage generated by RNS. Nitrite from food sources and saliva is deposited in the stomach, where the low pH generates acidified nitrite that can be quickly reduced to the gaseous RNS NO, which causes DNA damage and has potent antimicrobial activity (Fig. 4) (192, 193). *V. cholerae* copes with RNS by expressing *hmpA*, which encodes an enzyme responsible for destroying NO. Deletion of this gene attenuated colonization in the presence, but not absence, of NO (194). The involvement of HmpA in survival in the stomach indicates that RNS cause DNA damage in this environment. Conversely, loss of genes associated with reactive oxygen species had no effect on survival, indicating that RNS is the main source of DNA damage during *V. cholerae* infection (194).

After traversing through the stomach, *V. cholerae* must continue to cope with the presence of NO. In response to *V. cholerae* infection, epithelial cells in the small intestine express the gene that encodes NO synthase (iNOS), which can then generate NO (195). Evidence suggests that NO continues to induce DNA damage in the small intestine, and adaptation to this damage requires *hmpA* (196). In the adult mouse, *hmpA* deletion mutants had a colonization defect that was evident 3 days after inoculation, and infection was completely abrogated by day 7, indicating that HmpA is important for long-term colonization of the adult mouse in addition to mediating passage through the stomach (194, 196). A transcriptional regulator, NorR, is required for *hmpA* expression. Interestingly, expression of *norR* is not altered by the presence of NO, and NorR represses its own expression independently of NO. Competition experiments in iNOS-deficient mice revealed that HmpA and NorR are critical for responding to long-term challenge derived from iNOS in the adult mouse small intestine (196).

Additionally, disruption of *recO*, which encodes a protein involved in daughter strand gap repair, prevents the pathogen from mounting an ATR and causes a severe colonization defect in infant mice (190). Loss of *nfo*, encoding an endonuclease involved in base excision repair, and *mutS*, encoding a DNA mismatch repair protein, also led to colonization defects relative to wild type. Colonization defects of *nfo*, *mutS*, and *hmpA* mutants reached 50 to 60% just 3 hours postinoculation; however, these defects were rescued by neutralization of stomach acid in the infant mice, further bolstering the link between gastric acid and DNA damage (194). Additionally, these mutant strains did not have heightened sensitivity to a low-pH medium, indicating that DNA damage in the host is induced by RNS derived from acidified nitrite, rather than acid stress alone. The results detailed above indicate that not only are DNA repair mechanisms critical for successful passage through the gastric acid barrier, but they also facilitate long-term survival in the small intestine.

Responses to Challenges Encountered in the Intestine

After passage through the stomach, *V. cholerae* enters the small intestine, where it must survive additional stressors and overcome physical barriers to begin colonization. Here we discuss how *V. cholerae* survives exposure to bile salts, organic acids, and AMPs and how it penetrates the mucus layer to reach the epithelial cells. Once it accesses the epithelial cells, it attaches, multiplies, and begins the production of virulence factors. It is worth noting that *V. cholerae* likely must compete with commensal bacteria found in the host gut, but this process has not been studied and therefore is not discussed in detail.

Bile

Bile is an aqueous mixture whose primary function is to emulsify and solubilize lipids, and it acts as an antimicrobial agent by damaging the cell wall and disrupting cellular homeostasis. In *V. cholerae*, bile resistance commonly involves proteins required for lipopolysaccharide (LPS) synthesis, efflux pumps, porins, and Tol proteins (Fig. 5) (197). Mutations in the *V. cholerae* LPS biosynthesis genes *waaF*, *wavB*, and *galU* enhanced bile sensitivity (198, 199). *waaF* and *wavB* encode a

putative heptosyl II transferase and a putative 1-4-β-glycosyl transferase, respectively; these products are required to synthesize the core oligosaccharide, which is necessary for *V. cholerae* to survive in the presence of bile (198, 199). *galU* encodes a UDP-glucose-pyrophosphorylase, which is responsible for synthesizing UDP-glucose, a carbohydrate that is incorporated into LPS surface structures to enhance the organism's hydrophobic barrier (198, 200).

V. cholerae bile resistance is also dependent on the response of efflux pumps, which remove numerous types of harmful compounds from bacterial cells. Efflux pumps are paired with pore proteins, which form channels in the outer membrane that allow compounds to be pumped out of the cell. In *V. cholerae*, the pore protein TolC is required for bile resistance and colonization in an infant mouse model and is hypothesized to function as the outer membrane channel for efflux pump systems (201). The RND (resistance-nodulation-division) family efflux systems, VexAB and BreAB (formerly named VexCD), both contribute to bile resistance, though VexAB appears to confer resistance to a greater range of antimicrobial compounds, while BreAB appears to specifically confer resistance to certain bile acids and detergents (202). Additionally, the multidrug resistance pump system VceAB is involved in resistance to the bile salt deoxycholate (203).

Bile sensitivity is also affected by porins, such as OmpU and OmpT, which allow exogenous compounds to diffuse into the cell based on size. In response to bile, *V. cholerae* expression of *ompU* is increased. Replacement of *ompT* with *ompU* increases bile resistance, because the smaller channel size of OmpU encumbers bile flux into the cell (204).

Besides posing a challenge for *V. cholerae* to overcome, bile also serves as a signal for *V. cholerae* to regulate genes associated with biofilm formation and virulence, though different bile compounds appear to exert differential regulation of this process. Bile acids have been shown to trigger an increase

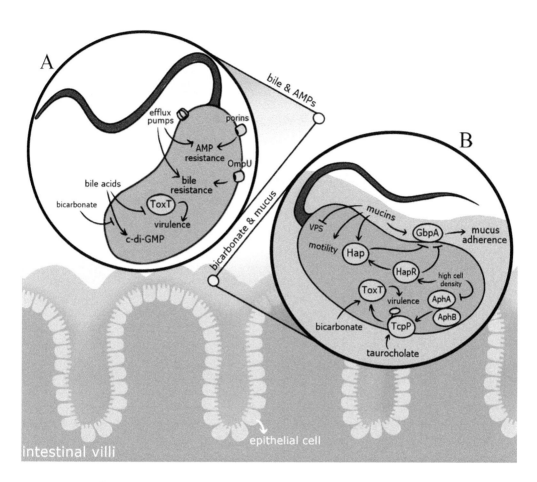

FIGURE 5 *V. cholerae* **adaptation to host signals in the small intestine. (A) In the intestinal lumen,** *V. cholerae* **encounters antimicrobial peptides and high concentrations of bile. Efflux pumps promote bile and AMP resistance by removing these compounds from the cell. Multiple porins, including OmpU and OmpT, contribute to AMP resistance. OmpU promotes bile resistance, because its relatively small channel size prevents bile compounds from entering the cell. Bile acids trigger an increase in the concentration of intracellular c-di-GMP; this response may be partially quenched by the low concentration of bicarbonate present in the intestinal lumen. Bile acids also interfere with the ability of the major virulence regulator ToxT to bind DNA, thus encumbering expression of virulence genes in the lumen. (B) Upon contacting the mucus layer,** *V. cholerae* **encounters mucins and high concentrations of bicarbonate. Mucins promote production of the GlcNac-binding protein GbpA, which is expressed on the cell surface and facilitates adhesion to the mucus layer. Mucins also promote production of Hap (hemagglutinin/protease), which breaks up mucus, thus facilitating penetration through the mucus layer. Hap downregulates GbpA, which may prevent the cell from continuing to adhere to the mucus layer as it penetrates through it. Additionally, mucins promote motility and downregulate** *vps* **genes, which may further foster movement through the mucus layer toward the epithelium. High cell density leads to activation of HapR, which downregulates GbpA production directly, as well as indirectly by promoting production of Hap. Virulence genes are activated when the high concentration of bicarbonate in the mucus layer enhances ToxT activity, as well as when the bile salt taurocholate promotes activation of TcpP.**

in the intracellular concentration of c-di-GMP, a signaling nucleotide that promotes biofilm formation and represses virulence genes (205). However, the effect of bile acids on c-di-GMP production was quenched by bicarbonate, which is produced by epithelial cells and secreted into the lumen of the small intestine to neutralize stomach acid (69, 206). Bile also influences the activity of a master virulence regulator, ToxT. *Cis*-palmitoleate, a fatty acid found in bile, binds to ToxT and reduces expression of its downstream virulence targets, *tcp* and *ctx*, by interfering with its ability to bind to DNA (207). Bicarbonate, which increases in concentration near the epithelial surface, enhances ToxT activity (206). Repression of ToxT activity by bile or activation by bicarbonate was shown to be dependent on a short, unstructured region of ToxT, which is proposed to bind to its negative or positive effectors and change conformation to enhance or reduce DNA binding (208). This supports a hypothesis in which bile components in the lumen bind to ToxT and hold it in its inactive confirmation until it enters the mucus layer of the intestine, where increasing levels of bicarbonate activate ToxT and expression of virulence factors as *V. cholerae* approaches epithelial cells (206, 208).

The bile salt taurocholate upregulates virulence by inducing formation of an intermolecular disulfide bond between two cysteine residues in the periplasmic domain of the transmembrane transcription factor TcpP (209). This disulfide bond formation allows for dimerization and activity of TcpP, which then activates virulence genes. TcpP is responsible for transcription of ToxT. Taurocholate additionally stimulates biofilm dispersal by degrading the biofilm matrix (210). Intriguingly, taurocholate activation of virulence was only observed in planktonic cells or in cells that were first abiotically dispersed from the biofilm in response to taurocholate (210). Thus, TcpP activation likely prepares the cell to produce further downstream virulence factors as it enters the

intestine and encounters the appropriate signals.

Antimicrobial peptides

V. cholerae must cope with AMPs in the small intestine. These peptides are part of the innate immune system and make up a diverse group of amphipathic molecules. AMPs have a variety of mechanisms for killing bacteria and often function by altering membrane permeability. As with other challenges in the host, bacteria have evolved a variety of mechanisms for coping with AMPs, including modification of LPS and export of AMPs from the cell (Fig. 5).

The acyltransferase MsbB aids in resistance to a wide variety of AMPs by facilitating modification of LPS (211). An *msbB* mutant was attenuated for colonization in the infant mouse, indicating that *msbB* is important for resistance to AMPs found in the infant mouse gut. The cathelin-related AMP CRAMP is prevalent in the infant mouse intestine, and loss of *msbB* was shown to significantly increase CRAMP sensitivity (211, 212). CRAMP is similar to the human AMP LL-37, indicating that MsbB may play a comparable role in human infection (213). The lipid A LPS moiety of *msbB* mutants is underacylated compared to wild-type LPS, which suggests that acylation of LPS provides resistance to mammalian AMPs, or alternatively, underacylation causes secondary membrane disruption that negatively impacts *V. cholerae* AMP resistance. Further studies are needed to distinguish between these two possibilities.

Various forms of LPS modification are involved in *V. cholerae* resistance to polymyxin B, an AMP produced by bacteria (211, 214, 215). Loss of *msbB* significantly decreases polymyxin B resistance in the El Tor biotype, indicating that lipid A acylation is critical for resistance to this AMP (211). MsbA/LpxN adds secondary hydroxylated acyl chains to the lipid A portion of LPS and mediates polymyxin B resistance (214). AlmG, AlmF, and AlmE are required to modify LPS with glycine and diglycine residues, and loss of *almG* strongly increases polymyxin B sensitivity (215). CarR, the response regulator of the two-component system CarRS, directly binds to and activates transcription at the *almEFG* promoter (216, 217). Though CarRS is known to be negatively regulated by high calcium levels, which naturally fluctuate in the aquatic environment, further study is needed to identify *in vivo* signals sensed by CarS that may be responsible for *in vivo* CarRS activity and *alm* gene expression (90). Though *alm* genes were shown to be dispensable for colonization of the infant mouse, these enzymes may confer resistance to AMPs unique to the human gut (217). The importance of lipid A modification, which could contribute to AMP resistance by modifying the cell surface charge and/or by altering the membrane fluidity of the cell, highlights the role of LPS in protecting *V. cholerae* from antimicrobial compounds.

Efflux pumps can export AMPs, and loss of any of *V. cholerae*'s six RND efflux systems caused heightened sensitivity to antimicrobial compounds. The *vexB* mutant was most sensitive to AMPs, indicating that the VexAB efflux system is the major contributor to AMP resistance. Furthermore, RND mutants mimic the AMP-sensitive phenotype of a *tolC* mutant, suggesting that these efflux systems work in conjunction with the pore protein TolC to remove AMPs from the cell (218).

Porins also have a role in *V. cholerae* resistance to AMPs. The OmpU and OmpT porins contribute to resistance to polymyxin B and BPI (bactericidal/permeability-increasing), an antimicrobial protein expressed on the surface of human gastrointestinal tract epithelial cells (219). *In vitro* studies revealed that loss of *toxR* increases killing by a BPI derivative known as P2 by 100-fold relative to wild type, and this activity was due to ToxR's role in regulating expression of the porins *ompU* and *ompT* (220). OmpU is primarily responsible for mediating P2 resistance in the mid-log phase and stationary phases, while OmpT plays a role in this process during the stationary phase (220). OmpU controls AMP resistance via a pathway that includes the alternative sigma factor RpoE. It has been proposed that AMP-induced membrane perturbations cause an OmpU conformational change that allows the porin to bind DegS, a periplasmic protease responsible for activating RpoE (219). This alternative sigma factor stimulates repair of AMP-induced membrane damage by triggering the extracytoplasmic stress response, which includes periplasmic protein folding chaperones such as the thiol:disulfide interchange proteins DsbA and DsbD and outer membrane components such as lipoproteins (221).

Mucus barrier

V. cholerae must navigate the thick coating of mucus that lines the small intestine. This viscous secretion serves as part of the body's innate immune system by preventing pathogens from contacting and colonizing the intestinal surface. Complex glycoproteins called mucins are the primary constituents of mucus and are responsible for its viscosity. Upon entering the small intestine, *V. cholerae* contacts and adheres to the mucosal lining (Fig. 5) (222). *gbpA*, which encodes a chitin-binding protein, is important for this adherence (105). GbpA binds the chitin monomer *N*-acetyl-D-glucosamine (GlcNac), which is a common constituent of human intestinal mucins (223). Most of the GbpA produced by *V. cholerae* is secreted, with a minor fraction remaining on the cell surface and facilitating adhesion. Experiments performed in the infant mouse suggest that coordinated interactions between GbpA and mucin facilitate the initial stage of *V. cholerae* intestinal adherence (105). GbpA binds to mucins and triggers a signaling cascade that stimulates the transcription of host genes associated with production of secreted mucins. Concomitantly, *V. cholerae* exposure to mucins stimulates transcription and production of GbpA. The increased levels of GbpA, especially on the bacterial surface, facilitate adherence to the intestinal mucus layer

(105). Additional factors are then needed to facilitate penetration through the mucus layer and attachment to host cells.

A soluble zinc-dependent metalloprotease known as Hap (hemagglutinin/protease) is required for *V. cholerae* to penetrate the host mucus layer (224). Hap, encoded by *hapA*, has both mucinolytic and cytotoxic activity and is required for *V. cholerae* to translocate through a mucin-containing gel in a column assay (224). Mucin stimulates Hap expression and production, which then facilitates breakdown of mucus and penetration to the intestinal surface. Hap also degrades GbpA, suggesting that production of Hap upon mucin binding stimulates degradation of both GbpA and mucin, allowing the cells to move through the mucus layer (225). The QS master regulator HapR represses *gbpA* expression and activates *hapA* expression, suggesting that cell division and increasing cell density after mucus attachment promote degradation of mucin by Hap and prevent production of new GbpA from hampering movement through the mucin (224, 225). Additionally, mucin activates *hapA* expression independently of HapR. Bile salts and growth at 37°C promote Hap production, but not expression, indicating that these factors control posttranscriptional modifications of *hapA* (224). Together, evidence suggests a model in which mucin and HapR stimulate Hap-dependent mucosal breakdown.

Mucin also stimulates *V. cholerae* motility and represses VPS production. VPS is capable of binding to mucin, and mutants that over-express VPS are attenuated for colonization in the distal intestine of the infant mouse, likely because they do not have the ability to migrate quickly through the mucus layer (226). Thus, the concomitant increase in motility and decrease in *vps* expression in response to mucin indicates that *V. cholerae* maximizes movement through the mucus layer. Experiments performed in mucin-containing columns indicated that the *V. cholerae* polar flagellum breaks as the organism migrates through mucin, and the loss of flagellar

proteins triggers a pathway that leads to inhibition of *hapR* transcription and expression of virulence genes (170). This study indicated that the flagellum is required for initial penetration into the mucin but that *V. cholerae* utilizes flagellar-independent motion to move in mucin. Alternatively, it was proposed that flagellar breakage may occur closely enough to the intestinal epithelium that the organism is still able to colonize and express virulence genes.

Intestinal cell contact and the production of virulence factors

After penetrating the mucus layer in the small intestine, *V. cholerae* attaches to epithelial cells, forms microcolonies, and produces the virulence factors that cause the disease cholera. Here we discuss mechanisms impacting localization in the intestine and the induction of key virulence factors upon cell contact.

The two main virulence factors produced by *V. cholerae* are TCP and cholera toxin. TCP is a type IV pilus that facilitates colonization of the intestinal epithelium (227). Cholera toxin's five B subunits bind to the surface of epithelial cells, and then a portion of the A subunit penetrates into the host cells and alters host cell signal transduction pathways leading to constitutive cyclic AMP production, leading to profuse secretion of chloride and water into the gut lumen while preventing Na^+ absorption (228). Production of TCP and cholera toxin, as well as other virulence factors, depends on two transmembrane transcriptional regulators, ToxR/ToxS and TcpP/TcpH, as well as the cytoplasmic regulators AphAB and ToxT (229–233). ToxR and TcpP directly activate expression of ToxT, the most downstream transcriptional regulator of the virulence regulatory cascade. *tcpPH* expression is modulated by AphAB, which binds to the promoter region of *tcpPH* and activates its expression (233). TcpH inhibits degradation of TcpP, which works with ToxR to bind to the *toxT* promoter and activate ToxT expression (234, 235). ToxT undergoes conformational changes depending on signals encountered in the stomach and small intestine; when in its active conformation, ToxT promotes production of TCP and cholera toxin by binding directly to the *tcpA* and *ctx* promoter regions and displacing the nucleoid-associated protein, H-NS, which acts as a silencer of virulence gene expression (64, 207, 236). Experiments performed with the intestinal epithelial cell line INT 407 indicate that contact with host cells results in strong induction of major virulence genes *ctxAB*, *tcpA*, and *toxT* (Fig. 6) (237). This response is triggered by strong induction of *vieA*, which encodes a PDE that degrades c-di-GMP via its EAL domain; furthermore, the VieA's EAL domain was required for induction of *toxT* in response to host cell contact (237). These results indicate that host cell contact following mucosal penetration results in virulence gene expression.

EXIT FROM THE HOST

An important stage in the *V. cholerae* life cycle is its exit from the host, which contributes to the fast-moving nature of cholera outbreaks by facilitating transmission to a new host or redepositing high numbers of bacteria into aquatic reservoirs. At this stage, *V. cholerae* must detach from epithelial cells to exit the small intestine and be shed in stool, where it is again exposed to drastic changes in its environment. In this section we discuss what is known about *V. cholerae* exit and survival strategies late in infection, as well as factors contributing to environmental fitness and virulence after *V. cholerae* is shed in stool.

Mucosal Escape Response

During late-stage infection, *V. cholerae* initiates a mucosal escape response that allows it to exit the host. During this process, regulation of virulence factors changes within the population, and only a portion of the exiting cells continue to express virulence factors (Fig. 6). These responses are thought to enhance the ability of *V. cholerae* to transition back into environmental reservoirs or facilitate reentry into a new human host and are discussed in greater detail below.

V. cholerae utilizes a genetic program controlled by RpoS, the starvation/stationary phase alternative sigma factor, to detach and migrate from the epithelial surface into the lumen of the intestine (238). As observed in a rabbit ileal loop model, wild-type *V. cholerae* cells leave the epithelial surface several hours into infection when cells would be expected to enter the stationary phase of growth, while strains lacking *rpoS* are much more likely to remain on the epithelium. RpoS positively controls production of HapR, which is also required for this transition (238). Whole-genome expression profiling studies have demonstrated that RpoS controls the expression of genes involved in flagellar assembly and chemotaxis; some of these genes are also under the control of HapR, suggesting that high cell density and nutrient limitation leads to RpoS-dependent activation of a motility program, termed the mucosal escape response (238). The mucosal escape response represents a distinct phase in the *V. cholerae* infection cycle that prepares *V. cholerae* for exit from the host and entry into the environment or for transmission to a new host. During this process, other complex genetic and physiological changes take place, including the differential downregulation of virulence gene expression (238).

While the *tcp* and *ctxAB* genes are highly expressed early in the infectious cycle in bacteria adjacent to epithelial surfaces, later in infection significant heterogeneity in virulence gene expression is observed. The *tcp* and *ctxAB* genes are controlled by an epigenetic bistable switch that causes the *V. cholerae* population to undergo bifurcation as it enters the stationary phase and prepares for the mucosal escape response (35). One subpopulation continued to express *tcp* and

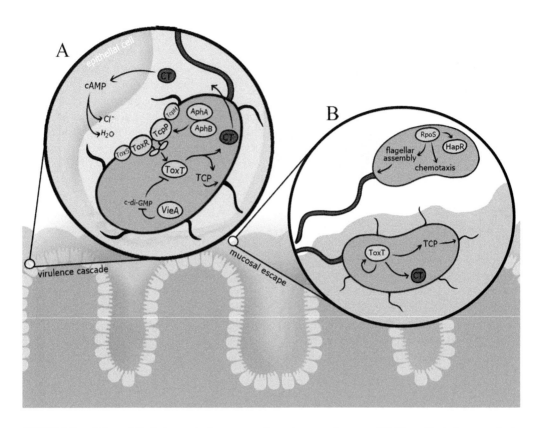

FIGURE 6 Regulation of *V. cholerae* virulence cascade and mucosal escape. (A) When *V. cholerae* contacts host epithelial cells, expression of the PDE VieA is upregulated, resulting in a decrease in intracellular c-di-GMP concentration. In turn, low c-di-GMP concentration induces expression of *toxT*, which controls the production of *V. cholerae*'s major virulence factors, toxin coregulated pilus (TCP) and cholera toxin (CT). Production of TCP and CT also depends on two transmembrane transcriptional regulators, ToxR and TcpP, as well as the cytoplasmic regulators AphAB and ToxT. TCP is a type IV pilus that facilitates colonization of the intestinal epithelium, while CT is a secreted toxin that causes constitutive cyclic AMP production in host epithelial cells, leading to profuse secretion of chloride and water into the gut lumen. (B) During later stages of infection, as the population density increases and cells reach the stationary phase, production of the starvation/stationary phase alternative sigma factor RpoS and the quorum sensing master regulator HapR are induced. These regulators trigger flagellar assembly and chemotaxis, which foster exit from the host. Additionally, the population of *V. cholerae* cells in the small intestine becomes bifurcated; half of the cells continue to show high expression of virulence genes (represented by the bottom cell), while the other half shows downregulation of virulence genes.

ctxAB genes, while the other subpopulation has decreased expression of these virulence genes. The master regulator of virulence, ToxT, plays a key role in this differential expression of virulence and dimerizes to promote expression of *tcp* genes and its own expression in a positively controlled regulatory feedback loop. This expression is hypersensitive to the number of ToxT dimers

in the cell and can be repressed by the cAMP-CRP complex, which forms during entry into stationary phase. Thus, only a fraction of the cells continue to express virulence genes as they enter stationary growth phase, and bifurcation within the population occurs (35). Intriguingly, TCP has self-aggregating properties, and expression of TCP was shown to be higher in bacterial aggregates, suggesting that this subpopulation may contribute to both aggregation and hyperinfectivity of *V. cholerae* shed in patient stool (35). It has been suggested that the bistable control of virulence gene expression contributes to the transmission and allows a subpopulation of shed bacteria to be prepared for reentry and infection in a new host (35).

Expression profiles of *V. cholerae* during infection using infant mouse and infant rabbit infection models have been determined using RNA-Seq. In both the infant mouse and infant rabbit models, 39 genes were found to be upregulated, while 478 genes were induced in one animal, indicating that there is minimum overlap in the expression profiles. These differences may be due to differences between infection microenvironments in these infection models (239). Over 400 genes have been identified as being critical to *V. cholerae in vivo* fitness, including the virulence factors described above, genes involved in metabolism, resistance to bile, T6SS, and synthesis of the second messenger molecule cyclic AMP-GMP (c-AMP-GMP) (172). While the significance of many of these genes is still being explored, it is evident that *V. cholerae* must initiate a complex and multifaceted cellular response to adapt to and survive in the host environment.

Survival During Late-Stage Infection and Dissemination from the Host

In addition to the two genetic programs described above, *V. cholerae* prepares for exit from the host by regulating a number of genes involved in metabolism, biofilm formation, and motility during late-stage infection and after being shed from the host. Here we discuss genes upregulated during late infection and their potential roles in environmental survival and transmission, as well as the hyperinfective state of cells shed in patient stool. We further explore factors influencing hyperinfectivity and describe what is known about this unique state.

Late-stage infection

During the late stages of infection *V. cholerae* prepares for dissemination and enters a unique physiological state that primes it to cope with nutrient limitations in the environment. Processes that are upregulated include recycling of amino acids, proteins, and cell wall components, which help the organism to conserve energy by making use of compounds that are already available in the cell (108). Furthermore, late-stage infection prepares *V. cholerae* to cope with carbon limitation by utilizing alternative carbon sources. VC1926, which encodes a predicted activator of C4-dicarboxylate transport, prepares the pathogen to make use of succinate. The product of VC_A0744, a glycerol kinase, is involved in glycine metabolism. Succinate and glycine may be components of dissolved organic matter in aquatic environments, indicating that *V. cholerae* prepares to scavenge nutrients after dissemination. The operon containing VC0612-3 encodes chitin degradation enzymes; its induction in late-stage infection prepares the pathogen to make use of chitin, a nutrient that is highly available in aquatic environments, but not in the human host. Only a small subset of mutants lacking late-stage genes were shown to be attenuated for infection in the infant mouse, and the attenuated phenotypes were all specific to late-stage infection. Conversely, late-stage genes were critical for prolonged survival in pond water, indicating that late-stage infection genes likely have functions in dissemination and environmental survival, but not host infection (240).

Gene regulation during late-stage infection also appears to regulate *V. cholerae* motility and biofilm formation by modulating levels of the signaling nucleotide c-di-GMP (111, 240). During late infection, the transcriptional regulator PhoB becomes activated, which then induces expression of the *acgAB* operon. *acgA* encodes an active EAL PDE, while *acgB* encodes an active DGC. When acgA and acgB are overproduced, the net result is decreased c-di-GMP levels and increased motility compared to wild type (111). However, the opposing activities of AcgA and AcgB may function by controlling fine-scale differences in c-di-GMP concentration in spatially localized modules, allowing them to regulate specific downstream processes. Late-stage infection was also shown to induce expression of three genes encoding DGCs, which are responsible for producing c-di-GMP (240). Each of these DGCs was shown to be capable of c-di-GMP synthesis, and loss of all three genes greatly diminished survival in pond water after 24 hours. Late-stage induction of enzymes that synthesize and degrade c-di-GMP suggests that motility and biofilm formation are tightly controlled during this time, and further studies are needed to determine if these enzymes have specific downstream functions or if they regulate net c-di-GMP concentration in the population. Many of the genes induced during late infection impact *V. cholerae*'s ability to survive when they are released in patient stool, where they may either transition back into the aquatic environment or be transmitted to a new host.

Hyperinfectivity

Stool-derived *V. cholerae* exhibits enhanced infectivity; this phenotype persists for up to 5 hours after shedding, even after dilution in nutrient-poor pond water. Shedding of hyperinfective bacteria in patient stool is predicted to impact the epidemic spread of cholera by lowering the infectious dose required to cause disease. Transcriptional profiling of *V. cholerae* isolated from patient stool revealed that genes required for nutrient acquisition and motility were upregulated, while genes required for chemotaxis were downregulated (12). It is interesting to note that nonchemotactic mutants of *V. cholerae* showed increased infectivity compared to wild type. These mutants also showed altered localization within the host; wild-type *V. cholerae* localizes primarily to the distal portion of the small intestine, while nonchemotactic mutants colonize evenly throughout the small intestine (241). It has been proposed that chemotaxis guides the cells to areas that are optimal for virulence gene expression, but survival is reduced by suboptimal conditions or host immune defenses, and/or the increased area of colonization allows nonchemotactic mutants to reach higher numbers. Because recently shed cells were highly motile, it was proposed that motility in the absence of chemotaxis aids in dissemination from the host and reentry into aquatic environments. Alternatively, repression of chemotaxis may promote shedding from the GI tract by dampening *V. cholerae*'s attraction to the intestinal epithelia (12, 242).

However, while some *V. cholerae* were highly motile after shedding, cholera patient stools also contained biofilm-like aggregates that were demonstrated to be hyperinfective relative to planktonic cells from the same stool samples (34). Formation of these aggregates appears to require VPS, because elimination of *vps* genes ablated aggregation *in vitro* and in rabbit ileal loops (147). This supports a hypothesis that VPS contributes to the biofilm-like aggregates identified in cholera stool, in addition to clumping observed from TCP production or mucus adhesion. Further studies have shown that growth in a biofilm, even in the absence of passage through a host, induces hyperinfectivity (31). Cells derived from biofilms, whether intact or dispersed, are hyperinfective relative to planktonic cells, indicating that the structure of biofilm has little or no effect on a strain's infectivity. Rather, growth in a biofilm induces a transient physiological state that enhances colonization, suggesting that conditions associated with biofilm formation act as triggers to prepare the cells for host infection (31). Intriguingly, QS-deficient *hapR* deletion mutants exhibited a colonization defect in an infant mouse model; however, this defect was only observed when the infectious dose was introduced in a biofilm rather than in a planktonic state. This result may be due to the inability of cells to detach from the biofilm in the absence of HapR and indicates that transitioning between the biofilm and planktonic state is critical for colonization, and the absence of this ability attenuates the hyperinfectivity of biofilms (56). Collectively, these studies revealed that hyperinfectivity plays an important role in the initiation and persistence of cholera.

CONCLUSION

As this chapter has demonstrated, *V. cholerae* is exposed to a wide variety of signals and challenges throughout its life cycle. Transmission of the pathogen between hosts is a multifactorial process influenced by the quantity and infectivity of bacterial cells upon host entry, as well as the mechanisms used to withstand harsh conditions in the host and the environment.

It is known that *V. cholerae* must survive a number of fluctuating, and sometimes severe, environmental conditions and then must adapt to the vastly different conditions encountered during infection of the host. A number of survival strategies appear to be unique to each environment, while others are utilized in both. Utilization of chitin as an energy source is vital to *V. cholerae* survival, evolution, and transmission in the aquatic environment but is not available during infection of the human host. In contrast, the T6SS is utilized in competition against other bacteria and as a defense against predation in the aquatic environment, but it may also be used in the host as protection against macrophages and gut commensal bacteria. Advantages provided by one environment can also prepare this pathogen for entry into the other. For example, biofilm formation in the aquatic environment contributes to hyperinfectivity in the human host, while glycogen acquisition and storage during infection increases *V. cholerae* survival in nutrient poor aquatic environments once it has been shed in stool. These and other factors influence transmission and the severity of cholera outbreaks, which are additionally impacted by growth on zooplankton, favorable environmental conditions, shedding in patient stool, bacteriophage concentrations, and acquired immunity in hosts followed by the rapid evolution of new pathogenic forms of *V. cholerae*. The relationships between pathogen, host, and the aquatic environment are therefore intricately linked, each contributing to the survival, transmission, and infectivity of *V. cholerae*.

ACKNOWLEDGMENTS

Jenna G. Conner and Jennifer K. Teschler contributed equally to this chapter. We thank Jay Zhu for his helpful comments on this document, Lynette Cegelski for generously sharing the biofilm image depicted in Fig. 1, and Adam Alpine for his assistance with Fig. 1. We would also like to acknowledge the members of the Yildiz lab for their useful input and contributions.

This work was supported by the National Institutes of Health grants AI102584, AI114261, and AI055987.

CITATION

Conner JG, Teschler JK, Jones CJ, Yildiz FH. 2016. Staying alive: *Vibrio cholerae's* cycle of environmental survival, transmission, and dissemination. Microbiol Spectrum 4(2):VMBF-0015-2015.

REFERENCES

1. **World Health Organization.** 2012. *TDR Global Report for Research on Infectious Diseases of Poverty.* http://www.who.int/tdr/publications/global_report/en/.
2. **Ali M, Lopez AL, You YA, Kim YE, Sah B, Maskery B, Clemens J.** 2012. The global burden of cholera. *Bull World Health Organ* **90:**209–218A.
3. **Kaper JB, Morris JG, Levine MM.** 1995. Cholera. *Clin Microbiol Rev* **8:**48–86.
4. **Charles RC, Ryan ET.** 2011. Cholera in the 21st century. *Curr Opin Infect Dis* **24:**472–477.
5. **Chin C-S, Sorenson J, Harris JB, Robins WP, Charles RC, Jean-Charles RR, Bullard J,**

Webster DR, Kasarskis A, Peluso P, Paxinos EE, Yamaichi Y, Calderwood SB, Mekalanos JJ, Schadt EE, Waldor MK. 2011. The origin of the Haitian cholera outbreak strain. *N Engl J Med* **364**:33–42.

6. **Nguyen BM, Lee JH, Cuong NT, Choi SY, Hien NT, Anh DD, Lee HR, Ansaruzzaman M, Endtz HP, Chun J, Lopez AL, Czerkinsky C, Clemens JD, Kim DW.** 2009. Cholera outbreaks caused by an altered *Vibrio cholerae* O1 El Tor biotype strain producing classical cholera toxin B in Vietnam in 2007 to 2008. *J Clin Microbiol* **47**:1568–1571.

7. **Mason PR.** 2009. Zimbabwe experiences the worst epidemic of cholera in Africa. *J Infect Dev Ctries* **3**:148–151.

8. **Alam M, Sultana M, Nair GB, Sack RB, Sack DA, Siddique AK, Ali A, Huq A, Colwell RR.** 2006. Toxigenic *Vibrio cholerae* in the aquatic environment of Mathbaria, Bangladesh. *Appl Environ Microbiol* **72**:2849–2855.

9. **Faruque SM, Albert MJ, Mekalanos JJ.** 1998. Epidemiology, genetics, and ecology of toxigenic *Vibrio cholerae*. *Microbiol Mol Biol Rev* **62**:1301–1314.

10. **Huq A, Sack RB, Nizam A, Longini IM, Nair GB, Ali A, Morris JG, Khan MNH, Siddique AK, Yunus M, Albert MJ, Sack DA, Colwell RR.** 2005. Critical factors influencing the occurrence of *Vibrio cholerae* in the environment of Bangladesh. *Appl Environ Microbiol* **71**:4645–4654.

11. **Weil AA, Khan AI, Chowdhury F, Larocque RC, Faruque ASG, Ryan ET, Calderwood SB, Qadri F, Harris JB.** 2009. Clinical outcomes in household contacts of patients with cholera in Bangladesh. *Clin Infect Dis* **49**:1473–1479.

12. **Merrell DS, Butler SM, Qadri F, Dolganov NA, Alam A, Cohen MB, Calderwood SB, Schoolnik GK, Camilli A.** 2002. Host-induced epidemic spread of the cholera bacterium. *Nature* **417**:642–645.

13. **Chowdhury F, Khan AI, Harris JB, LaRocque RC, Chowdhury MI, Ryan ET, Faruque ASG, Calderwood SB, Qadri F.** 2008. A comparison of clinical and immunologic features in children and older patients hospitalized with severe cholera in Bangladesh. *Pediatr Infect Dis J* **27**:986–992.

14. **Harris JB, LaRocque RC, Chowdhury F, Khan AI, Logvinenko T, Faruque ASG, Ryan ET, Qadri F, Calderwood SB.** 2008. Susceptibility to *Vibrio cholerae* infection in a cohort of household contacts of patients with cholera in Bangladesh. *PLoS Negl Trop Dis* **2**: e221. doi:10.1371/journal.pntd.0000221.

15. **Harris JB, Khan AI, LaRocque RC, Dorer DJ, Chowdhury F, Faruque ASG, Sack DA, Ryan ET, Qadri F, Calderwood SB.** 2005. Blood group, immunity, and risk of infection with *Vibrio cholerae* in an area of endemicity. *Infect Immun* **73**:7422–7427.

16. **Holmner A, Mackenzie A, Krengel U.** 2010. Molecular basis of cholera blood-group dependence and implications for a world characterized by climate change. *FEBS Lett* **584**:2548–2555.

17. **Glass RI, Holmgren J, Haley CE, Khan MR, Svennerholm AM, Stoll BJ, Belayet Hossain KM, Black RE, Yunus M, Barua D.** 1985. Predisposition for cholera of individuals with O blood group. Possible evolutionary significance. *Am J Epidemiol* **121**:791–796.

18. **Barua D, Paguio AS.** 1977. ABO blood groups and cholera. *Ann Hum Biol* **4**:489–492.

19. **Mukhopadhyay AK, Takeda Y, Nair GB.** 2014. Cholera outbreaks in the El Tor biotype era and the impact of the new El Tor variants, p 17–47. *In* Nair GB, Takeda Y (ed), *Cholera Outbreaks.* Springer, Heidelberg, Germany.

20. **Faruque AS, Fuchs GJ, Albert MJ.** 1996. Changing epidemiology of cholera due to *Vibrio cholerae* O1 and O139 Bengal in Dhaka, Bangladesh. *Epidemiol Infect* **116**:275–278.

21. **Faruque SM, Chowdhury N, Kamruzzaman M, Ahmad QS, Faruque ASG, Salam MA, Ramamurthy T, Nair GB, Weintraub A, Sack DA.** 2003. Reemergence of epidemic *Vibrio cholerae* O139, Bangladesh. *Emerg Infect Dis* **9**:1116–1122.

22. **Safa A, Nair GB, Kong RYC.** 2010. Evolution of new variants of *Vibrio cholerae* O1. *Trends Microbiol* **18**:46–54.

23. **Grim CJ, Hasan NA, Taviani E, Haley B, Chun J, Brettin TS, Bruce DC, Detter JC, Han CS, Chertkov O, Challacombe J, Huq A, Nair GB, Colwell RR.** 2010. Genome sequence of hybrid *Vibrio cholerae* O1 MJ-1236, B-33, and CIRS101 and comparative genomics with *V. cholerae. J Bacteriol* **192**:3524–3533.

24. **Kanungo S, Sah BK, Lopez AL, Sung JS, Paisley AM, Sur D, Clemens JD, Nair GB.** 2010. Cholera in India: an analysis of reports, 1997–2006. *Bull World Health Organ* **88**:185–191.

25. **Siddique AK, Nair GB, Alam M, Sack DA, Huq A, Nizam A, Longini IM, Qadri F, Faruque SM, Colwell RR, Ahmed S, Iqbal A, Bhuiyan NA, Sack RB.** 2010. El Tor cholera with severe disease: a new threat to Asia and beyond. *Epidemiol Infect* **138**:347–352.

26. **Piarroux R, Barrais R, Faucher B, Haus R, Piarroux M, Gaudart J, Magloire R, Didier R.** 2011. Understanding the cholera epidemic, Haiti. *Emerg Infect Dis* **17**:1161–1167.

27. **Wai SN, Mizunoe Y, Takade A, Kawabata SI, Yoshida SI.** 1998. *Vibrio cholerae* O1 strain

TSI-4 produces the exopolysaccharide materials that determine colony morphology, stress resistance, and biofilm formation. *Appl Environ Microbiol* **64:**3648–3655.

28. **Beyhan S, Yildiz FH.** 2007. Smooth to rugose phase variation in *Vibrio cholerae* can be mediated by a single nucleotide change that targets c-di-GMP signalling pathway. *Mol Microbiol* **63:**995–1007.

29. **Matz C, McDougald D, Moreno AM, Yung PY, Yildiz FH, Kjelleberg S.** 2005. Biofilm formation and phenotypic variation enhance predation-driven persistence of *Vibrio cholerae*. *Proc Natl Acad Sci USA* **102:**16819–16824.

30. **Tamplin ML, Gauzens AL, Huq A, Sack DA, Colwell RR.** 1990. Attachment of *Vibrio cholerae* serogroup O1 to zooplankton and phytoplankton of Bangladesh waters. *Appl Environ Microbiol* **56:**1977–1980.

31. **Tamayo R, Patimalla B, Camilli A.** 2010. Growth in a biofilm induces a hyperinfectious phenotype in *Vibrio cholerae*. *Infect Immun* **78:**3560–3569.

32. **Huq A, Xu B, Chowdhury MA, Islam MS, Montilla R, Colwell RR.** 1996. A simple filtration method to remove plankton-associated *Vibrio cholerae* in raw water supplies in developing countries. *Appl Environ Microbiol* **62:**2508–2512.

33. **Colwell RR, Huq A, Islam MS, Aziz KMA, Yunus M, Khan NH, Mahmud A, Sack RB, Nair GB, Chakraborty J, Sack DA, Russek-Cohen E.** 2003. Reduction of cholera in Bangladeshi villages by simple filtration. *Proc Natl Acad Sci USA* **100:**1051–1055.

34. **Faruque SM, Biswas K, Udden SMN, Ahmad QS, Sack DA, Nair GB, Mekalanos JJ.** 2006. Transmissibility of cholera: *in vivo*-formed biofilms and their relationship to infectivity and persistence in the environment. *Proc Natl Acad Sci USA* **103:**6350–6355.

35. **Nielsen AT, Dolganov NA, Rasmussen T, Otto G, Miller MC, Felt SA, Torreilles S, Schoolnik GK.** 2010. A bistable switch and anatomical site control *Vibrio cholerae* virulence gene expression in the intestine. *PLoS Pathog* **6:**e1001102. doi:10.1371/journal.ppat.1001102.

36. **Watnick PI, Kolter R.** 1999. Steps in the development of a *Vibrio cholerae* El Tor biofilm. *Mol Microbiol* **34:**586–595.

37. **Utada AS, Bennett RR, Fong JCN, Gibiansky ML, Yildiz FH, Golestanian R, Wong GCL.** 2014. *Vibrio cholerae* use pili and flagella synergistically to effect motility switching and conditional surface attachment. *Nat Commun* **5:**4913.

38. **Yildiz FH, Schoolnik GK.** 1999. *Vibrio cholerae* O1 El Tor: identification of a gene cluster required for the rugose colony type, exopolysaccharide production, chlorine resistance, and biofilm formation. *Proc Natl Acad Sci USA* **96:**4028–4033.

39. **Lauga E, DiLuzio WR, Whitesides GM, Stone HA.** 2006. Swimming in circles: motion of bacteria near solid boundaries. *Biophys J* **90:**400–412.

40. **Kojima S, Yamamoto K, Kawagishi I, Homma M.** 1999. The polar flagellar motor of *Vibrio cholerae* is driven by an Na+ motive force. *J Bacteriol* **181:**1927–1930.

41. **Reichhardt C, Fong JCN, Yildiz F, Cegelski L.** 2015. Characterization of the *Vibrio cholerae* extracellular matrix: a top-down solid-state NMR approach. *Biochim Biophys Acta* **1848:** 378–383.

42. **Berk V, Fong JCN, Dempsey GT, Develioglu ON, Zhuang X, Liphardt J, Yildiz FH, Chu S.** 2012. Molecular architecture and assembly principles of *Vibrio cholerae* biofilms. *Science* **337:**236–239.

43. **Fong JCN, Karplus K, Schoolnik GK, Yildiz FH.** 2006. Identification and characterization of RbmA, a novel protein required for the development of rugose colony morphology and biofilm structure in *Vibrio cholerae*. *J Bacteriol* **188:**1049–1059.

44. **Fong JCN, Yildiz FH.** 2007. The *rbmBCDEF* gene cluster modulates development of rugose colony morphology and biofilm formation in *Vibrio cholerae*. *J Bacteriol* **189:**2319–2330.

45. **Seper A, Fengler VHI, Roier S, Wolinski H, Kohlwein SD, Bishop AL, Camilli A, Reidl J, Schild S.** 2011. Extracellular nucleases and extracellular DNA play important roles in *Vibrio cholerae* biofilm formation. *Mol Microbiol* **82:**1015–1037.

46. **Fong JCN, Syed KA, Klose KE, Yildiz FH.** 2010. Role of *Vibrio* polysaccharide (*vps*) genes in VPS production, biofilm formation and *Vibrio cholerae* pathogenesis. *Microbiology* **156:**2757–2769.

47. **Yildiz F, Fong J, Sadovskaya I, Grard T, Vinogradov E.** 2014. Structural characterization of the extracellular polysaccharide from *Vibrio cholerae* O1 El-Tor. *PLoS One* **9:**e86751. doi:10.1371/journal.pone.0086751.

48. **Johnson TL, Fong JC, Rule C, Rogers A, Yildiz FH, Sandkvist M.** 2014. The type II secretion system delivers matrix proteins for biofilm formation by *Vibrio cholerae*. *J Bacteriol* **196:**4245–4252.

49. **Beyhan S, Bilecen K, Salama SR, Casper-Lindley C, Yildiz FH.** 2007. Regulation of rugosity and biofilm formation in *Vibrio cholerae*: comparison of VpsT and VpsR

regulons and epistasis analysis of *vpsT*, *vpsR*, and *hapR*. *J Bacteriol* **189:**388–402.

50. **Yildiz FH, Dolganov NA, Schoolnik GK.** 2001. VpsR, a member of the response regulators of the two-component regulatory systems, is required for expression of *vps* biosynthesis genes and EPS(ETr)-associated phenotypes in *Vibrio cholerae* O1 El Tor. *J Bacteriol* **183:**1716–1726.

51. **Yildiz FH, Liu XS, Heydorn A, Schoolnik GK.** 2004. Molecular analysis of rugosity in a *Vibrio cholerae* O1 El Tor phase variant. *Mol Microbiol* **53:**497–515.

52. **Krasteva PV, Fong JCN, Shikuma NJ, Beyhan S, Navarro MVAS, Yildiz FH, Sondermann H.** 2010. *Vibrio cholerae* VpsT regulates matrix production and motility by directly sensing cyclic di-GMP. *Science* **327:**866–868.

53. **Zamorano-Sánchez D, Fong JCN, Kilic S, Erill I, Yildiz FH.** 2015. Identification and characterization of VpsR and VpsT binding sites in *Vibrio cholerae*. *J Bacteriol* **197:**1221–1235.

54. **Yang M, Frey EM, Liu Z, Bishar R, Zhu J.** 2010. The virulence transcriptional activator AphA enhances biofilm formation by *Vibrio cholerae* by activating expression of the biofilm regulator VpsT. *Infect Immun* **78:**697–703.

55. **Hammer BK, Bassler BL.** 2003. Quorum sensing controls biofilm formation in *Vibrio cholerae*. *Mol Microbiol* **50:**101–104.

56. **Zhu J, Mekalanos JJ.** 2003. Quorum sensing-dependent biofilms enhance colonization in *Vibrio cholerae*. *Dev Cell* **5:**647–656.

57. **Waters CM, Lu W, Rabinowitz JD, Bassler BL.** 2008. Quorum sensing controls biofilm formation in *Vibrio cholerae* through modulation of cyclic di-GMP levels and repression of *vpsT*. *J Bacteriol* **190:**2527–2536.

58. **Tsou AM, Liu Z, Cai T, Zhu J.** 2011. The VarS/VarA two-component system modulates the activity of the *Vibrio cholerae* quorum-sensing transcriptional regulator HapR. *Microbiology* **157:**1620–1628.

59. **Lenz DH, Bassler BL.** 2007. The small nucleoid protein Fis is involved in *Vibrio cholerae* quorum sensing. *Mol Microbiol* **63:**859–871.

60. **Shikuma NJ, Fong JCN, Odell LS, Perchuk BS, Laub MT, Yildiz FH.** 2009. Overexpression of VpsS, a hybrid sensor kinase, enhances biofilm formation in *Vibrio cholerae*. *J Bacteriol* **191:**5147–5158.

61. **Liang W, Pascual-Montano A, Silva AJ, Benitez JA.** 2007. The cyclic AMP receptor protein modulates quorum sensing, motility and multiple genes that affect intestinal colonization in *Vibrio cholerae*. *Microbiology* **153:**2964–2975.

62. **Liu Z, Hsiao A, Joelsson A, Zhu J.** 2006. The transcriptional regulator VqmA increases expression of the quorum-sensing activator HapR in *Vibrio cholerae*. *J Bacteriol* **188:**2446–2453.

63. **Liu Z, Stirling FR, Zhu J.** 2007. Temporal quorum-sensing induction regulates *Vibrio cholerae* biofilm architecture. *Infect Immun* **75:**122–126.

64. **Stonehouse EA, Hulbert RR, Nye MB, Skorupski K, Taylor RK.** 2011. H-NS binding and repression of the *ctx* promoter in *Vibrio cholerae*. *J Bacteriol* **193:**979–988.

65. **Wang H, Ayala JC, Silva AJ, Benitez JA.** 2012. The histone-like nucleoid structuring protein (H-NS) is a repressor of *Vibrio cholerae* exopolysaccharide biosynthesis (*vps*) genes. *Appl Environ Microbiol* **78:**2482–2488.

66. **Beyhan S, Tischler AD, Camilli A, Yildiz FH.** 2006. Transcriptome and phenotypic responses of *Vibrio cholerae* to increased cyclic di-GMP level. *J Bacteriol* **188:**3600–3613.

67. **Cockerell SR, Rutkovsky AC, Zayner JP, Cooper RE, Porter LR, Pendergraft SS, Parker ZM, McGinnis MW, Karatan E.** 2014. *Vibrio cholerae* NspS, a homologue of ABC-type periplasmic solute binding proteins, facilitates transduction of polyamine signals independent of their transport. *Microbiology* **160:**832–843.

68. **Beyhan S, Odell LS, Yildiz FH.** 2008. Identification and characterization of cyclic diguanylate signaling systems controlling rugosity in *Vibrio cholerae*. *J Bacteriol* **190:**7392–7405.

69. **Koestler BJ, Waters CM.** 2014. Bile acids and bicarbonate inversely regulate intracellular cyclic di-GMP in *Vibrio cholerae*. *Infect Immun* **82:**3002–3014.

70. **Townsley L, Yildiz FH.** 2015. Temperature affects c-di-GMP signaling and biofilm formation in *Vibrio cholerae*. *Environ Microbiol*. [Epub ahead of print.] doi:10.1111/1462-2920.12799.

71. **Pratt JT, Tamayo R, Tischler AD, Camilli A.** 2007. PilZ domain proteins bind cyclic diguanylate and regulate diverse processes in *Vibrio cholerae*. *J Biol Chem* **282:**12860–12870.

72. **Sudarsan N, Lee ER, Weinberg Z, Moy RH, Kim JN, Link KH, Breaker RR.** 2008. Riboswitches in eubacteria sense the second messenger cyclic di-GMP. *Science* **321:**411–413.

73. **Srivastava D, Hsieh M-L, Khataokar A, Neiditch MB, Waters CM.** 2013. Cyclic di-GMP inhibits *Vibrio cholerae* motility by repressing induction of transcription and inducing extracellular polysaccharide production. *Mol Microbiol* **90:**1262–1276.

74. **Liang W, Silva AJ, Benitez JA.** 2007. The cyclic AMP receptor protein modulates colonial mor-

phology in *Vibrio cholerae*. *Appl Environ Microbiol* **73:**7482–7487.

75. **Fong JCN, Yildiz FH.** 2008. Interplay between cyclic AMP-cyclic AMP receptor protein and cyclic di-GMP signaling in *Vibrio cholerae* biofilm formation. *J Bacteriol* **190:**6646–6659.

76. **Das B, Pal RR, Bag S, Bhadra RK.** 2009. Stringent response in *Vibrio cholerae*: genetic analysis of *spoT* gene function and identification of a novel (p)ppGpp synthetase gene. *Mol Microbiol* **72:**380–398.

77. **Raskin DM, Judson N, Mekalanos JJ.** 2007. Regulation of the stringent response is the essential function of the conserved bacterial G protein CgtA in *Vibrio cholerae*. *Proc Natl Acad Sci USA* **104:**4636–4641.

78. **He H, Cooper JN, Mishra A, Raskin DM.** 2012. Stringent response regulation of biofilm formation in *Vibrio cholerae*. *J Bacteriol* **194:**2962–2972.

79. **Kapfhammer D, Karatan E, Pflughoeft KJ, Watnick PI.** 2005. Role for glycine betaine transport in *Vibrio cholerae* osmoadaptation and biofilm formation within microbial communities. *Appl Environ Microbiol* **71:**3840–3847.

80. **Shikuma NJ, Yildiz FH.** 2009. Identification and characterization of OscR, a transcriptional regulator involved in osmolarity adaptation in *Vibrio cholerae*. *J Bacteriol* **191:**4082–4096.

81. **Shikuma NJ, Davis KR, Fong JNC, Yildiz FH.** 2013. The transcriptional regulator, CosR, controls compatible solute biosynthesis and transport, motility and biofilm formation in *Vibrio cholerae*. *Environ Microbiol* **15:**1387–1399.

82. **Mueller RS, Beyhan S, Saini SG, Yildiz FH, Bartlett DH.** 2009. Indole acts as an extracellular cue regulating gene expression in *Vibrio cholerae*. *J Bacteriol* **191:**3504–3516.

83. **Hung DT, Zhu J, Sturtevant D, Mekalanos JJ.** 2006. Bile acids stimulate biofilm formation in *Vibrio cholerae*. *Mol Microbiol* **59:**193–201.

84. **Houot L, Chang S, Pickering BS, Absalon C, Watnick PI.** 2010. The phosphoenolpyruvate phosphotransferase system regulates *Vibrio cholerae* biofilm formation through multiple independent pathways. *J Bacteriol* **192:**3055–3067.

85. **Ymele-Leki P, Houot L, Watnick PI.** 2013. Mannitol and the mannitol-specific enzyme IIB subunit activate *Vibrio cholerae* biofilm formation. *Appl Environ Microbiol* **79:**4675–4683.

86. **Igarashi K, Kashiwagi K.** 2000. Polyamines: mysterious modulators of cellular functions. *Biochem Biophys Res Commun* **271:**559–564.

87. **McGinnis MW, Parker ZM, Walter NE, Rutkovsky AC, Cartaya-Marin C, Karatan E.** 2009. Spermidine regulates *Vibrio cholerae* biofilm formation via transport and signaling pathways. *FEMS Microbiol Lett* **299:**166–174.

88. **Karatan E, Duncan TR, Watnick PI.** 2005. NspS, a predicted polyamine sensor, mediates activation of *Vibrio cholerae* biofilm formation by norspermidine. *J Bacteriol* **187:**7434–7443.

89. **Kierek K, Watnick PI.** 2003. Environmental determinants of *Vibrio cholerae* biofilm development. *Appl Environ Microbiol* **69:**5079–5088.

90. **Bilecen K, Yildiz FH.** 2010. Identification of a calcium-controlled negative regulatory system affecting *Vibrio cholerae* biofilm formation. *Environ Microbiol* **11:**2015–2029.

91. **Huq A, Small EB, West PA, Huq MI, Rahman R, Colwell RR.** 1983. Ecological relationships between *Vibrio cholerae* and planktonic crustacean copepods. *Appl Environ Microbiol* **45:**275–283.

92. **Islam MS, Jahid MIK, Rahman MM, Rahman MZ, Islam MS, Kabir MS, Sack DA, Schoolnik GK.** 2007. Biofilm acts as a microenvironment for plankton-associated *Vibrio cholerae* in the aquatic environment of Bangladesh. *Microbiol Immunol* **51:**369–379.

93. **Meibom KL, Li XB, Nielsen AT, Wu C-Y, Roseman S, Schoolnik GK.** 2004. The *Vibrio cholerae* chitin utilization program. *Proc Natl Acad Sci USA* **101:**2524–2529.

94. **Kirn TJ, Jude BA, Taylor RK.** 2005. A colonization factor links *Vibrio cholerae* environmental survival and human infection. *Nature* **438:**863–866.

95. **Meibom KL, Blokesch M, Dolganov NA, Wu C-Y, Schoolnik GK.** 2005. Chitin induces natural competence in *Vibrio cholerae*. *Science* **310:**1824–1827.

96. **Blokesch M.** 2012. Chitin colonization, chitin degradation and chitin-induced natural competence of *Vibrio cholerae* are subject to catabolite repression. *Environ Microbiol* **14:**1898–1912.

97. **Broza M, Gancz H, Halpern M, Kashi Y.** 2005. Adult non-biting midges: possible windborne carriers of *Vibrio cholerae* non-O1 non-O139. *Environ Microbiol* **7:**576–585.

98. **Nahar S, Sultana M, Naser MN, Nair GB, Watanabe H, Ohnishi M, Yamamoto S, Endtz H, Cravioto A, Sack RB, Hasan NA, Sadique A, Huq A, Colwell RR, Alam M.** 2011. Role of shrimp chitin in the ecology of toxigenic *Vibrio cholerae* and cholera transmission. *Front Microbiol* **2:**260.

99. **Li X, Roseman S.** 2004. The chitinolytic cascade in *Vibrios* is regulated by chitin oligosaccharides and a two-component chitin catabolic sensor/kinase. *Proc Natl Acad Sci USA* **101:**627–631.

100. **Yamamoto S, Mitobe J, Ishikawa T, Wai SN, Ohnishi M, Watanabe H, Izumiya H.** 2014.

Regulation of natural competence by the orphan two-component system sensor kinase ChiS involves a non-canonical transmembrane regulator in *Vibrio cholerae. Mol Microbiol* **91:**326–347.

101. **Dalia AB, Lazinski DW, Camilli A.** 2014. Identification of a membrane-bound transcriptional regulator that links chitin and natural competence in *Vibrio cholerae. MBio* **5:**e01028-13. doi:10.1128/mBio.01028-13.

102. **Yamamoto S, Izumiya H, Mitobe J, Morita M, Arakawa E, Ohnishi M, Watanabe H.** 2011. Identification of a chitin-induced small RNA that regulates translation of the *tfoX* gene, encoding a positive regulator of natural competence in *Vibrio cholerae. J Bacteriol* **193:**1953–1965.

103. **Lo Scrudato M, Blokesch M.** 2013. A transcriptional regulator linking quorum sensing and chitin induction to render *Vibrio cholerae* naturally transformable. *Nucleic Acids Res* **41:**3644–3658.

104. **Wong E, Vaaje-Kolstad G, Ghosh A, Hurtado-Guerrero R, Konarev PV, Ibrahim AFM, Svergun DI, Eijsink VGH, Chatterjee NS, van Aalten DMF.** 2012. The *Vibrio cholerae* colonization factor GbpA possesses a modular structure that governs binding to different host surfaces. *PLoS Pathog* **8:**e1002373. doi:10.1371/journal.ppat.1002373.

105. **Bhowmick R, Ghosal A, Das B, Koley H, Saha DR, Ganguly S, Nandy RK, Bhadra RK, Chatterjee NS.** 2008. Intestinal adherence of *Vibrio cholerae* involves a coordinated interaction between colonization factor GbpA and mucin. *Infect Immun* **76:**4968–4977.

106. **Mondal M, Nag D, Koley H, Saha DR, Chatterjee NS.** 2014. The *Vibrio cholerae* extracellular chitinase ChiA2 is important for survival and pathogenesis in the host intestine. *PLoS One* **9:**e103119. doi:10.1371/journal.pone.0103119.

107. **Bourassa L, Camilli A.** 2009. Glycogen contributes to the environmental persistence and transmission of *Vibrio cholerae. Mol Microbiol* **72:**124–138.

108. **Kamp HD, Patimalla-Dipali B, Lazinski DW, Wallace-Gadsden F, Camilli A.** 2013. Gene fitness landscapes of *Vibrio cholerae* at important stages of its life cycle. *PLoS Pathog* **9:**e1003800. doi:10.1371/journal.ppat.1003800.

109. **Baker CS, Morozov I, Suzuki K, Romeo T, Babitzke P.** 2002. CsrA regulates glycogen biosynthesis by preventing translation of *glgC* in *Escherichia coli. Mol Microbiol* **44:**1599–1610.

110. **Pratt JT, Ismail AM, Camilli A.** 2010. PhoB regulates both environmental and virulence gene expression in *Vibrio cholerae. Mol Microbiol* **77:**1595–1605.

111. **Pratt JT, McDonough E, Camilli A.** 2009. PhoB regulates motility, biofilms, and cyclic di-GMP in *Vibrio cholerae. J Bacteriol* **191:**6632–6642.

112. **Von Krüger WMA, Lery LMS, Soares MR, de Neves-Manta FS, Batista e Silva CM, Neves-Ferreira AGDC, Perales J, Bisch PM.** 2006. The phosphate-starvation response in *Vibrio cholerae* O1 and *phoB* mutant under proteomic analysis: disclosing functions involved in adaptation, survival and virulence. *Proteomics* **6:**1495–1511.

113. **Von Kruger WMA, Humphreys S, Ketley JM.** 1999. A role for the PhoBR regulatory system homologue in the *Vibrio cholerae* phosphate-limitation response and intestinal colonization. *Microbiology* **145:**2463–2475.

114. **Jahid IK, Silva AJ, Benitez JA.** 2006. Polyphosphate stores enhance the ability of *Vibrio cholerae* to overcome environmental stresses in a low-phosphate environment. *Appl Environ Microbiol* **72:**7043–7049.

115. **Mey AR, Wyckoff EE, Kanukurthy V, Fisher CR, Payne SM.** 2005. Iron and fur regulation in *Vibrio cholerae* and the role of fur in virulence. *Infect Immun* **73:**8167–8178.

116. **Wyckoff EE, Mey AR, Leimbach A, Fisher CF, Payne SM.** 2006. Characterization of ferric and ferrous iron transport systems in *Vibrio cholerae. J Bacteriol* **188:**6515–6523.

117. **Andrews SC, Robinson AK, Rodríguez-Quiñones F.** 2003. Bacterial iron homeostasis. *FEMS Microbiol Rev* **27:**215–237.

118. **Crosa JH, Walsh CT.** 2002. Genetics and assembly line enzymology of siderophore biosynthesis in bacteria. *Microbiol Mol Biol Rev* **66:**223–249.

119. **Keating TA, Marshall CG, Walsh CT.** 2000. Reconstitution and characterization of the *Vibrio cholerae* vibriobactin synthetase from VibB, VibE, VibF, and VibH. *Biochemistry* **39:**15522–15530.

120. **Li N, Zhang C, Li B, Liu X, Huang Y, Xu S, Gu L.** 2012. Unique iron coordination in iron-chelating molecule vibriobactin helps *Vibrio cholerae* evade mammalian siderocalin-mediated immune response. *J Biol Chem* **287:**8912–8919.

121. **Occhino DA, Wyckoff EE, Henderson DP, Wrona TJ, Payne SM.** 1998. *Vibrio cholerae* iron transport: haem transport genes are linked to one of two sets of *tonB, exbB, exbD* genes. *Mol Microbiol* **29:**1493–1507.

122. **Butterton JR, Stoebner JA, Payne SM, Calderwoodl SB.** 1992. Cloning, sequencing, and transcriptional regulation of *viuA*, the gene encoding the ferric vibriobactin receptor of *Vibrio cholerae. J Bacteriol* **174:**3729–3738.

123. **Wyckoff EE, Valle A, Smith SL, Payne SM.** 1999. A multifunctional ATP-binding cassette transporter system from *Vibrio cholerae* transports vibriobactin and enterobactin. *J Bacteriol* **181:**7588–7596.

124. **Mey AR, Wyckoff EE, Oglesby AG, Rab E, Taylor RK, Payne SM.** 2002. Identification of the *Vibrio cholerae* enterobactin receptors VctA and IrgA: IrgA is not required for virulence. *Infect Immun* **70:**3419–3426.

125. **Butterton JR, Calderwoodl SB.** 1994. Identification, cloning, and sequencing of a gene required for ferric vibriobactin utilization by *Vibrio cholerae*. *J Bacteriol* **176:**5631–5638.

126. **Sigel SP, Stoebner JA, Payne SM.** 1985. Iron-vibriobactin transport system is not required for virulence of *Vibrio cholerae*. *Infect Immun* **47:**360–362.

127. **Wyckoff EE, Payne SM.** 2011. The *Vibrio cholerae* VctPDGC system transports catechol siderophores and a siderophore-free iron ligand. *Mol Microbiol* **81:**1446–1458.

128. **Acosta N, Pukatzki S, Raivio TL.** 2015. The *Vibrio cholerae* Cpx envelope stress response senses and mediates adaptation to low iron. *J Bacteriol* **197:**262–276.

129. **Stoebner JA, Payne SM.** 1988. Iron-regulated hemolysin production and utilization of heme and hemoglobin by *Vibrio cholerae*. *Infect Immun* **56:**2891–2895.

130. **Henderson DP, Payne SM.** 1994. Characterization of the *Vibrio cholerae* outer membrane heme transport protein HutA: sequence of the gene, regulation of expression, and homology to the family of TonB-dependent proteins. *J Bacteriol* **176:**3269–3277.

131. **Mey AR, Payne SM.** 2001. Haem utilization in *Vibrio cholerae* involves multiple TonB-dependent haem receptors. *Mol Microbiol* **42:**835–849.

132. **Pflughoeft KJ, Kierek K, Paula I, Watnick PI.** 2003. Role of ectoine in *Vibrio cholerae* osmoadaptation. *Appl Environ Microbiol* **69:**5919–5927.

133. **Lobitz B, Beck L, Huq A, Wood B, Fuchs G, Faruque ASG, Colwell R.** 2000. Climate and infectious disease: use of remote sensing for detection of *Vibrio cholerae* by indirect measurement. *Proc Natl Acad Sci* **97:**1438–1443.

134. **Lama JR, Seas CR, León-Barúa R, Gotuzzo E, Sack RB.** 2004. Environmental temperature, cholera, and acute diarrhoea in adults in Lima, Peru *J Health Popul Nutr* **22:**399–403.

135. **Louis VR, Russek-Cohen E, Choopun N, Rivera ING, Gangle B, Jiang SC, Rubin A, Patz JA, Huq A, Colwell RR.** 2003. Predictability of *Vibrio cholerae* in Chesapeake Bay. *Appl Environ Microbiol* **69:**2773–2785.

136. **Lipp EK, Huq A, Colwell RR.** 2002. Effects of global climate on infectious disease: the cholera model. *Clin Microbiol Rev* **15:**757–770.

137. **Stauder M, Vezzulli L, Pezzati E, Repetto B, Pruzzo C.** 2010. Temperature affects *Vibrio cholerae* O1 El Tor persistence in the aquatic environment via an enhanced expression of GbpA and MSHA adhesins. *Environ Microbiol Rep* **2:**140–144.

138. **Weber GG, Kortmann J, Narberhaus F, Klose KE.** 2014. RNA thermometer controls temperature-dependent virulence factor expression in *Vibrio cholerae*. *Proc Natl Acad Sci USA* **111:**14241–14246.

139. **Datta PP, Bhadra RK.** 2003. Cold shock response and major cold shock proteins of *Vibrio cholerae*. *Appl Environ Microbiol* **69:**6361–6369.

140. **Asakura H, Ishiwa A, Arakawa E, Makino S, Okada Y, Yamamoto S, Igimi S.** 2007. Gene expression profile of *Vibrio cholerae* in the cold stress-induced viable but non-culturable state. *Environ Microbiol* **9:**869–879.

141. **Colwell RR, Brayton PR, Grimes DJ, Roszak DB, Huq SA, Palmer LM.** 1985. Viable but non-culturable *Vibrio cholerae* and related pathogens in the environment: implications for release of genetically engineered microorganisms. *Nat Biotechnol* **3:**817–820.

142. **Ayrapetyan M, Williams TC, Oliver JD.** 2014. Bridging the gap between viable but non-culturable and antibiotic persistent bacteria. *Trends Microbiol* **23:**7–13.

143. **Faruque SM, Islam MJ, Ahmad QS, Faruque ASG, Sack DA, Nair GB, Mekalanos JJ.** 2005. Self-limiting nature of seasonal cholera epidemics: role of host-mediated amplification of phage. *Proc Natl Acad Sci USA* **102:**6119–6124.

144. **Jubair M, Morris JG, Ali A.** 2012. Survival of *Vibrio cholerae* in nutrient-poor environments is associated with a novel "persister" phenotype. *PLoS One* **7:**e45187. doi:10.1371/journal.pone.0045187.

145. **Chaiyanan S, Huq A, Maugel T, Colwell RR.** 2001. Viability of the nonculturable *Vibrio cholerae* O1 and O139. *Syst Appl Microbiol* **24:**331–341.

146. **Hood MA, Guckert JB, White DC, Deck F.** 1986. Effect of nutrient deprivation on lipid, carbohydrate, DNA, RNA, and protein levels in *Vibrio cholerae*. *Appl Envir Microbiol* **52:**788–793.

147. **Kamruzzaman M, Udden SMN, Cameron DE, Calderwood SB, Nair GB, Mekalanos JJ, Faruque SM.** 2010. Quorum-regulated biofilms enhance the development of conditionally viable, environmental *Vibrio cholerae*. *Proc Natl Acad Sci USA* **107:**1588–1593.

148. Colwell RR, Brayton P, Herrington D, Tall B, Huq A, Levine MM. 1996. Viable but non-culturable *Vibrio cholerae* O1 revert to a cultivable state in the human intestine. *World J Microbiol Biotechnol* **12:**28–31.

149. Wai SN, Moriya T, Kondo K, Misumi H, Amako K. 1996. Resuscitation of *Vibrio cholerae* O1 strain TSI-4 from a viable but nonculturable state by heat shock. *FEMS Microiology Lett* **136:**187–191.

150. Oh YT, Park Y, Yoon MY, Bari W, Go J, Min KB, Raskin DM, Lee K-M, Yoon SS. 2014. Cholera toxin production during anaerobic trimethylamine N-oxide respiration is mediated by stringent response in *Vibrio cholerae*. *J Biol Chem* **289:**13232–13242.

151. Zheng J, Ho B, Mekalanos JJ. 2011. Genetic analysis of anti-amoebae and anti-bacterial activities of the type VI secretion system in *Vibrio cholerae*. *PLoS One* **6:**e23876. doi:10.1371/journal.pone.0023876.

152. Pukatzki S, Ma AT, Sturtevant D, Krastins B, Sarracino D, Nelson WC, Heidelberg JF, Mekalanos JJ. 2006. Identification of a conserved bacterial protein secretion system in *Vibrio cholerae* using the *Dictyostelium* host model system. *Proc Natl Acad Sci USA* **103:**1528–1533.

153. Pukatzki S, Ma AT, Revel AT, Sturtevant D, Mekalanos JJ. 2007. Type VI secretion system translocates a phage tail spike-like protein into target cells where it cross-links actin. *Proc Natl Acad Sci USA* **104:**15508–15513.

154. MacIntyre DL, Miyata ST, Kitaoka M, Pukatzki S. 2010. The *Vibrio cholerae* type VI secretion system displays antimicrobial properties. *Proc Natl Acad Sci USA* **107:**19520–19524.

155. Basler M, Pilhofer M, Henderson GP, Jensen GJ, Mekalanos JJ. 2012. Type VI secretion requires a dynamic contractile phage tail-like structure. *Nature* **483:**182–186.

156. Brooks TM, Unterweger D, Bachmann V, Kostiuk B, Pukatzki S. 2013. Lytic activity of the *Vibrio cholerae* type VI secretion toxin VgrG-3 is inhibited by the antitoxin TsaB. *J Biol Chem* **288:**7618–7625.

157. Miyata ST, Kitaoka M, Brooks TM, McAuley SB, Pukatzki S. 2011. *Vibrio cholerae* requires the type VI secretion system virulence factor VasX to kill *Dictyostelium discoideum*. *Infect Immun* **79:**2941–2949.

158. Miyata ST, Unterweger D, Rudko SP, Pukatzki S. 2013. Dual expression profile of type VI secretion system immunity genes protects pandemic *Vibrio cholerae*. *PLoS Pathog* **9:**e1003752. doi:10.1371/journal.ppat.1003752.

159. Dong TG, Ho BT, Yoder-Himes DR, Mekalanos JJ. 2013. Identification of T6SS-dependent effector and immunity proteins by Tn-seq in *Vibrio cholerae*. *Proc Natl Acad Sci USA* **110:**2623–2628.

160. Unterweger D, Miyata ST, Bachmann V, Brooks TM, Mullins T, Kostiuk B, Provenzano D, Pukatzki S. 2014. The *Vibrio cholerae* type VI secretion system employs diverse effector modules for intraspecific competition. *Nat Commun* **5:**3549.

161. Unterweger D, Kitaoka M, Miyata ST, Bachmann V, Brooks TM, Moloney J, Sosa O, Silva D, Duran-Gonzalez J, Provenzano D, Pukatzki S. 2012. Constitutive type VI secretion system expression gives *Vibrio cholerae* intra- and interspecific competitive advantages. *PLoS One* **7:**e48320. doi:10.1371/journal.pone.0048320.

162. Kitaoka M, Miyata ST, Brooks TM, Unterweger D, Pukatzki S. 2011. VasH is a transcriptional regulator of the type VI secretion system functional in endemic and pandemic *Vibrio cholerae*. *J Bacteriol* **193:**6471–6482.

163. Dong TG, Mekalanos JJ. 2012. Characterization of the RpoN regulon reveals differential regulation of T6SS and new flagellar operons in *Vibrio cholerae* O37 strain V52. *Nucleic Acids Res* **40:**7766–7775.

164. Zheng J, Shin OS, Cameron DE, Mekalanos JJ. 2010. Quorum sensing and a global regulator TsrA control expression of type VI secretion and virulence in *Vibrio cholerae*. *Proc Natl Acad Sci USA* **107:**21128–21133.

165. Ishikawa T, Rompikuntal PK, Lindmark B, Milton DL, Wai SN. 2009. Quorum sensing regulation of the two *hcp* alleles in *Vibrio cholerae* O1 strains. *PLoS One* **4:**e6734. doi:10.1371/journal.pone.0006734.

166. Shao Y, Bassler BL. 2014. Quorum regulatory small RNAs repress type VI secretion in *Vibrio cholerae*. *Mol Microbiol* **92:**921–930.

167. Borgeaud S, Metzger LC, Scrignari T, Blokesch M. 2015. The type VI secretion system of *Vibrio cholerae* fosters horizontal gene transfer. *Science* **347:**63–67.

168. Syed KA, Beyhan S, Correa N, Queen J, Liu J, Peng F, Satchell KJF, Yildiz F, Klose KE. 2009. The *Vibrio cholerae* flagellar regulatory hierarchy controls expression of virulence factors. *J Bacteriol* **191:**6555–6570.

169. Bernard CS, Brunet YR, Gavioli M, Lloubès R, Cascales E. 2011. Regulation of type VI secretion gene clusters by sigma54 and cognate enhancer binding proteins. *J Bacteriol* **193:**2158–2167.

170. Liu Z, Miyashiro T, Tsou A, Hsiao A, Goulian M, Zhu J. 2008. Mucosal penetration primes *Vibrio cholerae* for host colonization by

repressing quorum sensing. *Proc Natl Acad Sci USA* **105:**9769–9774.

171. **Ishikawa T, Sabharwal D, Bröms J, Milton DL, Sjöstedt A, Uhlin BE, Wai SN.** 2012. Pathoadaptive conditional regulation of the type VI secretion system in *Vibrio cholerae* O1 strains. *Infect Immun* **80:**575–584.

172. **Fu Y, Waldor MK, Mekalanos JJ.** 2013. Tn-Seq analysis of *Vibrio cholerae* intestinal colonization reveals a role for T6SS-mediated antibacterial activity in the host. *Cell Host Microbe* **14:**652–663.

173. **Ma AT, Mekalanos JJ.** 2010. *In vivo* actin cross-linking induced by *Vibrio cholerae* type VI secretion system is associated with intestinal inflammation. *Proc Natl Acad Sci USA* **107:**4365–4370.

174. **Sun S, Kjelleberg S, McDougald D.** 2013. Relative contributions of *Vibrio* polysaccharide and quorum sensing to the resistance of *Vibrio cholerae* to predation by heterotrophic protists. *PLoS One* **8:**e56338. doi:10.1371/journal.pone.0056338.

175. **Sun S, Tay QXM, Kjelleberg S, Rice SA, McDougald D.** 2015. Quorum sensing-regulated chitin metabolism provides grazing resistance to *Vibrio cholerae* biofilms. *ISME J* **9:**1812–1820.

176. **Vaitkevicius K, Lindmark B, Ou G, Song T, Toma C, Iwanaga M, Zhu J, Tuck S, Wai SN, Andersson A, Hammarstro M.** 2006. A *Vibrio cholerae* protease needed for killing of *Caenorhabditis elegans* has a role in protection from natural predator grazing. *Proc Natl Acad Sci USA* **103:**9280–9285.

177. **Erken M, Weitere M, Kjelleberg S, McDougald D.** 2011. *In situ* grazing resistance of *Vibrio cholerae* in the marine environment. *FEMS Microbiol Ecol* **76:**504–512.

178. **Lutz C, Erken M, Noorian P, Sun S, McDougald D.** 2013. Environmental reservoirs and mechanisms of persistence of *Vibrio cholerae*. *Front Microbiol* **4:**375.

179. **Jensen MA, Faruque SM, Mekalanos JJ, Levin BR.** 2006. Modeling the role of bacteriophage in the control of cholera outbreaks. *Proc Natl Acad Sci USA* **103:**4652–4657.

180. **Faruque SM, Naser I Bin, Islam MJ, Faruque ASG, Ghosh AN, Nair GB, Sack DA, Mekalanos JJ.** 2005. Seasonal epidemics of cholera inversely correlate with the prevalence of environmental cholera phages. *Proc Natl Acad Sci USA* **102:**1702–1707.

181. **Nelson EJ, Chowdhury A, Flynn J, Schild S, Bourassa L, Shao Y, LaRocque RC, Calderwood SB, Qadri F, Camilli A.** 2008. Transmission of *Vibrio cholerae* is antagonized by lytic phage and entry into the aquatic environment. *PLoS Pathog* **4:**e1000187. doi:10.1371/journal.ppat.1000187.

182. **Zahid MSH, Udden SMN, Faruque ASG, Calderwood SB, Mekalanos JJ, Faruque SM.** 2008. Effect of phage on the infectivity of *Vibrio cholerae* and emergence of genetic variants. *Infect Immun* **76:**5266–5273.

183. **Seed KD, Faruque SM, Mekalanos JJ, Calderwood SB, Qadri F, Camilli A.** 2012. Phase variable O antigen biosynthetic genes control expression of the major protective antigen and bacteriophage receptor in *Vibrio cholerae* O1. *PLoS Pathog* **8:**e1002917. doi:10.1371/journal.ppat.1002917.

184. **Waldor MK, Mekalanos JJ.** 1996. Lysogenic conversion by a filamentous phage encoding cholera toxin. *Science* **272:**1910–1914.

185. **Angelichio MJ, Spector J, Waldor MK, Camilli A.** 1999. *Vibrio cholerae* intestinal population dynamics in the suckling mouse model of infection. *Infect Immun* **67:**3733–3739.

186. **Miller CJ, Drasar BS, Feachem RG.** 1984. Response of toxigenic *Vibrio cholerae* 01 to physico-chemical stresses. *J Hyg* **93:**475–495.

187. **Swenson GJ, Stochastic J, Bolander FF, Long RA.** 2012. Acid stress response in environmental and clinical strains of enteric bacteria. *Front Biol* **7:**495–505.

188. **Merrell DS, Camilli A.** 1999. The *cadA* gene of *Vibrio cholerae* is induced during infection and plays a role in acid tolerance. *Mol Microbiol* **34:**836–849.

189. **Kovacikova G, Lin W, Skorupski K.** 2010. The LysR-type virulence activator AphB regulates the expression of genes in *Vibrio cholerae* in response to low pH and anaerobiosis. *J Bacteriol* **192:**4181–4191.

190. **Merrell DS, Hava DL, Camilli A.** 2002. Identification of novel factors involved in colonization and acid tolerance of *Vibrio cholerae*. *Mol Microbiol* **43:**1471–1491.

191. **Angelichio MJ, Merrell DS, Camilli A.** 2004. Spatiotemporal analysis of acid adaptation-mediated *Vibrio cholerae* hyperinfectivity. *Infect Immun* **72:**2405–2407.

192. **Lundberg JO, Weitzberg E, Lundberg JM, Alving K.** 1994. Intragastric nitric oxide production in humans: measurements in expelled air. *Gut* **35:**1543–1546.

193. **Fang FC.** 1997. Perspectives series: host/pathogen interactions. Mechanisms of nitric oxide-related antimicrobial activity. *J Clin Invest* **99:**2818–2825.

194. **Davies BW, Bogard RW, Dupes NM, Gerstenfeld TA, Simmons LA, Mekalanos JJ.** 2011. DNA damage and reactive nitrogen

species are barriers to *Vibrio cholerae* colonization of the infant mouse intestine. *PLoS Pathog* **7**:e1001295. doi:10.1371/journal.ppat.1001295.

195. **Qadri F, Raqib R, Ahmed F, Rahman T, Wenneras C, Kumar Das S, Alam NH, Mathan MM, Svennerholm AM.** 2002. Increased levels of inflammatory mediators in children and adults infected with *Vibrio cholerae* O1 and O139. *Clin Vaccine Immunol* **9**:221–229.

196. **Stern AM, Hay AJ, Liu Z, Desland FA, Zhang J, Zhong Z, Zhu J.** 2012. The NorR regulon is critical for *Vibrio cholerae* resistance to nitric oxide and sustained colonization of the intestines. *MBio* **17**:e00013-12. doi:10.1128/mBio.00013-12.

197. **Begley M, Gahan CGM, Hill C.** 2005. The interaction between bacteria and bile. *FEMS Microbiol Rev* **29**:625–651.

198. **Nesper J, Lauriano CM, Klose KE, Kapfhammer D, Kraiss A, Reidl J.** 2001. Characterization of *Vibrio cholerae* O1 El Tor *galU* and *galE* mutants: influence on lipopolysaccharide structure, colonization, and biofilm formation. *Infect Immun* **69**:435–445.

199. **Nesper J, Schild S, Lauriano CM, Kraiss A, Klose KE, Reidl J.** 2002. Role of *Vibrio cholerae* O139 surface polysaccharides in intestinal colonization. *Infect Immun* **70**:5990–5996.

200. **Heinrichs DE, Yethon JA, Whitfield C.** 1998. Molecular basis for structural diversity in the core regions of the lipopolysaccharides of *Escherichia coli* and *Salmonella enterica*. *Mol Microbiol* **30**:221–232.

201. **Bina JE, Mekalanos JJ.** 2001. *Vibrio cholerae tolC* is required for bile resistance and colonization. *Infect Immun* **69**:4681–4685.

202. **Bina JE, Provenzano D, Wang C, Bina XR, Mekalanos JJ.** 2006. Characterization of the *Vibrio cholerae vexAB* and *vexCD* efflux systems. *Arch Microbiol* **186**:171–181.

203. **Colmer JA, Fralick JA, Hamood AN.** 1998. Isolation and characterization of a putative multidrug resistance pump from *Vibrio cholerae*. *Mol Microbiol* **27**:63–72.

204. **Wibbenmeyer JA, Provenzano D, Landry CF, Klose KE, Delcour AH.** 2002. *Vibrio cholerae* OmpU and OmpT porins are differentially affected by bile. *Infect Immun* **70**:121–126.

205. **Koestler BJ, Waters CM.** 2013. Exploring environmental control of cyclic di-GMP signaling in *Vibrio cholerae* by using the *ex vivo* lysate cyclic di-GMP assay (TELCA). *Appl Environ Microbiol* **79**:5233–5241.

206. **Abuaita BH, Withey JH.** 2009. Bicarbonate induces *Vibrio cholerae* virulence gene expression by enhancing ToxT activity. *Infect Immun* **77**:4111–4120.

207. **Lowden MJ, Skorupski K, Pellegrini M, Chiorazzo MG, Taylor RK, Kull FJ.** 2010. Structure of *Vibrio cholerae* ToxT reveals a mechanism for fatty acid regulation of virulence genes. *Proc Natl Acad Sci USA* **107**:2860–2865.

208. **Thomson JJ, Plecha SC, Withey JH.** 2015. A small unstructured region in *Vibrio cholerae* ToxT mediates the response to positive and negative effectors and ToxT proteolysis. *J Bacteriol* **197**:654–668.

209. **Yang M, Liu Z, Hughes C, Stern AM, Wang H, Zhong Z, Kan B, Fenical W, Zhu J.** 2013. Bile salt-induced intermolecular disulfide bond formation activates *Vibrio cholerae* virulence. *Proc Natl Acad Sci USA* **110**:2348–2353.

210. **Hay AJ, Zhu J.** 2015. Host intestinal signal-promoted biofilm dispersal induces *Vibrio cholerae* colonization. *Infect Immun* **83**:317–323.

211. **Matson JS, Yoo HJ, Hakansson K, Dirita VJ.** 2010. Polymyxin B resistance in El Tor *Vibrio cholerae* requires lipid acylation catalyzed by MsbB. *J Bacteriol* **192**:2044–2052.

212. **Ménard S, Förster V, Lotz M, Gütle D, Duerr CU, Gallo RL, Henriques-Normark B, Pütsep K, Andersson M, Glocker EO, Hornef MW.** 2008. Developmental switch of intestinal antimicrobial peptide expression. *J Exp Med* **205**:183–193.

213. **Pestonjamasp VK, Huttner KH, Gallo RL.** 2001. Processing site and gene structure for the murine antimicrobial peptide CRAMP. *Peptides* **22**:1643–1650.

214. **Hankins JV, Madsen JA, Giles DK, Childers BM, Klose KE, Brodbelt JS, Trent MS.** 2011. Elucidation of a novel *Vibrio cholerae* lipid A secondary hydroxy-acyltransferase and its role in innate immune recognition. *Mol Microbiol* **81**:1313–1329.

215. **Hankins JV, Madsen JA, Giles DK, Brodbelt JS, Trent MS.** 2012. Amino acid addition to *Vibrio cholerae* LPS establishes a link between surface remodeling in Gram-positive and Gram-negative bacteria. *Proc Natl Acad Sci USA* **109**:8722–8727.

216. **Herrera CM, Crofts AA, Henderson JC, Pingali SC, Davies BW, Stephen M.** 2014. The *Vibrio cholerae* VprA-VprB two-component system controls virulence through endotoxin modification. *MBio* **5**:e02283. doi:10.1128/mBio.02283-14.

217. **Bilecen K, Fong JCN, Cheng A, Jones CJ, Zamorano-Sánchez D, Yildiz FH.** 2015. Polymyxin B resistance and biofilm formation in

Vibrio cholerae is controlled by the response regulator CarR. *Infect Immun* **83:**1199–1209.

218. **Bina XR, Provenzano D, Nguyen N, Bina JE.** 2008. *Vibrio cholerae* RND family efflux systems are required for antimicrobial resistance, optimal virulence factor production, and colonization of the infant mouse small intestine. *Infect Immun* **76:**3595–3605.

219. **Mathur J, Davis BM, Waldor MK.** 2007. Antimicrobial peptides activate the *Vibrio cholerae* sigmaE regulon through an OmpU-dependent signalling pathway. *Mol Microbiol* **63:**848–858.

220. **Mathur J, Waldor MK.** 2004. The *Vibrio cholerae* ToxR-regulated porin OmpU confers resistance to antimicrobial peptides. *Infect Immun* **72:**3577–3583.

221. **Ding Y, Davis BM, Waldor MK.** 2004. Hfq is essential for *Vibrio cholerae* virulence and downregulates sigma expression. *Mol Microbiol* **53:**345–354.

222. **Yamamoto T, Yokota T.** 1988. Electron microscopic study of *Vibrio cholerae* 01 adherence to the mucus coat and villus surface in the human small intestine. *Infect Immun* **56:**2753–2759.

223. **Robbe C, Capon C, Coddeville B, Michalski J.** 2004. Structural diversity and specific distribution of O-glycans in normal human mucins along the intestinal tract. *Biochem J* **316:**307–316.

224. **Silva AJ.** 2003. Haemagglutinin/protease expression and mucin gel penetration in El Tor biotype *Vibrio cholerae*. *Microbiology* **149:**1883–1891.

225. **Jude BA, Martinez RM, Skorupski K, Taylor RK.** 2009. Levels of the secreted *Vibrio cholerae* attachment factor GbpA are modulated by quorum-sensing-induced proteolysis. *J Bacteriol* **191:**6911–6917.

226. **Liu Z, Wang Y, Liu S, Sheng Y, Rueggeberg K-G, Wang H, Li J, Gu FX, Zhong Z, Kan B, Zhu J.** 2015. *Vibrio cholerae* represses polysaccharide synthesis to promote motility in mucosa. *Infect Immun* **83:**1114–1121.

227. **Thelin KH, Taylor RK.** 1996. Toxin-coregulated pilus, but not mannose-sensitive hemagglutinin, is required for colonization by *Vibrio cholerae* O1 El Tor biotype and O139 strains. *Infect Immun* **64:**2853–2856.

228. **Ganguly NK, Kaur T.** 1996. Mechanism of action of cholera toxin & other toxins. *Indian J Med Res* **104:**28–37.

229. **Herrington BYDA, Hall RH, Losonsky G, Mekalanos JJ, Taylor IRK, Levine MM.** 1988. Toxin, toxin co-regulated pili, and the *toxR* regulon are essential for *Vibrio cholerae* pathogenesis in humans. *J Exp Med* **168:**1487–1492.

230. **Häse CC, Mekalanos JJ.** 1998. TcpP protein is a positive regulator of virulence gene expression in *Vibrio cholerae*. *Proc Natl Acad Sci USA* **95:**730–734.

231. **Dirita VJ, Parsott C, Jander G, Mekalanos JJ.** 1991. Regulatory cascade controls virulence in *Vibrio cholerae*. *Proc Natl Acad Sci USA* **88:**5403–5407.

232. **Skorupski K, Taylor RK.** 1999. A new level in the *Vibrio cholerae* ToxR virulence cascade: AphA is required for transcriptional activation of the *tcpPH* operon. *Mol Microbiol* **31:**763–771.

233. **Kovacikova G, Skorupski K.** 1999. A *Vibrio cholerae* LysR homolog, AphB, cooperates with AphA at the *tcpPH* promoter to activate expression of the ToxR virulence cascade. *J Bacteriol* **181:**4250–4256.

234. **Haas BL, Matson JS, DiRita VJ, Biteen JS.** 2014. Single-molecule tracking in live *Vibrio cholerae* reveals that ToxR recruits the membrane-bound virulence regulator TcpP to the *toxT* promoter. *Mol Microbiol* **96:**4–13.

235. **Beck NA, Krukonis ES, DiRita VJ.** 2004. TcpH influences virulence gene expression in *Vibrio cholerae* by inhibiting degradation of the transcription activator TcpP. *J Bacteriol* **186:**8309–8316.

236. **Nye MB, Pfau JD, Skorupski K, Taylor RK.** 2000. *Vibrio cholerae* H-NS silences virulence gene expression at multiple steps in the ToxR regulatory cascade. *J Bacteriol* **182:**4295–4303.

237. **Dey AK, Bhagat A, Chowdhury R.** 2013. Host cell contact induces expression of virulence factors and VieA, a cyclic di-GMP phosphodiesterase, in *Vibrio cholerae*. *J Bacteriol* **195:**2004–2010.

238. **Nielsen AT, Dolganov NA, Otto G, Miller MC, Wu CY, Schoolnik GK.** 2006. RpoS controls the *Vibrio cholerae* mucosal escape response. *PLoS Pathog* **2:**e109.

239. **Mandlik A, Livny J, Robins WP, Ritchie JM, Mekalanos JJ, Waldor MK.** 2011. RNA-Seq-based monitoring of infection-linked changes in *Vibrio cholerae* gene expression. *Cell Host Microbe* **10:**165–174.

240. **Schild S, Tamayo R, Nelson EJ, Qadri F, Calderwood SB, Camilli A.** 2007. Genes induced late in infection increase fitness of *Vibrio cholerae* after release into the environment. *Cell Host Microbe* **2:**264–277.

241. **Lee SH, Butler SM, Camilli A.** 2001. Selection for *in vivo* regulators of bacterial virulence. *Proc Natl Acad Sci USA* **98:**6889–6894.

242. **Butler SM, Nelson EJ, Chowdhury N, Faruque SM, Calderwood SB, Camilli A.** 2006. Cholera stool bacteria repress chemotaxis to increase infectivity. *Mol Microbiol* **60:**417–426.

HOST CELL ENSLAVEMENT BY INTRACELLULAR BACTERIA

Hijacking and Use of Host Lipids by Intracellular Pathogens

22

ALVARO TOLEDO[1] and JORGE L. BENACH[1]

INTRODUCTION

"Lipids" is the inclusive name for a complex group of molecules composed predominantly of carbon, hydrogen, and oxygen (also nitrogen and phosphorus) that are insoluble in water but soluble in organic solvents. They are characterized as being hydrophobic or amphiphilic. Lipids include fatty acids, glycerolipids, glycerophospholipids, sphingolipids, glycolipids, sterols, polyketides, and prenol lipids. The structures of the lipids discussed in this review are shown in Fig. 1. The functions of lipids were thought to be limited to being structural components of cell membranes and to being the main form of energy storage in cells. Aside from these important functions, lipids participate in key biological processes that include signaling, organization of the membrane, and trafficking from the membrane to the cytosol. In addition, lipid disorders are key to the pathogenesis of cardiovascular diseases and other metabolic disorders.

Lipids have had a large historical role in infection, first with pore-forming toxins using cholesterol for insertion and with AB toxins that use more complex lipids as their binding receptor. While microbes require lipids either synthesized or acquired for their biological functions, it has become apparent

[1]Department of Molecular Genetics and Microbiology, Stony Brook University, Center for Infectious Diseases at the Center for Molecular Medicine, Stony Brook, NY 11794.

Virulence Mechanisms of Bacterial Pathogens, 5th edition
Edited by Indira T. Kudva, Nancy A. Cornick, Paul J. Plummer, Qijing Zhang, Tracy L. Nicholson, John P. Bannantine, and Bryan H. Bellaire
© 2016 American Society for Microbiology, Washington, DC
doi:10.1128/microbiolspec.VMBF-0001-2014

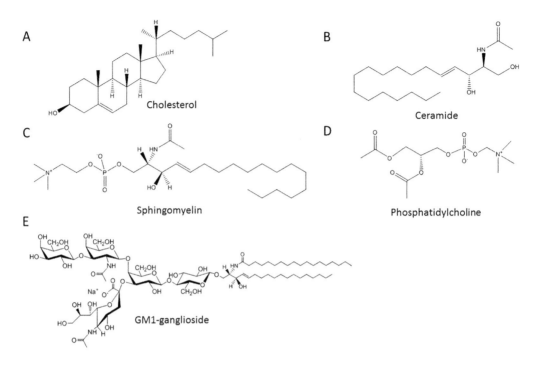

FIGURE 1 Structure of (A) cholesterol, (B) ceramide, (C) sphingomyelin, (D) phosphatidylcholine, and (E) GM1 ganglioside.

that there is a critical interplay between microbes and cells that require lipids. Specifically, this interplay is most important in the entry process of microbes into the cells and thereafter in the maintenance of their intracellular niches. In the last decade, an increasing number of studies have shown how microbes target and exploit different host lipids involved in a variety of functions. There is a large body of literature documenting the use of lipid microdomains by viruses for entry into the cells (see references 1 and 2 for reviews on this topic). Entry mechanisms using cell membrane lipids are also increasingly documented for bacteria, fungi, and protozoa. Following entry, lipids continue to be essential for the completion of the intracellular life cycle of the microbes. Incorporation of lipids within a cell environment can protect microorganisms from the effects of an acidified phagolysosomal compartment. Some pathogens can avoid the deleterious acidification of the phagolyso-

some through recruitment of host cell lipids, allowing the organisms to use a hostile environment and convert it into one where they can multiply and grow.

As mentioned earlier, the use of lipid molecules on the membranes of cells by a large variety of both DNA and RNA viruses has been amply documented. Likewise, the field of bacterial toxins utilizing lipid microdomains as binding sites in target cells has been reviewed exhaustively (3). Thus, the aim of this review is to summarize in a comprehensive manner the different strategies that bacteria use to exploit host lipids and hijack the cellular machinery to infect, survive, multiply, and disseminate in the host. In addition, we will review the importance of host lipid acquisition by extracellular pathogens. Even after narrowing down the scope of this chapter, we have found that the topic that we have chosen has been the subject of several excellent reviews that we have used as models for our own (4–9).

Some bacteria recruit cholesterol, sphingolipids, and phospholipids directly from the host. Although the list of prokaryotes that incorporate cholesterol and sphingolipids is growing, bacteria in general do not have the cellular tools to synthesize these lipids, but many have evolved the enzymatic machinery required to modify them. Prokaryotes incorporate host lipids for different reasons, and these can include cell permeability, membrane fluidity, energy or nutrient sources, and signaling processes. Bacteria can also modify and rearrange their lipid composition in the membrane in response to different conditions such as stress, temperature changes, or other types of stimuli.

In this chapter, we will review lipid incorporation by bacteria that are extracellular and bacteria that are either facultative or obligate intracellular organisms. The use of lipids is different between the two groups. For example, intracellular bacteria use host lipids to avoid phagosome maturation and to multiply in the intracellular niche, whereas extracellular bacteria incorporate lipids in their membrane, where they play a structural role. Nonetheless, lipids, particularly cholesterol, are increasingly recognized in bacteria (Table 1), and their lipidome is of both biological and pathogenesis interest. Mass spectrometry techniques have been developed and applied to study the lipidome of bacteria and to evaluate their changes under different conditions (10–12). This is of special importance for pathogens of the genus *Mycobacterium* that contain 60% of cellular dry weight

corresponding to lipids and can change their membrane lipid profile in response to stress condition such as pH (10). Lipids contribute to the impermeability of the cell wall, increasing the virulence of the *Mycobacterium tuberculosis* organism. Likewise, *Borrelia burgdorferi*, the agent of Lyme disease, and *Helicobacter pylori*, the causative agent of gastritis and peptic ulcer disease, incorporate cholesterol and modify it into glycolipids. Specifically, *B. burgdorferi* assembles the cholesterol and cholesterol glycolipids into lipid microdomains that resemble eukaryotic lipid rafts.

Cholesterol is an essential structural component of the cell membrane of vertebrates, and it is required for membrane integrity and fluidity. In eukaryotic cells, cholesterol and sphingolipids are the main components of membrane microdomains known as lipid rafts (13–15; for review see reference 16). These microdomains are characterized by being more tightly packed than the surrounding bilayer and enriched with proteins involved in signaling and other fundamental biological processes (17), including receptor clustering and lateral sorting of proteins, such as glycosylphosphatidylinositol (GPI)–anchored proteins and lipoproteins (18, 19), endocytosis, exocytosis, vesicle formation, and budding (20–22). Part of this review will focus on the use of eukaryotic lipid rafts by bacteria. This is a rapidly growing area of bacterial pathogenesis that affects entry as well as downstream events after the bacteria are internalized. Use of lipid rafts as points of attachment and entry of bacteria is shared by both Gram-positive and Gram-negative organisms and also by extra- and intracellular species. The importance of this association is evidenced by earlier reviews of the topic (23, 24).

The use of lipid receptors for bacterial toxins has been established for years. In this review, we have not included toxin use for adhering to lipid domains on the surface of the target cells because a significant literature on this topic exists. Instead, our focus is on the use of lipid rafts as entry points into

TABLE 1 Bacterial pathogens that incorporate cholesterol

Species	Reference
Anaplasma phagocytophilum	100
Borrelia burgdorferi (Lyme disease)	144, 145
Borrelia hermsii (relapsing fever)	215
Brachyspira hyodysenteriae	216, 217
Ehrlichia chaffeensis	100
Helicobacter pylori	218–220
Mycoplasma spp.	221, 222
Mycobacterium spp.	123

cells. There is significant information that distills a common theme that at least some bacteria show a marked preference for attaching to lipid microdomains to initiate entry into the cells. Not all the literature is in agreement, however, because some of the procedures that are used to remove cholesterol, and therefore show inhibition of entry, can create a number of unforeseen effects that could complicate the interpretation of results.

Infection of eukaryotic cells with bacterial pathogens includes the adhesion of the pathogen to surface lipid receptors (lipid rafts) of the cell. The attachment process can continue with the recruitment of proteins to the entry site, which in turn can assist in the remodeling of the membrane and the development of signal transduction required for internalization of the pathogen (such as actin polymerization). Once internalized, the bacteria in the phagosome will need to recruit lipids that are necessary for their nutrition and in some instances to avoid phagosome fusion with lysosomes to escape the degradation of the pathogen. In this review, we will present evidence for all parts and stages of this process. Splitting the process into entry, membrane reorganization, and acquisition of lipids is somewhat arbitrary because the entire process is a continuum. However, for the purposes of this review each will be considered separately.

BACTERIAL USE OF HOST LIPIDS FOR ENTRY INTO CELLS

A number of bacterial organisms have an obligate intracellular existence, notably, the chlamydiae and the rickettsiae. The others are facultative intracellular bacteria. Obviously, adaptations for entry by obligate organisms are critical for their survival, and these adaptations represent the strong association between the parasitic prokaryote and its eukaryotic cell host. The *Chlamydiaceae* are obligate intracellular bacteria, and significant research has been conducted regarding the use of lipids for cell entry by species of this genus. *Chlamydia trachomatis* is the most commonly reported sexually transmitted agent and also the most common of all notifiable infections (25, 26). *C. trachomatis* infects the lower genital tract of men as an agent of urethritis, prostatitis, and epididymitis (27–29) and cervicitis, salpingitis, and pelvic inflammatory disease in women (30–32). This species is also a major cause of trachoma and conjunctivitis in developing countries (33, 34). There is an enlarging clinical spectrum for *C. trachomatis* such as being a cofactor for HIV infection (35). *Chlamydophila* (Chlamydia) *pneumoniae* is responsible for outbreaks of community-acquired pneumonia, pharyngitis, and bronchitis (36). In addition, *C. pneumonia* has been reported to be involved in the development of atherosclerosis (37–39). Collectively, these diseases are a major global public health problem.

The chlamydiae have a unique dimorphic life cycle. The elementary body is the infecting stage and infects preferentially mucosal epithelial cells. The reticulate body is the dividing stage within large phagosomes known as inclusions (40). There are some important aspects that have been worked out for the entry of these bacteria into cells. These organisms promote the reorganization of actin, and early tyrosine phosphorylation is common across *Chlamydia* species and is associated with entry. Chlamydia secretes proteins into the host cell through a type III secretion system (TTSS) that can contribute to their internalization. One such translocated protein is Tarp (translocated actin-recruiting phosphoprotein), and it is phosphorylated with a critical role in the actin-driven uptake of the bacteria (41). Small GTPases of the Rho (42, 43) and ARF family (44) have also been shown to be important in actin-dependent internalization.

The infection starts with the internalization of the elementary bodies, and it involves interactions between chlamydial ligands and receptors on the surface of the cell. Proteoglycans have been possible candidates for initial contact of the elementary bodies with the cell surface, and this association may be a charge-driven interaction. A number of studies of *Chlamydia* point to lipid rafts as the site of entry in the cell and for subsequent internalization of the elementary bodies (42, 45, 46). Experiments using methyl-β-cyclodextrin (45–47) as an agent for cholesterol depletion or other cholesterol sequestering reagents (45, 48, 49) have shown that elementary bodies attach to cells at sites of high cholesterol concentration. Some studies have shown that *Chlamydia* enters the cell through membrane areas rich in GM1, a lipid raft marker (42), and colocalizes with caveolin-1 and caveolin-2 (48, 50). *C. pneumoniae*, an agent of respiratory infections in humans, and *Chlamydia psittaci*, a pathogen of birds that can also infect humans, each enter host cells after attachment to lipid rafts rich in cholesterol. Attachment to lipid rafts is not universal, however. While *C. trachomatis* serovars E and F also use lipid rafts to enter host cells, lipid rafts with associated caveolin were not used for entry of *C. trachomatis* serovars A-C (49).

Signaling molecules that are involved in bacterial entry into cells also partition in lipid rafts (51–53). It appears that Cdc42 and Rac (both small GTPases of the Rho family involved in morphological changes, migration, and actin polymerization) are translocated to lipid rafts in response to lipopolysaccharide (52), and these are also important in the entry of the elementary bodies. *C. trachomatis* has a number of serovars that behave differently on entry of the cells, and this emphasizes the individuality of these variants. Serovars A and C (associated with trachoma) are not inhibited by the removal of cholesterol; rather, they enter the cells through clathrin-mediated endocytosis (49). Likewise, the approaches of entry for serovars E and K remain unclear since different research groups reached different conclusions (47, 49). These biological distinctions between chlamydial species as well as between *C. trachomatis* serovars are reflected in the interaction with host cells

and the route of entry and could be due to the localization of the cell surface molecules used by different species/serovars to enter cells.

Brucella spp. are Gram-negative, facultative intracellular bacteria of medical and veterinary importance. These organisms replicate within a phagosome inside phagocytic cells as well as other cells. Inhibition of phagosome fusion with the lysosome appears to promote intracellular survival. Lipid raft disruption by filipin, methyl-β-cyclodextrin, and cholera toxin interfered with the entry process. Thus, lipid rafts may provide a portal of entry for Brucella into murine macrophages under nonopsonic conditions, thus allowing phagosome-lysosome fusion inhibition, which in turn promotes intracellular survival (54). Several approaches were used to show that plasma membrane cholesterol of macrophages is required for the VirB-dependent internalization of *B. abortus* and also contributed to the establishment of bacterial infection in mice after entry (55). The entry of *B. abortus* into macrophages was found to be more complex through the use of the class A scavenger receptor in addition to the requirement for location of this receptor within lipid rafts (56). The entry of *Brucella ovis and Brucella canis* into macrophages was mediated by a class A scavenger receptor, cholesterol, and ganglioside GM1 (57). The entry of *Brucella* spp. through membrane microdomains that contain cholesterol requires other protein receptors that have to be associated with the lipid structures. The association of proteins with lipid microdomains as portals of entry into cells is frequent among facultative intracellular bacteria.

Bordetella bronchiseptica, which is closely related to the agent of pertussis is an important veterinary pathogen, adhered to host cells at GM1-enriched lipid raft microdomains. BteA, a cytotoxic effector protein delivered by the TTSS of this bacterium, colocalized to lipid rafts as well, and disruption of the lipid rafts reduced its cytotoxicity. This study is significant in that it identified a 130–amino acid lipid raft targeting domain at the N-terminus of BteA (58).

Francisella tularensis is a Gram-negative facultative, intracellular zoonotic pathogen capable of infecting many different living organisms from protozoa to humans. *F. tularensis* was found to attach to cholesterol-rich lipid rafts in association with caveolin 1 for entry into mouse macrophages. Treatment of the mouse macrophages with cholera toxin and with phosphatidylinositol phospholipase C to inhibit attachment or destabilize the lipid rafts by removal of GPI-anchored proteins inhibited entry of *F. tularensis* and thereafter inhibited its intracellular proliferation (59).

Gram-negative enteric species (*Salmonella*, *Shigella*) use lipid microdomains rich in cholesterol for attachment to and entry into cells of the alimentary canal. A molecular complex involving proteins of both the host, CD44, the hyaluronan receptor, and *Shigella*, the invasin IpaB, is enriched in lipid rafts containing cholesterol and sphingolipids. This study also demonstrated the accumulation of cholesterol and raft-associated proteins at the *Shigella* entry site, and depletion of cholesterol and sphingolipids resulted in decreased invasion (60). Using cells that are deficient in the formation of lipid rafts, a recent study showed that cholesterol is not essential for invasion and intracellular replication by *Salmonella enterica* serovar Typhimurium and *C. trachomatis*, but entry of *Coxiella burnetii* into the host cell was impaired, indicating that cholesterol is important for this species (61).

Although not an intracellular enteric bacterium, *H. pylori* has effector molecules that use lipid microdomains for attachment. The vacuolating toxin (VacA) of *H. pylori* intoxicates cells. Treatment of target cells with cholesterol-depleting agents interfered with the internalization or intracellular localization of VacA and reduced vacuolation. The study concluded that VacA associates with lipid rafts for entry into the cells and is important for downstream cytotoxicity (62). Another effector from *H. pylori* requires lipid rafts for attachment. Delivery of CagA into epithelial cells by the bacterial type IV secretion system (T4SS) is mediated in a cholesterol-dependent manner (63). The α(5)β(1) integrin is found in lipid rafts and is a known ligand for attachment and translocation of CagA leading to cytoskeletal rearrangements. Integrin α(5)β(1) and the cholesterol-rich microdomains at the host cell surface are required for NOD1 recognition of peptidoglycan and subsequent induction of NF-κB-dependent responses to *H. pylori*. These results demonstrated that lipid rafts are a novel platform for delivery of bacterial effectors (CagA) to target the cells (64).

Infection with *Pseudomonas aeruginosa*, a Gram-negative bacterium, targets the respiratory system of susceptible individuals. Essentially opportunistic, *P. aeruginosa* is a dangerous bacterium that causes serious complications in patients with cystic fibrosis and neutropenia. In addition, *P. aeruginosa* infects the eyes and the skin in burn patients. It is unclear whether infection of macrophages with this bacterium prolongs or shortens the infection. However, understanding the molecular mechanisms of ingestion by these cells has provided important clues about its pathogenesis. Recently, lipid rafts that contain sphingolipids and cholesterol have been shown to be important for the initial interaction of the bacterium with the cell membrane. A number of studies have documented the predilection for the lipid microdomains for binding of *P. aeruginosa*.

On contact with cells, *P. aeruginosa* increased the enzymatic activity of the acid sphingomyelinase of macrophages, and this resulted in the release of ceramide into sphingolipid-rich rafts. The increase of ceramide led to the reorganization of the rafts into larger signaling platforms that are required to internalize *P. aeruginosa*. Once inside, the bacterium can induce apoptosis and regulate the cytokine response, which are both necessary to initiate the innate immune response. Failure to generate ceramide-enriched membrane platforms leads to a dysfunctional inflammatory response with resulting cytokine release and irreversible sepsis of mice. This study demonstrated that reorganization of the lipid rafts by incorporation of ceramide is essential for the initiation of cell defenses against this organism (65).

P. aeruginosa is a frequent cause of eye infections, particularly after corneal injury through the use of contact lenses. Lipid raft formation was evaluated *in vivo* in rabbit corneas with and without contact lens use. In addition, a human corneal epithelial cell line was used to detect lipid raft formation following infection with *P. aeruginosa*. Contact lens use in rabbits resulted in lipid raft formation. Likewise, the bacteria displayed preferential attachment to lipid rafts and to lipid raft aggregation, which in turn facilitated internalization by the cells (66). *P. aeruginosa* enters corneal epithelial cells *in vitro* via membrane microdomains or lipid rafts. In addition to lipid microdomains, *P. aeruginosa* has utilized the cystic fibrosis transmembrane conductance regulator (CFTR) for bacterial entry. A study to determine colocalization of the CFTR with or within lipid rafts was conducted using corneal cells expressing wild-type or Δ CFTR infected with this organism. *P. aeruginosa* and CFTR colocalized with the lipid rafts, leading to the conclusion that this bacterium enters human corneal epithelial cells via lipid rafts containing CFTR (67). Another study focused on the utilization of lipid rafts and specific proteins to facilitate the entry of *P. aeruginosa* into alveolar macrophages. Lyn, a member of the Src family tyrosine kinases, is mainly a negative regulator in B lymphocytes and is instrumental in ingestion. It appears that phagocytosis is initiated by lipid rafts and is dependent on Lyn. Blocking of Lyn and effectors of cholesterol synthesis inhibited ingestion of *P. aeruginosa* by alveolar macrophages. Moreover, both Lyn and lipid rafts followed the bacterium inside the cell, where they exerted various host defense functions (68).

P. aeruginosa uses a novel approach to deliver virulence factors without actually attaching to the cell. This organism uses outer membrane vesicles for the long-distance delivery of bacterial effectors into the host cell cytoplasm. The outer membrane vesicles deliver their protein cargo by fusing with lipid rafts in the host plasma membrane. This fusion process has also been used by *B. burgdorferi*, and it is essentially based on a lipid-lipid interaction. The *P. aeruginosa* virulence factors enter the host cell via Neural Wiskott-Aldrich syndrome protein (N-WASP)-mediated actin trafficking and thereafter migrate to other locations within the cell where they can affect the biology of the cell. The outer membrane vesicle route provides for a coordinated delivery system of bacterial effectors. The lipid rafts of the cell constitute the fusion platform to initiate the infection (69).There are other organisms that have been reported to use lipid microdomains for entry or attachment to cells, and these are summarized in Table 2.

BACTERIAL USE OF HOST LIPIDS FOR INTRACELLULAR GROWTH

The studies of acquisition of host lipids into phagosomes to maintain the growth and viability of intracellular bacteria represent major advances in both cell biology and microbiology. However, these studies are uneven in their representation of the various intracellular bacterial species. A large amount of work has been done on the acquisition and transport of lipids by the *Chlamydiae*, and its review summarizes a great chapter in bacterial pathogenesis.

After entry, the elementary bodies are bound into the inclusion which is derived from the host plasma membrane. The elementary bodies differentiate into reticulate bodies and begin to replicate. The inclusion avoids fusion with lysosomes and is transported to the Golgi region. During this period of chlamydial growth and replication, the inclusion is an active partner, and it interacts with different cellular compartments and trafficking pathways to acquire nutrients.

TABLE 2 Bacteria species that use lipid rafts to enter the host cell

Species and use	Reference
Porphyromonas gingivalis uses lipid rafts of macrophages for entry	223
Campylobacter promotes the translocation of gut commensals across the intestinal epithelium via a lipid raft transcellular process	224
Campylobacter jejuni invades epithelial cells through lipid rafts	225
Removing cholesterol from host cells decreases infectivity of *Legionella pneumophila*	226
Streptococcus suis inhibits ingestion through destabilization of macrophage lipid rafts	227
Streptococcus pneumonia uses lipid rafts to invade red blood cells	228
Group B *Streptococcus* uses lipid rafts to invade endometrial cells	229
Encapsulated group B *Streptococcus* enters dendritic cells through lipid rafts and clathrin-mediated endocytosis	230
Anthrax toxin uses a lipid-raft-mediated clathrin process for endocytosis	231
Ehrlichia chaffeensis and *Anaplasma phagocytophilum* intracellular infection involve cholesterol-rich lipid rafts	102

Chlamydia requires lipids from the host cell for survival and has developed different mechanisms to recruit sphingolipids and cholesterol from within the inclusion. The Golgi apparatus provides the main network for vesicular transport of lipids in host cells. Nonvesicular transport of lipids is modulated by cytosolic lipid transfer proteins. *Chlamydia* has developed diverse strategies to use vesicular and nonvesicular pathways for the acquisition of lipids. The *Chlamydiae* bacteria have the biochemical machinery to synthesize phosphatididylethanolamine, phosphatidylglycerol and phosphatidylserine (70, 71). Nonetheless, the membranes of *C. trachomatis* have substantial amounts of lipids derived from the host cells, notably sphingomyelin and cholesterol (70–72). Since this organism does not have the ability to synthesize these lipids, it must obtain them from the host (73). Specifically, the *Chlamydia* require sphingomyelin (74, 75).

Lipid recruitment may be mediated by host proteins in the membrane of the inclusion. Although it has not been defined yet how the host proteins are associated with the inclusion membrane, it has been proposed that some inclusion proteins could be responsible for the binding (76). Inclusion proteins are abundant in the membrane of the inclusion (i.e., phagosome), and over 50 such proteins have been characterized (77); a secondary structure characteristic in the

form of bilobed hydrophobic domains has been found to target inclusion proteins to the inclusion membrane (78).

Ceramide, the precursor of sphingomyelin and cholesterol, is acquired through Golgi-dependent processes, and a number of studies indicate that these processes are used effectively by the *Chlamydia* to locate these lipids in the inclusion membrane (72, 79–82). This is possible because there is a close association between the inclusion and the Golgi complex where sphingomyelin is synthesized. Ceramide is converted to sphingomyelin in the Golgi and subsequently accumulates within the inclusion membrane as early as 2 h postinfection (79, 80). To accomplish this, *C. trachomatis* intercepts an exocytic pathway by fusing vesicles containing sphingomyelin exiting the trans-Golgi in transit to the plasma membrane, and this is a common feature of several *Chlamydia* species (83, 84). Treatment of infected cells with a pharmacological inhibitor of the assembly of multivesicular bodies delayed the development of the inclusion and inhibited the acquisition of sphingomyelin and cholesterol (85). However, Golgi-dependent pathways appear to be specific to only certain lipids, because other lipids are not intercepted (86).

Chlamydia can utilize the ceramide-transfer protein (CERT) to promote the trafficking of ceramide from the endoplasmic reticulum to the inclusion membrane for subsequent conversion to sphingomyelin (82, 87). Subsequent studies showed that IncD (an inclusion membrane protein) can mediate the recruitment of CERT (88). It appears that the CERT-IncD interaction is very important and specific, because a non-human strain that infects guinea pigs, *Chlamydia caviae*, lacks IncD and does not recruit CERT to the inclusion membrane (87). However, as mentioned earlier, there are many pathways that the *Chlamydiae* use to incorporate lipids onto the inclusion membranes. Although the CERT pathway is important and specific, *C. caviae* can still incorporate sphingomyelin despite its lack of utilization of the CERT-IncD pathway (83).

Inhibition of CERT activity resulted in a decrease in the acquisition of sphingomyelin onto the inclusion membrane (82). This intriguing observation suggests that CERT binds ceramide at the endoplasmic reticulum to the inclusion, where it assembled into sphingomyelin. Alternatively, CERT can transfer ceramide to the Golgi, where it is converted to sphingomyelin and subsequently transferred to the nearby inclusion by vesicular traffic (82).

Dysfunction of organelles also enhances lipid uptake by the *Chlamydia* within the inclusion. Sphingomyelin incorporation into the inclusion increased as a result of Golgi fragmentation. The Golgi is fragmented into mini-stacks that surround the inclusion, leading to enhancement of *C. trachomatis* replication. Mini-stack formation is mediated by host, Golgin-84, and chlamydia, chlamydial protease like activity factor (CPFA), proteases (89). This is a unique means of lipid acquisition, where the bacteria and the host cell have a role in the degradation of the organelle (90, 91).

An increasing number of studies are linking specific proteins for translocation to the inclusion membranes, where they could play important roles in lipid acquisition, and some of these proteins can bind lipids directly. *Chlamydia* can acquire sphingomyelin by co-opting a subset of Golgi trafficking proteins including Arf1 GTPase (92) and GBF1 (82), a regulator of Arf1-dependent vesicular trafficking, and both are essential for inclusion membrane growth and stability. A small interfering RNA screen identified Src family kinases in the acquisition of sphingomyelin (93). The possibility of lipid acquisition pathways involving Incs and Rab GTPases has been explored, indicating that the latter are recruited to the inclusion membrane (94, 95). Rab-GTPases 6, 11, and 14 are key regulators of the Golgi apparatus; *Chlamydia* subverts the Golgi structure to enhance its intracellular development, presumably by mobilizing the Golgi fragments (91, 96). SNARE proteins can be instrumental in the fusion with host vesicles for acquisition of lipids (97).

Chlamydia acquires cholesterol from a low-density lipoprotein (LDL) pathway and from *de novo* synthesis (72). Lipid droplets have also been implicated as a source of neutral lipids. Lipid droplets are most obvious at the periphery of the inclusion and are translocated into the phagosome at IncA-rich sites (98, 99).

Anaplasma phagocytophilum is a Gram-negative, tick-borne bacterium that contains cholesterol in its outer membrane but does not produce lipid A. This bacterium occupies a unique niche within neutrophils and is an obligate intracellular microbe. *A. phagocytophilum* cannot synthesize cholesterol, so it has to acquire cholesterol directly from its host cells or from the medium (100). Cholesterol is required for growth of *A. phagocytophilum* in HL-60 cells, the preferred laboratory cell for cultivation of this organism. Even more important, high serum levels of cholesterol enhance *A. phagocytophilum* infection in the mouse model (101). This obligate intracellular bacterium uses cholesterol not only for growth and survival, but also uses it to enter host cells through caveolae or lipid rafts. The phagosome membrane maintains caveolin-1 throughout infection, indicating that there is a need for continuing acquisition of cholesterol (102). The manner by which *A. phagocytophilum* acquires cholesterol involves the use of the host cell pathway for uptake of this lipid. The source of cholesterol required for *A. phagocytophilum* replication is derived from serum LDL rather than from cholesterol synthesized by the cells themselves. *A. phagocytophilum* uses the host LDL uptake pathway and the LDL receptor mRNA regulatory system to acquire cholesterol in the phagosome to enhance its growth. *Anaplasma* acquires host cholesterol derived exclusively from serum LDLs, because infection with this bacterium can be blocked using pharmacological inhibitors of the LDL-CHOL vesicular transport pathway. These results demonstrate a unique evolutionary adaptation of *A. phagocytophilum* for the acquisition of cholesterol by upregulating low-density receptors. These findings also illustrate how *A. phagocytophilum* hijacks host cell cholesterol pathways for its own benefit (103).

C. burnetii is an obligate intracellular Gram-negative bacterial pathogen and the causative agent of Q fever. The genus *Coxiella* is closest to the *Legionella* but has several important differences. One important difference is that *C. burnetii* helps in the development of a parasitophorous vacuole that is required for replication. Intracellular vacuolar pathogens such as *C. burnetii* require lipids for both normal bacterial functions as well as formation of the acidic vacuole surrounding the bacteria. Host-derived cholesterol is necessary for the creation and maintenance of the vacuole, and its incorporation has been established by positive staining with filipin for the lipid raft marker, flotillin, showing that the vacuolar membranes are enriched in cholesterol and contain lipid raft microdomains (104). Inhibition experiments using pharmacological agents that inhibit uptake of cholesterol altered the morphology of the vacuoles and partially inhibited *C. burnetii* replication. The formation of vacuoles was inhibited after treatment of cells with inhibitors of cholesterol uptake and synthesis. This study concluded that *C. burnetii* interferes with cholesterol metabolism and that cholesterol is required

for intracellular replication (104). Using Chinese hamster ovary cells as a model, it was shown that the vacuoles of these cells infected with *C. burnetii* are rich in cholesterol, which is essential for growth of this organism in these cells (105). Unlike other organisms that incorporate lipids, *C. burnetii* can acquire lipids through both synthesis and utilization of host cell pools. The *C. burnetii* genome encodes enzymes for the synthesis of fatty acids and phospholipids, but *C. burnetii* also requires sterols for the biogenesis of the vacuoles. *C. burnetii* lacks enzymes for *de novo* cholesterol biosynthesis, but it encodes a sterol reductase homolog. This enzyme occurs infrequently in prokaryotes, and it reduces sterol double bonds in the final step of cholesterol biosynthesis. Working with the *Coxiella* gene in a yeast system, it was demonstrated that the sterol reductase of this organism was active and was likely to act on host sterols during *C. burnetii* intracellular growth (106).

This bacterium lacks the synthetic machinery to generate cholesterol. Yet it is known that *C. burnetii* utilizes host cell lipids for creation of the vacuole, implying that it can manipulate the cell's lipid-signaling pathways to support the intracellular location, for example, effectors secreted by *C. burnetii*. The T4SS of this organism may be involved in the utilization of cell lipids. A recent review considers all aspects of lipid utilization by this species (107). A new model system was used to assess cholesterol requirements in infection of mouse embryonic fibroblasts with *C. burnetii*, *S.* Typhimurium, and *C. trachomatis*. A cell line deficient in sterol reductase, and hence unable to complete cholesterol biosynthesis, was used to determine the role of cholesterol in infection with the three pathogens. Infection of the sterol reductase–deficient cells by *S.* Typhimurium and *C. trachomatis* was unaltered, whereas *C. burnetii* entry was significantly decreased, suggesting a role for lipid rafts in the ingestion of this bacterium. All three pathogens established residence in their respective vacuoles and replicated normally in the sterol reductase–deficient fibroblasts, except that the *C. burnetii* vacuoles were abnormal. While this study argued that cholesterol is not essential for invasion and replication by *S.* Typhimurium and *C. trachomatis*, it appears to be critical for invasion and growth of *Coxiella* (61).

Studies with *F. tularensis* also showed that cholesterol and caveolin-1 were incorporated into *Francisella*-containing vesicles during entry and the initial phase of intracellular trafficking inside the host cell (59). *F. tularensis* also can invade nonphagocytic cells, notably hepatocytes (108). *Francisella novicida* uses clathrin- and cholesterol-dependent mechanisms to invade hepatocytes. Clathrin accessory proteins AP-2 and Eps15, but not caveolin, colocalized with invading *F. novicida*. Caveolin was thus not required for the organism to enter hepatocytes. These results demonstrate that members of the same genus can utilize diverse entry pathways (109).

A ubiquitous early step in infection of humans and animals by enteric bacterial pathogens such as *Salmonella* spp., *Shigella* spp., and enteropathogenic *Escherichia coli* (EPEC) is the translocation of virulence effector proteins into mammalian cells via specialized TTSSs. Translocated effectors subvert the host cytoskeleton and stimulate signaling to promote bacterial internalization or survival. Target cell plasma membrane cholesterol is central to pathogen-host cross-talk, but the precise nature of its critical contribution remains unknown.

The uptake of *Listeria monocytogenes*, the Gram-positive agent of listeriosis, by nonphagocytic cells is accomplished by an assembled complex involving the bacterial proteins internalin and InlB and their host cell receptors E-cadherin and hepatocyte growth factor receptor (HGF-R)/Met, respectively. Through the use of lipid raft markers such as acyl-modified and GPI-anchored proteins, GM1 ganglioside, as well as cholesterol depletion, it was found that the presence of E-cadherin in lipid domains was necessary for initial interaction with internalin to promote bacterial entry. However, the initial interaction of InlB with HGF-R did not require membrane cholesterol. Downstream events after entry required cholesterol for F-actin polymerization (110). Listeriolysin O, a pore-forming toxin of *L. monocytogenes*, intercalates into cholesterol-rich membranes of target cells. However, this toxin also assists in the clustering of the lipid rafts. Evidence provided by the clustering of GPI-anchored proteins in membranes after listeriolysin treatment strengthened its role in the clustering of lipid rafts (111).

Enterohemorrhagic *E. coli* (EHEC) O157:H7 and EPEC O127:H6 can bind to intestinal epithelium at attaching-effacing lesions that undergo cytoskeletal rearrangements and loss of microvilli. The cholesterol requirement was documented for EPEC (112), and *E. coli* (type 1 fimbriated) invades uroepithelial cells via lipid rafts (113). Cholesterol depletion of epithelial and fibroblast cells resulted in inhibition of cytoskeletal rearrangement after exposure to both EHEC and EPEC, an effect that was restored by the addition of exogenous cholesterol. There were some differences in attachment by the two types of *E. coli*. Adherence to epithelial cells was reduced following cholesterol depletion in EPEC, but not in EHEC, bacteria (114). Likewise, extracting or changing membrane-bound cholesterol with methyl-β-cyclodextrin or filipin inhibited the entry of Dr-positive IH11128 *E. coli* into epithelial cells (115).

S. Typhimurium inhibits phagolysosome fusion and survives in a late endosome-like vacuole. Salmonella infection induces cholesterol accumulation in the vacuoles of both macrophages and epithelial cells and is dependent on intracellular replication. GPI-anchored protein CD55 is also recruited to the vacuole, suggesting an important role for cholesterol use (116). Enteroinvasive *Shigella* also uses a molecular complex involving proteins from the host, CD44, the hyaluronan receptor, and the bacterial invasin IpaB, that partition in lipid rafts. Cholesterol accumulated at the entry site of the *Shigella* organism and its depletion resulted in decreased invasion of the cells. In addition, cells that are deficient in sphingolipids had decreased invasion by the bacteria. These results pointed to a role for lipid microdomains in shigellosis (60). Shiga-toxigenic *E. coli* O113:H21 require lipid rafts to invade colonic epithelium (117).

Using *in vitro* cholesterol-binding assays provided a demonstration that two TTSS translocon molecules from *Salmonella* (SipB) and *Shigella* (IpaB) bound cholesterol with high affinity. Cholesterol depletion reduced the translocation of these molecules into cells, demonstrating a cholesterol-dependent association of the bacterial TTSS translocon with lipid rafts in the cell membrane (118). The presence of cholesterol on the host cell surface was essential for contact-mediated activation and TTSS-induced hemolysis. Purified detergent-resistant membranes and liposomes with a composition similar to lipid rafts activated the TTSS (119).

Mycobacteria are facultative intracellular pathogens that can survive inside macrophages. Cholesterol is essential for uptake of *Mycobacteria* by these cells by accumulation at the site of entry. Furthermore, once ingested, cholesterol mediates phagosome survival (120). When given a cholesterol-rich diet, tubercular patients cleared the bacilli from the sputum significantly faster (121). *Mycobacterium avium* induced lipid raft formation in mouse-derived macrophage cell lines, and the internalized organisms required cell-membrane-derived cholesterol. Follow-up experiments showed that mycobacterial lipids of high polarity interact with lipid rafts from the host cell (122). *M. tuberculosis* can use cholesterol as a sole carbon source. The gene cluster *mce4* encodes for a cholesterol import system. Cholesterol is not required for infection of mice or for growth in macrophages, but it appears to be essential for persistence in the lungs (123).

Extracellular bacteria also incorporate lipids, and specifically in the case of *Mycoplasma* spp., *B. burgdorferi*, and *H. pylori*, it is cholesterol that is prominently incorporated.

Sterol incorporation by *Mycoplasma* has been documented for a long time (124, 125). Similar to *Borrelia* and *Helicobacter*, the *Mycoplasma* spp. are not intracellular organisms and can modify free cholesterol into a glycolipid, specifically a cholesteryl-glucoside (126, 127). *Mycoplasma* can acquire cholesterol directly from serum lipoproteins (128). The distribution of lipids in the membrane also appears to be in segregated domains, reminiscent of lipid rafts in *Mycoplasma gallisepticum* (129). The uptake of cholesterol and phospholipids by several species of *Mycoplasma* is mediated by protein receptors, presumably for lipoproteins, and also by direct binding to membrane phospholipids and by existing glycolipids as well (130). The lipids of *Mycoplasma* are involved in cell fusion. These organisms attach to eukaryotic cells through a filamentous tip with specific protein adhesins, known as the tip organelle. Two proteins, P1 and P30, are involved in adhesion, and their removal abolishes binding (131, 132), and the consequences of adhesion in the pathogenesis of *Mycoplasma* infection are well known. In addition to this protein-mediated mechanism of adhesion, *Mycoplasma* can fuse with the target cells through an unesterified cholesterol-dependent process. *Mycoplasma* species adapted to grow without cholesterol supplements cannot fuse with cells (133). Fusion of the *Mycoplasma* also appears to be influenced by choline glycolipids, but their roles are not well established (134). The outcome of fusion may be to translocate effectors into the cell. The association of lipids with *Mycoplasma* spp. has been the topic of several excellent and comprehensive reviews beginning more than 50 years ago (135–137).

USE OF HOST LIPIDS BY EXTRACELLULAR BACTERIA

Borrelia burgdorferi is an extracellular tick-borne bacterium that causes Lyme disease. The spirochete requires an external cholesterol source for growth and multiplication since it cannot synthesize cholesterol. *Borrelia* represents an interesting example among bacterial pathogens that incorporate host lipids, since so far, it has been the only prokaryote described to have cholesterol-rich microdomains (Fig. 2) with all the hallmarks of eukaryotic lipid rafts (138). The membrane of *B. burgdorferi* contains phosphatidylcholine, phosphatidylglycerol, and lipoproteins (139–141). In addition, it has free cholesterol and two cholesterol glycolipids, acylated cholesteryl galactoside (ACGal) and cholesteryl galactoside (CGal), as well as a noncholesterol glycolipid, monogalactosyl diacylglycerol (MGalD) (142–145). Early studies established a link between the spirochete and host lipid by showing how *B. burgdorferi* elicits an antibody response in infected rats that targeted the host gangliosides (146). The basis of this cross-reaction is likely the presence of cholesterol glycolipids, specifically the beta linkage between the galactose and the cholesterol

group. The first evidence that *B. burgdorferi* has lipid raft microdomains in its membrane came from the study of the mechanism of the complement-independent antibody CB2. This antibody targets the outer surface lipoprotein OspB, and its bactericidal action was shown to be dependent on the presence of cholesterol glycolipids and cholesterol (147). Further analysis of these cholesterol glycolipids showed that they had an uneven distribution on the membrane of the spirochete, forming clusters or microdomains (Fig. 2). In addition, the number and size of these microdomains were shown to be temperature-dependent, and they were present in both culture- and mouse-derived spirochetes (147). Subsequent studies using biochemical approaches showed that *Borrelia* microdomains have all the hallmarks of eukaryotic lipid rafts despite lacking sphingolipids (138). In addition, cholesterol substitution experiments with live spirochetes using a range of sterols with dif-

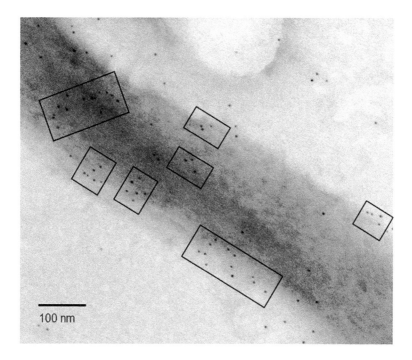

FIGURE 2 Negative-stain transmission electron microscopy image showing the localization of lipid rafts in *Borrelia burgdorferi*. Cholesterol glycolipids were detected by an antibody conjugated to 6-nm gold particles. From reference 137. Bar represents 100 nm.

ferent lipid raft formation properties showed that sterols that support raft formation were necessary and sufficient for the formation of *B. burgdorferi* membrane microdomains. Also, these sterols supported a higher number of detergent resistance membranes and were critical for membrane integrity (138).

Traditionally, studies of lipid rafts have used membrane models, and in this sense experiments using live *Borrelia* represent an opportunity to study the properties and dynamics of lipid rafts in a live organism. The role of lipid rafts in *Borrelia* are not yet known, but there are selective proteins including proteins that are tightly regulated during infection (148) and that play important roles in the life cycle of the bacterium. Therefore, it is possible that *B. burgdorferi* lipid rafts share functional roles with eukaryotic lipid rafts. Although lipid rafts contain a subset of specific proteins, little is known about the contribution of proteins to the actual lipid raft structure. A recent study addressed the structural contribution of selective proteins to lipid rafts in *B. burgdorferi*, showing that raft-associated lipoproteins contribute to lipid raft formation, whereas nonassociated raft proteins do not (149). *B. burgdorferi* needs to recruit cholesterol to form the glycolipids that are subsequently exported to the membrane, where they form lipid rafts. This bacterium establishes a crosstalk with the eukaryotic cell that results in the exchange of antigen and lipids. *B. burgdorferi* not only acquires cholesterol from epithelial cells by direct contact, but it also has the ability to recruit cholesterol from host-derived vesicles (150). In both cases, the acquisition of cholesterol in *B. burgdorferi* is time dependent (150), and it is glycosylated by undetermined bacterial enzymes (151) to make one of the most prominent glycolipids in the spirochete membrane, cholesteryl galactoside, which can be acylated to form acyl-cholesteryl galactoside. The mechanism by which *B. burgdorferi* acquires cholesterol from the host cell has not been defined yet, but it has been hypothesized that it could

be through lipid raft–lipid raft interactions between the spirochete and the host cell (150).

Although *H. pylori* is not an intracellular organism, it is one of the growing number of bacteria that incorporate cholesterol. Cholesterol incorporation by this agent is followed by the conversion of free cholesterol into a glucosyl-cholesterol complex. Cholesteryl glucosides are infrequent in bacteria. Moreover, those in *H. pylori* have an α-glycosidic linkage, which is unusual for natural glycosides. Sugar incorporation is attained by a glucosylation of the free hydroxyl group of cholesterol. Three kinds of glycolipids have been identified to be cholesteryl glucosides. Two of them were determined to be cholesteryl-α-D-glucopyranoside and cholesteryl-6-O-tetrade-canoyl-α-D-glucopyranoside, and the plausible structure of the third one was identified as cholesteryl-6-O-phosphatidyl-a-D-glucopyranoside. This last structure contains a phosphate-linked cholesteryl glycoside that is also unique to this organism. The affinity of *H. pylori* for cholesterol has been known for a long time (152), and this affinity is specific because this organism does not bind other steroids, and other common bacterial pathogens do not bind cholesterol (153). Furthermore, cholesterol supplementation is essential for the growth of *H. pylori* in culture, allowing it to avoid the use of serum (154).

Cholesterol acquisition by *Helicobacter* spp. is not well understood. One phospholipid of *H. pylori*, phosphatidylethanolamine, can bind free cholesterol, cholesterol esters, and a methyl-β-cyclodextrin-free cholesterol complex. In contrast, *E. coli* (which is not known to incorporate cholesterol as used as a control) had significantly less affinity for free cholesterol than *H. pylori*. This study disclosed that the fatty acid composition of phosphatidylethanolamine of *H. pylori* was important in binding sterols (155). Curiously, *H. pylori* senses cholesterol in the environment and displays a chemotactic response to areas of greater cholesterol concentrations. This organism can also acquire cholesterol directly from cell membranes, and does so by destroying the cell lipid rafts (156).

As mentioned, *H. pylori* acquires cholesterol from its environment and glycosylates to form glucosyl-cholesterol. This complex is incorporated into the membrane by an α-glucosyltransferase (157) and has been shown to have important effects on the viability and integrity of this bacterium. In a study to determine the role of cholesterol in antibiotics and antimicrobial peptides, it was found that bacteria grown in the absence of cholesterol were significantly more susceptible to the action of these agents (158). The glucosyl-cholesterol complex can be beneficial to *H. pylori*, because this bacterium can glucosylate toxic sterols and integrate the complex into the membrane without harming the organism. In contrast, mutants of the glucosyl transferase are killed by toxic sterols (159). Cholesterol in *H. pylori* modifies the membranes so that colonization of the gastric mucosa and expression of Lewis antigen are not impaired (160).

The cytotoxin-associated gene A (CagA) is the prominent virulence factor of *H. pylori*. It is translocated into cells by the T4SS encoded by the Cag pathogenicity island. Colonization of the gastric mucosa leads to chronic gastritis and development of disease that is dependent on the T4SS and the ability to incorporate cholesterol derived from the host. In addition, CagA is an indicator of gastric cancer risk because it interferes with numerous cell-signaling pathways (161). Cholesteryl glucosides promote the formation of functional T4SS, and mutants of components of the pathogenicity island have impaired activities of their T4SS that can be restored by complementation. Glucosyl cholesterol synthesized by *H. pylori* collects around host-pathogen contact sites and promotes the formation of a functional T4SS and, therefore, *H. pylori* infection (162).

Cholesterol incorporation by *H. pylori* also has important consequences for the innate and adaptive immune responses. Free cholesterol and glucosylated cholesterols in the

β-linkage (provided exogenously) promote enhanced phagocytosis, whereas cholesteryl-α-glucosides, the natural form in this organism, protect it from ingestion by phagocytes. The presence of the glucosylating enzyme assists this bacterium in evading several arms of the immune system (156).

HOST LIPIDS AS A SOURCE OF ENERGY

As mentioned before, intracellular pathogens can use a variety of lipids for different purposes including surviving in the phagosome and multiplying, among other functions. In addition, there are bacterial pathogens that can also recruit and use host lipids as a carbon source and for energy. Moreover, they can hijack the host lipid metabolism to create suitable reservoirs that facilitate the persistence of the pathogen in the human host. Several intracellular pathogens are known to do this, most notably but not exclusively, members of the genera *Mycobacterium*, including the human pathogens *M. tuberculosis* and *Mycobacterium leprae*.

There has been evidence since the 1950s that *M. tuberculosis* uses host lipids as the primary carbon source *in vivo* (163). There are other *Mycobacterium* species, as well as other bacteria including *C. burnetii* and *Vibrio cholera* that feed on host lipids, but classically, *M. tuberculosis* has been illustrated as the prototype organism to explain how pathogens exploit and utilize host lipid as a carbon and energy source. *M. tuberculosis* and other members of the genus are unique organisms regarding their lipid composition and metabolism. *M. tuberculosis* possesses a large variety of diverse lipids, including glycolipids, mycolic acids, and polyketides in the cell wall (164), which are encoded in the genome along with genes for their biosynthesis, some of them shared with distantly related organisms including plants and animals as well as other bacteria (165). Moreover, the genome of *M. tuberculosis* has an overrepresentation of genes related to fatty acid metabolism, with approximately 250 distinct enzymes (165). The enzymes that direct the degraded fatty acid products to different pathways influence the phenotype of the bacterium in different mouse models (166–168).

Cholesterol is another prominent host lipid recruited by *M. tuberculosis* and used as a carbon source. Indeed, *M. tuberculosis* encodes a cholesterol import system that allows the bacterium to recruit cholesterol and grow even if cholesterol is the only available source of carbon and energy (123). Even though *M. tuberculosis* does not require cholesterol for infection of mice or to grow in resting macrophages, it is essential for persistence in chronically infected animals and activated macrophages (169). However, in the context of lipids and carbon metabolism, the most striking characteristic of *M. tuberculosis* is its plasticity, because it can use multiple lipid energy sources available in the host. Rather than relying on a single source, this organism cocatabolizes multiple carbon sources (170). The adaptability of the carbon metabolism pathways is key for the adaptation of this bacterium to the intracellular niche in the macrophage, and it has been associated with its pathogenicity (170).

M. tuberculosis obtains fatty acids through the action of phospholipase C, an enzyme that hydrolyzes phospholipids, resulting in the release of fatty acids. The bacterium has four phospholipase C proteins encoded in four genes; three of them (*plcA*, *plcB*, and *plcC*) are in an operon, whereas *plcD* is located in a distant genomic region (165). Phospholipase C proteins are associated with the cell wall through a lipid anchor and have been associated with the controlled degradation of phospholipids from the phagosomal membrane to obtain fatty acids that are subsequently used as a carbon and energy source. Phospholipases C are required for virulence (171), and the polymorphisms of the enzymes have been associated with differential virulence in clinical isolates (172).

Although several proteins have been involved in the transport of fatty acids (173) and *M. tuberculosis* possesses homologs of Fad proteins (174), the mechanisms by which the bacterium transports fatty acids to the cytoplasm are not well established. In addition, *M. tuberculosis* has an ABC transporter encoded in the *mce4* operon that is dedicated to the transport of cholesterol and is essential for persistence in chronically infected animals and activated macrophages (123). Interestingly, there are genes involved in lipid metabolism located near the *mce4* operon that function in concert with the transporter (175).

Mycobacterium spp. have adapted to feed on lipids. Cholesterol is an abundant compound in the membrane of eukaryotes, and it is metabolized by *M. tuberculosis* through a specific pathway that was identified by studying the catabolism of cholesterol in species of the related actinomycete *Rhodococcus* (176). All the genes need for the catabolism of cholesterol in *Rhodococcus* spp. were found in an 82-gene cluster in *M. tuberculosis* and *Mycobacterium bovis* (176). Despite the presence of these pathways, *M. tuberculosis* does not require cholesterol for infection in mice or to grow in resting macrophages; rather, it is essential for persistence in chronically infected animals and activated macrophages (169). In addition, *M. tuberculosis* can grow even if cholesterol is the only source of carbon and energy available (123).

Using cholesterol comes with a price for *M. tuberculosis* since the degradation of the cholesterol rings and acyl side chain by β-oxidation generates propionyl-CoA (177), a toxic compound that needs to be metabolized. However, *M. tuberculosis* has developed different strategies to metabolize propionyl-CoA that allow the bacterium not only to eliminate the toxic metabolite but also to use it as an energy source or as a building block for cell wall synthesis. To obtain energy from propionyl-CoA, *M. tuberculosis* can incorporate the metabolite into the methyl citrate cycle that converts propionyl-CoA into pyruvate and succinate, and these are subsequently used in the tricarboxylic acid cycle to produce energy (178). This is possibly due to the methyl-isocitrate lyase enzymatic activity that isocitrate lyase enzymes have in *M. tuberculosis*. Also, to obtain energy, propionyl-CoA can be transformed into methylmalonyl-CoA, through the action of the propionyl-CoA carboxylase, and be incorporated into the vitamin B_{12}–dependent methylmalonyl pathway that results in the production of succinyl-CoA that is used also in the tricarboxylic acid cycle (179). Lastly, *M. tuberculosis* can use a third pathway to metabolize propionyl-CoA and utilize it as a building block for the cell wall (180). The bacterium achieves this through the action of a polyketide synthase that converts propionyl-CoA into methylmalonyl-CoA.

M. tuberculosis metabolizes fatty acids through two pathways: the β-oxidation cycle and the glyoxylate shunt. In the β-oxidation cycle, the fatty acids are broken down to produce acetyl-CoA. Although the β-oxidation cycle only requires five enzymes, *M. tuberculosis* has approximately 100 genes whose products are involved in the cycle and appear to have redundant enzymes for each reaction (181). This redundancy has been associated with the ability of the bacterium to adapt to different environments during infection by switching its metabolism. The glyoxylate shunt is an anabolic pathway essential for carbon synthesis; it converts acetyl-CoA to succinate for the synthesis of carbohydrates, and it is widespread among prokaryotes.

To better understand the pathogenesis of *M. tuberculosis*, scientists have studied these pathways (Fig. 3). The principal pathway for carbon synthesis is the glyoxylate shunt. However, since the β-oxidation pathway has an enzyme redundancy, the study of

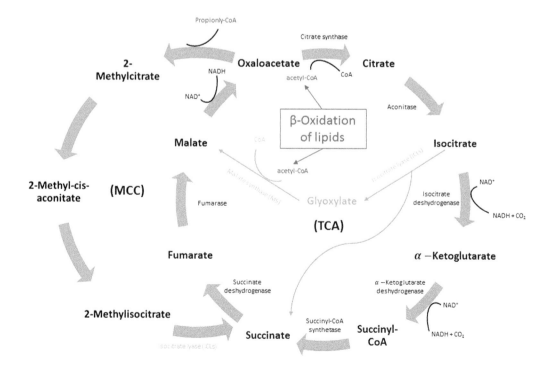

FIGURE 3 Schematic representation of the tricarboxylic acid and methyl citrate cycles. In green, the glyoxylate shunt, a variation of the tricarboxylic acid cycle.

this pathway has proven to be cumbersome. Initial protein and genetic studies of *Mycobacterium* spp. showed that the glyoxylate shunt enzymes, isocitrate lyases (ICLs), were upregulated during infection in macrophages (182, 183). *M. tuberculosis* has two isocitrate lyase homologous genes, *icl1* and *icl2*, but only one, *icl1*, complements a *Mycobacterium smegmatis icl* mutant for growth on C_2 carbon sources (183) and therefore was the first to be characterized. The construction of an *M. tuberculosis* mutant that lacked *icl1* showed that the mutation affects the survival of the bacterium in activated macrophages, while in mice, the *icl1* mutation had a negative effect in the persistence of *M. tuberculosis*, but it did not affect growth during the acute phase of the infection (168).

More recently, the role of *icl2* in infection and growth was addressed using a genetic approach to generate single and double *icl* mutants, proving that ICL2 in conjunction with ICL1 is also important for growth and virulence. Mutations of both *icl* genes resulted in a severe survival defect in resting macrophages and complete clearance from activated macrophages. Also, double *icl* mutants were rapidly eliminated from the lungs of infected mice. Together, these results indicated that ICL1 and ICL2 are jointly required for both *in vivo* and *in vitro* growth and virulence and that the glyoxylate cycle is essential for *M. tuberculosis* (184). However, the isocitrate lyase activity is not the only enzymatic activity that ICLs have involving fatty acid and cholesterol metabolism. ICLs also have a methylisocitrate lyase enzymatic activity, which is involved in the clearance of the propionyl-CoA, a product of the beta-oxidation of odd-chain fatty acids that is toxic for *M. tuberculosis* (185). The biochemical mechanisms responsible for the dramatic phenotype observed in the *icl* mutants were unclear since ICLs were associated with both the ability to incorporate carbon from fatty acids through their ICL activity and the detoxification of propionyl-CoA metabolites

through their MCL activity. A recent study shed some light using chemogenetic and metabolomics approaches and concluded that the methylcitrate cycle was responsible for the requirement of ICLs for the survival of *M. tuberculosis* (186). In addition, this study established a connection between propionate metabolism and membrane bioenergetics (186). ICLs have been associated with other functions that are not directly related to fatty acid metabolism, including antibiotic tolerance (187) and hypoxia (188), but that will not be reviewed here.

Malate synthase (MS) is the second enzyme of the glyoxylate cycle and mediates the production of malate through the condensation of glyoxylate with an acetyl group. MS requires magnesium to function (189); indeed, a Mg^{2+}-centered reaction mechanism in which glyoxylate binds first to enzymes has been proposed in *M. tuberculosis* (190). In addition to its role in the glyoxylate cycle, MS may participate in the pathogenesis of *M. tuberculosis* since it has adapted to bind laminin and fibronectin (191). Moreover, MS in *M. tuberculosis* is secreted by an undefined mechanism and enhances the adherence of the bacterium to lung epithelial cells *in vitro* (191). Lastly, there is increasing interest in these enzymes due to the important roles that they have in the survival of *M. tuberculosis* during infection. Pharmacological inhibitors targeting both MS and ICLs to inhibit the ability of the bacterium to use host lipids and persist would be a fruitful avenue for therapy of tuberculosis (192–195).

During infection, *M. tuberculosis* as well as other organisms such as *C. burnetii* can alter the host lipid metabolism to create an environment that allows these intracellular pathogens to survive. Such alterations are examples of the manner whereby these pathogens hijack the metabolism of the host. For example, after the adaptive immune system develops, *M. tuberculosis* can survive and persist for decades in a dormant stage within a characteristic, and pathological, structure of mononuclear cells known as a granulomas. In approximately 10% of the cases, the infection will reactivate. Granulomas are basically a collection of immune cells, including different types of macrophages such as multinucleated giant cells, epithelioid cells, and foamy cells, surrounded by a rim of lymphocytes. One of the characteristics of the granuloma is the presence of the foamy cells. These are macrophages enriched with lipid droplets (196, 197). The foamy macrophages are a secure reservoir for the bacterium and facilitate the persistence of *M. tuberculosis* in the host (196). *M. tuberculosis* inside the foamy macrophages imports fatty acids derived from host triacylglycerol and uses it as a carbon and energy source during latency (198). The mechanism by which *M. tuberculosis* manipulates the host cell metabolism is not completely understood. Nonetheless, several microbial compounds have been reported to induce differentiation of foamy macrophages.

During the infectious process, *M. tuberculosis* cross-talks with macrophages, reshaping host cell transcription (199) and reprogramming its lipid metabolism (200, 201). A recent study showed that the bacterium diverts the glycolytic pathway cell toward ketone body synthesis in the foamy cells. This dysregulation enables feedback activation of the anti-lipolytic G protein–coupled receptor GPR109A, leading to perturbations in lipid homeostasis and consequent accumulation of lipid bodies in the macrophage (202). Other mycobacterial molecules have been shown to be involved in the accumulation of lipid in foamy cells, including lipoarabinomannan, mycolic acids and ESAT-6, a secreted virulence factor (203).

Recently, a new experimental model for foamy cells using *M. avium* and bone marrow–derived mouse macrophages was proposed. In this model, the infected macrophages are exposed to very-low-density lipoprotein as a lipid source. The results showed that macrophages acquired a foamy appearance and suggest that triacylglycerol is essential for the formation of intracytoplasmic lipid inclu-

sions. In addition, the lipid transfer occurs by *Mycobacterium*-induced fusion of lipid bodies and phagosomes. Moreover, this process is reversible since upon removal of very-low-density lipoprotein, both lipid bodies and intracytoplasmic lipid inclusions decrease and *M. avium* starts to divide at the same levels as those found in the control macrophages (204).

C. burnetii is also a good example of host metabolic reprograming. Cholesterol is an essential component of the parasitophorous vacuole. Also, *Coxiella* relies on host cholesterol for replication, and inhibition of the cholesterol uptake or biosynthesis results in the partial inhibition of the bacterium replication and alteration of the vacuolar morphology. *Coxiella*-infected cells have 75% more cholesterol, and this is coincident with the upregulation of host cell genes involved in cholesterol biosynthesis and exogenous cholesterol uptake (104), suggesting that a cholesterol increase in the infected cell is required for optimal bacterial replication.

DISSEMINATION

Bacterial pathogens not only recruit and use host lipids during infection, but also target them through pore-forming proteins and phospholipase enzymes that destabilize the vacuole and host cell membranes. These processes allow the intracellular pathogens to escape the phagosome and ultimately to escape the host cell and disseminate, which are essential processes for bacterial survival and proliferation. We will not review the extensive work on pore-forming proteins and phospholipases in this chapter because it would be off-topic, but we will summarize some findings that we feel are relevant.

Gram-positive bacteria including *Streptococcus pneumoniae*, *Streptococcus pyogenes*, *L. monocytogenes*, and many *Clostridium* species produce cholesterol-dependent cytolysins. The cholesterol-dependent cytolysins are a family of β-barrel toxins that require the presence of cholesterol for pore formation; members of this family include listeriolysin, streptolysin, pneumolysin, and perfringolysin. Listeriolysin O mediates the rupture of the phagosomal membrane, allowing *L. monocytogenes* to reach the cytosol, its niche, where its activity is tightly regulated to ensure the stability of the cell membrane (205). Similarly, perfringolysin O allows *Clostridium perfringens* to escape the phagosome and persist in host tissues (206). Streptolysin O serves two important functions in *S. pyogenes*: it mediates the formation of pores in the phagolysosomal membrane and translocate the toxin NAD-glycohydrolase to the cytosol (207). Lastly, pneumolysin, produced by *S. pneumonia*, has several functions including cytosolic lysis (208), colonization (209), and survival, by interfering with the host immune response (210).

Bacterial phospholipases are enzymes that break down phospholipids, affecting the integrity of the membrane. Several bacteria species have enzymes with phospholipase activity. For example, *C. perfringens* has a phospholipase C that is involved in phagosomal escape. Phospholipases have also been associated with increased virulence; acquisition of bacteriophage encoding a phospholipase, SlaA, by a group A *Streptococcus* was shown to be associated with a dramatic increase of the virulence (211). However, phospholipases can also affect the survival of the bacteria. This is the case for *Legionella pneumophila* phospholipase PlaA, whose activity ultimately kills the host cell and degrades the bacteria in the absence of SdhA (212). Phospholipase activity is not an exclusive trait of intracellular pathogens; some extracellular pathogens also have it. For example, *P. aeruginosa* produces a phospholipase enzyme, ExoU, that enhance virulence and dissemination (213). Importantly, a recent study showed that phospholipases are not only host-virulent factors, since they can serve as specific antibacterial effectors by degrading phosphatidylethanolamine (214).

ACKNOWLEDGMENTS

This work was supported in part by NIH grants AI-027044 and U54-AI-057158.

CITATION

Toledo A, Benach JL. 2015. Hijacking and use of host lipids by intracellular pathogens. Microbiol Spectrum 3(6):VMBF-0001-2014.

REFERENCES

1. **Mercer J, Schelhaas M, Helenius A.** 2010. Virus entry by endocytosis. *Annu Rev Biochem* **79:**803–833.
2. **Cossart P, Helenius A.** 2014. Endocytosis of viruses and bacteria. *Cold Spring Harb Perspect Biol* **6:** pii: a016972.
3. **Tweten RK, Parker MW, Johnson AE.** 2001. The cholesterol-dependent cytolysins. *Curr Top Microbiol Immunol* **257:**15–33.
4. **Rosenberger CM, Brumell JH, Finlay BB.** 2000. Microbial pathogenesis: lipid rafts as pathogen portals. *Curr Biol* **10:**R823–R825.
5. **Duncan MJ, Shin JS, Abraham SN.** 2002. Microbial entry through caveolae: variations on a theme. *Cell Microbiol* **4:**783–791.
6. **Manes S, del Real G, Martinez AC.** 2003. Pathogens: raft hijackers. *Nat Rev Immunol* **3:** 557–568.
7. **Lafont F, van der Goot FG.** 2005. Bacterial invasion via lipid rafts. *Cell Microbiol* **7:**613–620.
8. **Abraham SN, Duncan MJ, Li G, Zaas D.** 2005. Bacterial penetration of the mucosal barrier by targeting lipid rafts. *J Invest Med* **53:**318–321.
9. **van der Meer-Janssen YP, van Galen J, Batenburg JJ, Helms JB.** 2010. Lipids in host-pathogen interactions: pathogens exploit the complexity of the host cell lipidome. *Progr Lipid Res* **49:**1–26.
10. **Sabareesh V, Singh G.** 2013. Mass spectrometry based lipid(ome) analyzer and molecular platform: a new software to interpret and analyze electrospray and/or matrix-assisted laser desorption/ionization mass spectrometric data of lipids: a case study from *Mycobacterium tuberculosis*. *J Mass Spectrom* **48:**465–477.
11. **Layre E, Moody DB.** 2013. Lipidomic profiling of model organisms and the world's major pathogens. *Biochimie* **95:**109–115.
12. **Benamara H, Rihouey C, Abbes I, Ben Mlouka MA, Hardouin J, Jouenne T, Alexandre S.**

2014. Characterization of membrane lipidome changes in *Pseudomonas aeruginosa* during biofilm growth on glass wool. *PloS One* **9**: e108478. doi:10.1371/journal.pone.0108478.

13. **Simons K, Ikonen E.** 1997. Functional rafts in cell membranes. *Nature* **387**:569–572.

14. **Brown DA, London E.** 1998. Structure and origin of ordered lipid domains in biological membranes. *J Membr Biol* **164**:103–114.

15. **Brown RE.** 1998. Sphingolipid organization in biomembranes: what physical studies of model membranes reveal. *J Cell Sci* **111**(Pt 1):1–9.

16. **Brown DA, London E.** 1998. Functions of lipid rafts in biological membranes. *Annu Rev Cell Dev Biol* **14**:111–136.

17. **Simons K, Toomre D.** 2000. Lipid rafts and signal transduction. *Nat Rev Mol Cell Biol* **1**:31–39.

18. **Brown DA, Rose JK.** 1992. Sorting of GPI-anchored proteins to glycolipid-enriched membrane subdomains during transport to the apical cell surface. *Cell* **68**:533–544.

19. **Epand RM.** 2008. Proteins and cholesterol-rich domains. *Biochim Biophys Acta* **1778**:1576–1582.

20. **Huttner WB, Zimmerberg J.** 2001. Implications of lipid microdomains for membrane curvature, budding and fission. *Curr Opin Cell Biol* **13**:478–484.

21. **Nichols B.** 2003. Caveosomes and endocytosis of lipid rafts. *J Cell Sci* **116**:4707–4714.

22. **Salaun C, James DJ, Chamberlain LH.** 2004. Lipid rafts and the regulation of exocytosis. *Traffic* **5**:255–264.

23. **Zaas DW, Duncan M, Rae Wright J, Abraham SN.** 2005. The role of lipid rafts in the pathogenesis of bacterial infections. *Biochim Biophys Acta* **1746**:305–313.

24. **Riethmuller J, Riehle A, Grassme H, Gulbins E.** 2006. Membrane rafts in host-pathogen interactions. *Biochim Biophys Acta* **1758**:2139–2147.

25. **Spiteri G.** 2013. *Sexually Transmitted Infections in Europe 2011.* European Center for Disease Prevention and Control, Stockholm. http://ecdc.europa.eu/en/publications/_layouts/forms/Publication_DispForm.aspx?List=4f55ad51-4aed-4d32-b960-af70113dbb90&ID=898.

26. **Centers for Disease Control and Prevention.** 2011. *Sexually Transmitted Disease Surveillance 2010.* CDC, Atlanta, GA. http://www.cdc.gov/std/stats10/.

27. **Workowski KA, Berman S, Centers for Disease Control and Prevention.** 2010. Sexually transmitted diseases treatment guidelines, 2010. *MMWR Recomm Rep* **59**:1–110.

28. **Taylor-Robinson D.** 1998. Chlamydia trachomatis as a probable cause of prostatitis. *Int J STD AIDS* **9**:779.

29. **Ostaszewska I, Zdrodowska-Stefanow B, Badyda J, Pucilo K, Trybula J, Bulhak V.** 1998. Chlamydia trachomatis: probable cause of prostatitis. *Int J STD AIDS* **9**:350–353.

30. **Marrazzo JM.** 2005. Mucopurulent cervicitis: no longer ignored, but still misunderstood. *Infect Dis Clin North Am* **19**:333–349, viii.

31. **Sweet RL.** 2012. Pelvic inflammatory disease: current concepts of diagnosis and management. *Curr Infect Dis Rep.* [Epub ahead of print.]

32. **Rours GI, Duijts L, Moll HA, Arends LR, de Groot R, Jaddoe VW, Hofman A, Steegers EA, Mackenbach JP, Ott A, Willemse HF, van der Zwaan EA, Verkooijen RP, Verbrugh HA.** 2011. *Chlamydia trachomatis* infection during pregnancy associated with preterm delivery: a population-based prospective cohort study. *Eur J Epidemiol* **26**:493–502.

33. **Munoz B, West S.** 1997. Trachoma: the forgotten cause of blindness. *Epidemiol Rev* **19**:205–217.

34. **Baneke A.** 2012. Review: targeting trachoma: strategies to reduce the leading infectious cause of blindness. *Travel Med Infect Dis* **10**:92–96.

35. **Cohen MS, Hoffman IF, Royce RA, Kazembe P, Dyer JR, Daly CC, Zimba D, Vernazza PL, Maida M, Fiscus SA, Eron JJ Jr.** 1997. Reduction of concentration of HIV-1 in semen after treatment of urethritis: implications for prevention of sexual transmission of HIV-1. AIDSCAP Malawi Research Group. *Lancet* **349**:1868–1873.

36. **Kuo CC, Jackson LA, Campbell LA, Grayston JT.** 1995. *Chlamydia pneumoniae* (TWAR). *Clin Microbiol Rev* **8**:451–461.

37. **Grayston JT, Kuo CC, Coulson AS, Campbell LA, Lawrence RD, Lee MJ, Strandness ED, Wang SP.** 1995. *Chlamydia pneumoniae* (TWAR) in atherosclerosis of the carotid artery. *Circulation* **92**:3397–3400.

38. **Laurila AL, Von Hertzen L, Saikku P.** 1997. *Chlamydia pneumoniae* and chronic lung diseases. *Scand J Infect Dis Suppl* **104**:34–36.

39. **Chen J, Zhu M, Ma G, Zhao Z, Sun Z.** 2013. *Chlamydia pneumoniae* infection and cerebrovascular disease: a systematic review and meta-analysis. *BMC Neurol* **13**:183.

40. **Moulder JW.** 1991. Interaction of chlamydiae and host cells *in vitro. Microbiol Rev* **55**:143–190.

41. **Clifton DR, Fields KA, Grieshaber SS, Dooley CA, Fischer ER, Mead DJ, Carabeo RA, Hackstadt T.** 2004. A chlamydial type III translocated protein is tyrosine-phosphorylated at the site of entry and associated with recruitment of actin. *Proc Natl Acad Sci USA* **101**:10166–10171.

42. **Subtil A, Wyplosz B, Balana ME, Dautry-Varsat A.** 2004. Analysis of *Chlamydia caviae* entry sites and involvement of Cdc42 and Rac activity. *J Cell Sci* **117:**3923–3933.

43. **Carabeo RA, Grieshaber SS, Hasenkrug A, Dooley C, Hackstadt T.** 2004. Requirement for the Rac GTPase in *Chlamydia trachomatis* invasion of non-phagocytic cells. *Traffic* **5:**418–425.

44. **Balana ME, Niedergang F, Subtil A, Alcover A, Chavrier P, Dautry-Varsat A.** 2005. ARF6 GTPase controls bacterial invasion by actin remodelling. *J Cell Sci* **118:**2201–2210.

45. **Korhonen JT, Puolakkainen M, Haveri A, Tammiruusu A, Sarvas M, Lahesmaa R.** 2012. *Chlamydia pneumoniae* entry into epithelial cells by clathrin-independent endocytosis. *Microb Pathog* **52:**157–164.

46. **Jutras I, Abrami L, Dautry-Varsat A.** 2003. Entry of the lymphogranuloma venereum strain of *Chlamydia trachomatis* into host cells involves cholesterol-rich membrane domains. *Infect Immun* **71:**260–266.

47. **Gabel BR, Elwell C, van Ijzendoorn SC, Engel JN.** 2004. Lipid raft-mediated entry is not required for *Chlamydia trachomatis* infection of cultured epithelial cells. *Infect Immun* **72:**7367–7373.

48. **Norkin LC, Wolfrom SA, Stuart ES.** 2001. Association of caveolin with *Chlamydia trachomatis* inclusions at early and late stages of infection. *Exp Cell Res* **266:**229–238.

49. **Stuart ES, Webley WC, Norkin LC.** 2003. Lipid rafts, caveolae, caveolin-1, and entry by *Chlamydiae* into host cells. *Exp Cell Res* **287:**67–78.

50. **Webley WC, Norkin LC, Stuart ES.** 2004. Caveolin-2 associates with intracellular chlamydial inclusions independently of caveolin-1. *BMC Infect Dis* **4:**23.

51. **Gruenheid S, Finlay BB.** 2003. Microbial pathogenesis and cytoskeletal function. *Nature* **422:**775–781.

52. **Fessler MB, Arndt PG, Frasch SC, Lieber JG, Johnson CA, Murphy RC, Nick JA, Bratton DL, Malcolm KC, Worthen GS.** 2004. Lipid rafts regulate lipopolysaccharide-induced activation of Cdc42 and inflammatory functions of the human neutrophil. *J Biol Chem* **279:**39989–39998.

53. **Brumell JH, Grinstein S.** 2003. Role of lipid-mediated signal transduction in bacterial internalization. *Cell Microbiol* **5:**287–297.

54. **Naroeni A, Porte F.** 2002. Role of cholesterol and the ganglioside GM(1) in entry and short-term survival of *Brucella suis* in murine macrophages. *Infect Immun* **70:**1640–1644.

55. **Watarai M, Makino S, Michikawa M, Yanagisawa K, Murakami S, Shirahata T.** 2002. Macrophage plasma membrane cholesterol contributes to *Brucella abortus* infection of mice. *Infect Immun* **70:**4818–4825.

56. **Kim S, Watarai M, Suzuki H, Makino S, Kodama T, Shirahata T.** 2004. Lipid raft microdomains mediate class A scavenger receptor-dependent infection of *Brucella abortus*. *Microb Pathog* **37:**11–19.

57. **Martin-Martin AI, Vizcaino N, Fernandez-Lago L.** 2010. Cholesterol, ganglioside GM1 and class A scavenger receptor contribute to infection by *Brucella ovis* and *Brucella canis* in murine macrophages. *Microbes Infect* **12:**246–251.

58. **French CT, Panina EM, Yeh SH, Griffith N, Arambula DG, Miller JF.** 2009. The *Bordetella* type III secretion system effector BteA contains a conserved N-terminal motif that guides bacterial virulence factors to lipid rafts. *Cell Microbiol* **11:**1735–1749.

59. **Tamilselvam B, Daefler S.** 2008. *Francisella* targets cholesterol-rich host cell membrane domains for entry into macrophages. *J Immunol* **180:**8262–8271.

60. **Lafont F, Tran Van Nhieu G, Hanada K, Sansonetti P, van der Goot FG.** 2002. Initial steps of *Shigella* infection depend on the cholesterol/sphingolipid raft-mediated CD44-IpaB interaction. *EMBO J* **21:**4449–4457.

61. **Gilk SD, Cockrell DC, Luterbach C, Hansen B, Knodler LA, Ibarra JA, Steele-Mortimer O, Heinzen RA.** 2013. Bacterial colonization of host cells in the absence of cholesterol. *PLoS Pathog* **9:**e1003107. doi:10.1371/journal.ppat.1003107.

62. **Schraw W, Li Y, McClain MS, van der Goot FG, Cover TL.** 2002. Association of *Helicobacter pylori* vacuolating toxin (VacA) with lipid rafts. *J Biol Chem* **277:**34642–34650.

63. **Lai CH, Chang YC, Du SY, Wang HJ, Kuo CH, Fang SH, Fu HW, Lin HH, Chiang AS, Wang WC.** 2008. Cholesterol depletion reduces *Helicobacter pylori* CagA translocation and CagA-induced responses in AGS cells. *Infect Immun* **76:**3293–3303.

64. **Hutton ML, Kaparakis-Liaskos M, Turner L, Cardona A, Kwok T, Ferrero RL.** 2010. *Helicobacter pylori* exploits cholesterol-rich microdomains for induction of NF-kappaB-dependent responses and peptidoglycan delivery in epithelial cells. *Infect Immun* **78:**4523–4531.

65. **Grassme H, Jendrossek V, Riehle A, von Kurthy G, Berger J, Schwarz H, Weller M, Kolesnick R, Gulbins E.** 2003. Host defense against *Pseudomonas aeruginosa* requires ceramide-rich membrane rafts. *Nat Med* **9:**322–330.

66. **Yamamoto N, Yamamoto N, Petroll MW, Cavanagh HD, Jester JV.** 2005. Internalization of *Pseudomonas aeruginosa* is mediated by lipid rafts in contact lens-wearing rabbit and cultured human corneal epithelial cells. *Invest Ophthalmol Vis Sci* **46:**1348–1355.

67. **Zaidi T, Bajmoczi M, Zaidi T, Golan DE, Pier GB.** 2008. Disruption of CFTR-dependent lipid rafts reduces bacterial levels and corneal disease in a murine model of *Pseudomonas aeruginosa* keratitis. *Invest Ophthalmol Vis Sci* **49:**1000–1009.

68. **Kannan S, Audet A, Huang H, Chen LJ, Wu M.** 2008. Cholesterol-rich membrane rafts and Lyn are involved in phagocytosis during *Pseudomonas aeruginosa* infection. *J Immunol* **180:** 2396–2408.

69. **Bomberger JM, Maceachran DP, Coutermarsh BA, Ye S, O'Toole GA, Stanton BA.** 2009. Long-distance delivery of bacterial virulence factors by *Pseudomonas aeruginosa* outer membrane vesicles. *PLoS Pathog* **5:**e1000382. doi:10.1371/journal.ppat.1000382.

70. **Wylie JL, Hatch GM, McClarty G.** 1997. Host cell phospholipids are trafficked to and then modified by *Chlamydia trachomatis*. *J Bacteriol* **179:**7233–7242.

71. **Hatch GM, McClarty G.** 1998. Phospholipid composition of purified *Chlamydia trachomatis* mimics that of the eucaryotic host cell. *Infect Immun* **66:**3727–3735.

72. **Carabeo RA, Mead DJ, Hackstadt T.** 2003. Golgi-dependent transport of cholesterol to the *Chlamydia trachomatis* inclusion. *Proc Natl Acad Sci USA* **100:**6771–6776.

73. **Stephens RS, Kalman S, Lammel C, Fan J, Marathe R, Aravind L, Mitchell W, Olinger L, Tatusov RL, Zhao Q, Koonin EV, Davis RW.** 1998. Genome sequence of an obligate intracellular pathogen of humans: *Chlamydia trachomatis*. *Science* **282:**754–759.

74. **Robertson DK, Gu L, Rowe RK, Beatty WL.** 2009. Inclusion biogenesis and reactivation of persistent *Chlamydia trachomatis* requires host cell sphingolipid biosynthesis. *PLoS Pathog* **5:** e1000664. doi:10.1371/journal.ppat.1000664.

75. **van Ooij C, Kalman L, van I, Nishijima M, Hanada K, Mostov K, Engel JN.** 2000. Host cell-derived sphingolipids are required for the intracellular growth of *Chlamydia trachomatis*. *Cell Microbiol* **2:**627–637.

76. **Valdivia RH.** 2008. Chlamydia effector proteins and new insights into chlamydial cellular microbiology. *Curr Opin Microbiol* **11:**53–59.

77. **Li Z, Chen C, Chen D, Wu Y, Zhong Y, Zhong G.** 2008. Characterization of fifty putative inclusion membrane proteins encoded in the *Chlamydia trachomatis* genome. *Infect Immun* **76:**2746–2757.

78. **Bannantine JP, Griffiths RS, Viratyosin W, Brown WJ, Rockey DD.** 2000. A secondary structure motif predictive of protein localization to the chlamydial inclusion membrane. *Cell Microbiol* **2:**35–47.

79. **Hackstadt T, Scidmore MA, Rockey DD.** 1995. Lipid metabolism in *Chlamydia trachomatis*-infected cells: directed trafficking of Golgi-derived sphingolipids to the chlamydial inclusion. *Proc Natl Acad Sci USA* **92:**4877–4881.

80. **Hackstadt T, Rockey DD, Heinzen RA, Scidmore MA.** 1996. *Chlamydia trachomatis* interrupts an exocytic pathway to acquire endogenously synthesized sphingomyelin in transit from the Golgi apparatus to the plasma membrane. *EMBO J* **15:**964–977.

81. **Beatty WL.** 2008. Late endocytic multivesicular bodies intersect the chlamydial inclusion in the absence of CD63. *Infect Immun* **76:** 2872–2881.

82. **Elwell CA, Jiang S, Kim JH, Lee A, Wittmann T, Hanada K, Melancon P, Engel JN.** 2011. *Chlamydia trachomatis* co-opts GBF1 and CERT to acquire host sphingomyelin for distinct roles during intracellular development. *PLoS Pathog* **7:**e1002198. doi:10.1371/journal.ppat.1002198.

83. **Rockey DD, Fischer ER, Hackstadt T.** 1996. Temporal analysis of the developing *Chlamydia psittaci* inclusion by use of fluorescence and electron microscopy. *Infect Immun* **64:**4269–4278.

84. **Wolf K, Hackstadt T.** 2001. Sphingomyelin trafficking in *Chlamydia pneumoniae*-infected cells. *Cell Microbiol* **3:**145–152.

85. **Beatty WL.** 2006. Trafficking from CD63-positive late endocytic multivesicular bodies is essential for intracellular development of *Chlamydia trachomatis*. *J Cell Sci* **119:**350–359.

86. **Moore ER, Fischer ER, Mead DJ, Hackstadt T.** 2008. The chlamydial inclusion preferentially intercepts basolaterally directed sphingomyelin-containing exocytic vacuoles. *Traffic* **9:**2130–2140.

87. **Derre I, Swiss R, Agaisse H.** 2011. The lipid transfer protein CERT interacts with the *Chlamydia* inclusion protein IncD and participates to ER-*Chlamydia* inclusion membrane contact sites. *PLoS Pathog* **7:**e1002092. doi:10.1371/journal. ppat.1002092.

88. **Agaisse H, Derre I.** 2014. Expression of the effector protein IncD in *Chlamydia trachomatis* mediates recruitment of the lipid transfer protein CERT and the endoplasmic reticulum-resident protein VAPB to the inclusion membrane. *Infect Immun* **82:**2037–2047.

89. Christian JG, Heymann J, Paschen SA, Vier J, Schauenburg L, Rupp J, Meyer TF, Hacker G, Heuer D. 2011. Targeting of a chlamydial protease impedes intracellular bacterial growth. *PLoS Pathog* **7:**e1002283. doi:10.1371/journal.ppat.1002283.

90. Heuer D, Rejman Lipinski A, Machuy N, Karlas A, Wehrens A, Siedler F, Brinkmann V, Meyer TF. 2009. *Chlamydia* causes fragmentation of the Golgi compartment to ensure reproduction. *Nature* **457:**731–735.

91. Rejman Lipinski A, Heymann J, Meissner C, Karlas A, Brinkmann V, Meyer TF, Heuer D. 2009. Rab6 and Rab11 regulate *Chlamydia trachomatis* development and golgin-84-dependent Golgi fragmentation. *PLoS Pathog* **5:**e1000615. doi:10.1371/journal.ppat.1000615.

92. Moorhead AM, Jung JY, Smirnov A, Kaufer S, Scidmore MA. 2010. Multiple host proteins that function in phosphatidylinositol-4-phosphate metabolism are recruited to the chlamydial inclusion. *Infect Immun* **78:**1990–2007.

93. Mital J, Hackstadt T. 2011. Role for the SRC family kinase Fyn in sphingolipid acquisition by chlamydiae. *Infect Immun* **79:**4559–4568.

94. Rzomp KA, Scholtes LD, Briggs BJ, Whittaker GR, Scidmore MA. 2003. Rab GTPases are recruited to chlamydial inclusions in both a species-dependent and species-independent manner. *Infect Immun* **71:**5855–5870.

95. Cortes C, Rzomp KA, Tvinnereim A, Scidmore MA, Wizel B. 2007. *Chlamydia pneumoniae* inclusion membrane protein Cpn0585 interacts with multiple Rab GTPases. *Infect Immun* **75:**5586–5596.

96. Capmany A, Damiani MT. 2010. *Chlamydia trachomatis* intercepts Golgi-derived sphingolipids through a Rab14-mediated transport required for bacterial development and replication. *PloS One* **5:**e14084. doi:10.1371/journal.pone.0014084.

97. Moore ER, Mead DJ, Dooley CA, Sager J, Hackstadt T. 2011. The trans-Golgi SNARE syntaxin 6 is recruited to the chlamydial inclusion membrane. *Microbiology* **157:**830–838.

98. Kumar Y, Cocchiaro J, Valdivia RH. 2006. The obligate intracellular pathogen *Chlamydia trachomatis* targets host lipid droplets. *Curr Biol* **16:**1646–1651.

99. Cocchiaro JL, Kumar Y, Fischer ER, Hackstadt T, Valdivia RH. 2008. Cytoplasmic lipid droplets are translocated into the lumen of the *Chlamydia trachomatis* parasitophorous vacuole. *Proc Natl Acad Sci USA* **105:**9379–9384.

100. Lin M, Rikihisa Y. 2003. *Ehrlichia chaffeensis* and *Anaplasma phagocytophilum* lack genes for lipid A biosynthesis and incorporate cholesterol for their survival. *Infect Immun* **71:**5324–5331.

101. Xiong Q, Wang X, Rikihisa Y. 2007. High-cholesterol diet facilitates *Anaplasma phagocytophilum* infection and up-regulates macrophage inflammatory protein-2 and CXCR2 expression in apolipoprotein E-deficient mice. *J Infect Dis* **195:**1497–1503.

102. Lin M, Rikihisa Y. 2003. Obligatory intracellular parasitism by *Ehrlichia chaffeensis* and *Anaplasma phagocytophilum* involves caveolae and glycosylphosphatidylinositol-anchored proteins. *Cell Microbiol* **5:**809–820.

103. Xiong QM, Lin MQ, Rikihisa Y. 2009. Cholesterol-dependent *Anaplasma phagocytophilum* exploits the low-density lipoprotein uptake pathway. *PLoS Pathog* **5:**e1000329. doi:10.1371/journal.ppat.1000329.

104. Howe D, Heinzen RA. 2006. *Coxiella burnetii* inhabits a cholesterol-rich vacuole and influences cellular cholesterol metabolism. *Cell Microbiol* **8:**496–507.

105. Howe D, Heinzen RA. 2005. Replication of *Coxiella burnetii* is inhibited in CHO K-1 cells treated with inhibitors of cholesterol metabolism. *Ann N Y Acad Sci* **1063:**123–129.

106. Gilk SD, Beare PA, Heinzen RA. 2010. *Coxiella burnetii* expresses a functional Delta24 sterol reductase. *J Bacteriol* **192:**6154–6159.

107. Gilk SD. 2012. Role of lipids in *Coxiella burnetii* infection. *Adv Exp Med Biol* **984:**199–213.

108. Rasmussen JW, Cello J, Gil H, Forestal CA, Furie MB, Thanassi DG, Benach JL. 2006. Mac-1+ cells are the predominant subset in the early hepatic lesions of mice infected with *Francisella tularensis*. *Infect Immun* **74:**6590–6598.

109. Law HT, Lin AE, Kim Y, Quach B, Nano FE, Guttman JA. 2011. *Francisella tularensis* uses cholesterol and clathrin-based endocytic mechanisms to invade hepatocytes. *Sci Rep* **1:**192.

110. Seveau S, Bierne H, Giroux S, Prevost MC, Cossart P. 2004. Role of lipid rafts in E-cadherin—and HGF-R/Met—mediated entry of *Listeria monocytogenes* into host cells. *J Cell Biol* **166:**743–753.

111. Gekara NO, Weiss S. 2004. Lipid rafts clustering and signalling by listeriolysin O. *Biochem Soc Trans* **32:**712–714.

112. Allen-Vercoe E, Waddell B, Livingstone S, Deans J, DeVinney R. 2006. Enteropathogenic *Escherichia coli* Tir translocation and pedestal formation requires membrane cholesterol in the absence of bundle-forming pili. *Cell Microbiol* **8:**613–624.

113. Duncan MJ, Li G, Shin JS, Carson JL, Abraham SN. 2004. Bacterial penetration of bladder epithelium through lipid rafts. *J Biol Chem* **279:**18944–18951.

114. **Riff JD, Callahan JW, Sherman PM.** 2005. Cholesterol-enriched membrane microdomains are required for inducing host cell cytoskeleton rearrangements in response to attaching-effacing *Escherichia coli. Infect Immun* **73:**7113–7125.

115. **Kansau I, Berger C, Hospital M, Amsellem R, Nicolas V, Servin AL, Bernet-Camard MF.** 2004. Zipper-like internalization of Dr-positive *Escherichia coli* by epithelial cells is preceded by an adhesin-induced mobilization of raft-associated molecules in the initial step of adhesion. *Infect Immun* **72:**3733–3742.

116. **Catron DM, Sylvester MD, Lange Y, Kadekoppala M, Jones BD, Monack DM, Falkow S, Haldar K.** 2002. The *Salmonella*-containing vacuole is a major site of intracellular cholesterol accumulation and recruits the GPI-anchored protein CD55. *Cell Microbiol* **4:**315–328.

117. **Rogers TJ, Thorpe CM, Paton AW, Paton JC.** 2012. Role of lipid rafts and flagellin in invasion of colonic epithelial cells by Shiga-toxigenic *Escherichia coli* O113:H21. *Infect Immun* **80:**2858–2867.

118. **Hayward RD, Cain RJ, McGhie EJ, Phillips N, Garner MJ, Koronakis V.** 2005. Cholesterol binding by the bacterial type III translocon is essential for virulence effector delivery into mammalian cells. *Mol Microbiol* **56:**590–603.

119. **van der Goot FG, Tran van Nhieu G, Allaoui A, Sansonetti P, Lafont F.** 2004. Rafts can trigger contact-mediated secretion of bacterial effectors via a lipid-based mechanism. *J Biol Chem* **279:**47792–47798.

120. **Gatfield J, Pieters J.** 2000. Essential role for cholesterol in entry of mycobacteria into macrophages. *Science* **288:**1647–1650.

121. **Perez-Guzman C, Vargas MH, Quinonez F, Bazavilvazo N, Aguilar A.** 2005. A cholesterol-rich diet accelerates bacteriologic sterilization in pulmonary tuberculosis. *Chest* **127:**643–651.

122. **Maldonado-Garcia G, Chico-Ortiz M, Lopez-Marin LM, Sanchez-Garcia FJ.** 2004. High-polarity *Mycobacterium avium*-derived lipids interact with murine macrophage lipid rafts. *Scand J Immunol* **60:**463–470.

123. **Pandey AK, Sassetti CM.** 2008. Mycobacterial persistence requires the utilization of host cholesterol. *Proc Natl Acad Sci USA* **105:**4376–4380.

124. **Edward DG, Fitzgerald WA.** 1951. Cholesterol in the growth of organisms of the pleuropneumonia group. *J Gen Microbiol* **5:**576–586.

125. **Argaman M, Razin S.** 1965. Cholesterol and cholesterol esters in *Mycoplasma. J Gen Microbiol* **38:**153–160.

126. **Smith PF, Mayberry WR.** 1968. Identification of the major glycolipid from *Mycoplasma* sp.,

127. **Smith PF.** 1971. Biosynthesis of cholesteryl glucoside by *Mycoplasma gallinarum. J Bacteriol* **108:**986–991.

128. **Slutzky GM, Razin S, Kahane I, Eisenberg S.** 1977. Cholesterol transfer from serum lipoproteins to *Mycoplasma* membranes. *Biochemistry* **16:**5158–5163.

129. **Rottem S, Verkleij AJ.** 1982. Possible association of segregated lipid domains of *Mycoplasma gallisepticum* membranes with cell resistance to osmotic lysis. *J Bacteriol* **149:**338–345.

130. **Razin S, Efrati H, Kutner S, Rottem S.** 1982. Cholesterol and phospholipid uptake by mycoplasmas. *Rev Infect Dis* **4**(Suppl):S85–S92.

131. **Inamine JM, Denny TP, Loechel S, Schaper U, Huang CH, Bott KF, Hu PC.** 1988. Nucleotide sequence of the P1 attachment-protein gene of *Mycoplasma pneumoniae. Gene* **64:**217–229.

132. **Dallo SF, Chavoya A, Baseman JB.** 1990. Characterization of the gene for a 30-kilodalton adhesion-related protein of *Mycoplasma pneumoniae. Infect Immun* **58:**4163–4165.

133. **Tarshis M, Salman M, Rottem S.** 1993. Cholesterol is required for the fusion of single unilamellar vesicles with *Mycoplasma capricolum. Biophys J* **64:**709–715.

134. **Deutsch J, Salman M, Rottem S.** 1995. An unusual polar lipid from the cell membrane of *Mycoplasma fermentans. Eur J Biochem* **227:**897–902.

135. **Dybvig K, Voelker LL.** 1996. Molecular biology of mycoplasmas. *Annu Rev Microbiol* **50:**25–57.

136. **Murray HW, Masur H, Senterfit LB, Roberts RB.** 1975. The protean manifestations of *Mycoplasma pneumoniae* infection in adults. *Am J Med* **58:**229–242.

137. **Baseman JB, Tully JG.** 1997. Mycoplasmas: sophisticated, reemerging, and burdened by their notoriety. *Emerg Infect Dis* **3:**21–32.

138. **LaRocca TJ, Pathak P, Chiantia S, Toledo A, Silvius JR, Benach JL, London E.** 2013. Proving lipid rafts exist: membrane domains in the prokaryote *Borrelia burgdorferi* have the same properties as eukaryotic lipid rafts. *PLoS Pathog* **9:**e1003353. doi:10.1371/journal.ppat.1003353.

139. **Belisle JT, Brandt ME, Radolf JD, Norgard MV.** 1994. Fatty acids of *Treponema pallidum* and *Borrelia burgdorferi* lipoproteins. *J Bacteriol* **176:**2151–2157.

140. **Jones JD, Bourell KW, Norgard MV, Radolf JD.** 1995. Membrane topology of *Borrelia burgdorferi* and *Treponema pallidum* lipoproteins. *Infect Immun* **63:**2424–2434.

strain J as 3,4,6-triacyl-beta-glucopyranose. *Biochemistry* **7:**2706–2710.

141. **Radolf JD, Goldberg MS, Bourell K, Baker SI, Jones JD, Norgard MV.** 1995. Characterization of outer membranes isolated from *Borrelia burgdorferi*, the Lyme disease spirochete. *Infect Immun* **63:**2154–2163.

142. **Stubs G, Fingerle V, Wilske B, Gobel UB, Zahringer U, Schumann RR, Schroder NW.** 2009. Acylated cholesteryl galactosides are specific antigens of borrelia causing Lyme disease and frequently induce antibodies in late stages of disease. *J Biol Chem* **284:**13326–13334.

143. **Stubs G, Fingerle V, Zahringer U, Schumann RR, Rademann J, Schroder NW.** 2011. Acylated cholesteryl galactosides are ubiquitous glycolipid antigens among *Borrelia burgdorferi* sensu lato. *FEMS Immunol Med Microbiol* **63:**140–143.

144. **Ben-Menachem G, Kubler-Kielb J, Coxon B, Yergey A, Schneerson R.** 2003. A newly discovered cholesteryl galactoside from *Borrelia burgdorferi*. *Proc Natl Acad Sci USA* **100:**7913–7918.

145. **Schroder NW, Schombel U, Heine H, Gobel UB, Zahringer U, Schumann RR.** 2003. Acylated cholesteryl galactoside as a novel immunogenic motif in *Borrelia burgdorferi* sensu stricto. *J Biol Chem* **278:**33645–33653.

146. **Garcia-Monco JC, Seidman RJ, Benach JL.** 1995. Experimental immunization with *Borrelia burgdorferi* induces development of antibodies to gangliosides. *Infect Immun* **63:**4130–4137.

147. **LaRocca TJ, Crowley JT, Cusack BJ, Pathak P, Benach J, London E, Garcia-Monco JC, Benach JL.** 2010. Cholesterol lipids of *Borrelia burgdorferi* form lipid rafts and are required for the bactericidal activity of a complement-independent antibody. *Cell Host Microbe* **8:**331–342.

148. **Coleman JL, Crowley JT, Toledo AM, Benach JL.** 2013. The HtrA protease of *Borrelia burgdorferi* degrades outer membrane protein BmpD and chemotaxis phosphatase CheX. *Mol Microbiol* **88:**619–633.

149. **Toledo A, Crowley JT, Coleman JL, LaRocca TJ, Chiantia S, London E, Benach JL.** 2014. Selective association of outer surface lipoproteins with the lipid rafts of *Borrelia burgdorferi*. *mBio* **5:**e00899-14. doi:10.1128/mBio.00899-14.

150. **Crowley JT, Toledo AM, LaRocca TJ, Coleman JL, London E, Benach JL.** 2013. Lipid exchange between *Borrelia burgdorferi* and host cells. *PLoS Pathog* **9:**e1003109. doi:10.1371/journal.ppat.1003109.

151. **Ostberg Y, Berg S, Comstedt P, Wieslander A, Bergstrom S.** 2007. Functional analysis of a lipid galactosyltransferase synthesizing the major envelope lipid in the Lyme disease spirochete *Borrelia burgdorferi*. *FEMS Microbiol Lett* **272:**22–29.

152. **Ansorg R, Muller KD, von Recklinghausen G, Nalik HP.** 1992. Cholesterol binding of *Helicobacter pylori*. *Zentralbl Bakteriol* **276:**323–329.

153. **Trampenau C, Muller KD.** 2003. Affinity of *Helicobacter pylori* to cholesterol and other steroids. *Microb Infect* **5:**13–17.

154. **Jimenez-Soto LF, Rohrer S, Jain U, Ertl C, Sewald X, Haas R.** 2012. Effects of cholesterol on *Helicobacter pylori* growth and virulence properties *in vitro*. *Helicobacter* **17:**133–139.

155. **Shimomura H, Hosoda K, Hayashi S, Yokota K, Hirai Y.** 2012. Phosphatidylethanolamine of *Helicobacter pylori* functions as a steroid-binding lipid in the assimilation of free cholesterol and 3beta-hydroxl steroids into the bacterial cell membrane. *J Bacteriol* **194:**2658–2667.

156. **Wunder C, Churin Y, Winau F, Warnecke D, Vieth M, Lindner B, Zahringer U, Mollenkopf HJ, Heinz E, Meyer TF.** 2006. Cholesterol glucosylation promotes immune evasion by *Helicobacter pylori*. *Nat Med* **12:**1030–1038.

157. **Lebrun AH, Wunder C, Hildebrand J, Churin Y, Zahringer U, Lindner B, Meyer TF, Heinz E, Warnecke D.** 2006. Cloning of a cholesterol-alpha-glucosyltransferase from *Helicobacter pylori*. *J Biol Chem* **281:**27765–27772.

158. **McGee DJ, George AE, Trainor EA, Horton KE, Hildebrandt E, Testerman TL.** 2011. Cholesterol enhances *Helicobacter pylori* resistance to antibiotics and LL-37. *Antimicrob Agents Chemother* **55:**2897–2904.

159. **Shimomura H, Hosoda K, McGee DJ, Hayashi S, Yokota K, Hirai Y.** 2013. Detoxification of 7-dehydrocholesterol fatal to *Helicobacter pylori* is a novel role of cholesterol glucosylation. *J Bacteriol* **195:**359–367.

160. **Hildebrandt E, McGee DJ.** 2009. *Helicobacter pylori* lipopolysaccharide modification, Lewis antigen expression, and gastric colonization are cholesterol-dependent. *BMC Microbiol* **9:**258.

161. **Odenbreit S, Puls J, Sedlmaier B, Gerland E, Fischer W, Haas R.** 2000. Translocation of *Helicobacter pylori* CagA into gastric epithelial cells by type IV secretion. *Science* **287:**1497–1500.

162. **Wang HJ, Cheng WC, Cheng HH, Lai CH, Wang WC.** 2012. *Helicobacter pylori* cholesteryl glucosides interfere with host membrane phase and affect type IV secretion system function during infection in AGS cells. *Mol Microbiol* **83:**67–84.

163. **Bloch H, Segal W.** 1956. Biochemical differentiation of *Mycobacterium tuberculosis* grown *in vivo* and *in vitro*. *J Bacteriol* **72:**132–141.

164. **Kolattukudy PE, Fernandes ND, Azad AK, Fitzmaurice AM, Sirakova TD.** 1997. Biochemistry and molecular genetics of cell-wall lipid biosynthesis in mycobacteria. *Mol Microbiol* **24:**263–270.

165. **Cole ST, Brosch R, Parkhill J, Garnier T, Churcher C, Harris D, Gordon SV, Eiglmeier K, Gas S, Barry CE 3rd, Tekaia F, Badcock K, Basham D, Brown D, Chillingworth T, Connor R, Davies R, Devlin K, Feltwell T, Gentles S, Hamlin N, Holroyd S, Hornsby T, Jagels K, Krogh A, McLean J, Moule S, Murphy L, Oliver K, Osborne J, Quail MA, Rajandream MA, Rogers J, Rutter S, Seeger K, Skelton J, Squares R, Squares S, Sulston JE, Taylor K, Whitehead S, Barrell BG.** 1998. Deciphering the biology of *Mycobacterium tuberculosis* from the complete genome sequence. *Nature* **393:**537–544.

166. **Liu K, Yu J, Russell DG.** 2003. pckA-deficient *Mycobacterium bovis* BCG shows attenuated virulence in mice and in macrophages. *Microbiology* **149:**1829–1835.

167. **Marrero J, Rhee KY, Schnappinger D, Pethe K, Ehrt S.** 2010. Gluconeogenic carbon flow of tricarboxylic acid cycle intermediates is critical for *Mycobacterium tuberculosis* to establish and maintain infection. *Proc Natl Acad Sci USA* **107:**9819–9824.

168. **McKinney JD, Honer zu Bentrup K, Munoz-Elias EJ, Miczak A, Chen B, Chan WT, Swenson D, Sacchettini JC, Jacobs WR Jr, Russell DG.** 2000. Persistence of *Mycobacterium tuberculosis* in macrophages and mice requires the glyoxylate shunt enzyme isocitrate lyase. *Nature* **406:**735–738.

169. **Sassetti CM, Rubin EJ.** 2003. Genetic requirements for mycobacterial survival during infection. *Proc Natl Acad Sci USA* **100:**12989–12994.

170. **de Carvalho LP, Fischer SM, Marrero J, Nathan C, Ehrt S, Rhee KY.** 2010. Metabolomics of *Mycobacterium tuberculosis* reveals compartmentalized co-catabolism of carbon substrates. *Chem Biol* **17:**1122–1131.

171. **Raynaud C, Guilhot C, Rauzier J, Bordat Y, Pelicic V, Manganelli R, Smith I, Gicquel B, Jackson M.** 2002. Phospholipases C are involved in the virulence of *Mycobacterium tuberculosis*. *Mol Microbiol* **45:**203–217.

172. **Viana-Niero C, de Haas PE, van Soolingen D, Leao SC.** 2004. Analysis of genetic polymorphisms affecting the four phospholipase C (plc) genes in *Mycobacterium tuberculosis* complex clinical isolates. *Microbiology* **150:**967–978.

173. **Trivedi OA, Arora P, Sridharan V, Tickoo R, Mohanty D, Gokhale RS.** 2004. Enzymic activation and transfer of fatty acids as acyl-adenylates in mycobacteria. *Nature* **428:**441–445.

174. **Jackson M, Stadthagen G, Gicquel B.** 2007. Long-chain multiple methyl-branched fatty acid-containing lipids of *Mycobacterium tuberculosis*: biosynthesis, transport, regulation and biological activities. *Tuberculosis* **87:**78–86.

175. **Joshi SM, Pandey AK, Capite N, Fortune SM, Rubin EJ, Sassetti CM.** 2006. Characterization of mycobacterial virulence genes through genetic interaction mapping. *Proc Natl Acad Sci USA* **103:**11760–11765.

176. **Van der Geize R, Yam K, Heuser T, Wilbrink MH, Hara H, Anderton MC, Sim E, Dijkhuizen L, Davies JE, Mohn WW, Eltis LD.** 2007. A gene cluster encoding cholesterol catabolism in a soil actinomycete provides insight into *Mycobacterium tuberculosis* survival in macrophages. *Proc Natl Acad Sci USA* **104:**1947–1952.

177. **Yang X, Nesbitt NM, Dubnau E, Smith I, Sampson NS.** 2009. Cholesterol metabolism increases the metabolic pool of propionate in *Mycobacterium tuberculosis*. *Biochemistry* **48:**3819–3821.

178. **Munoz-Elias EJ, Upton AM, Cherian J, McKinney JD.** 2006. Role of the methylcitrate cycle in *Mycobacterium tuberculosis* metabolism, intracellular growth, and virulence. *Mol Microbiol* **60:**1109–1122.

179. **Savvi S, Warner DF, Kana BD, McKinney JD, Mizrahi V, Dawes SS.** 2008. Functional characterization of a vitamin B12-dependent methylmalonyl pathway in *Mycobacterium tuberculosis*: implications for propionate metabolism during growth on fatty acids. *J Bacteriol* **190:**3886–3895.

180. **Russell DG, VanderVen BC, Lee W, Abramovitch RB, Kim MJ, Homolka S, Niemann S, Rohde KH.** 2010. *Mycobacterium tuberculosis* wears what it eats. *Cell Host Microbe* **8:**68–76.

181. **Williams KJ, Boshoff HI, Krishnan N, Gonzales J, Schnappinger D, Robertson BD.** 2011. The *Mycobacterium tuberculosis* beta-oxidation genes echA5 and fadB3 are dispensable for growth *in vitro* and *in vivo*. *Tuberculosis* **91:**549–555.

182. **Graham JE, Clark-Curtiss JE.** 1999. Identification of *Mycobacterium tuberculosis* RNAs synthesized in response to phagocytosis by human macrophages by selective capture of transcribed sequences (SCOTS). *Proc Natl Acad Sci USA* **96:**11554–11559.

183. **Honer Zu Bentrup K, Miczak A, Swenson DL, Russell DG.** 1999. Characterization of activity and expression of isocitrate lyase in *Mycobacterium avium* and *Mycobacterium tuberculosis*. *J Bacteriol* **181:**7161–7167.

184. **Munoz-Elias EJ, McKinney JD.** 2005. *Mycobacterium tuberculosis* isocitrate lyases 1 and 2 are jointly required for *in vivo* growth and virulence. *Nat Med* **11:**638–644.

185. **Gould TA, van de Langemheen H, Munoz-Elias EJ, McKinney JD, Sacchettini JC.** 2006. Dual role of isocitrate lyase 1 in the glyoxylate and methylcitrate cycles in *Mycobacterium tuberculosis*. *Mol Microbiol* **61:**940–947.

186. **Eoh H, Rhee KY.** 2014. Methylcitrate cycle defines the bactericidal essentiality of isocitrate lyase for survival of *Mycobacterium tuberculosis* on fatty acids. *Proc Natl Acad Sci USA* **111:**4976–4981.

187. **Nandakumar M, Nathan C, Rhee KY.** 2014. Isocitrate lyase mediates broad antibiotic tolerance in *Mycobacterium tuberculosis*. *Nat Commun* **5:**4306.

188. **Eoh H, Rhee KY.** 2013. Multifunctional essentiality of succinate metabolism in adaptation to hypoxia in *Mycobacterium tuberculosis*. *Proc Natl Acad Sci USA* **110:**6554–6559.

189. **Dixon GH, Kornberg HL, Lund P.** 1960. Purification and properties of malate synthetase. *Biochim Biophys Acta* **41:**217–233.

190. **Quartararo CE, Blanchard JS.** 2011. Kinetic and chemical mechanism of malate synthase from *Mycobacterium tuberculosis*. *Biochemistry* **50:**6879–6887.

191. **Kinhikar AG, Vargas D, Li H, Mahaffey SB, Hinds L, Belisle JT, Laal S.** 2006. *Mycobacterium tuberculosis* malate synthase is a laminin-binding adhesin. *Mol Microbiol* **60:**999–1013.

192. **May EE, Leitao A, Tropsha A, Oprea TI.** 2013. A systems chemical biology study of malate synthase and isocitrate lyase inhibition in *Mycobacterium tuberculosis* during active and NRP growth. *Comput Biol Chem* **47:**167–180.

193. **Bauza A, Quinonero D, Deya PM, Frontera A.** 2014. Long-range effects in anion-pi interactions: their crucial role in the inhibition mechanism of *Mycobacterium tuberculosis* malate synthase. *Chemistry* **20:**6985–6990.

194. **Kratky M, Vinsova J, Novotna E, Mandikova J, Wsol V, Trejtnar F, Ulmann V, Stolarikova J, Fernandes S, Bhat S, Liu JO.** 2012. Salicylanilide derivatives block *Mycobacterium tuberculosis* through inhibition of isocitrate lyase and methionine aminopeptidase. *Tuberculosis* **92:**434–439.

195. **Sriram D, Yogeeswari P, Senthilkumar P, Dewakar S, Rohit N, Debjani B, Bhat P, Veugopal B, Pavan VV, Thimmappa HM.** 2009. Novel phthalazinyl derivatives: synthesis, antimycobacterial activities, and inhibition of *Mycobacterium tuberculosis* isocitrate lyase enzyme. *Med Chem* **5:**422–433.

196. **Peyron P, Vaubourgeix J, Poquet Y, Levillain F, Botanch C, Bardou F, Daffe M, Emile JF, Marchou B, Cardona PJ, de Chastellier C, Altare F.** 2008. Foamy macrophages from tuberculous patients' granulomas constitute a nutrient-rich reservoir for *M. tuberculosis* persistence. *PLoS Pathog* **4:**e1000204. doi:10.1371/journal.ppat.1000204.

197. **Russell DG, Cardona PJ, Kim MJ, Allain S, Altare F.** 2009. Foamy macrophages and the progression of the human tuberculosis granuloma. *Nat Immunol* **10:**943–948.

198. **Daniel J, Maamar H, Deb C, Sirakova TD, Kolattukudy PE.** 2011. *Mycobacterium tuberculosis* uses host triacylglycerol to accumulate lipid droplets and acquires a dormancy-like phenotype in lipid-loaded macrophages. *PLoS Pathog* **7:**e1002093. doi:10.1371/journal.ppat.1002093.

199. **Tailleux L, Waddell SJ, Pelizzola M, Mortellaro A, Withers M, Tanne A, Castagnoli PR, Gicquel B, Stoker NG, Butcher PD, Foti M, Neyrolles O.** 2008. Probing host pathogen cross-talk by transcriptional profiling of both *Mycobacterium tuberculosis* and infected human dendritic cells and macrophages. *PLoS One* **3:**e1403. doi:10.1371/journal.pone.0001403.

200. **Kim MJ, Wainwright HC, Locketz M, Bekker LG, Walther GB, Dittrich C, Visser A, Wang W, Hsu FF, Wiehart U, Tsenova L, Kaplan G, Russell DG.** 2010. Caseation of human tuberculosis granulomas correlates with elevated host lipid metabolism. *EMBO Mol Med* **2:**258–274.

201. **Podinovskaia M, Lee W, Caldwell S, Russell DG.** 2013. Infection of macrophages with *Mycobacterium tuberculosis* induces global modifications to phagosomal function. *Cell Microbiol* **15:**843–859.

202. **Singh V, Jamwal S, Jain R, Verma P, Gokhale R, Rao KV.** 2012. *Mycobacterium tuberculosis*-driven targeted recalibration of macrophage lipid homeostasis promotes the foamy phenotype. *Cell Host Microbe* **12:**669–681.

203. **Neyrolles O.** 2014. Mycobacteria and the greasy macrophage: getting fat and frustrated. *Infect Immun* **82:**472–475.

204. **Caire-Brandli I, Papadopoulos A, Malaga W, Marais D, Canaan S, Thilo L, de Chastellier C.** 2014. Reversible lipid accumulation and associated division arrest of *Mycobacterium avium* in lipoprotein-induced foamy macrophages may resemble key events during latency and reactivation of tuberculosis. *Infect Immun* **82:**476–490.

205. **Schnupf P, Portnoy DA.** 2007. Listeriolysin O: a phagosome-specific lysin. *Microb Infect* **9:**1176–1187.

206. **O'Brien DK, Melville SB.** 2004. Effects of *Clostridium perfringens* alpha-toxin (PLC) and perfringolysin O (PFO) on cytotoxicity to macrophages, on escape from the phagosomes of macrophages, and on persistence of *C. perfringens* in host tissues. *Infect Immun* **72:**5204–5215.

207. **Bastiat-Sempe B, Love JF, Lomayesva N, Wessels MR.** 2014. Streptolysin O and NAD-glycohydrolase prevent phagolysosome acidification and promote group a streptococcus survival in macrophages. *mBio* **5:**e01690-14. doi:10.1128/mBio.01690-14.

208. **Baba H, Kawamura I, Kohda C, Nomura T, Ito Y, Kimoto T, Watanabe I, Ichiyama S, Mitsuyama M.** 2001. Essential role of domain 4 of pneumolysin from *Streptococcus pneumoniae* in cytolytic activity as determined by truncated proteins. *Biochem Biophys Res Commun* **281:**37–44.

209. **Rubins JB, Paddock AH, Charboneau D, Berry AM, Paton JC, Janoff EN.** 1998. Pneumolysin in pneumococcal adherence and colonization. *Microb Pathog* **25:**337–342.

210. **Cockeran R, Anderson R, Feldman C.** 2002. The role of pneumolysin in the pathogenesis of *Streptococcus pneumoniae* infection. *Curr Opin Infect Dis* **15:**235–239.

211. **Sitkiewicz I, Nagiec MJ, Sumby P, Butler SD, Cywes-Bentley C, Musser JM.** 2006. Emergence of a bacterial clone with enhanced virulence by acquisition of a phage encoding a secreted phospholipase A2. *Proc Natl Acad Sci USA* **103:**16009–16014.

212. **Creasey EA, Isberg RR.** 2012. The protein SdhA maintains the integrity of the *Legionella*-containing vacuole. *Proc Natl Acad Sci USA* **109:**3481–3486.

213. **Sitkiewicz I, Stockbauer KE, Musser JM.** 2007. Secreted bacterial phospholipase A2 enzymes: better living through phospholipolysis. *Trends Microbiol* **15:**63–69.

214. **Russell AB, LeRoux M, Hathazi K, Agnello DM, Ishikawa T, Wiggins PA, Wai SN, Mougous JD.** 2013. Diverse type VI secretion phospholipases are functionally plastic antibacterial effectors. *Nature* **496:**508–512.

215. **Livermore BP, Bey RF, Johnson RC.** 1978. Lipid metabolism of *Borrelia hermsi. Infect Immun* **20:**215–220.

216. **Plaza H, Whelchel TR, Garczynski SF, Howerth EW, Gherardini FC.** 1997. Purified outer membranes of *Serpulina hyodysenteriae* contain cholesterol. *J Bacteriol* **179:**5414–5421.

217. **Trott DJ, Alt DP, Zuerner RL, Wannemuehler MJ, Stanton TB.** 2001. The search for *Brachyspira* outer membrane proteins that interact with the host. *Anim Health Res Rev* **2:**19–30.

218. **Haque M, Hirai Y, Yokota K, Oguma K.** 1995. Lipid profiles of *Helicobacter pylori* and *Helicobacter mustelae* grown in serum-supplemented and serum-free media. *Acta Med Okayama* **49:**205–211.

219. **Hirai Y, Haque M, Yoshida T, Yokota K, Yasuda T, Oguma K.** 1995. Unique cholesteryl glucosides in *Helicobacter pylori*: composition and structural analysis. *J Bacteriol* **177:**5327–5333.

220. **Inamoto Y, Hamanaka S, Hamanaka Y, Nagate T, Kondo I, Takemoto T, Okita K.** 1995. Lipid composition and fatty acid analysis of *Helicobacter pylori. J Gastroenterol* **30:**315–318.

221. **Rodwell AW.** 1963. The steroid growth-requirement of *Mycoplasma mycoides. J Gen Microbiol* **32:**91–101.

222. **Razin S, Tully JG.** 1970. Cholesterol requirement of mycoplasmas. *J Bacteriol* **102:**306–310.

223. **Wang M, Hajishengallis G.** 2008. Lipid raft-dependent uptake, signalling and intracellular fate of *Porphyromonas gingivalis* in mouse macrophages. *Cell Microbiol* **10:**2029–2042.

224. **Kalischuk LD, Inglis GD, Buret AG.** 2009. *Campylobacter jejuni* induces transcellular translocation of commensal bacteria via lipid rafts. *Gut Pathog* **1:**2.

225. **Konkel ME, Samuelson DR, Eucker TP, Shelden EA, O'Loughlin JL.** 2013. Invasion of epithelial cells by *Campylobacter jejuni* is independent of caveolae. *Cell Commun Signal* **11:**100.

226. **Amer AO, Swanson MS.** 2005. Autophagy is an immediate macrophage response to *Legionella pneumophila. Cell Microbiol* **7:**765–778.

227. **Houde M, Gottschalk M, Gagnon F, Van Calsteren MR, Segura M.** 2012. *Streptococcus suis* capsular polysaccharide inhibits phagocytosis through destabilization of lipid microdomains and prevents lactosylceramide-dependent recognition. *Infect Immun* **80:**506–517.

228. **Yamaguchi M, Terao Y, Mori-Yamaguchi Y, Domon H, Sakaue Y, Yagi T, Nishino K, Yamaguchi A, Nizet V, Kawabata S.** 2013. *Streptococcus pneumoniae* invades erythrocytes and utilizes them to evade human innate immunity. *PloS One* **8:**e77282. doi:10.1371/journal.pone.0077282.

229. **Goluszko P, Popov V, Wen J, Jones A, Yallampalli C.** 2008. Group B streptococcus exploits lipid rafts and phosphoinositide 3-kinase/Akt signaling pathway to invade human endometrial cells. *Am J Obstet Gynecol* **199:**548.e-9.

230. **Lemire P, Houde M, Segura M.** 2012. Encapsulated group B *Streptococcus* modulates dendritic cell functions via lipid rafts and clathrin-mediated endocytosis. *Cell Microbiol* **14:**1707–1719.

231. **Abrami L, Liu S, Cosson P, Leppla SH, van der Goot FG.** 2003. Anthrax toxin triggers endocytosis of its receptor via a lipid raft-mediated clathrin-dependent process. *J Cell Biol* **160:**321–328.

23

Contrasting Lifestyles Within the Host Cell

ELIZABETH DI RUSSO CASE[1] and JAMES E. SAMUEL[1]

INTRODUCTION

Bacterial pathogens that adopt an intracellular lifestyle often avoid many challenges that are faced by their extracellular counterparts. However, upon entering the host cell, they have a new set of trials with which to contend. Upon phagocytic uptake or entry by receptor-mediated endocytosis, they immediately traffic to a degradative subcellular compartment. Successful intracellular pathogens have adopted different strategies to avoid trafficking of their initial phagosome along the endocytic pathway to fusion with the lysosome, a subcellular compartment that has specifically evolved to degrade them. In this chapter, we will compare the different molecular mechanisms employed by four intracellular pathogens that have adopted distinct vacuolar niches and lifestyles. Many vacuolar pathogens alter their initial phagosomal compartment to stall or exit the endocytic pathway and thereby avoid elimination. Yet a few species require at least some interaction with lysosomes for completion of their infectious cycle. In this chapter, we will compare the strategies employed by *Mycobacterium* and *Chlamydia* to avoid lysosomal fusion with those of *Brucella*, whose vacuole interacts with lysosomes

[1]Department of Microbial Pathogenesis and Immunology, College of Medicine, Texas A&M Health Sciences Center, Bryan, TX 77807.
Virulence Mechanisms of Bacterial Pathogens, 5th edition
Edited by Indira T. Kudva, Nancy A. Cornick, Paul J. Plummer, Qijing Zhang, Tracy L. Nicholson, John P. Bannantine, and Bryan H. Bellaire
© 2016 American Society for Microbiology, Washington, DC
doi:10.1128/microbiolspec.VMBF-0014-2015

transiently, and *Coxiella*, a bacterium adapted to growth in a compartment that closely resembles a terminal phagolysosome.

The Benefits of an Intracellular Lifestyle

Pathogens that live within a eukaryotic host cell obtain several benefits of a relatively protected niche. One important advantage of living within a host cell is evasion of acquired immunity. Once inside the confines of a eukaryotic cell, the pathogen is no longer susceptible to complement or neutralizing antibodies. Another benefit of this lifestyle derives from the fact that few bacterial species have evolved to live within a host cell, and even fewer within a professional phagocytic cell such as a macrophage. Pathogens that have adapted to this environment experience limited competition from other resident bacteria for nutrients. In fact, the intracellular environment can provide so many vital nutrients to a pathogen that they often have minimal genomes, saving coding capacity and energy for the expression of essential "housekeeping" genes, and virulence factors promoting its infectivity.

The Hazards of an Intracellular Lifestyle

Once a bacterium is taken up into a cell either by phagocytosis or receptor-mediated endocytosis, it begins to traffic along the endocytic pathway toward lysosomal fusion and destruction. Intracellular pathogens have adopted two main strategies to avoid the mature phagolysosome: modify the vacuole to create a replicative niche or escape and replicate within the cytosol. Whether a bacterium remains in the phagosome or escapes, it must contend with the host's defenses. Cytosolic pathogens such as *Listeria*, *Shigella*, *Rickettsia*, and *Francisella* rapidly escape the initial phagosome and thereby avoid lysosomal fusion (1). However, once in the cytosol, a pathogen must evade xenophagy, a selective form of autophagy that serves as an innate immune defense against cytosolic

pathogens (2). Bacteria that remain within the phagosome can avoid xenophagic killing, provided their vacuole remains intact. Taking up residence in a pathogen-tailored vacuole therefore provides a comfortable and protected compartment within a host cell if phagocytic maturation is quickly curtailed.

The Mature Phagosome Is a Dangerous Place for Most Intracellular Pathogens

In eukaryotic cells, the specific mechanism of particle internalization depends on the size of the individual item that is consumed. Phagocytosis generally refers to particles >0.5 μm in size, while smaller objects are taken up by receptor-mediated endocytosis or pinocytosis. Phagocytosis requires the extrusion of membrane for capture, whereas endocytosed particles submerge into the host cell in response to the binding of a ligand to a specific host receptor. Although the initial signaling events and structural changes at the membrane differ between these uptake processes, there are many common features of the phagocytic maturation pathway that follows (3).

The phagosomal maturation pathway is characterized by membrane changes in lipid content and the small GTPases that associate with them (Fig. 1). After a phagosome separates from the membrane, the small GTPase, Rab5, and vacuolar-sorting protein-34 (VPS 34) are recruited to its membrane. VPS 34, a class III PI3K, generates phagosomal phosphatidylinositol-3-phosphate (PtdIns3P) (4), identifying the vacuole as a phagosome/early endosome, distinct from the PtdIns(4,5)P_2- and PtdIns(4)P-enriched plasma membrane (5). Early endosome antigen-1 (EEA1), a Rab5 effector, binds to the PtdIns3P as well as Rab5 and facilitates endosome fusion (6). The early endosome is slightly acidified (7), but a further reduction in pH is achieved later with the recruitment of vacuolar (V) type ATPases. Rab5 is then exchanged for Rab7 in a process that appears to be regulated by SAND-1/Mon1 (8, 9) and requires

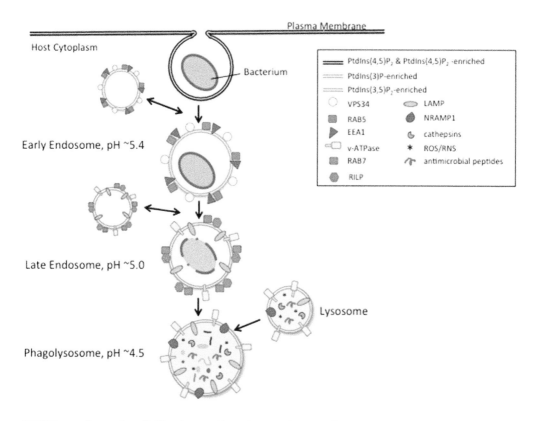

FIGURE 1 **Endosomal trafficking is coordinated by exchanges of lipids and Rab-GTPases. The normal endosomal pathway is illustrated here with major regulatory factors highlighted at each step. After uptake of a cargo, the phagosome fuses with early endosomes, acquiring Rab5, its effector EEA1, and VPS34, which coordinate the change in lipid profile of the endosomal membrane. Soon after, the compartment fuses with late endosomes, and Rab5 is exchanged for Rab7 and its effector RILP. LAMP and V-ATPases are also characteristic of the late endosome. Finally, the late endosome fuses with lysosomes, at which point the compartment is fully matured and highly degradative.**

lysosome-associated membrane proteins (LAMP) 1 and 2 (10).

With the swap of Rab5 for Rab7, the early endosome transitions to a late endosome. The late endosome acquires V-ATPases, which pump protons across the phagosomal membrane, dropping the vacuolar pH to approximately 5.0, making it an increasingly less hospitable place. The vacuoles also acquire RILP (Rab7-interacting lysosomal protein), a Rab7 effector that is required for trafficking of late endosomes to the perinuclear region and subsequent fusion with lysosomes (11). In addition to changes in associated Rabs and their effectors, the lipid profile of late endo-

somes is distinct from that of early endosomes. Late endosomes and lysosomes are enriched in $PtdIns(3,5)P_2$, the result of conversion of PtdIns3P by PtdIns(3)P5-kinase.

Upon maturation of the phagosome into a phagolysosome, the pH drops to approximately 4.5, activating proteolytic cathepsins and contributing to the generation of deadly reactive oxygen species (ROS) (12). In addition to these microbicidal contents, the lysosome also harbors antimicrobial peptides, NO^-, and natural resistance–associated macrophage protein 1 (NRAMP1), which ejects Zn^+ and Mn^+ from the lysosome to preserve its low pH and deprive any microbes from essential cofactors (13). Most pathogens that have adapted to life within a host vacuole have to act quickly to halt trafficking or otherwise tailor their environment to avoid destruction; maturation can occur within 18 minutes of uptake (14).

To Fuse or Not to Fuse

Many intracellular pathogens have successfully adopted a vacuolar lifestyle. However, the points at which these pathogen-tailored vacuoles depart from the endocytic pathway are diverse and species-specific. Most vacuolar pathogens have evolved mechanisms to avoid lysosomal fusion by arresting trafficking through the endocytic pathway, as exemplified by *Mycobacterium tuberculosis*. The *Chlamydia trachomatis* inclusion diverges from the pathway early on, modifying its vacuole so that it resembles an exocytic vacuole. Several intracellular bacteria allow acidification. *Brucella* requires a transient drop in vacuolar pH to activate the expression and secretion of key virulence factors and complete its infection cycle. In contrast, *Coxiella burnetii* has evolved to require sustained interaction with the lysosome to complete its developmental cycle. Over the course of this chapter, we will discuss the specific adaptations these four pathogens have evolved to create a hospitable niche inside a host vacuole.

M. TUBERCULOSIS

Tuberculosis is a leading cause of death worldwide, with 2 to 3 million fatal cases annually. These deaths represent a global burden on public health, since over 1 billion people are latently infected with the etiologic agent of tuberculosis, *M. tuberculosis* (15). While the vast majority of these individuals are asymptomatic for much of their life, they have a small chance (about 10%) of eventually developing active disease. The morbidity and mortality associated with *M. tuberculosis* has

been amplified by the pandemic of HIV/AIDS patients with *M. tuberculosis* complex (MTBC) infection, of which *M. tuberculosis* is a member (16). Additionally, the slow-growing and chronic nature of the infection has led to widespread hypervirulent multidrug-resistant and extremely drug resistant cases that are challenging to treat and strain public health systems worldwide (17). The MTBC also includes *Mycobacterium bovis*, from which the Calmette and Guerin (BCG) vaccine is derived. By evolution through a common ancestor, MTBC members can be compared genomically with respect to 14 regions of difference (RD-14) that help to identify specific virulence-associated regions (16). For the majority of comparisons across intracellular bacterial models, we highlight findings from the virulent isolate, H37Rv, for lifestyle and intracellular trafficking studies.

M. tuberculosis Colonizes Macrophages and Persists Inside Structurally Complex Granulomas

Macrophages and monocytes are the principally infected cells during *M. tuberculosis* infection and have been the most common cell types for intracellular trafficking studies. Once inside the macrophage, *M. tuberculosis* arrests phagosomal maturation at a very early stage, thereby avoiding degradation and enabling its intracellular replication within this compartment (18). Infected alveolar macrophages initiate cellular responses by nearby epithelial cells that recruit more macrophages to the infection site, creating a granuloma within the infected lung. These infection foci function as sites of chronic inflammation and provide a mechanism for bacterial spread as the newly arriving macrophages provide a growing niche for replication (19). Eventually, acquired immunity can control the bacterial growth until necrosis develops. *M. tuberculosis* released from necrotic cells inside the granuloma can replicate rapidly in the extracellular space, and it is these bacteria that are transmitted to a new host. As a result, the dynamics of the *M. tuberculosis* lifestyle is complicated by stage of infection, activation status of the host cell, and the ensuing inflammatory response. For this discussion, we will focus primarily on resident macrophages as replication sites for *M. tuberculosis*.

Macrophage Infection by *M. tuberculosis* Is Characterized by an Arrest of Phagosomal Maturation

M. tuberculosis avoids digestion by lysosomal enzymes by halting its progression along the phagosomal pathway at the early endosome stage (Fig. 2) (20, 21). In doing so, it specifi-

cally excludes V-ATPase from its vacuole and disables fusogenicity with late endosomes and lysosomes. The result is a parasitophorous vacuole of near-neutral pH that is exclusive of ROS and degradative enzymes. While the *Mycobacterium*-containing phagosomal compartment (MCP) evades fusion with degradative endosomal compartments, it retains the ability to interact with early endosomes, which provide the bacteria with essential nutrients for replication. *M. tuberculosis* orchestrates its trafficking arrest through the production of several key virulence factors that interfere with calcium flux, host membrane fusion events, and

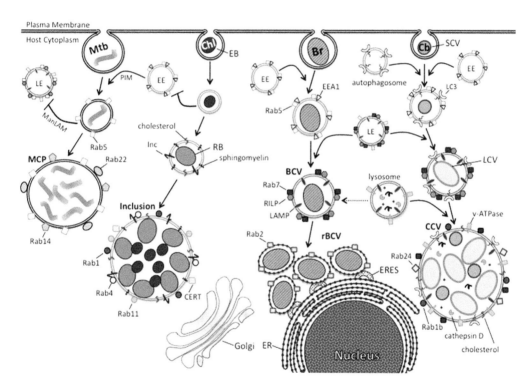

FIGURE 2 Intracellular pathogens have evolved distinct trafficking pathways to arrive within their ideal replicative niche. Intracellular trafficking pathways are shown for *Mycobacterium tuberculosis* (Mtb), *Chlamydia* (Chl), *Brucella* (Br), and *Coxiella burnetii* (Cb). Key regulatory factors, such as Rab-GTPases, lipids, and bacterial factors are shown. *M. tuberculosis* fuses with early endosomes (EE) but inhibits fusion with late endosomes (LE) and replicates in a compartment (MCP) that is stalled at an early point along the endocytic pathway. Chl traffics away from the endosomal pathway and escapes to replicate in a Golgi-associated Inclusion. Br allows EE and LE fusion as well as limited lysosomal fusion before trafficking to the ER to replicate in rBCVs (replicative *Brucella*-containing vacuoles). Cb interacts with EE, autophagosomes, and LE and allows lysosomal fusion to arrive in the CCV (*Coxiella*-containing vacuole), which resembles a terminal phagolysosome.

recruitment of inducible nitrous oxide synthase (iNOS) (18).

Lipoarabinomannan (LAM) arrests phagosomal maturation and prevents acidification of the MCP

M. tuberculosis begins the invasion process by interaction with several distinct receptors, but uptake of complement-opsonized bacteria by complement receptors represents its main route of entry (22, 23). Cholesterol-rich lipid domains may also drive selective entry and likely affect the signaling response to attachment as well as MCP formation (24). Soon after entry, the early endosome containing *M. tuberculosis* acquires Rab5, but Rab7 is altered or absent (25, 26). This block in the canonical trafficking pathway is the result of two converging signaling pathways that are regulated by *M. tuberculosis* LAM (18). LAM is a glycosylated phosphatidylinositol that is conserved among MTBC members, with the exception of the heterogeneous nature of its sugar cap. The LAM of *M. tuberculosis* has a cap of mannose and is therefore referred to as ManLAM. While ManLAM affects two different signaling pathways, the net effect of its activities is the exclusion of V-ATPase on the MCP.

The maturation block coordinated by ManLAM has two arms, one that affects calcium signaling and one that inhibits recruitment of EEA1. ManLAM contributes to the absence of VPS34 on the MCP by inhibiting an increase in cytosolic Ca^{2+} in response to *M. tuberculosis* infection (27). In macrophages, an increase cytosolic Ca^{2+} levels, as a response to phagocytosis, activates calmodulin to associate with Ca^{2+}/calmodulin protein kinase CaMKII, an essential factor for phagolysosome maturation (28). This signaling cascade is responsible for the recruitment of VPS34 to the phagosome, which generates the PtdIns3P necessary for EEA1 binding (27). ManLAM may also inhibit association of EEA1 through the activation of p38 MAP kinase (29). Activation of p38 mitogen-activated protein kinase reduces levels of Rab5 on early

endosomes and likewise levels of EEA1 (30). EEA1, a membrane tethering molecule, serves as a binding partner for syntaxin 6, a soluble NSF attachment protein receptor (SNARE) that delivers V-ATPase and cathepsins from the *trans*-Golgi network to endosomes (31). Through the complementary effects of ManLAM on macrophage signal transduction and membrane trafficking, the MCP is protected from acidification and lysosomal hydrolases.

M. tuberculosis uses multiple strategies to impede phagosomal maturation

In addition to the expression of ManLAM, *M. tuberculosis* employs other virulence factors in an effort to preserve the early endosomal qualities of the MCP. Another lipid produced by *M. tuberculosis*, called trehalose dimycolate (TDM), can delay phagosomal acidification via an unknown mechanism (32). In addition to lipids, a variety of protein "effectors" have been identified, via transposon mutant library screens, as being involved in arresting phagosomal maturation. Ndk is a nucleoside diphosphate kinase which is secreted into growth medium and is cytotoxic to macrophages (33). Based on *in vitro* and biochemical data, Ndk appears to dephosphorylate cellular Rab7-GTP and Rab5-GTP, thereby preventing Rab7-dependent heterotypic fusion of the MCP. PtpA is a low-molecular-weight tyrosine phosphatase that dephosphorylates VPS33B, a host protein involved in regulation of membrane fusion in the endocytic pathway. PtpA also binds to the H subunit of V-ATPase, inhibiting its ability to acidify vacuoles (34). These examples of *M. tuberculosis* products that participate in the regulation of intracellular trafficking of the MCP are only a subset of the identified bacterial factors that may play a role in this complex process.

M. tuberculosis evades iNOS through interactions with the host actin cytoskeleton

In addition to acidification and lysosomal hydrolases, *M. tuberculosis* also avoids the

ROS and reactive nitrogen species (RNS) that normally accompany phagosomal maturation in macrophages. iNOS synthesizes NO$^-$ gas on the cytosolic face of the phagosomal membrane, which then diffuses through the membrane into the phagosomal lumen. The apposition of iNOS to the phagosome is actin-dependent, and *M. tuberculosis* interference with the actin cytoskeleton prevented iNOS from contacting the MCP (35). Building on these observations, Davis et al. found that the scaffolding protein EBP50, which normally links iNOS to the actin cytoskeleton and regulates its localization, was rapidly lost from the *M. tuberculosis*–containing phagosomes (36). Keeping iNOS at a distance from the MCP excludes NO$^-$ from the phagosome, protecting *M. tuberculosis* from its harmful effects.

The *M. tuberculosis* lipid PIM counteracts, in part, the effects of ManLAM

ManLAM significantly reduces the fusogenicity of the MCP by the mechanisms detailed above. However, *M. tuberculosis* is capable of bypassing the restrictions that ManLAM sets in place through the production of another bacterial glycosylated phosphatidylinositol called PIM (phosphatidylinositol mannoside). PIM specifically stimulates homotypic fusion of the MCP with early endosomes in a Rab-dependent manner (37). PIM's effect is insensitive to inhibition of PtdIns3P, and the result is a membrane fusion pathway that is independent of that particular host lipid (27). The significance of this bypass pathway is that it solves the problem of how *M. tuberculosis* acquires iron, via transferrin, through interaction with early endosomes (38).

Mycobacterium Expresses Several Virulence Factors that Impart Resistance to Its Host's Oxidative Burst

While *M. tuberculosis* manages to evade interaction with the lysosome of macrophages, it must still contend with the oxidative burst induced by invading its host cell. There are sev-

eral proteins that either directly or indirectly contribute to the ability of *M. tuberculosis* to resist this form of macrophage-mediated killing. Additionally, the integrity of the mycobacterial lipid-rich cell wall may protect *M. tuberculosis* from ROS/RNS.

Several *M. tuberculosis* proteins directly detoxify ROS and RNS

M. tuberculosis employs many classical mediators of ROS/RNS resistance by directly deactivating them during infection. Alkyl hydroperoxidase C (AhpC), an enzyme that reduces organic peroxides, has been shown to exhibit peroxynitrite reductase activity *in vitro* (39). Mutants of this gene show increased susceptibility to peroxynitrite in resting macrophages compared to wild type *M. tuberculosis*, but this difference was nullified upon activation with interferon-γ (IFN-γ) (40). Another detoxifying enzyme that is important for *M. tuberculosis* survival is KatG, which degrades hydrogen peroxide to water and oxygen. KatG mutants of *M. tuberculosis* are attenuated in mice and guinea pigs (41, 42). TpX, a thiol peroxidase, is required for optimal replication in both activated and resting macrophages. A *tpx* mutant was not attenuated in iNOS$^{-/-}$ mice, which exhibit a modest oxidative burst, indicating that TpX is indispensable for resistance to RNS and ROS (43). The outer membrane lipoprotein SodC, which bestows *M. tuberculosis* with the ability to dismutate extracellular superoxide, was also found to promote survival within IFN-γ activated macrophages (44). Having these enzymes in its arsenal is a requirement for *M. tuberculosis* virulence.

Resistance to ROS/RNS is indirectly supplied by other *M. tuberculosis* virulence factors

Several *M. tuberculosis* proteins or other virulence factors, such as the lipid-rich cell wall, provide resistance to ROS and RNS without directly detoxifying them. Acr2 is one such protein whose expression is upregulated by the bacterium under various conditions of stress, including oxidative stress (16). While the molecular chaperone Acr2 is not absolutely essential to the pathogenic program of *M. tuberculosis*, deletion mutants exhibit a protracted disease progression (45). The role of the hypothetical gene *Rv2136c* in resistance to low pH, heat shock, and ROS, among other stressors, was identified as part of a transposon mutant screen (46). The transposon mutant also displayed attenuation in a mouse infection with regard to its ability to persist in the lung and spleen. The specific function of this protein is unknown, but it has homology to a peptidoglycan synthesis gene in *Escherichia coli*. Other genes of interest identified in the screen include *Rv2224c* and *ponA2*, which had more modest infection defects but are also predicted to play a role in cell wall synthesis or maintenance. These proteins that impart oxidative stress relief via prevention or repair of damage also play an important role in the survival and therefore pathogenesis of *M. tuberculosis*.

The primary survival strategy of *M. tuberculosis* is to quickly stall the progression of its internalized phagosome before it becomes too hostile to inhabit. It orchestrates a delicate balance between blocking of phagosomal fusogenicity with the ability to interact with early endosomes as a source of essential nutrients. While the arrested phagosome is free of degradative cathepsins and excludes acidifying V-ATPase, the niche that *M. tuberculosis* occupies is not devoid of host defenses. *M. tuberculosis* counters the vigorous oxidative burst of the infected macrophage by direct detoxification and indirectly through the expression of protective chaperones. These extremely effective pathogenic attributes have been fine-tuned over the course of millennia, because the relationship *M. tuberculosis* has with its host is truly ancient.

CHLAMYDIA

Two main species of *Chlamydiae* cause the majority of human disease. *Chlamydia tra-* *chomatis* is the causative agent of the most commonly reported sexually transmitted bacterial infection in the United States (47). It is also responsible for the blinding disease of trachoma, common in the developing world. *Chlamydophila pneumoniae* frequently causes community-acquired pneumonia and has been identified as a risk factor for atherosclerosis and asthma (48, 49). Another species, *Chlamydophila psittaci*, is known to cause a zoonotic fever carried by psittacine birds that is transmitted by aerosol and contrasts as an intracellular model. Psittacosis is a severe pulmonary infection that is difficult to treat, and therefore it has been proposed to have potential for use as a biological weapon (50).

Chlamydia Has a Biphasic Developmental Cycle

These Gram-negative obligate intracellular parasites have a characteristic developmental cycle that alternates between two disparate morphologies. The small, extracellular, infectious but metabolically inactive form is termed the elementary body (EB) (Fig. 2). The metabolically active reticulate body (RB) is larger and noninfectious and is found exclusively inside host cells. Upon attachment to its host cell, the EB induces its uptake by injection of a type III secreted effector called TARP, which remodels host actin at the site of entry (51). Once inside the host cell, the EB is contained within a specialized parasitophorous vacuole, called the inclusion. EBs rapidly differentiate into RBs and begin to replicate by binary fission within the inclusion. The bacteria continue to replicate while actively modifying the inclusion by inserting bacterial proteins (Incs) and incorporating host lipids as they traffic to the microtubule organizing center of the cell. The infection cycle completes between 48 and 72 hours later when the RBs asynchronously differentiate back into their infectious form and are released from the host cell by either lysis or a process called extrusion (52).

Over the course of the intracellular phase of chlamydial development, the bacteria are known to subvert a wide variety of host cell functions. Actin is remodeled at the entry site of EBs (51, 53, 54), and the host cytoskeleton is used to build a supporting scaffold for the growing inclusion (55). The lipid composition of the inclusion membrane is changed quickly after the infection is initiated, and the chlamydiae themselves incorporate host lipids into their membranes (56, 57). Rab GTPases that identify recycling endosomes and endoplasmic reticulum (ER)–Golgi trafficking pathways are recruited to the inclusion, and interactions with many host cell organelles have been documented, including the Golgi apparatus, mitochondria, lipid droplets, and multivesicular bodies (58). *Chlamydiae* are also known to interfere with host cell signaling to inhibit apoptosis and promote survival and to block innate immune signaling (59). All of these functions create a parasitophorous vacuole that is separate from the endocytic pathway, thereby evading lysosomal fusion while at the same time allowing acquisition of essential nutrients and replication within a protected niche.

Chlamydiae Depart the Endocytic Pathway Early in Infection

In contrast to *Mycobacterium*, which arrests phagocytic trafficking at an early point in the pathway, the chlamydial inclusion diverges from it completely to evade destruction and create a hospitable environment for replication. Nascent inclusions do not acquire transferrin receptor, EEA1, mannose 6 phosphate receptor, or LAMP1 following EB uptake. In fact, the vesicles containing endocytosed EBs are nonfusogenic with endocytic vacuoles, including recycling endosomes (60). Inclusions do not acidify and do not acquire V-ATPases (61, 62), despite the fact that they can be found in close apposition to lysosomes (63). Regulation of these early trafficking events of the chlamydial inclusion requires *de novo* protein synthesis, because chloramphenicol

treatment results in an increase in lysosomal fusion. Orchestrating the inclusion's escape involves the co-opting of the host's microtubule network, changing the lipid content of the vacuolar membrane, and recruiting specific Rab GTPases associated with recycling endosomes and ER-Golgi transport. The end result is a parasitophorous vacuole that operates as a unique pathogen-constructed organelle.

The host cytoskeleton is co-opted by *Chlamydia* for the duration of its infectious cycle

As soon as an EB is irreversibly attached to its host cell, it begins to use the host cytoskeleton to its advantage. EBs translocate the type III secretion effector TARP (translocated actin-recruiting phosphoprotein) across the host cell membrane to nucleate actin polymerization at the site of entry (51, 53, 54). *C. trachomatis* TARP is also known to activate Rac1, a master regulator of lamellipodium formation (64, 65). This initial actin remodeling induced by TARP is transient, and while the mechanisms governing the subsequent actin depolymerization are not understood, *Chlamydia* expresses two potential regulators for this process: CT166, an inhibitor of Rac1 (66, 67), and CT694, which results in an AHNAK-dependent loss of actin stress fibers (68).

While the actin rearrangements induced by EB attachment are quickly undone, *Chlamydiae* continue to appropriate the host cytoskeleton to support inclusion development. Following entry, the nascent inclusion is trafficked in a dynein-dependent but dynactin-independent manner to the peri-Golgi region of the host cell (69). Once there, the inclusion maintains an intimate association with the microtubule organizing center. Mital et al. identified cholesterol-rich microdomains on the inclusion membrane that appear to serve as platforms for signaling through Src-family kinases and interaction with centrosomes and dynein (70). Once at the microtubule organizing center, the growing inclusion requires a dynamic cytoskeletal scaffold for stabilization (55, 71). The structural integrity maintained by this framework may prevent leakage of inclusion contents into the host cytosol, which might otherwise alert the host cell's innate immune system.

The actin cytoskeleton has a final role to play in the infection cycle as it facilitates extrusion, one of two egress processes described for *Chlamydia* (52). During extrusion, the unbroken inclusion is ejected from the host cell through the plasma membrane, leaving the host cell intact. Pharmacological inhibitors revealed that extrusion requires Wiskott-Aldrich syndrome protein, myosin II, Rho GTPase, and actin polymerization (52). A recent study demonstrated that the myosin phosphatase pathway is also involved in extrusion, because siRNA depletion of myosin IIA/IIB, MLC2, and MLCK significantly reduced detectable extrusion events (72). The fate of an extruded inclusion is unknown, but it has been speculated that this release method may facilitate chlamydial persistence or spread to more distant sites of infection (52)

The inclusion incorporates host lipids that typify exocytic compartments

The lipid content of a eukaryotic vacuole is highly regulated and helps to define the identity of that specific subcellular compartment. In contrast to *Mycobacterium*, which halts endocytic trafficking by retaining the PtdIns(3)P on its phagosome, *Chlamydia* rapidly incorporates other host-derived lipids into its inclusion membrane, helping to identify it as an organelle separate from the endocytic pathway (73).

The first study to demonstrate host lipid acquisition by the inclusion membrane demonstrated that sphingomyelin generated from a fluorescent precursor (C6-NBD-ceramide) in the Golgi accumulated in the parasitophorous vacuole as soon as 2 hours postinfection, and the lipid was also incorporated into the bacteria themselves (57). Since then, it has been shown that *Chlamydia* intercept

sphingomyelin trafficking from the Golgi to the plasma membrane (56, 74, 75), as well as from vesicles trafficking basolaterally (76). Additionally, *Chlamydia* co-opts CERT, a host protein that regulates ceramide traffic from the ER to the Golgi, through binding to chlamydial inclusion membrane protein IncD. CERT interacts with the inclusion membrane to regulate sphingomyelin incorporation (77, 78).

Additional host lipids have been detected in the inclusion membrane, including cholesterol (79), phosphatidic acid (80), and PtdIns (4)P (81). PtdIns(4)P is an identifying lipid component of the Golgi apparatus, and two of its associated regulatory proteins, OCRL1 and PIK4IIα, are also inclusion-localized. Interestingly, depletion of either of these proteins in host cells results in decreased chlamydial infection (81). Other pathways for lipid acquisition include interactions with multivesicular bodies and lipid droplets (82, 83). By changing the lipid profile of the inclusion from that of a PtdIns(3)P-rich endosome to that resembling a Golgi-derived vesicle, the inclusion can avoid termination within a lysosome.

The chlamydial inclusion interacts with many host Rab GTPases

In addition to remodeling its lipid profile, *Chlamydia* recruits to the inclusion Rab GTPases that are characteristic of recycling endosomes and vesicles involved in transport to and from the Golgi apparatus. Rab GTPases, like membrane lipid content, also have an important role in organelle identification. Rabs tightly control maturation of phagosomes, with Rab5 and Rab7 being among the most important players in the process. Rab5 regulates fusion of early endosomes and early phagosomes and is replaced as phagosomes mature by Rab7, which regulates fusion of late endosomes with lysosomes (12). As *Chlamydia* quickly exits the phagocytic pathway, the inclusion membrane does not associate with either Rab5 or Rab7. Rather, the Rabs of recycling endosomes

(Rab4 and Rab11) and ER to Golgi transport (Rab1) are recruited to the inclusion (84). While the association of Rabs 1, 4, and 11 with the inclusion are universal to *Chlamydiae*, some species-specific interactions have also been described. Golgi-associated Rabs 6 and 14 appear only on the inclusions of *C. trachomatis*. Rab10, which is a regulator of ER dynamics and post-Golgi transport, is found only on the inclusions of *C. pneumoniae* (84, 85). The mechanisms by which Rab GTPases are recruited to the inclusion membrane are not well defined, but a few chlamydial inclusion membrane proteins (Incs) have been shown to bind Rabs. *C. trachomatis* CT229, a member of the Inc family of chlamydial proteins, interacts directly with Rab4-GTP in a number of assays, including two-hybrid binding and pull-down experiments (86). A *C. pneumoniae* Inc, Cpn0585, is capable of interacting with Rabs 1, 10, and 11 (87).

The specific Rabs that have been observed on the inclusion membrane not only identify the vacuole as a compartment apart from the endocytic pathway, but also enable interaction with host vesicles and organelles that support chlamydial growth and replication. Rabs 6, 11, and 14 coordinate acquisition of Golgi-derived lipids from the host cell (88, 89). *Chlamydiae* depend on host cell transferrin as a source of iron for growth. Concurrent inhibition of Rab4 and Rab11, which coordinate transferrin recycling to the host plasma membrane, resulted in decreased chlamydial replication and an accumulation of transferrin-containing vesicles adjacent to the inclusion (90). Rab11 is involved in the generation of multivesicular bodies, which have also been observed interacting with inclusions. Inhibition of their trafficking to the inclusion decreases lipid incorporation and bacterial replication (80, 82, 91). Mitochondria have long been associated with chlamydial inclusions (92, 93), and at least in the case of *Chlamydophila caviae*, interaction with them is essential for replication (94). This is not surprising, because *Chlamydia* relies on the host cell for ATP (95, 96).

The chlamydial replicative niche is thus characterized by its early departure from the endocytic pathway to escape the terminal lysosome and rapid association with the Golgi to acquire nutrients. While much is known about how *Chlamydia* actively remodels the inclusion to create a replicative niche, there is still much to discover, because many of the predicted Incs encoded within the chlamydial genome lack functional assignments (97, 98). The co-opting of host cytoskeleton by the inclusion provides structural integrity as it quickly takes up the bulk of the host cell's volume while at the same time provides a network for trafficking away from destruction and reception of host cell cargoes that provide necessary nutrients. Modification of the inclusion membrane further disguises the vacuole as a host organelle that is separate from the endocytic pathway. It is an elegant example of how to successfully hide from the host within one of its cells.

BRUCELLA

While *Brucellae* are known to infect a wide range of host species, there are three that cause the majority of human infection: *Brucella melitensis* (primarily associated with goats and sheep), *Brucella suis* (swine) and *Brucella abortus* (cattle). Humans are incidental hosts for these pathogens, but brucellosis is among the world's most common zoonoses, with over an estimated 500,000 new cases each year (99). The disease is highly infectious, requiring only 10 to 100 organisms to establish an infection via aerosol (100). While inhalation of the pathogen is certainly an important source of human infection, it is also commonly acquired through ingestion of contaminated animal products, particularly unpasteurized dairy (101). After passing through the mucus membranes to infect phagocytic cells, *Brucella* establishes a protected intracellular niche. As discussed above, an intracellular lifestyle allows a pathogen to evade immune surveillance, and this is particularly important for *Brucella*, which often becomes chronically associated with its host (101, 102). The infection begins with flu-like symptoms and is characterized by an undulant fever and night sweats. If left untreated, *Brucella* can disseminate via infected phagocytic cells to many different tissues and organs within the body.

Brucella Transitions Between Three Subcellular Compartments to Complete Its Infectious Cycle

Upon entry, *Brucella* begins an intracellular journey in which it will traffic through the endocytic pathway to the ER for replication and then an autophagosome-like compartment for egress. First, intracellular trafficking of *Brucella* to a replicative compartment is dependent on its LPS status, because only the smooth (virulent) variants with full-length O-antigen can avoid phagocytic maturation and destruction. However, it should be noted that even virulent *Brucella* are often killed within the phagolysosomes of macrophages, since fewer than 10% of the internalized bacteria survive to establish a replicative *Brucella*-containing vacuole (rBCV) (Fig. 2) (103). In contrast to *Mycobacterium* and *Chlamydia*, once internalized, the parasitophorous vacuole traffics along the endocytic pathway, acquiring early (104), as well as late, endosomal markers (105). There is even some limited interaction with host lysosomes, and the BCV acidifies transiently (106). After about 8 hours postinfection, the acidification of the BCV activates expression of the VirB-dependent type IV secretion system (T4SS) (107), named for its homology to the *Agrobacterium tumefaciens* virulence locus, directing the vacuole's escape from the endocytic pathway to set up an ER-associated rBCV (108, 109). It is within this compartment that *Brucella* replicates for up to 48 hours postinfection. Following replication, a subpopulation of *Brucella* traffics to a new subcellular compartment resembling an autophagosome, the aBCV (105). The precise signals

that induce aBCV formation are not understood, but these tertiary vacuoles appear to enhance the spread of *Brucella* to neighboring cells for a second round of infection. *Brucella* may also exit host cells as rough mutants that sporadically arise within the rBCV, causing host cell cytotoxicity and lysis. The released bacteria, an assortment of smooth and rough *Brucella*, then seed a new round of infection (110).

Trafficking to the ER Requires the Coordination of Several Bacterial and Host Cell Factors

Many host factors required for efficient *Brucella* replication have been identified, including Rho-family GTPases, SNARES, PtdIns(3) kinases, cytoskeletal proteins, and IRE1α, a kinase that regulates the unfolded protein response (UPR) and autophagosome formation (111). *Brucella* coordinates its trafficking through the secretion of a number of virulence factors and expression of proteins to resist the transient acidification of the BCV. Once it reaches the confines of the ER and has successfully evaded the terminal phagolysosome, it is safe to begin replication.

Endosomal trafficking of *Brucella* ends with acidification of the BCV

Unlike the other intracellular pathogens discussed in the first part of this chapter, *Brucella* stays within the endocytic trafficking pathway until it reaches a late stage. Smooth, nonopsonized *Brucella* entry into murine macrophages is dependent on lipid rafts (112), PtdIns(3) kinase (113), and TLR4 (114), and it fails to activate macrophages. Rough mutants, which lack O-antigen, enter cells independently of lipid rafts and are rapidly killed within activated macrophages (115–117). However, naturally rough *Brucella ovis* and *Brucella canis* are capable of lipid-raft-dependent entry (118), so there must be additional factors that regulate *Brucella* entry. Similar to *Chlamydia*, entry is also dependent on the host actin cytoskeleton. The small GTPase,

CDC42, which regulates actin polymerization through interaction with Wiskott-Aldrich syndrome protein, is recruited to and activated at the entry site (113).

Endosomal trafficking of the BCV proceeds with acquisition of early endosomal markers EEA1 and Rab5 (104, 108). Their association with the BCV is transient, because they are rapidly exchanged for the late endosomal markers Rab7, RILP, and LAMP1 (106). Acquisition of Rab7 and RILP are required for normal intracellular trafficking of *Brucella*, since expression of a dominant-negative Rab7 or overexpression of RILP interfered with conversion of the BCV to an ER-derived vacuole. As they traffic along the endosomal pathway, the BCV allow limited lysosomal fusion. Fusion with lysosomes can be observed up to about 12 hours postinfection, at which point the BCV loses its late endosomal markers. This study also confirmed that *Brucella* requires acidification for completion of its infectious cycle, because pharmacological inhibition of V-ATPases resulted in a dramatic decrease in viable bacteria (106, 108). This is likely because acidification is required for the activation of T4SS gene expression, which is crucial for setting up the rBCV (106–109, 119, 120).

Adaptations to resist degradation upon lysosomal fusion

Like *Chlamydia*, *Brucella* has evolved to escape destruction by trafficking away from the endocytic pathway before it can be degraded, but not before the BCV fuses with lysosomes. First, it should be noted that lysosomal fusion of the BCV is well controlled by the bacteria, and significantly less fusion occurs with virulent *Brucella* than with heat-killed bacteria (106). Cyclic-β-1,2-glucan, a critical virulence factor, has a role in decreasing lysosomal fusion by depletion of BCV membrane cholesterol (121). Nevertheless, the lumen of the BCV is acidified and does contain degradative enzymes. To mitigate the risk of destruction during this transition, *Brucellae* express several proteins to aid in resistance to the drop in pH, oxidative and nitrosative damage, and antimicrobial peptides (122).

Multiple *Brucella* proteins have been identified as having a role in acid resistance. HdeA, a homolog of the *E. coli* acid-resisting periplasmic chaperone, imparts acid resistance *in vitro* (123). CydB was found to contribute to both acid tolerance and resistance to ROS (124). Disruption of the *cydB* gene demonstrated that cytochrome *bd* ubiquinol oxidase is required for intracellular survival and virulence. *Brucellae* also express a functional urease that protects the bacteria from extremely low pH and is presumed to allow safe passage of the bacteria through the gastrointestinal tract after ingestion, but it is not required for virulence in cultured cells (125).

Reduced pH is certainly not the only hazard that intracellular *Brucella* encounters, because ROS and RNS are key defense mechanisms employed by infected phagocytic cells. In fact, ROS and nitric oxide production have been shown to be important for microbicidal activity against *Brucella* in macrophages (126). SodC, a Cu/Zn superoxide dismutase that counteracts ROS production, is required by *B. abortus* for survival within macrophages and virulence in a mouse model of infection (127). To resist the deleterious effects of RNS, *Brucella* generate nitric oxide reductase to detoxify NO within macrophages (128, 129). *Brucella* also enlist AhpC, a peroxiredoxin that is primarily involved in scavenging endogenous ROS generated by *Brucella* metabolism (130), to impart some resistance to peroxynitrite (122).

Finally, the lysosomes of macrophages contain cationic antimicrobial peptides called defensins that pose a threat to bacteria by creating pores in their outer membranes (12). The BvRS two-component regulatory system controls the expression of genes responsible for the acylation status of lipid A (131). Without this important modification of LPS, BvRS mutants are more susceptible to destruction by cationic antimicrobial peptides due to their altered membrane properties. It is evident that *Brucellae* have evolved many solutions to the problem of requiring lysosomal fusion for replication by expressing proteins that impart resistance to the myriad hazards encountered during endocytic trafficking.

The carefully coordinated transition to the ER begins the replicative phase of the *Brucella* infection

In epithelial cells, prior to ER fusion, the BCV has a short-lived association with autophagosomes. The BCVs acquire the autophagosome marker monodansylcadaverine and have a multilamellar appearance (104, 132). An autophagy-related protein IRE1α, is required for *Brucella* replication at this stage (111). IRE1α is a kinase that regulates the host UPR as well as the generation of ER-derived autophagosomes. Its role in autophagy induction was highlighted as part of the ER-fusion process, because other kinases involved in the UPR were not found to be important for *Brucella* replication in that study (111). However, this autophagic transition prior to ER fusion is not observed in macrophages. Interestingly, the UPR is induced in *Brucella*-infected macrophages and is required for efficient replication (133). The microtubule-associated *Brucella* protein TcpB has been identified as playing an important role in UPR induction in these cells. It is not surprising that the UPR is induced by *Brucella* infection, because a major reorganization of the ER is required for replication, but the idea that *Brucella* may actively induce the process is intriguing.

Brucella–ER fusion, which is required for bacterial replication, is carefully coordinated by secreted virulence factors. BCV–ER fusion requires the small GTPase Rab2, which is part of a multiprotein complex that regulates vesicular trafficking from the Golgi to the ER. Inhibition of Rab2 results in retention of LAMP1 on BCVs (134). A *Brucella* type IV secretion effector RicA has been implicated in initiating Rab2 recruitment through its interactions with the small GTPase (135, 136). Another *Brucella*-secreted protein, CstA, which interacts with the ER exit site–associated protein Sec24A, has recently been discovered as having a role in ER fusion of the BCV. Deletion mutants of *cstA* have delayed trafficking to the ER relative to wild type *B. abortus* (137). Secretion of CstA into cell culture supernatants appears to be dependent on flagellar genes, not type IV secretion, but more work must be done to confirm its secretion in infected cells. Several other type IV substrates have been identified as ER-localized during infection. *Brucella* effectors BspA, BspB, and BspF disrupt the host secretory pathway and inhibit host protein secretion (138). While deletion of these individual effectors does not significantly affect *Brucella* replication, the triple deletion mutant *ΔbspABF* displays reduced intracellular replication and virulence in a mouse model of chronic infection (138).

As BCVs lose fusogenicity with lysosomes, they progressively merge with the ER and acquire markers of this new subcellular compartment that is pH-neutral and represents a safe haven for replication. BCVs initially contact the ER at ER exit sites through interactions with the Sar1/COPII complex (139). Inhibition of Sar1 prevents BCV-ER fusion and results in a block in replication. Other ER-specific proteins found on rBCVs include calnexin, calreticulin, and Sec61 (104, 108). The rBCV membrane is also studded with ribosomes. The ER-targeted RNA-interference screen that identified IRE1α also found 29 other novel host ER proteins to be important for virulence, including important regulators of vesicular trafficking and host protein biosynthesis, as well as cytoskeletal proteins (111). As *Brucella* replicates in this new compartment, the rBCV membrane septates with the bacteria, so they continue to reside singly in tight vacuoles as the host cell fills with bacteria.

Following the replicative phase, egress from the host cells is poorly characterized, but two complementary hypotheses describing an exit route for *Brucella* have been proposed. Starr et al. described the formation of the late autophagosome-like aBCV, which appears to promote the spread of Brucella to neighboring uninfected cells (105). aBCV formation was observed at 72 hours postinfection, when rBCVs appear to transition back into a LAMP1-positive subcellular compartment and lose the ER marker calreticulin. Although the cells that harbor aBCVs make up a subset of the infected cell population, those cells had a tendency to form reinfection foci within the monolayer, suggesting that aBCVs offer a mode of egress for *Brucella* (105). Another method of host cell exit may involve a change in the LPS status of replicating *Brucella*. Spontaneous dissociation of smooth *Brucella* to rough mutants with truncated LPS O-antigen has been observed during infection of murine macrophages. Rough *Brucella* are cytotoxic to macrophages and cause host cell lysis. A recent report demonstrated that the subpopulation of rough mutants that arises during infection with *B. melitensis* enhances cell-to-cell spread of the bacteria by causing host cell lysis and release of smooth *Brucella* along with the sporadic rough mutants (110). Neither exit mechanism excludes the other, nor would it be surprising to find that like *Chlamydia*, *Brucella* uses more than one exit strategy.

Brucella has a unique strategy for setting up its replicative niche. Although trafficking to ER-derived replicative vacuoles is not specific to *Brucella*, the fact that it allows lysosomal fusion prior to arriving in this protected compartment is fairly distinctive. Utilizing the acidic environment of the late endosome as a signal to activate virulence genes and coordinate its escape to the ER is not without risk. Recall that over 90% of the bacteria that attempt to colonize macrophages meet an untimely demise. For the remaining 10%, the tools that *Brucella* employs to resist destruction are effective and allow it to hide within phagocytic cells for protracted periods of time, making brucellosis a particularly unpleasant disease to contract.

COXIELLA

C. burnetii is a Gram-negative, naturally obligate intracellular pathogen that causes Q fever in humans, a flu-like illness that is generally self-limiting and readily resolves without antibiotics. The organism has an extremely wide zoonotic host range that spans mammals, arthropods, fish, and avian species. *C. burnetii* RSA439 a clonal isolate that is avirulent and has a rough LPS phenotype (phase II), can be studied in a biosafety level 2 environment. *C. burnetii* isolates cause either acute or chronic disease, and phylogenetic studies show that they cluster into three clades corresponding to their clinical presentation. Experimental animal models support the hypothesis that there are three specific pathotypes of *Coxiella* (140). Recent outbreaks have highlighted the continually emerging nature of this pathogen (141), and the significant impact of *Coxiella* on U.S. military personnel in Iraq and Afghanistan demonstrates the endemic nature of the disease (142).

Coxiella Alternates Between Two Morphologies During Its Developmental Lifecycle

The highly infectious nature of *C. burnetii* is partially due to its ability to survive in the environment for long periods of time in its metabolically inactive, small cell variant (SCV) form. Replication in a range of developmental stages is similar in design, but not in mechanism, to that described for *Chlamydia*. In the current model, SCVs are predominantly extracellular, and while they are environmentally resistant, they are incapable of replication. After SCVs invade host cells, they transition to the metabolically active large cell variant (LCV) form following the acidification of the *Coxiella*-containing vacuole (CCV). The percentage of *Coxiella* organisms in the CCV that have transitioned to LCVs approaches 80% after 1 hour of infection, and by 16 hours the CCV contains exclusively LCVs (143, 144). LCVs replicate in an expanding CCV for 4 to 7 days, transitioning back to SCVs at later stages of the infection cycle, generating stable extracellular forms for future rounds of infection.

Completion of the *Coxiella* Infection Cycle Requires Replication in a Phagolysosome-Like Compartment

Unlike the vacuolar pathogens discussed to this point, *Coxiella* allows phagosomal trafficking to proceed all the way to lysosomal fusion. Development of the CCV involves a combination of normal phagosomal trafficking and pathogen-directed manipulation of host processes. The end result is a niche that represents a hostile environment to most other pathogens and is therefore free of competitors.

Adhesion and invasion

After aerosol transmission, *C. burnetii* targets alveolar macrophages and passively enters these cells by actin-dependent phagocytosis (145, 146). Recent studies using T4SS mutants that have no defect in their ability to infect either phagocytic or nonphagocytic cells (147, 148) support the hypothesis that entry into phagocytic cells proceeds via host-driven actin-dependent phagocytosis. Virulent *C. burnetii* binds to phagocytic cells (monocytes/macrophages) using $\alpha_V\beta_3$ integrin as the main receptor and are taken up into the cell via a Rac1-dependent phagocytosis that depends on membrane ruffling (149, 150).

Histopathologic analysis in both animal models of pneumonia and in humans with atypical pneumonia caused by *C. burnetii* primarily identified monocyte/macrophage infection, but epithelial and endothelial cell infection has also been reported (151). Nonphagocytic cells do not usually engulf large particles, but intracellular pathogens can invade after direct contact through a zippering of bacterial ligands to host cell receptors. While the identities of the host receptors for *Coxiella* on nonprofessional phagocytes remain to be determined, the mechanism of

entry also appears to be dependent on actin rearrangement (145). Recently, a *Coxiella* protein that is required for invasion of epithelial cells was identified. Mutants in CBU1260, which encodes the invasin OmpA, exhibit an epithelial cell-specific entry defect (173). Interestingly, attachment to epithelial cells is unaffected by mutation of CBU1260, indicating that binding and entry of *Coxiella* are independent processes. Despite the invasion defect observed in nonphagocytic cells, actin rearrangement is unaffected by mutation of CBU1260 in THP-1 macrophages, highlighting again the host-driven nature of phagocytic uptake of *Coxiella*.

In a variety of tissue culture models *C. burnetii* phase variants exhibit distinct uptake kinetics whereby avirulent phase II bacteria are more readily internalized than fully virulent phase I bacteria (145, 146). However, both variants replicate with similar kinetics within an indistinguishable, proteolytically active CCV in a variety of tissue culture cell lines (152), which is important to note, because the majority of studies that examine intracellular trafficking have used the avirulent phase II *C. burnetii* (153).

Trafficking from the phagosome to the CCV

Phagocytosis results in the formation of the phagosome, which matures into a phagolysosome following a series of highly ordered and regulated fusion and fission events (12). The maturation of the CCV essentially follows the general phagocytic pathway, terminating in a compartment that strongly resembles a mature phagolysosome (140). After internalization, the nascent CCV is similar in size to an endosome, and it traffics through the pathway described above as indicated by the sequential recruitment of Rab5 and Rab7 (Fig. 2) (153). A hallmark of *Coxiella* infection is a marked expansion in CCV size during maturation, prior to when the majority of LCV replication begins, resulting in an extremely spacious vacuole at early stages of infection. Functional inhibition of both Rab5 and Rab7 by overexpression of dominant negative forms of these proteins impairs large vacuole formation (153). Furthermore, formation of a spacious CCV is dependent on de novo *C. burnetii* protein synthesis, as well as secretion of T4SS effectors across the CCV membrane into the host cytoplasm (147, 154). Indeed, a growing number of *Coxiella* T4SS substrates are known to be required for CCV expansion, and several effectors have recently been shown to localize the CCV membrane during infection (155). However, in the absence of protein synthesis, small CCVs still acquire LAMP proteins and acidify, suggesting that acquisition of LAMPs and acidification are a consequence of the normal progression of phagosomal trafficking (156).

Coxiella is unlike the intracellular pathogens discussed so far, which disrupt the endosomal cascade or arrest maturation of the phagosome, thereby avoiding lysosomal fusion (157). In the case of *C. burnetii* infection, lysosomal enzymes including cathepsin D and acid phosphatase, accumulate within the CCV by 1 to 2 hours postinfection (144), a protracted time course compared to the 15 minutes required for phagosomes harboring inert particles. The observed delay is dependent upon *C. burnetii* protein synthesis, suggesting it is a pathogen-induced process (144, 158, 159). While the delay in lysosomal fusion of the CCV requires bacterial protein synthesis, the T4SS is an unlikely mediator of the process, because secretion is not detected until at least 8 hours postinfection (148). There is some evidence that interaction with the autophagy pathway contributes to this delayed phagosomal maturation (153). Autophagy serves as an innate host defense against many intracellular pathogens (160), and as early as 5 minutes after internalization, the phase II CCV is decorated with the autophagy marker microtubule-associated protein light-chain 3 (Fig. 2) (153, 161). However, *C. burnetii* may benefit from this early interaction with autophagosomes as autophagy induction in infected cells increases CCV size (162).

Survival inside a degradative vacuole

C. burnetii has adapted to replicate in the very compartment that *Mycobacterium*, *Chlamydia*, and *Brucella* have evolved to avoid. In fact, the metabolic activity of *Coxiella* is activated in response to the reduced pH of the nascent CCV (143, 144). As mentioned above, the CCV acquires degradative cathepsin D as well as acid phosphatase soon after infection (144). Other normally bactericidal contents of a lysosome include ROS and RNS, and *Coxiella* may employ various strategies to resist these deadly host defenses against infection (163). Upon host cell invasion, *Coxiella* upregulates transcription of stress response genes, which may serve to protect its DNA from the damaging effects of ROS (164). To supplement its SOS response, the *Coxiella* genome encodes several genes that enable the bacterium to resist the damaging effects of oxidative stress. An acid phosphatase, encoded by CBU0335, can suppress ROS production in neutrophils by preventing the assembly of host NADPH phagocyte oxidase (165), a major generator of superoxide radicals. *Coxiella* also expresses ROS scavenging systems for the direct detoxification of superoxide. *C. burnetii* encodes a functional cytoplasmic FeSOD (CBU1708) that complemented a double *sodA sodC* mutant strain of *E. coli* under conditions of oxidative stress (166). Other gene products that may take part in ROS scavenging include a periplasmic Cu/ZnSOD (CBU1822) and two alkyl hydroperoxide reductases, AhpC1 (CBU1706) and AhpC2D (CBU1477-1478). Resistance to acid may also be imparted by the expression of a large number of basic proteins, because close to 45% of *C. burnetii* proteins have a predicted pI $\geq$ 9 (167). While *C. burnetii* certainly has a cohort of genetic tools that may impart resistance to damaging phagolysosomal contents, they are not likely to be their first line of defense. A study by Brennan et al. illustrated that *C. burnetii* infection is well-controlled by the host's oxidative burst (168). As a stealth pathogen, it is probably *Coxiella*'s ability to infect macrophages without alerting the innate immune response that serves as its primary mechanism to avoid killing due to oxidative stress.

Expansion of the CCV into a spacious and replication competent compartment

The CCV enlarges dramatically between 8 hours and 2 days postinfection and can occupy nearly the entire space of the host cell (169). In the case of multiply infected cells, the formation of a large CCV is due to homotypic fusion of several smaller CCVs, while the expansion of the compartment proceeds through heterotypic fusion with autophagic, endocytic, and lysosomal vesicles (154, 156). The development of the CCVs not only requires bacterial protein synthesis (156), but several host proteins are also necessary. The actin cytoskeleton supports CCV development, and treatment with actin-depolymerizing agents results in the formation of only small CCVs (170). Additionally, *C. burnetii* infection activates several host cell kinases, including protein kinase C, protein kinase A, and myosin light chain kinase, all of which are required for the establishment and maintenance of the CCV (171). The parasitophorous vacuole also interacts with the early secretory pathway, because Rab1b accumulates on the CCV membrane, an interaction which is required for the formation of the large CCV (Fig. 2) (172). Interaction with the ER through the early secretory pathway may provide another source of membrane for the formation of a spacious CCV (172). The large number of cellular processes that are coordinated during *Coxiella* infection suggest that many virulence factors that direct the formation of the CCV remain to be identified.

C. burnetii is a unique bacterium in that it is specifically adapted to infect immune cells that are employed to destroy invading pathogens. Not only does it infect a particularly restrictive cell type, but it replicates within a niche that is especially hostile toward bacteria in general. It utilizes the low pH of the CCV to activate its metabolism, as well as its pathogenic program of type IV secreted substrates. It has adapted to resist the toxic ROS and RNS, as well as the degradative enzymes resident within lysosomes. Life in a CCV affords *Coxiella* some very important benefits in the form of acquired immune evasion and reduced competition from other pathogens. However, it is little wonder why other pathogens have evolved to avoid growth under these same conditions.

CONCLUSION

Intracellular pathogens have evolved many unique and elegant strategies for survival within host cells. Entry via phagocytosis does not necessarily sentence a pathogen to death in a phagolysosome. Some bacteria manage to break free of their phagosome to replicate in the nutrient-rich cytosol. For those that spend the duration of their intracellular life inside a vacuole, there are myriad ways to customize the replicative niche. The problem of lysosomal fusion can be avoided by stalling trafficking, as in the case of *M. tuberculosis*, or by diverting the vacuole from the endocytic pathway entirely, like *Chlamydia* and *Brucella*. For *C. burnetii*, lysosomal fusion is not avoided but is required for metabolic activation and replication. Whenever a pathogen adapts to a specific intracellular niche, its lifestyle is shaped by the innate immune defenses therein. For bacteria that replicate primarily in phagocytic cells, such as *M. tuberculosis* and *Coxiella*, the oxidative burst is a major evolutionary driver. Although they each inhabit and replicate in very different subcellular compartments, *M. tuberculosis*, *Chlamydia*, *Brucella*, and *Coxiella* are all very successful pathogens that can serve as valuable tools to enlighten our knowledge of host cell trafficking and immunity.

ACKNOWLEDGMENTS

We are grateful to Erin van Schaik for helpful discussions and critical reading of the manuscript.

This review was supported by grants from the Defense Threat Reduction Agency (DTRA) and the National Institute of Allergy and Infectious Diseases (NIAID) grant RO1AI090142 to J. Samuel. Any opinions, findings, and conclusions or recommendations expressed in this material are those of the author(s) and do not necessarily reflect the views of the funding agencies.

CITATION

Case EDR, Samuel JE. 2016. Contrasting lifestyles within the host cell. Microbiol Spectrum 4(1):VMBF-0014-2015.

REFERENCES

1. **Fredlund J, Enninga J.** 2014. Cytoplasmic access by intracellular bacterial pathogens. *Trends Microbiol* **22:**128–137.

2. **Gomes LC, Dikic I.** 2014. Autophagy in antimicrobial immunity. *Mol Cell* **54:**224–233.

3. **Kinchen JM, Ravichandran KS.** 2008. Phagosome maturation: going through the acid test. *Nat Rev Mol Cell Biol* **9:**781–795.

4. **Vieira OV, Botelho RJ, Rameh L, Brachmann SM, Matsuo T, Davidson HW, Schreiber A, Backer JM, Cantley LC, Grinstein S.** 2001. Distinct roles of class I and class III phosphatidyl-inositol 3-kinases in phagosome formation and maturation. *J Cell Biol* **155:**19–25.

5. **Di Paolo G, De Camilli P.** 2006. Phosphoinositides in cell regulation and membrane dynamics. *Nature* **443:**651–657.

6. **Simonsen A, Lippe R, Christoforidis S, Gaullier J-M, Brech A, Callaghan J, Toh B-H, Murphy C, Zerial M, Stenmark H.** 1998. EEA1 links PI(3)K function to Rab5 regulation of endosome fusion. *Nature* **394:**494–498.

7. **Hackam DJ, Rotstein OD, Zhang W-J, Demaurex N, Woodside M, Tsai O, Grinstein S.** 1997. Regulation of phagosomal acidification: differential targeting of Na$^+$/H$^+$ exchangers, Na$^+$/K$^+$-ATPases, and vacuolar-type H$^+$-ATPases. *J Biol Chem* **272:**29810–29820.

8. **Kinchen JM, Ravichandran KS.** 2010. Identification of two evolutionarily conserved genes regulating processing of engulfed apoptotic cells. *Nature* **464:**778–782.

9. **Poteryaev D, Datta S, Ackema K, Zerial M, Spang A.** 2010. Identification of the switch in early-to-late endosome transition. *Cell* **141:**497–508.

10. **Huynh KK, Eskelinen EL, Scott CC, Malevanets A, Saftig P, Grinstein S.** 2007. LAMP proteins are required for fusion of lysosomes with phagosomes. *EMBO J* **26:**313–324.

11. **Harrison RE, Bucci C, Vieira OV, Schroer TA, Grinstein S.** 2003. Phagosomes fuse with late endosomes and/or lysosomes by extension of membrane protrusions along microtubules: role of Rab7 and RILP. *Mol Cell Biol* **23:**6494–6506.

12. **Flannagan RS, Jaumouillé V, Grinstein S.** 2012. The cell biology of phagocytosis. *Annu Rev Pathol* **7:**61–98.

13. **Jabado N, Jankowski A, Dougaparsad S, Picard V, Grinstein S, Gros P.** 2000. Natural resistance to intracellular infections: natural resistance–associated macrophage protein 1 (Nramp1) functions as a pH-dependent manganese transporter at the phagosomal membrane. *J Exp Med* **192:**1237–1248.

14. **Yates RM, Hermetter A, Russell DG.** 2005. The kinetics of phagosome maturation as a function of phagosome/lysosome fusion and acquisition of hydrolytic activity. *Traffic* **6:**413–420.

15. **Zumla A, Raviglione M, Hafner R, von Reyn CF.** 2013. Tuberculosis. *N Engl J Med* **368:**745–755.

16. **Forrellad MA, Klepp LI, Gioffre A, Sabio y Garcia J, Morbidoni HR, de la Paz Santangelo M, Cataldi AA, Bigi F.** 2013. Virulence factors of the *Mycobacterium tuberculosis* complex. *Virulence* **4:**3–66.

17. **Matteelli A, Roggi A, Carvalho AC.** 2014. Extensively drug-resistant tuberculosis: epidemiology and management. *Clin Epidemiol* **6:**111–118.

18. **Vergne I, Chua J, Singh SB, Deretic V.** 2004. Cell biology of *Mycobacterium tuberculosis* phagosome. *Annu Rev Cell Dev Biol* **20:**367–394.

19. **Cambier CJ, Falkow S, Ramakrishnan L.** 2014. Host evasion and exploitation schemes of *Mycobacterium tuberculosis*. *Cell* **159:**1497–1509.

20. **Clemens DL, Horwitz MA.** 1995. Characterization of the *Mycobacterium tuberculosis* phagosome and evidence that phagosomal maturation is inhibited. *J Exp Med* **181:**257–270.

21. **Via LE, Deretic D, Ulmer RJ, Hibler NS, Huber LA, Deretic V.** 1997. Arrest of mycobacterial phagosome maturation is caused by a block in vesicle fusion between stages controlled by Rab5 and Rab7. *J Biol Chem* **272:**13326–13331.

22. **Kang BK, Schlesinger LS.** 1998. Characterization of mannose receptor-dependent phagocytosis mediated by *Mycobacterium tuberculosis* lipoarabinomannan. *Infect Immun* **66:**2769–2777.

23. **Ernst JD.** 1998. Macrophage receptors for *Mycobacterium tuberculosis*. *Infect Immun* **66:** 1277–1281.

24. **Gatfield J, Pieters J.** 2000. Essential role for cholesterol in entry of mycobacteria into macrophages. *Science* **288:**1647–1650.

25. **Clemens DL, Lee BY, Horwitz MA.** 2000. *Mycobacterium tuberculosis* and *Legionella pneumophila* phagosomes exhibit arrested maturation despite acquisition of Rab7. *Infect Immun* **68:**5154–5166.

26. **Clemens DL, Lee BY, Horwitz MA.** 2000. Deviant expression of Rab5 on phagosomes containing the intracellular pathogens *Mycobacterium tuberculosis* and *Legionella pneumophila* is associated with altered phagosomal fate. *Infect Immun* **68:**2671–2684.

27. **Vergne I, Chua J, Deretic V.** 2003. Tuberculosis toxin blocking phagosome maturation inhibits a novel Ca^{2+}/calmodulin-PI3K hVPS34 cascade. *J Exp Med* **198:**653–659.

28. **Malik ZA, Denning GM, Kusner DJ.** 2000. Inhibition of Ca(2+) signaling by *Mycobacterium tuberculosis* is associated with reduced phagosome-lysosome fusion and increased survival within human macrophages. *J Exp Med* **191:**287–302.

29. **Fratti RA, Chua J, Deretic V.** 2003. Induction of p38 mitogen-activated protein kinase reduces early endosome autoantigen 1 (EEA1) recruitment to phagosomal membranes. *J Biol Chem* **278:**46961–46967.

30. **Cavalli V, Vilbois F, Corti M, Marcote MJ, Tamura K, Karin M, Arkinstall S, Gruenberg J.** 2001. The stress-induced MAP kinase p38 regulates endocytic trafficking via the GDI: Rab5 complex. *Mol Cell* **7:**421–432.

31. **Fratti RA, Chua J, Vergne I, Deretic V.** 2003. *Mycobacterium tuberculosis* glycosylated phosphatidylinositol causes phagosome maturation arrest. *Proc Natl Acad Sci USA* **100:**5437–5442.

32. **Indrigo J, Hunter RL Jr, Actor JK.** 2003. Cord factor trehalose 6,6'-dimycolate (TDM) mediates trafficking events during mycobacterial infection of murine macrophages. *Microbiology* **149:**2049–2059.

33. **Sun J, Wang X, Lau A, Liao TY, Bucci C, Hmama Z.** 2010. Mycobacterial nucleoside diphosphate kinase blocks phagosome maturation in murine RAW 264.7 macrophages. *PLoS One* **5:**e8769. doi:10.1371/journal.pone.0008769.

34. **Wong D, Bach H, Sun J, Hmama Z, Av-Gay Y.** 2011. *Mycobacterium tuberculosis* protein tyrosine phosphatase (PtpA) excludes host vacuolar-H^+-ATPase to inhibit phagosome acidification. *Proc Natl Acad Sci USA* **108:**19371–19376.

35. **Miller BH, Fratti RA, Poschet JF, Timmins GS, Master SS, Burgos M, Marletta MA, Deretic V.** 2004. Mycobacteria inhibit nitric oxide synthase recruitment to phagosomes during macrophage infection. *Infect Immun* **72:** 2872–2878.

36. **Davis AS, Vergne I, Master SS, Kyei GB, Chua J, Deretic V.** 2007. Mechanism of inducible nitric oxide synthase exclusion from mycobacterial phagosomes. *PLoS Pathog* **3:**e186.

37. **Vergne I, Fratti RA, Hill PJ, Chua J, Belisle J, Deretic V.** 2004. *Mycobacterium tuberculosis* phagosome maturation arrest: mycobacterial phosphatidylinositol analog phosphatidylinositol mannoside stimulates early endosomal fusion. *Mol Biol Cell* **15:**751–760.

38. **Clemens DL, Horwitz MA.** 1996. The *Mycobacterium tuberculosis* phagosome interacts with early endosomes and is accessible to exogenously administered transferrin. *J Exp Med* **184:**1349–1355.

39. **Chauhan R, Mande SC.** 2001. Characterization of the *Mycobacterium tuberculosis* H37Rv alkyl hydroperoxidase AhpC points to the importance of ionic interactions in oligomerization and activity. *Biochem J* **354:**209–215.

40. **Master SS, Springer B, Sander P, Boettger EC, Deretic V, Timmins GS.** 2002. Oxidative stress response genes in *Mycobacterium tuberculosis*: role of ahpC in resistance to peroxynitrite and stage-specific survival in macrophages. *Microbiology* **148:**3139–3144.

41. **Heym B, Stavropoulos E, Honore N, Domenech P, Saint-Joanis B, Wilson TM, Collins DM, Colston MJ, Cole ST.** 1997. Effects of overexpression of the alkyl hydroperoxide reductase AhpC on the virulence and isoniazid resistance of *Mycobacterium tuberculosis*. *Infect Immun* **65:** 1395–1401.

42. **Li Z, Kelley C, Collins F, Rouse D, Morris S.** 1998. Expression of katG in *Mycobacterium tuberculosis* is associated with its growth and persistence in mice and guinea pigs. *J Infect Dis* **177:**1030–1035.

43. **Hu Y, Coates AR.** 2009. Acute and persistent *Mycobacterium tuberculosis* infections depend on the thiol peroxidase TpX. *PLoS One* **4:**e5150.

44. **Piddington DL, Fang FC, Laessig T, Cooper AM, Orme IM, Buchmeier NA.** 2001. Cu,Zn superoxide dismutase of *Mycobacterium tuberculosis* contributes to survival in activated macrophages that are generating an oxidative burst. *Infect Immun* **69:**4980–4987.

45. **Stewart GR, Newton SM, Wilkinson KA, Humphreys IR, Murphy HN, Robertson BD, Wilkinson RJ, Young DB.** 2005. The stress-responsive chaperone alpha-crystallin

2 is required for pathogenesis of *Mycobacterium tuberculosis*. *Mol Microbiol* **55:**1127–1137.

46. **Vandal OH, Roberts JA, Odaira T, Schnappinger D, Nathan CF, Ehrt S.** 2009. Acid-susceptible mutants of *Mycobacterium tuberculosis* share hypersusceptibility to cell wall and oxidative stress and to the host environment. *J Bacteriol* **191:**625–631.

47. **Johnson NB, Hayes LD, Brown K, Hoo EC, Ethier KA, Centers for Disease Control and Prevention.** 2014. CDC National Health Report: leading causes of morbidity and mortality and associated behavioral risk and protective factors: United States, 2005-2013. *MMWR Surveill Summ* **63**(Suppl 4):3–27.

48. **Hahn DL, Schure A, Patel K, Childs T, Drizik E, Webley W.** 2012. *Chlamydia pneumoniae*-specific IgE is prevalent in asthma and is associated with disease severity. *PLoS One* **7:** e35945. doi:10.1371/journal.pone.0035945.

49. **Honarmand H.** 2013. Atherosclerosis induced by *Chlamydophila pneumoniae*: a controversial theory. *Interdisc Perspect Infect Dis* **2013:**941392.

50. **Harkinezhad T, Geens T, Vanrompay D.** 2009. *Chlamydo-philapsittaci* infections in birds: a review with emphasis on zoonotic consequences. *Vet Microbiol* **135:**68–77.

51. **Clifton DR, Fields KA, Grieshaber SS, Dooley CA, Fischer ER, Mead DJ, Carabeo RA, Hackstadt T.** 2004. A chlamydial type III translocated protein is tyrosine-phosphorylated at the site of entry and associated with recruitment of actin. *Proc Natl Acad Sci USA* **101:** 10166–10171.

52. **Hybiske K, Stephens RS.** 2007. Mechanisms of host cell exit by the intracellular bacterium *Chlamydia*. *Proc Natl Acad Sci USA* **104:**11430–11435.

53. **Clifton DR, Dooley CA, Grieshaber SS, Carabeo RA, Fields KA, Hackstadt T.** 2005. Tyrosine phosphorylation of the chlamydial effector protein Tarp is species specific and not required for recruitment of actin. *Infect Immun* **73:**3860–3868.

54. **Jewett TJ, Fischer ER, Mead DJ, Hackstadt T.** 2006. Chlamydial TARP is a bacterial nucleator of actin. *Proc Natl Acad Sci USA* **103:**15599–15604.

55. **Kumar Y, Valdivia RH.** 2008. Actin and intermediate filaments stabilize the *Chlamydia trachomatis* vacuole by forming dynamic structural scaffolds. *Cell Host Microbe* **4:**159–169.

56. **Hackstadt T, Rockey D, Heinzen R, Scidmore M.** 1996. *Chlamydia trachomatis* interrupts an exocytic pathway to acquire endogenously synthesized sphingomyelin in transit from the Golgi apparatus to the plasma membrane. *EMBO J* **15:**964–977.

57. **Hackstadt T, Scidmore MA, Rockey DD.** 1995. Lipid metabolism in *Chlamydia trachomatis*-infected cells: directed trafficking of Golgi-derived sphingolipids to the chlamydial inclusion. *Proc Natl Acad Sci USA* **92:**4877–4881.

58. **Damiani MT, Gambarte Tudela J, Capmany A.** 2014. Targeting eukaryotic Rab proteins: a smart strategy for chlamydial survival and replication. *Cell Microbiol* **16:**1329–1338.

59. **Bastidas RJ, Elwell CA, Engel JN, Valdivia RH.** 2013. Chlamydial intracellular survival strategies. *Cold Spring Harbor Perspect Med* **3:**a010256.

60. **Scidmore MA, Fischer ER, Hackstadt T.** 2003. Restricted fusion of *Chlamydia trachomatis* vesicles with endocytic compartments during the initial stages of infection. *Infect Immun* **71:**973–984.

61. **Heinzen RA, Scidmore MA, Rockey DD, Hackstadt T.** 1996. Differential interaction with endocytic and exocytic pathways distinguish parasitophorous vacuoles of *Coxiella burnetii* and *Chlamydia trachomatis*. *Infect Immun* **64:**796–809.

62. **Schramm N, Bagnell CR, Wyrick PB.** 1996. Vesicles containing *Chlamydia trachomatis* serovar L2 remain above pH 6 within HEC-1B cells. *Infect Immun* **64:**1208–1214.

63. **Ouellette SP, Dorsey FC, Moshiach S, Cleveland JL, Carabeo RA.** 2011. Chlamydia species-dependent differences in the growth requirement for lysosomes. *PLoS One* **6:**e16783. doi:10.1371/journal.pone.0016783.

64. **Carabeo RA, Dooley CA, Grieshaber SS, Hackstadt T.** 2007. Rac interacts with Abi-1 and WAVE2 to promote an Arp2/3-dependent actin recruitment during chlamydial invasion. *Cell Microbiol* **9:**2278–2288.

65. **Lane BJ, Mutchler C, Al Khodor S, Grieshaber SS, Carabeo RA.** 2008. Chlamydial entry involves TARP binding of guanine nucleotide exchange factors. *PLoS Pathog* **4:**e1000014. doi:10.1371/journal.ppat.1000014.

66. **Belland RJ, Scidmore MA, Crane DD, Hogan DM, Whitmire W, McClarty G, Caldwell HD.** 2001. *Chlamydia trachomatis* cytotoxicity associated with complete and partial cytotoxin genes. *Proc Natl Acad Sci USA* **98:**13984–13989.

67. **Thalmann J, Janik K, May M, Sommer K, Ebeling J, Hofmann F, Genth H, Klos A.** 2010. Actin re-organization induced by *Chlamydia trachomatis* serovar D: evidence for a critical role of the effector protein CT166 targeting Rac. *PLoS One* **5:**e9887. doi:10.1371/journal.pone.0009887.

68. **Hower S, Wolf K, Fields KA.** 2009. Evidence that CT694 is a novel *Chlamydia trachomatis* T3S substrate capable of functioning during invasion or early cycle development. *Mol Microbiol* **72:**1423–1437.

69. **Grieshaber SS, Grieshaber NA, Hackstadt T.** 2003. *Chlamydia trachomatis* uses host cell dynein to traffic to the microtubule-organizing center in a p50 dynamitin-independent process. *J Cell Sci* **116:**3793–3802.

70. **Mital J, Miller NJ, Fischer ER, Hackstadt T.** 2010. Specific chlamydial inclusion membrane proteins associate with active Src family kinases in microdomains that interact with the host microtubule network. *Cell Microbiol* **12:**1235–1249.

71. **Campbell S, Richmond SJ, Yates PS.** 1989. The effect of *Chlamydia trachomatis* infection on the host cell cytoskeleton and membrane compartments. *J Gen Microbiol* **135:**2379–2386.

72. **Lutter EI, Barger AC, Nair V, Hackstadt T.** 2013. *Chlamydia trachomatis* inclusion membrane protein CT228 recruits elements of the myosin phosphatase pathway to regulate release mechanisms. *Cell Rep* **3:**1921–1931.

73. **Elwell CA, Engel JN.** 2012. Lipid acquisition by intracellular *Chlamydiae*. *Cell Microbiol* **14:**1010–1018.

74. **Rockey DD, Fischer ER, Hackstadt T.** 1996. Temporal analysis of the developing *Chlamydia psittaci* inclusion by use of fluorescence and electron microscopy. *Infect Immun* **64:** 4269–4278.

75. **Wolf K, Hackstadt T.** 2001. Sphingomyelin trafficking in *Chlamydia pneumoniae*-infected cells. *Cell Microbiol* **3:**145–152.

76. **Moore ER, Fischer ER, Mead DJ, Hackstadt T.** 2008. The chlamydial inclusion preferentially intercepts basolaterally directed sphingomyelin-containing exocytic vacuoles. *Traffic* **9:**2130–2140.

77. **Derre I, Swiss R, Agaisse H.** 2011. The lipid transfer protein CERT interacts with the *Chlamydia* inclusion protein IncD and participates to ER-*Chlamydia* inclusion membrane contact sites. *PLoS Pathog* **7:**e1002092. doi:10.1371/journal.ppat.1002092.

78. **Elwell CA, Jiang S, Kim JH, Lee A, Wittmann T, Hanada K, Melancon P, Engel JN.** 2011. *Chlamydia trachomatis* co-opts GBF1 and CERT to acquire host sphingomyelin for distinct roles during intracellular development. *PLoS Pathog* **7:**e1002198. doi:10.1371/journal.ppat.1002198.

79. **Carabeo RA, Mead DJ, Hackstadt T.** 2003. Golgi-dependent transport of cholesterol to the *Chlamydia trachomatis* inclusion. *Proc Natl Acad Sci* **100:**6771–6776.

80. **Beatty WL.** 2008. Late endocytic multivesicular bodies intersect the chlamydial inclusion in the absence of CD63. *Infect Immun* **76:**2872–2881.

81. **Moorhead AM, Jung JY, Smirnov A, Kaufer S, Scidmore MA.** 2010. Multiple host proteins that function in phosphatidylinositol-4-phosphate metabolism are recruited to the chlamydial inclusion. *Infect Immun* **78:**1990–2007.

82. **Beatty WL.** 2006. Trafficking from CD63-positive late endocytic multivesicular bodies is essential for intracellular development of *Chlamydia trachomatis*. *J Cell Sci* **119:**350–359.

83. **Kumar Y, Cocchiaro J, Valdivia RH.** 2006. The obligate intracellular pathogen *Chlamydia trachomatis* targets host lipid droplets. *Curr Biol* **16:**1646–1651.

84. **Rzomp KA, Scholtes LD, Briggs BJ, Whittaker GR, Scidmore MA.** 2003. Rab GTPases are recruited to chlamydial inclusions in both a species-dependent and species-independent manner. *Infect Immun* **71:**5855–5870.

85. **Brumell JH, Scidmore MA.** 2007. Manipulation of rab GTPase function by intracellular bacterial pathogens. *Microbiol Mol Biol Rev* **71:**636–652.

86. **Rzomp KA, Moorhead AR, Scidmore MA.** 2006. The GTPase Rab4 interacts with *Chlamydia trachomatis* inclusion membrane protein CT229. *Infect Immun* **74:**5362–5373.

87. **Cortes C, Rzomp KA, Tvinnereim A, Scidmore MA, Wizel B.** 2007. *Chlamydia pneumoniae* inclusion membrane protein Cpn0585 interacts with multiple Rab GTPases. *Infect Immun* **75:** 5586–5596.

88. **Capmany A, Leiva N, Damiani MT.** 2011. Golgi-associated Rab14, a new regulator for *Chlamydia trachomatis* infection outcome. *Commun Integr Biol* **4:**590–593.

89. **Rejman Lipinski A, Heymann J, Meissner C, Karlas A, Brinkmann V, Meyer TF, Heuer D.** 2009. Rab6 and Rab11 regulate *Chlamydia trachomatis* development and golgin-84-dependent Golgi fragmentation. *PLoS Pathog* **5:**e1000615. doi:10.1371/journal.ppat.1000615.

90. **Ouellette SP, Carabeo RA.** 2010. A functional slow recycling pathway of transferrin is required for growth of *Chlamydia*. *Front Microbiol* **1:**112.

91. **Robertson DK, Gu L, Rowe RK, Beatty WL.** 2009. Inclusion biogenesis and reactivation of persistent *Chlamydia trachomatis* requires host cell sphingolipid biosynthesis. *PLoS Pathog* **5:** e1000664. doi:10.1371/journal.ppat.1000664.

92. **Matsumoto A, Bessho H, Uehira K, Suda T.** 1991. Morphological studies of the association of mitochondria with chlamydial inclusions

and the fusion of chlamydial inclusions. *J Electron Microsc* **40**:356–363.

93. **Peterson EM, de la Maza LM.** 1988. *Chlamydia* parasitism: ultrastructural characterization of the interaction between the chlamydial cell envelope and the host cell. *J Bacteriol* **170**:1389–1392.

94. **Derre I, Pypaert M, Dautry-Varsat A, Agaisse H.** 2007. RNAi screen in *Drosophila* cells reveals the involvement of the Tom complex in *Chlamydia* infection. *PLoS Pathog* **3**:1446–1458. doi:10.1371/journal.ppat.003015.

95. **McClarty G, Tipples G.** 1991. *In situ* studies on incorporation of nucleic acid precursors into *Chlamydia trachomatis* DNA. *J Bacteriol* **173**: 4922–4931.

96. **McClarty G, Fan H.** 1993. Purine metabolism by intracellular *Chlamydia psittaci*. *J Bacteriol* **175**:4662–4669.

97. **Bannantine JP, Griffiths RS, Viratyosin W, Brown WJ, Rockey DD.** 2000. A secondary structure motif predictive of protein localization to the chlamydial inclusion membrane. *Cell Microbiol* **2**:35–47.

98. **Dehoux P, Flores R, Dauga C, Zhong G, Subtil A.** 2011. Multi-genome identification and characterization of *Chlamydiae*-specific type III secretion substrates: the Inc proteins. *BMC Genomics* **12**:109.

99. **Franco MP, Mulder M, Gilman RH, Smits HL.** 2007. Human brucellosis. *Lancet Infect Dis* **7**:775–786.

100. **Bossi P, Tegnell A, Baka A, Van Loock F, Hendriks J, Werner A, Maidhof H, Gouvras G.** 2004. Bichat guidelines for the clinical management of brucellosis and bioterrorism-related brucellosis. *Euro Surveill* **9**:E15–E16. http://www.eurosurveillance.org/ViewArticle. aspx?ArticleId=506.

101. **Seleem MN, Boyle SM, Sriranganathan N.** 2010. Brucellosis: a re-emerging zoonosis. *Vet Microbiol* **140**:392–398.

102. **Gomez G, Adams LG, Rice-Ficht A, Ficht TA.** 2013. Host-*Brucella* interactions and the *Brucella* genome as tools for subunit antigen discovery and immunization against brucellosis. *Front Cell Infect Microbiol* **3**:17.

103. **von Bargen K, Gorvel JP, Salcedo SP.** 2012. Internal affairs: investigating the *Brucella* intracellular lifestyle. *FEMS Microbiol Rev* **36**:533–562.

104. **Pizarro-Cerda J, Meresse S, Parton RG, van der Goot G, Sola-Landa A, Lopez-Goni I, Moreno E, Gorvel JP.** 1998. *Brucella abortus* transits through the autophagic pathway and replicates in the endoplasmic reticulum of nonprofessional phagocytes. *Infect Immun* **66**:5711–5724.

105. **Starr T, Child R, Wehrly TD, Hansen B, Hwang S, Lopez-Otin C, Virgin HW, Celli J.** 2012. Selective subversion of autophagy complexes facilitates completion of the *Brucella* intracellular cycle. *Cell Host Microbe* **11**:33–45.

106. **Starr T, Ng TW, Wehrly TD, Knodler LA, Celli J.** 2008. *Brucella* intracellular replication requires trafficking through the late endosomal/lysosomal compartment. *Traffic* **9**:678–694.

107. **Boschiroli ML, Ouahrani-Bettache S, Foulongne V, Michaux-Charachon S, Bourg G, Allardet-Servent A, Cazevieille C, Lavigne JP, Liautard JP, Ramuz M, O'Callaghan D.** 2002. Type IV secretion and *Brucella* virulence. *Vet Microbiol* **90**:341–348.

108. **Celli J, de Chastellier C, Franchini DM, Pizarro-Cerda J, Moreno E, Gorvel JP.** 2003. *Brucella* evades macrophage killing via VirB-dependent sustained interactions with the endoplasmic reticulum. *J Exp Med* **198**:545–556.

109. **Comerci DJ, Martinez-Lorenzo MJ, Sieira R, Gorvel JP, Ugalde RA.** 2001. Essential role of the VirB machinery in the maturation of the *Brucella abortus*-containing vacuole. *Cell Microbiol* **3**:159–168.

110. **Pei J, Kahl-McDonagh M, Ficht TA.** 2014. *Brucella* dissociation is essential for macrophage egress and bacterial dissemination. *Front Cell Infect Microbiol* **4**:23.

111. **Qin QM, Pei J, Ancona V, Shaw BD, Ficht TA, de Figueiredo P.** 2008. RNAi screen of endoplasmic reticulum-associated host factors reveals a role for IRE1α in supporting *Brucella* replication. *PLoS Pathog* **4**:e1000110. doi:10.1371/journal.ppat.1000110.

112. **Naroeni A, Porte F.** 2002. Role of cholesterol and the ganglioside GM(1) in entry and short-term survival of *Brucella suis* in murine macrophages. *Infect Immun* **70**:1640–1644.

113. **Guzman-Verri C, Chaves-Olarte E, von Eichel-Streiber C, Lopez-Goni I, Thelestam M, Arvidson S, Gorvel JP, Moreno E.** 2001. GTPases of the Rho subfamily are required for *Brucella abortus* internalization in nonprofessional phagocytes: direct activation of Cdc42. *J Biol Chem* **276**:44435–44443.

114. **Pei J, Turse JE, Ficht TA.** 2008. Evidence of *Brucella abortus* OPS dictating uptake and restricting NF-kappaB activation in murine macrophages. *Microbes Infect* **10**:582–590.

115. **Pei J, Ficht TA.** 2004. *Brucella abortus* rough mutants are cytopathic for macrophages in culture. *Infect Immun* **72**:440–450.

116. **Porte F, Naroeni A, Ouahrani-Bettache S, Liautard JP.** 2003. Role of the *Brucella suis* lipopolysaccharide O antigen in phagosomal genesis and in inhibition of phagosome-

lysosome fusion in murine macrophages. *Infect Immun* **71**:1481–1490.

117. **Rittig MG, Kaufmann A, Robins A, Shaw B, Sprenger H, Gemsa D, Foulongne V, Rouot B, Dornand J.** 2003. Smooth and rough lipopolysaccharide phenotypes of *Brucella* induce different intracellular trafficking and cytokine/chemokine release in human monocytes. *J Leukoc Biol* **74**:1045–1055.

118. **Martin-Martin AI, Vizcaino N, Fernandez-Lago L.** 2010. Cholesterol, ganglioside GM1 and class A scavenger receptor contribute to infection by *Brucella ovis* and *Brucella canis* in murine macrophages. *Microbes Infect* **12**:246–251.

119. **Hong PC, Tsolis RM, Ficht TA.** 2000. Identification of genes required for chronic persistence of *Brucella abortus* in mice. *Infect Immun* **68**:4102–4107.

120. **Sieira R, Comerci DJ, Sanchez DO, Ugalde RA.** 2000. A homologue of an operon required for DNA transfer in *Agrobacterium* is required in *Brucella abortus* for virulence and intracellular multiplication. *J Bacteriol* **182**:4849–4855.

121. **Arellano-Reynoso B, Lapaque N, Salcedo S, Briones G, Ciocchini AE, Ugalde R, Moreno E, Moriyon I, Gorvel JP.** 2005. Cyclic beta-1,2-glucan is a *Brucella* virulence factor required for intracellular survival. *Nat Immunol* **6**:618–625.

122. **Roop RM 2nd, Gaines JM, Anderson ES, Caswell CC, Martin DW.** 2009. Survival of the fittest: how *Brucella* strains adapt to their intracellular niche in the host. *Med Microbiol Immunol* **198**:221–238.

123. **Valderas MW, Alcantara RB, Baumgartner JE, Bellaire BH, Robertson GT, Ng WL, Richardson JM, Winkler ME, Roop RM 2nd.** 2005. Role of HdeA in acid resistance and virulence in *Brucella abortus* 2308. *Vet Microbiol* **107**:307–312.

124. **Endley S, McMurray D, Ficht TA.** 2001. Interruption of the cydB locus in *Brucella abortus* attenuates intracellular survival and virulence in the mouse model of infection. *J Bacteriol* **183**:2454–2462.

125. **Bandara AB, Contreras A, Contreras-Rodriguez A, Martins AM, Dobrean V, Poff-Reichow S, Rajasekaran P, Sriranganathan N, Schurig GG, Boyle SM.** 2007. *Brucella suis* urease encoded by ure1 but not ure2 is necessary for intestinal infection of BALB/c mice. *BMC Microbiol* **7**:57.

126. **Jimenez de Bagues MP, Dudal S, Dornand J, Gross A.** 2005. Cellular bioterrorism: how *Brucella* corrupts macrophage physiology to promote invasion and proliferation. *Clin Immunol* **114**:227–238.

127. **Gee JM, Valderas MW, Kovach ME, Grippe VK, Robertson GT, Ng WL, Richardson JM, Winkler ME, Roop RM 2nd.** 2005. The *Brucella abortus* Cu,Zn superoxide dismutase is required for optimal resistance to oxidative killing by murine macrophages and wild-type virulence in experimentally infected mice. *Infect Immun* **73**:2873–2880.

128. **Haine V, Dozot M, Dornand J, Letesson JJ, De Bolle X.** 2006. NnrA is required for full virulence and regulates several *Brucella melitensis* denitrification genes. *J Bacteriol* **188**:1615–1619.

129. **Loisel-Meyer S, Jimenez de Bagues MP, Basseres E, Dornand J, Kohler S, Liautard JP, Jubier-Maurin V.** 2006. Requirement of norD for *Brucella suis* virulence in a murine model of *in vitro* and *in vivo* infection. *Infect Immun* **74**:1973–1976.

130. **Steele KH, Baumgartner JE, Valderas MW, Roop RM 2nd.** 2010. Comparative study of the roles of AhpC and KatE as respiratory antioxidants in *Brucella abortus* 2308. *J Bacteriol* **192**:4912–4922.

131. **Manterola L, Moriyon I, Moreno E, Sola-Landa A, Weiss DS, Koch MH, Howe J, Brandenburg K, Lopez-Goni I.** 2005. The lipopolysaccharide of *Brucella abortus* BvrS/BvrR mutants contains lipid A modifications and has higher affinity for bactericidal cationic peptides. *J Bacteriol* **187**: 5631–5639.

132. **Pizarro-Cerda J, Moreno E, Sanguedolce V, Mege JL, Gorvel JP.** 1998. Virulent *Brucella abortus* prevents lysosome fusion and is distributed within autophagosome-like compartments. *Infect Immun* **66**:2387–2392.

133. **Smith JA, Khan M, Magnani DD, Harms JS, Durward M, Radhakrishnan GK, Liu YP, Splitter GA.** 2013. *Brucella* induces an unfolded protein response via TcpB that supports intracellular replication in macrophages. *PLoS Pathog* **9**:e1003785. doi:10.1371/journal.ppat.1003785.

134. **Fugier E, Salcedo SP, de Chastellier C, Pophillat M, Muller A, Arce-Gorvel V, Fourquet P, Gorvel JP.** 2009. The glyceraldehyde-3-phosphate dehydrogenase and the small GTPase Rab 2 are crucial for *Brucella* replication. *PLoS Pathog* **5**: e1000487. doi:10.1371/journal.ppat.1000487.

135. **de Barsy M, Jamet A, Filopon D, Nicolas C, Laloux G, Rual JF, Muller A, Twizere JC, Nkengfac B, Vandenhaute J, Hill DE, Salcedo SP, Gorvel JP, Letesson JJ, De Bolle X.** 2011. Identification of a *Brucella* spp. secreted effector specifically interacting with human small GTPase Rab2. *Cell Microbiol* **13**:1044–1058.

136. **Nkengfac B, Pouyez J, Bauwens E, Vandenhaute J, Letesson JJ, Wouters J, De**

Bolle X. 2012. Structural analysis of *Brucella abortus* RicA substitutions that do not impair interaction with human Rab2 GTPase. *BMC Biochem* **13**:16.

137. **de Barsy M, Mirabella A, Letesson JJ, De Bolle X.** 2012. A *Brucella abortus* cstA mutant is defective for association with endoplasmic reticulum exit sites and displays altered trafficking in HeLa cells. *Microbiology* **158**:2610–2618.

138. **Myeni S, Child R, Ng TW, Kupko JJ 3rd, Wehrly TD, Porcella SF, Knodler LA, Celli J.** 2013. *Brucella* modulates secretory trafficking via multiple type IV secretion effector proteins. *PLoS Pathog* **9**:e1003556. doi:10.1371/journal.ppat.1003556.

139. **Celli J, Salcedo SP, Gorvel JP.** 2005. *Brucella* coopts the small GTPase Sar1 for intracellular replication. *Proc Natl Acad Sci USA* **102**:1673–1678.

140. **van Schaik EJ, Chen C, Mertens K, Weber MM, Samuel JE.** 2013. Molecular pathogenesis of the obligate intracellular bacterium *Coxiella burnetii*. *Nat Rev Microbiol* **11**:561–573.

141. **Enserink M.** 2010. Infectious diseases. Questions abound in Q-fever explosion in the Netherlands. *Science* **327**:266–267.

142. **White B, Brooks T, Seaton RA.** 2013. Q fever in military and paramilitary personnel in conflict zones: case report and review. *Travel Med Infect Dis* **11**:134–137.

143. **Coleman SA, Fischer ER, Howe D, Mead DJ, Heinzen RA.** 2004. Temporal analysis of *Coxiella burnetii* morphological differentiation. *J Bacteriol* **186**:7344–7352.

144. **Howe D, Mallavia LP.** 2000. *Coxiella burnetii* exhibits morphological change and delays phagolysosomal fusion after internalization by J774A.1 cells. *Infect Immun* **68**:3815–3821.

145. **Baca OG, Klassen DA, Aragon AS.** 1993. Entry of *Coxiella burnetii* into host cells. *Acta Virol* **37**:143–155.

146. **Tujulin E, Macellaro A, Lilliehook B, Norlander L.** 1998. Effect of endocytosis inhibitors on *Coxiella burnetii* interaction with host cells. *Acta Virol* **42**:125–131.

147. **Beare PA, Gilk SD, Larson CL, Hill J, Stead CM, Omsland A, Cockrell DC, Howe D, Voth DE, Heinzen RA.** 2011. Dot/Icm type IVB secretion system requirements for *Coxiella burnetii* growth in human macrophages. *MBio* **2**:e00175-00111. doi:10.1128/mBio.00175-11.

148. **Carey KL, Newton HJ, Luhrmann A, Roy CR.** 2011. The *Coxiella burnetii* Dot/Icm system delivers a unique repertoire of type IV effectors into host cells and is required for intracellular replication. *PLoS Pathog* **7**:e1002056. doi:10.1371/journal.ppat.1002056.

149. **Capo C, Lindberg FP, Meconi S, Zaffran Y, Tardei G, Brown EJ, Raoult D, Mege JL.** 1999. Subversion of monocyte functions by *Coxiella burnetii*: impairment of the cross-talk between alphavbeta3 integrin and CR3. *J Immunol* **163**:6078–6085.

150. **Dellacasagrande J, Ghigo E, Machergui-El S Hammami, Toman R, Raoult D, Capo C, Mege J-L.** 2000. Alpha vbeta 3 integrin and bacterial lipopolysaccharide are involved in *Coxiella burnetii*-stimulated production of tumor necrosis factor by human monocytes. *Infect Immun* **68**:5673–5678.

151. **Russell-Lodrigue KE, Zhang GQ, McMurray DN, Samuel JE.** 2006. Clinical and pathologic changes in a guinea pig aerosol challenge model of acute Q fever. *Infect Immun* **74**:6085–6091.

152. **Howe D, Shannon JG, Winfree S, Dorward DW, Heinzen RA.** 2010. *Coxiella burnetii* phase I and II variants replicate with similar kinetics in degradative phagolysosome-like compartments of human macrophages. *Infect Immun* **78**:3465–3474.

153. **Romano PS, Gutierrez MG, Beron W, Rabinovitch M, Colombo MI.** 2007. The autophagic pathway is actively modulated by phase II *Coxiella burnetii* to efficiently replicate in the host cell. *Cell Microbiol* **9**:891–909.

154. **Howe D, Melnicâakova J, Barâak I, Heinzen RA.** 2003. Fusogenicity of the *Coxiella burnetii* parasitophorous vacuole. *Ann N Y Acad Sci* **990**:556–562.

155. **Larson CL, Beare PA, Voth DE, Howe D, Cockrell DC, Bastidas RJ, Valdivia RH, Heinzen RA.** 2015. *Coxiella burnetii* effector proteins that localize to the parasitophorous vacuole membrane promote intracellular replication. *Infect Immun* **83**:661–670.

156. **Howe D, Melnicâakovâa J, Barâak I, Heinzen RA.** 2003. Maturation of the *Coxiella burnetii* parasitophorous vacuole requires bacterial protein synthesis but not replication. *Cell Microbiol* **5**:469–480.

157. **Flannagan RS, Cosio G, Grinstein S.** 2009. Antimicrobial mechanisms of phagocytes and bacterial evasion strategies. *Nat Rev Microbiol* **7**:355–366.

158. **Oh YK, Alpuche-Aranda C, Berthiaume E, Jinks T, Miller SI, Swanson JA.** 1996. Rapid and complete fusion of macrophage lysosomes with phagosomes containing *Salmonella typhimurium*. *Infect Immun* **64**:3877–3883.

159. **Swanson MS, Fernandez-Moreira E.** 2002. A microbial strategy to multiply in macrophages: the pregnant pause. *Traffic* **3**:170–177.

160. **Levine B, Mizushima N, Virgin HW.** 2011. Autophagy in immunity and inflammation. *Nature* **469**:323–335.

161. Beron W, Gutierrez MG, Rabinovitch M, Colombo MI. 2002. *Coxiella burnetii* localizes in a Rab7-labeled compartment with autophagic characteristics. *Infect Immun* **70**:5816–5821.

162. Gutierrez MG, Vazquez CL, Munafo DB, Zoppino FC, Beron W, Rabinovitch M, Colombo MI. 2005. Autophagy induction favours the generation and maturation of the *Coxiella*-replicative vacuoles. *Cell Microbiol* **7**:981–993.

163. Criscitiello MF, Dickman MB, Samuel JE, de Figueiredo P. 2013. Tripping on acid: trans-kingdom perspectives on biological acids in immunity and pathogenesis. *PLoS Pathog* **9**:e1003402. doi:10.1371/journal.ppat.1003402.

164. Mertens K, Lantsheer L, Ennis DG, Samuel JE. 2008. Constitutive SOS expression and damage-inducible AddAB-mediated recombinational repair systems for *Coxiella burnetii* as potential adaptations for survival within macrophages. *Mol Microbiol* **69**:1411–1426.

165. Hill J, Samuel JE. 2011. *Coxiella burnetii* acid phosphatase inhibits the release of reactive oxygen intermediates in polymorphonuclear leukocytes. *Infect Immun* **79**:414–420.

166. Heinzen RA, Frazier ME, Mallavia LP. 1992. *Coxiella burnetii* superoxide dismutase gene: cloning, sequencing, and expression in *Escherichia coli*. *Infect Immun* **60**:3814–3823.

167. Seshadri R, Paulsen IT, Eisen JA, Read TD, Nelson KE, Nelson WC, Ward NL, Tettelin H, Davidsen TM, Beanan MJ, Deboy RT, Daugherty SC, Brinkac LM, Madupu R, Dodson RJ, Khouri HM, Lee KH, Carty HA, Scanlan D, Heinzen RA, Thompson HA, Samuel JE, Fraser CM, Heidelberg JF. 2003. Complete genome sequence of the Q-fever pathogen *Coxiella burnetii*. *Proc Natl Acad Sci USA* **100**:5455–5460.

168. Brennan RE, Russell K, Zhang G, Samuel JE. 2004. Both inducible nitric oxide synthase and NADPH oxidase contribute to the control of virulent phase I *Coxiella burnetii* infections. *Infect Immun* **72**:6666–6675.

169. Roman MJ, Crissman HA, Samsonoff WA, Hechemy KE, Baca OG. 1991. Analysis of *Coxiella burnetii* isolates in cell culture and the expression of parasite-specific antigens on the host membrane surface. *Acta Virol* **35**:503–510.

170. Aguilera M, Salinas R, Rosales E, Carminati S, Colombo MI, Beron W. 2009. Actin dynamics and Rho GTPases regulate the size and formation of parasitophorous vacuoles containing *Coxiella burnetii*. *Infect Immun* **77**:4609–4620.

171. Hussain SK, Broederdorf LJ, Sharma UM, Voth DE. 2011. Host kinase activity is required for *Coxiella burnetii* parasitophorous vacuole formation. *Front Microbiol* **1**:137.

172. Campoy EM, Zoppino FC, Colombo MI. 2011. The early secretory pathway contributes to the growth of the *Coxiella*-replicative niche. *Infect Immun* **79**:402–413.

173. Martinez E, Cantet F, Fava L, Norville I, Bonazzi M. 2014. Identification of OmpA, a *Coxiella burnetti* protein involved in host cell invasion, by multi-phenotypic high-content screening. *PLoS Pathog* **10**:p.e.1004013.

Intracellular Growth of Bacterial Pathogens: The Role of Secreted Effector Proteins in the Control of Phagocytosed Microorganisms

24

VALÉRIE POIRIER[1] and YOSSEF AV-GAY[1]

INTRODUCTION

Of the 56 million deaths reported worldwide in 2012, approximately 15 million are directly related to infectious diseases (1). The majority of annual deaths are related to bacterial infections such as tuberculosis, yellow and typhoid fever, cholera, shigellosis, pneumonia, etc. (1). Morbidity and mortality rates are highest in developing countries, where large numbers of infants and children count among the victims (2). In developed nations, infectious disease mortality falls most heavily on indigenous and disadvantaged minorities (3). The control of bacterial infectious diseases worldwide is an important task. Although antibiotics revolutionized the treatment of bacterial infections, increased resistance and the emergence of multidrug-resistant strains increasingly reduce their efficacy. This trend promotes an urgent need for better understanding of bacterial pathogenicity and resistance mechanisms, which will assist novel therapeutic and vaccination strategies.

To avoid destruction by host cells, a variety of evolutionarily unrelated bacteria have developed strategies to grow and replicate inside the host. These infectious bacteria are designated as intracellular pathogens and manipulate host responses to their advantage in unique ways. A widespread bacterial

[1]Division of Infectious Diseases, Department of Medicine, University of British Columbia, Vancouver, BC V6H 3Z6 Canada.

Virulence Mechanisms of Bacterial Pathogens, 5th edition
Edited by Indira T. Kudva, Nancy A. Cornick, Paul J. Plummer, Qijing Zhang, Tracy L. Nicholson, John P. Bannantine, and Bryan H. Bellaire
© 2016 American Society for Microbiology, Washington, DC
doi:10.1128/microbiolspec.VMBF-0003-2014

693

pathogenesis trait is the synthesis and secretion of numerous proteins into the cytoplasm or membrane of the host via specialized secretion systems. These secreted macromolecules, referred to as virulence factors or effectors, facilitate bacterial pathogenesis by manipulating host cellular processes to enhance bacterial colonization and survival within the infected host, and suppress host cell defenses (4–7).

BACTERIAL SECRETION SYSTEMS

The export of bacterial effectors occurs via secretion systems which are specialized protein translocation systems that enable transport of substrate molecules after production within the bacterium (8). These systems mediate intraspecies passage of genetic material, such as antibiotic resistance genes, as well as transfer of virulence factors across cellular membranes into the cytoplasm of the host. Consequently, secretion systems facilitate aspects of the infection process such as bacterial entry into the host cell, intracellular survival, and spreading of the pathogen to neighboring host cells (9).

These secretion systems have been categorized into six evolutionary and functionally related groups, namely type I to VI secretion systems (10). However, some species of Gram-positive bacteria use alternative protein secretion systems collectively called the type VII secretion system (10). The emphasis of this chapter is placed on bacterial macromolecules involved in manipulating phagosomal trafficking that are secreted by the membrane-associated transporter complexes type III, IV, and VII secretion systems. However, although not discussed in detail, we note that *Listeria* species export virulence factors via a general secretory pathway, the SecA2 secretion system (11).

Type III, IV, and VII Secretion Systems

Gram-negative bacteria possess a cell envelope composed of two membranes: an inner and an outer membrane (12). To manipulate host cells, these bacteria have developed an export system, the type III secretion system (T3SS), capable of transporting effector proteins across three membranes: the two membranes of the bacterial cell envelope and the cell membrane of the targeted cell (7). The T3SS has a needle-like shape that allows effectors to be exported across both bacterial membranes and into the cytoplasm of the targeted cell without being exposed to the extracellular milieu (13). Strains possessing T3SS include *Salmonella*, *Shigella*, and *Yersinia* species which are capable of controlling trafficking events in the phagosome, the cellular compartment formed by the fusion of the cell membrane around the invading pathogen.

The bacterial type IV secretion system (T4SS) is a membrane-associated transporter used by several Gram-positive and Gram-negative bacteria. This transporter is related to bacterial conjugation because it can transfer genetic material to other bacterial cells by horizontal gene transfer. The T4SS exports virulence factors into mammalian cells (5, 6). Several human pathogens such as *Legionella*, *Brucella*, and *Coxiella* species possess the T4SS and achieve intracellular survival by inhabiting vacuoles from the endocytic pathway (6).

The type VII secretion system (T7SS) distantly resembles T4SS (14) and is found in certain species of Gram-positive bacteria. The particularity of this specialized secretion system is its ability to ensure transport of virulence factors across the complex cell wall of acid-fast *Mycobacterium* species (15). Mycobacteria have a distinctive cell envelope structure that is characterized by an exceptionally hydrophobic, impermeable and thick layer, termed the mycomembrane. The unique features of the membrane are due to the presence of mycolic acids, which are large branched-chain fatty acids. In mycobacteria, the T7SS includes the ESX 1 to 5 secretion systems, some of which are essential for virulence and take active roles in macrophage escape and cell-to-cell spread

(16, 17). Despite the absence of the myco-membrane typical of *Mycobacterium* species, Gram-positive bacteria such as *Streptomyces* and *Listeria* species also possess a T7SS (10).

PHAGOSOME MATURATION

Upon engulfment by a phagocyte, microorganisms are trapped in an organelle derived from the plasma membrane, termed the phagosome. Phagosomes acquire microbicidal features that enable them to kill and digest engulfed microbes through a process known as phagosome maturation. Phagosome maturation includes a variety of fusion and fission events with compartments of the endocytic pathway whereby the contents of the phagosome are gradually delivered to lysosomes for degradation (18). Phagosome maturation radically alters the composition of the phagosome, converting it into a potent microbicidal organelle (18). As illustrated in Fig. 1, phagosomes containing foreign particles, such as invading microorganisms, interact with the endosomal pathway, allowing for the exchange of solute materials and membrane components between phagosomes and endosomes. Sequential interactions with endosomal compartments and lysosomes yield mature phagolysosomes that are markedly acidic due to the reduction in phagosomal pH resulting from the acquisition of vacuolar H+-ATPase (V-ATPase) pumps (18). These

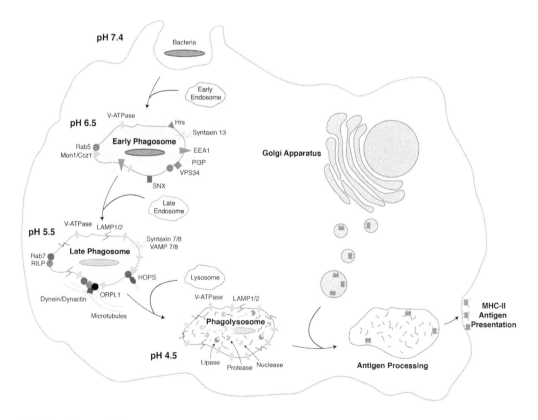

FIGURE 1 Stages of phagosome maturation. During phagocytosis, the phagosome undergoes a series of fusion and fission events with vesicles of the endocytic pathway, culminating in the formation of the phagolysosome. Maturation of the phagosome involves gradual decrease in pH and acquisition of antimicrobial properties, leading to the digestion of the invader and presentation of antigens on the surface of the phagocyte by MHC-II molecules.

fusion events modify the function of the phagosome to reflect the content of the lysosome, which is highly oxidative and enriched with hydrolytic enzymes (18). Invading microorganisms are ultimately degraded, and their peptides are presented on the surface of the phagocyte to initiate an adaptive immune response (19).

Although phagocytosis normally results in the eradication of microorganisms, some pathogens have developed strategies to interfere with phagosome maturation and use phagocytes as niches for survival and growth. Different stages of phagosome maturation can be targeted by different microorganisms: the fusion of the phagosome with early and late endosomes, the fusion with lysosomes, the acidification of the phagosome, the redirection of the phagosome to a nondigestive route, etc. These events create an alcove suited for bacterial replication.

While the list of effector macromolecules secreted by pathogens suggested to cross-talk with host proteins or specific host pathways is growing, the precise mechanisms of communication that allow pathogens to interfere with defined host proteins (e.g., signaling and metabolic proteins), and to survive and replicate within the hostile environment of the host, are still very limited and poorly understood. In this chapter, the current knowledge of a subset of bacterial pathogen effectors involved in altering the phagosome to circumvent pathogen destruction is summarized (Table 1). Each step of the phagosome maturation process is examined individually, and the effectors of selected pathogens involved in interfering with this process are described. In particular, effectors secreted by the Gram-negative bacteria are characterized: *Legionella*, which causes the acute lung disease Legionnaires' disease (*Legionella pneumophila*) (20), *Salmonella*, responsible for the localized small intestine disease salmonellosis (*Salmonella enterica*) and systemic disease typhoid fever (*Salmonella typhi*), *Shigella*, the causative agent of the small intestine disease shigellosis (*Shigella dysen-*

teriae, Shigella flexneri, Shigella sonnei), and *Yersinia*, the agent responsible for the black death, or bubonic/pneumonic plague (*Yersinia pestis*). Moreover, effectors secreted by the Gram-positive bacterium are enumerated: *Listeria*, responsible for listeriosis, an infection of the central nervous system or the small intestine (*Listeria monocytogenes*), and the acid-fast actinomycete *Mycobacterium*, the causative agent of diseases such as tuberculosis (*Mycobacterium tuberculosis*) (21). Identifying these effectors and their modes of action is essential to understanding the pathogenesis of diseases and how pathogens manipulate the defense mechanisms of the host to their advantage.

Targeting Phagosome-Endosome Fusion

As illustrated in Fig. 1 and described in detail in Fig. 2, the metamorphosis of the phagosomal membrane occurs after engulfment of the invader. Changes begin immediately and are coordinated by Rab GTPases, a family of molecular switches, which alternate between an active (GTP-bound) and an inactive (GDP-bound) state. Their activity is controlled by Rab GDP dissociation inhibitors, guanine nucleotide exchange factors (GEFs), and GTPase-activating proteins (22). Once activated, Rab molecules regulate host vesicular and membrane transport processes by modulating membrane structure and function (22).

Upon phagosome biogenesis, the pathogen-containing phagosome recruits the early endosomal marker, Rab5, which coordinates traffic between the phagosome and early endosomes (18). Rab5 recruits effector molecules such as the class III phosphatidylinositol 3-kinase vacuolar protein sorting 34 (VPS34) (23). VPS34 catalyzes the production of the lipid regulator phosphatidylinositol 3-phosphate (PI3P) from phosphatidylinositol (PI) (23). PI3P, in turn, is a phagosomal membrane tag that signals phagosomes to progress down the phagolysosome biogenesis pathway (24). To achieve fusion of the early phagosome with endosomes, PI3P affects the localization and function of specific proteins involved in membrane trafficking, endosomal protein sorting, and multisubunit enzyme assembly at the membrane (25). These proteins include early endosome antigen 1 (EEA1), p40 subunit of the NADPH oxidase, and hepatocyte growth factor-regulated tyrosine kinase substrate (Hrs) (24, 26, 27). EEA1 facilitates docking and fusion of the early phagosome with early organelles of the endocytic pathway via interaction with syntaxin 13, a soluble *N*-ethylmaleimide-sensitive factor attachment protein receptor (SNARE) protein (28). SNAREs assemble downstream of tethering molecules and drive fusion of membranes (29).

Following the fusion with early endosomes, the phagosome acquires the late endosomal marker, Rab7, which prompts fusion of the early phagosome with late endosomes and the acquisition of additional factors contributing to microbicidal functions, such as the integral membrane proteins lysosome-associated membrane proteins 1/2 (LAMP1 and LAMP2) and V-ATPases (18). The presence of additional V-ATPase pumps in the late phagosome further acidifies the organelle (luminal pH $\sim$ 5.5).

Pathogenic mycobacterial species inhibit fusion of the phagosome with endosomes. The *M. tuberculosis* cell wall glycolipid mannosylated lipoarabinomannan (ManLAM) is secreted into the host cytoplasm (30) and inhibits intracellular calcium (Ca^{2+}) levels, resulting in the disruption of phagosome maturation (31). Ca^{2+} is an essential cell signaling molecule, and increases in intracellular Ca^{2+} following infection lead to the accumulation of the small GTPase Rab5 in the phagosomal membrane. As seen in Fig. 2, upon secretion of ManLAM, intracellular Ca^{2+} is reduced and Rab5 only partially localizes to the phagosomal membrane. The recruitment of Rab5's effector VPS34 to the phagosomal membrane is consequently hindered. Since PI3P is partly excluded from the phagosome, PI3P-binding proteins, such as EEA1, only accumulate in small amounts (32). Thus, ManLAM reduces the fusion of

the phagosome with early endosomes and the delivery of the endosomal cargo between them (33).

Partial PI3P exclusion mediated by ManLAM is not sufficient to cause complete inhibition of phagosome and endosome fusion. *M. tuberculosis* secretes an acid phosphatase termed secreted acid phosphatase of *M. tuberculosis* (SapM), which hydrolyzes host PI3P into PI (32). Dephosphorylation of PI3P into PI prevents PI3P accumulation at the phagosomal membrane, impeding EEA1 recruitment and fusion with endosomes (32). The means by which ManLAM and SapM are able to cross the phagosomal membrane and gain access to the cytoplasmic face of the phagosome, where they prevent intracellular Ca^{2+} levels from rising and hydrolyze PI3P, remains a conundrum (32).

Legionella species are also able to inhibit fusion of the phagosome with endosomes. The *L. pneumophila* effectors VipD and VipA interfere with early and late endosomal transport, respectively. VipD tightly binds to the GTP-bound form of the early endosomal markers Rab5 and Rab22a, limiting interactions with downstream effector molecules and inhibiting endocytic trafficking (34). VipA possesses a coiled-coil region and is suspected of interacting with host proteins that also contain coiled-coil regions such as SNAREs and EEA1 (Fig. 2) (35).

Salmonella species, such as *S. enterica*, promote fusion of the phagosome with endosomes but inhibit fusion with lysosomes. Interestingly, *S. enterica* promotes fusion of the phagosome with endosomes by secreting the effectors *Salmonella* outer protein B/E (SopB and SopE), which recruit the small GTPase Rab5 to the phagosomal membrane and activate it by subverting inactive GDP-bound Rab5 for active GTP-bound Rab5 (Fig. 2) (36–38). In addition, studies have shown that SopE promotes retaining Rab5 on the phagosome by stimulating GDP to GTP nucleotide exchange of Rho GTPases (39). Retaining active Rab5 on the phagosomal membrane thus promotes fusion of the

TABLE 1 Host physiological events and substrates targeted by effectors secreted by *Legionella*, *Listeria*, *Mycobacterium*, *Salmonella*, *Shigella*, and *Yersinia* species

Biological event targeted	Pathogen	Bacterial effector	Host target	Refs.
Endosomal trafficking	*Mycobacterium tuberculosis*	ManLAM	Reduces intracellular Ca^{2+} concentration	31
		SapM	Hydrolyzes PI3P into PI	32
	Legionella pneumophila	VipD	Interacts with GTP-Rab5 and GTP-Rab22a	34
		VipA	Interacts with EEA1 and SNAREs	35
	Salmonella enterica	SopB	Recruits Rab5	36
		SopE	Recruits and activates Rab5	37, 38
Phagosome and lysosome fusion	*S. enterica*	SifA	Uncouples Rab7 from RILP	45
		SipC	Inactivates Hook3	46
		SopB	Hydrolyzes PI(4,5)P$_2$ into PI5P, reducing the recruitment of Rab8, Rab13, Rab23, and Rab35	48
	M. tuberculosis	PtpA	Dephosphorylates VPS33B	49
		EsxG/H	Form a complex that targets Hrs, a component of the ESCRT machinery.	51
		EspB	Inhibits phagolysosome fusion when cosecreted with ESAT-6 and CFP-10	53
		Cord factor	Creates a steric block to fusion and/or increases the hydration force between two phospholipid bilayers	56
	Yersinia pestis	Unknown	Resides and replicates in a phagolysosome-like vacuole	63, 64
Phagosome acidification	*M. tuberculosis*	PtpA	Binds subunit H of V-ATPase and prevents assembly of the proton pump	66
	L. pneumophila	SidK	Binds subunit A of V-ATPase and inhibits ATP hydrolysis and proton translocation	67
	Yersinia pseudotuberculosis	Unknown	Decreases the activity of the V-ATPase pump	59
	S. enterica	SseB/C/D	Forms a complex that helps in the translocation of T3SS effectors across the bacterial membrane	69
Cytoskeleton remodeling	*S. enterica*	SipA	Catalyzes actin polymerization and bundling of actin filaments. Stabilizes SifA via its actin modification effects	71, 74
		SipC	Bundles and nucleates actin filaments	73
		SseI	Interacts with filamin A and promotes cross-linking of F-actin by filamin A	72
		SspH2	Interacts with filamin A and promotes cross-linking of F-actin by filamin A	72
		SpvB	Depolymerizes and disrupts the actin cytoskeleton by modifying G-actin	75
		SopB	Indirectly recruits SNX3, which forms tubules for the movement of the phagosome to the perinuclear region	76
		PipB2	Interacts with kinesin-1 and forms Sifs	81
		SifA	Interacts with SKIP, forms Sifs, promotes phagosomal tubulation, and uncouples Rab7 from RILP	45, 76, 81, 84
		SseJ	Interacts with SKIP and GTPase RhoA and promotes phagosomal tubulation	84

		SseF/G	Participates in the dynein-mediated movement of the phagosome along microtubules; serves as a scaffold for Sif formation	87, 88
	L. pneumophila	VipA	Binds actin and enhances its polymerization	89
	Mycobacterium marinum	Unknown	Recruits WASp and induces the formation of actin tails	90
	Listeria monocytogenes	ActA	Mimics WASp to induce actin polymerization	92
	Shigella flexneri	IcsA	Recruits neural WASp to induce actin polymerization	93
Vacuolar membrane lysis	*M. marinum*	Unknown	Escapes from the phagosome	90
	S. flexneri	IpgD	Hydrolyzes PI(4,5)P$_2$ into PI5P, which recruits EGFR and Rab11-positive vacuoles	94–96
		IpaB	Forms pores in the vacuole membrane	97, 98
		IpaC	Disrupts the integrity of the phospholipid bilayer of vesicles	97
		IpaH7.8	Promotes bacterial phagosome escape	100
	L. monocytogenes	LLO	Forms pores in the vacuole membrane	101
		PI/PC-PLC	Causes the breakdown of the vacuole membrane	102
Phagosomal Membrane Remodeling	*L. pneumophila*	SidF	Hydrolyzes PI(3,4)P$_2$ and PI(3,4,5)P$_3$ into PI4P and PI(4,5)P$_2$	105
		LidA	Recruits Rab1	108
		DrrA/SidM	Recruits and converts inactive GDP-Rab1 into active GTP-Rab1 and maintains it on the phagosomal membrane; AMPylates Rab1	108, 111, 112
		LepB	Converts active GTP-Rab1 into inactive GDP-Rab1 and releases it from the phagosomal membrane	114
		SidD	DeAMPylates Rab1	115
		AnkX	Catalyzes the attachment of a phosphocholine moiety (phosphocholination) to GTPases Rab1 and Rab35	116, 117
		Lem3	Reverses post-translationnal modification (dephosphocholination) on Rab1	119
		RalF	Recruits ARF1 to the membrane and activates it	120
		SidJ	Modulates host processes to redirect the recruitment of ER-derived vesicles to the phagosome	123
		SidP	Hydrolyzes PI3P and PI(3,5)P$_2$ promoting the evasion of the endocytic pathway by the phagosome	124
		SidC	Acts as a tethering factor for the recruitment of ER-derived vesicles to the phagosome	122
		SetA	Binds PI3P and impairs vesicular trafficking via its glycosyltransferase activity	125

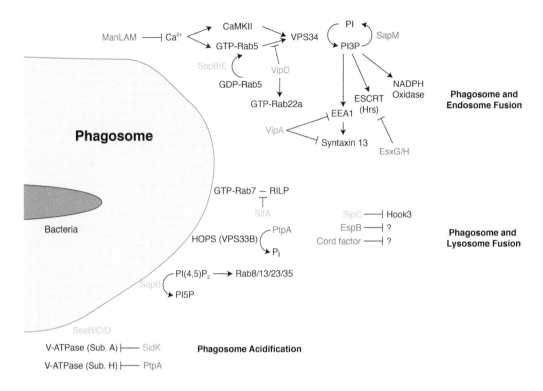

FIGURE 2 Microbial effectors interfering with intracellular trafficking and acidification events. Orange proteins represent *Legionella* virulence factors; pink, *Mycobacterium* virulence factors; and blue, *Salmonella* virulence factors.

phagosome with early endosomes via the recruitment of VPS34, as previously described, and explains the relatively large membrane-bound vesicle size in which *Salmonella* resides (40). Moreover, previous studies have demonstrated that phagosomes containing pathogenic *Listeria* and *Mycobacterium* species are enriched in Rab5, thereby inhibiting their transport to lysosomes (41, 42). Thus, the prolonged period of time spent in the mildly acidic early phagosome may account for blocking transport of the *Salmonella*-containing phagosome to lysosomes and *Salmonella*'s survival.

Targeting Phagosome-Lysosome Fusion

The mature phagosome is the ultimate microbicidal and degradative organelle. To complete phagosome maturation, the small GTPase Rab7 recruits Rab-interacting lyso-somal protein (RILP) and oxysterol-binding protein–related protein 1L (ORP1L) to the late phagosome (Fig. 1) (18). RILP is a dynein adaptor, and ORP1L regulates the binding of RILP to dynein. Together, RILP and ORPL1 interact with the dynein-dynactin molecular motor and coordinate microtubule-dependent vesicular trafficking of the late phagosome to the microtubule organizing center, a perinuclear region near the Golgi apparatus, where fusion with lysosomes occurs (18). Rab7 also associates with the homotypic fusion and vacuole protein sorting (HOPS) complex, a large multimeric tethering factor essential for vesicle fusion (43). The HOPS complex is composed of VPS11, VPS16, VPS18, VPS33B, VPS39, and VPS41 (18). The HOPS complex is needed during the tethering and docking stages of vesicle fusion between the phagosome and the lysosomes (44), where it regulates the assembly of SNARE molecules such as syntaxin 7 and vesicle-associated membrane protein 7 at the phagosomal membrane (18). Phagolysosome fusion permits the exchange of cytosolic contents such as hydrolases (nucleases, lipases, proteases, etc.), and additional LAMP1/2 proteins and V-ATPase pumps (Fig. 1) (18). The phagolysosome possesses a strong acidic luminal (pH ~ 4.5) which, along with the action of hydrolytic enzymes and oxidants, contributes to the degradation of microorganisms. Lastly, the phagolysosome subsequently fuses with Golgi vesicles carrying major histocompatibility class II molecules for antigen processing and presentation (18).

Late endocytic and lysosomal markers are often the targets of choice for pathogens because inhibition or inactivation of these targets guards bacteria from exposure to microbicidal compounds. As illustrated in Fig. 2, the *Salmonella* effectors *Salmonella*-induced filaments A (SifA) and *Salmonella* invasion protein C (SipC) block phagolysosome fusion by uncoupling Rab7 from RILP (45) and inactivating Hook3, a mammalian protein implicated in cellular trafficking (46), respectively. In addition to recruiting the small GTPase Rab5 to the phagosome, the SopB effector acts as a PI phosphatase. PI lipids are important regulators of cellular processes such as cell signaling, cytoskeleton remodeling, and membrane trafficking (47). SopB alters the PI composition of the phagosomal membrane by hydrolyzing phosphatidylinositol 4,5-bisphosphate ($PI[4,5]P_2$) into phosphatidylinositol 5-phosphate (PI5P), reducing the recruitment of Rab8, Rab13, Rab23, and Rab35 while preventing phagolysosome fusion (48).

Pathogenic *Mycobacterium* species interfere with phagolysosome fusion by secreting effectors which have been shown to interact with the host proteins PtpA, EsxG, EsxH, EspB, and cord factor (Fig. 2). The low-molecular-weight tyrosine phosphatase, protein tyrosine phosphatase A (PtpA), translocates to the host cytosol, where it dephosphorylates VPS33B (49). As a member of the HOPS complex,

VPS33B plays a key role in the regulation of vesicle trafficking and membrane fusion in the endocytic pathway (50). Dephosphorylation of VPS33B by PtpA disrupts the assembly of the HOPS complex and translates directly into phagosome maturation arrest and avoidance of proteolytic degradation (49). EsxG and EsxH are secreted by mycobacteria and target the component of the host endosomal sorting complexes required for transport (ESCRT) machinery, Hrs (51). The ESCRT machinery directs cargo destined for degradation to lysosomes (52). However, the combined action of EsxG and EsxH disrupts ESCRT function and impairs phagolysosome fusion, preventing delivery of *M. tuberculosis* to the lysosome (51). In addition, the EspB effector, when combined with other mycobacterial antigens, increases phagosome maturation inhibition (53). Indeed, cosecretion of EspB with the 6-kDa early secretory antigenic target (ESAT-6) and 10-kDa culture filtrate protein (CFP-10) enhances inhibition of phagosome maturation and promotes survival of the pathogen (53). However, the mechanism of action which allows EspB to prevent phagolysosome fusion and its target remains unknown.

Finally, cord factor is the most abundant glycolipid found in the mycobacterial cell wall, and it interferes with phagolysosome fusion (54). Cord factor consists of the disaccharide trehalose covalently bound to two mycolic acid residues, which in turn are anchored to the bacterial membrane by the hydrophobic component. Such molecules have been observed to confer fusion inhibition of phospholipid bilayers (55). In agreement with this, cord factor is thought to act as a barrier and prevent the fusion of phospholipid vesicles such as phagosomes and lysosomes. The mechanism by which cord factor is transferred from the bacterial cell to the phagosomal membrane, and how it blocks phagolysosome fusion, remains unclear. However, phagolysosome fusion inhibition is believed to be due to cord factor creating a steric block to fusion and/or increasing the hydration force (56).

Yersinia's primary niche for replication is extracellular. Thus, *Yersinia* synthesizes a large number of effectors that block phagocytosis and promote extracellular growth. In spite of this antiphagocytotic effort, a significant amount of its microbial population is engulfed by macrophages (57). The ability of *Yersinia* to replicate in macrophages remains a disputed issue despite several studies supporting this claim (58–60). Unlike other intracellular pathogens which have developed multiple strategies to inhibit phagoysosome fusion (61, 62), certain strains of *Yersinia* have been reported to reside within the phagolysosome (63). These results indicate that, as observed in *Salmonella* infection, the *Yersinia*-containing phagosome acquires lysosomal markers before being excluded from the lysosomal pathway (64). Transient interactions with lysosomes may be mandatory for remodeling the phagosome into a replication-permissive vacuole. Over the years, considerable attention has been given to how *Yersinia* manipulates the functions of macrophages from the outside, but little is known about the modes of action behind the intracellular subversion of macrophage function.

Inhibition of Phagosomal Acidification

The impressive destructive capacity of the phagolysosome is attributed to the concerted effort of molecules, such as hydrolytic enzymes and oxidants, plus the acidification of the phagosome. The acidification of the phagosome is generated by the V-ATPase pump, a protein complex that controls phagosome acidification by transporting protons across membranes (65). The acidification of the phagolysosome serves several purposes: it restricts microbial growth, it activates lysosomal hydrolases whose activity is optimal at low pH, and intraphagosomal protons are used to produce reactive oxygen species which are important antimicrobial ammunition for phagocytes (18).

Given the importance of phagosome acidification, it is not surprising that several

pathogens have developed strategies to block phagosome acidification by targeting the proton pump, allowing them to remain in a relatively neutral pH where they can survive. As seen in Fig. 2, the *M. tuberculosis* secreted phosphatase PtpA directly interferes with phagosome acidification by blocking the assembly of the macrophage's V-ATPase pump (66). Specifically, PtpA binds to subunit H of the pump and excludes the pump from the phagosomal membrane, resulting in diminished phagosome acidification (66). In a similar manner, the *L. pneumophila* protein SidK interacts with subunit A of the V-ATPase pump and inhibits ATP hydrolysis and proton translocation, resulting in a fairly neutral pH inside the phagosome (67).

Yersinia has also been shown to prevent acidification of phagolysosomes. Unlike pathogenic mycobacteria, which inhibit acidification of the phagosome by excluding the proton pump from the phagosomal membrane, *Y. pseudotuberculosis* attenuates the activity of the V-ATPase pump (59). To date, however, no *Yersinia* effectors inhibiting phagosomal acidification have been identified.

Contrary to *Mycobacterium*, *Legionella*, or *Yersinia* species, *Salmonella* species do not interfere with phagosome acidification. Instead, they adapt to the lower phagosomal pH. *Salmonella*'s adaptive response involves activation of acid tolerance genes which help the bacterium cope with the acidic pH (68). Upon exposure to the acidic environment, *Salmonella* secretes secreted system effector B/C/D (SseB, SseC, and SseD) to its surface, where they form a complex and participate in the translocation of T3SS effectors (see below) across the bacterial membrane (69).

SURVIVAL STRATEGIES OF INTRACELLULAR PATHOGENS BEYOND PHAGOSOME MATURATION ARREST

To avoid prolonged exposure to the harsh environment of the phagolysosome, intracellular pathogens have developed alternative survival strategies. In addition to prevention of phagosome maturation or acidification, some pathogens, such as *Salmonella* and *Chlamydia*, relocalize the phagosome outside of the endocytic pathway where they can replicate. Others, exemplified by *Shigella* and *Listeria*, escape the phagosome before fusion with lysosomes and replicate in the host cytoplasm. Alternatively, *Legionella* forces the remodeling of the phagosomal membrane into a replicative-permissive vacuole (70). These numerous strategies suggest several ways to circumvent the killing capacity of the phagosomal pathway.

Cytoskeleton Remodeling

After blocking the digestive endocytic pathway, certain pathogens require the localization of the phagosome to areas of the cell where acquisition of nutrients or membrane components from organelles occurs. To establish a replication-permissive vacuole, pathogens manipulate actin polymerization and form an intermediate filament network around the phagosome, allowing for the rerouting of the pathogen-containing phagosome.

To replicate, *Salmonella* must localize to the microtubule organizing center near the Golgi apparatus. This migration is ensured by the formation of an actin network around the phagosome (71). As illustrated in Fig. 3, the effectors *Salmonella* invasion protein (Sip) AC, secretion system effector I (SseI), *Salmonella*-secreted protein H2 (SspH2), and *Salmonella* plasmid virulence protein B (SpvB) take active roles in the formation of this network (72). SipA and SipC cause actin condensation and cytoskeletal rearrangements by bundling and nucleating actin

Phagosomal Membrane Remodeling

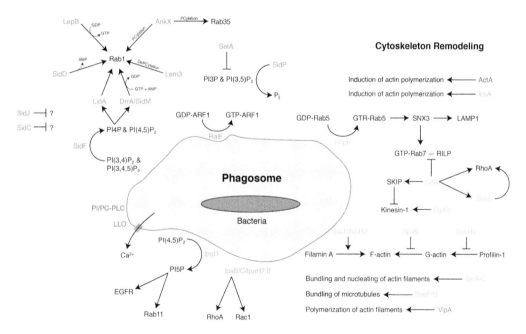

Vacuolar Membrane Lysis

FIGURE 3 Cytoskeleton remodeling, vacuolar membrane lysis, and phagosomal membrane remodeling by microbial pathogens. Orange proteins represent *Legionella* virulence factors; red, *Listeria* virulence factors; blue, *Salmonella* virulence factors; and green, *Shigella* virulence factors.

filaments (71, 73, 74), while both SseI and SspH2 interact with the host actin cross-linking protein filamin A for cross-linking F-actin (72). The cross-linking of F-actin is important for remodeling the cytoskeleton for modulation of cell shape and motility and for vesicle and organelle movement. Moreover, SspH2 interacts with profilin-1, another actin-binding protein, and thus prevents the interaction of profilin-1 with G-actin and alters the rate of actin polymerization (72). The redistribution of the phagosome away from the perinuclear region occurs by the depolymerization and disruption of the actin cytoskeleton of the host cell. Termination of actin polymerization is carried by the SpvB effector, which post-translationally modifies G-actin monomers, preventing their polymerization into F-actin filaments (75).

The proper positioning of the *Salmonella*-containing phagosome near the Golgi apparatus is dependent on the formation of tubules from the phagosome. The SopB effector is required early in infection to recruit Rab5 to the early phagosome (36). Rab5 subsequently recruits sorting nexin 3 (SNX3), an important regulator of membrane trafficking, which contributes to the recruitment of Rab7 and LAMP1 to the phagosome (Fig. 3). SNX3 also promotes the formation of tubules and the movement of the phagosome (76).

Upon localization of the phagosome near the Golgi apparatus, phagosome maturation stops, replication of the pathogen is initiated, and specialized filamentous membrane structures named *Salmonella*-induced filaments (Sifs) form. Sifs are derived from late endosomes, because they contain late endocytic markers such as LAMP1 and V-ATPase (77). They extend from the surface of the phagosome along microtubules to the cell periphery, where they recruit host Rab9 and Rab11 which regulate fusion with Golgi-derived vesicles (78, 79). Sifs also contribute to the localization of endocytic compartments to the cell periphery for nutrient acquisition, the movement of bacteria from cell to cell, and the enlargement of the phagosome to accommodate growing numbers of replicating bacteria (80).

The formation of Sifs is principally dependent on two effectors, PipB2 and SifA (80, 81), and to a lesser extent on SseJ, SseF, and SseG (Fig. 3) (82). On the one hand, PipB2 promotes the outward, or anterograde, movement of the phagosome by recruiting host kinesin-1 to the phagosomal membrane (81). Kinesin-1 is a microtubule motor complex that transports intracellular cargo to the cell periphery (83). On the other hand, SifA, necessary for the stability of the phagosome, promotes the movement of the phagosome toward the perinuclear region (80). In contrast to PipB2, SifA downregulates the recruitment of kinesin-1 by interacting with the host protein SifA kinesin-interacting protein (SKIP) (81). SKIP binds kinesin-1 and regulates kinesin-1 levels at the phagosomal membrane (84). The formation of Sifs requires a balance between the activities of PipB2 and SifA, and this balance is influenced by the actin-binding protein SipA, which stabilizes SifA via its actin-modulatory effects (74). Thus, the counteracting functions of PipB2 and SifA suggest that opposing as well as complementary activities of *Salmonella* effectors are required for Sif formation. Moreover, in a parallel pathway, the SifA-mediated uncoupling of Rab7 from RILP is also believed to facilitate the extension of tubules from the phagosome as SifA binding to Rab7 displaces RILP/dynein-dynactin from Sifs (45).

In cooperation with SifA, the effector SseJ also contributes to Sif formation by controlling the dynamics of the phagosome. Upon recruitment by SifA, SKIP and the small GTPase RhoA form a complex with SseJ which promotes the induction of tubular filaments from the phagosomal membrane (85). The exact mechanism of tubulation induction is currently unknown. The small GTPase RhoA, known to participate in the regulation of microtubule dynamics, regulates kinesin-1 binding to the microtubule and, therefore, kinesin-1-mediated transport

(86). SseF and SseG participate in the dynein-mediated movement of the phagosome along microtubules. Indeed, SseF and SseG colocalize with microtubules, induce their bundling, which serves as a scaffold for Sif formation, and control the positioning of the phagosome by modulating the activity of dynein on the phagosome (87). In addition to their role in Sif formation, SseF and SseG also promote the aggregation of endosomal vesicles into tubules and recruit Golgi-derived vesicles to the phagosome, indicating that interactions with the secretory pathway are required for intracellular replication (88).

Legionella also secretes effectors that interfere with host cell organelle trafficking pathways. *In vitro* studies have shown that the effector VipA colocalizes with early endosomes and host cell actin filaments and causes a direct enhancement of microfilament polymerization (89). This helps isolate the phagosome from the endocytic pathway and enables the pathogen to escape degradation.

Lastly, cytoskeleton remodeling has also been observed in the *Mycobacterium* species *Mycobacterium marinum*, a pathogen of fish and frogs. *M. marinum* escapes the phagosome and is free in the host cytoplasm, where it manipulates the actin filament network of the host to induce the formation of actin tails. The use of actin-based motility propels the pathogen through the cell cytoplasm to the cell periphery or into neighboring cells. This behavior has only been observed in this specific *Mycobacterium* species (90). In a similar fashion, *Listeria* and *Shigella* also utilize the host actin assembly machinery to move within the host and spread between host cells (91). During normal actin remodeling in host cells, members of the Wiskott-Aldrich syndrome protein (WASp) family activate the actin-related protein 2/3 (Arp2/3) complex. *Listeria* and *Shigella* have both developed mechanisms to induce actin polymerization by activating the Arp2/3 complex. As shown in Fig. 3, *Listeria* releases ActA (92), which mimics WASp, and *Shigella*

secretes IcsA (93), which recruits neural WASp to the bacterial surface. Both host proteins activate the Arp2/3 complex (91). The mechanism by which *M. marinum* induces actin polymerization remains incomplete, but studies have shown that *M. marinum* recruits WASp to its surface, and its mode of action shares more similarities to that of *Shigella* than *Listeria* (90).

Lysis of the Vacuolar Membrane

Shigella, *Listeria*, and *M. marinum* have all developed mechanisms enabling them to lyse the membrane of the vacuole in which they reside, permitting their escape into the host cytoplasm. The mechanism by which *M. marinum* escapes the phagosome remains unknown. During infection, *Shigella* secretes the PI phosphatase IpgD, which changes the lipid composition of the early endosomal membrane (Fig. 3). IpgD dephosphorylates $PI(4,5)P_2$ to produce PI5P (94). PI5P recruits epidermal growth factor receptor (EGFR) to the membrane, and prolonged signaling via EGFR slows down phagosome maturation and impairs lysosomal degradation (95). In addition, PI5P also recruits Rab11-positive vacuoles to the phagosome, aiding in the process of vacuolar rupture (96). During the late phagosomal stage *Shigella* releases IpaB and IpaC, two virulence factors that facilitate membrane lysis. In particular, IpaB forms pores within membranes, while IpaC disrupts membrane integrity (97, 98). The specific mechanism by which pores are formed remains to be discovered, but it is suggested to involve host signaling as the small GTPases RhoA and Rac1 are recruited to the lysing vacuoles (99). In addition to IpaB and IpaC, IpaH7.8 has been suggested to promote bacterial phagosomal escape, but its participation in this process is controversial (100). As previously described, once the pathogen escapes into the cytoplasm, it releases effectors that cause actin polymerization reorganization to facilitate its intracellular motility inside the host cell.

Listeria also perforates the phagosomal membrane and escapes into the cytoplasm in a process mediated by the secretion of listeriolysin O (101). In addition, *Listeria* releases the phospholipases phosphatidylinositol phospholipase C and phosphatidylcholine phospholipase C, which also contribute to phagosomal membrane breakdown (Fig. 3) (102).

Membrane Remodeling of the *Legionella*-Containing Phagosome

To bypass the conventional endocytic maturation route, *Legionella* has developed the ability to modify the composition of the phagosomal membrane into a replicative-permissive compartment analogous to endoplasmic reticulum (ER)–derived vesicles (103). This remodeling process is unique to *Legionella* and occurs in sequential steps soon after phagocytosis. First, the bacterium intercepts early secretory vesicles from the ER and associates them with the phagosome. These ER vesicles then fuse to each other to form a large structure surrounding the phagosome (103, 104). The second stage involves the elimination of the phagosomal membrane allowing *Legionella* to replicate in this new ER-like compartment (103).

To allow fusion with ER-derived vesicles, the *Legionella*-harboring phagosome first remodels its own membrane via a process that involves PI metabolism (103). *Legionella* secretes SidF, a phosphoinositide 3-phosphatase, which hydrolyzes $PI(3,4)P_2$ and $PI(3,4,5)P_3$, the two PI species generated on the phagosome upon phagocytosis, into PI4P and $PI(4,5)P_2$ (Fig. 3) (105). As a result, the lipid composition of the phagosome resembles that of the Golgi apparatus, an appealing site for ER-derived vesicles.

The SidF-mediated conversion of the phagosome into a PI4P enriched organelle anchors LidA and DrrA/SidM, two effectors that promote the recruitment of ER-derived vesicles and fusion with the phagosome (106, 107). As illustrated in Fig. 3, LidA and DrrA/

SidM recruit early secretory vesicles to the phagosome via interaction with the host GTPase Rab1, which plays a distinct role in the maturation of phagosomes (108). Rab1 is necessary for the fusion of ER-derived vesicles with the Golgi apparatus (109), conferring an ER-like membrane to the phagosomes (110). The DrrA/SidM effector performs two covalent modifications on Rab1; its GEF domain recruits Rab1 to the phagosome and converts inactive GDP-bound Rab1 into active GTP-bound Rab1 (111), and its nucleotidyltransferase domain transfers an adenosine monophosphate (AMPylation) to a tyrosine residue on Rab1, which contributes to maintaining it on the phagosomal membrane and disrupting vesicular transport (112). Active Rab1 then recruits host-tethering factors to the phagosomal membrane and facilitates membrane fusion with ER-derived vesicles (110). Rab1 activity is also regulated by LepB, a GTPase-activating protein (113). However, unlike DrrA/SidM, LepB regulates the removal of Rab1 from membranes by binding to GTP-bound Rab1 and promoting GTP hydrolysis, which results in inactivated Rab1 (114). SidD also functions as an antagonist of DrrA/SidM, contributing to its release from the membrane (Fig. 3) (115).

The effector ankyrin repeat-containing protein X (AnkX), a phosphorylcholine transferase, also modifies the small GTPase Rab1. It does so by catalyzing the attachment of a phosphocholine moiety (PCylation) to a serine residue of Rab1 (116). This covalent modification interferes with the GTPase activity of Rab1, preventing it from interacting with cellular effectors and impeding microtubule-dependent vesicular transport between specific membranes (117). PCylation of Rab1 may inhibit fusion of early secretory events involving vesicular transport on microtubules with ER-derived vesicles (117). AnkX also attaches a phosphocholine moiety to Rab35, a member of the Rab1 family which regulates the sorting of cargo from early endosomes. Modulation of Rab35 function results in enlarged early endosomes (118). Thus, phosphocholination of Rab1 and Rab35 by AnkX is necessary for disrupting the activities of host membrane transport proteins and for efficient inhibition of the acquisition of the endosomal marker LAMP1 (117).

To counteract AnkX-mediated modification on Rab1, *Legionella* secretes Lem3, a dephosphorylcholinase, which reverses the post-translational modification on Rab1, making it more accessible to GEFs such as DrrA/SidM (119). Another *Legionella* effector that is important in the remodeling of the membrane is RalF. RalF is essential for recruiting the host GTPase ADP-ribosylation factor 1 (ARF1) to the phagosome and activating it via its ARF GEF activity (120). ARF1 is an enticing target for *Legionella* because it regulates transport of vesicles between the ER and Golgi apparatus (121).

Other *Legionella* effectors that have been shown to redirect the recruitment of ER-derived vesicles to the phagosome include SidJ, SidP, SidC, and subversion of eukaryotic traffic protein A (SetA) (122–124). SidJ redirects the recruitment of ER-derived vesicles to the *Legionella* phagosome (123). SidP is a PI phosphatase that hydrolyzes PI3P and PI(3,5)P$_2$, promoting the evasion of the endocytic pathway by the phagosome (124). SidC anchors to the membrane via binding of PI4P, a marker of secretory-vesicle trafficking (106), and SidC is suggested to function as a bacterial tethering factor as *Legionella* lacking the *sidC* gene alter the recruitment of ER-derived vesicles to the phagosome (122). The exact mechanisms by which SidJ, SidP, and SidC recruit ER-derived vesicles, and the identity of their host targets, remain unknown. Lastly, SetA, a glycosyltransferase, modifies vesicular trafficking by attaching glucose moieties to conserved threonine residues within the catalytic region of host targets (125). SetA also anchors to the phagosomal membrane by binding to PIs (125). The effect of this modification remains unknown, but it is suggested to involve disruption of host targets and signaling events. The rerouting of ER-derived vesicles to the surface of phagosomes harboring *Legionella* is suggested as a potential downstream effect of glycosylation catalyzed by SetA (126).

CONCLUDING REMARKS

To perpetuate their reign, several infectious agents highjack circulating macrophages which paradoxically serve as both the first line of defense against microbial infections as well as the pathogens' natural habitat. In this review, we show that the ability of Gram-negative *Legionella*, *Salmonella*, *Shigella*, and *Yersinia*, as well as the acid-fast actinomycete *Mycobacterium*, to circumvent the phagocytes' bactericidal activity and perturb the host killing machinery is mediated by effectors injected into the cytoplasm of the host by specialized secretion systems. These secreted virulence factors confer remarkable resilience to pathogens by exerting functional redundancy with each other and facilitating and maximizing host cell invasion, replication, and intracellular survival.

The host-pathogen interactome is a recent field of study and requires further scrutiny. Much remains unknown regarding the cellular functions of the effectors implicated, their host targets, and their mechanisms of action. Understanding the approach and dynamics by which microbial proteins execute their functions will greatly increase our understanding of the mechanisms employed by pathogens to alter host cell physiology. The characterization of bacterial secreted proteins continues to be a major focus of future research. Newly acquired knowledge is crucial for the development of vaccines and therapeutic intervention against established and emerging infectious diseases.

ACKNOWLEDGMENTS

Funding for this study was provided by the Canadian Institute of Health Research Operating Grant MOP-106622, the British Columbia

Lung Association, and the TB Veterans Association. We thank Stefan Szary for his help with illustrations and Joseph Chao and Jeffrey Helm for their useful comments.

CITATION

Poirier V, Av-Gay Y. 2015. Intracellular growth of bacterial pathogens: the role of secreted effector proteins in the control of phagocytosed microorganisms. Microbiol Spectrum 3(6):VMBF-0003-2014.

REFERENCES

1. **World Health Organization.** 2015. *The Top 10 Causes of Death*. Fact sheet No. 310. http://www.who.int/mediacentre/factsheets/fs310/en/.
2. **Guerrant RL, Blackwood BL.** 1999. Threats to global health and survival: the growing crises of tropical infectious diseases: our "unfinished agenda." *Clin Infect Dis* **28:**966–986.
3. **Butler JC, Crengle S, Cheek JE, Leach AJ, Lennon D, O'Brien KL, Santosham M.** 2001. Emerging infectious diseases among indigenous peoples. *Emerg Infect Dis* **7**(Suppl 3)**:**554–555.
4. **Bliska JB, Copass MC, Falkow S.** 1993. The *Yersinia pseudotuberculosis* adhesin YadA mediates intimate bacterial attachment to and entry into HEp-2 cells. *Infect Immun* **61:**3914–3921.
5. **Cascales E, Christie PJ.** 2003. The versatile bacterial type IV secretion systems. *Nat Rev Microbiol* **1:**137–149.
6. **Backert S, Meyer TF.** 2006. Type IV secretion systems and their effectors in bacterial pathogenesis. *Curr Opin Microbiol* **9:**207–217.
7. **Saier MHJ.** 2006. Protein secretion systems in Gram-negative bacteria. *Microbe* **1:**414–419.
8. **Yen M-R, Peabody CR, Partovi SM, Zhai Y, Tseng Y-H, Saier MHJ.** 2002. Protein-translocating outer membrane porins of Gram-negative bacteria. *Biochim Biophys Acta* **1562:**6–31.
9. **Thanassi DG, Bliska JB, Christie PJ.** 2012. Surface organelles assembled by secretion systems of Gram-negative bacteria: diversity in structure and function. *FEMS Microbiol Rev* **36:**1046–1082.
10. **Abdallah AM, Gey van Pittius NC, Champion PA, Cox J, Luirink J, Vandenbroucke-Grauls CM, Appelmelk BJ, Bitter W.** 2007. Type VII secretion: mycobacteria show the way. *Nat Rev Microbiol* **5:**883–891.
11. **Lenz LL, Mohammadi S, Geissler A, Portnoy DA.** 2003. SecA2-dependent secretion of autolytic enzymes promotes *Listeria monocytogenes* pathogenesis. *Proc Natl Acad Sci USA* **100:**12432–12437.
12. **Stanier RY, Adelberg EA, Ingraham JL.** 1976. *The Microbial World*, 4th ed. Prentice-Hall, Englewood Cliffs, NJ.
13. **Coombes BK, Finlay BB.** 2005. Insertion of the bacterial type III translocon: not your average needle stick. *Trends Microbiol* **13:**92–95.
14. **Bitter W, Houben EN, Bottai D, Brodin P, Brown EJ, Cox JS, Derbyshire K, Fortune SM, Gao LY, Liu J, Gey van Pittius NC, Pym AS, Rubin EJ, Sherman DR, Cole ST, Brosch R.** 2009. Systematic genetic nomenclature for type VII secretion systems. *PLoS Pathog* **5:**e1000507. doi:10.1371/journal.ppat.1000507.
15. **Stanley SA, Raghavan S, Hwang WW, Cox JS.** 2003. Acute infection and macrophage subversion by *Mycobacterium tuberculosis* require a specialized secretion system. *Proc Natl Acad Sci USA* **100:**13001–13006.
16. **Guinn KM, Hickey MJ, Mathur SK, Zakel KL, Grotzke JE, Lewinsohn DM, Smith S, Sherman DR.** 2004. Individual RD1-region genes are required for export of ESAT-6/CFP-10 and for virulence of *Mycobacterium tuberculosis*. *Mol Microbiol* **51:**359–370.
17. **Abdallah AM, Verboom T, Hannes F, Safi M, Strong M, Eisenberg D, Musters RJ, Vandenbroucke-Grauls CM, Appelmelk BJ, Luirink J, Bitter W.** 2006. A specific secretion system mediates PPE41 transport in pathogenic mycobacteria. *Mol Microbiol* **62:**667–679.
18. **Flannagan RS, Jaumouillé V, Grinstein S.** 2012. The cell biology of phagocytosis. *Annu Rev Pathol* **7:**61–98.
19. **Sturgill-Koszycki S, Schlesinger PH, Chakraborty P, Haddix PL, Collins HL, Fok AK, Allen RD, Gluck SL, Heuser J, Russell DG.** 1994. Lack of acidification in *Mycobacterium* phagosomes produced by exclusion of the vesicular proton-ATPase. *Science* **263:**678–681.
20. **Fraser DW, Tsai TR, Orenstein W, Parkin WE, Beecham HJ, Sharrar RG, Harris J, Mallison GF, Martin SM, McDade JE, Shepard CC, Brachman PS.** 1977. Legionnaires' disease: description of an epidemic of pneumonia. *N Engl J Med* **297:**1189–1197.
21. **Baess I.** 1979. Deoxyribonucleic acid relatedness among species of slowly-growing mycobacteria. *Acta Pathol Microbiol Scand B* **87:**221–226.
22. **Stenmark H.** 2009. Rab GTPases as coordinators of vesicle traffic. *Nat Rev Mol Cell Biol* **10:**513–525.

23. **Christoforidis S, Miaczynska M, Ashman K, Wilm M, Zhao L, Yip SC, Waterfield MD, Backer JM, Zerial M.** 1999. Phosphatidylinositol-3-OH kinases are Rab5 effectors. *Nat Cell Biol* **1:**249–252.

24. **Fratti RA, Backer JM, Gruenberg J, Corvera S, Deretic V.** 2001. Role of phosphatidylinositol 3-kinase and Rab5 effectors in phagosomal biogenesis and mycobacterial phagosome maturation arrest. *J Cell Biol* **154:**631–644.

25. **Lemmon MA.** 2003. Phosphoinositide recognition domains. *Traffic* **4:**201–213.

26. **Ellson C, Davidson K, Anderson K, Stephens LR, Hawkins PT.** 2006. PtdIns3P binding to the PX domain of p40phox is a physiological signal in NADPH oxidase activation. *EMBO J* **25:**4468–4478.

27. **Vieira OV, Harrison RE, Scott CC, Stenmark H, Alexander D, Liu J, Gruenberg J, Schreiber AD, Grinstein S.** 2004. Acquisition of Hrs, an essential component of phagosomal maturation, is impaired by mycobacteria. *Mol Cell Biol* **24:**4593–4604.

28. **McBride HM, Rybin V, Murphy C, Giner A, Teasdale R, Zerial M.** 1999. Oligomeric complexes link Rab5 effectors with NSF and drive membrane fusion via interactions between EEA1 and syntaxin 13. *Cell* **98:**377–386.

29. **Jahn R, Scheller RH.** 2006. SNAREs-engines for membrane fusion. *Nat Rev Mol Cell Biol* **7:**631–643.

30. **Chatterjee D, Khoo KH.** 1998. Mycobacterial lipoarabinomannan: an extraordinary lipoheteroglycan with profound physiological effects. *Glycobiology* **8:**113–120.

31. **Malik ZA, Denning GM, Kusner DJ.** 2000. Inhibition of Ca2+ signalling by *Mycobacterium tuberculosis* is associated with reduced phagosome-lysosome fusion and increased survival within human macrophages. *J Exp Med* **191:**287–302.

32. **Vergne I, Chua J, Lee HH, Lucas M, Belisle J, Deretic V.** 2005. Mechanism of phagolysosome biogenesis block by viable *Mycobacterium tuberculosis*. *Proc Natl Acad Sci USA* **102:**4033–4038.

33. **Simonsen A, Gaullier JM, D'Arrigo A, Stenmark H.** 1999. The Rab5 effector EEA1 interacts directly with syntaxin-6. *J Biol Chem* **274:**28857–28860.

34. **Ku B, Lee KH, Park WS, Yang CS, Ge J, Lee SG, Cha SS, Shao F, Heo WD, Jung JU, Oh BH.** 2012. VipD of *Legionella pneumophila* targets activated Rab5 and Rab22 to interfere with endosomal trafficking in macrophages. *PLoS Pathog* **8:** e1003082. doi:10.1371/journal.ppat.1003082.

35. **Shohdy N, Efe JA, Emr SD, Shuman HA.** 2005. Pathogen effector protein screening in yeast identifies *Legionella* factors that interfere with membrane trafficking. *Proc Natl Acad Sci USA* **102:**4866–4871.

36. **Mallo GV, Espina M, Smith AC, Terebiznik MR, Alemán A, Finlay BB, Rameh LE, Grinstein S, Brumell JH.** 2008. SopB promotes phosphatidylinositol 3-phosphate formation on *Salmonella* vacuoles by recruiting Rab5 and Vps34. *J Cell Biol* **182:**741–752.

37. **Madan R, Krishnamurthy G, Mukhopadhyay A.** 2008. SopE-mediated recruitment of host Rab5 on phagosomes inhibits *Salmonella* transport to lysosomes. *Methods Mol Biol* **445:**417–437.

38. **Mukherjee K, Parashuraman S, Raje M, Mukhopadhyay A.** 2001. SopE acts as an Rab5-specific nucleotide exchange factor and recruits non-prenylated Rab5 on *Salmonella*-containing phagosomes to promote fusion with early endosomes. *J Biol Chem* **276:**23607–23615.

39. **Hardt WD, Chen LM, Schuebel KE, Bustelo XR, Galán JE.** 1998. *S. typhimurium* encodes an activator of Rho GTPases that induces membrane ruffling and nuclear responses in host cells. *Cell* **93:**815–826.

40. **Alpuche-Aranda CM, Racoosin EL, Swanson JA, Miller SI.** 1994. *Salmonella* stimulate macrophage macropinocytosis and persist within spacious phagosomes. *J Exp Med* **179:** 601–608.

41. **Alvarez-Dominguez C, Barbieri AM, Berón W, Wandinger-Ness A, Stahl PD.** 1996. Phagocytosed live *Listeria monocytogenes* influences Rab5-regulated *in vitro* phagosome-endosome fusion. *J Biol Chem* **271:**13834–13843.

42. **Via LE, Deretic D, Ulmer RJ, Hibler NS, Huber LA, Deretic V.** 1997. Arrest of mycobacterial phagosome maturation is caused by a block in vesicle fusion between stages controlled by Rab5 and Rab7. *J Biol Chem* **272:**13326–13331.

43. **Darsow T, Reider SE, Emr SD.** 1997. A multi-specificity syntaxin homologue, Vam3p, essential for autophagic and biosynthetic protein transport to the vacuole. *J Cell Biol* **138:**517–529.

44. **Price A, Wickner W, Ungermann C.** 2000. Proteins needed for vesicle budding from the golgi complex are also required for the docking step of homotypic vacuole fusion. *J Cell Biol* **148:**1223–1229.

45. **Harrison RE, Brumell JH, Khandani A, Bucci C, Scott CC, Jiang X, Finlay BB, Grinstein S.** 2004. *Salmonella* impairs RILP recruitment to Rab7 during maturation of invasion vacuoles. *Mol Biol Cell* **15:**3146–3154.

46. **Shotland Y, Krämer H, Groisman EA.** 2003. The *Salmonella* SpiC protein targets

the mammalian Hook3 protein function to alter cellular trafficking. *Mol Microbiol* **49:** 1565–1576.

47. **Di Paolo G, De Camilli P.** 2006. Phospho-inositides in cell regulation and membrane dynamics. *Nature* **443:**651–657.

48. **Marcus SL, Knodler LA, Finlay BB.** 2002. *Salmonella enterica* serovar Typhimurium effector SigD/SopB is membrane-associated and ubiquitinated inside host cells. *Cell Microbiol* **4:**435–446.

49. **Bach H, Papavinasasundaram KG, Wong D, Hmama Z, Av-Gay Y.** 2008. *Mycobacterium tuberculosis* virulence is mediated by PtpA dephosphorylation of human vacuolar protein sorting 33B. *Cell Host Microbe* **3:**316–322.

50. **Banta LM, Robinson JS, Klionsky DJ, Emr SD.** 1988. Organelle assembly in yeast: characterization of yeast mutants defective in vacuolar biogenesis and protein sorting. *J Cell Biol* **107:**1369–1383.

51. **Mehra A, Zahra A, Thompson V, Sirisaengtaksin N, Wells A, Porto M, Köster S, Penberthy K, Kubota Y, Dricot A, Rogan D, Vidal M, Hill DE, Bean AJ, Philips JA.** 2013. *Mycobacterium tuberculosis* type VII secreted effector EsxH targets host ESCRT to impair trafficking. *PLoS Pathog* **9:** e1003734. doi:10.1371/journal.ppat.1003734.

52. **Katzmann DJ, Odorizzi G, Emr SD.** 2002. Receptor downregulation and multivesicular-body sorting *Nat Rev Mol Cell Biol* **3:**893–905.

53. **Xu J, Laine O, Masciocchi M, Manoranjan J, Smith J, Du SJ, Edwards N, Zhu X, Fenselau C, Gao LY.** 2007. A unique mycobacterium ESX-1 protein co-secretes with CFP-10/ESAT-6 and is necessary for inhibiting phagosome maturation. *Mol Microbiol* **66:**3787–3800.

54. **Hunter RL, Olsen MR, Jagannath C, Actor JK.** 2006. Multiple roles of cord factor in the pathogenesis of primary, secondary, and cavitary tuberculosis, including a revised description of the pathology of secondary disease. *Ann Clin Lab Sci* **36:**371–386.

55. **Hoekstra D, Düzgünes N, Wilschut J.** 1985. Agglutination and fusion of globoside GL-4 containing phospholipid vesicles mediated by lectins and calcium ions. *Biochemistry* **24:**565–572.

56. **Spargo BJ, Crowe LM, Ioneda T, Beaman BL, Crowe JH.** 1991. Cord factor (alpha,alpha-trehalose 6,6′-dimycolate) inhibits fusion between phospholipid vesicles. *Proc Natl Acad Sci USA* **88:**737–740.

57. **Rosqvist R, Bölin I, Wolf-Watz H.** 1988. Inhibition of phagocytosis in *Yersinia pseudotuberculosis*: a virulence plasmid-encoded ability involving the Yop2b protein. *Infect Immun* **56:**2139–2143.

58. **Pujol C, Bliska JB.** 2003. The ability to replicate in macrophages is conserved between *Yersinia pestis* and *Yersinia pseudotuberculosis*. *Infect Immun* **71:**5892–5829.

59. **Tsukano H, Kura F, Inoue S, Sato S, Izumiya H, Yasuda T, Watanabe H.** 1999. *Yersinia pseudotuberculosis* blocks the phagosomal acidification of B10.A mouse macrophages through the inhibition of vacuolar H(+)-ATPase activity. *Microb Pathog* **27:**253–263.

60. **Tabrizi SN, Robins-Browne RM.** 1992. Influence of a 70 kilobase virulence plasmid on the ability of *Yersinia enterocolitica* to survive phagocytosis *in vitro*. *Microb Pathog* **13:**171–179.

61. **Finlay BB, Falkow S.** 1997. Common themes in microbial pathogenicity revisited. *Microbiol Mol Biol Rev* **61:**136169.

62. **Duclos S, Desjardins M.** 2000. Subversion of a young phagosome: the survival strategies of intracellular pathogens. *Cell Microbiol* **2:**365–377.

63. **Straley SC, Harmon PA.** 1984. *Yersinia pestis* grows within phagolysosomes in mouse peritoneal macrophages. *Infect Immun* **45:**655–659.

64. **Holden DW.** 2002. Trafficking of the *Salmonella* vacuole in macrophages. *Traffic* **3:**161–169.

65. **Hackam DJ, Rotstein OD, Zhang WJ, Demaurex N, Woodside M, Tsai O, Grinstein S.** 1997. Regulation of phagosomal acidification. Differential targeting of Na+/H+ exchangers, Na+/K+-ATPases, and vacuolar-type H+-ATPases. *J Biol Chem* **272:**29810–29820.

66. **Wong D, Bach H, Hmama Z, Av-Gay Y.** 2011. *Mycobacterium tuberculosis* protein tyrosine phosphatase A disrupts phagosome acidification by exclusion of host vacuolar H+-ATPase. *Proc Natl Acad Sci USA* **108:**19371–196.

67. **Xu L, Shen X, Bryan A, Banga S, Swanson MS, Luo ZQ.** 2010. Inhibition of host vacuolar H+-ATPase activity by a *Legionella pneumophila* effector. *PLoS Pathog* **6:**e1000822. doi:10.1371/journal.ppat.1000822.

68. **Prost LR, Daley ME, Le Sage V, Bader MW, Le Moual H, Klevit RE, Miller SI.** 2007. Activation of the bacterial sensor kinase PhoQ by acidic pH. *Mol Cell* **26:**165–174.

69. **Nikolaus T, Deiwick J, Rappl C, Freeman JA, Schröder W, Miller SI, Hensel M.** 2001. SseBCD proteins are secreted by the type III secretion system of *Salmonella* pathogenicity island 2 and function as a translocon. *J Bacteriol* **183:**6036–6045.

70. **Scott CC, Botelho RJ, Grinstein S.** 2003. Phagosome maturation: a few bugs in the system. *J Membr Biol* **193:**137–152.

71. Méresse S, Unsworth KE, Habermann A, Griffiths G, Fang F, Martínez-Lorenzo MJ, Waterman SR, Gorvel JP, Holden DW. 2001. Remodelling of the actin cytoskeleton is essential for replication of intravacuolar *Salmonella*. *Cell Microbiol* **3**:567–577.

72. Miao EA, Brittnacher M, Haraga A, Jeng RL, Welch MD, Miller SI. 2003. *Salmonella* effectors translocated across the vacuolar membrane interact with the actin cytoskeleton. *Mol Microbiol* **48**:401–415.

73. Hayward RD, Koronakis V. 1999. Direct nucleation and bundling of actin by the SipC protein of invasive *Salmonella*. *EMBO J* **18**:4926–4934.

74. Brawn LC, Hayward RD, Koronakis V. 2007. *Salmonella* SPI1 effector SipA persists after entry and cooperates with a SPI2 effector to regulate phagosome maturation and intracellular replication. *Cell Host Microbe* **1**:63–75.

75. Lesnick ML, Reiner NE, Fierer J, Guiney DG. 2001. The *Salmonella* spvB virulence gene encodes an enzyme that ADP-ribosylates actin and destabilizes the cytoskeleton of eukaryotic cells. *Mol Microbiol* **39**:1464–1470.

76. Braun V, Wong A, Landekic M, Hong WJ, Grinstein S, Brumell JH. 2010. Sorting nexin 3 (SNX3) is a component of a tubular endosomal network induced by *Salmonella* and involved in maturation of the *Salmonella*-containing vacuole. *Cell Microbiol* **12**:1352–1367.

77. Drecktrah D, Levine-Wilkinson S, Dam T, Winfree S, Knodler LA, Schroer TA, Steele-Mortimer O. 2008. Dynamic behavior of *Salmonella*-induced membrane tubules in epithelial cells. *Traffic* **9**:2117–2129.

78. Rajashekar R, Liebl D, Seitz A, Hensel M. 2008. Dynamic remodeling of the endosomal system during formation of *Salmonella*-induced filaments by intracellular *Salmonella enterica*. *Traffic* **9**:2100–2116.

79. Husebye H, Aune MH, Stenvik J, Samstad E, Skjeldal F, Halaas O, Nilsen NJ, Stenmark H, Latz E, Lien E, Mollnes TE, Bakke O, Espevik T. 2010. The Rab11a GTPase controls Toll-like receptor 4-induced activation of interferon regulatory factor-3 on phagosomes. *Immunity* **33**:583–596.

80. Beuzón CR, Méresse S, Unsworth KE, Ruíz-Albert J, Garvis S, Waterman SR, Ryder TA, Boucrot E, Holden DW. 2000. *Salmonella* maintains the integrity of its intracellular vacuole through the action of SifA. *EMBO J* **19**:3235–3249.

81. Henry T, Couillault C, Rockenfeller P, Boucrot E, Dumont A, Schroeder N, Hermant A, Knodler LA, Lecine P, Steele-Mortimer O, Borg JP, Gorvel JP, Méresse S. 2006. The *Salmonella* effector protein PipB2 is a linker for kinesin-1. *Proc Natl Acad Sci USA* **103**:13497–13502.

82. Kuhle V, Hensel M. 2002. SseF and SseG are translocated effectors of the type III secretion system of *Salmonella* pathogenicity island 2 that modulate aggregation of endosomal compartments. *Cell Microbiol* **4**:813–824.

83. Vale RD, Reese TS, Sheetz MP. 1985. Identification of a novel force-generating protein, kinesin, involved in microtubule-based motility. *Cell* **42**:39–50.

84. Boucrot E, Henry T, Borg JP, Gorvel JP, Méresse S. 2005. The intracellular fate of *Salmonella* depends on the recruitment of kinesin. *Science* **308**:1174–1178.

85. Ohlson MB, Huang Z, Alto NM, Blanc MP, Dixon JE, Chai J, Miller SI. 2008. Structure and function of *Salmonella* SifA indicate that its interactions with SKIP, SseJ, and RhoA family GTPases induce endosomal tubulation. *Cell Host Microbe* **4**:434–446.

86. Cai D, McEwen DP, Martens JR, Meyhofer E, Verhey KJ. 2009. Single molecule imaging reveals differences in microtubule track selection between kinesin motors. *PLoS Biol* **7**:e1000216. doi:10.1371/journal.pbio.1000216.

87. Kuhle V, Jäckel D, Hensel M. 2004. Effector proteins encoded by *Salmonella* pathogenicity island 2 interfere with the microtubule cytoskeleton after translocation into host cells. *Traffic* **5**:356–370.

88. Kuhle V, Abrahams GL, Hensel M. 2006. Intracellular *Salmonella enterica* redirect exocytic transport processes in a *Salmonella* pathogenicity island 2-dependent manner. *Traffic* **7**:716–730.

89. Franco IS, Shohdy N, Shuman HA. The *Legionella pneumophila* effector VipA is an actin nucleator that alters host cell organelle trafficking. *PLoS Pathog* **8**:e1002546. doi:10.1371/journal.ppat.1002546.

90. Stamm LM, Morisaki JH, Gao LY, Jeng RL, McDonald KL, Roth R, Takeshita S, Heuser J, Welch MD, Brown EJ. 2003. *Mycobacterium marinum* escapes from phagosomes and is propelled by actin-based motility. *J Exp Med* **198**:1361–1368.

91. Goldberg MB. 2001. Actin-based motility of intracellular microbial pathogens. *Microbiol Mol Biol Rev* **65**:595–626.

92. Moors MA, Levitt B, Youngman P, Portnoy DA. 1999. Expression of listeriolysin O and ActA by intracellular and extracellular *Listeria monocytogenes*. *Infect Immun* **67**:131–139.

93. Goldberg MB, Theriot JA, Sansonetti PJ. 1994. Regulation of surface presentation of

IcsA, a *Shigella* protein essential to intracellular movement and spread, is growth phase dependent. *Infect Immun* **62**:5664–5668.

94. **Niebuhr K, Giuriato S, Pedron T, Philpott DJ, Gaits F, Sable J, Sheetz MP, Parsot C, Sansonetti PJ, Payrastre B.** 2002. Conversion of PtdIns(4,5)P(2) into PtdIns(5)P by the *S. flexneri* effector IpgD reorganizes host cell morphology. *EMBO J* **21**:5069–5078.

95. **Ramel D, Lagarrigue F, Pons V, Mounier J, Dupuis-Coronas S, Chicanne G, Sansonetti PJ, Gaits-Iacovoni F, Tronchère H, Payrastre B.** 2011. *Shigella flexneri* infection generates the lipid PI5P to alter endocytosis and prevent termination of EGFR signaling. *Sci Signal* **4**:ra61.

96. **Mellouk N, Weiner A, Aulner N, Schmitt C, Elbaum M, Shorte SL, Danckaert A, Enninga J.** 2014. *Shigella* subverts the host recycling compartment to rupture its vacuole. *Cell Host Microbe* **16**:517–530.

97. **Blocker A, Gounon P, Larquet E, Niebuhr K, Cabiaux V, Parsot C, Sansonetti P.** 1999. The tripartite type III secreton of *Shigella flexneri* inserts IpaB and IpaC into host membranes. *J Cell Biol* **147**:683–693.

98. **High N, Mounier J, Prévost MC, Sansonetti PJ.** 1992. IpaB of *Shigella flexneri* causes entry into epithelial cells and escape from the phagocytic vacuole. *EMBO J* **11**:1991–1999.

99. **Mounier J, Laurent V, Hall A, Fort P, Carlier MF, Sansonetti PJ, Egile C.** 1999. Rho family GTPases control entry of *Shigella flexneri* into epithelial cells but not intracellular motility. *J Cell Sci* **112**:2069–2080.

100. **Fernandez-Prada CM, Hoover DL, Tall BD, Hartman AB, Kopelowitz J, Venkatesan MM.** 2000. *Shigella flexneri* IpaH(7.8) facilitates escape of virulent bacteria from the endocytic vacuoles of mouse and human macrophages. *Infect Immun* **68**:3608–3619.

101. **Portnoy DA, Jacks PS, Hinrichs DJ.** 1988. Role of hemolysin for the intracellular growth of *Listeria monocytogenes*. *J Exp Med* **167**:1459–1471.

102. **Smith GA, Marquis H, Jones S, Johnston NC, Portnoy DA, Goldfine H.** 1995. The two distinct phospholipases C of *Listeria monocytogenes* have overlapping roles in escape from a vacuole and cell-to-cell spread. *Infect Immun* **63**:4231–4237.

103. **Tilney LG, Harb OS, Connelly PS, Robinson CG, Roy CR.** 2001. How the parasitic bacterium *Legionella pneumophila* modifies its phagosome and transforms it into rough ER: implications for conversion of plasma membrane to the ER membrane. *J Cell Sci* **114**:4637–4650.

104. **Kagan JC, Roy CR.** 2002. *Legionella* phagosomes intercept vesicular traffic from endoplasmic reticulum exit sites. *Nat Cell Biol* **4**:945–954.

105. **Hsu F, Zhu W, Brennan L, Tao L, Luo ZQ, Mao Y.** 2012. Structural basis for substrate recognition by a unique *Legionella* phosphoinositide phosphatase. *Proc Natl Acad Sci USA* **109**:13567–13572.

106. **Weber SS, Ragaz C, Reus K, Nyfeler Y, Hilbi H.** 2006. *Legionella pneumophila* exploits PI(4)P to anchor secreted effector proteins to the replicative vacuole. *PLoS Pathog* **2**:e46.

107. **Conover GM, Derré I, Vogel JP, Isberg RR.** 2003. The *Legionella pneumophila* LidA protein: a translocated substrate of the Dot/Icm system associated with maintenance of bacterial integrity. *Mol Microbiol* **48**:305–321.

108. **Machner MP, Isberg RR.** 2006. Targeting of host Rab GTPase function by the intravacuolar pathogen *Legionella pneumophila*. *Dev Cell* **11**:47–56.

109. **Moyer BD, Allan BB, Balch WE.** 2001. Rab1 interaction with a GM130 effector complex regulates COPII vesicle cis–Golgi tethering. *Traffic* **2**:268–276.

110. **Kagan JC, Stein MP, Pypaert M, Roy CR.** 2004. *Legionella* subvert the functions of Rab1 and Sec22b to create a replicative organelle. *J Exp Med* **199**:1201–1211.

111. **Murata T, Delprato A, Ingmundson A, Toomre DK, Lambright DG, Roy CR.** 2006. The *Legionella pneumophila* effector protein DrrA is a Rab1 guanine nucleotide-exchange factor. *Nat Cell Biol* **8**:971–977.

112. **Müller MP, Peters H, Blümer J, Blankenfeldt W, Goody RS, Itzen A.** 2010. The *Legionella* effector protein DrrA AMPylates the membrane traffic regulator Rab1b. *Science* **329**:946–949.

113. **Chen J, de Felipe KS, Clarke M, Lu H, Anderson OR, Segal G, Shuman HA.** 2004. *Legionella* effectors that promote nonlytic release from protozoa. *Science* **303**:1358–1361.

114. **Ingmundson A, Delprato A, Lambright DG, Roy CR.** 2007. *Legionella pneumophila* proteins that regulate Rab1 membrane cycling. *Nature* **450**:365–369.

115. **Tan Y, Luo ZQ.** 2011. *Legionella pneumophila* SidD is a deAMPylase that modifies Rab1. *Nature* **475**:506–509.

116. **Mukherjee S, Liu X, Arasaki K, McDonough J, Galán JE, Roy CR.** 2011. Modulation of Rab GTPase function by a protein phosphocholine transferase. *Nature* **477**:103–106.

117. **Pan X, Lührmann A, Satoh A, Laskowski-Arce MA, Roy CR.** 2008. Ankyrin repeat proteins comprise a diverse family of bacterial type IV effectors. *Science* **320**:1651–1654.

118. **Allaire PD, Marat AL, Dall'Armi C, Di Paolo G, McPherson PS, Ritter B.** 2010. The Connecdenn DENN domain: a GEF for Rab35 mediating cargo-specific exit from early endosomes. *Mol Cell* **37:**370–382.

119. **Tan Y, Arnold RJ, Luo ZQ.** 2011. *Legionella pneumophila* regulates the small GTPase Rab1 activity by reversible phosphorylcholination. *Proc Natl Acad Sci USA* **108:**21212–21217.

120. **Nagai H, Kagan JC, Zhu X, Kahn RA, Roy CR.** 2002. A bacterial guanine nucleotide exchange factor activates ARF on *Legionella* phagosomes. *Science* **295:**679–682.

121. **Robinson CG, Roy CR.** 2006. Attachment and fusion of endoplasmic reticulum with vacuoles containing *Legionella pneumophila*. *Cell Microbiol* **8:**793–805.

122. **Ragaz C, Pietsch H, Urwyler S, Tiaden A, Weber SS, Hilbi H.** 2008. The *Legionella pneumophila* phosphatidylinositol-4 phosphate-binding type IV substrate SidC recruits endo-plasmic reticulum vesicles to a replication-permissive vacuole. *Cell Microbiol* **10:**2416–2433.

123. **Liu Y, Luo ZQ.** 2007. The *Legionella pneumophila* effector SidJ is required for efficient recruitment of endoplasmic reticulum proteins to the bacterial phagosome. *Infect Immun* **75:**592–603.

124. **Toulabi L, Wu X, Cheng Y, Mao Y.** 2013. Identification and structural characterization of a *Legionella* phosphoinositide phosphatase. *J Biol Chem* **288:**24518–24527.

125. **Jank T, Böhmer KE, Tzivelekidis T, Schwan C, Belyi Y, Aktories K.** 2012. Domain organization of *Legionella* effector SetA. *Cell Microbiol* **14:**852–868.

126. **Heidtman M, Chen EJ, Moy MY, Isberg RR.** 2009. Large-scale identification of *Legionella pneumophila* Dot/Icm substrates that modulate host cell vesicle trafficking pathways. *Cell Microbiol* **11:**230–248.

Cellular Exit Strategies of Intracellular Bacteria

25

KEVIN HYBISKE[1] and RICHARD STEPHENS[2]

INTRODUCTION

Many infectious microbes spend all or some of their time within a host in an intracellular niche. Consequently, to maintain survival as a species these pathogens have evolved diverse mechanisms for overcoming a critical biological challenge they all face: how to exit the host cell. Historically, experimental research into the strategies adopted by intracellular pathogens to accomplish this task has been lacking, and many of our presumptions about how pathogens exit, or egress, from host cells were therefore largely speculative and unsupported by experimental data. Some explanations for our collective lack of knowledge include the difficulty of working with some of these organisms, especially in light of their often complex developmental growth cycles, the complexity and variation of the host cell types targeted by bacteria (exit mechanisms may be very different in macrophages than epithelial cells, for example), and the inadequacies of genetic manipulation of some bacteria. Finally, the general question of host cell exit has simply been overlooked by the field; earlier infection events such as attachment or entry

[1]Division of Allergy and Infectious Diseases, Department of Medicine, University of Washington, Seattle, WA 98195; [2]Program in Infectious Diseases, School of Public Health, University of California, Berkeley, Berkeley, CA 94720.
Virulence Mechanisms of Bacterial Pathogens, 5th edition
Edited by Indira T. Kudva, Nancy A. Cornick, Paul J. Plummer, Qijing Zhang, Tracy L. Nicholson, John P. Bannantine, and Bryan H. Bellaire
© 2016 American Society for Microbiology, Washington, DC
doi:10.1128/microbiolspec.VMBF-0002-2014

are far easier to understand and investigate experimentally and have therefore attracted much of researchers' attention.

Fortunately, recent years have witnessed a sea change for this key theme of microbial pathogenesis that has been fueled by methodological advances, technical leaps in experimental manipulation of previously intractable organisms, and an emerging appreciation for the critical role microbial exit plays in pathogenesis, as well as our collective failure to understand it. Cellular exit has proven to be a highly regulated biological mechanism and is a marvelous example of convergent evolution by bacteria and parasitic pathogens.

Many significant discoveries have been made in recent years, and these findings have illuminated the diverse strategies adopted by intracellular pathogens for facilitating their exit from cells. Although a complete understanding of bacterial exit from host cells and cell-to-cell spread is lacking, the increasing rate of discoveries from recent years has revealed clear themes in this critical event for intracellular bacteria (1, 2). The general strategies available to intracellular bacteria for escaping the confines of a host cell can be most easily conceptualized as (i) lysis of the host cell (Table 1), (ii) nonlytic exit of free bacteria (Table 2), and (iii) release into membrane-encased compartments (Table 3). Microbial exit can be destructive or nondestructive, proinflammatory or immunologically silent, exclusively pathogen-directed or accomplished by engaging host signaling pathways, and can result in free organisms or membrane-bound bacteria once outside the host cell. As for other pathogenic processes, a deeper understanding of the molecular aspects of how intracellular pathogens control and promote their exit from host cells is expected to provide new insight into host cell biology, signaling pathways, and the precise strategies exploited by pathogens to manipulate these networks. A lack of knowledge about specific molecular factors and mediators of these processes remains an issue, however. Further challenges in exper-

imentation or for synergizing themes regarding microbial exit include the host models used, developmental stages of some pathogens, host cell targets (for which preferences may be promiscuous), and possible shifts in host cell preference during the course of infection by a given bacteria.

It should be expected that intracellular pathogens have evolved a diverse array of strategies for promoting their escape from the many host cell niches they inhabit, and experimental data are consistent with this notion. What we also observe, when looking at microbial exit from a broad perspective, is overlap in some of the underlying molecular mechanisms exploited by these pathogens. The high prevalence of some exit pathways suggests that there may be a finite pool of natural processes in the host cell that can be targeted by pathogens for promoting their exit. This is an argument for the strong evolutionary pressures that shape their development—in that not all possible solutions for initiating host cell escape are equally productive or beneficial to the microbe. The convergent evolution of shared strategies also underscores the strong evolutionary requirement for efficiently accomplishing this event, as well as its importance in the natural history of microbial infections. It is especially critical for pathogens to transmit to new hosts—truly the most important bottleneck for any intracellular pathogen—and likely a key determinant in the evolutionary development of strategies for accomplishing host cell exit.

This chapter will summarize our current understanding of the varied strategies used by intracellular bacteria and some eukaryotic parasites to escape host cells. A key theme that will be highlighted throughout this discussion is the evolutionary foundation for development of individual exit strategies. Intracellular pathogens are faced with many selective pressures in their natural history of infection, and although intracellular survival and growth are prerequisites, the primary goal for any intracellular pathogen is to successfully transmit to a new host. Where

TABLE 1 Lysis exit strategies[a]

Organism	Exit strategy	Intracellular	Host cell	Niche	Cell death?	Inflammatory?	Virulence factors	Host targets
Bacteria								
Chlamydia	Lysis	Obligate	Columnar epithelia	Vacuole	Yes	Expected	Cysteine proteases, possibly CPAF	Unknown
Brucella	Lysis	Facultative	Macrophages	Vacuole	Yes	Unknown	Unknown	Unknown
Mycobacterium marinum	Necroptosis	Facultative	Macrophages	Cytoplasm	Yes	Yes	Unknown	RIP1, RIP3, ROS, cyclophilin D, ceramide
Francisella	Pyroptosis	Facultative	Macrophages, neutrophils	Cytoplasm	Yes	Yes	Bacterial DNA	AIM2 inflammasome
Legionella pneumophila	Pyroptosis	Facultative	Macrophages	Vacuole	Yes	Yes	Flagellin	NLRC4 and NLRP3 inflammasomes
Listeria monocytogenes	Pyroptosis	Facultative	Macrophages, epithelial cells	Cytoplasm	Yes	Yes	Flagellin, LLO, DNA	NLRC4, NLRP3 and AIM2 inflammasomes
Salmonella	Pyroptosis	Facultative	Macrophages	Vacuole	Yes	Yes	SPI-1 and SPI-2 T3SS, flagellin, PrgJ	NLRC4 and NLRP3 inflammasomes
Shigella flexneri	Pyroptosis	Facultative	Macrophages, epithelial cells	Cytoplasm	Yes	Yes	MxiH, MxiI, IpaB	NLRC4 and NLRP3 inflammasomes
Burkholderia	Pyroptosis	Facultative	Macrophages	Cytoplasm	Yes	Yes	BsaK	NLRC4 and NLRP3 inflammasomes
Salmonella	Apoptosis	Facultative	Epithelial cells	Vacuole	Yes	Likely no	SPI-2 T3SS	Casp-3 and Casp-8
Francisella tularensis	Apoptosis	Facultative	Macrophages, neutrophils	Cytoplasm	Yes	No	Unknown	Intrinsic activation
Mycobacteria	Apoptosis	Facultative	Macrophages	Cytoplasm	Yes	Likely no	ESX1 secretion	Unknown
Brucella abortus	Autophagy-associated	Facultative	Macrophages	Vacuole	Mix	Mix	Unknown	Autophagy initiation proteins, PI3K
Parasites								
Toxoplasma gondii	Lysis	Obligate	Many	Vacuole	Yes	Expected	TgPLP1, CDPK1	Calpain
Plasmodium	Lysis	Obligate	Red blood cells	Vacuole	Yes	Expected	Cysteine proteases, including PfSUB1 and DPAP3; kinase PfCDPK5, SERA3, LISP1	Calpain, membrane and cytoskeleton-associated proteins (e.g., tropomyosin, adducin)
Trypanosoma cruzi	Lysis	Obligate	Many	Cytoplasm	Yes	Expected	Cruzipain or other proteases	Unknown
Leishmania	Apoptosis	Facultative	Neutrophils, macrophages	Cytoplasm	Yes	Yes	Unknown	Unknown

[a]Abbreviations: CPAF, chlamydial protease/proteasome-like activity factor; ROS, reactive oxygen species; NLRC4, Nod-like receptor family caspase recruitment domain-containing protein 4; NLRP, NLR family, pyrin domain containing 3; LLO, listeriolysin O; AIM2, absent in melanoma 2; SPI, *Salmonella* pathogenicity island; T3SS, type III secretion system; TgPLP1, *Toxoplasma* perforin-like protein 1.

TABLE 2 Cell-free expulsion exit strategies

Organism	Exit strategy	Intracellular	Host cell	Niche	Cell death?	Inflammatory?	Virulence factors	Host targets
Bacteria								
Legionella pneumophila	Exocytosis	Facultative	Amoeba	Vacuole	No	Unknown	LepA, LepB	Unknown
Porphyromonas gingivalis	Exocytosis	Facultative	Gingival epithelia	Vacuole	No	Unknown	Unknown	Rab11, RalA, actin, microtubules, exocyst
Mycobacteria	Ejection	Facultative	Amoeba	Cytoplasm	No	Unknown	ESX1 secretion	Actin, RacH
Brucella abortus	Autophagy-associated	Facultative	Macrophages	Vacuole	Mix	Mix	Unknown	Autophagy initiation proteins; PI3K
Parasites								
Cryptococcus neoformans	Vomocytosis	Facultative	Macrophages	Vacuole	No	No	Phospholipase B1 (CnPlb1)	Actin, Arp2/3, WASH[a]

[a]Abbreviation: WASH, Wiskott-Aldrich syndrome protein.

applicable, we will emphasize whether bacteria are obligate intracellular or facultative and also the nature of their preferred host cell target and intracellular niche (e.g., vacuole, cytoplasm, modified phagosome). All of these factors are critical in shaping the unique microenvironment for each pathogen and determining the requirements and challenges they face when the need arises to exit their respective niches.

LYSIS

For many intracellular pathogens, inducing lysis of the host cell represents the most direct means of exiting a vacuole or cell. Historically, lysis of cells was believed to be a physical or mechanical consequence of an increasing intracellular bacterial burden, for example, due to outward physical pressures on the cell membrane. Focused studies in recent years have definitively demonstrated that this is not true; rather, lysis is a pathogen-direct biological process. The predominance of this strategy in nature may be attributable to the relative ease by which pathogens can acquire the ability to lyse their resident host cells. Frequently this is accomplished by a single gene, e.g., a pore-forming toxin, protease, or pathogen-associated molecular pattern. Microbe-triggered lysis of host cells can be conceptualized as direct action—mediated by factors that compromise membrane integrity by forming pores or weakening membrane-associated cytoskeletal proteins—or indirect action through activation of host cell death pathways.

Pathogen-induced cell lysis not only results in viable escape for the microbe, but it is also routinely associated with pro-inflammatory outcomes. Nonapoptotic rupture of host cells leads to release of intracellular debris and molecules, which can exacerbate the level of inflammation in infected tissue. Furthermore, the inflammatory cell death pathway, known as pyroptosis, is mechanistically distinct from apoptosis and leads to even further aggrava-

TABLE 3 Membrane-encased exit strategies[a]

Organism	Exit strategy	Intracellular	Host cell	Niche	Cell death?	Inflammatory?	Virulence factors	Host targets
Bacteria								
Chlamydia	Extrusion	Obligate	Columnar epithelia	Vacuole	No	Unknown	T3SS	Actin, formins, septins, myosin II, Rho GTPase
Ehrlichia	Protrusion	Obligate	Macrophages	Cytoplasm	No	No	Unknown	Actin, N-WASP
Rickettsia	Protrusion	Obligate	Endothelial cells	Cytoplasm	No	No	Sca2	Actin
Burkholderia pseudomallei	Protrusion	Facultative	Macrophages, epithelia	Cytoplasm	No	No	BimA, BimC	Actin
Listeria monocytogenes	Protrusion	Facultative	Macrophages, epithelia	Cytoplasm	No	No	ActA, InlC, LLO, PI-PLC, PC-PLC	Actin, Arp2/3, ezrin, CD44, CSNK1A1, Tuba, Rho GTPases, formins
Mycobacterium marinum	Protrusion	Facultative	Macrophages	Cytoplasm	No	No	Unknown	Actin, WASP, N-WASP, Arp2/3
Shigella flexneri	Protrusion	Facultative	Epithelial cells	Cytoplasm	No	No	IcsA, VirA, VirG	Actin, Dia1, myosin X, E-cadherin, Toca-1
Orientia tsutsugamushi	Budding	Obligate	Macrophages, endothelial cells	Cytoplasm	No	Unknown	Unknown	Possibly lipid rafts
Parasites								
Plasmodium	Extrusion	Obligate	Hepatocyte	Vacuole	Probably	No	Unknown	Unknown

[a]Abbreviations: T3SS, type III secretion system; N-WASP, neuronal Wiskott-Aldrich syndrome protein; LLO, listeriolysin O; PI-PLC, phosphatidylinositol-phospholipase C; PC-PLC, phosphatidylcholine-phospholipase C.

tion of local inflammatory responses through the activation and secretion of proinflammatory cytokines and chemokines. Pyroptosis could be an evolutionary example of mutual benefit to host and bacterium—the bacteria wins by escaping and gaining the opportunity to transmit, and the host wins by removing a favorable cellular niche (macrophage) from the pathogen. Alternatively, the promotion of additional inflammatory events by pyroptosis may be beneficial to the bacteria, for example through recruitment of susceptible macrophages or dendritic cells that are the preferred target cell for the bacteria.

For some bacteria, the proteins used to initially lyse their resident vacuole are secondarily exploited to subsequently lyse the host plasma membrane. Also frequently, checks are in place to ensure that these lytic factors are inactivated upon vacuole breakdown. Many of the strategies used by intracellular pathogens for lysing host cells are additionally used to disrupt pathogen-containing vacuoles; in fact, the role of lytic factors is better understood in the context of vacuole disruption.

Pore-Forming Proteins

Bacterial utilization of pore-forming proteins for disruption of intracellular vacuoles is well understood (3–8). Subsequent use of this strategy for lysis of host plasma membranes, however, is less prevalent, and concrete examples have been described only for intracellular protozoan parasites (9). In fact, in several instances bacterial pore-forming proteins are regulated such that they are inactive after bacteria and toxins have gained access to the cytosol of host cells (10, 11).

The best example of pore-forming proteins as a microbial exit mechanism is the *Toxoplasma* perforin-like protein 1 (TgPLP1), a secreted perforin-like protein of the intracellular protozoan pathogen *Toxoplasma gondii* that displays structural features necessary for pore formation (12–15). Egress of intracellular *T. gondii* tachyzoites appears to

be a synchronized event that is morphologically characterized by parasite penetration through the vacuole and cell at discrete protruding foci.

Through key contributions made by several laboratories, a clear picture has emerged of how *T. gondii* triggers this process (Fig. 1). Immediately prior to egress, elevation in levels of abscisic acid, as a direct consequence of parasite replication, leads to the production of the second messenger cyclic ADP-ribose, which in turn elevates the level of calcium concentration in the parasite (16). This signaling is thought to be the natural triggering signal

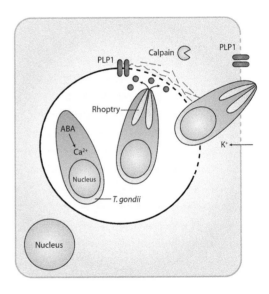

FIGURE 1 **Pore-forming proteins mediate the exit of *Toxoplasma gondii*. Exit signals for *T. gondii* originate within the parasite and consist of elevations in abscisic acid (ABA) leading to increases in intraparasite calcium concentrations. Calcium spikes induce protein secretion by *Toxoplasma* rhoptry organelles, including the pore-forming protein TgPLP1. Insertion of PLP1 in the vacuole membrane causes its disruption, and PLP1 insertion in the host plasma membrane causes further disruption of ionic gradients, including potassium. Host calpains are also activated during this process, and they play key roles in degrading cytoskeletal proteins and complexes that are normally important for maintaining vacuole membrane integrity. Successful exit of *T. gondii* parasites is accomplished by penetration of motile parasites through these weakened membranes.**

for *T. gondii* egress. Microneme secretion is Ca^{2+}-dependent; Ca^{2+} ionophores can trigger these events artificially. Elevated calcium levels in turn induce rhoptry secretion, and one key effector is the TgPLP1, which is secreted into the vacuole lumen from parasite organelles called rhoptries. TgPLP1 destabilizes the parasitophorous vacuole membrane and perhaps other host membranes (12). In addition to TgPLP1, release of calcium from the host endoplasmic reticulum results in activation of host calpains that assist egress by cleaving cytoskeletal proteins important for membrane stability (17). TgPLP1 likely also disrupts ion gradients in the host cell, and the parasite may sense this damage to host plasma membranes; for example, the parasite can sense drops in intracellular potassium levels (15).

Despite the ease and utility of inserting pore-forming proteins into host plasma membranes, there are few examples of this strategy being used by intracellular bacteria to exit cells in nature. The intracellular parasite *Leishmania amazonensis* encodes a pore-forming protein, leishporin, which may facilitate parasite escape from vacuoles and host cells (9, 18). In addition, the bacterium *Brucella abortus* has been reported to lyse macrophages by a cytotoxic mechanism, potentially by a pore-forming protein (19). The lack of further examples is somewhat puzzling given the higher frequency of adoption of pore-forming proteins for vacuole lysis, and thus indirectly, the availability of these pathogenic factors in the microbial gene pool. There may be poorly understood fitness costs associated with the expression of pore-forming proteins, such as the loss of a nutrient pool or the loss of a protected niche.

Proteases

Chlamydia spp. have long been known to lyse their host cells at the end of their developmental growth cycle, but only recently have molecular determinants of this process been revealed (20–22). Exploitation of combina-

tions of cysteine protease inhibitors revealed that *Chlamydia*-induced host cell lysis is a sequential process that is critically dependent on cysteine proteases (20) (Fig. 2). The initial event in this exit pathway is rupture of the chlamydial inclusion; this step can be blocked by treatment of cells with cysteine protease inhibitors (20). Rupture of the nucleus follows, even though other host organelles are preserved. Approximately 10 to 15 minutes after vacuole dissolution, integrity of the host plasma membrane is compromised by a mechanism that requires intracellular calcium signaling (20).

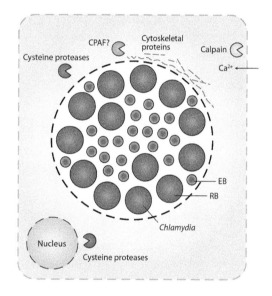

FIGURE 2 Lysis of *Chlamydia*-infected cells by cysteine proteases. Cysteine proteases are activated at late stages of *Chlamydia* developmental growth in cells; protease identities are unknown but may be bacterial, host, or both. Cysteine protease activity is required to degrade proteins essential for maintaining *Chlamydia* vacuole integrity. The secreted chlamydial serine protease CPAF plays a role in degradation of intermediate filaments that associate with the chlamydial vacuole and may play a role in host cell lysis. After degradation of the vacuole, host nuclei are permeabilized, possibly by cysteine proteases. Lysis of the host plasma membrane is mediated by intracellular calcium signaling, calpain, and potentially additional proteases. Abbreviations: EB, elementary body; RB, reticulate body.

Although the exact nature of the putative chlamydial factors and host targets remains unknown, preliminary data argue for the activity of *Chlamydia* cysteine proteases in mediating the proteolytic events (K. Hybiske, unpublished data). Furthermore, recent experiments using mutagenized strains of *Chlamydia trachomatis* suggest that the secreted chlamydial serine protease chlamydial protease/proteasome-like activity factor (CPAF) may play an important role in intracellular membrane permeabilization, including targeting intermediate filaments on the cytoplasmic face of the inclusion membrane (23). In the context of microbial exit, proteases are thought to act by degrading membrane proteins or membrane-associated cytoskeletal proteins that result in weakening the membrane bilayer integrity and ultimately in the formation of large holes and cell destruction (24).

A similar, two-step proteolytic lysis process has been characterized for the release of *Plasmodium* parasites from red blood cells. This exit strategy occurs during the blood stage of infection and is among the better examples of the adaptation of pathogen proteases for promoting host membrane breakdown and pathogen escape (25, 26). Rupture of *Plasmodium*-infected red blood cells is a two-step process, consisting of lysis of the parasitophorous vacuole membrane and host plasma membrane (27, 28). The mechanism requires parasite-secreted proteases and calcium-dependent proteases, including the proteases DPAP3 and PfSUB1 (29, 30), and a plant-like calcium-dependent protein kinase PfCDPK5 (31). Important host proteins in *Plasmodium*-induced cell lysis include calpain (17, 32) and a wide array of membrane and cytoskeleton-associated proteins (most notably tropomyosin and adducin) whose targeted removal is believed to weaken red blood cell membrane stability (32). *Plasmodium* exit from hepatocytes may also be dependent on parasite-secreted proteases (33, 34).

Similar to pore-forming proteins, examples of the adoption of proteases by intracellular pathogens as a singular mechanism for promoting their cellular escape is limited. In addition to the examples discussed above, another is the protozoan parasite *Trypanosoma cruzi*, for which a key role for parasitic proteases, notably cruzipain, has been shown for parasite egress (35). The involvement of proteases in microbial exit is widespread, yet these proteins appear to mostly play accessory roles in exit strategies, rather than function as exclusive players.

Pyroptosis

Pyroptosis is a caspase-1 dependent, inflammatory programmed cell death pathway that is primarily operative in macrophages (36, 37). The end result of pyroptosis is lytic death of the cell and the release of processed proinflammatory cytokines IL-1β and IL-18; these cytokines elicit widespread effects on fever and IFN-γ levels in the host (38). Although pyroptosis may not be a pathogen-directed mechanism per se, the process is unilaterally triggered by microbial factors and facilitates the release of bacteria from the host cell. Consequently, pyroptosis can be considered a viable and productive exit strategy by exploitation of a host cell response pathway. It may be in the best interest of some bacteria to spread to new phagocytic cells, and therefore connecting cellular exit to a proinflammatory burst would be in line with this strategy by recruiting new host cells to the bacteria.

Many bacteria have been shown to exploit this cellular mechanism as a strategy for egress: *Burkholderia*, *Francisella tularensis*, *Legionella pneumophila*, *Listeria monocytogenes*, *Salmonella*, and *Shigella flexneri* (39–41). *L. monocytogenes* represents a prime example of pyroptosis activation by intracellular bacteria, and it can accomplish this through multiple pathways (Fig. 3). Once in the cytosol of infected macrophages, shedding of flagellin monomers from *Listeria* activates the Nod-like receptor family caspase recruitment domain-containing protein 4 (NLRC4)

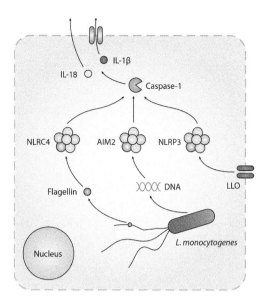

FIGURE 3 Induction of pyroptosis and host cell lysis by *Listeria monocytogenes*. Once in the cytosol of a host cell, three discrete microbial factors of *Listeria* are capable of activating inflammasomes, subsequent activation of caspase-1, and downstream processing and secretion of IL-1α and IL-18. Flagellin monomers that are sloughed off from *Listeria* flagella trigger activation of the canonical NLRC4 (Nod-like receptor family caspase recruitment domain-containing protein 4) inflammasome. DNA that is released from infrequent lysis of intracellular *Listeria* is recognized by the absent-in-melanoma-2 (AIM2) inflammasome. Listeriolysin O (LLO), the pore-forming protein secreted by *Listeria*, is capable of activating the NLRP3 inflammasome. Pyroptosis leads to host cell death and the release of *Listeria* from the host cell.

inflammasome, and DNA released from lysed bacteria can activate the absent-in-melanoma-2 inflammasome (42–44). Furthermore, it has been shown that treatment of cells with purified listeriolysin O protein alone can activate the NLR family, pyrin domain containing 3 (NLRP3) inflammasome, a situation that has context for a cellular infection (45).

The underlying themes for pyroptosis activation are reasonably conserved for other intracellular bacteria. *Burkholderia* spp., upon escape from their vacuole into the cytoplasm, activate the NLRC4 inflammasome via the type III secretion system rod protein BsaK of *Burkholderia*; furthermore, infection can activate the NLRP3 inflammasome by an undefined agonist/mechanism (46, 47). *S. flexneri*, after rapidly escaping into the cytoplasm of macrophages or intestinal epithelial cells, can activate inflammasome-based caspase-1 secretion. The MxiI rod protein and the needle protein MxiH of *Shigella* can trigger NLRC4 inflammasome activation (47–49) and is a process that also requires the type III secretion system and the secreted effector IpaB (50, 51). *F. tularensis* occasionally autolyses in the cytosol of macrophages, thereby releasing DNA that triggers absent-in-melanoma-2 inflammasome activation (52, 53). *L. pneumophila* and *Salmonella* both activate inflammasomes through inadvertent secretion of flagellin into the cytosol of the host cell from their resident vacuoles, by a *Salmonella* pathogenicity island 1–dependent type III secretion system and SipB mechanism for *Salmonella* (54–56) and Dot-Icm type IV secretion for *Legionella* (40, 57, 58). *Salmonella* can also elicit a delayed SPI-2-dependent activation of NLRC4 and NLRP3 inflammasomes (36, 59). Finally, and perhaps related, the necrotic death of macrophages infected with *Mycobacterium tuberculosis* has been reported to require NLRP3 inflammasome activation (60); and the necroptosis of macrophages infected with *Mycobacterium marinum* has been demonstrated, as a direct consequence of high levels of TNF-α production and mediated by RIP1/RIP3-dependent reactive oxygen species signaling (61).

Apoptosis

Intracellular pathogens have evolved numerous mechanisms for delaying or halting apoptosis as a means of establishing their intracellular niche, promoting their survival, and avoiding immune-based clearance (62, 63). For some bacteria the induction of apoptosis—either intentionally or by accident—results in host cell escape, and therefore apoptosis represents a viable exit strategy. Furthermore, many bacteria that were originally thought to elicit pro-apoptotic responses have since been reclassified as pro-pyroptotic based on updated research findings.

The induction of apoptosis by intracellular bacteria is likely temporally and host cell dependent, and therefore it is a great challenge to ascribe specific functions of apoptosis-based exit to a pathogen in the context of an *in vivo* infection. Apoptosis is a well-characterized cellular process, however, and in light of this many inferences can be drawn about what apoptotic escape could mean for the pathogen and host. First, the infected host cell is killed and bacteria are liberated within membrane-encased apoptotic bodies. Apoptotic bodies traditionally express externalized phosphatidylserine on their outer membrane leaflets; these signals mark apoptotic bodies for engulfment and clearance by phagocytic cells. This fate could be shared by bacteria that are released from cells by apoptosis, although this idea has not been explored experimentally. Another impact on infection is the noninflammatory nature of apoptosis, an outcome which can be potentially beneficial to the pathogen and host.

Most examples of bacterial induction of apoptosis are incompletely defined. *F. tularensis* has been shown to be capable of activating the intrinsic apoptotic pathway in macrophages (Fig. 4). This classical activation of apoptosis consists of cytochrome c release from mitochondria and sequential activation of initiator and effector caspase-3 and caspase-9 (64, 65). Apoptotic host cell death has been demonstrated for other intracellular bacteria, including intestinal epithelial cells infected with *Salmonella enterica* (59, 66) and *Mycobacterium avium*–infected macrophages (67). In some instances a role for apoptosis has been connected to pathogen dissemination. Apoptosis was found to functionally mediate the spread of *M. marinum* in granulomas; apoptotic activation was dependent on *Mycobacteria* ESX-1 secretion (68). Furthermore, *Leishmania* spp. have evolved

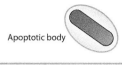

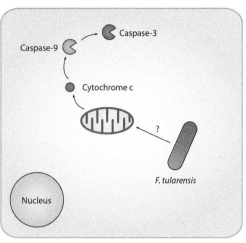

FIGURE 4 Activation of intrinsic apoptosis and host cell death by *Francisella tularensis*. Intracellular *F. tularensis* is capable of activating the intrinsic pathway of apoptosis in host cells. The microbial factors of *Francisella* that induce apoptosis signaling have not been identified; however, infection results in cytochrome c release from mitochondria, followed by caspase-9 and caspase-3 activation. Ultimately, cellular substrates are cleaved by caspases, and host membranes bleb into apoptotic bodies which may contain bacteria. Whether *Francisella*, or other bacteria that trigger apoptotic death, reside exclusively in apoptotic bodies or if they have free access to the extracellular space upon host death is unclear.

to exploit apoptosis as a strategy for dissemination, specifically for the neutrophil to dendritic cell transfer of *Leishmania major* (69), neutrophil to macrophage transfer of *L. major* (70), and macrophage to macrophage transfer of *L. amazonensis* (71). Finally, the role of autophagy in microbial pathogenesis has become an emergent theme, and there is mechanistic overlap between autophagy and apoptosis in some contexts. As an example, *B. abortus* has been shown to engage autophagy-associated factors in host cells in a manner that directly affects the ability of *Brucella* to spread to new cells (72).

CELL-FREE EXPULSIVE ESCAPE

A distinctive theme of microbial exit by cell-free expulsion is to leave without killing the host cell and in a fully cell-free state. Simplistically, this strategy can be conceptualized as entry in reverse. There is no consensus in the field regarding this category or how to classify it; semantically, we have chosen the term expulsion because it best describes the direct release of free microorganisms into the extracellular space. Importantly, host cells remain intact and potentially devoid of any bacterial load after this mechanism of bacteria exit. Another key theme is that this manner of exit likely occurs without activation of proinflammatory signaling. It is reasonable to postulate that the evolutionary pressures that shaped this strategy were a need to transmit without inflammatory exacerbation and not to be compartmentalized in a host membrane.

Exocytosis

Exocytosis is a conserved eukaryotic cellular process for the secretion of secreted molecules and surface membrane proteins derived from intracellular vacuoles, endosomes, and secretory vesicles. The timing and specificity of exocytic membrane fusion is primarily mediated by paired interactions between membrane-bound soluble *N*-ethylmaleimide-sensitive factor attachment protein receptor proteins (73). During infection of its natural amoeba hosts, *L. pneumophila* can exit by a nonlytic mechanism that is morphologically similar to exocytosis (74, 75) (Fig. 5). This mechanism was shown to be critically dependent on the Icm/Dot type IV secretion system and the secreted proteins LepA and LepB. LepA and LepB are large-molecular-weight coiled-coil proteins whose function remains unknown, and their secretion into the host cell cytoplasm is dependent on host actin polymerization (74). It was proposed that these proteins may enable *Legionella* to commandeer a protozoan exocytic pathway,

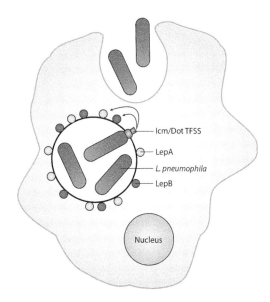

FIGURE 5 Exit of *Legionella pneumophila* from amoeba by exocytosis. From inside a vacuole of an infected amoeboid host, *L. pneumophila* secretes two known effector proteins into the host cytosol, LepA and LepB, which are directly responsible for promoting the fusion of the *Legionella*-containing vacuole with the amoeba plasma membrane. This exocytic process results in the free release of bacteria into the extracellular space and leaves the host cell intact. Both effector proteins are secreted by the *Legionella* Icm/Dot type IV secretion system, and thereafter they are recruited to the vacuole membrane.

normally utilized for the expulsion of food waste (75).

Porphyromonas gingivalis can exit gingival epithelial cells by an exocytosis mechanism of pathogen-containing endosome fusion with the plasma membrane (76, 77). Nonlytic exit of *P. gingivalis* has been described as an exocytosis-like strategy that is dependent on a range of host factors, including Rab11, RalA, actin, microtubules, and protein components of the exocyst complex (78).

Adding breadth to exocytosis as a strategy, *Cryptococcus neoformans* can exit macrophages by a nonlytic mechanism called "vomocytosis" (79–85). In this mechanism, phagosomes containing *C. neoformans* homotypically fuse into a giant vacuole; the vacuole subsequently fuses

with the host plasma membrane to expel a
large number of organisms. The molecular
mechanism involves a secreted phospholipase (SEC14) (86) and interactions with the
actin cytoskeleton, including the Arp2/3 complex and Wiskott-Aldrich syndrome protein
(WASH) (84, 87).

Ejection

M. marinum, and to a lesser extent *M. tuberculosis*, were recently discovered to exit from
the amoeba *Dictyostelium* by a process
termed the "ejectosome" (88) (Fig. 6). This
process is nonlytic and consists of the formation of a barrel-shaped actin pore-like
structure on the host plasma membrane.
Through this conduit, cytosolic mycobacteria
traverse the host cell membrane and escape
the intracellular space of the cell. The actin-
associated machinery involved with ejectosome formation was shown to be dependent
on mycobacterial ESX-1 (type VII) secretion
by *Mycobacterium* and the host factors RacH,
Myosin IB, and coronin, but not Arp2/3 (88).
Actin tails are rarely associated with bacteria
exiting cells by the ejectosome mechanism.
Multiple ejectosomes were found to cluster
at host cell membranes, and the process of
bacteria traversal was associated with membrane deformations. It was postulated that
the release of mycobacteria through ejectosomes might be aided by ejectile mechanical
forces (88).

Mycobacteria are the only bacteria that
have been shown to utilize this exit strategy.
Bacterial exit through specialized interactions with the host actin cytoskeleton, however, appears to have widespread adoption by
intracellular pathogens and will be discussed
in the next section. A final example that may
relate to ejection concerns cell-to-cell spread
of the microsporidia pathogen *Nematocida
parisii*. This pathogen has been described to
induce actin cytoskeletal rearrangements as
part of its mechanism for nonlytic exit and
cell-to-cell spread through intestinal epithelial cells during infections in *C. elegans* (89).

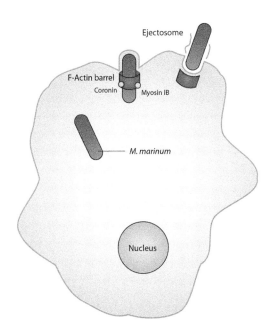

FIGURE 6 Ejection of *Mycobacterium marinum*
from amoeba. Through a mechanism that requires
myosin IB coronin, and type VII secreted protein
(s) by the bacteria, *M. marinum* can induce the
formation of an actin barrel-like structure on the
amoeba plasma membrane. Through this large
pore-like structure, *M. marinum* can traverse the
cell membrane and exit from the cell. Although
permeability is transiently formed on the amoeba
membrane, it reseals to keep the host cell intact
after the event is completed.

MEMBRANE-ENCASED ESCAPE

This exit strategy encompasses the apparent
need of some intracellular pathogens to depart the host cell without causing host cell
lysis and, importantly, to remain encased by
host membranes. Broadly, this strategy covers
the packaged release of numerous microorganisms (exemplified by *Chlamydia*) and
the protrusion of individual bacteria by actin-
mediated propulsion (exemplified by *Listeria*).
In the case of the former, it has been proposed
that membrane-encased exit could confer advantages to the pathogen, for example, facilitating immune evasion. Because these exit
strategies are noninflammatory, another likely
advantageous outcome is to avoid additional

recruitment of innate immune cells enabling immune evasion coupled to dissemination within the host. It can be argued that during the coevolutionary history of these pathogens with their respective hosts, it is in the bacteria's best interest not to elicit additional pro-inflammatory responses, which would be the case with promoting host cell lysis. Another common theme of membrane-encased exit is the critical participation of interactions with the actin cytoskeleton.

Extrusion

Upon completion of their intracellular developmental growth in epithelial cells, *Chlamydia* spp. can exit their host by either inducing vacuole and host cell lysis or by a membrane-encased release called extrusion (20). These processes are equivalently active *in vitro*. The frequency of extrusion for infections *in vivo* is unknown; however, its presence has been documented (90). Extrusion of *Chlamydia* is a nondestructive exit strategy wherein type III secreted proteins by *Chlamydia* engage host cytoskeleton and actomyosin contraction signaling pathways to promote the pinching of the chlamydial inclusion into a released compartment containing infectious *Chlamydia* that are encased by vacuole and host plasma membranes (Fig. 7) (20, 91, 92). Both lysis and extrusion are bacteria-driven processes (91), so it appears that *Chlamydia* organisms make a concerted choice in many instances to exit cells by nondestructive extrusion.

Extrusion requires an inordinate investment of energy and resources to orchestrate, most likely more than any of the other exit strategies discovered to date. What advantages, then, does it confer to *Chlamydia* during infection in a host? Membrane encasement of extracellular *Chlamydia* should provide physical protection against antibacterial factors released around inflammatory foci of infection, perhaps as a means of immune evasion. Furthermore, because they frequently contain mitochondria and host cytoplasm, extrusions provide a finite supply of nutrients to sustain

prolonged chlamydial growth and development even while these bacteria are outside host cells (K. Hybiske, unpublished data). Extrusions in tissue culture become permeabilized within hours, after which released bacteria readily infect new epithelial cells (K. Hybiske, unpublished data). It is also

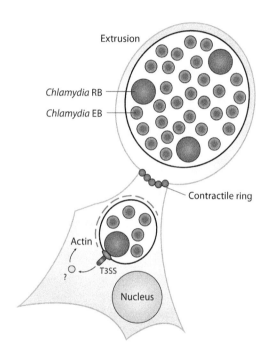

FIGURE 7 Extrusion of *Chlamydia* from host cells. Chlamydial extrusion is a complex process that is orchestrated from bacteria residing in a vacuole. This mechanism consists of a large portion of the bacteria-containing vacuole pinching off and releasing from the host cell. The host cell remains intact upon completion of this exit strategy and can even retain a residual *Chlamydia* vacuole after the extruded body is released. Extrusion appears to be initiated by unidentified secreted *Chlamydia* proteins that are secreted across the vacuole membrane and into the host cytosol by type III secretion. Polymerization of nascent actin filaments on the vacuole membrane is required for extrusion formation. The pinching step is mediated by actomyosin contraction and Rho GTPase signaling pathways. A hypothesized contractile ring may form on the vacuole membrane to give rise to the major contraction event that occurs on both the vacuole and host cell. Abbreviations: EB, elementary body; RB, reticulate body.

likely that *in vivo* extrusions function as a dissemination vehicle, for example, to navigate away from proinflammatory foci and to other tissues. Support for this notion comes from recent findings concerning the active engulfment of *Chlamydia* extrusions by macrophages and dendritic cells and the preservation of these structures and the bacteria they contain once inside phagocytes (K. Hybiske, unpublished data). Finally, *Chlamydia pneumoniae* is capable of exiting host cells by extrusion (K. Hybiske, unpublished data), and these microorganisms have long been connected with inflammatory arterial lesions and associations with macrophages delivering organisms from the lung to arterial sites (93, 94).

Another example of extrusion as a dissemination strategy comes from *Plasmodium*. Liver stage parasites of *Plasmodium falciparum* and related rodent species use extrusion to exit hepatocytes and transition to the symptomatic blood stage of malaria. Malarial extrusions, or merosomes, have been shown *in vivo* to carry parasites into the bloodstream and microvasculature of the airways (95–99). During *Plasmodium* extrusion the host cell does not remain intact after the event; rather, it detaches from neighboring cells (95). This is a key distinction from chlamydial extrusion, in which the host cell remains viable and intact after the event. Also unlike chlamydial extrusions, malarial extrusions maintain asymmetric distribution of phosphatidylserine in their outer membrane; this may allow nascent merosomes to avoid phagocytic clearance (95).

Actin-Based Protrusion

After their escape into the host cytoplasm, some bacteria that recruit host actin polymerization machinery for actin-based motility exploit this mechanism further to push outward from the host cell and into a neighboring cell as a means of cell-to-cell spread (100–102). *L. monocytogenes* best exemplifies the mechanisms associated with this exit strategy (Fig. 8). *Listeria*, like the other

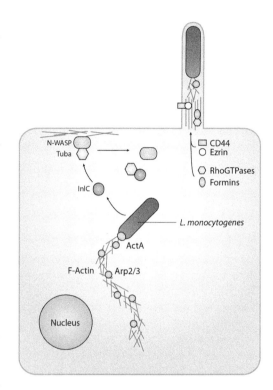

FIGURE 8 **Actin-based protrusion of *Listeria monocytogenes*. *Listeria* can disseminate to neighboring cells by protruding out of its infected host cell as long filopodia projections and into an adjacent cell. This process is largely derived from mechanisms responsible for the formation of polar actin comet tails on *Listeria* and other bacteria; however, additional molecules are required for actin-based motility to lead to filopodial protrusions. *Listeria* secretes InlC, a protein which binds to the host protein Tuba and sequesters it away from neuronal Wiskott-Aldrich syndrome protein (N-WASP). This results in destabilized cortical actin structures of cell membranes. At these vulnerable membrane regions, *Listeria* protrudes outward into long, membrane-bound filopodia, using Arp2/3- and formin-based actin polymerization as the propulsive force. It is critical for *Listeria* actin tails in protrusions to maintain interactions with the plasma membrane through ezrin and membrane proteins such as CD44.**

bacteria that use actin-based protrusion to spread from cell to cell, targets the host Arp2/3 protein complex for induction of y-branched actin polymerization on one pole of the bacterium. This manipulation of host F-actin nucleation is mediated by the *Listeria* protein ActA; actin nucleation and the subsequent formation of actin tails via ActA leads to intracellular motility of *Listeria*. This motility can form filopodia-like structures when the bacterium pushes into the host plasma membrane (103–105). Filopodia containing *Listeria* can be engulfed by neighboring cells, leading to direct cell-to-cell transfer of the bacteria (104, 106). The *Listeria* protein InlC has been shown to be essential for protrusion; InlC binds to the host protein Tuba to disengage Tuba from neuronal Wiskott-Aldrich syndrome protein (N-WASP), thereby weakening actin cortical tension at the plasma membrane and enhancing the capacity for membrane protrusions to form (107). Additional host factors required include formins and Rho GTPases, which promote bundled actin structures at the base of protrusions (108) and the host protein ezrin, a member of the ezrin-radixin-moesin family, which connects actin filaments to plasma membrane proteins such as CD44 (106, 109).

Once a protrusion has been internalized by a neighboring cell, *Listeria* must escape from a double membrane encasement to gain access to the cytosol of the newly infected cell, thus completing cell-to-cell transfer. *Listeria* accomplishes this through the coordinated and sequential activity of two phospholipases, phosphatidylinositol-phospholipase C and phosphatidylcholine-phospholipase C, and a secreted pore-forming protein (listeriolysin O) (8, 110–112). The human casein kinase 1 alpha also plays a role in the transition of protrusions to vacuoles in the cell that receives it (113).

Numerous other intracellular bacteria have evolved this strategy for cellular exit and spread, and a common theme is the expression and secretion of bacterial factors that mimic host proteins with key roles in nucleating actin filaments. *S. flexneri* expresses a protein, IcsA, that activates N-WASP and Arp2/3-mediated actin polymerization to form comet tails, and the bacteria also has

the ability to switch to a formin-mediated mechanism (114–118). *Rickettsia* secretes an actin nucleator, Sca2, that mimics formin proteins to produce long, unbranched actin tails (119, 120). *Mycobacteria* possesses a mechanism for exploiting WASP, N-WASP, and Arp2/3-mediated actin polymerization for motility and cell-to-cell spread (121, 122). *Burkholderia pseudomallei* and *Ehrlichia* have similar strategies for actin-based protrusion, with less well-characterized mechanisms (123–126).

Budding

Orientia tsutsugamushi, a member of the scrub group of *Rickettsia*, exits endothelial cells by a slow budding process in which individual bacteria are released within plasma membrane–encased compartments (Fig. 9) (127–133). Unlike extrusions of *Chlamydia* or *Plasmodium*, membrane-encased *Orientia* contains single organisms, much like budding viral particles. The mechanism behind this process is entirely unknown; however, a role for lipid rafts in targeting *Orientia* to the host plasma membrane was implicated (127). The eventual fate of budded *Orientia* appears to be phagocytosis by new cells, thus highlighting the role of this exit strategy for *Orientia* dissemination.

THE EVOLUTION OF EXIT

The spectrum of mechanisms for microbial pathogen escape from their host cells can be appreciated by viewing through the lens of adaptive evolution and reproductive success. For pathogens, reproductive success requires survival, growth, persistence (often requiring dissemination within the host), and transmission to new hosts or environments (134). For intracellular microbial pathogens of eukaryotic cells, a means of exit from their cell is additionally required for evolutionary progress.

Exit from infected cells is necessary for dissemination to uninfected cells and tissues within the host niche. This is not a trivial

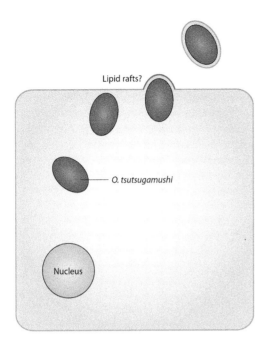

FIGURE 9 **Exit of *Orientia tsutsugamushi* by budding release. The escape of *O. tsutsugamushi* from host cells is mediated by a budding process that releases individual bacteria out of the cell and encased by host membranes. The underlying molecular mechanisms are poorly understood, but there is evidence that *Orientia* may target lipid raft domains at the plasma membrane as sites for bud formation and egress.**

challenge, because the landscape of the host is complex, involving tissue architecture, innate protective mechanisms, and adaptive immune responses. Exit is also required for organisms to transmit to new susceptible hosts by establishing within-host persistence concomitant with optimizing transmission opportunities between hosts. Because both within-host and between-host transmission are required for reproductive success, adaptive evolution for unique cellular exit pathways represents a fundamental evolutionary keystone. Microbial pathogens have found effective solutions to these complex challenges through step-wise evolutionary processes.

The mechanisms for generating the genetic diversity necessary for natural selection are mutation, recombination of existing genes, and acquisition of new genes by horizontal gene transfer, especially by mobile genetic elements. Facultative intracellular pathogens often obtain sets of virulence genes by horizontal gene transfer, thereby making large adaptive leaps by a single genetic event. In contrast, obligate intracellular pathogens are fundamentally sequestered from intercourse with other diverse sets of microorganisms, and adaptive evolution is dependent upon point mutations and reshuffling of DNA. Thus, the evolutionary pathways for pathogens that are obligate intracellular pathogens may have taken significantly longer than those for facultative intracellular pathogens that can replicate in environments outside of a eukaryotic cell. *Salmonella* is an example of a facultative intracellular pathogen that has acquired complete sets of virulence genes by horizontal gene transfer of pathogenicity islands (135). *Chlamydia*, in contrast, is an obligate intracellular pathogen whose genetic diversity has been limited to mutation and recombination of intracellular genes (136).

The time frame for the evolution of pathogenesis and virulence is tens of thousands of years for *Salmonella* (137) and hundreds of millions of years for *Chlamydia* (136, 138). Nevertheless, the foundation for the selective adaptation of virulence factors is the hereditary legacy of the evolutionary design by early pathogens that provided the substrates for virulence capacities that subsequently were shared among modern ancestors. For example, it has been hypothesized that the evolutionary progenitor of the type III secretion virulence system originated from the adaptive selection and modification of separate components of flagellar system genes by *Chlamydia*-like organisms during their interactions within their ancient intracellular niche (139, 140). One consequence of a longer time of evolution is the opportunity for a more sophisticated or mechanistically complex adaptation.

Cellular entry is a prerequisite for exit, and microbial organisms first entered cells by nonselective host-cell-initiated vacuolar uptake mechanisms such as phagocytosis, without a means for exit. This becomes a dead end for the microorganism, yet it remains a chronic fate because they serve as a digestive nutrient for the predatory host cell. The first evolutionary challenges following entry are managing the hurdles of finding mechanisms for intracellular survival, growth, and persistence. Microbial pathogens have either remained within their intracellular entry vacuole or acquired the means to exit the vacuole and reside in the host cell cytoplasm. Although intracellular survival and growth are complex enterprises in their own right, they appear typically independent of the mechanisms of exit. The earliest method of cellular exit was to persist long enough within the host cell until the host cell dies, thereby liberating surviving microbes. These capabilities of entry and persistence provided the time to acquire pathogen-directed mechanisms of cellular manipulation and exit, but because of the selective bottleneck of transmission, exit must be coordinated with growth and persistence to optimize the pathogen's reproductive success.

One strategy of exit, and quite likely the earliest to evolve, is to promote and facilitate the inevitable death of the host cell. To achieve this goal, pathogens have taken advantage of a selection of cytotoxins that could be acquired from the existing gene pool, repurposed from other pathogenic mechanisms, or by incidental exploitation of preexisting host cell lytic pathways such as apoptosis or pyroptosis. An alternative method of exit is to transit out of the cell by a nonlethal mechanism, leaving the host cell viable. This requires an additional level of cell biological sophistication; however, as diverse as the evolutionary trajectories are, common, evolutionarily convergent themes emerge. One such theme is the role of actin in these expulsive mechanisms. Opportunities during the microbe–host cell evolutionary relationship to exploit actin polymerization result from the promiscuity

of actin assembly machinery to be exploited at discrete steps in the pathway that can be intersected by a variety of microbial molecules. This convergent theme is evidenced by actin-mediated motility and cellular exit for bacteria (e.g., *Listeria*, *Shigella*, *Rickettsia*, *Mycobacterium*, *Burkholderia*), viruses (e.g., vaccinia), fungi (e.g. *C. neoformans*), and parasites (e.g., microsporidia [*Nematocida parisii*]), each with a different microbial actin-assembly-initiating molecule.

A final exit strategy is for pathogens to extrude out of the host cell within a host-membrane-encased compartment, best typified by the release of *Chlamydia* and *Plasmodium*. This mechanism represents the ultimate level of mechanistic sophistication based on our current knowledge, because it requires pathogen manipulation of many host signaling networks and cellular processes coordinated and regulated over a longer temporal scale. Evolutionary pressures leading to the independent development of extrusion by *Chlamydia* and malarial parasites likely surround the need to navigate host immune defenses while traversing the extracellular microenvironment.

The evolutionary pathways that define the natural history of intracellular pathogens are diverse and are facilitated by gene pool opportunities for acquisition of virulence components. Nevertheless, even a single nucleotide polymorphism is sufficient to define a pathogenesis and virulence determinant. For example, tissue tropism by *C. trachomatis* is the function of a single gene mutation that alters the mutually exclusive reproductive success within either the eye or the genital tract (141). The success of pathogens is not limited by the genetic mechanisms available because even organisms with limited access to gene pools have through adaptive mutation become highly successful in their respective hosts. Rather, it is the ultimate necessity of transmission that defines the selective opportunities for pathogen evolution, especially for highly adapted obligate pathogens. The complexities and elegance of some cellular exit strategies, such as extrusion, evolved by pathogens are a direct consequence of in-tracellular pathogens learning to parse the cellular mechanisms of their host to enable co-option of host cell functions. Thus, the multiplicities of mechanistic development from the outcome of host cell death to the cultivation of its host cell resulting in non-destructive cellular exit are a function of effective transmission and hence reproductive success. Future opportunities for research are expected to reveal the intricacies of the pathogen's orchestration of the host cell that promote a balance of the needs of the pathogen to optimize its evolutionary fitness.

CITATION

Hybiske K, Stephens R. 2015. Cellular exit strategies of intracellular bacteria. Microbiol Spectrum 3(6):VMBF-0002-2014.

REFERENCES

1. **Hybiske K, Stephens RS.** 2008. Exit strategies of intracellular pathogens. *Nat Rev Microbiol* **6:**99–110.

2. **Friedrich N, Hagedorn M, Soldati-Favre D, Soldati T.** 2012. Prison break: pathogens' strategies to egress from host cells. *Microbiol Mol Biol Rev* **76:**707–720.

3. **Beauregard KE, Lee KD, Collier RJ, Swanson JA.** 1997. pH-dependent perforation of macrophage phagosomes by listeriolysin O from *Listeria monocytogenes. J Exp Med* **186:**1159–1163.

4. **Glomski IJ, Gedde MM, Tsang AW, Swanson JA, Portnoy DA.** 2002. The *Listeria monocytogenes* hemolysin has an acidic pH optimum to compartmentalize activity and prevent damage to infected host cells. *J Cell Biol* **156:**1029–1038.

5. **High H, Mounier J, Prevost MC, Sansonetti PJ.** 1992. IpaB of *Shigella flexneri* causes entry into epithelial cells and escape from the phagocytic vacuole. *EMBO J* **11:**1991–1999.

6. **Schnupf P, Portnoy DA.** 2007. Listeriolysin O: a phagosome-specific lysin. *Microbes Infect* **9:**1176–1187.

7. **Schnupf P, Hofmann J, Norseen J, Glomski IJ, Schwartzstein H, Decatur AL.** 2006. Regulated translation of listeriolysin O controls virulence of *Listeria monocytogenes. Mol Microbiol* **61:**999–1012.

8. **Alberti-Segui C, Goeden KR, Higgins DE.** 2007. Differential function of *Listeria monocytogenes* listeriolysin O and phospholipases C in vacuolar dissolution following cell-to-cell spread. *Cell Microbiol* **9:**179–195.

9. **Almeida-Campos FR, Noronha FS, Horta MF.** 2002. The multitalented pore-forming proteins of intracellular pathogens. *Microbes Infect* **4:**741–750.

10. **Andrews NW, Abrams CK, Slatin SL, Griffiths G.** 1990. A *T. cruzi*-secreted protein immunologically related to the complement component C9: evidence for membrane pore-forming activity at low pH. *Cell* **61:**1277–1287.

11. **Schuerch DW, Wilson-Kubalek EM, Tweten RK.** 2005. Molecular basis of listeriolysin O pH dependence. *Proc Natl Acad Sci USA* **102:**12537–12542.

12. **Kafsack BF, Pena JD, Coppens I, Ravindran S, Boothroyd JC, Carruthers VB.** 2009. Rapid membrane disruption by a perforin-like protein facilitates parasite exit from host cells. *Science* **323:**530–533.

13. **Black MW, Boothroyd JC.** 2000. Lytic cycle of *Toxoplasma gondii. Microbiol Mol Biol Rev* **64:**607–623.

14. **Black MW, Arrizabalaga G, Boothroyd JC.** 2000. Ionophore-resistant mutants of *Toxoplasma gondii* reveal host cell permeabilization as an early event in egress. *Mol Cell Biol* **20:**9399–9408.

15. **Moudy R, Manning TJ, Beckers CJ.** 2001. The loss of cytoplasmic potassium upon host cell breakdown triggers egress of *Toxoplasma gondii. J Biol Chem* **276:**41492–41501.

16. **Nagamune K, Hicks LM, Fux B, Brossier F, Chini EN, Sibley LD.** 2008. Abscisic acid controls calcium-dependent egress and development in *Toxoplasma gondii. Nature* **451:**207–210.

17. **Chandramohanadas R, Davis PH, Beiting DP, Harbut MB, Darling C, Velmourougane G, Lee MY, Greer PA, Roos DS, Greenbaum DC.** 2009. Apicomplexan parasites co-opt host calpains to facilitate their escape from infected cells. *Science* **324:**794–797.

18. **Noronha F, Cruz JS, Beirão P, Horta MF.** 2000. Macrophage damage by *Leishmania amazonensis* cytolysin: evidence of pore formation on cell membrane. *Infect Immun* **68:**4578–4584.

19. **Pei J, Kahl-McDonagh M, Ficht TA.** 2014. *Brucella* dissociation is essential for macrophage egress and bacterial dissemination. *Front Cell Infect Microbiol* **4:**23.

20. **Hybiske K, Stephens RS.** 2007. Mechanisms of host cell exit by the intracellular bacterium *Chlamydia. Proc Natl Acad Sci USA* **104**:11430–11435.

21. **Campbell S, Richmond SJ, Yates P.** 1989. The development of *Chlamydia trachomatis* inclusions within the host eukaryotic cell during interphase and mitosis. *J Gen Microbiol* **135:** 1153–1165.

22. **Neeper ID, Patton DL, Kuo CC.** 1990. Cinematographic observations of growth cycles of *Chlamydia trachomatis* in primary cultures of human amniotic cells. *Infect Immun* **58**:2042–2047.

23. **Snavely EA, Kokes M, Dunn JD, Saka HA, Nguyen BD, Bastidas RJ, McCafferty DG, Valdivia RH.** 2014. Reassessing the role of the secreted protease CPAF in *Chlamydia trachomatis* infection through genetic approaches. *Pathog Dis* **71**:336–351.

24. **Liu X, Van Vleet T, Schnellmann RG.** 2004. The role of calpain in oncotic cell death. *Annu Rev Pharmacol Toxicol* **44**:349–370.

25. **Blackman MJ.** 2008. Malarial proteases and host cell egress: an 'emerging'' cascade. *Cell Microbiol* **10**:1925–1934.

26. **Rosenthal PJ.** 2011. Falcipains and other cysteine proteases of malaria parasites. *Adv Exp Med Biol* **712**:30–48.

27. **Wickham ME, Culvenor JG, Cowman AF.** 2003. Selective inhibition of a two-step egress of malaria parasites from the host erythrocyte. *J Biol Chem* **278**:37658–37663.

28. **Glushakova S, Yin D, Li T, Zimmerberg J.** 2005. Membrane transformation during malaria parasite release from human red blood cells. *Curr Biol* **15**:1645–1650.

29. **Yeoh S, O'Donnell RA, Koussis K, Dluzewski AR, Ansell KH, Osborne SA, Hackett F, Withers-Martinez C, Mitchell GH, Bannister LH, Bryans JS, Kettleborough CA, Blackman MJ.** 2007. Subcellular discharge of a serine protease mediates release of invasive malaria parasites from host erythrocytes. *Cell* **131**:1072–1083.

30. **Arastu-Kapur S, Ponder EL, Fonović UP, Yeoh S, Yuan F, Fonović M, Grainger M, Phillips CI, Powers JC, Bogyo M.** 2008. Identification of proteases that regulate erythrocyte rupture by the malaria parasite *Plasmodium falciparum. Nat Chem Biol* **4**:203–213.

31. **Dvorin JD, Martyn DC, Patel SD, Grimley JS, Collins CR, Hopp CS, Bright AT, Westenberger S, Winzeler E, Blackman MJ, Baker DA, Wandless TJ, Duraisingh MT.** 2010. A plant-like kinase in *Plasmodium falciparum* regulates parasite egress from erythrocytes. *Science* **328**:910–912.

32. **Millholland MG, Chandramohanadas R, Pizzarro A, Wehr A, Shi H, Darling C, Lim CT, Greenbaum DC.** 2011. The malaria parasite progressively dismantles the host erythrocyte cytoskeleton for efficient egress. *Mol Cell Proteomics* **10**:M111.010678.

33. **Ishino T, Boisson B, Orito Y, Lacroix C, Bischoff E, Loussert C, Janse C, Ménard R, Yuda M, Baldacci P.** 2009. LISP1 is important for the egress of *Plasmodium berghei* parasites from liver cells. *Cell Microbiol* **11**:1329–1339.

34. **Schmidt-Christensen A, Sturm A, Horstmann S, Heussler V.** 2008. Expression and processing of *Plasmodium berghei* SERA3 during liver stages. *Cell Microbiol* **10**:1723–1734.

35. **Costales J, Rowland EC.** 2007. A role for protease activity and host-cell permeability during the process of *Trypanosoma cruzi* egress from infected cells. *J Parasitol* **93**:1350–1359.

36. **Broz P, Monack DM.** 2011. Molecular mechanisms of inflammasome activation during microbial infections. *Immunol Rev* **243**:174–190.

37. **Hagar JA, Miao EA.** 2014. Detection of cytosolic bacteria by inflammatory caspases. *Curr Opin Microbiol* **17**:61–66.

38. **Moltke von J, Ayres JS, Kofoed EM, Chavarría-Smith J, Vance RE.** 2013. Recognition of bacteria by inflammasomes. *Annu Rev Immunol* **31**:73–106.

39. **Knodler LA, Vallance BA, Celli J, Winfree S, Hansen B, Montero M, Steele-Mortimer O.** 2010. Dissemination of invasive *Salmonella* via bacterial-induced extrusion of mucosal epithelia. *Proc Natl Acad Sci USA* **107**:17733–17738.

40. **Silveira TN, Zamboni DS.** 2010. Pore formation triggered by *Legionella* spp. is an Nlrc4 inflammasome-dependent host cell response that precedes pyroptosis. *Infect Immun* **78**:1403–1413.

41. **Santic M, Pavokovic G, Jones S, Asare R, Kwaik YA.** 2010. Regulation of apoptosis and anti-apoptosis signalling by *Francisella tularensis. Microbes Infect* **12**:126–134.

42. **Sauer JD, Witte CE, Zemansky J, Hanson B, Lauer P, Portnoy DA.** 2010. *Listeria monocytogenes* triggers AIM2-mediated pyroptosis upon infrequent bacteriolysis in the macrophage cytosol. *Cell Host Microbe* **7**:412–419.

43. **Rathinam VA, Jiang Z, Waggoner SN, Sharma S, Cole LE, Waggoner L, Vanaja SK, Monks BG, Ganesan S, Latz E, Hornung V, Vogel SN, Szomolanyi-Tsuda E, Fitzgerald KA.** 2010. The AIM2 inflammasome is essential for host defense against cytosolic bacteria and DNA viruses. *Nat Immunol* **11**:395–402.

44. **Wu J, Fernandes-Alnemri T, Alnemri ES.** 2010. Involvement of the AIM2, NLRC4, and NLRP3 inflammasomes in caspase-1 activation by *Listeria monocytogenes. J Clin Immunol* **30**:693–702.

45. Meixenberger K, Pache F, Eitel J, Schmeck B, Hippenstiel S, Slevogt H, N'Guessan P, Witzenrath M, Netea MG, Chakraborty T, Suttorp N, Opitz B. 2010. *Listeria monocytogenes*-infected human peripheral blood mononuclear cells produce IL-1beta, depending on listeriolysin O and NLRP3. *J Immunol* **184:**922–930.

46. Aachoui Y, Leaf IA, Hagar JA, Fontana MF, Campos CG, Zak DE, Tan MH, Cotter PA, Vance RE, Aderem A, Miao EA. 2013. Caspase-11 protects against bacteria that escape the vacuole. *Science* **339:**975–978.

47. Miao EA, Mao DP, Yudkovsky N, Bonneau R, Lorang CG, Warren SE, Leaf IA, Aderem A. 2010. Innate immune detection of the type III secretion apparatus through the NLRC4 inflammasome. *Proc Natl Acad Sci USA* **107:**3076–3080.

48. Zhao Y, Yang J, Shi J, Gong Y-N, Lu Q, Xu H, Liu L, Shao F. 2011. The NLRC4 inflammasome receptors for bacterial flagellin and type III secretion apparatus. *Nature* **477:**596–600.

49. Yang J, Zhao Y, Shi J, Shao F. 2013. Human NAIP and mouse NAIP1 recognize bacterial type III secretion needle protein for inflammasome activation. *Proc Natl Acad Sci USA* **110:**14408–14413.

50. Chen Y, Smith MR, Thirumalai K, Zychlinsky A. 1996. A bacterial invasin induces macrophage apoptosis by binding directly to ICE. *EMBO J* **15:**3853–3860.

51. Hilbi H, Moss JE, Hersh D, Chen Y, Arondel J, Banerjee S, Flavell RA, Yuan J, Sansonetti PJ, Zychlinsky A. 1998. *Shigella*-induced apoptosis is dependent on caspase-1 which binds to IpaB. *J Biol Chem* **273:**32895–32900.

52. Fernandes-Alnemri T, Yu J-W, Juliana C, Solorzano L, Kang S, Wu J, Datta P, McCormick M, Huang L, McDermott E, Eisenlohr L, Landel CP, Alnemri ES. 2010. The AIM2 inflammasome is critical for innate immunity to *Francisella tularensis*. *Nat Immunol* **11:**385–393.

53. Jones JW, Kayagaki N, Broz P, Henry T, Newton K, O'Rourke K, Chan S, Dong J, Qu Y, Roose-Girma M, Dixit VM, Monack DM. 2010. Absent in melanoma 2 is required for innate immune recognition of *Francisella tularensis*. *Proc Natl Acad Sci USA* **107:**9771–9776.

54. Brennan MA, Cookson BT. 2000. *Salmonella* induces macrophage death by caspase-1-dependent necrosis. *Mol Microbiol* **38:**31–40.

55. Franchi L, Amer A, Body-Malapel M, Kanneganti T-D, Ozören N, Jagirdar R, Inohara N, Vandenabeele P, Bertin J, Coyle A, Grant EP, Núñez G. 2006. Cytosolic flagellin requires Ipaf for activation of caspase-1 and interleukin 1beta in *Salmonella*-infected macrophages. *Nat Immunol* **7:**576–582.

56. Miao EA, Alpuche-Aranda CM, Dors M, Clark AE, Bader MW, Miller SI, Aderem A. 2006. Cytoplasmic flagellin activates caspase-1 and secretion of interleukin 1beta via Ipaf. *Nat Immunol* **7:**569–575.

57. Ren T, Zamboni DS, Roy CR, Dietrich WF, Vance RE. 2006. Flagellin-deficient *Legionella* mutants evade caspase-1- and Naip5-mediated macrophage immunity. *PLoS Pathog* **2:**e18.

58. Molofsky AB, Byrne BG, Whitfield NN, Madigan CA, Fuse ET, Tateda K, Swanson MS. 2006. Cytosolic recognition of flagellin by mouse macrophages restricts *Legionella pneumophila* infection. *J Exp Med* **203:**1093–1104.

59. Fink SL, Cookson BT. 2007. Pyroptosis and host cell death responses during *Salmonella* infection. *Cell Microbiol* **9:**2562–2570.

60. Seto S, Tsujimura K, Horii T, Koide Y. 2013. Autophagy adaptor protein p62/SQSTM1 and autophagy-related gene Atg5 mediate autophagosome formation in response to *Mycobacterium tuberculosis* infection in dendritic cells. *PLoS One* **8:**e86017. doi:10.1371/journal.pone.0086017.

61. Roca FJ, Ramakrishnan L. 2013. TNF dually mediates resistance and susceptibility to mycobacteria via mitochondrial reactive oxygen species. *Cell* **153:**521–534.

62. Weinrauch Y, Zychlinsky A. 1999. The induction of apoptosis by bacterial pathogens. *Annu Rev Microbiol* **53:**155–187.

63. Gao LY, Kwaik YA. 2000. The modulation of host cell apoptosis by intracellular bacterial pathogens. *Trends Microbiol* **8:**306–313.

64. Lai XH, Golovliov I, Sjöstedt A. 2001. *Francisella tularensis* induces cytopathogenicity and apoptosis in murine macrophages via a mechanism that requires intracellular bacterial multiplication. *Infect Immun* **69:**4691–4694.

65. Lai X-H, Sjöstedt A. 2003. Delineation of the molecular mechanisms of *Francisella tularensis*-induced apoptosis in murine macrophages. *Infect Immun* **71:**4642–4646.

66. Paesold G, Guiney DG, Eckmann L, Kagnoff MF. 2002. Genes in the *Salmonella* pathogenicity island 2 and the *Salmonella* virulence plasmid are essential for *Salmonella*-induced apoptosis in intestinal epithelial cells. *Cell Microbiol* **4:**771–781.

67. Early J, Fischer K, Bermudez LE. 2011. *Mycobacterium avium* uses apoptotic macrophages as tools for spreading. *Microb Pathog* **50:**132–139.

68. Davis JM, Ramakrishnan L. 2009. The role of the granuloma in expansion and dissemination of early tuberculous infection. *Cell* **136:**37–49.

69. **Ribeiro-Gomes FL, Peters NC, Debrabant A, Sacks DL.** 2012. Efficient capture of infected neutrophils by dendritic cells in the skin inhibits the early anti-leishmania response. *PLoS Pathog* **8:**e1002536. doi:10.1371/journal.ppat.1002536.

70. **van Zandbergen G, Klinger M, Mueller A, Dannenberg S, Gebert A, Solbach W, Laskay T.** 2004. Cutting edge: neutrophil granulocyte serves as a vector for *Leishmania* entry into macrophages. *J Immunol* **173:**6521–6525.

71. **Real F, Florentino PTV, Reis LC, Ramos Sanchez EM, Veras PS, Goto H, Mortara RA.** 2014. Cell-to-cell transfer of *Leishmania amazonensis* amastigotes is mediated by immunomodulatory LAMP-rich parasitophorous extrusions. *Cell Microbiol* **16:**1549–1564.

72. **Starr T, Child R, Wehrly TD, Hansen B, Hwang S, López-Otin C, Virgin HW, Celli J.** 2012. Selective subversion of autophagy complexes facilitates completion of the *Brucella* intracellular cycle. *Cell Host Microbe* **11:**33–45.

73. **Chen YA, Scheller RH.** 2001. SNARE-mediated membrane fusion. *Nat Rev Mol Cell Biol* **2:**98–106.

74. **Chen J, Reyes M, Clarke M, Shuman HA.** 2007. Host cell-dependent secretion and translocation of the LepA and LepB effectors of *Legionella pneumophila*. *Cell Microbiol* **9:**1660–1671.

75. **Chen J, de Felipe KS, Clarke M, Lu H, Anderson OR, Segal G, Shuman HA.** 2004. *Legionella* effectors that promote nonlytic release from protozoa. *Science* **303:**1358–1361.

76. **Takeuchi H, Furuta N, Morisaki I, Amano A.** 2011. Exit of intracellular *Porphyromonas gingivalis* from gingival epithelial cells is mediated by endocytic recycling pathway. *Cell Microbiol* **13:**677–691.

77. **Yilmaz O, Verbeke P, Lamont RJ, Ojcius DM.** 2006. Intercellular spreading of *Porphyromonas gingivalis* infection in primary gingival epithelial cells. *Infect Immun* **74:**703–710.

78. **Takeuchi H, Furuta N, Amano A.** 2011. Cell entry and exit by periodontal pathogen via recycling pathway. *Commun Integr Biol* **4:**587–589.

79. **Ma H, Croudace JE, Lammas DA, May RC.** 2006. Expulsion of live pathogenic yeast by macrophages. *Curr Biol* **16:**2156–2160.

80. **Alvarez M, Casadevall A.** 2006. Phagosome extrusion and host-cell survival after *Cryptococcus neoformans* phagocytosis by macrophages. *Curr Biol* **16:**2161–2165.

81. **Alvarez M, Casadevall A.** 2007. Cell-to-cell spread and massive vacuole formation after *Cryptococcus neoformans* infection of murine macrophages. *BMC Immunol* **8:**16. doi:10.1186/1471-2172-8-16.

82. **Nicola AM, Robertson EJ, Albuquerque P, Derengowski LD, Casadevall A.** 2011. Nonlytic exocytosis of *Cryptococcus neoformans* from macrophages occurs *in vivo* and is influenced by phagosomal pH. *MBio* **2:**e00167-11. doi:10.1128/mBio.00167-11.

83. **Stukes S, Cohen HW, Casadevall A.** 2014. Temporal kinetics and quantitative analysis of *Cryptococcus neoformans* nonlytic exocytosis. *Infect Immun* **82:**2059–2067.

84. **Johnston SA, May RC.** 2010. The human fungal pathogen *Cryptococcus neoformans* escapes macrophages by a phagosome emptying mechanism that is inhibited by Arp2/3 complex-mediated actin polymerisation. *PLoS Pathog* **6:**e1001041. doi:10.1371/journal.ppat.1001041.

85. **Johnston SA, May RC.** 2012. *Cryptococcus* interactions with macrophages: evasion and manipulation of the phagosome by a fungal pathogen. *Cell Microbiol* **15:**403–411.

86. **Chayakulkeeree M, Johnston SA, Oei JB, Lev S, Williamson PR, Wilson CF, Zuo X, Leal AL, Vainstein MH, Meyer W, Sorrell TC, May RC, Djordjevic JT.** 2011. SEC14 is a specific requirement for secretion of phospholipase B1 and pathogenicity of *Cryptococcus neoformans*. *Mol Microbiol* **80:**1088–1101.

87. **Carnell M, Zech T, Calaminus SD, Ura S, Hagedorn M, Johnston SA, May RC, Soldati T, Machesky LM, Insall RH.** 2011. Actin polymerization driven by WASH causes V-ATPase retrieval and vesicle neutralization before exocytosis. *J Cell Biol* **193:**831–839.

88. **Hagedorn M, Rohde KH, Russell DG, Soldati T.** 2009. Infection by tubercular mycobacteria is spread by nonlytic ejection from their amoeba hosts. *Science* **323:**1729–1733.

89. **Estes KA, Szumowski SC, Troemel ER.** 2011. Non-lytic, actin-based exit of intracellular parasites from *C. elegans* intestinal cells. *PLoS Pathog* **7:**e1002227. doi:10.1371/journal.ppat.1002227.

90. **Doughri AM, Storz J, Altera KP.** 1972. Mode of entry and release of chlamydiae in infections of intestinal epithelial cells. *J Infect Dis* **126:**652–657.

91. **Chin E, Kirker K, Zuck M, James G, Hybiske K.** 2012. Actin recruitment to the *Chlamydia* inclusion is spatiotemporally regulated by a mechanism that requires host and bacterial factors. *PLoS One* **7:**e46949. doi:10.1371/journal.pone.0046949.

92. **Lutter EI, Barger AC, Nair V, Hackstadt T.** 2013. *Chlamydia trachomatis* inclusion membrane protein CT228 recruits elements of the myosin phosphatase pathway to regulate release mechanisms. *Cell Rep* **3:**1921–1931.

93. **Campbell LA, Kuo CC.** 2004. *Chlamydia pneumoniae*: an infectious risk factor for atherosclerosis? *Nat Rev Microbiol* **2**:23–32.

94. **Watson C, Alp NJ.** 2008. Role of *Chlamydia pneumoniae* in atherosclerosis. *Clin Sci* **114**: 509–531.

95. **Sturm A, Amino R, van de Sand C, Regen T, Retzlaff S, Rennenberg A, Krueger A, Pollok JM, Ménard R, Heussler V.** 2006. Manipulation of host hepatocytes by the malaria parasite for delivery into liver sinusoids. *Science* **313**:1287–1290.

96. **Tarun AS, Baer K, Dumpit RF, Gray S, Lejarcegui N, Frevert U, Kappe SH.** 2006. Quantitative isolation and *in vivo* imaging of malaria parasite liver stages. *Int J Parasitol* **36**:1283–1293.

97. **Baer K, Klotz C, Kappe SH, Schnieder T, Frevert U.** 2007. Release of hepatic *Plasmodium yoelii* merozoites into the pulmonary microvasculature. *PLoS Pathog* **3**:e171.

98. **Meis JF, Verhave JP, Jap PH, Meuwissen JH.** 1985. Fine structure of exoerythrocytic merozoite formation of *Plasmodium berghei* in rat liver. *J Protozool* **32**:694–699.

99. **Graewe S, Stanway RR, Rankin KE, Lehmann C, Deschermeier C, Hecht L, Froehlke U, Heussler V.** 2011. Hostile takeover by *Plasmodium*: reorganization of parasite and host cell membranes during liver stage egress. *PLoS Pathog* **7**:e1002224. doi:10.1371/journal.ppat.1002224.

100. **Carlsson F, Brown EJ.** 2006. Actin-based motility of intracellular bacteria, and polarized surface distribution of the bacterial effector molecules. *J Cell Physiol* **209**:288–296.

101. **Stevens JM, Galyov EE, Stevens MP.** 2006. Actin-dependent movement of bacterial pathogens. *Nat Rev Microbiol* **4**:91–101.

102. **Ireton K.** 2013. Molecular mechanisms of cell–cell spread of intracellular bacterial pathogens. *Open Biol* **3**:130079. doi:10.1098/rsob.130079.

103. **Portnoy DA, Auerbuch V, Glomski IJ.** 2002. The cell biology of *Listeria monocytogenes* infection: the intersection of bacterial pathogenesis and cell-mediated immunity. *J Cell Biol* **158**:409–414.

104. **Tilney LG, Portnoy DA.** 1989. Actin filaments and the growth, movement, and spread of the intracellular bacterial parasite, *Listeria monocytogenes*. *J Cell Biol* **109**:1597–1608.

105. **Kocks C, Marchand JB, Gouin E, d'Hauteville H, Sansonetti PJ, Carlier MF, Cossart P.** 1995. The unrelated surface proteins ActA of *Listeria monocytogenes* and IcsA of *Shigella flexneri* are sufficient to confer actin-based motility on *Listeria innocua* and *Escherichia coli* respectively. *Mol Microbiol* **18**:413–423.

106. **Robbins JR, Barth AI, Marquis H, de Hostos EL, Nelson WJ, Theriot JA.** 1999. *Listeria monocytogenes* exploits normal host cell processes to spread from cell to cell. *J Cell Biol* **146**:1333–1350.

107. **Rajabian T, Gavicherla B, Heisig M, Müller-Altrock S, Goebel W, Gray-Owen SD, Ireton K.** 2009. The bacterial virulence factor InlC perturbs apical cell junctions and promotes cell-to-cell spread of *Listeria*. *Nat Cell Biol* **11**:1212–1218.

108. **Fattouh R, Kwon H, Czuczman MA, Copeland JW, Pelletier L, Quinlan ME, Muise AM, Higgins DE, Brumell JH.** 2014. The diaphanous-related formins promote protrusion formation and cell-to-cell spread of *Listeria monocytogenes*. *J Infect Dis* **211**:1185–1195.

109. **Pust S, Morrison H, Wehland J, Sechi AS, Herrlich P.** 2005. *Listeria monocytogenes* exploits ERM protein functions to efficiently spread from cell to cell. *EMBO J* **24**:1287–1300.

110. **Gedde MM, Higgins DE, Tilney LG, Portnoy DA.** 2000. Role of listeriolysin O in cell-to-cell spread of *Listeria monocytogenes*. *Infect Immun* **68**:999–1003.

111. **Smith GA, Marquis H, Jones S, Johnston NC, Portnoy DA, Goldfine H.** 1995. The two distinct phospholipases C of *Listeria monocytogenes* have overlapping roles in escape from a vacuole and cell-to-cell spread. *Infect Immun* **63**:4231–4237.

112. **Gründling A, Gonzalez MD, Higgins DE.** 2003. Requirement of the *Listeria monocytogenes* broad-range phospholipase PC-PLC during infection of human epithelial cells. *J Bacteriol* **185**:6295–6307.

113. **Chong R, Squires R, Swiss R, Agaisse H.** 2011. RNAi screen reveals host cell kinases specifically involved in *Listeria monocytogenes* spread from cell to cell. *PLoS One* **6**:e23399. doi:10.1371/journal.pone.0023399.

114. **Bernardini ML, Mounier J, d'Hauteville H, Coquis-Rondon M, Sansonetti PJ.** 1989. Identification of icsA, a plasmid locus of *Shigella flexneri* that governs bacterial intra- and intercellular spread through interaction with F-actin. *Proc Natl Acad Sci USA* **86**:3867–3871.

115. **Fukumatsu M, Ogawa M, Arakawa S, Suzuki M, Nakayama K, Shimizu S, Kim M, Mimuro H, Sasakawa C.** 2012. *Shigella* targets epithelial tricellular junctions and uses a noncanonical clathrin-dependent endocytic pathway to spread between cells. *Cell Host Microbe* **11**:325–336.

116. **Bishai EA, Sidhu GS, Li W, Dhillon J, Bohil AB, Cheney RE, Hartwig JH, Southwick FS.** 2013. Myosin-X facilitates *Shigella*-induced

membrane protrusions and cell-to-cell spread. *Cell Microbiol* **15**:353–367.

117. **Sansonetti PJ, Mounier J, Prévost MC, Mège RM.** 1994. Cadherin expression is required for the spread of *Shigella flexneri* between epithelial cells. *Cell* **76**:829–839.

118. **Leung Y, Ally S, Goldberg MB.** 2008. Bacterial actin assembly requires toca-1 to relieve N-wasp autoinhibition. *Cell Host Microbe* **3**:39–47.

119. **Haglund CM, Choe JE, Skau CT, Kovar DR, Welch MD.** 2010. *Rickettsia* Sca2 is a bacterial formin-like mediator of actin-based motility. *Nat Cell Biol* **12**:1057–1063.

120. **Kleba B, Clark TR, Lutter EI, Ellison DW, Hackstadt T.** 2010. Disruption of the *Rickettsia rickettsii* Sca2 autotransporter inhibits actin-based motility. *Infect Immun* **78**:2240–2247.

121. **Stamm LM, Morisaki JH, Gao LY, Jeng RL, McDonald KL, Roth R, Takeshita S, Heuser J, Welch MD, Brown EJ.** 2003. *Mycobacterium marinum* escapes from phagosomes and is propelled by actin-based motility. *J Exp Med* **198**:1361–1368.

122. **Stamm LM, Pak MA, Morisaki JH, Snapper SB, Rottner K, Lommel S, Brown EJ.** 2005. Role of the WASP family proteins for *Mycobacterium marinum* actin tail formation. *Proc Natl Acad Sci USA* **102**:14837–14842.

123. **Kespichayawattana W, Rattanachetkul S, Wanun T, Utaisincharoen P, Sirisinha S.** 2000. *Burkholderia pseudomallei* induces cell fusion and actin-associated membrane protrusion: a possible mechanism for cell-to-cell spreading. *Infect Immun* **68**:5377–5384.

124. **Lu Q, Xu Y, Yao Q, Niu M, Shao F.** 2014. A polar-localized iron-binding protein determines the polar targeting of *Burkholderia* BimA autotransporter and actin tail formation. *Cell Microbiol* **17**:408–424.

125. **Stevens MP, Stevens JM, Jeng RL, Taylor LA, Wood MW, Hawes P, Monaghan P, Welch MD, Galyov EE.** 2005. Identification of a bacterial factor required for actin-based motility of *Burkholderia pseudomallei*. *Mol Microbiol* **56**:40–53.

126. **Thomas S, Popov VL, Walker DH.** 2010. Exit mechanisms of the intracellular bacterium *Ehrlichia*. *PLoS One* **5**:e15775. doi:10.1371/journal.pone.0015775.

127. **Kim MJ, Kim MK, Kang JS.** 2013. Involvement of lipid rafts in the budding-like exit of *Orientia tsutsugamushi*. *Microb Pathog* **63**:37–43.

128. **Urakami H, Tsuruhara T, Tamura A.** 1984. Electron microscopic studies on intracellular multiplication of *Rickettsia tsutsugamushi* in L cells. *Microbiol Immunol* **28**:1191–1201.

129. **Rikihisa Y, Ito S.** 1982. Entry of *Rickettsia tsutsugamushi* into polymorphonuclear leukocytes. *Infect Immun* **38**:343–350.

130. **Ewing EP, Takeuchi A, Shirai A, Osterman JV.** 1978. Experimental infection of mouse peritoneal mesothelium with scrub typhus rickettsiae: an ultrastructural study. *Infect Immun* **19**:1068–1075.

131. **Tamiya T (ed).** 1962. *Recent Advances in Studies of Tsutsugamushi Disease in Japan.* Medical Culture, Tokyo, Japan.

132. **Urakami H, Tsuruhara T, Tamura A.** 1983. Penetration of *Rickettsia tsutsugamushi* into cultured mouse fibroblasts (L cells): an electron microscopic observation. *Microbiol Immunol* **27**:251–263.

133. **Kadosaka T, Kimura E.** 2003. Electron microscopic observations of *Orientia tsutsugamushi* in salivary gland cells of naturally infected *Leptotrombidium pallidum* larvae during feeding. *Microbiol Immunol* **47**:727–733.

134. **Anderson RM, May RM.** 1982. Coevolution of hosts and parasites. *Parasitology* **85**(Pt 2):411–426.

135. **Ehrbar K, Hardt WD.** 2005. Bacteriophage-encoded type III effectors in *Salmonella enterica* subspecies 1 serovar Typhimurium. *Infect Genet Evol* **5**:1–9.

136. **Stephens RS, Myers G, Eppinger M, Bavoil PM.** 2009. Divergence without difference: phylogenetics and taxonomy of *Chlamydia* resolved. *FEMS Immunol Med Microbiol* **55**:115–119.

137. **Roumagnac P, Weill FX, Dolecek C, Baker S, Brisse S, Chinh NT, Le TA, Acosta CJ, Farrar J, Dougan G, Achtman M.** 2006. Evolutionary history of *Salmonella typhi*. *Science* **314**:1301–1304.

138. **Clarke IN.** 2011. Evolution of *Chlamydia trachomatis*. *Ann NY Acad Sci* **1230**:E11–E18.

139. **Stephens RS, Kalman S, Lammel C, Fan J, Marathe R, Aravind L, Mitchell W, Olinger L, Tatusov RL, Zhao Q, Koonin EV, Davis RW.** 1998. Genome sequence of an obligate intracellular pathogen of humans: *Chlamydia trachomatis*. *Science* **282**:754–759.

140. **Hueck CJ.** 1998. Type III protein secretion systems in bacterial pathogens of animals and plants. *Microbiol Mol Biol Rev* **62**:379–433.

141. **Fehlner-Gardiner C, Roshick C, Carlson JH, Hughes S, Belland RJ, Caldwell HD, McClarty G.** 2002. Molecular basis defining human *Chlamydia trachomatis* tissue tropism. A possible role for tryptophan synthase. *J Biol Chem* **277**:26893–26903.

TARGETED THERAPIES

Novel Targets of Antimicrobial Therapies

26

SARAH E. MADDOCKS[1]

INTRODUCTION: TRADITIONAL TREATMENTS AND CLASSICAL TARGETS

During the golden age of antibiotic discovery, from the 1930s through the 1960s, methods of antibiotic identification relied solely on scientific observation, and while chemical analogues such as amoxicillin, derived from penicillin, continued to be developed, they retained the same mechanisms of action and hence the same bacterial targets. Moreover, there are finite modifications that can ultimately be made to "old" classes of antibiotics. Consequently, only two new classes of antibiotics have been discovered in the past 40 years, and both entered the market early in the new millennium. The advent of the genomics revolution offered a new hope for the discovery of novel antimicrobial targets. Genomic strategies were utilized to identify potential antibacterial targets, namely those that, if inhibited, resulted in the death of the bacterium. Such targets were to be present in pathogenic strains of bacteria and absent from the human host; they could include metabolic pathways, receptor ligands, and virulence traits, to name a few. Despite the abundance of targets identified using this strategy, no new antibiotics have

[1]Department of Biomedical Sciences, Cardiff School of Health Sciences, Cardiff Metropolitan University, Western Avenue, Llandaff, Wales, CF5 2YB.
Virulence Mechanisms of Bacterial Pathogens, 5th edition
Edited by Indira T. Kudva, Nancy A. Cornick, Paul J. Plummer, Qijing Zhang, Tracy L. Nicholson, John P. Bannantine, and Bryan H. Bellaire
© 2016 American Society for Microbiology, Washington, DC
doi:10.1128/microbiolspec.VMBF-0018-2015

reached the marketplace as a result of the genomics approach. However, new antimicrobials with novel targets continue to be identified and contribute to the ongoing struggle against antimicrobial resistance that threatens to return humankind to a situation comparable to the preantibiotic era.

This article will describe and discuss some of the novel targets for emerging antimicrobial treatments, highlighting pivotal research on which our ability to continue to successfully treat bacterial infection relies.

COMBINATION APPROACHES TO TACKLE MULTIDRUG-RESISTANT BACTERIA

Combination therapies are widely used in medicine and have proved crucial for the treatment of infectious diseases, including, for example, *Mycobacterium tuberculosis*, which is treated using four simultaneously administered antibiotics. Monotherapies are increasingly inadequate, and several strategies are currently employed that combine either different classes of antibiotics or antibiotics with targeted adjuvants. Above all, the principal aim of this approach is to reduce the minimum inhibitory concentration or to resensitize resistant organisms. Often this involves inhibition of different targets within the same synthetic or metabolic pathways, inhibition of the same target within different pathways, or inhibition of unrelated targets within different pathways. One such example is the commercially available antibiotic combination co-amoxiclav, which utilizes a combination of amoxicillin, a beta-lactam antibiotic, with the beta-lactamase inhibitor clavulanic acid, which renders beta-lactamase-producing microorganisms susceptible to the action of the penicillin-derived antibiotic (1).

Antibiotics combined with adjuvants in this manner have increased efficacy, but the adjuvant itself is generally not bactericidal; this approach reduces the onset of antimicrobial resistance but does not affect a new cellular target *per se*. Two-component sensor–regulator proteins are ubiquitous among prokaryotes but, despite their high degree of conservation, are not essential for viability. As such, they have become attractive targets for adjuvants, especially due to the predominant role many of these systems have in antimicrobial resistance. Cell wall biosynthesis in *Staphylococcus aureus* is in part regulated by the VraSR system, which coordinates the expression of D-alanyl-D-lactate, a peptide that is incorporated into peptidoglycan (2). Additionally, VraSR also mediates resistance to beta-lactam and glycopeptide antibiotics; as such, expression of this system is induced by exposure to beta-lactams, glycopeptide, and bacitracin. Null-mutations of *vraSR* result in greatly enhanced susceptibility to antibiotics that disrupt cell wall biosynthesis, similarly if *vra*SR expression is inhibited resistance is also lessened (3, 4).

Natural and synthetic two-component inhibitors exist, and the RWJ-family and its derivatives are the best characterized. These inhibitors are hydrophobic tyramines which exhibit a broad spectrum of activity against Gram-positive microorganisms and are themselves inherently bactericidal (5). Analogues vary in their ability to inhibit bacterial growth, a characteristic that has been correlated with an ability to "jam" two-component systems. Mechanistically, such inhibitors appear to function by impairing auto-phosphorylation of sensor kinases, sometimes completely abolishing this function. Compounds are thought to disrupt the four-helix bundles required for dimerization, driving them apart to expose hydrophobic residues that result in misfolding or aggregation, with a subsequent loss of function. Synthetic two-component inhibitors are also known for Gram-negative microorganisms; for *Pseudomonas aeruginosa*, inhibition of the AlgR1R2 system results in reduced expression of alginate biosynthesis genes, but inhibitions of two-component sensor-regulators are not directly antimicrobial (6). It is supposed that inhibitors of this nature could be used in conjunction with antibiotics to treat infected cystic fibrosis patients, with the aim of rendering *P. aeruginosa* more susceptible to antimicrobial treatment by disruption of the secreted, protective alginate layer. However, despite the promise of two-component-system targeting compounds, step-wise training experiments have demonstrated that microorganisms readily evolve resistance to them (5).

ANTIBIOFILM AND ANTIADHESIVE STRATEGIES

Communities of bacteria growing as a biofilm are afforded protection from environmental stresses, including antimicrobial treatments, by virtue of the thick, exopolysaccharide layer that surrounds the biofilm and impedes the diffusion of antimicrobial compounds. Colonization of the host requires bacterial adhesion prior to proliferation, and it is understood that a vast majority of pathogens exist within the host, at the site of infection, as a biofilm which is often comprised of more than one species. Prophylactic measures that impede microbial adhesion have the capacity to limit microbial colonization and thus prevent infection; antiadhesive compounds, if appropriately targeted, also have the potential to disrupt already established biofilms, being highly beneficial for the treatment of chronic infections.

Cationic antimicrobial peptides are well known for their broad-spectrum lytic activity and low propensity to induce resistance. Aggregating within the bacterial cell-leaflet, these small peptides mediate widespread disruption of the bacterial cell, but not all antimicrobial peptides have the same efficacy, and some exhibit poor lytic properties. A subgroup of this type of cationic antimicrobial peptide has potent antiadhesive activity, inhibiting biofilm formation as well as disrupting established microbial communities (7). Studies of an archetypical nine-amino-acid, antibiofilm antimicrobial peptide (1037) identified a consensus sequence (FRIRVRV) subsequently found to be well conserved

among those antimicrobial peptides that were antiadhesive (8). Transcriptomics revealed that this peptide targeted expression of several genes associated with the expression of flagella, resulting in impaired swimming and swarming motility as well as biofilm formation. Interestingly, a preserved characteristic of antimicrobial peptides with antiadhesive activity is poor bactericidal efficacy. Subsequently, approaches have been implemented to synthesize hybrid peptides containing the peptide motif associated with antiadhesive activity that have good bactericidal activity but minimal hemolytic properties.

More comprehensive studies of so called antibiofilm antimicrobial peptides have confirmed that at least one peptide (1018) mediates biofilm impairment by targeting molecules involved in the bacterial cellular stress response (9). This peptide does not impair the growth of planktonic bacteria but inhibits biofilm growth as well as disrupting established biofilms comprised of either Gram-positive or Gram-negative microorganisms, including *P. aeruginosa*, *Klebsiella pneumonia*, *Acinetobacter baumannii*, and *S. aureus*. Specifically, this peptide was found to target (p)ppGpp, a vital signal required for biofilm formation, and it is believed to target intracellular (p)ppGpp for degradation (9). This means that peptide 1018 must traverse the cytoplasmic membrane and gain access to the cytoplasm. It is hypothesized that this peptide might also mediate expression of (p)ppGpp through the enzymes SpoT and RelA, which are fundamental to the stringent response.

High-throughput screening of natural (including fungal and plant extracts) and chemically synthesized small molecules has begun to lead the way in identifying small molecules that interfere with bacterial adhesion and biofilm growth. With *P. aeruginosa* used as a test organism, over 65,000 compounds have been screened to identify those that exclusively inhibit biofilm formation without impairing the growth of planktonic cells. Biofilm growth and detachment assays reported 30 such compounds that fell into this remit but did not shed light on possible cellular targets. Parallel screening of a different library comprising over 70,000 small molecules, identified *N*-(4-chloro-phenyl 0-2-{5-[4-(pyrrolidine-1-sulfonyl)-phenyl]-[1,3,4]oxodiazol-2-yl sulfanyl}-acetamide) (abbreviated to AL1) as a strongly antiadhesive compound that suppressed the assembly of type I pili in uropathogenic *Escherichia coli* (10). Bacteria exposed to this chemical were found to be devoid of type I pili, and subsequently pilus-dependent adhesion was abrogated. AL1 specifically targeted polymerization steps during the subunit incorporation cycle of the chaperone-usher pathway, specifically interaction between FimC and FimH; given the highly conserved nature of this pathway, it is likely that the effects observed for uropathogenic *E. coli* would be seen for other microorganisms. Activity of this molecule is believed not to be constrained only to *de novo* synthesis, because addition of AL1 to uropathogenic *E. coli* immediately disrupts adhesion, suggesting that it also targets preformed pili. Despite these advances in the discovery of antiadhesive/antibiofilm small molecules, it should be noted that currently, no approved drugs exist that specifically target biofilms.

Efflux pump inhibitors are a class of molecules whose major purpose is to impair the function of bacterial efflux pumps, which deal with removal of, for example, metabolic waste products, toxins, or antimicrobials (11). They have long been known to be efficacious against planktonic bacteria, and used in combination with other antibiotics, they can resensitize microorganisms to those antibiotics by preventing efflux from the cell. Such compounds do not possess antiadhesive properties but can impede biofilm development, and when a number of these molecules are administered together, they can completely abolish biofilm formation. Using *E. coli* as a model, it was documented that the expression of over 20 different efflux systems was highly upregulated in the biofilm mode of

growth. Their role in the bacterial biofilm lifestyle remains incompletely understood, but gene expression analysis showed that many were involved in multidrug resistance, suggesting that to some extent these targets were no different than those observed for planktonic microorganisms (12). Therefore, these efflux pump inhibitors could be successfully used in combination with antibiotics to remove biofilm. Conversely, biofilm development was disrupted by efflux pump inhibitors alone, in the absence of additional antibiotics, suggesting an alternative role for them in maintaining a healthy biofilm. In addition, it has been hypothesized that the high expression of efflux systems within the biofilm serves as a waste-removal strategy to prevent metabolite accumulation, so impairing these systems could result in biofilm disruption as a consequence of the build-up of toxic waste products (13).

Targeting iron metabolism within pathogenic microorganisms has been a long-debated strategy to attenuate virulence and impede microbial growth within the host (14). Evidence now suggests that this strategy could also be effective against biofilms and that by hijacking the iron-acquisition systems, biofilm bacteria can be effectively killed and biofilm development blocked (15). Gallium is a redox-inactive metal that can replace iron in a number of biological iron compounds, including siderophores (15–17). Metallocomplexes comprised of the siderophore desferrioxamine and gallium (in place of iron) effectively target bacterial siderophore uptake systems to transport toxic gallium to the cytoplasm; in this methodology the siderophore is likened to a Trojan horse, tricking the pathogen into taking up a lethal metal ion (18). While the toxic effects of such metal ions on the bacterial cell are known, the observed impairment of biofilm development has not been thoroughly described outside the scope of a reduction in bacterial numbers, so putative targets in this respect remain unknown, and the process might be mediated purely by toxicity.

TARGETING PATHOGENICITY AND VIRULENCE

A significant factor associated with the development of infection is an organism's ability to evade the immune system and damage the host. Targeting mechanisms of pathogenicity and virulence are attractive because they have the potential to render pathogens susceptible to host clearance mechanisms without killing them. Used alone or in combination with cidal therapies, antivirulence antimicrobials could have a place among traditional antimicrobial therapies, especially since current research suggests that resistance occurs less readily.

Numerous antivirulence strategies exist, but none as yet have entered the clinic. Such strategies are diverse in their approach and their mechanism of action and include small molecules that inhibit enzymatic activity, or biosynthesis of virulence factors, those that impede the expression of global regulators of known virulence traits, as well as inhibitors of quorum sensing (see below) (19). Small molecules have been utilized experimentally to inhibit the proteolytic activity of the lethal factor produced by *Bacillus anthracis*. In a mouse model the small molecule (2R)-2-[(4-fluoro-3-methylphenyl) sulfonylamino]-N-hydroxy-2-(tetrahydro-2H-pyran-4-yl)acetamide was found to offer a survival benefit of between 50 and 60% (Sterne strain in a BALB/c model) when administered as a monotherapy, with full protection from death when administered in combination with an antibiotic (20). The latter combination therapy shows the most promise for antivirulence antimicrobials, and it seems most likely that these therapies will be administered as a means of attenuation of virulence to promote clearance by the host, with additional low-dose antibiotic treatment to assist removal of vulnerable pathogens.

Chemical inhibitors of K capsular biosynthesis in *E. coli* have demonstrated similar efficacy with regard to attenuation and subsequent clearance of infection following antibiotic treatments (21). Innate immunity is impaired by capsular polysaccharide that impedes opsonization and recognition by the complement system. Despite the molecular target remaining unknown, screens of small molecules have identified candidates that impair early stage capsule biosynthesis, rendering pathogens susceptible to C3 complement and sensitizing them to antibiotic treatment.

Alternative antivirulence strategies target receptor-mediated pathogenicity mechanisms, such as the interaction between Shiga-like toxins, produced by enterohemorrhagic *E. coli* and its receptor, Gb3, found on the surface of epithelial cells (22). Enterohemorrhagic *E. coli* can result in serious diarrheal disease, culminating in hemolytic uremic syndrome (HUS), and antibiotic treatment is not advised, meaning that current treatment for infection is supportive. In *in vivo* mouse infection models Shiga-like toxin inhibitors neutralize toxicity by preventing adhesion to epithelial cells, resulting in protection against doses that are known to be fatal. At present, the precise mechanism remains unknown, but this strategy offers a means of attenuating infection and preventing the onset of hemolytic uremic syndrome.

Perturbations in the environment in which infection ensues can also impact pathogenicity and virulence, as has been demonstrated by the use of the micronutrient zinc. At high concentrations zinc is toxigenic to most organisms, including bacteria, but at low levels it can disrupt aggregation and biofilm formation as well as the expression of numerous virulence-associated genes, without damage to the host. These effects are not dissimilar to those observed with other micronutrients such as iron (23). Enteroaggregative *E. coli* has been used best to demonstrate these effects, where subinhibitory concentrations of zinc impaired both intracellular aggregation and the development of biofilm by this prolifically aggregative organism. Moreover, gene expression analysis indicated that this process was likely mediated via significantly reduced expression of the virulence-associated transcriptional regulator *aagR*. Reduced gene expression was initially observed 3 hours post-treatment and was maintained following removal of treatment, with a 30% reduction in gene expression still evident (24).

The versatility of antivirulence antimicrobials offers an abundance of possible avenues of scientific exploration and the development of novel antimicrobial treatments. However, the vastness of the field calls for a refined approach to avoid the emergence of an overwhelming situation in which the most promising or adaptable targets are overlooked. Large-scale analysis including phylogenetic profiling of proteomic clusters offers such clarity and has indeed successfully identified 17 potential candidates that are common to diverse human pathogens but which are uncommon in nonpathogenic microorganisms. Prospective antivirulence contenders identified using these methods include *mgtB* and *mntH*, both of which are involved in manganese transport, *sodC* (oxidative stress), the stringent response gene *sspB*, and the protoheme IX biosynthesis gene *hemY*, to name a few (25). The ubiquitous nature of these genes and their orthologues throughout the *Gammaproteobacteria* and *Firmicutes*, combined with their affiliation with virulence, makes them ideal. Consequently, these candidates could form the basis of a preliminary antivirulence design for therapies that could be efficacious against a large variety of pathogens, or several subgroups of similar organisms, much like current antibiotics (i.e., broad- and narrow-spectrum antibiotics).

PREVENTING MICROBIAL COMMUNICATION

One of the most intently studied antivirulence strategies involves jamming microbial communication. This approach has been pursued as a means of attenuating virulence, adhesion, and bacterial community development without impairing growth and survival, thus providing less selective pressure toward resistance. Quorum sensing occurs between bacteria of the same species and members of diverse species; thousands of natural quorum sensing inhibitory compounds have been screened and numerous synthetic analogues produced that have the potential to impair microbial communication. Three major quorum sensing targets have so far been utilized; these include inhibition of quorum sensing molecule synthesis, arrest of molecule–receptor interaction, and degradation of quorum sensing molecules (26).

The majority of quorum sensing inhibitors (QSIs) that impair synthesis of quorum sensing molecules have been developed using *P. aeruginosa* as a model microorganism. These include signal agonists that target LasR or MvfR. MvfR is a global quorum sensing regulator known to be nonessential for growth. Eight compounds that bind directly to the MvfR protein have been shown to impair quorum sensing and attenuate virulence in a mouse infection model, without reducing bacterial load (27). These compounds share structural similarity, and each possesses a benzamide–benzimidazole backbone. This provides the host with an advantage, making infection more likely to clear, or allows successful cotreatment with other bactericidal antimicrobials.

Anti–quorum sensing stratagems that target acyl-homoserine lactones produced primarily by Gram-negative microorganisms, as well as peptide quorum sensing molecules produced by Gram-positive microorganisms, have proved effective at impairing the expression of virulence factors *in vitro* as well as attenuating pathogenicity *in vivo*. Moreover, the autoinducer 3 system, known to mediate interspecies signaling, can similarly be impaired; for example, strategies to impede phosphorylation of QseC could potentially impede signaling between species as diverse as *E. coli*, *Salmonella* spp., and *Francisella tularensis*, to name a few. QseC is conserved in over 25 bacterial species, making it a diverse target for anti–quorum sensing approaches (28).

Molecule–receptor interaction is imperative for the bacterial response to the presence of quorum sensing molecules; targeting this aspect of quorum sensing relies on natural or synthetic signaling-molecule analogues that preferentially bind to receptors without stimulating an intracellular response signal (29). These general nonresponsive signal–receptor complexes block subsequent binding by quorum sensing molecules. LuxR-type receptor proteins have been well studied as potential candidates for this type of interference, and crystal structure analysis is likely to prove imperative for applicable inhibitor design. However, screening of natural compounds has revealed a number of efficacious analogues capable of inhibiting signaling in this manner (30).

Quorum sensing signal degradation is generally reliant on enzymes such as lactonases, acylases, or oxidoreductases (31). Lactonases tend to have a broad specificity for acyl homoserine lactones by virtue of the highly conserved lactone ring within these molecules. Acylases exhibit substrate specificity based on the chain length of the acyl moiety and tend not to be as broadly acting as lactonases. The least is known about the oxidoreductases, which work via oxidation of reduction of the acyl side chain.

Anti–quorum sensing treatments have the most potential to be used in combination with either other antimicrobials or surface antiseptics or disinfectants, due to their inherent tendency to disrupt biofilm formation. For example, biofilms of *P. aeruginosa* treated with a QSI appeared more susceptible to dispersal using a simple detergent such as sodium dodecyl sulfate (32). Despite their promise as novel new antimicrobial targets, QSIs also have their limitations. Primarily, they can interact with one another. QSIs that target LuxR result in transcriptional feedback which generates a nonlinear response to increases in inhibitor concentration (33). Moreover, competitive LuxR inhibitors can weakly activate LuxR, alone or in combination with other QSIs, leading to increased bacterial virulence. These models have focused only on Lux systems to date, but these types of transcriptional feedback effects could occur for any QSI that acts by interfering with transcriptional regulators.

Quorum sensing molecules can have a direct effect upon the host. The quorum sensing signal molecule of *P. aeruginosa*, N-(3-oxododecanoyl)-L-homoserine lactone (OdHL), modulates inflammation and immune responses in mammals by acting as a PPARδ inhibitor, preventing NF-κB gene expression and ultimately suppressing STAT3 activity (34). Consequently, the innate proinflammatory immune response is dampened, thus promoting a shift toward infection. QSIs, particularly LasR inhibitors, which have cross-reactivity with OdHL, administered appropriately as a prophylactic measure could prevent this process and promote immune clearance. As more work is undertaken to elucidate a place for QSIs in antimicrobial treatment, it is clear that an appropriate application must be considered, be this as part of a cotreatment or as a prophylactic measure; it is imperative that QSIs are administered at the right time and at the right dose to increase microbial susceptibility to the host immune response and other antibacterial agents.

NANO-FORMULATED ANTIBIOTICS

Nanomedicine, or nanotechnology, is a relatively new application in the field of medicine that exploits a novel means of delivery of antimicrobial compounds to microorganisms and may also target novel components of the bacterial cell. Nanoparticles are broadly defined as particles with at least one dimension that are smaller than 100 nm; their surface area and biological and chemical activity can be modified for a preferred application. Antimicrobials formulated as nanoparticles characteristically exhibit higher antimicrobial activity due in part to their polycationic or polyanionic nature, facilitating better interaction with the bacterial membrane; moreover there is a correlation between the size of a nanoparticle and its inherent antimicrobial activity, with smaller particles having the best efficacy (35).

To date, the majority of antimicrobial nanoparticles have been primarily metal-ion-based, with zinc and silver receiving the most attention (36). Metals are well documented for possessing antimicrobial activity, but those that have so far been developed as nanoparticles are more effective antimicrobials and are associated with a lower likelihood of the emergence of resistance when compared to their chemical counterparts (37). It is currently hypothesized that the antibacterial activity of nanoparticulate zinc oxide is facilitated by its electrostatic attraction to the negatively charged bacterial membrane, whereupon it likely results in altered permeability and eventual disruption of the cell envelope and subsequent death. However, silver nanoparticles are believed to mediate bacterial death via the production of reactive oxygen species such as hydroxyl radicals or superoxide, which catalyze extensive lipid peroxidation (38). Likely additional targets for metal-ion formulated nanoparticles include metal ion transporters and impairment of efflux pumps. The relative lack of specificity of these compounds makes them efficacious against a broad spectrum of pathogenic bacteria.

More recently, nanoparticulate formulations of common disinfectants such as chlorhexidine have been produced which can be deposited onto surfaces such as glass, titanium, and ethylene vinyl acetate (39–41). These particles exhibit antibiofilm activity and appear to be more efficacious than non-nano-formulated chlorhexidine against some of the most notorious health care– and wound-associated pathogens including *P. aeruginosa* and methicillin-resistant *S. aureus*. While the mechanism of action of chlorhexidine as a membrane-disrupting chemical is well de-

scribed, it is thought that additional targets might be involved or that the novel delivery mechanism itself might predispose organisms that ordinarily show good tolerance to chlorhexidine to its bactericidal properties.

Therefore, nano-formulated antibiotics deviate from traditional antibiotics that are chemically synthesized or biosynthesized and have a broad range of bacterial cell targets, which is advantageous with regard to the development of resistance. As such, they do not affect novel targets per se (that are currently known), but their novelty lies in their chemistry and delivery. By using nanotechnology, it might be possible in the future to reintroduce redundant antimicrobials or enable antimicrobials to be better internalized by bacteria.

INTERFERING WITH RNA

Small RNA (sRNA) profiling of pathogens has enabled the rapid identification of potential targets for antimicrobial therapeutics. At between 50 to 500 nucleotides in length, these are naturally occurring genetic regulatory elements that govern posttranslational expression of a wide variety of bacterial genes (42). sRNAs are involved in the bacterial response to "challenging" conditions, including antimicrobial treatment. Studies with methicillin-resistant *S. aureus* using RNA sequencing technology have identified an sRNA profile for this organism following exposure to antibiotics, which has provided a framework to investigate the potential of sRNA-targeted or sRNA-mediated antimicrobial therapies.

The postantibiotic treatment sRNA profile for methicillin-resistant *S. aureus* revealed 195 sRNAs, some of which had a role in general metabolic processes and others which constituted a critical component of the antibiotic resistance response. Some of these novel ribo-targets were associated with expression of *gyrA* and *mecA*, both of which are involved in the expression of antibiotic resistance traits and provide an opportunity to explore the benefits of manipulating sRNA targets to resensitize microorganisms to antimicrobial treatment (43).

Similar studies with multidrug-resistant isolates of *Pseudomonas putida* treated with rifampicin, tetracycline, ciprofloxacin, ampicillin, kanamycin, spectinomycin, and gentamicin identified 138 new sRNA targets that were related to genes encoding antibiotic resistance traits. Crucially, the observed relationship between mRNA and sRNA expression emphasizes the importance of such targets, which are thought to play a critical role in fine-tuning the antimicrobial response (44).

A different strategy also making use of sRNA-based technologies has utilized phage delivery systems to silence or knock down antibiotic-resistant phenotypes in *E. coli*. In this case sRNAs were specifically designed to impair the translation of mRNA transcribed from either kanamycin-resistance or chloramphenicol-resistance cassettes and successfully restored sensitivity to both of these antibiotics within populations that were demonstrated previously to be resistant to treatment with kanamycin or chloramphenicol (45). While proof of principle was applied only to *E. coli*, this strategy has the potential to be applied to numerous multidrug-resistant pathogens for which there are known phage.

This shotgun approach to sRNA antisense screening has the potential to reveal large numbers of novel antimicrobial targets and has proved successful for *S. aureus*, *E. coli*, and *P. aeruginosa*. Despite this, therapies that utilize or target sRNAs remain in the early stages of development. However, much like other targeted strategies, nonessential genes such as those that encode virulence factors could be targeted to attenuate pathogens without providing the selective pressure that favors resistance.

TOXICOGENOMICS

There are a plethora of novel antimicrobial targets with remarkable potential as targets for antimicrobial therapies. Strategies to best exploit them continue to be developed, but numerous barriers lie in the way. Finding a balance between the therapeutic dose to have efficacy against pathogens and toxicity within the host is a challenge that can be addressed by traditional toxicology and toxicogenomics. Toxicogenomics assesses combined information regarding gene and protein activity within a particular cell, tissue, or organism (46). Transcriptomic and proteomic approaches are employed to gather this type of data to elucidate mechanisms involved in the presentation of toxicity, and in this manner molecular expression profiles can be obtained following exposure to a given toxin. This can predict genetic susceptibility.

The application of toxicogenomics for the screening of new antimicrobial compounds is clear, but it also has the potential to be used to identify mechanisms of toxicity for novel antimicrobials in bacteria and indeed to facilitate the rapid identification of potential new targets that could be exploited (47). Systematic strategies to enable effectual antimicrobial candidates remain a challenge, and the toxicogenomic approach can identify developable contenders early on while eliminating ineffective ones. Furthermore, this kind of approach could provide a profile of targets that could form the basis of a library of antimicrobial targets for an informed assessment of new antimicrobial candidates.

SUMMARY AND CONCLUDING REMARKS

Novel targeted antimicrobial therapies are critical to triumph in the relentless race against the evolution of antimicrobial resistance. A directed approach to recognize specific targets is shrewd, but it remains imperative to ensure that consideration is given to appropriate targets that are not likely to encourage rapid emergence of resistance. Comprehensive, inclusive methodologies are paramount to establish a pool of suitable antimicrobial targets that provide little evolutionary pressure for survival and if used appropriately can extend the life-time for which they are effective. Combination therapies are attractive and are often significantly more effective, offering an antimicrobial approach akin to the hurdle technologies used by the food industry. Importantly, a sustained commitment to identify and augment such targeted approaches, in whatever form they may take, should not lose momentum against a backdrop of an impending antimicrobial crisis.

CITATION

Maddocks SE. 2016. Novel targets of antimicrobial therapies. Microbiol Spectrum 4(2): VMBF-0018-2015.

REFERENCES

1. **Bryan J.** 2011. Still going at 30: co-amoxiclav. *Pharm J* **286:**762.
2. **Belcheva A, Golemi-Kotra D.** 2008. A close up view of the VraSR two-component system. *J Biol Chem* **283:**12354–12364.
3. **Boyle-Vavra S, Yin S, Sun Jo D, Montgomery CP, Duam RS.** 2013. VraT/YvqF is required for methicillin resistance and activation of the VraSR a regulon in *Staphylococcus aureus*. *Antimicrob Agents Chemother* **57:**83–95.
4. **Utaida S, Dunman PM, Macapagal D, Murphy E, Projan SJ, Singh VK, Jayaswal RK, Wilkinson BJ.** 2003. Genome-wide transcriptional profiling of the response of *Staphylococcus aureus* to cell-wall-active antibiotics reveals a cell-wall-stress stimulon. *Microbiol* **149:**2719–2732.
5. **Barrett JF, Goldschmidt RM, Lawrence LE, Foleno B, Chen R, Demers JP, Johnson S, Kanojia R, Fernandez J, Bernstein J, Licata L, Huang S, Hlasta DJ, Macielag MJ, Ohemeng K, Frechette R, Frosco MB, Klaubert DH, Whiteley JM, Wang L, Hoch JA.** 1998. Antibacterial agents that inhibit two-component signal transduction systems. *Proc Natl Acad Sci USA* **95:**5317–5322.
6. **Roychoudhury S, Zielinski NA, Ninfa AJ, Allen NE, Jungheim LN, Nicas TI, Chakrabarty AM.** 1993. Inhibitors of two-component signal transduction systems: inhibition of alignate gene activation in *Pseudomonas aeruginosa*. *Proc Natl Acad Sci USA* **90:**965–969.
7. **Park S, Park Y, Hahm K.** 2011. The role of anti-microbial peptides in preventing multi

8. drug-resistant bacterial infections and biofilm formation. *Int J Mol Sci* **12:**5971–5992.
8. **Xu W, Zhu X, Tan T, Li W, Shan A.** 2014. Design of embedded-hybrid anti-microbial peptides with enhanced cell selectivity and anti-biofilm activity. *PLoS One* **9:**e98935. doi:10.1371/journal.pone.0098935.
9. **Fuente-Nunez C, Reffuvielle F, Haney EF, Strauss SK, Hancock REW.** 2014. Broad-spectrum anti-biofilm peptide that targets a cellular stress response. *PLoS Pathog* **10:** e1004152. doi:10.1371/journal.ppat.1004152.
10. **Lo AWH, Water K, Gane PJ, Chan AWE, Steadman D, Stevens K, Selwood DL, Waksman G, Remaut H.** 2014. Suppression of type 1 pillus assembly in uropathogenic *Escherichia coli* by chemical inhibition of subunit polymerization. *J Antimicrob Chemother* **69:** 1017–1026.
11. **Kvist M, Hancock V, Klemm P.** 2008. Inactivation of effluent pumps abolishes bacterial biofilm formation. *App Env Microbiol* **23:**7376–7382.
12. **Zhang L, Mah T.** 2008. Invovlement of a novel efflux system in biofilm-specific resistance to antibiotics. *Appl Environ Microbiol* **74:**7376–7382.
13. **Poole K.** 2005. Efflux-mediated antimicrobial resistance. *J Antimicrob Chemother* **56:**20–51.
14. **Nairz M, Haschka D, Demetz E, Weiss G.** 2014. Iron at the interface of immunity and infection. *Front Pharmacol* **16:**152.
15. **Frangipani E, Bonchi C, Minandri F, Imperi F, Visca P.** 2014. Pyochelin potentiates the inhibitory activity of gallium on *Pseudomonas aeruginosa*. *Antimicrob Agents Chemother* **58:**5572–5575.
16. **Oglesby-Sherrouse AG, Djapgne L, Nguyen AT, Vasil AL, Vasil ML.** 2014. The complex interplay of iron, biofilm formation, and mucoidy affecting antimicrobial resistance of *Pseudomonas aeruginosa*. *Pathog Dis* **70:**307–320.
17. **Ross-Gillespie A, Weigert M, Brown SP, Kummerli R.** 2014. Gallium-mediated siderophore quenching as an evolutionary robust antibacterial treatment. *Evol Med Public Health* **1:**18–29.
18. **Kelson AB, Carnevali M, Truong-Le V.** 2013. Gallium-based anti-infectives: targeting microbial iron-uptake mechanisms. *Curr Opin Pharmacol* **13:**707–716.
19. **Banin E, Lozinski A, Brady KM, Berenshtein E, Butterfield PW, Moshe M, Chevion M, Greenberg EP, Banin E.** 2008. The potential of desferrioxamine-gallium as an anti-*Pseudomonas* therapeutic agent. *Proc Natl Acad Sci USA* **43:** 16761–16766.

20. **Escaich S.** 2008. Antivirulence as a new antibacterial approach for chemotherapy. *Curr Opin Chem Biol* **12**:400–408.

21. **Moayeri M, Crown D, Jiao G, Kim S, Johnson A, Leysath C, Leppla SH.** 2013. Small-molecule inhibitors of lethal factor protease activity protect against anthrax infection. *Antimicrob Agents Chemother* **57**:4139–4145.

22. **Goller C, Seed PC.** 2010. High-throughput identification of chemical inhibitors of *E. coli* group 2 capsule biogenesis as anti-virulence agents. *PLoS One* **5**:e11642. doi:10.1371/journal.pone.0011642.

23. **Pacheco AR, Sperandio V.** 2012. Shiga toxin in enterohaemorrhagic *E. coli*: regulation and novel anti-virulence strategies. *Front Cell Infect Microbiol* **2**:81.

24. **Medeiros P, Bolick DT, Roche JK, Norohna F, Pinheiro C, Kolling GL, Lima A, Guerrant RL.** 2013. The micronutrient zinc inhibits EAEC strain 042 adherence, biofilm formation, virulence gene expression, and epithelial cytokines responses benefitting the infected host. *Virulence* **4**:624–633.

25. **Stubbed CJ, Duffield ML, Cooper IA, Ford DC, Gans JD, Karlyshev AV, Lingard B, Oyston PCF, de Rochefort A, Song J, Wren BW, Titball RW, Wolonsky M.** 2009. Steps towards broad-spectrum therapeutics: discovering virulence-associated genes present in diverse human pathogens. *BMC Genomics* **10**:501.

26. **Njorage J, Sperandio V.** 2009. Jamming bacterial communication: new approaches for the treatment of infectious disease. *EMBO Mol Med* **1**:201–210.

27. **Starkey M, Lepine F, Maura D, Bandyopadhaya A, Lesic B, He J, Kitao T, Righi V, Milot S, Tzika A, Rahme L.** 2014. Identification of anti-virulence compounds that disrupt quorum-sensing regulated acute and persistent pathogenicity. *PLoS Pathog* **10**:e1004321. doi:10.1371/journal.ppat.1004321.

28. **Curtis MM, Russell R, Moreira CG, Adebesin AM, Wang C, Williams NS, Taussig R, Stewart D, Zimmern P, Lu B, Prasad RN, Zhu C, Rasko DA, Huntley JF, Falck JR, Sperandio V.** 2014. QseC inhibitors as an antivirulence approach for Gram-negative pathogens. *mBio* **5**:e02165-14. doi:10.1128/mBio.02165-14.

29. **Lasarre B, Frederie MJ.** 2013. Exploiting quorum sensing to confuse bacterial pathogens. *Microbiol Mol Biol Rev* **77**:73–111.

30. **Hentzer M, Givskov M.** 2003. Pharmacological inhibition of quorum sensing for the treatment of chronic bacterial infections. *J Clin Inv* **112**:1300–1307.

31. **Fetzner S.** 2014. Quorum quenching enzymes. *J Biotechnol* **201**:2–14.

32. **Cegelski L, Marshal GR, Eldridge GR, Hultgren SJ.** 2008. The biology and future prospects of antivirulence therapies. *Nat Rev Microbial* **6**:17–27.

33. **Anand R, Rai N, Thattai M.** 2013. Interactions among quorum sensing inhibitors. *PLoS One* **8**:e62254. doi:10.1371/journal.pone.0062254.

34. **Li H, Want L, Ye L, Mao Y, Xie X, Xia C, Chen J, Lu Z, Song J.** 2009. Influence of *Pseudomonas aeruginosa* quorum sensing signal molecule N-(3-oxododecanoyl) homoserine lactose on mast cells. *Med Microbiol Immunol* **189**:113–121.

35. **Shang L, Pornpattananangkul D, Hu CM, Huang CM.** 2010. Development of nano particles for anti-microbial drug delivery. *Curr Med Chem* **17**:585–594.

36. **Palanisamy NK, Ferina N, Amirulhusni AN, Mohd-Zain Z, Hussaini J, Ping LJ, Duairaj R.** 2014. Antibiofilm properties of chemically synthesized silver nano particles found against *Pseudomonas aeruginosa. J Nanobiotech* **12**:2.

37. **Azam A, Ahmed SA, Oves M, Khan MS, Habib SS, Memic A.** 2012. Antimicrobial activity of metal oxide nanoparticles against Gram-positive and Gram-negative bacteria: a comparative study. *Int J Nanomed* **12**:6003–6009.

38. **Prahu S, Poulose EK.** 2012. Silver nano particles: mechanism of anti-microbial action, synthesis, medical applications, and toxicity effects. *Int Nano Lett* **2**:32.

39. **Barbour ME, Maddocks SW, Wood NJ, Collins AM.** 2013. Synthesis, characterization and efficacy of antimicrobial chlorhexidine hexametaphosphate nanoparticles for applications in biomedical materials and consumer products. *Int J Nanomed* **8**:3507–3519.

40. **Hook ER, Owen OJ, Bellis CA, Holder JA, O'Sullivan DJ, Barbour ME.** 2014. Development of a novel antimicrobial-releasing glass ionomer cement functionalized with chlorhexidine hexametaphosphate nanoparticles. *J Nanobiotechnol* **12**:3–3.

41. **Wood NJ, Maddocks SE, Grady HJ, Collins AM, Barbour ME.** 2014. Functionalization of ethylene vinyl acetate with antimicrobial chlorhexidine hexametaphosphate nanoparticles. *Int J Nanomedicine* **9**:4145–4152.

42. **van Assche E, Van Piyvelde S, Vanderleyden J, Steenackers HP.** 2015. RNA-binding proteins involved in post-transcriptional regulation in bacteria. *Front Microbiol* **6**:141.

43. **Eyraud A, Tattevin P, Chabelskaya S, Feldon B.** 2014. A small RNA controls a protein regulator involved in antibiotic resistance in *Staphylococcus aureus. Nucleic Acids Res* **42**:4892–4905.

44. **Molina-Santiago C, Daddaoua A, Gomez-Lozano M, Udaono X, Molin S, Ramos JL.** 2015. Differential transcriptional response to antibiotics by *Pseudomonas putida* DOT-T1E. **17:**3251–3262.

45. **Libis VK, Bernheim AG, Basier C, Jaramillo-Rivera S, Deyell M, Aghoghogbe I, Atanaskovic I, Bencherif AC, Benony M, Koutsoubelis N, Lochner AC, Marinkovic ZS, Zahra S, Zegman Y, Lindner AB, Wintermute EH.** 2014. Silencing of antibiotic resistance in *E. coli* with engineered phage bearing small regulatory RNAs. *ACS Synth Biol* **3:**1003–1006.

46. **Ghosh S, Watson MA, Collins JL.** 2007. The relative transcription index: a gene expression based metric for prioritization of drug candidates. *Comb Chem High Throughput Screen* **10:**239–245.

47. **Sabir JS, Abu-Zinadah OA, Bora RS, Ahmed MM, Saini KS.** 2013. Role of toxicogenomics in the development of safe, efficacious and novel anti-microbial therapies. *Infect Disord Drug Targets* **13:**205–214.

Innovative Solutions to Sticky Situations: Antiadhesive Strategies for Treating Bacterial Infections

27

ZACHARY T. CUSUMANO,[1] ROGER D. KLEIN,[1] and SCOTT J. HULTGREN[1]

INTRODUCTION

The discovery of penicillin in 1928 and its subsequent introduction as a therapeutic in the 1940s sparked the antibiotic era, ushering in effective treatment options for many common bacterial infections (1). Following the end of World War II, several pharmaceutical companies including Bayer, Merck, and Pfizer became household names through the discovery and clinical success of a number of additional antibiotics, which were identified by screening soil samples for antimicrobial activity (1). Compounds identified during this screening became the founding members of many now-ubiquitous groups of antibiotics, including the tetracycline, rifamycin, quinolone, and aminoglycoside families. In the early 1970s, declining rates of novel antibiotic discovery from microbial sources shifted the onus of antimicrobial development to synthetic chemists, who were tasked with designing and screening new compounds based on known principles of antibiotic design. These synthetic chemists were faced with many practical challenges, including poor penetration into bacterial cells, bacterial enzymes, and/or efflux pumps that degrade or expel the compounds, respectively, innate resistance mechanisms, and the

[1]Department of Molecular Microbiology, Washington University School of Medicine, St. Louis, MO 63110.
Virulence Mechanisms of Bacterial Pathogens, 5th edition
Edited by Indira T. Kudva, Nancy A. Cornick, Paul J. Plummer, Qijing Zhang, Tracy L. Nicholson, John P. Bannantine, and Bryan H. Bellaire
© 2016 American Society for Microbiology, Washington, DC
doi:10.1128/microbiolspec.VMBF-0023-2015

requirement of high concentrations of some compounds that result in toxic side effects (2, 3).

As the difficulty of novel antimicrobial discovery increased and the incidence of vaccine-preventable disease continued to fall, the apparent ease and speed with which most infections were cured decreased the incentives driving antimicrobial development. As a result, for-profit drug companies shifted their foci away from the development of antimicrobials and toward drugs designed to treat chronic, noncommunicable diseases. Indeed, the increase in patient life expectancy, brought on in part by the decrease in deaths from infectious diseases, coupled with the rising prevalence of metabolic diseases, dramatically increased the population of patients requiring treatment for cancer, diabetes, and hyperlipidemia. In contrast to the 5- to 7-day treatment course for most antibiotic infections, chronic diseases require constant medication, providing pharmaceutical companies with a much higher return on investment. Investigation into these more lucrative therapeutic areas largely halted the research and development of new antimicrobials by for-profit companies (2, 3). Concurrently, resistance to existing antimicrobials has continued to rise as a result of their sustained misuse in both agriculture and clinical settings (4, 5), propelling us into a postantibiotic era defined by dwindling treatment options for many common infections. Recently, the CDC has recognized several pathogens as "urgent" or "serious" threats, including *Clostridium difficile*, carbapenem-resistant *Enterobacteriaceae*, multidrug-resistant *Pseudomonas aeruginosa*, vancomycin-resistant *Enterococcus*, and others (6). The prevalence of these pathogens and their associated morbidity and mortality has highlighted the need for the identification of new canonical antibiotics and innovative therapeutic strategies to fight what were once considered easily curable bacterial infections.

Currently, common antibiotics function by inhibiting or disrupting important bacterial cellular processes, including cell wall synthesis, RNA transcription, DNA replication, and protein synthesis needed for cell viability. While this has resulted in the development of effective broad-spectrum antibiotics, it has also generated a strong selective pressure that fosters development of bacterial resistance. To circumvent this problem, researchers have begun targeting specific virulence mechanisms critical to the ability of specific bacteria to cause disease (7–9). These "antivirulence" therapeutics are designed to neutralize pathogenesis and promote efficient clearance by the host immune system without affecting overall bacterial viability. It is believed that targeting these nonessential processes will weaken the selective pressure currently driving the development of resistance, increasing the effective therapeutic lifetime of these drugs (10). Additionally, the specific targeting of pathogenic bacteria eliminates the nonspecific killing of the beneficial human microbiota, which occurs during broad-spectrum antibiotic therapy (11–14). Recent research into the role of the human microbiota in human health and disease has led to our understanding of the microbiota as a bacterial organ within the host that trains the immune system and provides essential metabolic functions for the host. Perturbation of this system has been linked to significant decreases in overall health and a plethora of numerous disease complications (15). Thus, regular insults to the human microbiota through antibiotic treatment can result in a detrimental state of dysbiosis (16). To overcome resistance and protect the commensal microbiota, researchers are actively pursuing antibiotic-sparing therapeutic strategies to target and disrupt pathways related to virulence but not to general bacterial viability (9, 10, 17).

Antivirulence Therapies

Bacterial virulence factors are defined by their role in pathogen replication and formation of the disease state within the host environment. These bacterial determinants can provide a fitness advantage by mediating a variety of processes, including evasion of the host immune system, extraction of required nutrients from the host, or colonization of a particular niche. Toxins, cytolysins, bacterial secretion systems, and proteases are a few common examples of such factors that have been the subject of intensive investigation. To date, many successful examples of antivirulence therapeutic studies have focused on abrogating the effectiveness of toxins, be it through direct inhibition of activity, delivery, or attachment to the host cell (18–20). One such study utilized a glycomimetic approach to inhibit Shiga toxin's recognition of the host receptor, globotriaosylceramide, which has proven to be effective *in vitro* and in animal models of enterohemorrhagic *Escherichia coli* infections (21, 22). Similarly, the monoclonal antibody raxibacumab targets the protective antigen component of anthrax toxin (23) and was approved by the FDA in 2012 for protection against and treatment of inhaled anthrax (23–25). Despite this great promise, however, only a handful of antivirulence therapeutics have made it to human clinical trials to date.

In addition to secreted factors, investigators have also targeted virulence factors on the cellular surface. Two such targets, the polysaccharide capsule and flagellar appendages of *E. coli*, have been studied extensively for their role in phagocytosis of bacteria by host immune cells and bacterial chemotaxis and motility, respectively (26, 27). Structures mediating bacterial adhesion have also proven to be promising antivirulence targets, because nearly all bacterial pathogens utilize specific adhesion modalities to colonize biotic and abiotic surfaces (28–32). This adhesion is required to resist the natural clearance mechanisms of the host, including high liquid flow rates on mucosal surfaces in the gastrointestinal, upper-respiratory, and genito-urinary tracts. Thus, the importance of adhesion in establishing an infection makes it one of the most attractive targets for new therapeutics.

BACTERIAL ADHESIVE STRATEGIES

Pili

Pili (or fimbriae) are long proteinaceous filaments that are utilized by both Gram-negative and Gram-positive bacteria to adhere to host surfaces while maintaining a separation between the cell membranes, preventing the electrostatic repulsion that occurs as a result of the net negative charge found on the surface of both the bacteria and host. Pili are generally composed of hundreds or thousands of repeating protein subunits interacting covalently (in the case of Gram-positive bacteria) or noncovalently (in the case of Gram-negative bacteria) to form the shaft of the pilus. For both Gram-negative and Gram-positive bacteria to interact with the host, additional protein subunits are often incorporated into the pilus, including tip adhesins that mediate stereochemically specific interactions with a host receptor (33). Like lectins, adhesin domains frequently recognize oligosaccharides found on glycoproteins or glycolipids (34). The specificity of these interactions often dictates a pathogen's tropism for a particular host tissue. In addition to cell surface carbohydrate receptors, some pili also interact with proteinaceous components of the basement membrane or extracellular matrix and may bind the collagen, fibronectin, and fibrinogen found extensively throughout the host (30, 35). Despite a common overall function of Gram-negative and Gram-positive pili of mediating attachment, the structure and biosynthetic machinery required to generate these adhesive structures vary drastically (28) (Fig. 1).

Chaperone usher pathway (CUP) pili

Members of the CUP family of pili have been extensively characterized in Gram-negative bacteria. CUP pili are a diverse set of homologous appendages distributed throughout the *Enterobacter* genus. A recent analysis identified 458 CUP pili operons, which represent 38 distinct CUP pilus types based on usher phylogeny in *Escherichia* alone (36, 37).

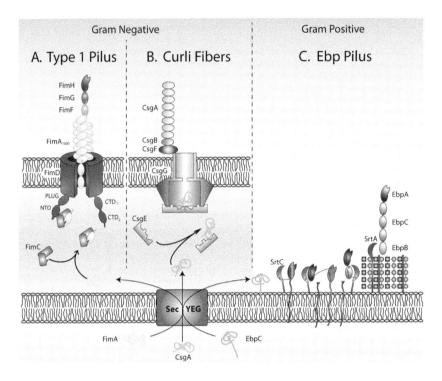

FIGURE 1 **Comparison of structure and assembly mechanism of common extracellular adhesive organelles. (A) Following translocation through the SecYEG apparatus, the FimA structural subunits are bound by the FimC chaperone via the donor strand complementation reaction before delivery to the FimD usher, which catalyzes a donor strand exchange reaction that links subunits of the growing pilus. (B) In the periplasmic space, soluble CsgA binds the CsgE chaperone, which delivers it to the CsgG pore for secretion to the outer membrane. From there, its folding and polymerization is nucleated by CsgB, which is anchored to the outer membrane by the CsgF assembly factor. (C) Ebp pilus subunits integrate themselves into the membrane, where the dedicated pilus assembly sortase, SrtC, cleaves the sorting sequence and facilitates the nucleophilic attack by a new incoming subunit. The fully assembled pilus is then integrated into the membrane by the housekeeping sortase, SrtA.**

CUP pili tipped with specific adhesins enable *E. coli* to bind to distinct ligands on host cells with stereochemical specificity. CUP pilus biogenesis is defined by the utilization of the eponymous chaperone and usher, which function to coordinate and catalyze pilus assembly. CUP chaperones are localized to the bacterial periplasm and consist of two immunoglobulin (Ig) domains that are required for the folding and stability of the secreted pilin structural subunits. Each structural subunit is composed of an incomplete immunoglobulin fold lacking the C-terminal beta strand, which results in the presence of a hydrophobic grove with,

in the case of the well-studied Pap (P) pilus system, five defined hydrophobic pockets, termed P1 to P5. Chaperone-assisted folding of pilin domains occurs by a reaction termed donor strand complementation. During this process, a series of conserved exposed hydrophobic residues on the cognate chaperone's G1 strand are buried in the hydrophobic pockets comprising the groove of the pilus subunit, thus forming a complex in which the subunit's Ig fold is completed (38, 39). Incorporation of the chaperone's G1 β-strand occurs in a noncanonical parallel fashion, generating a stable yet high-energy intermediate.

Chaperone-subunit complexes are next targeted to the outer membrane, where they interact with the membrane-localized usher, which both catalyzes pilus assembly and acts as a gated pore (Fig. 1). Ushers contain five functional domains: a 24-stranded trans-membrane β-barrel translocation domain, a β-sandwich plug domain (PD) that resides in the pore of the TD in the apo-usher, an N-terminal periplasmic domain (NTD), and two C-terminal periplasmic domains (CTD1 and 2) (40–42). These domains function as components of a molecular machine that catalyzes pilus biogenesis and secretes pili across the outer membrane. The crystal structures of both an usher-chaperone-adhesin ternary complex in the well-studied type 1 pilus system (FimCDH) and a fimbrial tip (FimFGH) in complex with the chaperone and usher have been solved (41, 43). Binding of the chaperone-adhesin complex to the usher results in translocation of the PD into the periplasmic space (40, 41) and a conformational change in the translocation domain from the apo, kidney-shaped conformation (52 x 28 Å) to a circular form (44 x 36 Å). This conformational change likely facilitates the extrusion of folded pilins (~20 to 25 Å in diameter) across the outer membrane. After translocation into the periplasmic space, the PD mediates a high-affinity interaction with the NTD of the usher (41, 44). Thus, the PD gates the translocation domain such that, in the absence of pili, the PD prevents large molecules from flowing freely across the outer membrane (45). The PD, NTD, CTD1, and CTD2 work together in the assembly function of this molecular machine. Mutations in either NTD or CTDs or deletions of the PD completely inhibit pilus assembly, implicating their direct role in catalysis of pilus assembly (44, 46).

Polymerization of pilus subunits occurs via a process known as donor strand exchange (DSE) and is dependent upon a hydrophobic N-terminal extension encoded by all pilus subunits, excluding the adhesin. (45, 47–49). Pilus DSE occurs at the usher

when the chaperone is displaced, and an incoming subunit's N-terminal extension zips into the previously chaperone-bound groove of a nascently incorporated subunit at the growing terminus of the pilus (Fig. 2B and C). It is believed that interaction of the donated N-terminal extension with the vacant pocket of the acceptor pilus subunit results in initiation of a "zip-in-zip-out mechanism," displacing the chaperone's G1 β-strand and facilitating the final folding of the pilus subunit. This process is repeated for

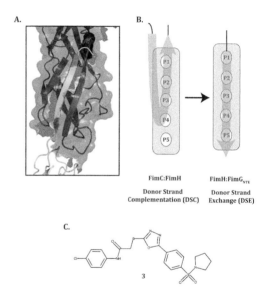

FIGURE 2 **Inhibitors of the donor strand exchange reaction between pilus subunits are able to abrogate pilus biogenesis. (A) Crystal structure of the FimG adaptor's donor strand exchange reaction with the pilin domain of the FimH adhesin (PDB ID code 3JWN). FimG donates its hydrophobic N-terminal beta strand to FimH, which is shown residing in the P5 pocket. (B) Schematic of the donor strand complementation and donor strand exchange pathways. The donor strand complementation reaction between the chaperone G1 strand and the bound pilin results in a noncanonical parallel fashion (left panel), while the zip-in, zip-out process underlying the DSE reactions results in the formation of an antiparallel, low-energy interaction (adapted from reference 240). (C) Chemical structure of compound 3, first identified from an *in silico* docking assay before further refinement in *in vitro* DSE assays.**

each round of subunit incorporation into the fiber such that every subunit in the pilus completes the Ig fold of its neighbor. In contrast to the chaperone's donated β-strand, which interacts in a parallel fashion, the incoming N-terminal extension binds in the canonical antiparallel fashion (Fig. 2B and C). This results in a folded pilin domain in a much lower energy state than its chaperone-bound form. It is believed that the transition from the chaperone-bound high-energy state to the NTE-bound low-energy state that occurs during DSE provides the energy necessary to drive pilus formation in the periplasmic space, which lacks ATP and is not coupled to the proton motive force (50).

Type 1 and pap pili: roles in urinary tract infections (UTIs)

CUP pili have been identified as key virulence determinants in murine UTIs, making them exciting targets for novel therapeutics. UTIs affect more than 150 million people annually and are a significant cause of morbidity in women throughout their lifespan, (51, 52). UTI is generally divided into two major diseases, demarcated by their location within the urinary tract. Infection and colonization of the bladder in healthy women is commonly referred to as uncomplicated cystitis. Upon introduction of bacteria into the bladder, bacteria can ascend the ureters and colonize the kidneys, causing pyelonephritis. The clinical sequelae of pyelonephritis are particularly concerning, because an uncontrolled bacterial infection in the renal pelvis and calyces can spread to the bloodstream, leading to sepsis and death.

Uropathogenic *E. coli* (UPEC) is the most common causative agent of UTI, responsible for 80 to 90% of all infections (53–55). UPEC tropism for the murine bladder is largely mediated via type 1 (fim) pili. The type 1 pilus adhesin, FimH, binds mannosylated uroplakins on the bladder surface and β1-3 integrin receptors throughout the bladder tissue. The rod of the type 1 pilus is composed of ~1,000 FimA protein subunits, which are wound in

a helical manner to create a force-sensitive cylindrical shaft (56). At the distal tip of the rod is a flexible fibrillum composed of two adaptor proteins, FimF and FimG, and the two-domain tip adhesin FimH (57). It is the lectin domain ($FimH_L$) of this adhesin that mediates interaction with host cell receptors and facilitates invasion of the bacteria into the uroepithelial cells, also called superficial facet cells (58). The pilin domain ($FimH_P$) interacts with the FimG adaptor. Once internalized, a single bacterium can rapidly replicate in the host cytoplasm to form a biofilm-like intracellular bacterial community (IBC) (58–60). Once these communities reach maturation, bacteria within the IBC disperse and flux out, becoming filamentous. These filamentous bacteria can then go on to adhere to and invade neighboring superficial facet cells, reinitiating IBC formation and the pathogenic cycle.

Following this acute pathogenic cycle, the outcome of UPEC bladder infection in naïve mice often resolves, leading to sterilization of the urine within days of inoculation. However, fairly frequently, this acute infection results in chronic cystitis, which is characterized by persistent high titer bacteriuria accompanied by chronic bladder inflammation. Clinical evidence of chronic inflammation in women suffering from recurrent UTIs (61, 62), as well as the observation of IBCs and bacterial filaments in women diagnosed with acute UTIs (63), supports the validity of the IBC pathogenic cycle and the ability of the mouse model to recapitulate human disease.

In contrast to colonization of the bladder, adherence to and infection of the kidneys is believed to occur primarily via interactions of P pili with Galα-4Gal-containing glycolipid receptors, which are expressed throughout the kidneys and ureters of mammals (64). Like the type 1 pilus, P pili are comprised of a rod generated from repeating major subunits (PapA) and a distal fibrillum tip containing minor pilins (PapK, PapE, and PapF) and the adhesin PapG (65, 66). To date, three alleles of PapG have been discovered, each mediating attachment to a slightly different host receptor and consequently determining host tropism (67–69). Human kidneys, for example, abundantly express the ligands for PapG-II, globoside, and as a result, human pyelonephritis usually involves colonization of UPEC that expresses PapG-II alleles. Conversely, PapG-III binds strongly to Forssman glycolipid, which is present in dog but not in human kidneys, and most cases of pyelonephritis in dogs involve UPEC encoding the PapG-III allele (67–69). Unfortunately, the lack of these receptors in small mammals, specifically mice, has limited the ability to dissect the molecular details of pathogenesis with regard to pyelonephritis. Nevertheless, the unique role of these pili in mediating tissue-specific tropism makes them excellent targets for preventing infection throughout the urinary tract.

Gram-positive pili

While pili expressed by Gram-negative bacteria have been extensively studied over the last several decades, the identification and characterization of pili from Gram-positive bacteria has occurred relatively recently. Although pili were observed in *Corynebacterium renale* as early as 1968 (70), the mechanism of biogenesis remained unknown until a decade ago, when work with *Corynebacterium diphtheriae* revealed the unique function of a pilus-specific sortase on the highly conserved pilus domain structure (71).

In Gram-positive bacteria, each pilus subunit domain contains a highly conserved sortase recognition motif (LPXTG) followed by a hydrophobic transmembrane domain and a positively charged C-terminal tail (72, 73). Pilus assembly is initiated by the Sec-dependent secretion of pilin subunits, which become anchored to the cytoplasmic membrane via their C-terminal hydrophobic membrane-spanning region (74). Subsequently, following insertion in the membrane, the pilus-dedicated sortase recognizes and cleaves between the threonine and glycine residues of the LPXTG

motif to produce an acyl-enzyme intermediate (75, 76). This intermediate is resolved by nucleophilic attack from an amino group on a specific lysine side chain from an incoming pilin subunit, resulting in the covalent attachment of the two pilin subunits (71, 77). The lysine responsible for the nucleophilic attack is located within a pilin motif whose sequence varies between pilus subtypes (72, 78). Repetition of this process results in growth of the pilus fiber from the base as sortase cleavage of each subsequent pilus subunit is resolved by nucleophilic attack by a newly incorporating subunit. Pilus assembly is terminated by a housekeeping sortase enzyme encoded outside the pilus operon, which covalently attaches the pilus to the cell wall through a final transpeptidation reaction (71) (Fig. 1). Similar to Gram-negative bacteria, minor subunits can be commonly found at the distal end of Gram-positive pili, including adhesins that mediate interactions with host receptors (79). Since their identification nearly 50 years ago, pili have been identified and implicated in diseases for several Gram-positive pathogens including *Streptococcus agalactiae* (80), *Streptococcus pneumonia* (81), and *Enterococcus faecalis* (82, 83).

Role of Ebp pilus in *Enterococcus* catheter-associated UTI (CAUTI)

The endocarditis- and biofilm-associated (Ebp) pilus is encoded by several Gram-positive bacteria including *E. faecalis* (84). *E. faecalis* is a leading cause of CAUTI, because its ability to adhere to both host and abiotic surfaces as well as its resistance to multiple antibiotics makes it difficult to prevent and treat (85, 86). A common feature of *E. faecalis* infections is their dependence on an abiotic surface, such as a catheter, to cause an infection (87). This reliance can be recapitulated in a mouse model of CAUTI using a small piece of silicone tubing to mimic catheterization in humans (88). Consistent with clinical findings, *E. faecalis* is rapidly cleared from the mouse bladder in the absence of a catheter.

Establishment of the mouse CAUTI model has allowed investigation of the molecular mechanisms of *E. faecalis* pathogenesis, identifying the unique interplay between the host and pathogen. Catheterization in mice stimulates a robust inflammatory response, increasing the levels of inflammatory cytokines while causing edema and the release of fibrinogen, a glycoprotein shown to adhere to implanted catheters (82, 89). Within 24 hours, the surface of the indwelling catheter is completely coated with fibrinogen (82). Many of these immunological findings have been demonstrated in humans and verified by a number of clinical studies, giving further credence to the robustness of the murine CAUTI model (90–92). Accumulation of fibrinogen on the urinary catheter provides a surface for the attachment of *E. faecalis*, which is mediated by the Ebp pilus and involves direct recognition of fibrinogen (82). Deletion of the pilus operon eliminates the ability of the bacteria to adhere to the catheter *in vivo* and abolishes the infection, demonstrating the essential role for the pilus in mediating attachment to the catheter and establishing disease (82, 83).

The Ebp pilus is composed of three proteins, EbpA, EbpB, and EbpC, and is encoded in the enterococcal genome as a single operon along with the pilus-dependent sortase, SrtC (Fig. 1) (93). The shaft of the pilus is comprised of a polymer of EbpC subunits, with EbpA localized at the distal tip of the pilus and EbpB at the base (93) (Fig. 1). Deletion of *ebpA* disrupted bacterial binding to fibrinogen *in vitro* and completely attenuated virulence *in vivo* (82, 83). The N-terminal region of EbpA, which contains a Von Willebrand factor A domain with a conserved metal-ion-dependent adhesion site (MIDAS) motif, is required for recognition of fibrinogen (82, 83). MIDAS motifs are commonly found in proteins responsible for mediating interactions with extracellular matrix proteins (94). Mutation of the MIDAS motif in *ebpA* eliminates binding to fibrinogen *in vitro* and phenocopies an *ebpA* mutant *in vivo* (82,

83). Together, this work has elucidated the molecular recognition of fibrinogen by EbpA, identifying it as a putative target for prevention and treatment of CAUTI.

Biofilm Formation

Biofilms are loosely defined as surface-associated microbial communities and have been shown to play a central role in bacterial persistence in both commensal environmental and pathogenic colonization of the host niches (95, 96). Biofilm formation is generally triggered by an environmental cue that initiates a change in the physiological state of the bacteria, drastically altering the biological properties of the bacteria compared to a planktonic state (97, 98). The expression of pili or nonpilus adhesins is considered central to this transition, because they allow bacteria to interact with cellular or abiotic surfaces and other bacteria during formation of the extracellular matrix, which often consists of both proteinaceous and polysaccharide components (78, 99, 100). Disruption of this adherence through genetic deletion of specific pili or adhesins completely abolishes biofilm formation in many bacterial systems (101–104).

Upon establishment, bacteria embedded within a biofilm are able to survive a number of environmental stresses, contributing to bacterial pathogenesis and disease in a variety of chronic infections (105). Encapsulation within a biofilm decreases bacterial susceptibility to changes in environmental pH and osmolarity while conferring resistance to phagocytosis, desiccation, and UV light (106). In addition, bacteria within biofilms are commonly recalcitrant to antibiotic treatment due to a number of mechanisms, including a decrease in antibiotic penetration, expression of antibiotic-modifying enzymes, and the formation of persister cells whose metabolic dormancy promotes the resistance of colonization (107, 108). Given the high association of biofilms with indwelling medical devices, the increased use of these devices has resulted in a concurrent increase in the incidence of chronic, antibiotic-resistant infections.

Curli

Curli were first described in *Salmonella* in 1989 and have been extensively studied in both *Salmonella* and *E. coli* (109). Curli fibers mediate the formation of bacterial biofilms and have also been to shown to interact with extracellular DNA as part of the biofilm. Although this interaction is not essential for biofilm formation (110), it has been shown to increase the rate of biofilm formation (111).

The biochemical and biophysical properties of curli fibers have long been known to mirror those of pathologic amyloids (112). Indeed, structural characterization has revealed that, like known amyloids, curli fibers are 4 to 12 nm wide, highly resistant to denaturation, possess a cross β-sheet structure, and bind to amyloid-specific dyes such as Congo red and thioflavin T (113). A variety of pathogenic, eukaryotic amyloids have been implicated in several neurodegenerative diseases, including Alzheimer's, Parkinson's, and Huntington's diseases, making prevention of amyloid formation therapeutically relevant. Identification of curli fibers as functional amyloids has opened up an interesting avenue of research focused on understanding the molecular mechanisms of curli assembly and the processes by which bacteria regulate the spatio-temporal formation of curli fibers (114–116). Ultimately, this approach may aid in the identification of novel therapeutics to target bacterial production of curli-associated biofilms while elucidating new treatment options for common neurodegenerative diseases. Further, Rapsinski et al. reported that extracellular DNA is bound tightly by bacterial amyloid fibrils during biofilm formation and that amyloid/DNA composites are powerful immune stimulators when injected into mice, leading to autoimmunity (111).

Curli assembly in bacteria is directed by a unique, highly regulated process (114–116) (Fig. 1). The extracellular curli fibers consist primarily of a major component, CsgA, and a minor component, CsgB (112). Formation of curli fibers requires the periplasmic assembly factor CsgE and outer membrane assembly factor CsgF, which both associate with the outer membrane channel protein CsgG (117, 118). Nine CsgG subunits form a 36-stranded β-barrel that traverses the lipid bilayer, forming a 0.9-nM channel through which CsgA, CsgB, and CsgF are secreted as disordered monomers (119, 120). Once secreted, CsgF associates with CsgG on the outside of the cell and anchors CsgB to the pore and/or outer membrane (117). CsgB in turn anchors curli fibers to the cell surface and nucleates CsgA polymerization (121–123). Deletion of CsgB or CsgF results in attenuation of curli formation and the release of CsgA monomers into the surrounding milieu (117, 123). CsgE is believed to function as a pore gating factor and curli-specific chaperone, sequestering unfolded CsgA subunits in the periplasm and facilitating their interactions with CsgG subunits within the pore (118, 120). Deletion of *csgE* attenuates curli formation and results in the promiscuous transport of proteins and small molecules through the CsgG pore (118).

Role of curli in biofilm formation and UPEC pathogenesis

Curli have been implicated in *E. coli* and *Salmonella* colonization of the gastrointestinal tract (124, 125) and, in the case of UPEC, promote infection. A *csgA* mutant or *csgB/csgG* double mutant are both attenuated during acute infection in a murine model of cystitis, suggesting that curli fibers contribute to UTI pathogenesis (126). This defect in virulence could be partially explained by the binding of curli fibers with the human antimicrobial peptide LL-37 and the murine ortholog, cathelicidin-related antimicrobial peptide (CRAMP) (127). This interaction is believed to sequester these peptides and attenuate their antimicrobial activity. Curli have also been implicated in the binding of several additional host proteins including the extracellular matrix protein fibronectin (128, 129).

Nonpili adhesins

In addition to pili and curli, bacteria have evolved a number of additional surface-associated proteins to interact with host cell receptors and aid in adhesion and invasion. The majority of these adhesins are anchored to the membrane through a transmembrane region or, in the case of Gram-positive bacteria, through attachment to the cell wall via the activity of a housekeeping sortase. Some of these adhesins recognize the cell adhesion molecules, which mediate specific interactions with other cells and with the extracellular matrix (130–132). One of the best-characterized nonpilus bacterial adhesins is the invasin protein from the Gram-negative pathogen *Yersinia enterocolitica*, which mediates high-affinity binding to a subset of β1-integrins, resulting in bacterial invasion (133, 134). Internalin, an adhesin from the Gram-positive pathogen *Listeria monocytogenes*, functions in a similar manner through the binding of E-cadherin (135).

In addition to recognition of cell adhesion molecules, many nonpilus adhesins contain lectin domains and function in a manner similar to the adhesins incorporated into pili: through the recognition of specific sugar moieties. Two well-characterized soluble adhesins from *P. aeruginosa* are LecA (PA-IL) and LecB (PA-IIL), which have been determined to make significant contributions to both biofilm formation and *Pseudomonas* pathogenesis (102, 103, 136).

Role of LecA and LecB adhesins in *P. aeruginosa* pathogenesis

P. aeruginosa is an opportunistic pathogen often associated with hospital-acquired infections and is the most common bacteria found in the sputum of patients with cystic fibrosis (CF) (137, 138). The presence of *P. aeruginosa* in the lower respiratory tract of CF patients is associated with poor lung function and a decreased quality of life and is the leading cause of mortality among CF patients (139). Following colonization of the airway, *P. aeruginosa* is believed to encapsulate itself in a biofilm, thus promoting its persistence by increasing resistance to antibiotic treatment and aiding in the ability to adapt to the harsh host environment (140, 141). Biofilm formation and the pathogenesis of *P. aeruginosa* have been shown to involve several virulence factors, including the type III secretion system and several adhesins (142). Investigation into the adhesive properties of *P. aeruginosa* revealed a significant role of the two soluble lectin domains, LecA and LecB, which were both found to contribute to the attachment of *P. aeruginosa* to the human lung epithelial cell line A549 (136, 143). LecA and LecB are tetrameric adhesins with four identical binding sites (144, 145). Although originally isolated from the cytoplasm of *P. aeruginosa*, these lectins have since been shown to accumulate on the outer membrane in high quantities (103, 146). Subsequent studies have determined that LecA has specificity for D-galactose and binds α-galactosyl residues found in the glycosphingolipids of the lung epithelial membranes (147, 148). Conversely, LecB has been demonstrated to recognize L-fucose and its derivatives and has high affinity for Lewis-a oligosaccharides (149). In addition to their role in bacterial adhesion to lung epithelial cells, both LecA and LecB have been shown to contribute to *in vitro* biofilm formation, likely by mediating contact with biotic and abiotic surfaces as well as initiating interactions with other bacterial cells (102, 103, 136).

In vivo analysis of *lecA* and *lecB* mutants has demonstrated a significantly decreased bacterial lung burden 16 hours following inoculation compared to wild-type bacteria. LecA and LecB were also found to mediate alveolar capillary barrier injury, facilitating the dissemination of *P. aeruginosa* into the bloodstream (136). This phenotype may be due in part to the cytotoxic effect seen by purified LecA in primary epithelial cells in culture (143). These varied and significant contributions of LecA and LecB to *P. aeruginosa* pathogenesis make them exciting therapeutic targets. Indeed, inhibition of LecA and LecB could have a 2-fold effect on *P. aeruginosa* pathogenesis, preventing adherence to epithelial cells to decrease invasion while disrupting preformed biofilms to render the pathogens more susceptible to antimicrobial therapy.

SMALL-MOLECULE ANTIVIRULENCE THERAPEUTICS

Inhibition of Pathogen Receptor Biogenesis

The assembly and anchoring of pili to the cell surface of pathogens requires the coordinated expression and interaction of several proteins. An understanding of the complexity of this assembly process has uncovered a plethora of targets for the disruption of adhesive strategies utilized by both Gram-negative and Gram-positive pathogens summarized in this section and Table 1.

Small-molecule inhibitors of CUP pili biogenesis

Pilicides were the first small molecules to be utilized for the inhibition of CUP assembly (150). They belong to a class of molecules known collectively as pyrisides. These compounds are based upon a bicyclic 2-pyridone scaffold that maintains a rigid, peptide-like

conformation that closely mimics a β-strand (Fig. 3A). Measurement of pilicide activity in culture revealed remarkable success in inhibiting the assembly of both P and type 1 pili as monitored via electron microscopy (150) (Fig. 3B) and as determined in a variety of *in vitro* assays, including hemagglutination, biofilm formation, and adherence to a bladder tissue cell line. Pilicides were originally designed to disrupt the formation of chaperone-subunit complexes by targeting the chaperone-subunit interface. However, X-ray crystallographic studies with the P pilus chaperone, PapD, in complex with pilicide 1 (see Table 1) determined that the pilicide was instead binding a conserved hydrophobic region on the chaperone known to interact with the N-terminal domain of the usher pore, suggesting a disruption of a key interaction between the chaperone-subunit complexes and the usher (150) (Fig. 3C). *In vitro* binding studies with the type 1 FimCH chaperone-subunit complex and the N-terminal domain of the FimD usher confirmed this hypothesis, because increasing concentrations of pilicide were shown to inhibit binding between these two species (150).

Continued development of pilicides has led to a detailed understanding of the structure-activity relationship of these compounds and has resulted in the synthesis of molecules with vastly improved inhibition of type 1 pilus biogenesis (151, 152). The most efficacious compounds inhibit type 1 pilus-mediated *E. coli* biofilm formation in the low μM and high nM range. One such pilicide, compound 2, was found to disrupt several virulence-associated pili, including type 1 pili, P pili, and S pili (153) (Fig. 3A), as well as flagellar motility (153). Growth of the cystitis isolate UTI89 in compound 2 results in a dramatic downregulation of the type 1 pilus genes. Type 1 pilus expression is controlled by inversion of the *fimS* promoter element, which can oscillate between phase ON and phase OFF orientations. Growth in compound 2 results in *fimS* orientating into the OFF phase. In

TABLE 1 Antiadhesive small molecules

Compound number	Synonyms	References
1	MP048, 2c	150
2	ec240	153
3	AL1	155
4	FN075	126
5	6e	170
6	Heptyl mannoside	180
7	5a	241
8	FIM-2238, 2ZFH238, 8e	181
9	FIM-4269, 4ZFH269, 8	188
10	7a	193
11	7b	193
12	19	194
13	4d	196

A.

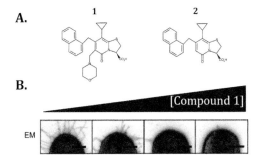

B.

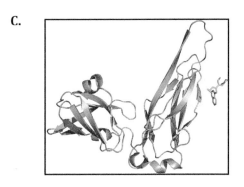

C.

FIGURE 3 **Small molecules known as "pilicides" disrupt pilus biogenesis. (A) Structures of two potent curlicides. Curlicide 1 disrupts type 1, P, and S pili. Curlicide 2 binds to the P pilus chaperone PapD, inhibiting its interaction with the PapC usher. (B) Electron micrographs demonstrating a loss of P pili on uropathogenic _Escherichia coli_ cells exposed to increasing concentrations of curlicide 2 (adapted from reference 150, with permission; copyright [2006] National Academy of Sciences, USA). (C) Crystal structure of the two-domain adhesin FimH complexed with pilicide (PDB ID code 2J7L).**

addition, it results in increased levels of the transcriptional regulators SfaB and PapB, which also promote the phase OFF orientation of the _fimS_ promoter (153). Thus, the potency of pilicide 2 is in part due to the unexpected mechanism of inducing a phase OFF orientation of the type 1 pilus promoter. Additionally, pilicide activity against Dr pili, another type of CUP pili known to play a role in pyelonephritis in mice and humans, has also been confirmed, further expanding the therapeutic potential of these compounds in targeting UTI (154). The exciting ability of

these compounds to target multiple CUP pili suggests that these compounds could demonstrate broad therapeutic coverage in the clinic. However, further testing of these compounds in animal models of infection along with pharmacological development will be required to solidify their role as a therapeutic.

In addition to the bicyclic 2-pyridone pilicides, another class of small-molecule compounds has been identified to target the P5 pocket of the FimH pilus subunit (155). This rationally designed molecule was developed to prevent the donor strand exchange reaction between FimH and the FimG rod adaptor (Fig. 2A and B). Because assembly of the pilus rod initiated by FimH binding to the usher complex followed by FimG incorporation is necessary for pilus biogenesis, abrogation of the FimH-FimG interaction completely abolishes pilus formation (156, 157). To identify such a molecule, a virtual screen was performed that measured _in silico_ docking of 2,000 compounds in the P5 pocket of FimH of the usher-bound FimCH protein structure (155). The top compounds from this screen were further examined in an _in vitro_ DSE assay, resulting in the identification of the most potent inhibitor, compound 3 (Fig. 2C) (155). This compound was found to completely inhibit type 1 pili expression when the bacteria were grown in the presence of a 200-μM compound. Interestingly, addition of compound 3 to growing bacterial cells rapidly resulted in the decrease of surface-localized pili, suggesting that this compound was capable of facilitating the disassembling and/or shedding of preformed pili (155). Based on the existing crystal structures and known mechanism of action, it is hypothesized that compound 3 may disrupt the anchoring of type 1 pili in the outer membrane by disrupting the terminal chaperone-subunit complex. Further verification of this mechanism of action, along with identification of the compound 3 binding site, will be necessary to continue the development of this compound as a therapeutic.

Small-molecule inhibitors of curli biogenesis

Another class of pyrisides has been shown to inhibit curli assembly. The 2-pyridone scaffold's modular nature allows for the manipulation of chemical activity through the substitution of various R groups onto the ring. When substituted compounds were screened for their ability to inhibit curli-dependent biofilms, it was found that replacement of a cyclopropyl group with a CF_3-phenyl substituent (Fig. 4A) inhibited curli fiber formation at a concentration of 250 µM (Fig. 4B) (126). To determine if this inhibition occurred during the ordered assembly of CsgA into amyloid fibers, various concentrations of compound 4 were added *in vitro* to purified CsgA (126). Compound 4 was able to completely prevent amyloid formation of purified CsgA when present in 5-fold excess. This inhibition is believed to occur via a direct interaction with soluble CsgA, thus preventing its transition into an amyloid-competent state prior to polymerization.

Interestingly, compound 4 has also been demonstrated to inhibit type 1 pilus biogenesis, suggesting its ability to inhibit multiple adhesive strategies utilized by UPEC to colonize the bladder and underscoring its promise as a therapeutic for UTI. Indeed, studies in a murine model of cystitis demonstrated that *E. coli* pretreated with compound 4 is significantly attenuated during infection when compared to untreated bacteria (126). Iterative rounds of synthetic chemistry and structural studies continue to provide further insight into the relationship between curlicide structure and potency (158). Additionally, structural similarities between curli fibers and other amyloid proteins have prompted investigators to test the inhibitory effects of curlicide compounds in other disease states. Indeed, specific curlicides have shown excellent efficacy in the *in vitro* inhibition of Aβ and α-synuclein polymerization, two amyloids associated with Alzheimer's and Parkinson's disease, respectively (159, 160). This ability to target amyloids in a nonspecific manner has provided generalizable insights at the molecular level into the process of amyloid formation. Further knowledge of aggregative mechanisms and their role in disease pathology will help inform the development of therapeutics that target specific regions vital to amyloid pathology.

A.

4

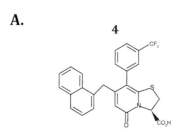

B.

[Compound 4]

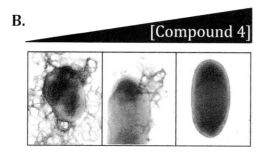

FIGURE 4 Curlicides inhibit biofilm formation. (A) Structure of the curlicide 4 compound. Curlicide compounds are based on 2-pyridine scaffold functionalized with a variety of substituents. (B) Inhibition of extracellular curli formation in the presence of increasing concentrations of curlicide 4 (adapted from reference 126).

Small-molecule inhibitors of sortase

Sortase enzymes play a unique role in Grampositive bacterial physiology and are essential for the virulence of many pathogens. Grampositive organisms encode up to four distinct classes of sortases that can be classified based on the substrates they act upon and the nucleophile they employ to resolve the acyl enzyme intermediate (76). The class A and B sortases are responsible for the covalent attachment of surface-anchored proteins to the cell wall. Thus, the pentaglycine crossbridge of the peptidoglycan precursor lipid II acts as the nucleophile in the transpeptidation reaction (161). Although they are structurally homologous to one another, the class A sortase (commonly referred to as the housekeeping sortase) acts on a majority of surface-associated proteins, while the class B sortase functions to specifically anchor heme transporters to the cell wall (162). Class C sortases are responsible for the covalent attachment of pilin subunits in the assembly of pili and are encoded in a pilus-specific manner within the pilus operons (71). Thus, while pilus biogenesis requires sortase C, anchoring of the pilus to the cell wall requires the activity of sortase A. Finally, the class D sortase mediates the attachment of envelope proteins to the cell wall and is believed to play a specific role in sporulation (163).

The conservation of the class A sortase and the integral nature of the process it facilitates have prompted investigators to aggressively pursue therapeutic inhibitors of sortase function. Indeed, virulence of Gram-positive pathogens, including *E. faecalis* and *Staphylococcus aureus*, is severely attenuated in animal models when the class A sortase is deleted (164, 165). These findings have resulted in the pursuit of many strategies to discover inhibitors of sortase A function, including screening of natural products, high-throughput screening of chemical libraries, and structure-based *in silico* screening of compounds (Table 2). While all of these inhibitors were originally screened against sortase A, further analysis demonstrated inhibition of both sortase B and C for many compounds, demonstrating the conservation of sortase protein structure and its mechanism of action.

The first major attempt to identify natural products with sortase inhibitory activity focused its efforts on the screening of extracts from 80 Korean medicinal plants (166). This work led to the identification of several compounds (summarized in Table 2) that demonstrate varying degrees of inhibition *in vitro* and *in vivo*. Most notable were the isoquinoline alkaloids from the rhizomes of

Coptis chinensis (167) and β-sitosterol-3-*O*-glucopyranoside from *Fritillaria verticillata*, which were determined to have an IC_{50} of 18.3 μg/mL and 15 μg/ml, respectively (168). These compounds demonstrated inhibition of sortase enzymatic activity *in vitro*, but their utilization in bacterial culture resulted in a growth defect (167, 168). Given that a *sortase A* mutant behaves similarly to wild type when grown in culture, these findings suggest that some compounds may target more than one cellular process, resulting in the measured pleiotropic effects. Future work will look to expand on these studies in an attempt to understand the mechanism of inhibition of sortase activity, such that specific inhibitors of sortase function can be identified and optimized for therapeutic use.

In addition to the screening of natural products, high-throughput screens of chemical libraries have led to the identification of several compounds that demonstrate both reversible and nonreversible inhibition of sortase activity. One class of inhibitors which demonstrated the most promise were the aryl β-amino(ethyl) ketones (AEEK) (169) (Table 1). These compounds irreversibly inhibit sortase A with an IC_{50} in the low micromolar range and have a simple, drug-like structure. Preliminary investigations into the structure-activity relationship have identified the value of anionic substituents in the para position on the aryl ring. Structural studies have also helped elucidate a model of inhibition, which involves the generation of an electrophilic intermediate that reacts with the catalytic cysteine, resulting in irreversible inactivation of the thiol active site (169). While these inhibitors hold promise, *in vivo* analysis of these compounds will be required for further verification.

Currently, the most successful class of sortase inhibitors has come from a rational design approach using the crystal structure of sortase A:substrate complex (PDB ID code 2KID) to virtually screen 300,000 compounds for putative binding to the active site (170) (Fig. 5A). From this screen, 105 compounds

TABLE 2 Antiadhesive strategies targeting the Gram-positive sortase^{a,b}

Inhibitor	Origin of inhibitor	IC$_{50}$ measured from in vitro assay	Surface protein measured during inhibition of sortase in culture	References
Methanethiosulfonate	Synthetic	N.D.	Seb anchoring	242
p-hydroxymercuribenzoic acid	Synthetic	N.D.	Seb anchoring	242
β-Sitosterol-3-O-glucopyranoside	Fritillaria verticillata (plant)	18 µg/ml	Binding to fibronectin	168
Berberine chloride	Callosobruchus chinensis (plant)	SrtA: 8.7 µg/ml; SrtB: 6.3 µg/ml	Binding to fibronectin	167, 243
Psammaplin A1	Aplysinella rhax (sponge)	SrtA: 39 µg/ml; SrtB: 23 µg/ml	Binding to fibronectin	243
Bromodeoxytopsentin	Topsentia genitrix (sponge)	19.4 µg/ml	Binding to fibronectin	244
Curcumin	Curcuma longa (plant)	13 µg/ml	Binding to fibronectin	245
Flavonoid phenols	Rhus verniciflua (bark) and natural products	SrtA: 37-52 µM; SrtB: 8-36 µM	Clumping	246
Diazo/chloromethyl ketone	Synthetic, substrate mimetic	N.D.	N.D.	247
3,3,3-trifluoro-1-(phenylsulfonyl)-1-propene	Synthetic	190 µM	Binding to fibronectin	248
Phosphinic-peptidomimetic	Synthetic, transition state mimic	10 Mm	N.D.	249
Diarylacrylonitrile	Small-molecule library	SrtA: 2.7 µg/ml; SrtB: 10 µg/ml	Binding to fibronectin	243, 250
Aryl β-amino(ethyl)ketones	Small-molecule library	SrtA: 4.8 µM; SrtB: 14 µM; SrtC: 15 µM	N.D.	169
3-(4-pyridinyl)-6-(2-sodiumsulfonatephenyl)[1,2,4]triazolo[3,4-b][1,3,4]thiadiazole] (5), see Table 1	Small-molecule library	Staphyloccocus aureus SrtA: 9.3 µM; Streptococcus pyogenes SrtA: 0.82 µM	Spa anchoring; Binding to fibrinogen	170

^{a}N.D., not determined
^{b}Adapted from reference 251

A.

B.

5

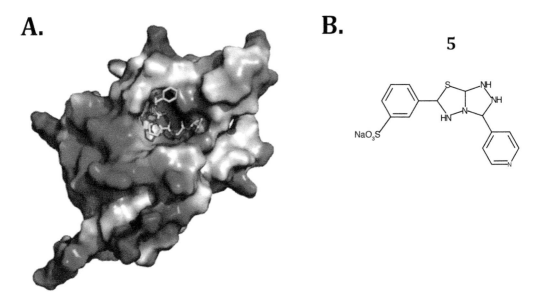

FIGURE 5 **Potent inhibitors of sortase A function. (A) X-ray crystal structure of sortase A from** *Staphylococcus aureus* **(PDB ID code 2KID) with** *in silico* **docking of compound 5, which binds directly to the active site of the enzyme (adapted from reference 170, with permission). (B) Structure of the sortase inhibitor compound 5, which inhibits sortase A from** *S. aureus* **with an** IC_{50} **of 9.3 µM and** *Streptococcus pyogenes* **with an** IC_{50} **of 0.82 µM.**

were selected for further *in vitro* characterization. Identification of a potent inhibitor of recombinant *S. aureus* sortase A activity followed by synthetic optimization produced compound 5 (Fig. 5B), which demonstrated an IC_{50} of 9.3 µM (170). This compound was found to inhibit sortase A in a reversible fashion and was demonstrated to directly bind to sortase A with a K_d = 8.8 µM. *In vivo* analysis of the influence of compound 5 on *S. aureus* in culture demonstrated no influence on growth but revealed a decrease in incorporation of cell wall–anchored proteins (170). One such protein showing decreased incorporation is protein A (SpA), which is known to aid bacterial subversion of phagocytosis by host immune cells by the binding the Fcγ and Fab domains of host immunoglobins (171). To determine compounds 5's potential as a therapeutic, the ability of intraperitoneal doses of the compound to protect mice from a lethal challenge of *S. aureus* was tested. These studies found that intraperitoneal dosing of compound 5 in mice

resulted in a significant increase in murine survival, demonstrating the anti-infective capabilities of sortase inhibitors (170). Interestingly, compound 5 was also found to inhibit the sortase from *Streptococcus pyogenes* with an IC_{50} of 0.82 µM, suggesting that it could have broad therapeutic use in the clinic (170). Further optimization of compound 5 and validation in additional animal models could make the targeting of sortase activity a legitimate therapeutic option.

Inhibition of Pathogen Binding by Receptor Analogs

Recognition of surface-exposed glycans by a pathogen is often characterized by a relatively weak association between the pathogen carbohydrate-binding domain (CBD) and the host glycoconjugate (34). To compensate for this relatively weak interaction, bacteria typically express multiple copies of the CBD to increase the avidity for the target and strengthen the interaction between the pathogen and the host. One strategy that is commonly employed to target this interaction involves the introduction of small "glycomimetics" to the system, which saturates the CBDs by imitating their natural ligand. This saturation weakens the pathogen's interaction with host tissue, increasing susceptibility to natural mechanical expulsion. The efficacy of this treatment approach is thus based on the generation of high-affinity glycomimetics that can outcompete the natural ligand for the CBD at physiologically plausible concentrations. To accomplish this task, both high-affinity monovalent as well as multivalent inhibitors have proven to hold great promise (Table 3).

FimH antagonists: mannosides

The type 1 pilus adhesin, FimH, mediates adherence of UPEC to the bladder epithelium and is essential for infection in a murine model of cystitis (172). The lectin domain of FimH has been demonstrated to mediate binding to several glycoproteins, including uroplakin Ia (UPIa), Tamm-Horsfall protein, and $\beta 1$ and $\alpha 3$ integrins (173–175). Recognition of this diverse set of host ligands occurs through a stereochemically specific interaction with mannose. Crystallographic studies of FimH complexed with a number of mannose derivatives have revealed the structural basis of mannose recognition on a molecular level. The FimH lectin domain (FimH$_L$) is composed of an 11-stranded elongated β-barrel with a jelly roll–like topology with a mannose-binding pocket located at the tip of the two-domain protein (176–178). This binding pocket is comprised of several residues, which make extensive hydrogen bonding and hydrophobic interactions with D-mannose. Outside of this pocket is a hydrophobic ridge, which includes two tyrosine residues that form the so-called tyrosine gate (Fig. 6A). Genetic analyses of hundreds of *fimH* sequences have found these distinct regions to be invariant, further arguing for their importance in the pathogenic cascade (177, 179). Indeed, interactions with the

tyrosine gate and other hydrophobic residues found within the ridge are believed to mediate the increase in affinity seen for many mannose-containing oligosaccharides, including Manα1,3Manβ1,4GlcNAcβ1,4GlcNAc (oligomannose-3). Crystallization of FimH$_L$ with oligomannose-3 confirmed this hypothesis and has directed the development of mannosides that initiate interactions with this hydrophobic ridge (180). Interestingly, one of the first mannosides, butyl α-D-mannoside, was initially identified when it was serendipitously copurified and crystallized with FimH$_L$ (178). This mannoside displayed a 15-fold increase in affinity compared to D-mannose, largely resulting from the hydrophobic interaction between the alkyl chain and the tyrosine gate (178).

Subsequent rounds of rational compound design and testing continued to examine the influence of alkyl chain length on affinity. In this manner, heptyl α-D-mannoside (compound 6) was identified as a lead compound, because its binding was shown to be 30-fold tighter than butyl α-D-mannoside and 600 times tighter than the natural ligand, D-mannose (Fig. 6B) (178). The therapeutic efficacy of this compound was tested in a murine model of cystitis, which demonstrated that incubation of UPEC with compound 6 prior to infection in mice resulted in a significant decrease in bacterial burden in the bladder 6 hours postinoculation (180). This was the first study demonstrating the utility of mannosides *in vivo*, highlighting the therapeutic potential of targeting FimH.

Since these initial findings, further development of mannosides has continued to focus on structure-based optimization of affinity. To exploit π-π stacking interactions with the tyrosine gate and interactions beyond the binding pocket, the alkyl chain was substituted with a variety of aromatic substituents. Ultimately, it was found that the affinity of biphenyl α-D-mannosides (compounds 7, 8, and 9) for FimH was much higher than aryl- or heptyl-mannose (compound 6), resulting in a new line of potent therapeutic candidates

TABLE 3 Antiadhesive strategies utilizing receptor and adhesin analogs[a]

Bacterium	Method of validation	Inhibitor	References
Receptor analogs			
Campylobacter jejuni	Murine gastrointestinal model	Fucosyloligosaccharides of human milk	252
Helicobacter pylori	Rhesus model	3-sialyllactose	253
Listeria monocytogenes	Human epithelial colorectal cell line	Xylo-oligosaccharides	254
Streptococcus pneumoniae	Rabbit and rat nasopharynx	6′-sialylneolactotetraose	255
Yersinia pestis	Human epithelial respiratory cell line	GalNAcβ1-3Gal and GalNAcβ1-4Gal	256
Streptococcus sobrinus	Rat oral cavity	Oxidized α1,6glucan	257
Streptococcus suis	Murine model of peritonitis	Tetravalent galabiose	258–262
Escherichia coli (type 1 pili)	Murine model of cystitis	Mannosides	181, 182, 188–190, 263–267
E. coli (P pili)	In vitro binding assay	Multivalent galabiose	268–270
E. coli (F1C pili)	In vitro binding assay	Multivalent GalNAcβ1-4Gal	271
Pseudomonas aeruginosa (LecA)	Murine model of lung infection	Galactosides	193, 272–276
P. aeruginosa (LecB)	Murine model of lung infection	Fucosides/mannosides	193, 195, 196, 277–279
Adhesin analogs			
Streptococcus mutans	Human studies monitoring recolonization of *S. mutans*	Full length streptococcal antigen (SA) I/II and 22 residue peptide	280, 281
Streptococcus gordonii	In vitro binding and biofilm assay	Peptides of the adhesin *Streptococcus gordonii* surface protein SspB	282
Enterotoxigenic *Escherichia coli*	Horse red blood cells and calf ileal enterocytes	Truncated versions of K99 pili	283
Gram-negative bacteria and *Staphylococcus aureus*	Multiple human tissue culture cell lines	MAM7	197, 200

[a]Adapted from references 284, 285.

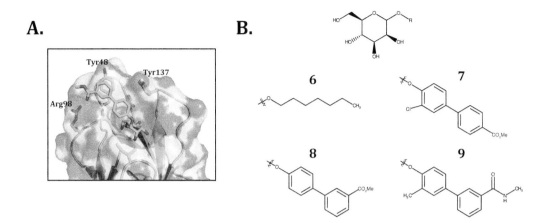

FIGURE 6 Mannosides are potent inhibitors of FimH binding. (A) Crystal structure of FimH complexed with mannoside 8, which binds to FimH with an affinity over 1 million times higher than its natural substrate, D-mannose (PDB ID code 3MCY). (B) Structure of a variety of mannosides, each rationally designed to increase affinity for FimH by interacting with the hydrophobic ridge outside of the mannose-binding pocket. Although heptyl α-D-mannoside 6 successfully bound FimH with a 600 times increased affinity when compared to D-mannoside, the biphenyl substituents ultimately proved to be the most effective compounds (7, 8, and 9).

(Fig. 6B). Further substitutions to these rings have focused on the addition of electron withdrawing groups to decrease the electron density of the aryl ring and increase π-π stacking (Fig. 6B). These charged residues have also been found to facilitate hydrogen bond formation with Arg98, which resides right outside the binding pocket (Fig. 6A). Additionally, it is believed that increased binding affinity of compounds can also be related to a decrease in conformational flexibility and thus a decrease in the entropic cost of binding (181–183).

Iterative refinement of these compounds has necessitated the use of multiple modalities to assess mannoside potency. Inhibition of epitope binding can be measured directly by examining the inhibition of the type 1–dependent hemagglutination of guinea pig red blood cells, which present mannosylated epitopes on the surface of the cell (181). Additional assays include inhibition of bacterial adherence to plastic plates that have been coated in mannosylated bovine serum albumin or inhibition of type 1–dependent adherence to human epithelial carcinoma bladder 5637 cells expressing mannosylated uroplakins (184, 185). Measurement of mannoside binding to $FimH_L$ can also be measured by isothermal titration calorimetry, differential scanning calorimetry, or biolayer interferometry. Comparative analyses of mannosides using a multitude of these distinct methods have consistently produced similar results, demonstrating that each assay measures aspects of mannoside affinity. Combined with structural studies, this research has led to the development of one of the most potent mannosides, compound 9 (Fig. 6B), which can inhibit FimH function in the nanomolar concentration range as measured by hemagglutination. Indeed, compound 9 is over 1 million times more potent than D-mannose as measured by hemagglutination.

Continued improvement of this potent compound and others has focused on improving their pharmacokinetic behavior through a number of approaches, including the use of bioisosteres, as well as the development of prodrugs (186, 187). The culmination of this work has led to the development of small, orally bioavailable compounds capable of preventing acute UTIs and treating chronic UTIs (188). Furthermore, prophylactic use of mannosides was found to significantly reduce bacterial burden in a murine model of CAUTI (189). Ongoing research continues to improve the pharmacokinetic behavior of these drugs to optimize their therapeutic potential in human disease.

While these efforts have largely been based around monovalent inhibition of FimH, other investigations have been directed at the development of multivalent compounds designed to interact with more than one FimH lectin domain. Attachment of compound 6 to a cyclodextrin core has resulted in compounds capable of binding multiple adhesins, thus increasing compound affinity relative to their monovalent counterparts (190). This increase in affinity has resulted in a significant improvement in the *in vivo* efficacy during acute UTI compared to the monovalent heptyl mannoside. However, delivery of these compounds was performed by transurethral administration (190), making their potential as a prophylactic tool or treatment in patients susceptible or suffering with a UTI uncertain.

Multivalent inhibitors of
P. aeruginosa LecA and LecB

Interaction of lectin domains with specific glycosidic ligands is often relatively weak and usually relies upon multiple interactions to increase the overall avidity. The affinity of LecA and LecB for monomeric galactose and fucose has been determined to be 87.5 µM and 3 µM, respectively (191, 192). However, several multivalent inhibitors have been found to bind in the nanomolar range, supporting the utility of a multivalent approach to lectin inhibition (Table 3). This "clustering" effect has been exploited in the design of multivalent glycoconjugate inhibitors of the LecA and LecB soluble adhesins from *P. aeruginosa*. These synthetic glycoclusters have utilized a variety of scaffolds including peptides (192), modified oligonucleotides (192), fullerenes (192), and trithiotriazine (192) with either

galactose or fucose attached to target LecA and LecB, respectively.

Two of the most thoroughly examined inhibitors of the LecA and LecB adhesins are the multivalent galactosylated and fucosylated calixarenes (193). These tetravalent compounds contain triethylene glycol linkers that are attached to the calixarene core and functionalized with either galactose (compound 11) or fucose (compound 10) at the distal tip (Fig. 7A). Measurements of the affinity of these compounds by isothermal titration calorimetry were able to demonstrate nanomolar K_ds of 48 and 176 nM for compounds 10 and 11, respectively (193). These experiments also demonstrated that these compounds functioned in a multivalent manner, as determined by analysis of the isothermal titration calorimetry measurements (193). Given the spacing between subunits within the tetrameric proteins and the length of the ethylene glycol linkers, structural analysis suggested that these inhibitors interacted with separate epitopes on individual tetrameric proteins. Binding to glycomimetic compounds was also found to correlate with *in vitro* bacterial phenotypes. Micromolar concentrations of either drug were found to significantly inhibit *P. aeruginosa* adherence to A549 epithelial cells, reducing binding to between 70 and 90% of wild type levels (193). Additionally, both compounds 10 and 11 were found to inhibit biofilm formation, albeit at the fairly high concentration of 5 mM (193). The efficacy of these compounds *in vivo* was also investigated by preincubating *P. aeruginosa* with compound prior to intranasal instillation in a mouse model of pneumonia. Incubation with either 1 or 5 mM of either compound resulted in a significant reduction in bacterial burden in the lung and was associated with decreased alveolar capillary permeability, which is directly correlated with *P. aeruginosa*–induced lung injury (193). Despite the high concentrations needed to obtain *in vivo* phenotypes, these studies validate this anti-LecA and -LecB approach, providing an impetus to continue biochemical

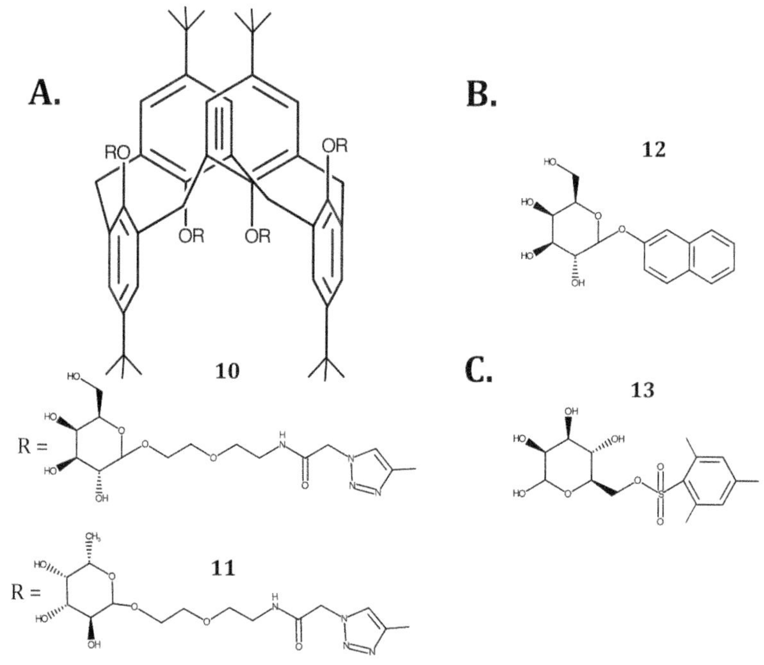

FIGURE 7 Inhibitors of soluble lectins LecA and LecB. (A) Structural depiction of the tetravalent calixarene scaffold, which can be functionalized with galactose and fucose moieties using triethylene glycol linkers to form compounds 11 and 10, respectively. (B) Monovalent inhibitor of LecA 12 binds with a K_d of 4.2 μM. (C) Monovalent inhibitor of LecB 13 activity binds with a K_d of 3.3 μM.

and pharmacokinetic optimization of these compounds as therapies for *P. aeruginosa* infections.

In addition to a multivalent approach, development of both divalent and monovalent inhibitors of LecA and LecB has also been attempted (Table 3). These efforts have involved modification of galactose and fucose with aglycon structures to generate additional contacts with protein residues outside of the binding pocket, thus increasing the affinity and specificity of the compound for their cognate lectin. In the case of LecA, aromatic aglycon structures have proved to be successful, especially those containing a naphthalene ring (Fig. 7B compound 12) (194). For LecB, optimization of the disaccharide substructure L-Fucβ1-GlcNAc from Lewis-a identified a relatively high-affinity molecule with a K_d = 290 nM (195). However, cross-reactivity of this compound with the lectin DC-SIGN, which is found on the sur-

face of macrophages and dendritic cells, was identified as a potentially harmful side effect (195). To circumvent this problem, additional compounds utilizing mannose in place of fucose have been generated. While LecB has a relatively low affinity for mannose compared to fucose, modification of C6 carbon on mannose has resulted in high-affinity compounds, with IC_{50} approaching the low μM range (Fig. 7C compound 13) (196). Continued development in this field will hopefully lead to new therapeutics for the treatment of *P. aeruginosa* infections.

Inhibition of Pathogen Binding by Adhesin Analogs

While the approaches described above have attempted to competitively inhibit adhesin binding by mimicking the adhesin's natural ligand, inhibition of adherence can also be achieved through delivery of adhesin analogs that compete with the bacteria for their natural receptor (Table 3). This approach often utilizes peptide-like inhibitors as opposed to the glycomimetics described above, but it requires the same stable, high-affinity interactions to be successful. Additionally, adhesin analogs must avoid disruption of the host cell function, which can occur with host cell receptor recognition.

MAM7, a peptide-like inhibitor of Gram-negative and Gram-positive infections

The Gram-negative outer membrane protein multivalent adhesion molecule 7 (MAM7) was first identified in the pathogen *Vibrio parahaemolyticus* and found to consist of a transmembrane motif followed by seven mammalian cell entry (mce) domains, all of which are required for attachment to cultured HeLa epithelial cells (197). Utilizing a bioinformatics approach, it was determined that MAM7, or its 6-mce domain counterpart MAM6, was highly conserved among Gram-negative pathogens but absent in Gram-positive bacteria (197). MAM7 is believed to mediate attachment to host cells via interactions with host fibronectin and the host membrane lipid phosphatidic acid and was shown to augment cell death mediated by the type III secretion system (197, 198). Interestingly, prior addition of nonpathogenic bacteria expressing MAM7 was able to ameliorate infection of cultured HeLa epithelial cells infected with a variety of Gram-negative pathogens, including additional *Vibrio* species, *Yersinia pseudotuberculosis*, enteropathogenic *E. coli*, *Klebsiella pneumoniae*, *Acinetobacter baumannii-calcoaceticus*, and *P. aeruginosa* (197, 199).

It has also been demonstrated that nonpathogenic bacteria expressing MAM7 or purified recombinant MAM7 immobilized on latex beads are able to prophylactically inhibit cytotoxicity in a tissue culture model of infection of either HeLa epithelial cells or 3T3 fibroblasts (197, 199). Delivery of MAM7 involved a 30-minute preincubation of the tissue culture cells with either the MAM7-expressing bacteria at a multiplicity of infection of 100 or the addition of MAM7-coated latex beads at a concentration of 7.5 mg protein/10^6 beads/well (199). This decrease in cytotoxicity results from a decrease in MAM-7-mediated adhesion, which is believed to occur primarily through competition with the pathogen's MAM7 homolog.

MAM7 can also be effective at outcompeting non-MAM7 adhesins for the same receptor. For example, *S. aureus* is known to interact with the extracellular glycoprotein fibronectin. Preincubation of HaCaT, human dermal fibroblast, or HeLa tissue culture cells with 500 nM of bead-coupled MAM7 significantly reduced attachment of *S. aureus* (200). This reduction is similar to that observed when beads coated with the staphylococcal fibronectin-binding protein (FnBPA) or the *S. pyogenes* fibronectin-binding protein F1 are preincubated with tissue culture cells prior to the introduction of *S. aureus* (200). It should be noted that treatment with F1- or FnBPA-coated beads disrupted host cell function, resulting in a delay in wound healing due to impaired matrix formation and cellular adhesion, even in the absence of a pathogen (200). Thus, MAM7 is uniquely able to prevent adherence of *S. aureus* without contaminant perturbation of the host cell environment. The broad coverage of MAM7 as an inhibitor of both Gram-positive and Gram-negative infections makes it an exciting candidate as a broad-spectrum antivirulence therapeutic. However, the size of MAM7 (~840 amino acids) and the lack of *in vivo* data still represent major obstacles to overcome in the course of development of this concept into a stable, high-affinity therapeutic.

INHIBITION OF PATHOGEN BINDING BY ANTIADHESION ANTIBODIES AND VACCINES

Adhesin-based vaccines have proven to be highly successful in the prevention of bacterial infections in a number of animal models (Table 4). This strategy relies upon vaccination with an essential adhesin required for colonization and disease. Generation of antibodies against the adhesin can result in disruption of adhesin-receptor interactions by occlusion of the binding pocket in an orthosteric manner. Alternatively, antibodies may disrupt binding via allosteric interactions by blocking a conformational change within the adhesin required for ligand recognition (201). Either of these mechanisms, when fully realized, result in the host's elimination of the pathogen by natural mechanisms. This protection has been seen following both active and passive vaccination, suggesting that the development of a monoclonal antibody may also be highly effective at treating active infections.

Vaccines for urinary tract infections

Elucidation of the role of type 1 pili and the FimH adhesin led to one of the first adhesin-based vaccines. Vaccination of mice with a truncated version of FimH corresponding to the lectin domain or with the FimC-FimH chaperone-adhesin complex produced high serum titers of anti-FimH IgG (202). These antibodies were also detectable in the urine and were shown to reduce colonization of the bladder mucosa by 99% following transurethral challenge in mice with a model UPEC strain (202). Independent *ex vivo* studies further verified that these antibodies were able to recognize FimH and prevent the binding of UPEC to human bladder epithelial cells (202). Protection of neutropenic mice from UTI by vaccination with FimH further demonstrated that elimination of bacteria was occurring independently of neutrophilic involvement, supporting the notion that protection occurs via inhibition of bacterial adhesion and subsequent mechanical elimination of UPEC strains (202).

Nonhuman primate trials subsequently demonstrated that immunization of monkeys with FimCH was found to be effective, generating a strong IgG response and preventing

infection in three out of four animals, compared to a 100% infection rate in the control group (203). Further, vaccination was found to have no impact on the *E. coli* niche in the gut microbiota, demonstrating the specific targeting of pathogenic *E. coli* in the urinary tract (203). Continued development of this vaccine has primarily been focused on inducing a greater immune stimulation in an attempt to increase the concentration of protective antibodies near the mucosal surface. To this end, investigators have attempted to fuse FimH to the flagellin FliC to stimulate a stronger acute inflammatory response (204). Similarly, coadministration of the FimC-FimH vaccine with a synthetic analogue of monophosphoryl lipid A has resulted in a phase 1 clinical trial that began in January 2014.

Adhesin-based vaccines for other uropathogens, including *Proteus mirabilis* and *E. faecalis*, have been shown to be successful in animal models. Vaccination with the adhesin capping the MR/P pilus from *P. mirabilis* was found to significantly reduce bladder bacterial burdens compared to unvaccinated controls (205). Additionally, vaccination with the pilus adhesin EbpA from *E. faecalis* reduced the bladder bacterial burden 1,000 times, representing a significant amount of protection against infection (82). Similar to the FimH vaccine, this protection was found to be specific to the adhesin, EbpA, and was demonstrated to disrupt EbpA's interaction with fibrinogen. Interestingly, vaccination with an EbpA construct lacking the metal-binding MIDAS motif necessary for fibrinogen recognition did not result in the production of protective antibodies (82).

Additional antiadhesive vaccine strategies

In addition to the straightforward adhesin-based vaccine strategies described above wherein soluble protein is introduced directly into the animal, investigators are also pursuing a number of alternative approaches designed to ensure that adhesins are properly

TABLE 4 Antiadhesive strategies utilizing antiadhesin vaccines or antibodies

Bacterium	Adhesin targeted	Details	References
Salmonella enterica serovar Typhi	T2544	Active and passive immunization provides limited protection	286
S. enterica serovar Typhi	SadA	Active vaccination provides limited protection	287
Enterotoxigenic *Escherichia coli* (ETEC)	K88ab, K88ac, FedA, and FedF	Vaccination of proteins expressed in live attenuated *Salmonella* Typhimurium strain	209, 210
Enterotoxigenic *E. coli*	FaeG major subunit of K88ac fimbriae	Active vaccination with heat-labile (LT) toxin and the A subunit of shiga toxin (STa) is protective	288
Enterohemorrhagic *E. coli*	Intimin	Active vaccination with fusion protein of intimin and two shiga toxin antigens provides protection	289
Uropathogenic *E. coli*	FimCH	Active and passive vaccination provides protection	202, 203
Pseudomonas aeruginosa	Type IV pilin adhesin	Generation of an effective antibody response relied on coupling of the N- and C-terminal to a carrier, provides protection against multiple strains	290
Proteus mirabilis	MrpH, MR/P pilus adhesin	Active vaccination as fusion with cholera toxin provides significant protection	205
Enterococcus faecalis	EbpA	Active vaccination of full length EbpA or its N-terminal provides protection	82
Bordetella pertussis	Hemagglutinin adhesin and pertactin	Both adhesins are included in the vaccine against whooping cough and function partly by inhibition of adhesion	291
Streptococcus mutans	Streptococcal antigen (SA) I/II	Application of a monoclonal antibody prevents tooth colonization	292, 293
Staphylococcus aureus	Clumping factor A, fibronectin-binding protein A, and fibronectin-binding protein B	Both active and passive vaccination provided protection against prosthetic-device infection	294
S. aureus	Collagen-binding protein (CNA)	DNA vaccine generated antibodies against CNA, but does not provide protection against intra-peritoneal infection	211
S. aureus	Clumping factor A (ClfA), fibronectin-binding protein (FnBPa)	DNA vaccine including the sortase enzyme provides strain-dependent protection	212
Streptococcus pneumoniae	Surface adhesin A and surface protein A	Intranasal vaccination reduced colonization	295

oriented and displayed in a physiologically relevant conformation for antibody generation. For example, development of a vaccine against the Gram-negative pathogen *Neisseria meningitidis* required the delivery of adhesin antigens encapsulated in outer membrane vesicles to ensure proper presentation. Previous attempts at vaccination had focused simply on the delivery of adhesins: NadA, factor H binding protein (fHBP) and *Neisseria* heparin binding antigen (NHBA) (206–208). Similarly, a vaccine against enterotoxigenic *E. coli* (ETEC) successfully developed for post-weaning pigs utilizes a *Salmonella enterica* serovar Typhimurium strain that expresses and displays the *E. coli* fimbrial components (K88ab, K88ac, FedA, and FedF) (209, 210). Although this vaccine is effective, additional care must be taken when vaccinating with live strains to ensure that no live, genetically modified bacteria are introduced into the environment.

Finally, some studies have been directed toward the development of DNA vaccines, which involve the direct delivery of DNA encoding the pathogen-derived antigen. Expression, processing, and presentation of a DNA antigen are believed to occur in a more efficient manner, leading to both a humoral and cellular response. DNA vaccines against adhesins from enterotoxigenic *E. coli*, *S. pneumoniae*, and *S. aureus* have been attempted with variable success (211–214). As a whole, the targeting of adhesin-receptor interactions through vaccination has shown great promise, leading to the successful development of several novel therapies for both Gram-negative and Gram-positive pathogens (Table 4).

DIETARY SUPPLEMENTS AND PROBIOTICS AS INHIBITORS OF BACTERIAL ADHESION

There are several cited examples of fruits, plants, and milk that possess the ability to inhibit bacterial adherence to a variety of tissues (Table 5) (215). Extraction and char-

acterization of the active constituents from these products suggest that they often function as receptor analogs or adhesin inhibitors. A number of extracted plant phenols have been shown to prevent attachment by a number of bacteria, including *Streptococcus mutans* and *Helicobacter pylori*, which are known to cause dental caries and gastric ulcers, respectively (216–218). However, the exact mechanism or active component of the majority of these inhibitors is unknown. Some of the most thoroughly studied extracts come from cranberries (*Vaccinium macrocarpon*), which have long been recognized for their possible preventative and therapeutic utility toward UTIs (219). Although some studies of elderly and young women suggested that regular intake of cranberry juice results in a significant reduction in bacteriuria, additional studies have not shown a significant difference (220–222). However, high-molecular-weight polyphenols extracted and purified from cranberry extracts have demonstrated the ability to inhibit bacterial binding of *E. coli* (223), *N. meningitidis* (224), and *S. mutans* (225) to host tissue *in vitro*. While the mechanism of inhibition in many of these cases has not yet been fully elucidated, in the case of UTIs it is possible that the high level of fructose present in most cranberry juices may bind to the FimH adhesin in type 1 pili and compete with the natural mannosylated receptors. However, this mechanism of action cannot explain the ability of cranberry extract to inhibit P pili–mediated adhesion *in vitro*, suggesting that multiple inhibitors may be present (226).

Milk from humans and other mammals has also been determined to contain a number of antibodies, glycoproteins, and oligosaccharides that inhibit or reduce bacterial binding (Table 5). A murine model of *H. pylori* infection revealed that the oligosaccharides Lewis-b and sialyl Lewis-x present in porcine milk have the ability to reduce colonization of the gastrointestinal tract through the inhibition of bacterial adherence to host receptors (227). Human milk oligosaccharides have also

TABLE 5 Antiadhesive strategies utilizing dietary supplements[a]

Plant	Active ingredient	Bacterium	References
Plant derivatives			
Camilla sinensis (green tea)	Green tea extract, (-) epicatechin gallate, (-) gallocatechin gallate	*Helicobacter pylori*, *Staphylococcus aureus*, *Porphyromonas gingivalis*	218
Vaccinium spp.	Cranberry polyphenols	*Escherichia coli*, *Neisseria meningitidis*, *Streptococcus mutans*, *H. pylori*	223–225
Curcuma longa (turmeric)	Essential oil components	*S. mutans*	296
Nidus vespae (honeycomb extract from *Polistes* spp.)	Chloroform/methanol fraction	*S. mutans*	297
Paullinia cupana (guarana)	Tannins	*Streptococcus mutans*	216
Psidium guajava	Guaijaverin	*S. mutans*	298
Vitis (red grape marc)	Polyphenols	*S. mutans*	217
Azadirachta indica (neem stick)	N.D.	*Streptococcus sanguis*	299
Gilanthus nivalis (snowdrop)	Mannose-sensitive lectin	*E. coli*	300
Gloiopeltis furcata and *Gigatina teldi* (seaweeds)	Sulfated polysaccharides	*Streptococcus sobrinus*	301
Melaphis chinensis	Gallotannin	*S. sanguis*	299
Persea americana (avocado)	Tannins	*S. mutans*	302
Legume storage proteins	Glycoprotein	*E. coli*	303
Milk constituents			
Human milk	Fucosyloligosaccharides	*E. coli*	304
Mammalian milk	Free oligosaccharides	*Neisseria meningitidis*	305
Human milk	Polymeric glycan	*Pseudomonas aeruginosa* and *Chromobacterium violaceum*	306
Human milk	Lactoferrins	*Shigella* spp.	307
Human milk	Caseins	*S. mutans*	308
Human milk	Caseinoglycopeptides	*H. pylori*	309
Human milk	Glycoprotein	*Staphylococcus aureus*	310
Human milk	Neutral oligosaccharides	*Streptococcus pneumonia* and *Haemophilus influenzae*	311
Human milk	Sialylated glycoproteins	*Mycoplasma pneumoniae*	312
Porcine milk	Glycosylated proteins	*H. pylori*	227
Human milk	Sialylated poly(N-acetyl lactosamine)	*Mycoplasma pneumoniae*	313
Human milk	Sialylated poly(N-acetyl lactosaminoglycans)	*Streptococcus suis*	314
Human milk	Sialyl-3'-Lac and sialylated glycoproteins	*E. coli* (S pili)	315
Human milk	Sialylgalactosides	*E. coli* (S pili)	316

[a] Adapted from references 284, 285.

been demonstrated to inhibit binding of the enteric pathogens *E. coli, Vibrio cholerae,* and *Salmonella fyris* to epithelial cell lines (228). This observation likely explains the correlation between protection against diarrhea and the quantity of oligosaccharides detected in breast milk (229). Taken together, the inhibition of bacterial adhesion by naturally occurring products in milk and plant tissue may represent an evolved approach to targeting bacterial adhesion as a host defense mechanism. Indeed, many attempts at inhibiting bacterial adhesion have been informed by investigation into the activity of naturally occurring products. Further screening of these natural products for inhibitors of bacterial binding will likely serve as an important source of novel therapeutics for targeting pathogen adherence.

Additional strategies to prevent adhesion and colonization by human pathogens have included the use of commensal or probiotic strains to reduce binding of detrimental microorganisms by saturating host surface receptors and eliminating pathogen-binding sites. This form of protection is known as colonization resistance (230). Interestingly, administration of antibiotics has been shown to perturb the beneficial commensal bacteria that generate this resistance, resulting in increased colonization of opportunistic pathogens (231). Probiotic bacteria can also compete with pathogens for vital nutrients required for growth, as well as influence production of host mucins that improve barrier function (232, 233). Ultimately, utilization of probiotics can function to prevent pathogen colonization through a diverse array of mechanisms.

SMALL-MOLECULE INHIBITORS OF ADHESIN EXPRESSION

In addition to interruption of protein complex assembly and inhibition of adhesin-receptor interactions, disruption of adhesin transcription is also a viable mechanism of preventing and treating bacterial infections. In many pathogens, regulation of adhesin transcription is integrated into large regulons that impact a number of additional virulence factors, including toxins and secretion systems. Expression of these regulatory networks is often controlled by a variety of cellular and environmental signals, including bacterial density. Detection of bacterial populations can occur by a number of mechanisms but often involves quorum sensing, a mode of bacterial communication utilized by several pathogens to regulate expression of growth and virulence factors as a function of population density. Quorum sensing typically involves the secretion of a small signaling molecule that accumulates in the extracellular space until a critical threshold is reached, resulting in the transcriptional upregulation of a number of virulence genes, including adhesins (234). There are a number of examples in which targeting and disruption of these regulatory pathways has prevented the expression of adhesins and other known virulence factors (235–238).

CONCLUDING REMARKS: THE ADVANTAGES OF TARGETING PATHOGEN ADHESIN

As the effectiveness of broad-spectrum antibiotics continues to decline at an alarming rate, the need for the development of novel antimicrobial agents has never been more immediate. The current paradigm of antibiotic discovery is largely based on continued expansion of existing classes of antibiotics to circumvent evolved bacterial resistance mechanisms. While this approach may provide short-term solutions, the strong selective pressure conferred by drugs that target vital cell processes will ultimately limit the effective lifetime of these derivatives. To mitigate this selective pressure, investigators are instead pursuing novel mechanisms of antimicrobial action that target virulence factors central to the bacterial pathogenic cascade.

These factors play a role in a variety of processes, beginning with the colonization of host niches and continuing with engagement of secretion systems, formation of biofilms, and others.

A necessary first step in the progression of many bacterial infections is adherence to host tissues in the niche targeted by the pathogen. There are many structurally distinct but functionally overlapping mechanisms by which bacteria mediate this adhesion. These mechanisms depend on the bacteria's location, identity, and local environment. As we continue to build our understanding of these systems at the molecular level, we will elucidate several new strategies for the targeting of these vital bacterial processes.

Further refinement of these antivirulence compounds, peptides, and vaccines will lead to the development of therapeutics that target pathogens in the niche in which they cause disease. By directing these strategies toward a diverse array of disease processes, investigators hope to provide clinicians with a formidable arsenal of tools for use against a wide variety of infections. The ability of these therapeutics to target pathogens within their specific host niches eliminates the concomitant disruption of the host commensal microbiota that commonly accompanies treatment with current, broad-spectrum antibiotics. This, in turn, eliminates the blooming of other pathogenic bacteria that can occur in states of host dysbiosis.

An additional advantage conferred by the utilization of therapeutics that target bacterial virulence rather than essential cellular metabolic processes is a possible reduction in the rate of antimicrobial resistance. It is conceivable that any mutations made to escape the therapeutic mechanism will result in a concomitant decrease in the ability of the adhesin to interact with its natural receptor. While this hypothesis has not yet been vigorously tested, this may represent a unique scenario wherein development of resistance to antiadhesive therapeutics may occur, but doing so will result in a significant attenuation of virulence.

Recent advances in the targeting of bacterial adhesion have come from *in silico* docking with solved protein structures. The ability to virtually screen thousands of compounds reduces costs and decreases the time necessary to identify promising targets. Thus, it is necessary to continue to pursue a structural understanding of host-pathogen interactions on a molecular level through NMR and X-ray crystallography to inform computational identification and rational design of potent and effective compounds. Additionally, consideration of the pharmacokinetic behavior of compounds early in their development will also be crucial in identifying successful antiadhesive approaches that will be conducive to a clinical setting.

Finally, while the development of small molecules and vaccines can provide exciting therapeutic options, their development is also fundamental to obtaining a clear and complete understanding of bacterial pathogenesis. As with genetic manipulation, these compounds provide investigators with molecular scalpels that can dissect host-pathogen interactions, allowing one to understand the contribution of these interactions to disease in animal models, as well as to identify putative host targets. Indeed, there are a number of examples in which chemical biology through the generation of molecular probes has aided in the study of bacterial pathogenesis (239). Ultimately, continued development of antiadhesive strategies will further our understanding of bacterial virulence as it relates to human disease and provide unique approaches to the treatment of infectious diseases.

ACKNOWLEDGMENTS

Scott Hultgren has an ownership interest in Fimbrion and may financially benefit if the company is successful in marketing the mannosides that are related to this research.

CITATION

Cusumano ZT, Klein RD, Hultgren SJ. 2016. Innovative solutions to sticky situations: antiadhesive strategies for treating bacterial infections. Microbiol Spectrum 4(2):VMBF-0023-2015.

REFERENCES

1. **Aminov RI.** 2010. A brief history of the antibiotic era: lessons learned and challenges for the future. *Front Microbiol* **1:**134.
2. **Cole ST.** 2014. Who will develop new antibacterial agents? *Philos Trans R Soc Lond B Biol Sci* **369:**20130430.
3. **Walsh C.** 2003. Where will new antibiotics come from? *Nat Rev Microbiol* **1:**65–70.
4. **Chang Q, Wang W, Regev-Yochay G, Lipsitch M, Hanage WP.** 2015. Antibiotics in agriculture and the risk to human health: how worried should we be? *Evol Appl* **8:**240–247.
5. **Palumbi SR.** 2001. Humans as the world's greatest evolutionary force. *Science* **293:**1786–1790.
6. **Hampton T.** 2013. Report reveals scope of US antibiotic resistance threat. *JAMA* **310:**1661–1663.
7. **Rasko DA, Sperandio V.** 2010. Anti-virulence strategies to combat bacteria-mediated disease. *Nat Rev Drug Discov* **9:**117–128.
8. **Barczak AK, Hung DT.** 2009. Productive steps toward an antimicrobial targeting virulence. *Curr Opin Microbiol* **12:**490–496.
9. **Lee YM, Almqvist F, Hultgren SJ.** 2003. Targeting virulence for antimicrobial chemotherapy. *Curr Opin Pharmacol* **3:**513–519.
10. **Allen RC, Popat R, Diggle SP, Brown SP.** 2014. Targeting virulence: can we make evolution-proof drugs? *Nat Rev Microbiol* **12:**300–308.
11. **Brown K, Valenta K, Fisman D, Simor A, Daneman N.** 2015. Hospital ward antibiotic prescribing and the risks of *Clostridium difficile* infection. *JAMA Intern Med* **175:**626–633.
12. **Dethlefsen L, Relman DA.** 2011. Incomplete recovery and individualized responses of the human distal gut microbiota to repeated antibiotic perturbation. *Proc Natl Acad Sci USA* **108**(Suppl 1)**:**4554–4561.
13. **Sekirov I, Tam NM, Jogova M, Robertson ML, Li Y, Lupp C, Finlay BB.** 2008. Antibiotic-induced perturbations of the intestinal microbiota alter host susceptibility to enteric infection. *Infect Immun* **76:**4726–4736.
14. **Ubeda C, Taur Y, Jenq RR, Equinda MJ, Son T, Samstein M, Viale A, Socci ND, van den Brink MR, Kamboj M, Pamer EG.** 2010. Vancomycin-resistant *Enterococcus* domination of intestinal microbiota is enabled by antibiotic treatment in mice and precedes bloodstream invasion in humans. *J Clin Invest* **120:**4332–4341.
15. **Keeney KM, Yurist-Doutsch S, Arrieta MC, Finlay BB.** 2014. Effects of antibiotics on human microbiota and subsequent disease. *Annu Rev Microbiol* **68:**217–235.
16. **Vangay P, Ward T, Gerber JS, Knights D.** 2015. Antibiotics, pediatric dysbiosis, and disease. *Cell Host Microbe* **17:**553–564.
17. **Clatworthy AE, Pierson E, Hung DT.** 2007. Targeting virulence: a new paradigm for antimicrobial therapy. *Nat Chem Biol* **3:**541–548.
18. **Turgeon Z, Jorgensen R, Visschedyk D, Edwards PR, Legree S, McGregor C, Fieldhouse RJ, Mangroo D, Schapira M, Merrill AR.** 2011. Newly discovered and characterized antivirulence compounds inhibit bacterial mono-ADP-ribosyltransferase toxins. *Antimicrob Agents Chemother* **55:**983–991.
19. **Kauppi AM, Nordfelth R, Uvell H, Wolf-Watz H, Elofsson M.** 2003. Targeting bacterial virulence: inhibitors of type III secretion in *Yersinia. Chem Biol* **10:**241–249.
20. **Kozel TR.** 2014. The road to toxin-targeted therapeutic antibodies. *MBio* **5:**e01477-14. doi:10.1128/mBio.01477-14.
21. **Nishikawa K, Matsuoka K, Kita E, Okabe N, Mizuguchi M, Hino K, Miyazawa S, Yamasaki C, Aoki J, Takashima S, Yamakawa Y, Nishijima M, Terunuma D, Kuzuhara H, Natori Y.** 2002. A therapeutic agent with oriented carbohydrates for treatment of infections by Shiga toxin-producing *Escherichia coli* O157:H7. *Proc Natl Acad Sci USA* **99:**7669–7674.
22. **Nishikawa K, Matsuoka K, Watanabe M, Igai K, Hino K, Hatano K, Yamada A, Abe N, Terunuma D, Kuzuhara H, Natori Y.** 2005. Identification of the optimal structure required for a Shiga toxin neutralizer with oriented carbohydrates to function in the circulation. *J Infect Dis* **191:**2097–2105.
23. **Migone TS, Subramanian GM, Zhong J, Healey LM, Corey A, Devalaraja M, Lo L, Ullrich S, Zimmerman J, Chen A, Lewis M, Meister G, Gillum K, Sanford D, Mott J, Bolmer SD.** 2009. Raxibacumab for the treatment of inhalational anthrax. *N Engl J Med* **361:**135–144.
24. **Kummerfeldt CE.** 2014. Raxibacumab: potential role in the treatment of inhalational anthrax. *Infect Drug Resist* **7:**101–109.

25. **Migone TS, Bolmer S, Zhong J, Corey A, Vasconcelos D, Buccellato M, Meister G.** 2015. Added benefit of raxibacumab to antibiotic treatment of inhalational anthrax. *Antimicrob Agents Chemother* **59:**1145–1151.

26. **Menard R, Schoenhofen IC, Tao L, Aubry A, Bouchard P, Reid CW, Lachance P, Twine SM, Fulton KM, Cui Q, Hogues H, Purisima EO, Sulea T, Logan SM.** 2014. Small-molecule inhibitors of the pseudaminic acid biosynthetic pathway: targeting motility as a key bacterial virulence factor. *Antimicrob Agents Chemother* **58:**7430–7440.

27. **Goller CC, Seed PC.** 2010. High-throughput identification of chemical inhibitors of *E. coli* group 2 capsule biogenesis as anti-virulence agents. *PLoS One* **5:**e11642. doi:10.1371/journal.pone.0011642.

28. **Proft T, Baker EN.** 2009. Pili in Gram-negative and Gram-positive bacteria: structure, assembly and their role in disease. *Cell Mol Life Sci* **66:**613–635.

29. **Boyle EC, Finlay BB.** 2003. Bacterial pathogenesis: exploiting cellular adherence. *Curr Opin Cell Biol* **15:**633–639.

30. **Chagnot C, Listrat A, Astruc T, Desvaux M.** 2012. Bacterial adhesion to animal tissues: protein determinants for recognition of extracellular matrix components. *Cell Microbiol* **14:**1687–1696.

31. **Ofek I, Beachey EH.** 1980. General concepts and principles of bacterial adherence, p 1–29. *In* Beachey EH (ed), *Bacterial Adherence, Receptors and Recognition*, vol. 6. Chapman and Hall, London.

32. **Ofek I, Doyle RJ.** 1994. *Bacterial Adhesion to Cells and Tissues*, pp 513–561. Chapman & Hall, New York.

33. **Jones CH, Jacob-Dubuisson F, Dodson K, Kuehn M, Slonim L, Striker R, Hultgren SJ.** 1992. Adhesin presentation in bacteria requires molecular chaperones and ushers. *Infect Immun* **60:**4445–4451.

34. **Dam TK, Brewer CF.** 2002. Thermodynamic studies of lectin-carbohydrate interactions by isothermal titration calorimetry. *Chem Rev* **102:**387–429.

35. **Rivera J, Vannakambadi G, Hook M, Speziale P.** 2007. Fibrinogen-binding proteins of Gram-positive bacteria. *Thromb Haemost* **98:**503–511.

36. **Nuccio SP, Baumler AJ.** 2007. Evolution of the chaperone/usher assembly pathway: fimbrial classification goes Greek. *Microbiol Mol Biol Rev* **71:**551–575.

37. **Wurpel DJ, Beatson SA, Totsika M, Petty NK, Schembri MA.** 2013. Chaperone-usher fimbriae of *Escherichia coli*. *PLoS One* **8:**e52835. doi:10.1371/journal.pone.0052835.

38. **Sauer FG, Futterer K, Pinkner JS, Dodson KW, Hultgren SJ, Waksman G.** 1999. Structural basis of chaperone function and pilus biogenesis. *Science* **285:**1058–1061.

39. **Barnhart MM, Pinkner JS, Soto GE, Sauer FG, Langermann S, Waksman G, Frieden C, Hultgren SJ.** 2000. PapD-like chaperones provide the missing information for folding of pilin proteins. *Proc Natl Acad Sci USA* **97:**7709–7714.

40. **Remaut H, Tang C, Henderson NS, Pinkner JS, Wang T, Hultgren SJ, Thanassi DG, Waksman G, Li H.** 2008. Fiber formation across the bacterial outer membrane by the chaperone/usher pathway. *Cell* **133:**640–652.

41. **Phan G, Remaut H, Wang T, Allen WJ, Pirker KF, Lebedev A, Henderson NS, Geibel S, Volkan E, Yan J, Kunze MB, Pinkner JS, Ford B, Kay CW, Li H, Hultgren SJ, Thanassi DG, Waksman G.** Crystal structure of the FimD usher bound to its cognate FimC-FimH substrate. *Nature* **474:**49–53.

42. **Ford B, Rego AT, Ragan TJ, Pinkner J, Dodson K, Driscoll PC, Hultgren S, Waksman G.** Structural homology between the C-terminal domain of the PapC usher and its plug. *J Bacteriol* **192:**1824–1831.

43. **Geibel S, Procko E, Hultgren SJ, Baker D, Waksman G.** 2013. Structural and energetic basis of folded-protein transport by the FimD usher. *Nature* **496:**243–246.

44. **Thanassi DG, Stathopoulos C, Dodson K, Geiger D, Hultgren SJ.** 2002. Bacterial outer membrane ushers contain distinct targeting and assembly domains for pilus biogenesis. *J Bacteriol* **184:**6260–6269.

45. **Volkan E, Kalas V, Pinkner JS, Dodson KW, Henderson NS, Pham T, Waksman G, Delcour AH, Thanassi DG, Hultgren SJ.** 2013. Molecular basis of usher pore gating in *Escherichia coli* pilus biogenesis. *Proc Natl Acad Sci USA* **110:**20741–20746.

46. **Mapingire OS, Henderson NS, Duret G, Thanassi DG, Delcour AH.** 2009. Modulating effects of the plug, helix, and N- and C-terminal domains on channel properties of the PapC usher. *J Biol Chem* **284:**36324–36333.

47. **Sauer FG, Pinkner JS, Waksman G, Hultgren SJ.** 2002. Chaperone priming of pilus subunits facilitates a topological transition that drives fiber formation. *Cell* **111:**543–551.

48. **Barnhart MM, Sauer FG, Pinkner JS, Hultgren SJ.** 2003. Chaperone-subunit-usher interactions required for donor strand exchange during bacterial pilus assembly. *J Bacteriol* **185:**2723–2730.

49. **Remaut H, Rose RJ, Hannan TJ, Hultgren SJ, Radford SE, Ashcroft AE, Waksman G.**

2006. Donor-strand exchange in chaperone-assisted pilus assembly proceeds through a concerted beta strand displacement mechanism. *Mol Cell* **22**:831–842.

50. **Jacob-Dubuisson F, Striker R, Hultgren SJ.** 1994. Chaperone-assisted self-assembly of pili independent of cellular energy. *J Biol Chem* **269**:12447–12455.

51. **Nicolle LE, Committee* ACG.** 2005. Complicated urinary tract infection in adults. *Can J Infect Dis Med Microbiol* **16**:349–360.

52. **Stamm WE, Norrby SR.** 2001. Urinary tract infections: disease panorama and challenges. *J Infect Dis* **183**:S1–S4.

53. **Griebling TL.** 2007. Urinary tract infection in women, p 587–620. *In* Litwin MS, Saigal CS (ed), *Urologic Diseases in Amerca.* U.S. Government Printing Office, Washington, DC.

54. **Foxman B.** 2014. Urinary tract infection syndromes: occurrence, recurrence, bacteriology, risk factors, and disease burden. *Infect Dis Clin North Am* **28**:1–13.

55. **Nielubowicz GR, Mobley HL.** 2010. Host-pathogen interactions in urinary tract infection. *Nat Rev Urol* **7**:430–441.

56. **Puorger C, Vetsch M, Wider G, Glockshuber R.** 2011. Structure, folding and stability of FimA, the main structural subunit of type 1 pili from uropathogenic *Escherichia coli* strains. *J Mol Biol* **412**:520–535.

57. **Jones CH, Pinkner JS, Roth R, Heuser J, Nicholes AV, Abraham SN, Hultgren SJ.** 1995. FimH adhesin of type 1 pili is assembled into a fibrillar tip structure in the *Enterobacteriaceae. Proc Natl Acad Sci USA* **92**:2081–2085.

58. **Anderson GG, Palermo JJ, Schilling JD, Roth R, Heuser J, Hultgren SJ.** 2003. Intracellular bacterial biofilm-like pods in urinary tract infections. *Science* **301**:105–107.

59. **Song J, Bishop BL, Li G, Grady R, Stapleton A, Abraham SN.** 2009. TLR4-mediated expulsion of bacteria from infected bladder epithelial cells. *Proc Natl Acad Sci USA* **106**:14966–14971.

60. **Allison KR, Brynildsen MP, Collins JJ.** 2011. Metabolite-enabled eradication of bacterial persisters by aminoglycosides. *Nature* **473**:216–220.

61. **Schlager TA, LeGallo R, Innes D, Hendley JO, Peters CA.** 2011. B cell infiltration and lymphonodular hyperplasia in bladder submucosa of patients with persistent bacteriuria and recurrent urinary tract infections. *J Urol* **186**:2359–2364.

62. **Hansson S, Hanson E, Hjalmas K, Hultengren M, Jodal U, Olling S, Svanborg-Eden C.** 1990. Follicular cystitis in girls with untreated asymp-tomatic or covert bacteriuria. *J Urol* **143**:330–332.

63. **Rosen DA, Hooton TM, Stamm WE, Humphrey PA, Hultgren SJ.** 2007. Detection of intracellular bacterial communities in human urinary tract infection. *PLoS Med* **4**:e329.

64. **Lanne B, Olsson BM, Jovall PA, Angstrom J, Linder H, Marklund BI, Bergstrom J, Karlsson KA.** 1995. Glycoconjugate receptors for P-fimbriated *Escherichia coli* in the mouse. An animal model of urinary tract infection. *J Biol Chem* **270**:9017–9025.

65. **Lund B, Lindberg F, Marklund BI, Normark S.** 1987. The PapG protein is the alpha-D-galactopyranosyl-(1-4)-beta-D-galactopyranose-binding adhesin of uropathogenic *Escherichia coli. Proc Natl Acad Sci USA* **84**:5898–5902.

66. **Dodson KW, Pinkner JS, Rose T, Magnusson G, Hultgren SJ, Waksman G.** 2001. Structural basis of the interaction of the pyelonephritic *E. coli* adhesin to its human kidney receptor. *Cell* **105**:733–743.

67. **Haslam DB, Baenziger JU.** 1996. Expression cloning of Forssman glycolipid synthetase: a novel member of the histo-blood group ABO gene family. *Proc Natl Acad Sci USA* **93**:10697–10702.

68. **Breimer ME, Karlsson KA.** 1983. Chemical and immunological identification of glycolipid-based blood group ABH and Lewis antigens in human kidney. *Biochim Biophys Acta* **755**:170–177.

69. **Breimer ME, Hansson GC, Leffler H.** 1985. The specific glycosphingolipid composition of human ureteral epithelial cells. *J Biochem* **98**:1169–1180.

70. **Yanagawa R, Otsuki K, Tokui T.** 1968. Electron microscopy of fine structure of *Corynebacterium renale* with special reference to pili. *Jpn J Vet Res* **16**:31–37.

71. **Ton-That H, Schneewind O.** 2003. Assembly of pili on the surface of *Corynebacterium diphtheriae. Mol Microbiol* **50**:1429–1438.

72. **Ton-That H, Marraffini LA, Schneewind O.** 2004. Sortases and pilin elements involved in pilus assembly of *Corynebacterium diphtheriae. Mol Microbiol* **53**:251–261.

73. **Ton-That H, Schneewind O.** 2004. Assembly of pili in Gram-positive bacteria. *Trends Microbiol* **12**:228–234.

74. **Fischetti VA, Pancholi V, Schneewind O.** 1990. Conservation of a hexapeptide sequence in the anchor region of surface proteins from Gram-positive cocci. *Mol Microbiol* **4**:1603–1605.

75. **Guttilla IK, Gaspar AH, Swierczynski A, Swaminathan A, Dwivedi P, Das A, Ton-That H.** 2009. Acyl enzyme intermediates in sortase-

catalyzed pilus morphogenesis in Gram-positive bacteria. *J Bacteriol* **191**:5603–5612.

76. **Schneewind O, Missiakas D.** 2014. Sec-secretion and sortase-mediated anchoring of proteins in Gram-positive bacteria. *Biochim Biophys Acta* **1843**:1687–1697.

77. **Kang HJ, Coulibaly F, Clow F, Proft T, Baker EN.** 2007. Stabilizing isopeptide bonds revealed in Gram-positive bacterial pilus structure. *Science* **318**:1625–1628.

78. **Mandlik A, Swierczynski A, Das A, Ton-That H.** 2008. Pili in Gram-positive bacteria: assembly, involvement in colonization and biofilm development. *Trends Microbiol* **16**:33–40.

79. **Vengadesan K, Narayana SV.** 2011. Structural biology of Gram-positive bacterial adhesins. *Protein Sci* **20**:759–772.

80. **Dramsi S, Caliot E, Bonne I, Guadagnini S, Prevost MC, Kojadinovic M, Lalioui L, Poyart C, Trieu-Cuot P.** 2006. Assembly and role of pili in group B streptococci. *Mol Microbiol* **60**:1401–1413.

81. **Barocchi MA, Ries J, Zogaj X, Hemsley C, Albiger B, Kanth A, Dahlberg S, Fernebro J, Moschioni M, Masignani V, Hultenby K, Taddei AR, Beiter K, Wartha F, von Euler A, Covacci A, Holden DW, Normark S, Rappuoli R, Henriques-Normark B.** 2006. A pneumococcal pilus influences virulence and host inflammatory responses. *Proc Natl Acad Sci USA* **103**:2857–2862.

82. **Flores-Mireles AL, Pinkner JS, Caparon MG, Hultgren SJ.** 2014. EbpA vaccine antibodies block binding of *Enterococcus faecalis* to fibrinogen to prevent catheter-associated bladder infection in mice. *Sci Transl Med* **6**:254ra127.

83. **Nielsen HV, Guiton PS, Kline KA, Port GC, Pinkner JS, Neiers F, Normark S, Henriques-Normark B, Caparon MG, Hultgren SJ.** 2012. The metal ion-dependent adhesion site motif of the *Enterococcus faecalis* EbpA pilin mediates pilus function in catheter-associated urinary tract infection. *MBio* **3**:e00177-00112. doi:10.1128/mBio.00177-12.

84. **Nallapareddy SR, Singh KV, Sillanpaa J, Garsin DA, Hook M, Erlandsen SL, Murray BE.** 2006. Endocarditis and biofilm-associated pili of *Enterococcus faecalis*. *J Clin Invest* **116**:2799–2807.

85. **Paganelli FL, Willems RJ, Leavis HL.** 2012. Optimizing future treatment of enterococcal infections: attacking the biofilm? *Trends Microbiol* **20**:40–49.

86. **Hollenbeck BL, Rice LB.** 2012. Intrinsic and acquired resistance mechanisms in enterococcus. *Virulence* **3**:421–433.

87. **Parker D, Callan L, Harwood J, Thompson D, Webb ML, Wilde M, Willson M.** 2009. Catheter-associated urinary tract infections: fact sheet. *J Wound Ostomy Continence Nurs.* http://www.wocn.org/news/67129/New-Fact-Sheet---Catheter-Associated-Urinary-Tract-Infections.htm.

88. **Guiton PS, Hung CS, Hancock L, Caparon MG, Hultgren SJ.** 2010. Enterococcal biofilm formation and virulence in an optimized murine model of foreign body-associated urinary tract infections. *Infect Immun* **78**:4166–4175.

89. **Guiton PS, Hannan TJ, Ford B, Caparon MG, Hultgren SJ.** 2013. *Enterococcus faecalis* overcomes foreign body-mediated inflammation to establish urinary tract infections. *Infect Immun* **81**:329–339.

90. **Delnay KM, Stonehill WH, Goldman H, Jukkola AF, Dmochowski RR.** 1999. Bladder histological changes associated with chronic indwelling urinary catheter. *J Urol* **161**:1106–1108; discussion 1108–1109.

91. **Peychl L, Zalud R.** 2008. Changes in the urinary bladder caused by short-term permanent catheter insertion. *Cas Lek Cesk* **147**:325–329. [In Czech.]

92. **Hart JA.** 1985. The urethral catheter: a review of its implication in urinary-tract infection. *Int J Nurs Stud* **22**:57–70.

93. **Nielsen HV, Flores-Mireles AL, Kau AL, Kline KA, Pinkner JS, Neiers F, Normark S, Henriques-Normark B, Caparon MG, Hultgren SJ.** 2013. Pilin and sortase residues critical for endocarditis- and biofilm-associated pilus biogenesis in Enterococcus faecalis. *J Bacteriol* **195**:4484–4495.

94. **Whittaker CA, Hynes RO.** 2002. Distribution and evolution of von Willebrand/integrin A domains: widely dispersed domains with roles in cell adhesion and elsewhere. *Mol Biol Cell* **13**:3369–3387.

95. **Wilson M.** 2001. Bacterial biofilms and human disease. *Sci Prog* **84**:235–254.

96. **Donlan RM, Costerton JW.** 2002. Biofilms: survival mechanisms of clinically relevant microorganisms. *Clin Microbiol Rev* **15**:167–193.

97. **O'Toole G, Kaplan HB, Kolter R.** 2000. Biofilm formation as microbial development. *Annu Rev Microbiol* **54**:49–79.

98. **Kierek-Pearson K, Karatan E.** 2005. Biofilm development in bacteria. *Adv Appl Microbiol* **57**:79–111.

99. **Kline KA, Dodson KW, Caparon MG, Hultgren SJ.** 2010. A tale of two pili: assembly and function of pili in bacteria. *Trends Microbiol* **18**:224–232.

100. **Van Houdt R, Michiels CW.** 2005. Role of bacterial cell surface structures in *Escherichia coli* biofilm formation. *Res Microbiol* **156**:626–633.

101. Konto-Ghiorghi Y, Mairey E, Mallet A, Dumenil G, Caliot E, Trieu-Cuot P, Dramsi S. 2009. Dual role for pilus in adherence to epithelial cells and biofilm formation in *Streptococcus agalactiae*. *PLoS Pathog* **5**:e1000422. doi:10.1371/journal.ppat.1000422.

102. Diggle SP, Stacey RE, Dodd C, Camara M, Williams P, Winzer K. 2006. The galactophilic lectin, LecA, contributes to biofilm development in *Pseudomonas aeruginosa*. *Environ Microbiol* **8**:1095–1104.

103. Tielker D, Hacker S, Loris R, Strathmann M, Wingender J, Wilhelm S, Rosenau F, Jaeger KE. 2005. *Pseudomonas aeruginosa* lectin LecB is located in the outer membrane and is involved in biofilm formation. *Microbiology* **151**:1313–1323.

104. Orndorff PE, Devapali A, Palestrant S, Wyse A, Everett ML, Bollinger RR, Parker W. 2004. Immunoglobulin-mediated agglutination of and biofilm formation by *Escherichia coli* K-12 require the type 1 pilus fiber. *Infect Immun* **72**:1929–1938.

105. Lebeaux D, Ghigo JM, Beloin C. 2014. Biofilm-related infections: bridging the gap between clinical management and fundamental aspects of recalcitrance toward antibiotics. *Microbiol Mol Biol Rev* **78**:510–543.

106. Costerton JW, Stewart PS, Greenberg EP. 1999. Bacterial biofilms: a common cause of persistent infections. *Science* **284**:1318–1322.

107. del Pozo JL, Patel R. 2007. The challenge of treating biofilm-associated bacterial infections. *Clin Pharmacol Ther* **82**:204–209.

108. Lewis K. 2008. Multidrug tolerance of biofilms and persister cells. *Curr Top Microbiol Immunol* **322**:107–131.

109. Olsen A, Jonsson A, Normark S. 1989. Fibronectin binding mediated by a novel class of surface organelles on *Escherichia coli*. *Nature* **338**:652–655.

110. Hung C, Zhou Y, Pinkner JS, Dodson KW, Crowley JR, Heuser J, Chapman MR, Hadjifrangiskou M, Henderson JP, Hultgren SJ. 2013. *Escherichia coli* biofilms have an organized and complex extracellular matrix structure. *MBio* **4**:e00645-13. doi:10.1128/mBio.00645-13.

111. Rapsinski GJ, Wynosky-Dolfi MA, Oppong GO, Tursi SA, Wilson RP, Brodsky IE, Tukel C. 2015. Toll-like receptor 2 and NLRP3 cooperate to recognize a functional bacterial amyloid, curli. *Infect Immun* **83**:693–701.

112. Chapman MR, Robinson LS, Pinkner JS, Roth R, Heuser J, Hammar M, Normark S, Hultgren SJ. 2002. Role of *Escherichia coli* curli operons in directing amyloid fiber formation. *Science* **295**:851–855.

113. Blanco LP, Evans ML, Smith DR, Badtke MP, Chapman MR. 2012. Diversity, biogenesis and function of microbial amyloids. *Trends Microbiol* **20**:66–73.

114. DePas WH, Chapman MR. 2012. Microbial manipulation of the amyloid fold. *Res Microbiol* **163**:592–606.

115. Evans ML, Chapman MR. 2014. Curli biogenesis: order out of disorder. *Biochim Biophys Acta* **1843**:1551–1558.

116. Wang X, Chapman MR. 2008. Curli provide the template for understanding controlled amyloid propagation. *Prion* **2**:57–60.

117. Nenninger AA, Robinson LS, Hultgren SJ. 2009. Localized and efficient curli nucleation requires the chaperone-like amyloid assembly protein CsgF. *Proc Natl Acad Sci USA* **106**:900–905.

118. Nenninger AA, Robinson LS, Hammer ND, Epstein EA, Badtke MP, Hultgren SJ, Chapman MR. 2011. CsgE is a curli secretion specificity factor that prevents amyloid fibre aggregation. *Mol Microbiol* **81**:486–499.

119. Robinson LS, Ashman EM, Hultgren SJ, Chapman MR. 2006. Secretion of curli fibre subunits is mediated by the outer membrane-localized CsgG protein. *Mol Microbiol* **59**:870–881.

120. Goyal P, Krasteva PV, Van Gerven N, Gubellini F, Van den Broeck I, Troupiotis-Tsaikali A, Jonckheere W, Pehau-Arnaudet G, Pinkner JS, Chapman MR, Hultgren SJ, Howorka S, Fronzes R, Remaut H. 2014. Structural and mechanistic insights into the bacterial amyloid secretion channel CsgG. *Nature* **516**:250–253.

121. Hammer ND, McGuffie BA, Zhou Y, Badtke MP, Reinke AA, Brannstrom K, Gestwicki JE, Olofsson A, Almqvist F, Chapman MR. 2012. The C-terminal repeating units of CsgB direct bacterial functional amyloid nucleation. *J Mol Biol* **422**:376–389.

122. Shu Q, Crick SL, Pinkner JS, Ford B, Hultgren SJ, Frieden C. 2012. The *E. coli* CsgB nucleator of curli assembles to beta-sheet oligomers that alter the CsgA fibrillization mechanism. *Proc Natl Acad Sci USA* **109**:6502–6507.

123. Hammer ND, Schmidt JC, Chapman MR. 2007. The curli nucleator protein, CsgB, contains an amyloidogenic domain that directs CsgA polymerization. *Proc Natl Acad Sci USA* **104**:12494–12499.

124. Saldana Z, Xicohtencatl-Cortes J, Avelino F, Phillips AD, Kaper JB, Puente JL, Giron JA. 2009. Synergistic role of curli and cellulose in cell adherence and biofilm formation of

attaching and effacing *Escherichia coli* and identification of Fis as a negative regulator of curli. *Environ Microbiol* **11**:992–1006.

125. **Oppong GO, Rapsinski GJ, Newman TN, Nishimori JH, Biesecker SG, Tukel C.** 2013. Epithelial cells augment barrier function via activation of the Toll-like receptor 2/ phosphatidylinositol 3-kinase pathway upon recognition of *Salmonella enterica* serovar Typhimurium curli fibrils in the gut. *Infect Immun* **81**:478–486.

126. **Cegelski L, Pinkner JS, Hammer ND, Cusumano CK, Hung CS, Chorell E, Aberg V, Walker JN, Seed PC, Almqvist F, Chapman MR, Hultgren SJ.** 2009. Small-molecule inhibitors target *Escherichia coli* amyloid biogenesis and biofilm formation. *Nat Chem Biol* **5**:913–919.

127. **Kai-Larsen Y, Luthje P, Chromek M, Peters V, Wang X, Holm A, Kadas L, Hedlund KO, Johansson J, Chapman MR, Jacobson SH, Romling U, Agerberth B, Brauner A.** 2010. Uropathogenic *Escherichia coli* modulates immune responses and its curli fimbriae interact with the antimicrobial peptide LL-37. *PLoS Pathog* **6**: e1001010. doi:10.1371/journal.ppat.1001010.

128. **Arnqvist A, Olsen A, Pfieffer J, Russel DG, Normark S.** 1992. The Crl protein activates cryptic genes for curli formation and fibronectin binding in *Escherichia coli*. *Mol Microbiol* **6**:2443–2453.

129. **Hammar M, Arnqvist A, Bian Z, Olsen A, Normark S.** 1995. Expression of two csg operons is required for production of fibronectin- and congo red-binding curli polymers in *Escherichia coli* K-12. *Mol Microbiol* **18**:661–670.

130. **Juliano RL.** 2002. Signal transduction by cell adhesion receptors and the cytoskeleton: functions of integrins, cadherins, selectins, and immunoglobulin-superfamily members. *Annu Rev Pharmacol Toxicol* **42**:283–323.

131. **Finlay BB.** 1997. Interactions of enteric pathogens with human epithelial cells. Bacterial exploitation of host processes. *Adv Exp Med Biol* **412**:289–293.

132. **Finlay BB, Cossart P.** 1997. Exploitation of mammalian host cell functions by bacterial pathogens. *Science* **276**:718–725.

133. **Schulte R, Kerneis S, Klinke S, Bartels H, Preger S, Kraehenbuhl JP, Pringault E, Autenrieth IB.** 2000. Translocation of *Yersinia entrocolitica* across reconstituted intestinal epithelial monolayers is triggered by *Yersinia* invasin binding to beta1 integrins apically expressed on M-like cells. *Cell Microbiol* **2**:173–185.

134. **Isberg RR, Leong JM.** 1990. Multiple beta 1 chain integrins are receptors for invasin, a protein that promotes bacterial penetration into mammalian cells. *Cell* **60**:861–871.

135. **Cossart P, Pizarro-Cerda J, Lecuit M.** 2003. Invasion of mammalian cells by *Listeria monocytogenes*: functional mimicry to subvert cellular functions. *Trends Cell Biol* **13**:23–31.

136. **Chemani C, Imberty A, de Bentzmann S, Pierre M, Wimmerova M, Guery BP, Faure K.** 2009. Role of LecA and LecB lectins in *Pseudomonas aeruginosa*-induced lung injury and effect of carbohydrate ligands. *Infect Immun* **77**:2065–2075.

137. **Fagon JY, Chastre J, Domart Y, Trouillet JL, Gibert C.** 1996. Mortality due to ventilator-associated pneumonia or colonization with *Pseudomonas* or *Acinetobacter* species: assessment by quantitative culture of samples obtained by a protected specimen brush. *Clin Infect Dis* **23**:538–542.

138. **Lyczak JB, Cannon CL, Pier GB.** 2002. Lung infections associated with cystic fibrosis. *Clin Microbiol Rev* **15**:194–222.

139. **Murray TS, Egan M, Kazmierczak BI.** 2007. *Pseudomonas aeruginosa* chronic colonization in cystic fibrosis patients. *Curr Opin Pediatr* **19**:83–88.

140. **Garcia-Medina R, Dunne WM, Singh PK, Brody SL.** 2005. *Pseudomonas aeruginosa* acquires biofilm-like properties within airway epithelial cells. *Infect Immun* **73**:8298–8305.

141. **Smith EE, Buckley DG, Wu Z, Saenphimmachak C, Hoffman LR, D'Argenio DA, Miller SI, Ramsey BW, Speert DP, Moskowitz SM, Burns JL, Kaul R, Olson MV.** 2006. Genetic adaptation by *Pseudomonas aeruginosa* to the airways of cystic fibrosis patients. *Proc Natl Acad Sci USA* **103**:8487–8492.

142. **Gellatly SL, Hancock RE.** 2013. *Pseudomonas aeruginosa*: new insights into pathogenesis and host defenses. *Pathog Dis* **67**:159–173.

143. **Bajolet-Laudinat O, Girod-de Bentzmann S, Tournier JM, Madoulet C, Plotkowski MC, Chippaux C, Puchelle E.** 1994. Cytotoxicity of *Pseudomonas aeruginosa* internal lectin PA-I to respiratory epithelial cells in primary culture. *Infect Immun* **62**:4481–4487.

144. **Cioci G, Mitchell EP, Gautier C, Wimmerova M, Sudakevitz D, Perez S, Gilboa-Garber N, Imberty A.** 2003. Structural basis of calcium and galactose recognition by the lectin PA-IL of *Pseudomonas aeruginosa*. *FEBS Lett* **555**:297–301.

145. **Mitchell E, Houles C, Sudakevitz D, Wimmerova M, Gautier C, Perez S, Wu AM, Gilboa-Garber N, Imberty A.** 2002. Structural basis for oligosaccharide-mediated adhesion of *Pseudomonas aeruginosa* in the lungs of cystic fibrosis patients. *Nat Struct Biol* **9**:918–921.

146. **Glick J, Garber N.** 1983. The intracellular localization of *Pseudomonas aeruginosa* lectins. *J Gen Microbiol* **129:**3085–3090.

147. **Chen CP, Song SC, Gilboa-Garber N, Chang KS, Wu AM.** 1998. Studies on the binding site of the galactose-specific agglutinin PA-IL from *Pseudomonas aeruginosa. Glycobiology* **8:**7–16.

148. **Lanne B, Ciopraga J, Bergstrom J, Motas C, Karlsson KA.** 1994. Binding of the galactose-specific *Pseudomonas aeruginosa* lectin, PA-I, to glycosphingolipids and other glycoconjugates. *Glycoconj J* **11:**292–298.

149. **Wu AM, Wu JH, Singh T, Liu JH, Tsai MS, Gilboa-Garber N.** 2006. Interactions of the fucose-specific *Pseudomonas aeruginosa* lectin, PA-IIL, with mammalian glycoconjugates bearing polyvalent Lewis(a) and ABH blood group glycotopes. *Biochimie* **88:**1479–1492.

150. **Pinkner JS, Remaut H, Buelens F, Miller E, Aberg V, Pemberton N, Hedenstrom M, Larsson A, Seed P, Waksman G, Hultgren SJ, Almqvist F.** 2006. Rationally designed small compounds inhibit pilus biogenesis in uropathogenic bacteria. *Proc Natl Acad Sci USA* **103:**17897–17902.

151. **Svensson A, Larsson A, Emtenas H, Hedenstrom M, Fex T, Hultgren SJ, Pinkner JS, Almqvist F, Kihlberg J.** 2001. Design and evaluation of pilicides: potential novel antibacterial agents directed against uropathogenic *Escherichia coli. Chembiochem* **2:**915–918.

152. **Chorell E, Pinkner JS, Phan G, Edvinsson S, Buelens F, Remaut H, Waksman G, Hultgren SJ, Almqvist F.** Design and synthesis of C-2 substituted thiazolo and dihydrothiazolo ring-fused 2-pyridones: pilicides with increased antivirulence activity. *J Med Chem* **53:**5690–5695.

153. **Greene SE, Pinkner JS, Chorell E, Dodson KW, Shaffer CL, Conover MS, Livny J, Hadjifrangiskou M, Almqvist F, Hultgren SJ.** 2014. Pilicide ec240 disrupts virulence circuits in uropathogenic *Escherichia coli. MBio* **5:**e02038. doi:10.1128/mBio.02038-14.

154. **Piatek R, Zalewska-Piatek B, Dzierzbicka K, Makowiec S, Pilipczuk J, Szemiako K, Cyranka-Czaja A, Wojciechowski M.** 2013. Pilicides inhibit the FGL chaperone/usher assisted biogenesis of the Dr fimbrial polyadhesin from uropathogenic *Escherichia coli. BMC Microbiol* **13:**131.

155. **Lo AW, Van de Water K, Gane PJ, Chan AW, Steadman D, Stevens K, Selwood DL, Waksman G, Remaut H.** 2014. Suppression of type 1 pilus assembly in uropathogenic *Escherichia coli* by chemical inhibition of subunit polymerization. *J Antimicrob Chemother* **69:**1017–1026.

156. **Munera D, Hultgren S, Fernandez LA.** 2007. Recognition of the N-terminal lectin domain of FimH adhesin by the usher FimD is required for type 1 pilus biogenesis. *Mol Microbiol* **64:**333–346.

157. **Nishiyama M, Ishikawa T, Rechsteiner H, Glockshuber R.** 2008. Reconstitution of pilus assembly reveals a bacterial outer membrane catalyst. *Science* **320:**376–379.

158. **Andersson EK, Bengtsson C, Evans ML, Chorell E, Sellstedt M, Lindgren AE, Hufnagel DA, Bhattacharya M, Tessier PM, Wittung-Stafshede P, Almqvist F, Chapman MR.** 2013. Modulation of curli assembly and pellicle biofilm formation by chemical and protein chaperones. *Chem Biol* **20:**1245–1254.

159. **Aberg V, Norman F, Chorell E, Westermark A, Olofsson A, Sauer-Eriksson AE, Almqvist F.** 2005. Microwave-assisted decarboxylation of bicyclic 2-pyridone scaffolds and identification of Abeta-peptide aggregation inhibitors. *Org Biomol Chem* **3:**2817–2823.

160. **Horvath I, Sellstedt M, Weise C, Nordvall LM, Krishna Prasad G, Olofsson A, Larsson G, Almqvist F, Wittung-Stafshede P.** 2013. Modulation of alpha-synuclein fibrillization by ring-fused 2-pyridones: templation and inhibition involve oligomers with different structure. *Arch Biochem Biophys* **532:**84–90.

161. **Mazmanian SK, Liu G, Ton-That H, Schneewind O.** 1999. *Staphylococcus aureus* sortase, an enzyme that anchors surface proteins to the cell wall. *Science* **285:**760–763.

162. **Maresso AW, Chapa TJ, Schneewind O.** 2006. Surface protein IsdC and sortase B are required for heme-iron scavenging of *Bacillus anthracis. J Bacteriol* **188:**8145–8152.

163. **Marraffini LA, Schneewind O.** 2006. Targeting proteins to the cell wall of sporulating *Bacillus anthracis. Mol Microbiol* **62:**1402–1417.

164. **Mazmanian SK, Liu G, Jensen ER, Lenoy E, Schneewind O.** 2000. *Staphylococcus aureus* sortase mutants defective in the display of surface proteins and in the pathogenesis of animal infections. *Proc Natl Acad Sci USA* **97:**5510–5515.

165. **Guiton P, Hung C, Kline K, Roth R, Kau A, Hayes E, Heuser J, Dodson K, Caparon M, Hultgren S.** 2009. Contribution of autolysin and sortase A during *Enterococcus faecalis* DNA-dependent biofilm development. *Infect Immun* **77:**3626–3638.

166. **Kim SW, Chang IM, Oh KB.** 2002. Inhibition of the bacterial surface protein anchoring transpeptidase sortase by medicinal plants. *Biosci Biotechnol Biochem* **66:**2751–2754.

167. **Kim SH, Shin DS, Oh MN, Chung SC, Lee JS, Oh KB.** 2004. Inhibition of the bacterial surface protein anchoring transpeptidase sortase

by isoquinoline alkaloids. *Biosci Biotechnol Biochem* **68:**421–424.

168. **Kim SH, Shin DS, Oh MN, Chung SC, Lee JS, Chang IM, Oh KB.** 2003. Inhibition of sortase, a bacterial surface protein anchoring transpeptidase, by beta-sitosterol-3-O-glucopyranoside from *Fritillaria verticillata*. *Biosci Biotechnol Biochem* **67:**2477–2479.

169. **Maresso AW, Wu R, Kern JW, Zhang R, Janik D, Missiakas DM, Duban ME, Joachimiak A, Schneewind O.** 2007. Activation of inhibitors by sortase triggers irreversible modification of the active site. *J Biol Chem* **282:**23129–23139.

170. **Zhang J, Liu H, Zhu K, Gong S, Dramsi S, Wang YT, Li J, Chen F, Zhang R, Zhou L, Lan L, Jiang H, Schneewind O, Luo C, Yang CG.** 2014. Antiinfective therapy with a small molecule inhibitor of *Staphylococcus aureus* sortase. *Proc Natl Acad Sci USA* **111:**13517–13522.

171. **Falugi F, Kim HK, Missiakas DM, Schneewind O.** 2013. Role of protein A in the evasion of host adaptive immune responses by *Staphylococcus aureus*. *MBio* **4:**e00575-13. doi:10.1128/mBio.00575-13.

172. **Ashkar AA, Mossman KL, Coombes BK, Gyles CL, Mackenzie R.** 2008. FimH adhesin of type 1 fimbriae is a potent inducer of innate antimicrobial responses which requires TLR4 and type 1 interferon signalling. *PLoS Pathog* **4:**e1000233. doi:10.1371/journal.ppat.1000233.

173. **Pak J, Pu Y, Zhang ZT, Hasty DL, Wu XR.** 2001. Tamm-Horsfall protein binds to type 1 fimbriated *Escherichia coli* and prevents *E. coli* from binding to uroplakin Ia and Ib receptors. *J Biol Chem* **276:**9924–9930.

174. **Wu XR, Sun TT, Medina JJ.** 1996. *In vitro* binding of type 1-fimbriated *Escherichia coli* to uroplakins Ia and Ib: relation to urinary tract infections. *Proc Natl Acad Sci USA* **93:**9630–9635.

175. **Eto DS, Jones TA, Sundsbak JL, Mulvey MA.** 2007. Integrin-mediated host cell invasion by type 1-piliated uropathogenic *Escherichia coli*. *PLoS Pathog* **3:**e100.

176. **Choudhury D, Thompson A, Stojanoff V, Langermann S, Pinkner J, Hultgren SJ, Knight SD.** 1999. X-ray structure of the FimC-FimH chaperone-adhesin complex from uropathogenic *Escherichia coli*. *Science* **285:**1061–1066.

177. **Hung C-S, Bouckaert J, Hung D, Pinkner J, Widberg C, De Fusco A, Auguste CG, Strouse B, Langerman S, Waksman G, Hultgren SJ.** 2002. Structural basis of tropism of *Escherichia coli* to the bladder during urinary tract infection. *Mol Microbiol* **44:**903–915.

178. **Bouckaert J, Berglund J, Schembri M, De Genst E, Cools L, Wuhrer M, Hung CS, Pinkner J, Slattegard R, Zavialov A, Choudhury D, Langermann S, Hultgren SJ, Wyns L, Klemm P, Oscarson S, Knight SD, De Greve H.** 2005. Receptor binding studies disclose a novel class of high-affinity inhibitors of the *Escherichia coli* FimH adhesin. *Mol Microbiol* **55:**441–455.

179. **Chen SL, Hung CS, Pinkner JS, Walker JN, Cusumano CK, Li Z, Bouckaert J, Gordon JI, Hultgren SJ.** 2009. Positive selection identifies an *in vivo* role for FimH during urinary tract infection in addition to mannose binding. *Proc Natl Acad Sci USA* **106:**22439–22444.

180. **Wellens A, Garofalo C, Nguyen H, Van Gerven N, Slattegard R, Hernalsteens JP, Wyns L, Oscarson S, De Greve H, Hultgren S, Bouckaert J.** 2008. Intervening with urinary tract infections using anti-adhesives based on the crystal structure of the FimH-oligomannose-3 complex. *PLoS One* **3:**e2040. doi:10.1371/journal.pone.0002040.

181. **Han Z, Pinkner JS, Ford B, Obermann R, Nolan W, Wildman SA, Hobbs D, Ellenberger T, Cusumano CK, Hultgren SJ, Janetka JW.** 2010. Structure-based drug design and optimization of mannoside bacterial FimH antagonists. *J Med Chem* **53:**4779–4792.

182. **Schwardt O, Rabbani S, Hartmann M, Abgottspon D, Wittwer M, Kleeb S, Zalewski A, Smiesko M, Cutting B, Ernst B.** 2011. Design, synthesis and biological evaluation of mannosyl triazoles as FimH antagonists. *Bioorg Med Chem* **19:**6454–6473.

183. **Klein T, Abgottspon D, Wittwer M, Rabbani S, Herold J, Jiang X, Kleeb S, Lüthi C, Scharenberg M, Bezençon J, Gubler E, Pang L, Smiesko M, Cutting B, Schwardt O, Ernst B.** 2010. FimH antagonists for the oral treatment of urinary tract infections: from design and synthesis to *in vitro* and *in vivo* evaluation. *J Med Chem* **53:**8627–8641.

184. **Abgottspon D, Rolli G, Hosch L, Steinhuber A, Jiang X, Schwardt O, Cutting B, Smiesko M, Jenal U, Ernst B, Trampuz A.** 2010. Development of an aggregation assay to screen FimH antagonists. *J Microbiol Methods* **82:**249–255.

185. **Scharenberg M, Abgottspon D, Cicek E, Jiang X, Schwardt O, Rabbani S, Ernst B.** 2011. A flow cytometry-based assay for screening FimH antagonists. *Assay Drug Dev Technol* **9:**455–464.

186. **Klein T, Abgottspon D, Wittwer M, Rabbani S, Herold J, Jiang X, Kleeb S, Luthi C, Scharenberg M, Bezencon J, Gubler E, Pang L, Smiesko M, Cutting B, Schwardt O,**

Ernst B. 2010. FimH antagonists for the oral treatment of urinary tract infections: from design and synthesis to *in vitro* and *in vivo* evaluation. *J Med Chem* **53:**8627–8641.

187. **Kleeb S, Pang L, Mayer K, Eris D, Sigl A, Preston RC, Zihlmann P, Sharpe T, Jakob RP, Abgottspon D, Hutter AS, Scharenberg M, Jiang X, Navarra G, Rabbani S, Smiesko M, Ludin N, Bezencon J, Schwardt O, Maier T, Ernst B.** 2015. FimH antagonists: bioisosteres to improve the *in vitro* and *in vivo* PK/PD profile. *J Med Chem* **58:**2221–2239.

188. **Cusumano CK, Pinkner JS, Han Z, Greene SA, Ford BA, Crowley JR, Henderson JP, Janetka JW, Hultgren SJ.** 2011. Treatment and prevention of urinary tract infection with orally active FimH inhibitors. *Sci Transl Med* **3:**109–115.

189. **Guiton PS, Cusumano CK, Kline KA, Dodson KW, Han Z, Janetka JW, Henderson JP, Caparon MG, Hultgren SJ.** 2012. Combinatorial small-molecule therapy prevents uropathogenic *Escherichia coli* catheter-associated urinary tract infections in mice. *Antimicrob Agents Chemother* **56:**4738–4745.

190. **Bouckaert J, Li Z, Xavier C, Almant M, Caveliers V, Lahoutte T, Weeks SD, Kovensky J, Gouin SG.** 2013. Heptyl alpha-D-mannosides grafted on a beta-cyclodextrin core to interfere with *Escherichia coli* adhesion: an *in vivo* multivalent effect. *Chemistry* **19:**7847–7855.

191. **Kadam RU, Bergmann M, Hurley M, Garg D, Cacciarini M, Swiderska MA, Nativi C, Sattler M, Smyth AR, Williams P, Camara M, Stocker A, Darbre T, Reymond JL.** 2011. A glycopeptide dendrimer inhibitor of the galactose-specific lectin LecA and of *Pseudomonas aeruginosa* biofilms. *Angew Chem Int Ed Engl* **50:**10631–10635.

192. **Perret S, Sabin C, Dumon C, Pokorna M, Gautier C, Galanina O, Ilia S, Bovin N, Nicaise M, Desmadril M, Gilboa-Garber N, Wimmerova M, Mitchell EP, Imberty A.** 2005. Structural basis for the interaction between human milk oligosaccharides and the bacterial lectin PA-IIL of *Pseudomonas aeruginosa*. *Biochem J* **389:**325–332.

193. **Boukerb AM, Rousset A, Galanos N, Mear JB, Thepaut M, Grandjean T, Gillon E, Cecioni S, Abderrahmen C, Faure K, Redelberger D, Kipnis E, Dessein R, Havet S, Darblade B, Matthews SE, de Bentzmann S, Guery B, Cournoyer B, Imberty A, Vidal S.** 2014. Antiadhesive properties of glycoclusters against *Pseudomonas aeruginosa* lung infection. *J Med Chem* **57:**10275–10289.

194. **Kadam RU, Garg D, Schwartz J, Visini R, Sattler M, Stocker A, Darbre T, Reymond**
JL. 2013. CH-pi "T-shape" interaction with histidine explains binding of aromatic galactosides to *Pseudomonas aeruginosa* lectin LecA. *ACS Chem Biol* **8:**1925–1930.

195. **Hauck D, Joachim I, Frommeyer B, Varrot A, Philipp B, Moller HM, Imberty A, Exner TE, Titz A.** 2013. Discovery of two classes of potent glycomimetic inhibitors of *Pseudomonas aeruginosa* LecB with distinct binding modes. *ACS Chem Biol* **8:**1775–1784.

196. **Hofmann A, Sommer R, Hauck D, Stifel J, Gottker-Schnetmann I, Titz A.** 2015. Synthesis of mannoheptose derivatives and their evaluation as inhibitors of the lectin LecB from the opportunistic pathogen *Pseudomonas aeruginosa*. *Carbohydr Res* **412:**34–42.

197. **Krachler AM, Ham H, Orth K.** 2011. Outer membrane adhesion factor multivalent adhesion molecule 7 initiates host cell binding during infection by Gram-negative pathogens. *Proc Natl Acad Sci USA* **108:**11614–11619.

198. **Krachler AM, Orth K.** 2011. Functional characterization of the interaction between bacterial adhesin multivalent adhesion molecule 7 (MAM7) protein and its host cell ligands. *J Biol Chem* **286:**38939–38947.

199. **Krachler AM, Mende K, Murray C, Orth K.** 2012. *In vitro* characterization of multivalent adhesion molecule 7-based inhibition of multidrug-resistant bacteria isolated from wounded military personnel. *Virulence* **3:**389–399.

200. **Hawley CA, Watson CA, Orth K, Krachler AM.** 2013. A MAM7 peptide-based inhibitor of *Staphylococcus aureus* adhesion does not interfere with *in vitro* host cell function. *PLoS One* **8:** e81216. doi:10.1371/journal.pone.0081216.

201. **Kisiela DI, Avagyan H, Friend D, Jalan A, Gupta S, Interlandi G, Liu Y, Tchesnokova V, Rodriguez VB, Sumida JP, Strong RK, Wu XR, Thomas WE, Sokurenko EV.** 2015. Inhibition and reversal of microbial attachment by an antibody with parasteric activity against the FimH adhesin of uropathogenic *E. coli*. *PLoS Pathog* **11:**e1004857. doi:10.1371/journal.ppat.1004857.

202. **Langermann S, Palaszynski S, Barnhart M, Auguste G, Pinkner JS, Burlein J, Barren P, Koenig S, Leath S, Jones CH, Hultgren SJ.** 1997. Prevention of mucosal *Escherichia coli* infection by FimH-adhesin-based systemic vaccination. *Science* **276:**607–611.

203. **Langermann S, Mollby R, Burlein JE, Palaszynski SR, Auguste CG, DeFusco A, Strouse R, Schenerman MA, Hultgren SJ, Pinkner JS, Winberg J, Guldevall L, Soderhall M, Ishikawa K, Normark S, Koenig S.** 2000. Vaccination with FimH adhesin protects cyno-

molgus monkeys from colonization and infection by uropathogenic *Escherichia coli. J Infect Dis* 181:774–778.

204. **Savar NS, Jahanian-Najafabadi A, Mahdavi M, Shokrgozar MA, Jafari A, Bouzari S.** 2014. *In silico* and *in vivo* studies of truncated forms of flagellin (FliC) of enteroaggregative *Escherichia coli* fused to FimH from uropathogenic *Escherichia coli* as a vaccine candidate against urinary tract infections. *J Biotechnol* 175:31–37.

205. **Li X, Erbe JL, Lockatell CV, Johnson DE, Jobling MG, Holmes RK, Mobley HL.** 2004. Use of translational fusion of the MrpH fimbrial adhesin-binding domain with the cholera toxin A2 domain, coexpressed with the cholera toxin B subunit, as an intranasal vaccine to prevent experimental urinary tract infection by *Proteus mirabilis. Infect Immun* 72:7306–7310.

206. **Su EL, Snape MD.** 2011. A combination recombinant protein and outer membrane vesicle vaccine against serogroup B meningococcal disease. *Expert Rev Vaccines* 10:575–588.

207. **Serruto D, Bottomley MJ, Ram S, Giuliani MM, Rappuoli R.** 2012. The new multicomponent vaccine against meningococcal serogroup B, 4CMenB: immunological, functional and structural characterization of the antigens. *Vaccine* 30(Suppl 2):B87–B97.

208. **Findlow J, Borrow R, Snape MD, Dawson T, Holland A, John TM, Evans A, Telford KL, Ypma E, Toneatto D, Oster P, Miller E, Pollard AJ.** 2010. Multicenter, open-label, randomized phase II controlled trial of an investigational recombinant meningococcal serogroup B vaccine with and without outer membrane vesicles, administered in infancy. *Clin Infect Dis* 51:1127–1137.

209. **Hur J, Lee JH.** 2012. Development of a novel live vaccine delivering enterotoxigenic *Escherichia coli* fimbrial antigens to prevent post-weaning diarrhea in piglets. *Vet Immunol Immunopathol* 146:283–288.

210. **Hur J, Stein BD, Lee JH.** 2012. A vaccine candidate for post-weaning diarrhea in swine constructed with a live attenuated *Salmonella* delivering *Escherichia coli* K88ab, K88ac, FedA, and FedF fimbrial antigens and its immune responses in a murine model. *Can J Vet Res* 76:186–194.

211. **Therrien R, Lacasse P, Grondin G, Talbot BG.** 2007. Lack of protection of mice against *Staphylococcus aureus* despite a significant immune response to immunization with a DNA vaccine encoding collagen-binding protein. *Vaccine* 25:5053–5061.

212. **Gaudreau MC, Lacasse P, Talbot BG.** 2007. Protective immune responses to a multi-gene DNA vaccine against *Staphylococcus aureus. Vaccine* 25:814–824.

213. **Alves AM, Lasaro MO, Almeida DF, Ferreira LC.** 2000. DNA immunisation against the CFA/I fimbriae of enterotoxigenic *Escherichia coli* (ETEC). *Vaccine* 19:788–795.

214. **Ferreira DM, Oliveira ML, Moreno AT, Ho PL, Briles DE, Miyaji EN.** 2010. Protection against nasal colonization with *Streptococcus pneumoniae* by parenteral immunization with a DNA vaccine encoding PspA (pneumococcal surface protein A). *Microb Pathog* 48:205–213.

215. **Signoretto C, Canepari P, Stauder M, Vezzulli L, Pruzzo C.** 2012. Functional foods and strategies contrasting bacterial adhesion. *Curr Opin Biotechnol* 23:160–167.

216. **Yamaguti-Sasaki E, Ito LA, Canteli VC, Ushirobira TM, Ueda-Nakamura T, Dias Filho BP, Nakamura CV, de Mello JC.** 2007. Antioxidant capacity and *in vitro* prevention of dental plaque formation by extracts and condensed tannins of *Paullinia cupana. Molecules* 12:1950–1963.

217. **Furiga A, Lonvaud-Funel A, Dorignac G, Badet C.** 2008. *In vitro* anti-bacterial and anti-adherence effects of natural polyphenolic compounds on oral bacteria. *J Appl Microbiol* 105:1470–1476.

218. **Lee JH, Shim JS, Chung MS, Lim ST, Kim KH.** 2009. *In vitro* anti-adhesive activity of green tea extract against pathogen adhesion. *Phytother Res* 23:460–466.

219. **Howell AB, Foxman B.** 2002. Cranberry juice and adhesion of antibiotic-resistant uropathogens. *JAMA* 287:3082–3083.

220. **Avorn J, Monane M, Gurwitz JH, Glynn RJ, Choodnovskiy I, Lipsitz LA.** 1994. Reduction of bacteriuria and pyuria after ingestion of cranberry juice. *JAMA* 271:751–754.

221. **Kontiokari T, Sundqvist K, Nuutinen M, Pokka T, Koskela M, Uhari M.** 2001. Randomised trial of cranberry-lingonberry juice and *Lactobacillus* GG drink for the prevention of urinary tract infections in women. *BMJ* 322:1571.

222. **Barbosa-Cesnik C, Brown MB, Buxton M, Zhang L, DeBusscher J, Foxman B.** 2011. Cranberry juice fails to prevent recurrent urinary tract infection: results from a randomized placebo-controlled trial. *Clin Infect Dis* 52:23–30.

223. **Liu Y, Pinzon-Arango PA, Gallardo-Moreno AM, Camesano TA.** 2010. Direct adhesion force measurements between *E. coli* and human uroepithelial cells in cranberry juice cocktail. *Mol Nutr Food Res* 54:1744–1752.

224. **Toivanen M, Huttunen S, Lapinjoki S, Tikkanen-Kaukanen C.** 2011. Inhibition of adhesion of *Neisseria meningitidis* to human epithelial cells by berry juice polyphenolic fractions. *Phytother Res* **25:**828–832.

225. **Yamanaka A, Kimizuka R, Kato T, Okuda K.** 2004. Inhibitory effects of cranberry juice on attachment of oral streptococci and biofilm formation. *Oral Microbiol Immunol* **19:**150–154.

226. **Foo LY, Lu Y, Howell AB, Vorsa N.** 2000. A-type proanthocyanidin trimers from cranberry that inhibit adherence of uropathogenic P-fimbriated *Escherichia coli*. *J Nat Prod* **63:**1225–1228.

227. **Gustafsson A, Hultberg A, Sjostrom R, Kacskovics I, Breimer ME, Boren T, Hammarstrom L, Holgersson J.** 2006. Carbohydrate-dependent inhibition of *Helicobacter pylori* colonization using porcine milk. *Glycobiology* **16:**1–10.

228. **Coppa GV, Zampini L, Galeazzi T, Facinelli B, Ferrante L, Capretti R, Orazio G.** 2006. Human milk oligosaccharides inhibit the adhesion to Caco-2 cells of diarrheal pathogens: *Escherichia coli, Vibrio cholerae,* and *Salmonella fyris*. *Pediatr Res* **59:**377–382.

229. **Morrow AL, Ruiz-Palacios GM, Jiang X, Newburg DS.** 2005. Human-milk glycans that inhibit pathogen binding protect breastfeeding infants against infectious diarrhea. *J Nutr* **135:**1304–1307.

230. **Buffie CG, Pamer EG.** 2013. Microbiota-mediated colonization resistance against intestinal pathogens. *Nat Rev Immunol* **13:**790–801.

231. **Britton RA, Young VB.** 2014. Role of the intestinal microbiota in resistance to colonization by *Clostridium difficile*. *Gastroenterology* **146:**1547–1553.

232. **Mack DR, Michail S, Wei S, McDougall L, Hollingsworth MA.** 1999. Probiotics inhibit enteropathogenic *E. coli* adherence *in vitro* by inducing intestinal mucin gene expression. *Am J Physiol* **276:**G941–G950.

233. **Candela M, Perna F, Carnevali P, Vitali B, Ciati R, Gionchetti P, Rizzello F, Campieri M, Brigidi P.** 2008. Interaction of probiotic *Lactobacillus* and *Bifidobacterium* strains with human intestinal epithelial cells: adhesion properties, competition against enteropathogens and modulation of IL-8 production. *Int J Food Microbiol* **125:**286–292.

234. **Miller MB, Bassler BL.** 2001. Quorum sensing in bacteria. *Annu Rev Microbiol* **55:**165–199.

235. **Starkey M, Lepine F, Maura D, Bandyopadhaya A, Lesic B, He J, Kitao T, Righi V, Milot S, Tzika A, Rahme L.** 2014. Identification of anti-virulence compounds that disrupt quorum-sensing regulated acute and persistent pathogenicity.

236. **Mayville P, Ji G, Beavis R, Yang H, Goger M, Novick RP, Muir TW.** 1999. Structure-activity analysis of synthetic autoinducing thiolactone peptides from *Staphylococcus aureus* responsible for virulence. *Proc Natl Acad Sci USA* **96:**1218–1223.

237. **Hentzer M, Wu H, Andersen JB, Riedel K, Rasmussen TB, Bagge N, Kumar N, Schembri MA, Song Z, Kristoffersen P, Manefield M, Costerton JW, Molin S, Eberl L, Steinberg P, Kjelleberg S, Hoiby N, Givskov M.** 2003. Attenuation of *Pseudomonas aeruginosa* virulence by quorum sensing inhibitors. *EMBO J* **22:**3803–3815.

238. **Manefield M, Rasmussen TB, Henzter M, Andersen JB, Steinberg P, Kjelleberg S, Givskov M.** 2002. Halogenated furanones inhibit quorum sensing through accelerated LuxR turnover. *Microbiology* **148:**1119–1127.

239. **Anthouard R, DiRita VJ.** 2015. Chemical biology applied to the study of bacterial pathogens. *Infect Immun* **83:**456–469.

240. **Steadman D, Lo A, Waksman G, Remaut H.** 2014. Bacterial surface appendages as targets for novel antibacterial therapeutics. *Future Microbiol* **9:**887–900.

241. **Pang L, Kleeb S, Lemme K, Rabbani S, Scharenberg M, Zalewski A, Schadler F, Schwardt O, Ernst B.** 2012. FimH antagonists: structure-activity and structure-property relationships for biphenyl alpha-D-mannopyranosides. *ChemMedChem* **7:**1404–1422.

242. **Ton-That H, Liu G, Mazmanian SK, Faull KF, Schneewind O.** 1999. Purification and characterization of sortase, the transpeptidase that cleaves surface proteins of *Staphylococcus aureus* at the LPXTG motif. *Proc Natl Acad Sci USA* **96:**12424–12429.

243. **Oh KB, Oh MN, Kim JG, Shin DS, Shin J.** 2006. Inhibition of sortase-mediated *Staphylococcus aureus* adhesion to fibronectin via fibronectin-binding protein by sortase inhibitors. *Appl Microbiol Biotechnol* **70:**102–106.

244. **Oh KB, Mar W, Kim S, Kim JY, Oh MN, Kim JG, Shin D, Sim CJ, Shin J.** 2005. Bis(indole) alkaloids as sortase A inhibitors from the sponge *Spongosorites* sp. *Bioorg Med Chem Lett* **15:**4927–4931.

245. **Park BS, Kim JG, Kim MR, Lee SE, Takeoka GR, Oh KB, Kim JH.** 2005. *Curcuma longa* L. constituents inhibit sortase A and *Staphylococcus aureus* cell adhesion to fibronectin. *J Agric Food Chem* **53:**9005–9009.

246. **Kang SS, Kim JG, Lee TH, Oh KB.** 2006. Flavonols inhibit sortases and sortase-mediated

PLoS Pathog **10:**e1004321. doi:10.1371/journal. ppat.1004321.

Staphylococcus aureus clumping to fibrinogen. *Biol Pharm Bull* **29:**1751–1755.

247. **Scott CJ, McDowell A, Martin SL, Lynas JF, Vandenbroeck K, Walker B.** 2002. Irreversible inhibition of the bacterial cysteine protease-transpeptidase sortase (SrtA) by substrate-derived affinity labels. *Biochem J* **366:**953–958.

248. **Frankel BA, Bentley M, Kruger RG, McCafferty DG.** 2004. Vinyl sulfones: inhibitors of SrtA, a transpeptidase required for cell wall protein anchoring and virulence in *Staphylococcus aureus*. *J Am Chem Soc* **126:**3404–3405.

249. **Kruger RG, Barkallah S, Frankel BA, McCafferty DG.** 2004. Inhibition of the *Staphylococcus aureus* sortase transpeptidase SrtA by phosphinic peptidomimetics. *Bioorg Med Chem* **12:**3723–3729.

250. **Oh KB, Kim SH, Lee J, Cho WJ, Lee T, Kim S.** 2004. Discovery of diarylacrylonitriles as a novel series of small molecule sortase A inhibitors. *J Med Chem* **47:**2418–2421.

251. **Maresso AW, Schneewind O.** 2008. Sortase as a target of anti-infective therapy. *Pharmacol Rev* **60:**128–141.

252. **Ruiz-Palacios GM, Cervantes LE, Ramos P, Chavez-Munguia B, Newburg DS.** 2003. *Campylobacter jejuni* binds intestinal H(O) antigen (Fuc alpha 1, 2Gal beta 1, 4GlcNAc), and fucosyloligosaccharides of human milk inhibit its binding and infection. *J Biol Chem* **278:**14112–14120.

253. **Mysore JV, Wigginton T, Simon PM, Zopf D, Heman-Ackah LM, Dubois A.** 1999. Treatment of *Helicobacter pylori* infection in rhesus monkeys using a novel antiadhesion compound. *Gastroenterology* **117:**1316–1325.

254. **Ebersbach T, Andersen JB, Bergstrom A, Hutkins RW, Licht TR.** 2012. Xylo-oligosaccharides inhibit pathogen adhesion to enterocytes in vitro. *Res Microbiol* **163:**22–27.

255. **Idanpaan-Heikkila I, Simon PM, Zopf D, Vullo T, Cahill P, Sokol K, Tuomanen E.** 1997. Oligosaccharides interfere with the establishment and progression of experimental pneumococcal pneumonia. *J Infect Dis* **176:**704–712.

256. **Thomas R, Brooks T.** 2006. Attachment of *Yersinia pestis* to human respiratory cell lines is inhibited by certain oligosaccharides. *J Med Microbiol* **55:**309–315.

257. **Wang Q, Singh S, Taylor KG, Doyle RJ.** 1996. Anti-adhesins of *Streptococcus sobrinus*. *Adv Exp Med Biol* **408:**249–262.

258. **Ohlsson J, Larsson A, Haataja S, Alajaaski J, Stenlund P, Pinkner JS, Hultgren SJ, Finne J, Kihlberg J, Nilsson UJ.** 2005. Structure-activity relationships of galabioside derivatives as inhibitors of *E. coli* and *S. suis* adhesins: nanomolar inhibitors of *S. suis* adhesins. *Org Biomol Chem* **3:**886–900.

259. **Branderhorst HM, Kooij R, Salminen A, Jongeneel LH, Arnusch CJ, Liskamp RM, Finne J, Pieters RJ.** 2008. Synthesis of multivalent *Streptococcus suis* adhesion inhibitors by enzymatic cleavage of polygalacturonic acid and 'click' conjugation. *Org Biomol Chem* **6:**1425–1434.

260. **Pieters RJ, Slotved HC, Mortensen HM, Arler L, Finne J, Haataja S, Joosten JA, Branderhorst HM, Krogfelt KA.** 2013. Use of tetravalent galabiose for inhibition of *Streptococcus suis* serotype 2 infection in a mouse model. *Biology (Basel)* **2:**702–718.

261. **Joosten JA, Loimaranta V, Appeldoorn CC, Haataja S, El Maate FA, Liskamp RM, Finne J, Pieters RJ.** 2004. Inhibition of *Streptococcus suis* adhesion by dendritic galabiose compounds at low nanomolar concentration. *J Med Chem* **47:**6499–6508.

262. **Haataja S, Tikkanen K, Nilsson U, Magnusson G, Karlsson KA, Finne J.** 1994. Oligosaccharide-receptor interaction of the Gal alpha 1-4Gal binding adhesin of *Streptococcus suis*. Combining site architecture and characterization of two variant adhesin specificities. *J Biol Chem* **269:**27466–27472.

263. **Han Z, Pinkner JS, Ford B, Chorell E, Crowley JM, Cusumano CK, Campbell S, Henderson JP, Hultgren SJ, Janetka JW.** 2012. Lead optimization studies on FimH antagonists: discovery of potent and orally bioavailable ortho-substituted biphenyl mannosides. *J Med Chem* **55:**3945–3959.

264. **Gouin SG, Wellens A, Bouckaert J, Kovensky J.** 2009. Synthetic multimeric heptyl mannosides as potent antiadhesives of uropathogenic *Escherichia coli*. *ChemMedChem* **4:**749–755.

265. **Klein T, Abgottspon D, Wittwer M, Rabbani S, Herold J, Jiang X, Kleeb S, Luthi C, Scharenberg M, Bezencon J, Gubler E, Pang L, Smiesko M, Cutting B, Schwardt O, Ernst B.** 2010. FimH antagonists for the oral treatment of urinary tract infections: from design and synthesis to *in vitro* and *in vivo* evaluation. *J Med Chem* **53:**8627–8641.

266. **Jiang X, Abgottspon D, Kleeb S, Rabbani S, Scharenberg M, Wittwer M, Haug M, Schwardt O, Ernst B.** 2012. Antiadhesion therapy for urinary tract infections: a balanced PK/PD profile proved to be key for success. *J Med Chem* **55:**4700–4713.

267. **Aronson M, Medalia O, Schori L, Mirelman D, Sharon N, Ofek I.** 1979. Prevention of colonization of the urinary tract of mice with

Escherichia coli by blocking of bacterial adherence with methyl alpha-D-mannopyranoside. *J Infect Dis* **139**:329–332.

268. **Salminen A, Loimaranta V, Joosten JA, Khan AS, Hacker J, Pieters RJ, Finne J.** 2007. Inhibition of P-fimbriated *Escherichia coli* adhesion by multivalent galabiose derivatives studied by a live-bacteria application of surface plasmon resonance. *J Antimicrob Chemother* **60**:495–501.

269. **Ohlsson J, Jass J, Uhlin BE, Kihlberg J, Nilsson UJ.** 2002. Discovery of potent inhibitors of PapG adhesins from uropathogenic *Escherichia coli* through synthesis and evaluation of galabiose derivatives. *Chembiochem* **3**:772–779.

270. **Larsson A, Ohlsson J, Dodson KW, Hultgren SJ, Nilsson U, Kihlberg J.** 2003. Quantitative studies of the binding of the class II PapG adhesin from uropathogenic *Escherichia coli* to oligosaccharides. *Bioorg Med Chem* **11**:2255–2261.

271. **Autar R, Khan AS, Schad M, Hacker J, Liskamp RM, Pieters RJ.** 2003. Adhesion inhibition of F1C-fimbriated *Escherichia coli* and *Pseudomonas aeruginosa* PAK and PAO by multivalent carbohydrate ligands. *Chembiochem* **4**:1317–1325.

272. **Cecioni S, Faure S, Darbost U, Bonnamour I, Parrot-Lopez H, Roy O, Taillefumier C, Wimmerova M, Praly JP, Imberty A, Vidal S.** 2011. Selectivity among two lectins: probing the effect of topology, multivalency and flexibility of "clicked" multivalent glycoclusters. *Chemistry* **17**:2146–2159.

273. **Cecioni S, Lalor R, Blanchard B, Praly JP, Imberty A, Matthews SE, Vidal S.** 2009. Achieving high affinity towards a bacterial lectin through multivalent topological isomers of calix[4]arene glycoconjugates. *Chemistry* **15**:13232–13240.

274. **Otsuka I, Blanchard B, Borsali R, Imberty A, Kakuchi T.** 2010. Enhancement of plant and bacterial lectin binding affinities by three-dimensional organized cluster glycosides constructed on helical poly(phenylacetylene) backbones. *Chembiochem* **11**:2399–2408.

275. **Chabre YM, Giguere D, Blanchard B, Rodrigue J, Rocheleau S, Neault M, Rauthu S, Papadopoulos A, Arnold AA, Imberty A, Roy R.** 2011. Combining glycomimetic and multivalent strategies toward designing potent bacterial lectin inhibitors. *Chemistry* **17**:6545–6562.

276. **Pertici F, Pieters RJ.** 2012. Potent divalent inhibitors with rigid glucose click spacers for *Pseudomonas aeruginosa* lectin LecA. *Chem Commun (Camb)* **48**:4008–4010.

277. **Marotte K, Preville C, Sabin C, Moume-Pymbock M, Imberty A, Roy R.** 2007. Synthesis and binding properties of divalent and trivalent clusters of the Lewis a disaccharide moiety to *Pseudomonas aeruginosa* lectin PA-IIL. *Org Biomol Chem* **5**:2953–2961.

278. **Morvan F, Meyer A, Jochum A, Sabin C, Chevolot Y, Imberty A, Praly JP, Vasseur JJ, Souteyrand E, Vidal S.** 2007. Fucosylated pentaerythrityl phosphodiester oligomers (PePOs): automated synthesis of DNA-based glycoclusters and binding to *Pseudomonas aeruginosa* lectin (PA-IIL). *Bioconjug Chem* **18**:1637–1643.

279. **Andreini M, Anderluh M, Audfray A, Bernardi A, Imberty A.** 2010. Monovalent and bivalent N-fucosyl amides as high affinity ligands for *Pseudomonas aeruginosa* PA-IIL lectin. *Carbohydr Res* **345**:1400–1407.

280. **Kelly CG, Younson JS, Hikmat BY, Todryk SM, Czisch M, Haris PI, Flindall IR, Newby C, Mallet AI, Ma JK, Lehner T.** 1999. A synthetic peptide adhesion epitope as a novel antimicrobial agent. *Nat Biotechnol* **17**:42–47.

281. **Younson J, Kelly C.** 2004. The rational design of an anti-caries peptide against *Streptococcus mutans*. *Mol Divers* **8**:121–126.

282. **Okuda K, Hanada N, Usui Y, Takeuchi H, Koba H, Nakao R, Watanabe H, Senpuku H.** 2010. Inhibition of *Streptococcus mutans* adherence and biofilm formation using analogues of the SspB peptide. *Arch Oral Biol* **55**:754–762.

283. **Jay CM, Bhaskaran S, Rathore KS, Waghela SD.** 2004. Enterotoxigenic K99+ *Escherichia coli* attachment to host cell receptors inhibited by recombinant pili protein. *Vet Microbiol* **101**:153–160.

284. **Ofek I, Hasty DL, Sharon N.** 2003. Anti-adhesion therapy of bacterial diseases: prospects and problems. *FEMS Immunol Med Microbiol* **38**:181–191.

285. **Cozens D, Read RC.** 2012. Anti-adhesion methods as novel therapeutics for bacterial infections. *Expert Rev Anti Infect Ther* **10**:1457–1468.

286. **Ghosh S, Chakraborty K, Nagaraja T, Basak S, Koley H, Dutta S, Mitra U, Das S.** 2011. An adhesion protein of *Salmonella enterica* serovar *Typhi* is required for pathogenesis and potential target for vaccine development. *Proc Natl Acad Sci USA* **108**:3348–3353.

287. **Raghunathan D, Wells TJ, Morris FC, Shaw RK, Bobat S, Peters SE, Paterson GK, Jensen KT, Leyton DL, Blair JM, Browning DF, Pravin J, Flores-Langarica A, Hitchcock JR, Moraes CT, Piazza RM, Maskell DJ, Webber**

MA, May RC, MacLennan CA, Piddock LJ, Cunningham AF, Henderson IR. 2011. SadA, a trimeric autotransporter from *Salmonella enterica* serovar Typhimurium, can promote biofilm formation and provides limited protection against infection. *Infect Immun* **79:**4342–4352.

288. **Zhang C, Zhang W.** 2010. *Escherichia coli* K88ac fimbriae expressing heat-labile and heat-stable (STa) toxin epitopes elicit antibodies that neutralize cholera toxin and STa toxin and inhibit adherence of K88ac fimbrial *E. coli. Clin Vaccine Immunol* **17:**1859–1867.

289. **Gao X, Cai K, Li T, Wang Q, Hou X, Tian R, Liu H, Tu W, Xiao L, Fang L, Luo S, Liu Y, Wang H.** 2011. Novel fusion protein protects against adherence and toxicity of enterohemorrhagic *Escherichia coli* O157:H7 in mice. *Vaccine* **29:**6656–6663.

290. **Sheth HB, Glasier LM, Ellert NW, Cachia P, Kohn W, Lee KK, Paranchych W, Hodges RS, Irvin RT.** 1995. Development of an antiadhesive vaccine for *Pseudomonas aeruginosa* targeting the C-terminal region of the pilin structural protein. *Biomed Pept Proteins Nucleic Acids* **1:**141–148.

291. **Greco D, Salmaso S, Mastrantonio P, Giuliano M, Tozzi AE, Anemona A, Ciofi degli Atti ML, Giammanco A, Panei P, Blackwelder WC, Klein DL, Wassilak SG.** 1996. A controlled trial of two acellular vaccines and one whole-cell vaccine against pertussis. Progetto Pertosse Working Group. *N Engl J Med* **334:**341–348.

292. **Ma JK, Hunjan M, Smith R, Lehner T.** 1989. Specificity of monoclonal antibodies in local passive immunization against *Streptococcus mutans. Clin Exp Immunol* **77:**331–337.

293. **Lehner T, Caldwell J, Smith R.** 1985. Local passive immunization by monoclonal antibodies against streptococcal antigen I/II in the prevention of dental caries. *Infect Immun* **50:**796–799.

294. **Arrecubieta C, Matsunaga I, Asai T, Naka Y, Deng MC, Lowy FD.** 2008. Vaccination with clumping factor A and fibronectin binding protein A to prevent *Staphylococcus aureus* infection of an aortic patch in mice. *J Infect Dis* **198:** 571–575.

295. **Briles DE, Ades E, Paton JC, Sampson JS, Carlone GM, Huebner RC, Virolainen A, Swiatlo E, Hollingshead SK.** 2000. Intranasal immunization of mice with a mixture of the pneumococcal proteins PsaA and PspA is highly protective against nasopharyngeal carriage of *Streptococcus pneumoniae. Infect Immun* **68:**796–800.

296. **Lee KH, Kim BS, Keum KS, Yu HH, Kim YH, Chang BS, Ra JY, Moon HD, Seo BR, Choi NY, You YO.** 2011. Essential oil of *Curcuma longa* inhibits *Streptococcus mutans* biofilm formation. *J Food Sci* **76:**H226–H230.

297. **Xiao J, Zuo Y, Liu Y, Li J, Hao Y, Zhou X.** 2007. Effects of nidus vespae extract and chemical fractions on glucosyltransferases, adherence and biofilm formation of *Streptococcus mutans. Arch Oral Biol* **52:**869–875.

298. **Prabu GR, Gnanamani A, Sadulla S.** 2006. Guaijaverin: a plant flavonoid as potential antiplaque agent against *Streptococcus mutans. J Appl Microbiol* **101:**487–495.

299. **Wolinsky LE, Mania S, Nachnani S, Ling S.** 1996. The inhibiting effect of aqueous *Azadirachta indica* (Neem) extract upon bacterial properties influencing *in vitro* plaque formation. *J Dent Res* **75:**816–822.

300. **Pusztai A, Grant G, Spencer RJ, Duguid TJ, Brown DS, Ewen SW, Peumans WJ, Van Damme EJ, Bardocz S.** 1993. Kidney bean lectin-induced *Escherichia coli* overgrowth in the small intestine is blocked by GNA, a mannose-specific lectin. *J Appl Bacteriol* **75:**360–368.

301. **Saeki Y.** 1994. Effect of seaweed extracts on *Streptococcus sobrinus* adsorption to saliva-coated hydroxyapatite. *Bull Tokyo Dent Coll* **35:**9–15.

302. **Staat RH, Doyle RJ, Langley SD, Suddick RP.** 1978. Modification of *in vitro* adherence of *Streptococcus mutans* by plant lectins. *Adv Exp Med Biol* **107:**639–647.

303. **Neeser JR, Koellreutter B, Wuersch P.** 1986. Oligomannoside-type glycopeptides inhibiting adhesion of *Escherichia coli* strains mediated by type 1 pili: preparation of potent inhibitors from plant glycoproteins. *Infect Immun* **52:**428–436.

304. **Newburg DS, Ruiz-Palacios GM, Altaye M, Chaturvedi P, Meinzen-Derr J, Guerrero Mde L, Morrow AL.** 2004. Innate protection conferred by fucosylated oligosaccharides of human milk against diarrhea in breastfed infants. *Glycobiology* **14:**253–263.

305. **Hakkarainen J, Toivanen M, Leinonen A, Frangsmyr L, Stromberg N, Lapinjoki S, Nassif X, Tikkanen-Kaukanen C.** 2005. Human and bovine milk oligosaccharides inhibit *Neisseria meningitidis* pili attachment *in vitro. J Nutr* **135:**2445–2448.

306. **Zinger-Yosovich KD, Iluz D, Sudakevitz D, Gilboa-Garber N.** 2010. Blocking of *Pseudomonas aeruginosa* and *Chromobacterium violaceum* lectins by diverse mammalian milks. *J Dairy Sci* **93:**473–482.

307. **Willer Eda M, Lima Rde L, Giugliano LG.** 2004. *In vitro* adhesion and invasion inhibition of *Shigella dysenteriae*, *Shigella flexneri* and *Shigella sonnei* clinical strains by human milk proteins. *BMC Microbiol* **4:**18.

308. **Danielsson Niemi L, Hernell O, Johansson I.** 2009. Human milk compounds inhibiting adhesion of mutans streptococci to host ligand-coated hydroxyapatite *in vitro*. *Caries Res* **43:**171–178.

309. **Stromqvist M, Falk P, Bergstrom S, Hansson L, Lonnerdal B, Normark S, Hernell O.** 1995. Human milk kappa-casein and inhibition of *Helicobacter pylori* adhesion to human gastric mucosa. *J Pediatr Gastroenterol Nutr* **21:**288–296.

310. **Mamo W, Froman G.** 1994. Adhesion of *Staphylococcus aureus* to bovine mammary epithelial cells induced by growth in milk whey. *Microbiol Immunol* **38:**305–308.

311. **Andersson B, Porras O, Hanson LA, Lagergard T, Svanborg-Eden C.** 1986. Inhibition of attachment of *Streptococcus pneumoniae* and *Haemophilus influenzae* by human milk and receptor oligosaccharides. *J Infect Dis* **153:**232–237.

312. **Roberts DD, Olson LD, Barile MF, Ginsburg V, Krivan HC.** 1989. Sialic acid-dependent adhesion of *Mycoplasma pneumoniae* to purified glycoproteins. *J Biol Chem* **264:**9289–9293.

313. **Loveless RW, Feizi T.** 1989. Sialo-oligosaccharide receptors for *Mycoplasma pneumoniae* and related oligosaccharides of poly-N-acetyllactosamine series are polarized at the cilia and apical-microvillar domains of the ciliated cells in human bronchial epithelium. *Infect Immun* **57:**1285–1289.

314. **Liukkonen J, Haataja S, Tikkanen K, Kelm S, Finne J.** 1992. Identification of N-acetylneuraminyl alpha 2-->3 poly-N-acetyllactosamine glycans as the receptors of sialic acid-binding *Streptococcus suis* strains. *J Biol Chem* **267:**21105–21111.

315. **Korhonen TK, Valtonen MV, Parkkinen J, Vaisanen-Rhen V, Finne J, Orskov F, Orskov I, Svenson SB, Makela PH.** 1985. Serotypes, hemolysin production, and receptor recognition of *Escherichia coli* strains associated with neonatal sepsis and meningitis. *Infect Immun* **48:**486–491.

316. **Schroten H, Plogmann R, Hanisch FG, Hacker J, Nobis-Bosch R, Wahn V.** 1993. Inhibition of adhesion of S-fimbriated *E. coli* to buccal epithelial cells by human skim milk is predominantly mediated by mucins and depends on the period of lactation. *Acta Paediatr* **82:**6–11.

The Role of Biotin in Bacterial Physiology and Virulence: a Novel Antibiotic Target for *Mycobacterium tuberculosis*

28

WANISA SALAEMAE,[1] GRANT W. BOOKER,[1,2] and STEVEN W. POLYAK[1,2]

TUBERCULOSIS AND THE RISE OF ANTIBIOTIC RESISTANCE

Tuberculosis (TB) is a global pandemic that ranks alongside HIV-AIDS and malaria as the leading cause of death by infectious disease, with the highest incidence rates observed in Southeast Asian, African, and Western Pacific countries (1). In 1993 the WHO declared TB to be a global health emergency and set the Millennium Development Goal of reducing the prevalence and mortality rates to 50% of those observed in 1990 by the 2015 deadline (2). Although the rates of new TB cases and mortality have declined over the past decade and are within reach of the 2015 target, the number of TB patients and the prevalence of drug-resistant strains are rising (3). Multidrug-resistant TB (MDR-TB) must be addressed now as a public health crisis to achieve the ambitious Millennium Development Goal target of complete elimination of TB as a public health concern by 2050 (4).

The worldwide TB epidemic has been aggravated by several factors such as the rising epidemic of HIV-AIDS coinfection (5), decreasing efficacy of the BCG vaccine (6), inadequate or inefficient administration of chemotherapies, and noncompliance of treatment (7). These factors have contributed to the rise

[1]Department of Molecular and Cellular Biology, School of Biological Science; [2]Center for Molecular Pathology, University of Adelaide, North Terrace Campus, Adelaide, South Australia 5005, Australia.
Virulence Mechanisms of Bacterial Pathogens, 5th edition
Edited by Indira T. Kudva, Nancy A. Cornick, Paul J. Plummer, Qijing Zhang, Tracy L. Nicholson, John P. Bannantine, and Bryan H. Bellaire
© 2016 American Society for Microbiology, Washington, DC
doi:10.1128/microbiolspec.VMBF-0008-2015

of drug-resistant *Mycobacterium tuberculosis* strains that are causative agents of MDR-TB (resistant to isoniazid and rifampicin) and extensively drug-resistant TB (resistant to isoniazid, rifampicin, fluoroquinolones, and second-line injectable drugs) (8, 9). In 2012, MDR-TB was found in 3.6% of new TB cases and 20% of treated TB patients. Approximately 10% of patients with MDR-TB go on to develop extensively drug-resistant TB (1). Of immense concern is the rise of totally drug-resistant TB strains, discovered in Italy (in 2007), Iran (in 2009), and India (in 2012) (10–13). This new definition has not yet been formally recognized by the WHO (3).

The development of novel TB antibiotics is a crucial component of an effective fight against this epidemic. Since rifampicin was approved in 1963, the only new antibiotic to combat TB has been Sirturo (bedaquiline), which was approved by the FDA in 2012 (14). This highlights a void in antibiotic discovery over the past decade. Sirturo inhibits mycobacterial ATP synthase, which is essential for energy production. This novel mechanism of action allows for the treatment of MDR-TB when combined with other therapies (15). The prevalence of drug-resistant TB will increasingly drive demand for novel antibiotics that are not circumvented by existing resistance mechanisms (15, 16). In addition, treatments targeting latent *M. tuberculosis* infection are highly desirable because only rifampicin and bedaquiline can address this stage of the life cycle (17). Targeting latent infection is challenging because the pathogen can invoke various mechanisms to evade host immune responses and antibiotic chemotherapy. Ideally, the desired properties of new treatments should feature (i) shortened treatment durations compared to the current 6 months minimum, (ii) unique mechanisms of action to address drug-resistant strains, (iii) good pharmacokinetics and bioavailability, (iv) reduced daily number of pills and dosing frequency to simplify treatment and increase patient compliance, (v) effectiveness for treating both active and latent phases of the tuberculi life cycle, and (vi) safe coadministration with nonrelated medications, e.g., antiviral drugs for patients with TB/HIV coinfection.

BIOTIN AND ITS ROLE IN MYCOBACTERIA

Biotin (also known as vitamin B7, vitamin H, or coenzyme R) is a water-soluble vitamin that is required for the growth and pathogenicity of *M. tuberculosis*. Biotin is an essential cofactor for the biotin-dependent enzymes that are involved in important metabolic pathways such as membrane lipid synthesis, replenishment of the tricarboxylic acid cycle, and amino acid metabolism (described further below) (18–22). Although biotin is essential for all living cells, only microorganisms, plants, and some fungi synthesize biotin *de novo* (23). Humans and other mammals lack this metabolic pathway, thereby relying on exogenous biotin obtained from dietary sources or from intestinal biotin-producing bacteria (24, 25). Biochemical and genetic studies suggest that *de novo* biosynthesis is the sole source of biotin in *M. tuberculosis* due to the lack of a high-affinity transporter through which to scavenge exogenous material. Several biotin transporters from *Eubacteria* and *Archaea* have recently been identified and characterized. The biotin transporter, BioY, which works in cooperation with an ATP-dependent energy-coupling system (BioMN), has been characterized in several bacterial species (26, 27). Alternatively, the elusive YigM transporter in *Escherichia coli* has finally been identified 42 years after the first reports on this transporter (28–38). A homologue of YigM, MadN, has also been identified in certain Gram-negative bacteria (28). Noteworthy genome annotation studies have failed to identify a BioY homologue in mycobacteria (26, 39). Likewise, our own nucleotide sequence analysis using online homology algorithms has not found a homologue of YigM or MadN in the *M. tuberculosis* genome.

Furthermore, inhibition of mycobacterial growth using the natural products amiclenomycin and actithiazic acid, which target biotin biosynthetic enzymes, strongly suggests that mycobacteria rely exclusively on *de novo* biotin synthesis (described in further detail later) (40–44). The inhibitory activity of amiclenomycin was not compromised unless the growth media was supplemented with high concentrations of biotin (>42 µM) (45). This concentration is at least 3 orders of magnitude higher than that normally found in human plasma (46, 47), suggesting that biotin can diffuse into mycobacterial cells at nonphysiological concentrations but is not imported via a high-affinity transporter. Hence, biotin biosynthesis is essential for *M. tuberculosis*, leading to the enzymes that synthesize biotin as promising drug targets for new antibiotics, and these are the subject of this review.

BIOTIN-DEPENDENT ENZYMES

The biotin-dependent enzymes are a family of enzymes that are found throughout the living world. Because these enzymes all require the biotin cofactor, they are commonly known as the biotin-dependent enzymes. Based on current literature and genome annotation studies, *M. tuberculosis* appears to have two classes of biotin-dependent enzymes: acyl-CoA carboxylases and pyruvate carboxylase (PC). These enzymes are positioned in key metabolic pathways that are required for mycobacterial growth and virulence, as discussed further below. All biotin-dependent enzymes function through a conserved reaction mechanism that requires biotin to bind and transfer carbon dioxide between metabolites in carboxylation, decarboxylation, and transcarboxylation reactions (24, 48). The biotin-dependent enzymes contain three highly conserved subunits required for catalysis, namely, biotin carboxylase, carboxyltransferase, and biotin carboxyl carrier protein (49–51). Biotin is covalently attached

to the biotin carboxyl carrier protein that oscillates between two partial reaction sites during catalysis. At the first site biotin is carboxylated through the activity of biotin carboxylase. The biotin carboxyl carrier domain–carboxybiotin complex then translocates to the sites of the transcarboxylase, where the CO_2 is transferred to the metabolic substrate. Without the attached biotin cofactor, these enzymes are inactive and unable to fulfill the important metabolic activities that are essential for bacterial survival.

Acyl-CoA Carboxylases (ACCs)

Bacterial ACCs are multisubunit enzymes composed of a homodimeric biotin carboxylase, a heteroligomer carboxyltransferase, and the biotin carboxyl carrier protein (52). Mycobacterial genomes contain three *accA* and six *accD* genes that encode the two subunits of the carboxyltransferase complex (53). These subunits are believed to combine in a variety of different assemblies to produce unique acyl-CoA carboxylases that can utilize various-length short chain acyl-CoAs as substrates including acetyl-CoA, propionyl-CoA, and butyryl-CoA (22, 54). Carboxylation of these substrates provides metabolites that feed into the fatty acid synthesis and polyketide synthesis pathways, resulting in the production of structurally diverse lipids such as mycolic acids and multimethyl-branched fatty acids (21). One of the important, intrinsic features of *M. tuberculosis* is the presence of a complex lipid bilayer that is primarily composed of mycolic acid in the mycobacterial cell envelope. It is estimated that lipids account for up to 60% of the mycobacterial dry cell weight (55), and 10% of the *M. tuberculosis* genome is devoted to fatty acid biosynthesis (56), reflecting its importance for bacterial physiology and pathogenicity. The complex nature of the cell envelope greatly enhances the mycobacteria's ability to resist chemical assault and survive hostile environments and limit its susceptibility to certain antibiotics (8, 9).

Some of the surface-exposed lipids have also been found to be important virulence factors unique to *M. tuberculosis*. Targeting fatty acid synthesis represents one of the most successful approaches to combating TB, as demonstrated by the clinical efficacy of the drugs isoniazid, ethionamide, and thiocarlide (11).

Of particular relevance is the first committed step in the fatty acid synthesis pathway that is catalyzed by the biotin-dependent enzyme acetyl-CoA carboxylase. Here the carboxylation of acetyl-CoA yields malonyl-CoA, which is required for fatty acid elongation. Hence, acetyl CoA carboxylase is an important metabolic enzyme that is positioned at a crucial regulatory point for fatty acid synthesis. This is highlighted by a mutagenesis study that showed that the genes encoding the subunits of ACC, namely, *accA3*, *accD4*, and *accD6*, are essential for the growth of *M. tuberculosis in vitro* (57). Fatty acid synthesis has been proposed as a promising pathway to target for the development of novel agents against certain bacterial pathogens (58–60), and a recent review focuses on efforts to specifically target acetyl-CoA carboxylase (52).

Pyruvate Carboxylase (PC)

PC catalyzes the synthesis of oxaloacetate through the fixation of CO_2 onto pyruvate. Because oxaloacetate is one of the intermediates in the tricarboxylic acid cycle, one role for PC is to replenish this pathway (61). It has traditionally been difficult to study metabolism in intracellular pathogens such as *M. tuberculosis* due to redundant pathways and the contribution of the host cell. Hence, biotin-dependent PC has not been as well explored as the ACCs. However, advances in technology together with access to mutant strains of *M. tuberculosis* have provided new insights into metabolic adaptation and the relationship between host and pathogen. Using isotopically labeled substrates coupled with mass spectrometry has allowed the study of metabolomics of bacteria cultured

inside host macrophages (62). A critical finding from these studies is that *M. tuberculosis* is capable of utilizing a variety of carbon substrates simultaneously, including CO_2 (63, 64). Moreover, macrophages are unable to fix CO_2 (62), suggesting that carbon fixation is potentially a novel target for anti-TB agents. The labeled amino acids aspartate, threonine, and methionine, all derived from the common precursor oxaloacetate, were all detected in infected macrophages that were cultured in ^{13}C bicarbonate, but not in uninfected macrophages.

PC is one of three enzymes present in *M. tuberculosis* that is capable of oxaloacetate production, with phosphoenol pyruvate carboxykinase (PEPCK) and malate dehydrogenase being the other two. PEPCK-deficient strains of mycobacteria have helped establish an essential role for this enzyme in the establishment and maintenance of *M. tuberculosis* infection in a mouse model (65). PEPCK also played a key role in the synthesis of aspartate, threonine, and methionine in the ^{13}C profiling study when a mutant *M. tuberculosis* strain was employed. However, PEPCK could only account for half of the amino acid production, suggesting a role for other enzymes in CO_2 fixation, such as PC. This work is important because the intracellular environment of the macrophage is hypoxic and CO_2 rich. Further exploration of the metabolic pathways required for survival inside cells and whole animals promises to yield new drug targets to combat TB.

PROTEIN BIOTINYLATION

The covalent attachment of biotin to protein, or "protein biotinylation", of biotin-dependent enzymes is a biotin and ATP-dependent reaction. Protein biotinylation is performed by biotin protein ligase (BPL; encoded by *birA*) (66). BPL is generally divided into three classes based on the divergent nature of the N-terminal domain, while the catalytic domain for catalyzing biotinylation is highly conserved in all classes. Class I BPLs, such as those from *M. tuberculosis*, are the smallest of the three BPL classes (67). These enzymes are composed of the catalytic module that is required to catalyze protein biotinylation (66, 68). Class II BPLs, such as those from *E. coli, Bacillus subtilis*, and *Staphylococcus aureus*, contain an N-terminal extension on the catalytic module that facilitates DNA binding, making these proteins truly bifunctional since they act as transcriptional repressors and catalyze protein biotinylation (69–72). Class III BPLs, found in mammals, yeast, and insects, also possess an extended N-terminal region that permits selective binding of certain protein substrates for biotinylation (73). Because protein biotinylation is essential for the activity of ACCs and PC, BPL has also been proposed as a promising target for anti-TB drug development (68). This work has recently been reviewed in (74).

VALIDATION OF BIOTIN BIOSYNTHESIS AS A TARGET FOR ANTI-TB DRUG DEVELOPMENT

Biotin biosynthesis has been proposed as a promising target for the development of new antibiotics due to its intimate association with membrane lipid synthesis (58–60). As described above, the products of lipid synthesis are key components of the cell membrane that play critical roles in bacterial survival and defense. Targeting enzymes involved in membrane lipid synthesis therefore inhibits bacterial growth and virulence. This approach is clinically validated by isoniazid that targets InhA in the fatty acid synthase II system (75, 76). Importantly, screening of drugs effective against latent *M. tuberculosis* has revealed that certain lipid biosynthetic enzymes can be targeted against tuberculi at this stage of the life cycle that is challenging to treat (77, 78). These data validate biotin biosynthesis as an excellent target for the development of new anti-TB

drugs that are able to combat both the active and latent stages of TB. The absence of a homologous pathway in humans and other mammals also adds to the appeal of this target for new antibiotics (18, 79).

Validation of biotin biosynthesis as a druggable anti-TB target is further supported by a number of genetic knockout studies. MMAR_2770 is the *Mycobacterium marinum* homologue of Rv1882c in *M. tuberculosis* and encodes a putative short chain dehydrogenase/reductase that is required for the early steps of the synthesis of the pimeloyl-thioester biotin precursor. Deletion of MMAR_2770 impaired the growth of *M. marinum* on blood agar unless supplemented with high concentrations of biotin (>1 μM) (80). The mutant also failed to establish an infection and colonize murine macrophages or zebra fish (80). In separate studies, disruption of *bioA* in the biotin biosynthetic operon impaired survival of *Mycobacterium smegmatis* during the stationary phase on carbon-depleted media (81, 82), while disruption of *bioF* and *bioB* debilitated the bacterial growth during and postinfection of murine macrophages (83). Likewise, genome-wide genetic screens revealed that *bioF, bioA*, and *bioB* are essential for virulence as shown by impeded growth of the deletion strains in murine macrophages (84). In addition, *bioF*$^{-/-}$ *M. tuberculosis* showed poor recovery from mouse lung and spleen in an infection challenge experiment (84). Together, these genetic studies further validate biotin biosynthesis as a key metabolic process during growth, infection, and survival in the latent life cycle of mycobacteria.

THE BIOTIN BIOSYNTHETIC PATHWAY

The biotin biosynthetic scheme can be divided into two stages: (i) synthesis of the pimelate precursor and (ii) the conserved metabolic pathway catalyzing the final four steps that yield biotin. Figure 1 shows the biotin biosynthetic pathway and the chemical

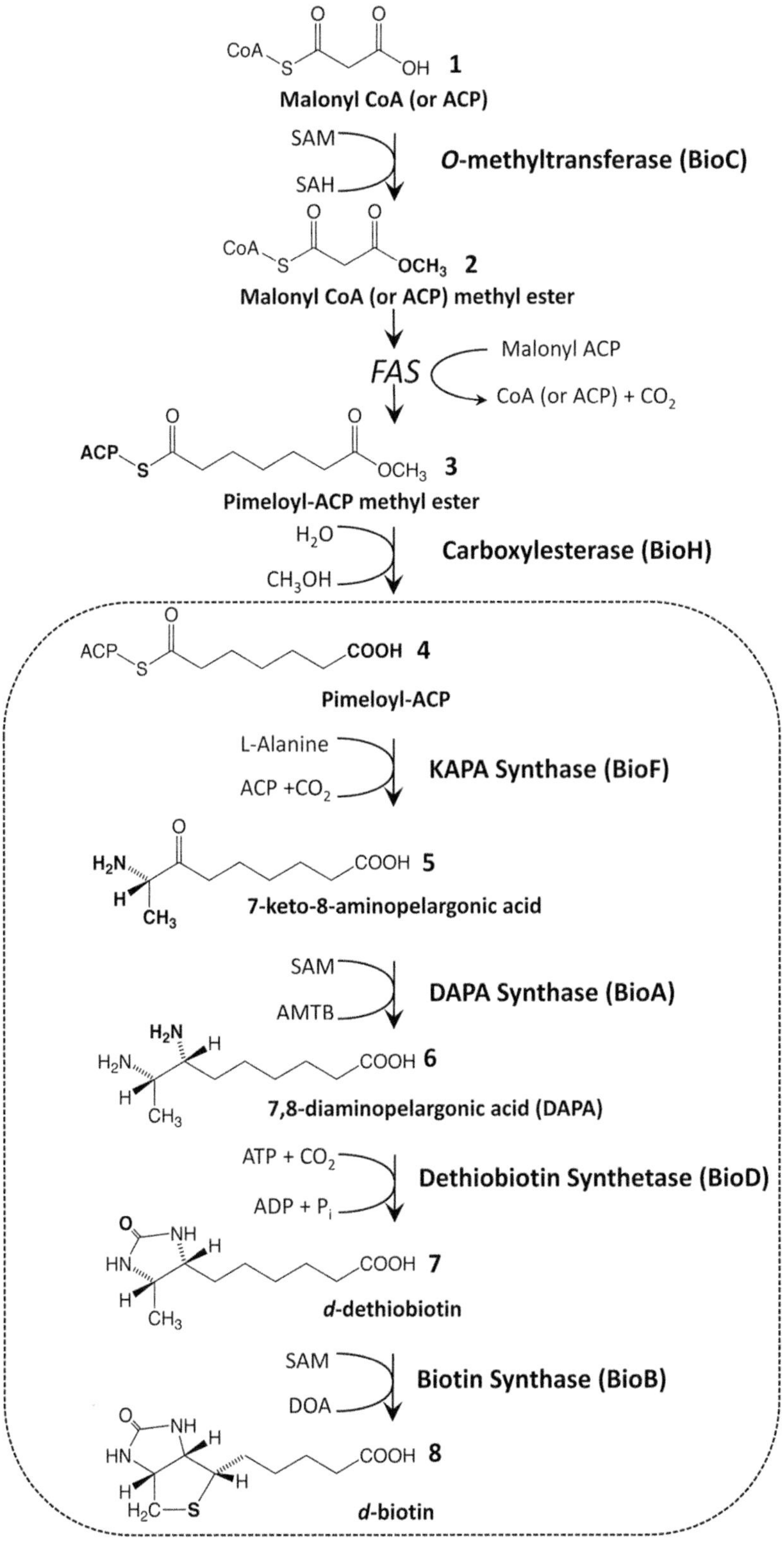

Malonyl CoA (or ACP) 1

SAM, SAH

***O*-methyltransferase (BioC)**

Malonyl CoA (or ACP) methyl ester 2

FAS — Malonyl ACP; CoA (or ACP) + CO_2

Pimeloyl-ACP methyl ester 3

H_2O, CH_3OH

Carboxylesterase (BioH)

Pimeloyl-ACP 4

L-Alanine, ACP + CO_2

KAPA Synthase (BioF)

7-keto-8-aminopelargonic acid 5

SAM, AMTB

DAPA Synthase (BioA)

7,8-diaminopelargonic acid (DAPA) 6

ATP + CO_2, ADP + P_i

Dethiobiotin Synthetase (BioD)

***d*-dethiobiotin 7**

SAM, DOA

Biotin Synthase (BioB)

***d*-biotin 8**

structures of the synthetic intermediates. The steps leading to the formation of a pimeloyl-thioester precursor (linked to either CoA or acyl carrier protein) are variable among biotin-producing organisms. The best-understood pathways are in *E. coli* (i.e., BioC-BioH pathway) and *B. subtilis* (i.e., BioI-BioW pathway) (reviewed in references 85, 86). The presence of BioC and BioH homologues in mycobacterial genomes suggests that *M. tuberculosis* employs the same pathway as *E. coli* (18, 80). Here, a 3-carbon malonyl-thioester (compound 1) is first methylated by the BioC-O-methyltransferase to produce methyl ester (compound 2), which serves as the precursor for two iterations of alkyl chain elongation using the fatty acid synthesis pathway, producing a 7-carbon pimeloyl–acyl carrier protein (ACP) methyl ester (compound 3). The methyl group of the pimeloyl-ACP methyl ester (compound 3) is then hydrolyzed by BioH carboxylesterase to generate the pimeloyl-ACP (compound 4) (85–87). Pimeloyl-ACP, rather than pimeloyl-CoA, is believed to be the physiological intermediate required in the subsequent conserved metabolic pathway (86).

Unlike the synthesis of the pimelate precursor (compound 3), the final four reactions in the pathway that assemble the bicyclic rings of biotin are highly conserved among microorganisms and plants. Pimeloyl-ACP (compound 4) is converted to biotin by the activities of 7-keto-8-aminopelargonic acid synthase (KAPAS), 7,8-diaminopelargonic acid synthase (DAPAS), dethiobiotin synthetase (DTBS), and biotin synthase (BS), which are encoded by *bioF*, *bioA*, *bioD*, and *bioB*, respectively (18, 88–90). Among biotin-producing organisms, *Saccharomyces cere-*

visiae is the only species reported that employs only the last three steps of the conserved metabolic pathway due to the presence of a 7-keto-8-aminopelargonic acid (KAPA) transporter (91, 92). Briefly, KAPAS converts pimeloyl-ACP (compound 4) to KAPA (compound 5) by using L-alanine as an amino donor and releasing ACP and CO_2 (93). At the antepenultimate step, DAPAS catalyzes the conversion of KAPA (compound 5) to 7,8-diaminopelargonic acid (DAPA) (compound 6) using S-adenosyl-L-methionine (SAM) as an amino group donor (90). Next, DTBS catalyzes closure of the ureido ring of dethiobiotin (DTB) (compound 7) from DAPA (compound 6) using CO_2 and ATP with the release of ADP and inorganic phosphate (90). Finally, closure of the thiophane ring of biotin (compound 8) by biotin synthase requires the insertion of a sulfur atom between the C6 carbon and the nonreactive methyl C9 of DTB (compound 7) (94).

STRUCTURAL BIOLOGY OF BIOTIN BIOSYNTHETIC ENZYMES

There has been much research activity in recent years to better understand biotin biosynthesis. This includes the determination of the X-ray crystal structures of these important biosynthetic enzymes. This data is invaluable in the rational design of inhibitors that target these enzymes. Indeed, researchers have employed structural biology to define the binding mechanism of ligands and products and to identify the chemical structures of reaction intermediates. These compounds provide starting points for medicinal chemistry. The following section

---

FIGURE 1 Biotin biosynthetic pathway. The proposed synthesis of biotin precursors and the conserved metabolic pathway (dashed box) are shown. The atoms modified in each step are highlighted in bold text. Abbreviations: ACP, acyl carrier protein; AaaS, acyl-ACP synthetase; AMTB, S-adenosyl-2-oxo-4-methylthiobutyric acid; DOA, 5′-deoxyadenosine; FAS, fatty acid synthesis; SAM, S-adenosyl-L-methionine; SAH, S-adenosylhomocysteine. Figure adapted from Lin and Cronan (85).

TABLE 1 Structural biology of biotin biosynthetic enzymes and crystallographic data for the biotin biosynthetic enzymes[a]

Protein	Ligands	Organism	PDB	Reference
BioH S82A	Pimeloyl-ACP methyl ester, in complex with acyl carrier protein	*Shigella flexneri*	4ETW	87
BioH	3-hydroxy-propanoic acid, ethylene glycol	*Escherichia coli*	1M33	97
BioH	Cl⁻, dihydroxyethyl ether	*Salmonella enterica*	4NMW	–
KAPAS	PLP, $(SO_4)^{2-}$	*E. coli*	1DJE	110
KAPAS	PLP, KAPA, $(SO_4)^{2-}$	*E. coli*	1DJ9	110
KAPAS	–	*E. coli*	1BS0	108
KAPAS	Trifluoroalanine	*E. coli*	2G6W	109
KAPAS	–	*Francisella tularensis*	4IW7	–
DAPAS	PLP, ethylene glycol, $(SO_4)^{2-}$, 1,3-benxothiazol-2-ylmethylamine	*Mycobacterium tuberculosis*	4CXR	114
DAPAS	PLP, KAPA, dihydroxyethyl ether, ethylene	*M. tuberculosis*	4CXQ	114
DAPAS	2B9, ethylene glycol	*M. tuberculosis*	4MQR	114
DAPAS	2B6, ethylene glycol, Cl⁻, imidazole	*M. tuberculosis*	4MQQ	114
DAPAS	2B1, ethylene glycol, dihydroxyethyl ether	*M. tuberculosis*	4MQP	114
DAPAS	PL8, dimethyl sulfoxide	*M. tuberculosis*	3TFU	117
DAPAS	PLP, dimethyl sulfoxide	*M. tuberculosis*	3TFT	117
DAPAS	PLP, adenosyl-ornitine	*M. tuberculosis*	3LV2	114
DAPAS	PLP	*M. tuberculosis*	3BVO	114
DAPAS Y17F	Na⁺	*E. coli*	1S0A	117
DAPAS Y144F	Na⁺	*E. coli*	1S09	118
DAPAS D147N	Na⁺	*E. coli*	1S08	118
DAPAS R253A	PLP, 2-propanol, Na⁺	*E. coli*	1S07	118
DAPAS R253K	Na⁺	*E. coli*	1S06	118
DAPAS	Trans-amiclenomycin, PLP, Na²⁺	*E. coli*	1MLZ	118
DAPAS	Cis-amiclenomycin, PLP, Na²⁺	*E. coli*	1MLY	118
DAPAS	PLP, K⁺	*E. coli*	1QJ5	112
DAPAS	PLP, KAPA, Na⁺	*E. coli*	1QJ3	112
DAPAS	PLP, Na⁺	*E. coli*	1DTY	–
DAPAS R391A	PLP, 2-propanol, Na⁺	*E. coli*	1MGV	113
DAPAS	PLP, KAPA	*Bacillus subtilis*	3DU4	90
DAPAS	–	*B. subtilis*	3DRD	90
DAPAS	PLP	*B. subtilis*	3DOD	90
DAPAS	Thiocyanate ion, Na⁺	*Chromobacterium violaceum*	4A6U	116
DAPAS	PLP	*C. violaceum*	4A6T	116
DAPAS and DTBS	L(+)-tartaric acid, PLP, DTB	*Arabidopsis thaliana*	4A0R	115
DTBS	CTP, $(SO_4)^{2-}$	*M. tuberculosis*	4WOP	125
DTBS	DTB, Mg²⁺, $(PO_4)^{2-}$	*M. tuberculosis*	3FPA	90
DTBS	KAPA, $(SO_4)^{2-}$	*M. tuberculosis*	3FMI	90
DTBS	DAPA carbamate	*M. tuberculosis*	3FMF	90
DTBS	–	*M. tuberculosis*	3FGN	90
DTBS	–	*E. coli*	1DTS	121
DTBS	$(SO_4)^{2-}$	*E. coli*	1DBS	121
DTBS	DAPA carbamate	*E. coli*	1DAI	120
DTBS	DAPA, AMP-PCP, Mn²⁺	*E. coli*	1DAH	120
DTBS	DAPA carbamate, AMP-PCP	*E. coli*	1DAG	120
DTBS	DAPA carbamate, ADP, Ca²⁺	*E. coli*	1DAF	120
DTBS	3-(1-aminoethyl)nonanedioic acid	*E. coli*	1DAE	120

(Continued on next page)

TABLE 1 Structural biology of biotin biosynthetic enzymes and crystallographic data for the biotin biosynthetic enzymes*a* *(Continued)*

Protein	Ligands	Organism	PDB	Reference
DTBS	ADP	*E. coli*	1DAD	120
DTBS	–	*E. coli*	1BYI	124
DTBS	DAPA, ATP, Mg^{2+}	*E. coli*	1A82	119
DTBS	ADP, DTB, Mg^{2+}, $(PO_4)^{2-}$	*E. coli*	1DAM	119
DTBS	ADP, Mg^{2+}, DAPA carbamate with aluminum Fl	*E. coli*	1BS1	119
DTBS	ADP, DAPA-PO_4, Mg^{2+}, $(PO_4)^{2-}$	*E. coli*	1DAK	119
DTBS	Cl^-	*Helicobacter pylori*	2QMO	123
DTBS	Ethylene glycol, GDP, $(PO_4)^{2-}$, Mg^{2+}	*H. pylori*	3QY0	123
DTBS	8-aminocaprylic acid, GDP, ethylene glycol, Mg^{2+}, $(PO_4)^{2-}$	*H. pylori*	3QXX	123
DTBS	Mg^{2+}, HNO3, adenylyl imidodiphosphate	*H. pylori*	3QXS	123
DTBS	GTP, Mg^{2+}, HNO_3, ethylene glycol	*H. pylori*	3QXJ	123
DTBS	8-aminocaprylic acid, ADP, Mg^{2+}, $(PO_4)^{2+}$, ethylene glycol	*H. pylori*	3QXH	123
DTBS	ATP, Mg^{2+}, HNO_3, ethylene glycol, glycerin	*H. pylori*	3QXC	123
DTBS	$(PO_4)^{2-}$, Mg^{2+}, HNO_3, Cl^-, 8-aminocaprylic acid	*H. pylori*	3MLE	123
DTBS	Acetate ion, Na^+	*F. tularensis*	3OF5	–
BS	[4Fe-4S], [2Fe-2S], SAM, DTB	*E. coli*	1R30	94

*a*Abbreviations: PDB, Protein Data Bank; ACP, acyl carrier protein; KAPAS, 7-keto-8-aminopelargonic acid synthase; KAPA, 7-keto-8-aminopelargonic acid; DAPAS, 7,8-diaminopelargonic acid synthase; PLP, pyridoxal 5′-phosphate; DTBS, dethiobiotin synthetase; BS, biotin synthase; SAM, S-adenosyl-L-methionine; DTB, dethiobiotin.

highlights key structural features of the biotin biosynthesis enzymes. This is followed by a detailed overview of efforts to develop inhibitors with utility in antibacterial research. Where possible, we highlight the impact of this work for TB research.

BioC-O-Methyltransferase (BioC)

BioC (EC 2.1.1.197, encoded by *bioC*) is a SAM-dependent methyltransferase (86). The native form of BioC from *E. coli* and *Bacillus cereus* is monomeric, with a molecular mass of ~31 kDa (95). No crystal structure of BioC has yet been reported. The function of BioC is to generate methyl ester (compound 2) by transferring a methyl group from SAM to the free carboxyl group of a malonyl-thioester (compound 1), which is linked to either CoA or ACP (Fig. 1) (86, 95). This methylation step is essential to neutralize the negative charge of the carboxyl group prior to interaction with the extremely hydrophobic active sites of the fatty acid synthesis enzymes (95).

Without BioC, the hydrophilic malonyl-thioester cannot enter fatty acid synthesis for assembling the pimelate moiety. Of note, malonyl-ACP was shown to be the preferred acceptor of methyl groups from SAM over malonyl-CoA (95) and is also an early precursor of the canonical fatty acid synthesis pathway (95). Therefore, the expression of BioC and its activity must be tightly controlled to avoid the depletion of the malonyl-ACP pool, causing impaired cell growth (95).

BioH Carboxylesterase

As described above, the fatty acid machinery is utilized during the biosynthesis of biotin (85, 86). Thus, the carboxyl group of the pimeloyl-ACP methyl ester (compound 3 in Fig. 1) must be liberated after two cycles of carbon elongation to leave the fatty acid synthesis machinery. Indeed, the free carboxyl group is further required for protein biotinylation by BPL (48). BioH carboxylesterase (BioH; EC 3.1.1.85), encoded by *bioH*, plays an

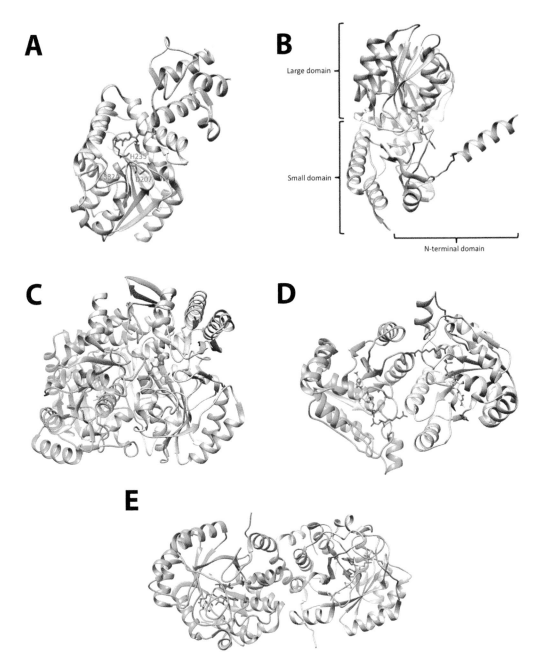

FIGURE 2 Structures of biotin biosynthetic enzymes. (A) The crystal structure of BioH S82A from *Shigella flexneri* is shown (gray ribbon) in complex with pimeloyl-ACP methyl ester (in purple) and an acyl carrier protein partner (in blue) (PDB 4ETW). Residues in the catalytic triad, namely, Ser82, Asp207, and His235 (in green), are located at the interface between the two domains. (B) One subunit of the *Escherichia coli* KAPAS homodimer is shown in complex with KAPA-PLP aldimine intermediate (shown in pink connected to blue, respectively) (PDB 1DJ9). The Mg^{2+} ion is shown in green. (C) The homodimer of DAPAS formed by two subunits, chain A (in gray) and chain B (in green). The enzyme was crystallized in complex with PLP cofactor (in blue) and KAPA substrate (in pink) (PDB 4CXQ). (D) The homodimer of DTBS is formed by two subunits: chain A (in gray) and chain B (in green). The structure of the mycobacterial enzyme has

essential role in the cleavage of the methyl ester (compound 3) producing the pimeloyl-ACP precursor (compound 4) required for KAPAS in the subsequent conserved biotin biosynthetic pathway (Fig. 1) (86, 87).

BioH is active as a monomeric protein of 28 kDa (96). It belongs to the hydrolase superfamily, a group of enzymes containing a classical Ser-His-Asp catalytic triad and a pentapeptide Gly-Xaa-Ser-Xaa-Gly motif (97–99). BioH is a carboxylesterase that can employ short acyl chains as substrates (97, 100). Three crystal structures of BioH have been determined from *E. coli*, *Shigella flexneri*, and *Salmonella enterica* (Table 1), showing a two-domain-containing protein (Fig. 2A) (87, 97). The large N-terminal domain possesses a Rossman fold consisting of a twisted seven-strand β-sheet in the middle sandwiched by five α-helices at both ends. Meanwhile, the small C-terminal domain consists of four α-helices. The catalytic triad in the active site is located at the interface between these two domains (87, 97). The overall structure of BioH is similar to bromoperoxidase (EC 1.11.1.10), aminopeptidase (EC 3.4.11.5), epoxide hydrolase (EC 3.3.2.3), haloalkane dehalogenase (EC3.8.1.5), and lyase (EC 4.2.1.39) (97). BioH captures the pimeloyl-ACP methyl ester (compound 3) substrate in association with an acyl carrier protein (Fig. 2A). The acyl carrier protein consists of four helices; the second helix (α2) interacts with the BioH small domain to facilitate the capture of the phosphopantetheine arm of the pimeloyl-ACP methyl ester substrate through Ser35 positioned at the N-terminus of the α2 helix (87). This acyl carrier protein-dependent complex is also found in other enzymes such as P450-BioI and castor desaturase (EC 1.14.99.6) (87, 101, 102).

Although various ACP-bound methyl ester compounds such as glutaryl (C5), adipyl (C6), suberyl (C8), and azelayl (C9) can interact with BioH, pimeloyl-ACP methyl ester (compound 3) (C7) is the preferred substrate. Its length is such that it can bind within the hydrophobic active site to reach the catalytic triad, and thus, it is hydrolyzed faster than unnatural substrates (87). Shorter carbon chains cannot span from the hydrophobic cavity to the catalytic triad, while longer alkyl chains cause steric clashes within the cavity. This suggests that the length of the substrate is critical for catalysis. The reaction mechanism of BioH has also been investigated in some detail. A recent study of *E. coli* BioH has revealed that the enzyme can ligate a variety of aldehydes and activated alkenes via a Baylis-Hillman reaction (103). Together, the combined knowledge of the productive carbon length of the ligand that is required for binding and the substrate promiscuity of BioH provides useful information for rational design of BioH inhibitors.

In certain BioC-containing bacteria BioH can be substituted with other biotin biosynthetic enzymes such as BioG, BioJ, and BioK to complement the growth of *E. coli* ΔBioH biotin auxotrophic strains on biotin-free medium (39, 104, 105). Although these enzymes share low sequence similarity to BioH, they belong to the same α,β-hydrolase family with associated esterase activity (104, 105). A recent study of BioJ demonstrated that the ΔBioJ strain of *Francisella novicida* had attenuated growth in minimal medium. Importantly, the replication of this mutant

---

been reported in complex with DAPA carbamate (PDB 3FMF) or CTP (PDB 4WOP). Two active sites are located at the interface between the subunits where each active site contains two adjacent binding pockets of DAPA carbamate (in red) and CTP (in yellow). (E) The crystal structure of BS was determined in complex with SAM (in orange) and DTB (in blue) (PDB 1R30). Each subunit, chain A (in gray) and chain B (in green), of the homodimer folds as a triosephosphate isomerase type (α/β)$_8$ barrel with extensions on the N- and C-terminal ends. BS contains one [4Fe-4S] and one [2Fe-2S] per monomer as highlighted in yellow.

strain is 5-fold lower than that of wild type after infection in murine bone marrow–derived macrophages, highlighting the importance of BioH-like enzymes for bacterial virulence (104).

7-Keto-8-Aminopelargonic Acid Synthase (KAPAS)

KAPAS (EC 2.3.1.47), which is encoded by *bioF* and is also known as 8-amino-7-oxononanoate synthase, catalyzes the first step of the conserved biotin biosynthetic pathway. It is classified as a type I pyridoxal 5′-phosphate (PLP or vitamin B6)–dependent enzyme in aminotransferase subclass II (85, 89). Unusually, there are two *bioF* genes in the genome of *M. tuberculosis*: *bioF* and a putative *bioF₂*, which are translated to 386 and 771 amino acid products, respectively (106). The function of an additional N-terminal extension on *bioF₂* is unclear, although it contains the putative conserved acetyl-transferase (GNAT) domain (accession: pfam13480), similar to enzymes in the N-acyl-transferase superfamily.

KAPAS converts a pimeloyl CoA (compound 4) to 7-keto-8-aminopelargonic acid (KAPA) (compound 5) using L-alanine as an amino donor and PLP as a cofactor. Unlike the homologues from other species that utilize only L-alanine, *M. tuberculosis* KAPAS can use both L-alanine and D-alanine as amino donor substrates (107). The mechanism of KAPAS is similar to those of other aminotransferase enzymes where the reaction proceeds through several intermediates, namely, an alanine-bound external aldimine complex, a quinonoid intermediate, a lysine-bound internal aldimine complex, and a 3-oxoacid aldimine complex. This leads to DAPA (compound 6) production via the addition of two carbons (C8, C9) and a nitrogen (N8) atom onto the pimeloyl-ACP substrate (compound 4) (Fig. 1) (85).

Currently, the structure of KAPAS from *M. tuberculosis* has not been determined. However, available structures of the *E. coli*

and *Francisella tularensis* orthologues determined in the apo and holo forms suggest that KAPAS is active as a homodimer (Table 1) (108–110). Each subunit assembles into three domains: (i) a small N-terminal domain composed of a three-stranded β-sheet, (ii) a large central domain containing a seven-stranded β-sheet, and (iii) a small C-terminal domain consisting of a four-stranded β-sheet with α-helices (89, 108) (Fig. 2B). The C4′ atom of PLP cofactor is covalently attached to the ε-amino group of a conserved Lys236 (numbering in *E. coli*) in the active site, positioning the PLP molecule at the interface between subunits (108, 110). Apart from Lys236, active site residues His133, Ser179, Asp204, His207, and Thr233 are also important for making direct contact with PLP (110, 111). These residues are highly conserved in all species, as well as other enzymes in the α-oxoamine synthase family (111). A Mg^{2+} ion is essential for coordination with the O3 and hydroxyl groups of Ser179, the N8′ of the KAPA intermediate, and two water molecules. A conformational change within the C-terminus upon KAPA binding results in movement of Arg349 to align antiparallel with Arg21 from the N-terminal domain, allowing these two arginine residues to H-bond with the carboxyl group of KAPA (110). In addition to H-bonding, the ligand is stabilized via hydrophobic interactions between the methylene chain of KAPA and Val79 from the subunit that interacts with PLP and with Tyr264 and Ile263 from the partner subunit. This molecular detail will provide powerful information for future structure-guided drug design.

7,8-Diaminopelargonic Acid Synthase (DAPAS)

DAPAS (EC 2.6.1.62), encoded by *bioA*, is also known as adenosylmethionine-8-amino-7-oxononanoate aminotransferase. DAPAS is analogous to KAPAS because both belong to the same subclass of the aminotransferase family (89). Briefly, DAPAS catalyzes the attachment of a nitrogen atom derived from SAM to KAPA (compound 5), which becomes the N7 moiety of biotin in DAPA (compound 6) (Fig. 1). The aminotransferase reaction of DAPAS is similar to KAPAS in that it proceeds through two partial reactions that require a PLP cofactor and an amino group donor. In contrast to KAPAS, which utilizes L-alanine, here SAM serves as the amino group donor (89, 112, 113). The first partial reaction catalyzes an aldimine from DAPAS and PLP that then interacts with SAM to generate the subsequent quinonoid, keta- mine, and then PMP (113). Following the second partial reaction, PMP interacts with KAPA substrate generating an intermediate in the reverse direction of the first partial reaction, i.e., ketamine, quinonoid, and then aldimine intermediates, before the release of the product DAPA and recycled PLP (107, 113). Interestingly, although the KAPA sub- strate has an amino group, it cannot serve as an amino donor in the DAPAS reaction (112). The interaction of DAPAS in the first partial reaction with PLP and KAPA, instead of SAM, is unproductive. This is explained by the crystal structure of DAPAS in complex with KAPA, which shows that the substrate N8 amino group in the substrate is orientated away from C4′ carbon of the PLP cofactor, thus preventing transamination and forma- tion of the aldimine intermediate (112). This structural data demonstrated specificity for the amino acid donor and revealed the important role of the C4′ carbon of the PLP cofactor for transamination. This finding paves the way to design inhibitors of DAPAS based on chemical analogues of the reaction intermediates such as the aldimine.

Crystal structures of DAPAS have been reported from *M. tuberculosis*, *E. coli*, *Arabi- dopsis thaliana*, *Chromobacterium violaceum*, and *B. subtilis* (Table 1) (43, 90, 112–118). The crystal structure of *M. tuberculosis* DAPAS in complex with PLP cofactor and KAPA sub- strate (Protein Data Bank [PDB] 4CXQ) showed that the active form of DAPAS is a homodimer with a molecular mass of ~46

kDa per monomer (Fig. 2C) (114). While there are a number of X-ray structures of *M. tuberculosis* DAPAS, most of the mech- anistic studies of DAPAS have been per- formed with the *E. coli* orthologue. As with other aminotransferases, a conserved lysine (Lys283 in *M. tuberculosis* DAPA) in the active site is essential for catalysis by forming an interaction with PLP. Upon the binding of KAPA, a conformational change repositions Arg400 such that it can H-bond with the carboxyl group of KAPA (90, 112, 114). The equivalent arginine is also important for bonding to the carboxyl group of DAPA, as shown by the 180-fold increase of K_m for DAPA in the R391A mutant (numbering in *E. coli*) compared to wild type (113). The amino group of KAPA H-bonds to the hydroxyl group of Tyr157, the carbonyl oxygen of Gly316, and the phosphate group of PLP with an additional hydrophobic interaction with the aromatic ring of Trp64 (114). Cur- rently, no crystal structure of DAPAS bound to SAM is available. However, SAM is pro- posed to bind the enzyme at the KAPA binding site. Based on mutagenesis studies of *E. coli* DAPAS, the R253A mutant in- creased the K_m for SAM by >3-fold higher than wild type, indicating that this conserved residue is important for SAM binding (118). These key residues provide useful structural information required for ligand binding and can be used in rational drug design.

Dethiobiotin Synthetase (DTBS)

DTBS (EC 6.3.3.3) is encoded by *bioD*. DTBS catalyzes the penultimate step of the biotin biosynthetic pathway to produce dethiobiotin (DTB) (compound 7) from DAPA (compound 6) using ATP and CO_2 (Fig. 1) (89). The DTBS reaction proceeds through three discrete steps: (i) formation of N7-DAPA carbamate, (ii) formation of carbamic phosphoric acid anhydride, and (iii) closure of the ureido ring of DTB with the release of inorganic phos- phate and ADP (119). Following the forma- tion of carbamic phosphoric acid anhydride, a tetrahedral intermediate is proposed to form before proceeding to the last step and closure of the ureido ring with the release of inorganic phosphate. However, this mechanism has not yet been verified by crystallographic studies (119, 120).

The structures of DTBS have been reported from *M. tuberculosis, E. coli, Helicobacter pylori,* and *F. tularensis* either in apo-form or in complex with ligands such as ATP, CTP, or DAPA (Table 1) (90, 119–125). Active DTBS is a homodimer with a molecular mass of ~46 kDa (Fig. 2D). The two active sites are placed at the interface between the two subunits in antiparallel directions 25 Å apart (124). Each subunit folds into a single α/β globular domain consisting of a seven-stranded parallel β sheet in the core surrounded by helices, similar to certain GTP-dependent enzymes such as adenylsuccinate synthase and p21ras (120, 124). Each active site contains adjacent binding pockets for DAPA and ATP substrates. The DAPA pocket is located in the dimer interface and is formed by amino acids from the two subunits, whereas the ATP pocket is composed of residues present within each of the individual monomers. Four amino acid residues (including Lys37, Thr41 from the first subunit, Leu146, and Asn147 from the partner subunit) (numbering in *M. tuberculosis*) are required for DAPA binding (124). Mutagenesis studies performed on *E. coli* DTBS revealed that mutation of Lys37 dramatically reduced k_{cat} to less than 0.9% of wild type and increased the K_m for DAPA by more than 100-fold. (126). Moreover, the phosphate-binding loop (P-loop; Gly8-Xaa9-Xaa10-Thr11-Xaa12-Xaa13-Gly14-Lys15-Thr16; numbering in *M. tuberculosis*) is crucial for H-bonding with the three phosphate groups of ATP. Binding of ATP to *E. coli* DTBS induces conformational changes in the phosphate-binding loop (120). In particular, the replacement of Thr11 with valine results in a 24,000-fold increase in the K_m for ATP, while Lys15 is a critical residue for both catalysis and ATP binding (K15Q 0.01% of

wild type k_{cat} and 1,800-fold higher K_m than wild type, respectively) (120, 126). These data suggest key residues for enzyme–ligand interaction that are useful for structure-based drug design.

Biotin Synthase (BS)

BS (EC 2.8.1.6), encoded by *bioB*, catalyzes the final step of the biotin biosynthetic pathway. Here a sulfur atom is inserted between the methyl carbons (C6 and C9) of DTB (compound 7), thus creating the thiophane ring and generating biotin (compound 8) (Fig. 1). BS belongs to a radical SAM (or AdoMet) superfamily that uses SAM for radical generation. BS contains three cysteines in a conserved eight-residue sequence motif (C-xxx-C-xx-C) that is necessary for binding of the [4Fe-4S]$^{2+/1+}$ cluster (127, 128). Only one structure of BS has been resolved, that from *E. coli* in complex with both SAM and DTB (Table 1) (94). Each subunit of the homodimer folds into a triosephosphate isomerase type (α/β)$_8$ barrel flanked with two helices at the N-terminus and nonstructured C-terminal region (Fig. 2E).

Two iron clusters are present within the protein; [2Fe-2S] is located deep within a barrel, while [4Fe-4S]$^{2+/1+}$ is positioned at the C-terminal end of the barrel. These iron-sulfur clusters serve different functions in BS. The [4Fe-4S]$^{2+/1+}$ cluster is involved in the extraction of a hydrogen atom from the methyl and methylene groups of DTB. The cluster is initially in the [4Fe-4S]$^{1+}$ state from the electron transfer system containing NADPH, flavodoxin, and ferredoxin (127, 129). The reduced [4Fe-4S]$^{1+}$ cluster catalyzes the reductive cleavage of SAM to generate a 5′-deoxyadenosyl radical and methionine. This radical can then extract one proton from each of C6 and C9 of the DTB substrate (127). As a result, this first half reaction requires two SAM equivalents per molecule of biotin formed. The dimer of BS has a single functional active site with a 2:1 stoichiometry of SAM:DTB per BS dimer

(127, 130). In the second half reaction, the [2Fe-2S] cluster has been proposed to close the thiophane ring of biotin by donating a sulfur atom (130, 131). Thus, BS itself appears to act as a substrate *in vitro* rather than as an enzyme by producing less than one molecule of biotin per molecule of BS protein (0.3 to 0.4 biotin equivalents/protein monomer) (132). *In vivo*, BS has an extremely modest catalysis rate of 10 to 60 turnovers per monomer, suggesting that a cellular mechanism exists to repair the [2Fe-2S] cluster (133, 134). A mitochondrial matrix protein, Isa2, has been proposed to play a role in the regeneration of the [2Fe-2S] cluster. BS is inactive in the *Isa* mutant strain of *S. cerevisiae*, leading to the failure of cell growth in minimum media or DTB supplementing media unless biotin is supplied (133).

Like other SAM-dependent enzymes, three conserved cysteine residues in the C-xxx-C-xx-C sequence motif contribute to ligand binding to BS. Indeed, the replacement of Cys53, Cys57, and Cys60 with alanine was shown to abolish the SAM reduction activity of *E. coli* BS in the [4Fe-4S]$^{2+/1+}$ cluster (135, 136). In addition, Cys97, Cys128, and Cys188 that do not belong to the motif and a conserved Arg260 are essential for binding of the [2Fe-2S] cluster (136, 137). These identified key residues provide structural information for further use in structure-guided drug design.

INHIBITORS OF BIOTIN BIOSYNTHETIC ENZYMES

A number of studies have investigated inhibitors of biotin biosynthetic enzymes for antibacterial drug discovery. For most of these studies, enzyme inhibitors have been designed using the chemical structures of the known substrates, reaction intermediates, or products. While most studies have characterized the *in vitro* properties of these compounds as enzyme inhibitors, the antibacterial activities of only a select few have

been reported (see below). Like other SAM-dependent methyltransferases, BioC is inhibited by chemical analogues of the SAM substrate (compound 9 in Fig. 3). Demethylated SAM, namely, *S*-adenosylhomocysteine (compound 10), is the product of the methyl transfer reaction catalyzed by BioC. *S*-adenosylhomocysteine inhibited BioC in a concentration-dependent manner, with 1 μM of S-adenosylhomocysteine reducing ~40% of the *E. coli* BioC activity (95). Sinefungin (compound 11), a natural antibiotic isolated from *Streptomyces griseolus*, has also been shown to inhibit BioC (95, 138). Sinefungin is a steric and electrostatic mimic of SAM but has greater potency than *S*-adenosylhomocysteine (138). It reduced ~60% of the enzyme activity at 0.1 μM and completely abolished activity at 1 μM (95).

The inhibition of KAPAS has also been pursued using chemical analogues of either

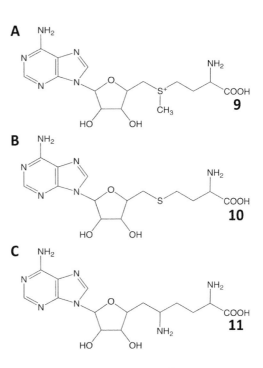

FIGURE 3 Chemical structures of BioC substrate and inhibitors. (A)*S*-adenosyl *L*-methionine substrate. **(B)***S*-adenosylhomocysteine product of BioC reaction. **(C) Sinefungin.**

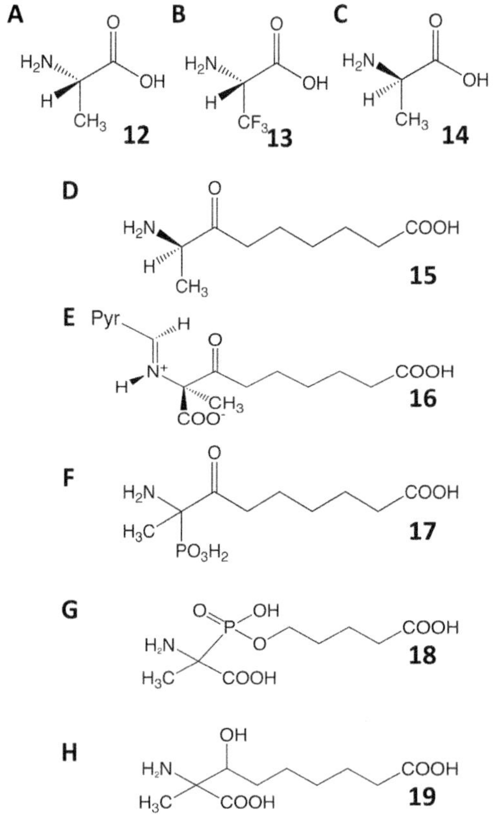

FIGURE 4 Chemical structures of KAPAS substrate, reaction intermediate, and inhibitors. (A) L-alanine. (B) L-trifluroalanine. (C) D-alanine. (D) D-KAPA. (E) The aldimine reaction intermediate. (F) (±)-8-amino-7-oxo-8-phosphonononaoic acid. (G) 4-carboxybutyl (1-amino-1-carboxyethyl) phosphate. (H) 2-amino-3-hydroxy-2-methylnonadioic acid. Abbreviation: Pyr, pyrimidine ring of the PLP cofactor.

L- and D-configurations (107). Interestingly, the product of the D-alanine-utilized reaction, D-KAPA (compound 15) (compare L-KAPA compound 5), was found to inhibit KAPAS (K_i = 115 μM) (107). Several analogues of the aldimine intermediate (compound 16), such as (±)-8-amino-7-oxo-8-phosphononononaoic acid (compound 17), 4-carboxybutyl-(1-amino-1-carboxyethyl)-phosphonate (compound 18), and 2-amino-3-hydroxy-2-methylnonadioic acid (compound 19) are also competitive inhibitors of E. coli KAPAS with respect to L-alanine, with K_i values of 7, 68, and 80 mM, respectively (92).

Amiclenomycin (Fig. 5), another suicide inhibitor isolated from Streptomyces spp.,

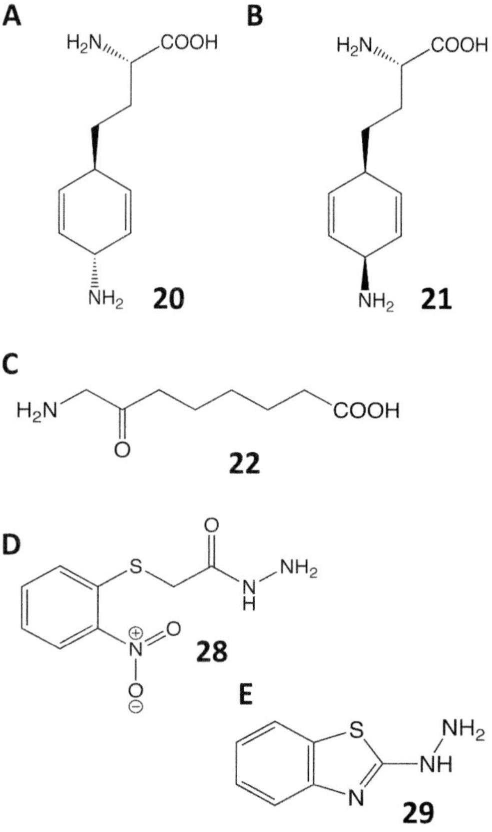

FIGURE 5 Chemical structures of DAPAS inhibitors. (A) Cis-amiclenomycin. (B) Trans-amiclenomycin. (C) 8-amino-7-oxooctanoic acid. (D) MAC13772. (E) Aryl hydrazine.

substrate, reaction intermediate, or products. The L-alanine substrate (compound 12) analogue L-trifluoroalanine (compound 13) (Fig. 4) is a slow suicide inhibitor of E. coli KAPAS ($t_{1/2}$ ~ 20 min) that covalently binds to the active site lysine and forms an irreversible 2-(pyridoximine phosphate) acetoyl protein addict (109). D-alanine (compound 14), which is the enantiomer of the native L-alanine substrate, was found to competitively inhibit the E. coli KAPAS with a K_i of 0.59 mM (92). In contrast, D-alanine is not a competitive inhibitor for M. tuberculosis KAPAS because the enzyme can utilize both showed inhibitory activity against DAPAS from *E. coli* and *M. tuberculosis* (K_i = 2 µM and 12 µM, respectively) (41–43, 139–142). The crystal structures of *E. coli* DAPAS in complex with amiclenomycin suggest that the inhibition of the enzyme is stereo-selective because the *cis*-isomer (compound 20) (PDB 1MLY) is active, while the *trans*-isomer (compound 21) (PDB 1MLZ) causes a steric hindrance at the active site that results in a significantly less potent inhibitor (43). The design of amiclenomycin analogs revealed that the *cis*-configuration, but not the amino acid moiety, is essential for inhibitory activity (44, 141). In addition to KAPAS, as mentioned above, D-KAPA (compound 15) (or [*R*]-KAPA) also showed inhibitory activity against *M. tuberculosis* DAPAS, with a K_i of 5.9 µM (107, 143). 8-amino-7-oxooctanoic acid (compound 22), an achiral

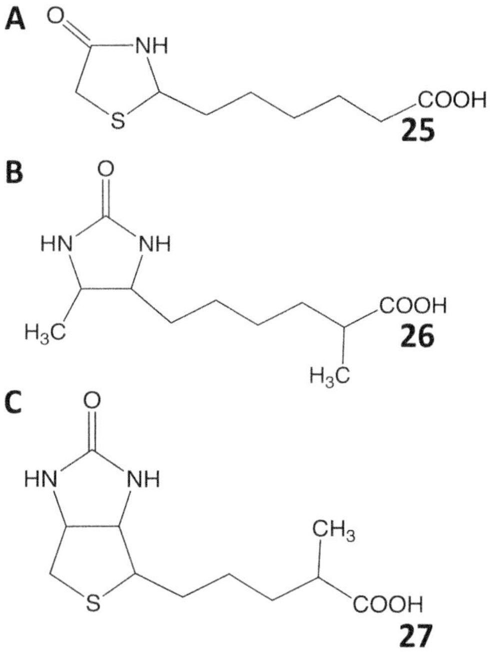

FIGURE 7 Chemical structures of BS inhibitors. (A) Actithiazic acid. (B) α-methyldethiobiotin. (C) α-methylbiotin.

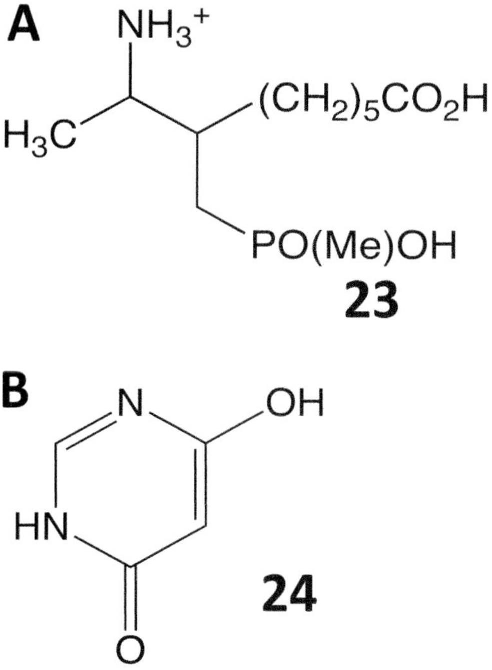

analog of the KAPA substrate, inhibited DAPAS, with a K_i of 4.2 µM (143).

To inhibit DTBS, a series of DAPA, DAPA carbamate, and ATP mimics have been rationally designed. For the purpose of herbicide development, a total of 54 compounds, such as phosphonic acid (compound 23) (Fig. 6), were synthesized and tested for inhibitory activity against *E. coli* DTBS, but none showed submillimolar inhibition constants (144). In a separate study using available X-ray data of ATP bound to *E. coli* DTBS, a pharmacophore was proposed and employed to design an inhibitor that targeted the ATP binding pocket. Consequently, 6-hydroxypyrimidin-4(3H)-one (compound 24) was synthesized and shown to have a K_i of 11 mM (145).

Finally, a number of BS inhibitors have also been reported. Actithiazic acid (compound 25) (Fig. 7) (also known as acidomycin) isolated from *Actinomyces virginiae*

FIGURE 6 Chemical structures of DTBS inhibitor. (A) A phosphate-based mimic of DAPA carbamate. (B) 6-hydroxypyrimidin-4(3H)-one (also known as 6-HP4).

and *Streptomyces* spp. inhibited BS from *E. coli* (K_i = 0.45 μM) and *M. tuberculosis* (no record of K_i; see the antibacterial activity discussed later) (146–149). α-methyldethiobiotin (compound 26) and α-methylbiotin (compound 27), isolated from *Streptomyces lydicus*, were also shown to inhibit the *E. coli* BS activity (K_i = 1.1 μM for α-methyldethiobiotin) (146, 150, 151).

The antibacterial activities for a select few of the above inhibitors that target DAPAS and BS have been investigated against several strains of mycobacteria. Amiclenomycin (compound 20) and actithiazic acid (compound 25) inhibit growth of *M. smegmatis* with MICs of 12.5 and 0.4 μg/ml, respectively, but failed to reduce the bacterial burden in a murine model of infection (42, 142, 146, 148, 149). Meanwhile, α-methyldethiobiotin (compound 26) and α-methylbiotin (compound 27) were found to effectively inhibit *Mycobacterium fortuitum*, *M. smegmatis*, *Mycobacterium avium*, *Mycobacterium phlei*, and *Mycobacterium salmoniphilum*, with MIC values of 0.8 to 80 μg/ml and 12.5 to 200 μg/ml, respectively (150). While the detailed structural information about these biosynthetic enzymes is very valuable, the application of structure-based rational-design strategies has so far resulted in compounds with inhibition constants in the micromolar to millimolar range and weak antibiotic activity. This suggests that new approaches are now required.

FUTURE DIRECTIONS FOR DRUG SCREENING

Phenotypic Screening

After a decade of target-based high-throughput screening campaigns to discover new classes of antibiotics, there has been a reversal back toward using the phenotypic, whole-cell screens that researchers favored during the golden era of antibiotic discovery (152–154). This is highlighted by the recent identification of a novel depsipeptide antibiotic isolated from soil-borne bacteria (155). By culturing the bacteria in their natural habitat, the researchers avoided the need to culture the microorganisms under laboratory conditions, where many species fail to grow. Indeed, identifying the appropriate conditions that mimic the natural environment in which bacteria are found is important for antibiotic susceptibility. Often the microniches that pathogenic bacteria colonize are deficient in nutrients, causing the bacteria to adapt their metabolic activities to support their requirement for various micronutrients, including biotin. This should be considered when performing whole-cell-based screens. Recently, a new inhibitor of biotin biosynthesis was identified using differential susceptibility under varying growth conditions (65). A primary screen was performed on a library of 30,000 compounds for molecules that inhibited growth of *E. coli* on limited nutrient media. The hits were subsequently reassayed using a defined medium supplemented with a mixture of amino acids, purines, pyrimidines, and vitamins. Those compounds that showed differential antibacterial susceptibility under nutrient-limited conditions, but not the deplete media, were selected for further characterization. Through this approach compound MAC13772 (compound 28) (Fig. 5) was identified as an inhibitor of biotin biosynthesis with antibacterial activity in the nutrient-limited broth (MIC 8 μg/ml) but not in media supplemented with 2 nM biotin. The antibacterial activity was reversed when media were supplemented with biotin, desthiobiotin, or DAPA, but not KAPA. Thus, the mechanism of action for this compound was proposed to be through inhibition of DAPAS and was subsequently confirmed through biochemical analysis. Similar consideration should be given to the growth conditions when screening for new antimycobacterials, given the hypoxic and nutrient-poor intracellular environments that the bacteria naturally colonize in human macrophages.

Fragment-Based Drug Discovery (FBDD)

FBDD has become a powerful approach for early-stage hit discovery over the past decade (156–159). This technique aims to identify small starting structures that can be optimized into drug-like compounds. FBDD has enjoyed success in drug discovery with one FDA approved drug (Zelboraf, also known as Vemurafenib), which is approved for melanoma treatment, and more than 10 compounds in clinical trials for treating leukemia, myeloma, coronary artery disease, chronic obstructive pulmonary disease, diabetes, and bacterial skin infections (160–162). Conceptually, FBDD is the discovery of small fragments that can bind to specific target sites. Fragments are defined by a "rule of three" with low molecular weight <300 Da, less than three hydrogen bond donors and acceptors, and cLogP < 3 (163). Once fragment hits have been identified, larger lead molecules with higher affinity can be created by growing or modifying the chemical structure of one fragment or by linking or merging two adjacent fragments (164–167). Fragments are preferable as starting points for hit to lead development, rather than larger (molecular weight ≤ 500) drug-like compounds obtained from conventional high-throughput screenings. First, the low molecular mass often results in fragments that have high ligand efficiency, where the binding affinity is calculated relative to the number of heavy atoms in the ligand (167–170). Second, fragment libraries can be chemically diverse such that they can probe chemical space more effectively than larger compounds (160, 171, 172). Last, fragments with less complexity can bind to various sites of the protein target such that screening a fragment library often leads to hit rates as high as 5 to 10% (160).

While FBDD has been emphasized in several fields of drug discovery, its application in the field of antibiotic discovery is still underutilized. The previous large-scale failure of hit identification from natural compound libraries, which have limited permeability through the mycobacterial cell envelope, restricts success in a target-based high throughput screening approach (153). However, a recent study of synthetic TB drugs and prodrugs suggests that many of the successful compounds that are reactive inside mycobacteria can be considered fragment-like (i.e., molecular weight ≤ 300), such as isoniazid, ethionamide, para-aminosalicylic acid, and pyrazinamide (173). Indeed, being a smaller compound with moderate lipophilicity (clogP < 3) seems to be a positive feature for penetration through the complex mycobacterial cell envelope (173). There is only one recent report of an inhibitor of *M. tuberculosis* DAPAS identified by FBDD, namely, aryl hydrazine (compound 29) (Fig. 5) (114). It competitively inhibited the enzyme with respect to SAM (K_i = 10.4 µM). The crystal structure (PDB 4MQP) revealed that the aryl hydrazine forms a reversible covalent adduct with the PLP cofactor bound to DAPAS. These successes suggest that fragment-based screening could be an excellent way to enhance current anti-TB drug discovery efforts, and using these methods to target the biotin biosynthesis pathway in *M. tuberculosis* is a particularly exciting and novel approach to finding new anti-TB agents.

ACKNOWLEDGMENTS

This work was supported by the National Health and Medical Research Council of Australia (applications APP1068885) and the Center of Molecular Pathology, University of Adelaide. W.S. was a recipient of the Royal Thai Government Scholarship. The authors acknowledge that they have no conflict of interest to declare.

CITATION

Salaemae W, Booker GW, Polyak SW. 2016. The role of biotin in bacterial physiology and virulence: a novel antibiotic target for *Mycobacterium tuberculosis*. Microbiol Spectrum 4(2):VMBF-0008-2015.

REFERENCES

1. **World Health Organization.** 2014. WHO Fact Sheet No 104. http://www.who.int/mediacentre/factsheets/fs104/en/.

2. **World Health Organization.** 2006. *The Global Plan to Stop TB 2006-2015.* Part I Strategic directions. WHO, Geneva Switzerland.

3. **World Health Organization.** 2012. "Totally drug-resistant" tuberculosis: a WHO consultation on the diagnostic definition and treatment options. http://www.who.int/tb/challenges/xdr/xdrconsultation/en/.

4. **World Health Organization.** 2015. *Global Tuberculosis Report 2014.* WHO, Geneva, Switzerland.

5. **Demissie M, Lemma E, Gebeyehu M, Lindtjorn B.** 2001. Sensitivity to anti-tuberculosis drugs in HIV-positive and -negative patients in Addis Ababa. *Scan J Infec Dis* **33:**914–919.

6. **Colditz G, Berkey C, Mosteller F, Brewer T, Wilson M, Burdick E, Fineberg H.** 1995. The efficacy of bacillus Calmette-Guerin vaccination of newborns and infants in the prevention of tuberculosis: meta-analyses of the published literature. *Pediatrics* **96:**29–35.

7. **Sandhu G.** 2011. Tuberculosis: current situation, challenges, and overview of its control programs in India. *J Glob Infec Dis* **3:**143–150.

8. **Ferguson L, Rhoads J.** 2009. Multidrug-resistant and extensively drug-resistant tuberculosis: the new face of an old disease. *J Am Acad Nurse Pract* **21:**603–609.

9. **Chopra P, Meena L, Singh Y.** 2003. New drug targets for *Mycobacterium tuberculosis. Ind J Med Res* **117:**1–9.

10. **Udwadia Z, Amale R, Ajbani K, Rodrigues C.** 2011. Totally drug-resistant tuberculosis in India. *Clin Infect Dis* **54:**579–581.

11. **Velayati A, Masjedi M, Farnia P, Tabarsi P, Ghanavi J, Ziazarifi A, Hoffner S.** 2009. Emergence of new forms of totally drug-resistant tuberculosis bacilli: super extensively drug-resistant tuberculosis or totally drug-resistant strains in Iran. *Chest* **136:**420–425.

12. **Rowland K.** 2012. Totally drug-resistant TB emerges in India. *Nature.* doi:10.1038/nature.2012.9797.

13. **Migliori G, De Iaco G, Besozzi G, Centis R, Cirillo D.** 2007. First tuberculosis cases in Italy resistant to all tested drugs. *Euro Surveil* **12:**E070517.1. http://www.eurosurveillance.org/ViewArticle.aspx?ArticleId=3194.

14. **US Food and Drug Administration.** 2012. *FDA news release.* http://www.fda.gov/NewsEvents/Newsroom/PressAnnouncements/ucm333695.htm.

15. **Koul A, Arnoult E, Lounis N, Guillemont J, Andries K.** 2011. The challenge of new drug discovery for tuberculosis. *Nature* **469:**483–490.

16. **Parida SK, Axelsson-Robertson R, Rao MV, Singh N, Master I, Lutckii A, Keshavjee S, Andersson J, Zumla S, Maeurer M.** 2014. Totally drug-resistant tuberculosis and adjunct therapies. *J Intern Med.* [Epub ahead of print.] doi:10.1111/joim.12264.

17. **Lanoix JP, Betoudji F, Nuermberger E.** 2014. Novel regimens identified in mice for treatment of latent tuberculosis infection in contacts of patients with multidrug-resistant tuberculosis. *Antimicrob Agents Chemother* **58:**2316–2321.

18. **Salaemae W, Azhar A, Booker G, Polyak S.** 2011. Biotin biosynthesis in *Mycobacterium tuberculosis*: physiology, biochemistry and molecular intervention. *Prot Cell* **2:**691–695.

19. **Park S, Klotzsche M, Wilson D, Boshoff H, Eoh H, Manjunatha U, Blumenthal A, Rhee K, Barry C III, Aldrich C, Ehrt S, Schnappinger D.** 2011. Evaluating the sensitivity of *Mycobacterium tuberculosis* to biotin deprivation using regulated gene expression. *PLoS Pathog* **7:**e1002264. doi:10.1371/journal.ppat.1002264.

20. **Eisenreich W, Dandekar T, Heesemann J, Goebel W.** 2010. Carbon metabolism of intracellular bacterial pathogens and possible links to virulence. *Nat Rev Microbiol* **8:**401–412.

21. **Takayama K, Wang C, Besra G.** 2005. Pathway to synthesis and processing of mycolic acids in *Mycobacterium tuberculosis. Clin Microbiol Rev* **18:**81–101.

22. **Gago G, Diacovich L, Arabolaza A, Tsai S, Gramajo H.** 2011. Fatty acid biosynthesis in actinomycetes. *FEMS Microbiol Rev* **35:**475–497.

23. **Roje S.** 2007. Vitamin B biosynthesis in plants. *Phytochemistry* **68:**1904–1921.

24. **Polyak S, Bailey L, Azhar A, Booker G.** 2012. Biotin (vitamin H or B7), p 65–93. *In* Betancourt A, Gaitan H (ed), *Micronutrients: Sources, Properties and Health Benefits.* Nova Science Publishers, New York, NY.

25. **Zewmpleni J, Wijeratne S, Hassan Y.** 2009. Biotin. *Biofactors* **35:**36–46.

26. **Hebblen P, Rodionov D, Alfandega A, Eitinger T.** 2007. Biotin uptake in prokaryotes by solute transporters with an optional ATP-binding cassette-containing module. *Proc Natl Acad Sci USA* **104:**2909–2914.

27. **Rodionov D, Hebblen P, Eudes A, ter Beek J, Rodionov I, Erkens E, Slotboom D, Gelfand M, Osterman A, Hanson A, Eitinger T.** 2009. A novel class of modular transporters for vitamins in prokaryotes. *J Bacteriol* **191:**42–51.

28. **Ringlstetter S.** 2010. Identification of the biotin transporter in *Escherichia coli*, biotinylation of

histones in *Saccharomyces cerevisiae* and analysis of biotin sensing in *Saccharomyces cerevisiae*. PhD thesis University Regensburg, Regensburg, Germany.

29. **Finkenwirth F, Kirsch F, Eitinger T.** 2014. A versatile *Escherichia coli* strain for identification of biotin transporters and for biotin quantification. *Bioengineered* **5:**129–132.

30. **Pai C.** 1972. Mutant of *Escherichia coli* with derepressed levels of the biotin biosynthetic enzymes. *J Bacteriol* **112:**1280–1287.

31. **Eisenberg M, Mee B, Prakash O, Eisenberg M.** 1975. Properties of alpha-dehydrobiotin-resistant mutants of *Escherichia coli* K-12. *J Bacteriol* **122:**66–72.

32. **Kondo H, Kazuta Y, Goto T.** 2000. Search for a microbial biotin transporter. *BioFactors* **11:**101–102.

33. **Cicmanec J, Lichstein H.** 1978. Uptake of extracellular biotin by *Escherichia coli* biotin prototrophs. *J Bacteriol* **133:**270–278.

34. **Pai C.** 1973. Biotin uptake in biotin regulatory mutant of *Escherichia coli*. *J Bacteriol* **116:**494–496.

35. **Piffeteau A, Gaudry M.** 1985. Biotin uptake: influx, efflux and countertransport in *Escherichia coli* k12. *Biochem Biophys Acta* **816:**77–82.

36. **Piffeteau A, Zamboni M, Gaudry M.** 1982. Biotin transport by a biotin-deficient strain of *Escherichia coli*. *Biochem Biophys Acta* **688:**29–36.

37. **Prakash O, Eisenberg M.** 1974. Active transport of biotin in *Escherichia coli* K-12. *J Bacteriol* **120:**785–791.

38. **Walker J, Altman E.** 2005. Biotinylation facilitates the uptake of large peptides by *Escherichia coli* and other Gram-negative bacteria. *Appl Environ Microbiol* **71:**1850–1855.

39. **Rodionov D, Mironov A, Gelfand M.** 2002. Conservation of the biotin regulon and the BirA regulatory signal in *Eubacteria* and *Archaea*. *Gen Res* **12:**1507–1516.

40. **Ogata K, Izumi Y, Tani Y.** 1973. The controlling action of actithiazic acid on the biosynthesis of biotin-vitamers by various microorganisms. *Agr Biol Chem* **37:**1079–1085.

41. **Okami Y, Kitahara T, Hamada M, Naganawa H, Kondo S, Maeda K, Takeuchi T, Umezawa H.** 1974. Studies on a new amino acid antibiotic, amiclenomycin. *J Antibiot* **27:**656–664.

42. **Kitahara T, Hotta K, Yoshida M, Okami Y.** 1975. Biological studies of amiclenomycin. *J Antibiot* (Tokyo) **28:**215–221.

43. **Sandmark J, Mann S, Marquet A, Schneider G.** 2002. Structural basis for the inhibition of the biosynthesis of biotin by the antibiotic amiclenomycin. *J Biol Chem* **277:**43352–43358.

44. **Mann S, Marquet A, Ploux O.** 2005. Inhibition of 7,8-diaminopelargonic acid aminotransferase by amiclenomycin and analogues. *Biochem Soc Trans* **33:**802–805.

45. **Okami Y, Kitahara T, Hamada M, Naganawa H, Kondo S.** 1974. Studies on a new amino acid antibiotic, amiclenomycin. *J Antibiot* (Tokyo) **27:**656–664.

46. **Mock D, Malik M.** 1992. Distribution of biotin in human plasma: most of the biotin is not bound to protein. *Am J Clin Nutr* **56:**427–432.

47. **Harthe C, Claustrat B.** 2003. A sensitive and practical competitive radioassay for plasma biotin. *Ann Clin Biochem* **40:**259–263.

48. **Polyak SW, Chapman-Smith A.** 2013. Biotin, p 221–225. *In* Lennarz WJ, Lane MD (ed), *Encyclopaedia of Biological Chemistry*, 2nd ed. Academic Press, London, UK.

49. **Kondo S, Nakajima Y, Sugio S, Yong-Biao J, Sueda S, Kondo H.** 2004. Structure of the biotin carboxylase subunit of pyruvate carboxylase from *Aquifex aeolicus* at 2.2 A resolution. *Acta Crystallogr D Biol Crystallogr* **60:**486–492.

50. **Yu L, Xiang S, Lasso G, Gil D, Valle M, Tong L.** 2009. A symmetrical tetramer for *S. aureus* pyruvate carboxylase in complex with coenzyme A. *Structure* **17:**823–832.

51. **Tong L.** 2013. Structure and function of biotin-dependent carboxylases. *Cell Mol Life Sci* **70:**863–891.

52. **Polyak S, Abell A, Wilce M, Zhang L, Booker G.** 2012. Structure, function and selective inhibition of bacterial acetyl-coa carboxylase. *Appl Microbiol Biotechnol* **93:**983–992.

53. **Kurth DG, Gago GM, de la Iglesia A, Bazet Lyonnet B, Lin TW, Morbidoni HR, Tsai SC, Gramajo H.** 2009. ACCase 6 is the essential acetyl-CoA carboxylase involved in fatty acid and mycolic acid biosynthesis in mycobacteria. *Microbiology* **155:**2664–2675.

54. **Arabolaza A, Shillito M, Lin T, Diacovich L, Melgar M, Pham H, Amick D, Gramajo H, Tsai S.** 2010. Crystal structures and mutational analyses of acyl-CoA carboxylase beta subunit of *Streptomyces coelicolor*. *Biochemistry* **49:**7367–7376.

55. **Sartain MJ, Dick DL, Rithner CD, Crick DC, Belisle JT.** 2011. Lipidomic analyses of *Mycobacterium tuberculosis* based on accurate mass measurements and the novel "Mtb LipidDB". *J Lipid Res* **52:**861–872.

56. **Minnikin D, Kremer L, Dover L, Besra G.** 2002. The methyl-branched fortifications of *Mycobacterium tuberculosis*. *Chem Biol* **9:**545–553.

57. **Sassetti CM, Boyd DH, Rubin EJ.** 2003. Genes required for mycobacterial growth defined by

high density mutagenesis. *Mol Microbiol* **48**:77–84.

58. **Wright H, Reynolds K.** 2007. Antibacterial targets in fatty acid biosynthesis. *Curr Opin Microbiol* **10**:447–453.

59. **Parsons J, Rock C.** 2011. Is bacterial fatty acid synthesis a valid target for antibacterial drug discovery? *Curr Opin Microbiol* **14**:544–549.

60. **Chan D, Vogel H.** 2010. Current understanding of fatty acid biosynthesis and the acyl carrier protein. *Biochemistry* **430**:1–19.

61. **Jitrapakdee S, St Maurice M, Rayment I, Cleland WW, Wallace JC, Attwood PV.** 2008. Structure, mechanism and regulation of pyruvate carboxylase. *Biochem J* **413**:369–387.

62. **Beste DJ, Noh K, Niedenfuhr S, Mendum TA, Hawkins ND, Ward JL, Beale MH, Wiechert W, McFadden J.** 2013. 13C-flux spectral analysis of host-pathogen metabolism reveals a mixed diet for intracellular *Mycobacterium tuberculosis*. *Chem Biol* **20**:1012–1021.

63. **de Carvalho LP, Fischer SM, Marrero J, Nathan C, Ehrt S, Rhee KY.** 2010. Metabolomics of *Mycobacterium tuberculosis* reveals compartmentalized co-catabolism of carbon substrates. *Chem Biol* **17**:1122–1131.

64. **Rhee KY, de Carvalho LP, Bryk R, Ehrt S, Marrero J, Park SW, Schnappinger D, Venugopal A, Nathan C.** 2011. Central carbon metabolism in *Mycobacterium tuberculosis*: an unexpected frontier. *Trends Microbiol* **19**:307–314.

65. **Zlitni S, Ferruccio LF, Brown ED.** 2013. Metabolic suppression identifies new antibacterial inhibitors under nutrient limitation. *Nat Chem Biol* **9**:796–804.

66. **Purushothaman S, Gupta G, Srivastava R, Ramu V, Surolia A.** 2008. Ligand specificity of group I biotin protein ligase of *Mycobacterium tuberculosis*. *PloS One* **3**:e2320. doi:10.1371/journal.pone.0002320.

67. **Pendini NR, Bailey LM, Booker GW, Wilce MC, Wallace JC, Polyak SW.** 2008. Microbial biotin protein ligases aid in understanding holocarboxylase synthetase deficiency. *Biochim Biophys Acta* **1784**:973–982.

68. **Duckworth B, Geders T, Tiwari D, Boshoff H, Sibbald P, Barry C, Schnappinger D, Finzel B, Aldrich C.** 2011. Bisubstrate adenylation inhibitors of biotin protein ligase from *Mycobacterium tuberculosis*. *Chem Biol* **18**:1432–1441.

69. **Chakravartty V, Cronan J.** 2012. Altered regulation of *Escherichia coli* biotin biosynthesis in BirA superrepressor mutant strains. *J Bacteriol* **194**:1113–1126.

70. **Henke S, Cronan J.** 2014. Successful conversion of the *Bacillus subtilis* BirA group II biotin protein ligase into a group I ligase. *PloS One* **9**:e96757. doi:10.1371/journal.pone.0096757.

71. **Pendini N, Yap M, Yap S, Polyak S, Cowieson N, Abell A, Booker G, Wallace J, Wilce J, Wilce M.** 2013. Structural characterization of *Staphylococcus aureus* biotin protein ligase and interaction partners: an antibiotic target. *Protein Sci* **22**:762–773.

72. **Soares da Costa TP, Yap MY, Perugini MA, Wallace JC, Abell AD, Wilce MC, Polyak SE, Booker GW.** 2014. Dual roles of F123 in protein homodimerization and inhibitor binding to biotin protein ligase from *Staphylococcus aureus*. *Mol Microbiol* **91**:110–120.

73. **Mayende L, Swift RD, Bailey LM, Soares da Costa TP, Wallace JC, Booker GW, Polyak SW.** 2012. A novel molecular mechanism to explain biotin-unresponsive holocarboxylase synthetase deficiency. *J Mol Med* (Berl) **90**:81–88.

74. **Paparella AS, Soares da Costa TP, Yap MY, Tieu W, Wilce MC, Booker GW, Abell AD, Polyak SW.** 2014. Structure guided design of biotin protein ligase inhibitors for antibiotic discovery. *Curr Top Med Chem* **14**:4–20.

75. **Marrakchi H, Laneelle G, Quemard A.** 2000. InhA, a target of the antituberculous drug isoniazid, is involved in a mycobacterial fatty acid elongation system, FAS-II. *Microbiology* **146**:289–296.

76. **Tonge P, Kisker C, Slayden R.** 2007. Development of modern InhA inhibitors to combat drug resistant strains of *Mycobacterium tuberculosis*. *Curr Top Med Chem* **7**:489–498.

77. **Singh G, Singh G, Jadeja D, Kaur J.** 2010. Lipid hydrolizing enzymes in virulence: *Mycobacterium tuberculosis* as a model system. *Crit Rev Microbiol* **36**:259–269.

78. **Deb C, Lee C, Dubey V, Daniel J, Abomoelak B, Sirakova T, Pawar S, Rogers L, Kolattukudy P.** 2009. A novel *in vitro* multiple-stress dormancy model for *Mycobacterium tuberculosis* generates a lipid-loaded, drug-tolerant, dormant pathogen. *PloS One* **4**:e6077. doi:10.1371/journal.pone.0006077.

79. **Ashkenazi T, Pinkert D, Nudelman A, Widberg A, Wexler B, Wittenbach V, Flint D, Nudelman A.** 2007. Aryl chain analogues of the biotin vitamers as potential herbicides. Part 3. *Pest Manag Sci* **63**:974–1001.

80. **Yu J, Niu C, Wang D, Li M, Teo W, Sun G, Wang J, Liu J, Gao Q.** 2011. MMAR_2770, a new enzyme involved in biotin biosynthesis, is essential for the growth of *Mycobacterium marinum* in macrophages and zebrafish. *Microbes Infect* **13**:33–41.

81. **Keer J, Smeulders Gray K, Williams H.** 2000. Mutants of *Mycobacterium smegmatis* im-

paired in stationary-phase survival. *Microbiology* **146:**2209–2217.

82. **Sassetti C, Boyd D, Rubin E.** 2001. Comprehensive identification of conditionally essential genes in mycobacteria. *Proc Natl Acad Sci USA* **98:**12712–12717.

83. **Rengarajan J, Bloom B, Rubin E.** 2005. Genome-wide requirements for *Mycobacterium tuberculosis* adaptation and survival in macrophages. *Proc Natl Acad Sci USA* **102:** 8327–8332.

84. **Sassetti C, Rubin E.** 2003. Genetic requirements for mycobacterial survival during infection. *Proc Natl Acad Sci USA* **100:**12989–12994.

85. **Lin S, Cronan J.** 2011. Closing in on complete pathways of biotin biosynthesis. *Mol BioSys* **7:**1811–1821.

86. **Lin S, Hanson R, Cronan J.** 2010. Biotin synthesis begins by hijacking the fatty acid synthetic pathway. *Nat Chem Biol* **6:**682–688.

87. **Agarwal V, Lin S, Lukk T, Nair S, Cronan J.** 2012. Structure of the enzyme-acyl carrier protein (ACP) substrate gatekeeper complex required for biotin synthesis. *Proc Natl Acad Sci USA* **109:**17406–17411.

88. **Cronan J, Lin S.** 2010. Synthesis of the alpha, omega-dicarboxylic acid precursor of biotin by the canonical fatty acid biosynthetic pathway. *Curr Opin Chem Biol* **15:**407–413.

89. **Schneider G, Lindqvist Y.** 2001. Structural enzymology of biotin biosynthesis. *FEBS Lett* **495:**7–11.

90. **Dey S, Lane J, Lee R, Rubin E, Sacchettini J.** 2010. Structural characterization of the *Mycobacterium tuberculosis* biotin biosynthesis enzymes 7,8-diaminopelargonic acid synthase and dethiobiotin synthetase. *Biochemistry* **49:**6746–6760.

91. **Phalip V, Kuhn I, Lemoine Y, Jeltsch J.** 1999. Characterization of the biotin biosynthesis pathway in *Saccharomyces cerevisiae* and evidence for a cluster containing BIO5, a novel gene involved in vitamer uptake. *Gene* **232:**43–51.

92. **Ploux O, Breyne O, Carillon S, Marquet A.** 1999. Slow-binding and competitive inhibition of 8-amino-7-oxopelargonate synthase, a pyridoxal-5′-phosphate-dependent enzyme involved in biotin biosynthesis, by substrate and intermediate analogs: kinetic and binding studies. *Eur J Biochem* **259:**63–70.

93. **Marquet A, Tse Sum Bui B, Florentin D.** 2001. Biosynthesis of biotin and lipoic acid. *Vitam Horm* **61:**51–101.

94. **Berkovitch F, Nicolet Y, Wan J, Jarrett J, Drennan C.** 2004. Crystal structure of biotin synthase, an S-adenosylmethionine-dependent radical enzyme. *Science* **303:**76–79.

95. **Lin S, Cronan J.** 2012. The BioC O-methyltransferase catalyzes methyl esterification of malonyl-acyl carrier protein, an essential step in biotin synthesis. *J Biol Chem* **287:**37010–37020.

96. **Flores H, Lin S, Contreras-Ferrat G, Cronan J, Morett E.** 2012. Evolution of a new function in an esterase: simple amino acid substitutions enable the activity present in the larger paralog, BioH. *Protein Eng Des Sel* **25:**387–395.

97. **Sanishvili R, Yakunin A, Laskowski R, Skarina T, Evdokimova E, Doherty-Kirby A, Lajoie G, Thornton J, Arrowsmith C, Savchenko A, Joachimiak A, Edwards A.** 2013. Genomics proteomics and bioinformatics: integrating structure, bioinformatics, and enzymology to discover function: BioH, a new carboxylesterase from *Escherichia coli. J Biol Chem* **278:**26039–26045.

98. **Shi Y, Pan Y, Li B, He W, She Q, Chen L.** 2013. Molecular cloning of a novel bioH gene from an environmental metagenome encoding a carboxylesterase with exceptional tolerance to organic solvents. *BMC Biotechnol* **13:**1–11.

99. **Tomczyk N, Nettleship J, Baxter R, Crichton H, Webster S, Campopiano D.** 2002. Purification and characterization of the BIOH protein from the biotin biosynthetic pathway. *FEBS Lett* **513:**299–304.

100. **Min-A K, Kim H, Oh J, Song B, Song J.** 2009. Gene cloning, expression, and characterization of a new carboxylesterase from *Serratia* sp. SES-01: comparison with *Escherichia coli* BioHe enzyme. *J Microbiol Biotechnol* **19:**147–154.

101. **Cryle M, Schlichting I.** 2008. Structural insights from a P450 carrier protein complex reveal how specificity is achieved in the P450BioI ACP complex. *Proc Natl Acad Sci USA* **105:**15696–15701.

102. **Guy J, Whittle E, Moche M, Lengqvist J, Lindqvist Y, Shanklin J.** 2011. Remote control of regioselectivity in acyl-acyl carrier protein-desaturases. *Proc Natl Acad Sci USA* **108:** 16594–16599.

103. **Jiang L, Yu H.** 2014. An example of enzymatic promiscuity: the Baylis-Hillman reaction catalyzed by a biotin esterase (BioH) from *Escherichia coli. Biotechnol Lett* **36:**99–103.

104. **Feng Y, Napier B, Manandhar M, Henke S, Weiss D, Cronan J.** 2014. A *Francisella* virulence factor catalyses an essential reaction of biotin synthesis. *Mol Microbiol* **91:**300–314.

105. **Shapiro M, Chakravartty V, Cronan J.** 2012. Remarkable diversity in the enzymes catalyzing the last step in synthesis of the pimelate moiety of biotin. *PloS One* **7:**e49440. doi:10.1371/journal.pone.0049440.

106. **Camus J, Pryor M, Medigue C, Cole S.** 2002. Re-annotation of the genome sequence of *Mycobacterium tuberculosis* H37Rv. *Microbiology* **148:**2967–2973.

107. **Bhor V, Sagarika D, Vasanthakumar G, Kumar O, Sinha S, Surolia A.** 2006. Enzyme catalysis and regulation: broad substrate stereospecificity of the *Mycobacterium tuberculosis* 7-keto-8-aminopelargonic acid synthase: spectroscopic and kinetic studies. *J Biol Chem* **281:**25076–25088.

108. **Alexeev D, Alexeeva M, Baxter R, Campopiano D, Webster S, Sawyer L.** 1998. The crystal structure of 8-amino-7-oxononanoate synthase: a bacterial PLP-dependent, acyl-CoA-condensing enzyme. *J Mol Biol* **284:**401–419.

109. **Alexeev D, Baxter R, Campopiano D, Kerbarh O, Sawyer L, Tomczyk N, Watt R, Webster S.** 2006. Suicide inhibition of alpha-oxamine synthases: structures of the covalent adducts of 8-amino-7-oxononanoate synthase with trifluoroanaline. *Org Biomol Chem* **4:**1209–1212.

110. **Webster S, Alexeev D, Campopiano D, Watt R, Alexeeva M, Sawyer L, Baxter R.** 2000. Mechanism of 8-amino-7-oxononanoate synthase: spectroscopic, kinetic, and crystallographic studies. *Biochemistry* **39:**516–528.

111. **Mann S, Ploux O.** 2011. Pyridoxal-5′-phosphate-dependent enzymes involved in biotin biosynthesis: structure, reaction mechanism and inhibition. *Biochim Biophys Acta* **1814:**1459–1466.

112. **Kack H, Sandmark J, Gibson K, Schneider G, Lindqvist Y.** 1999. Crystal structure of diaminopelargonic acid synthase: evolutionary relationships between pyridoxal-5′-phosphate-dependent enzymes. *J Mol Biol* **291:**857–876.

113. **Eliot A, Sandmark J, Schneider G, Kirsch J.** 2002. The dual-specific active site of 7,8-diaminopelargonic acid synthase and the effect of the R391A mutation. *Biochemistry* **41:**12582–12589.

114. **Dai R, Wilson D, Geders T, Aldrich C, Finzel B.** 2014. Inhibition of *Mycobacterium tuberculosis* transaminase BioA by aryl hydrazines and hydrazides. *Chembiochem* **15:**575–586.

115. **Cobessi D, Dumas R, Pautre V, Meinguet C, Ferrer J, Alban C.** 2012. Biochemical and structural characterization of the *Arabidopsis* bifunctional enzyme dethiobiotin synthetase-diaminopelargonic acid aminotransferase: evidence for substrate channeling in biotin synthesis. *Plant Cell* **24:**1608–1625.

116. **Humble M, Cassimjee K, Hakansson M, Kimbung Y, Walse B, Abedi V, Federsel H, Berglund P, Logan D.** 2012. Crystal structures of the *Chromobacterium violaceum* ω-transaminase reveal major structural rearrangements upon binding of coenzyme PLP. *FEBS J* **279:**779–792.

117. **Shi C, Geders T, Park S, Wilson D, Boshoff H, Abayomi O, Barry C III, Schnappinger D, Finzel B, Aldrich C.** 2011. Mechanism-based inactivation by aromatization of the transaminase BioA involved in biotin biosynthesis in *Mycobacterium tuberculosis*. *J Am Chem Soc* **133:**18194–18201.

118. **Sandmark J, Eliot A, Famm K, Schneider G, Kirsch J.** 2004. Conserved and nonconserved residues in the substrate binding site of 7,8-diaminopelargonic acid synthase from *Escherichia coli* are essential for catalysis. *Biochemistry* **43:**1213–1222.

119. **Kack H, Gibson K, Lindqvist Y, Schneider G.** 1998. Snapshot of a phosphorylated substrate intermediate by kinetic crystallography. *Proc Natl Acad Sci USA* **95:**5495–5500.

120. **Huang W, Jia J, Gibson K, Taylor W, Rendina A, Schneider G, Lindqvist Y.** 1995. Mechanism of an ATP-dependent carboxylase, dethiobiotin synthetase, based on crystallographic studies of complexes with substrates and a reaction intermediate. *Biochemistry* **34:**10985–10995.

121. **Huang W, Lindqvist Y, Schneider G, Gibson K, Flint D, Lorimer G.** 1994. Crystal-structure of an ATP-dependent carboxylase, dethiobiotin synthetase, at 1.65-angstrom resolution. *Structure* **2:**407–414.

122. **Alexeev D, Baxter R, Sawyer L.** 1994. Mechanistic implications and family relationships from the structure of dethiobiotin synthetase. *Structure* **2:**1061–1072.

123. **Porebski P, Klimecka M, Chruszcz M, Nicholls R, Murzyn K, Cuff M, Xu X, Cymborowski M, Murshudov G, Savchenko A, Edwards A, Minor W.** 2012. Structural characterization of *Helicobacter pylori* dethiobiotin synthetase reveals differences between family members. *FEBS J* **279:**1093–1105.

124. **Sandalova T, Schneider G, Kack H, Lindqvist Y.** 1999. Structure of dethiobiotin synthetase at 0.97 Å resolution. *Acta Crystallograph* **D55:**610–624.

125. **Salaemae W, Yap M, Wegener K, Booker GW, Wilce M, Polyak S.** 2015. Nucleotide triphosphate promiscuity in *Mycobacterium tuberculosis* dethiobiotin synthetase. *Tuberculosis* **95:**259–266.

126. **Yang G, Sandalova T, Lohman K, Lindqvist Y, Rendina A.** 1997. Active site mutants of *Escherichia coli* dethiobiotin synthetase: effects of mutations on enzyme catalytic and structural properties. *Biochemistry* **36:**4751–4760.

127. **Ugulava N, Frederick K, Jarrett J.** 2003. Control of adenosylmethionine-dependent radical generation in biotin synthase: a kinetic and thermodynamic analysis of substrate binding to active and inactive forms of BioB. *Biochemistry* **42:**2708–2719.

128. **Frey P, Hegeman A, Reed G.** 2006. Free radical mechanisms in enzymology. *Chem Rev* **106:** 3302–3316.

129. **Duschene K, Veneziano S, Silver S, Broderick J.** 2009. Control of radical chemistry in the AdoMet radical enzymes. *Curr Opin Chem Biol* **13:**74–83.

130. **Cosper M, Jameson G, Hernandez H, Krebs C, Huynh B, Johnson M.** 2004. Characterization of the cofactor composition of *Escherichia coli* biotin synthase. *Biochemistry* **43:**2007–2021.

131. **Booker S, Cicchillo R, Grove T.** 2007. Self-sacrifice in radical S-adenosylmethionine proteins. *Curr Opin Chem Biol* **11:**543–552.

132. **Tse Sum Bui B, Lotierzo M, Escalettes F, Florentin D, Marquet A.** 2004. Further investigation on the turnover of *Escherichia coli* biotin synthase with dethiobiotin and 9-mercaptodethiobiotin as substrates. *Biochemistry* **43:**16432–16441.

133. **Muhlenhoff U, Gerl M, Flauger B, Pirner H, Balser S, Richhardt N, Lill R, Stolz J.** 2007. The iron-sulfur cluster proteins Isa1 and Isa2 are required for the function but not for the de novo synthesis of the Fe/S clusters of biotin synthase in *Saccharomyces cerevisiae*. *Eukaryotic Cell* **6:**495–504.

134. **Choi-Rhee E, Cronan J.** 2005. Biotin synthase is catalytic *in vivo*, but catalysis engenders destruction of the protein. *Chem Biol* **12:**461–468.

135. **Choudens S, Sanakis Y, Hewitson K, Roach P, Munck E, Fontecave M.** 2002. Reductive cleavage of S-adenosylmethionine by biotin synthase from *Escherichia coli*. *J Biol Chem* **277:**13449–13454.

136. **Hewitson K, Choudens S, Sanakis Y, Shaw N, Baldwin J, Munck E, Roach P, Fontecave M.** 2002. The iron-sulfur center of biotin synthase: site-directed mutants. *J Biol Inorg Chem* **7:**83–93.

137. **Broach R, Jarrett J.** 2006. Role of the [2Fe-2S]2+ cluster in biotin synthase: mutagenesis of the atypical metal ligand arginine 260. *Biochemistry* **45:**14166–14174.

138. **Borchardt R, Eiden L, Wu B, Rutledge C.** 1979. Sinefungin, a potent inhibitor or S-adenosylmethionine. Protein O-methyltransferase. *Biochem Biophys Res Commun* **89:**919–924.

139. **Mann S, Carillon S, Breyne O, Marquet A.** 2002. Total synthesis of amiclenomycin, an inhibitor of biotin biosynthesis. *Chem Eur J* **8:**439–450.

140. **Mann S, Carillon S, Breyne O, Duhayon C, Hamon L, Marquet A.** 2002. Synthesis and stereochemical assignments of cis- and trans-1-amino-4-ethylcyclohexa-2,5-diene as models for amiclenomycin. *Eur J Org Chem* **2002:**736–744.

141. **Mann S, Florentin D, Lesage D, Drujon T, Ploux O, Marquet A.** 2003. Inhibition of diamino pelargonic acid aminotransferase, an enzyme of the biotin biosynthetic pathway, by amiclenomycin: a mechanistic study. *Helvetica Chimica Acta* **86:**3836–3850.

142. **Mann S, Ploux O.** 2006. 7,8-Diaminopelargonic acid aminotransferase from *Mycobacterium tuberculosis*, a potential therapeutic target. Characterization and inhibition studies. *FEBS J* **273:**4778–4789.

143. **Mann S, Colliandre L, Labesse G, Ploux O.** 2009. Inhibition of 7,8-diaminopelargonic acid aminotransferase from *Mycobacterium tuberculosis* by chiral and achiral analogs of its substrate: biological implications. *Biochimie* **91:**826–834.

144. **Rendina A, Taylor W, Gibson K, Lorimer G, Rayner D, Lockett B, Kranis K, Wexler B, Marcovici-Mizrahi D, Nudelman A, Nudelman A, Marsilii E, Chi H, Wawrzak Z, Calabrese J, Huang W, Jia J, Schneider G, Lindqvist Y, Yang G.** 1999. The design and synthesis of inhibitors of dethiobiotin synthetase as potential herbicides. *Pesticide Sci* **55:**236–247.

145. **Alexeev D, Baxter R, Campopiano D, McAlpine R, McIver L, Sawyer L.** 1998. Rational design of an inhibitor of dethiobiotin synthetase: interaction of 6-hydroxypyrimidin-4 (3H)-one with the adenine base binding site. *Tetrahedron* **54:**15891–15898.

146. **Eisenberg M, Hsiung S.** 1982. Mode of action of the biotin antimetabolites actithiazic acid and alpha-methyldethiobiotin. *Antimicrob Agents Chemother* **21:**5–10.

147. **Schenck J, De Rose S.** 1952. Actithiazic acid. II. Isolation and characterization. *Biochem Biophys* **40:**263–269.

148. **Dhyse F, Hertz R.** 1958. The effects of actithiazic acid on egg white-induced biotin deficiency and upon the microbial formation of biotin vitamers in the rat. *Arch Biochem Biophys* **74:**7–16.

149. **Kwang K.** 1952. Actithiazic acid. IV. Pharmacological studies. *Antibiot Chemother* **9:**453–459.

150. **Hanka L, Martin D, Reineke L.** 1972. Two new antimetabolites of biotin: α-methyldethiobiotin and α-methylbiotin. *Antimicro Agents Chemother* **1:**135–138.

151. **Martin D, Hanka L, Reineke L.** 1971. New antimetabolite antibiotics related to biotin: α-

methyldethiobiotin and α-methylbiotin. *Tetrahedron Lett* **41**:3791–3794.

152. **Payne D, Gwynn M, Holmes D, Pompliano D.** 2007. Drugs for bad bugs: confronting the challenges of antibacterial discovery. *Nat Rev Drug Discov* **6**:29–40.

153. **Barry C, Boshoff H, Dartois V, Dick T, Ehrt S, Flynn J, Schnappinger D, Wilkinson R, Young D.** 2009. The spectrum of latent tuberculosis: rethinking the biology and intervention strategies. *Nat Rev Microbiol* **7**:845–855.

154. **Silver LL.** 2011. Challenges of antibacterial discovery. *Clin Microbiol Rev* **24**:71–109.

155. **Ling LL, Schneider T, Peoples AJ, Spoering AL, Engels I, Conlon BP, Mueller A, Schaberle TF, Hughes DE, Epstein S, Jones M, Lazarides L, Steadman VA, Cohen DR, Felix CR, Fetterman KA, Millett WP, Nitti AG, Zullo AM, Chen C, Lewis K.** 2015. A new antibiotic kills pathogens without detectable resistance. *Nature* **517**:455–459.

156. **Congreve M, Chessari G, Tisi D, Woodhead A.** 2008. Recent developments in fragment-based drug discovery. *J Med Chem* **51**:3661–3680.

157. **Erlanson D, McDowell R, O'Brien T.** 2004. Fragment-based drug discovery. *J Med Chem* **47**:3463–3482.

158. **Rees D, Congreve M, Murray C, Carr R.** 2004. Fragment-based lead discovery. *Nat Rev Drug Discov* **3**:660–672.

159. **Hajduk P, Greer J.** 2007. A decade of fragment-based drug design: strategic advances and lessons learned. *Nat Rev Drug Discov* **6**:211–219.

160. **Kumar A, Voet A, Zhang K.** 2012. Fragment based drug design: from experimental to computational approaches. *Curr Med Chem* **19**:5128–5147.

161. **Hughes T, Baldwin I, Churcher I.** 2011. Fragment-based drug discovery—from hit discovery to FDA approval: lessons learned and future challenge. *Internatl Drug Discov* **6**(5):34.

162. **US Food and Drug Administration.** 2011. *FY 2011 innovative drug approvals*, p 1–28. http://www.fda.gov/AboutFDA/ReportsManualsForms/Reports/ucm330502.htm.

163. **Congreve M, Robin C, Murray C, Jhoti H.** 2003. A 'rule of three' for fragment-based lead discovery? *Drug Discov Today* **8**:876–877.

164. **Chessari G, Woodhead A.** 2009. From fragment to clinical candidate: a historical perspective. *Drug Discov Today* **14**:668–675.

165. **Hopkins A, Groom C.** 2004. Ligand efficiency: a useful metric for drug selection. *Drug Discov Today* **9**:430–431.

166. **Fattori D, Squarcia A, Bartoli S.** 2008. Fragment-based approach to drug lead discovery: overview and advances in various techniques. *Drugs R D* **9**:217–227.

167. **Joseph-McCarthy D, Campbell A, Kern G, Moustakas D.** 2014. Fragment-based lead discovery and design. *J Chem Inf Model* **54**:693–704.

168. **Hann M, Leach A, Harper G.** 2001. Molecular complexity and its impact on the probability of finding leads for drug discovery. *J Chem Inf Comput Sci* **41**:856–864.

169. **Mochalkin I, Miller J, Narasimhan L, Thanabal V, Erdman P, Cox P, Prasad J, Lightle S, Huband M, Stover C.** 2009. Discovery of antibacterial biotin carboxylase inhibitors by virtual screening and fragment-based approaches. *ACS Chem Biol* **4**:473–483.

170. **Hopkins A, Keseru G, Leeson P, Rees D, Reynolds C.** 2014. The role of ligand efficiency metric in drug discovery. *Nat Rev Drug Discov* **13**:105–121.

171. **Fink T, Reymond J.** 2007. Virtual exploration of the chemical universe up to 11 atoms of C, N, O, F: assembly of 26.4 million structures (110.9 million stereoisomers) and analysis for new ring systems, stereochemistry, physicochemical properties, compound classes, and drug discovery. *J Chem Inf Model.* **47**:342–353.

172. **Blum L, Reymond J.** 2009. 970 million druglike small molecules for virtual screening in the chemical universe database GDB-13. *J Am Chem Soc* **131**:8732–8733.

173. **Gopal P, Dick T.** 2014. Reactive dirty fragments: implications for tuberculosis drug discovery. *Curr Opin Microbiol* **21**:7–12.

Recent Advances and Understanding of Using Probiotic-Based Interventions to Restore Homeostasis of the Microbiome for the Prevention/Therapy of Bacterial Diseases

29

JAN S. SUCHODOLSKI[1] and ALBERT E. JERGENS[2]

THE GASTROINTESTINAL MICROBIOME

The mammalian gastrointestinal (GI) tract is comprised of several hundred species of microorganisms including bacteria, archaea, fungi, bacteriophages, eukaryotic viruses, and protozoa. This complex and eclectic ecosystem is collectively known as the gut microbiota. Bacteria are by far the most abundant constituent of the microbiota; studies using DNA shotgun sequencing analysis have estimated that bacteria make up approximately 98% of all metagenomic sequences in fecal samples of various mammals (1, 2). The GI microbiota is acquired rapidly after birth and undergoes substantial compositional changes (from a more aerobic to a predominantly anaerobic flora) in the first 1 to 2 years of life before reaching a stable and symbiotic relationship with the host (3). It then remains dynamic but relatively stable throughout adulthood unless perturbed.

Microbes are much more abundant in number than cells of the host. It has been estimated that the number of bacterial cells is approximately 10 times as

[1]Gastrointestinal Laboratory, Department of Small Animal Clinical Sciences, College of Veterinary Medicine and Biomedical Sciences, Texas A&M University, College Station, TX 77845; [2]Department of Veterinary Clinical Sciences, College of Veterinary Medicine, Iowa State University, Ames, IA 50010.

Virulence Mechanisms of Bacterial Pathogens, 5th edition
Edited by Indira T. Kudva, Nancy A. Cornick, Paul J. Plummer, Qijing Zhang, Tracy L. Nicholson, John P. Bannantine, and Bryan H. Bellaire
© 2016 American Society for Microbiology, Washington, DC
doi:10.1128/microbiolspec.VMBF-0025-2015

many as host cells. This also has an influence on the metagenome of the host, because there are approximately 1,000-fold more microbial genes than human genes in any individual. This combination of host and microbial genes is referred to as the microbiome. This concept of the microbiome was first suggested by Joshua Lederberg, to "signify the ecological community of commensal, symbiotic and pathogenic microorganisms that literally share our body space" (4).

Because of the close proximity of the microbiome to the host, gut microbes are considered primarily beneficial for the health status of the host. The microbiome plays a crucial role in the development of intestinal immune responses, provides metabolites for host physiology, maintains intestinal gut barrier function, regulates intestinal motility, and protects against pathogenic bacteria (5).

In recent years, microbiome research has initially focused on characterizing bacterial inhabitants at different body sites in humans and animals. Considerable progress has been made in defining and understanding microbial communities due to advances in and decreased costs of large-scale genomic sequencing techniques, which are summarized in various NIH publications supported by the Human Microbiome Project (6). The newest area of microbiome research focuses on understanding the functional properties of the microbial-host gene interactions. This can be achieved either through the use of metagenomics (shotgun sequencing of fecal DNA or RNA) or through targeted/untargeted metabolomics (7–9). Also, the newest computational methods allow prediction of the functional properties of the microbiome from existing 16S rRNA gene sequencing data, thus avoiding a costly full metagenomic sequencing approach (10).

An understanding of changes in the composition and function of the microbiome, and it's deficiencies in disease, will allow the selection of novel therapeutic targets for probiotics and the potential novel therapeutic concept of postbiotics (i.e., bacterial metabolites).

Composition of Microbiota in Health and Disease

Various studies have described the composition of the intestinal microbiota in humans and different animal species. There is a remarkable similarity in gut microbiota, at least on higher phylogenetic levels, between humans and other mammals, especially monogastric animals. The most abundant cultivable groups are *Bacteroides*, *Clostridium*, *Lactobacillus*, *Bifidobacterium*, and *Enterobacteriaceae* spp. There is a clear gradient along the length of the GI tract, with an increase in total bacterial numbers as well as the number of bacterial species from the less populated and less diverse small intestinal microbiota to the highly populated colonic microbiota. Furthermore, the proximal intestine harbors more aerobes and facultative anaerobes, while the colon is occupied mostly by facultative and strict anaerobes. For example, *Proteobacteria*, including *Enterobacteriaceae*, make up ≥30% of bacteria in the small intestine but <1% in feces. There are also clear differences between the luminal and the mucosa-adherent microbiota. Early studies used bacterial culture to characterize the predominant bacterial groups in the GI tract. The most abundant cultivable groups were *Bacteroides*, *Clostridium*, *Lactobacillus*, *Bifidobacterium* spp., and *Enterobacteriaceae*. Because of this observation, much of the focus in probiotic research was placed on the investigation of lactic acid bacteria, such as *Lactobacillus*, *Bifidobacterium*, and *Streptococcus* spp., because they were believed to be the most abundant bacterial groups in the GI tract of mammals. However, with the advent of molecular-based techniques aimed at sequencing the 16S rRNA gene, a much more diverse gut microbiota has been identified, with other noncultivable bacterial groups recognized as having significant abundance within the GI tract.

The GI microbiota is dominated by members of the bacterial phyla *Bacteroidetes* and *Firmicutes*, with other members including the *Proteobacteria, Actinobacteria* (containing *Bifidobacterium* spp.), and *Fusobacteria.* The phyla *Spirochaetes, Tenericutes, Verrucomicrobia, Cyanobacteria,* and *Chloroflexi* are minor contributors to the overall microbiota. The *Firmicutes* are a diverse bacterial phylum consisting of *Clostridiales* and *Lactobacillales.* A major contributor to the makeup of the intestinal microbiota is the phylum *Firmicutes,* especially members of the *Clostridiales.* This order is comprised of many bacterial species, organized into different *Clostridium* clusters. Of those, *Clostridium* clusters XI, XIVa, and IV are the most abundant. All bacterial groups within the *Clostridium* clusters and *Bacteroidetes* are believed to be major contributors in the production of short chain fatty acids (SCFA) and other bacterial metabolites. The *Bifidobacterium* spp. are a minor part of the normal intestinal microbiota.

One important finding of microbiome research is the large variability in the microbiota composition between healthy individuals. Only an estimated 10% of phylotypes are shared between individuals. Initial studies in humans have suggested the presence of three distinct enterotypes (11); however, the presence of so-called enterogradients is now a more contemporary concept, because it has been shown that it is not possible to group each individual into categories with predominance of only a few genera (12). This observation, that there are various differences in the microbiome of individuals, is important, because it might explain the different interindividual responses to probiotic and prebiotic interventions. Interestingly, despite the huge variation in microbial communities between individuals, the metagenomes and the potential metabolic and functional properties that are encoded through the bacterial metagenomes are quite conserved across individuals. That is, although microbial taxonomic composition varied among healthy individuals, their collective metabolic functions remained remarkably stable within each body site (13).

Intestinal Microbiota in GI Disease

The close proximity between the intestinal microbiota and the host epithelial cells significantly impacts GI health, and an improper balance in the microbiota may contribute to acute or chronic disease. One way for enteric disease to develop is through transient colonization with a bacterial enteropathogen. Infections with specific pathogens (e.g., *Salmonella,* toxigenic *Clostridium difficile,* enterotoxigenic *Clostridium perfringens,* and *Campylobacter jejuni*) may profoundly perturb the GI epithelial barrier. Enteric pathogens can also produce neurotoxins, exotoxins, or enterotoxins that alter GI epithelial function. For example, bacterial toxins can stimulate mucosal fluid secretions, while villus effacement and loss of surface area will diminish mucosal absorptive capacity, resulting in diarrhea and changes in the community structure of the microbiota (14). Changes in the balance of the microbiota can also be impacted by various extrinsic factors (i.e., sudden dietary changes/dietary indiscretion, changes in the architecture of the intestine with subsequent changes in intestinal motility). These circumstances can lead to loss of normal protective microbiota and concurrent overgrowth by opportunistic resident bacterial groups. Such compositional changes in the microbiota negatively impact the proper function of the GI tract by compromising the intestinal barrier via damage to the intestinal brush border and enterocytes causing nutrient and vitamin malabsorption. An overgrowth in specific bacterial groups may also lead to increased competition for nutrients and vitamins along with deleterious changes in concentrations of various bacterial metabolites (e.g., SCFA concentrations, changes in ratios of primary and secondary bile acid concentrations) (15).

There is strong evidence that the resident intestinal microbiota is involved in the pathogenesis of inflammatory bowel diseases (IBDs) in humans and animal species (i.e., dogs and cats) (16–18). The current hypothesis about IBD involves interplay between the intestinal microbiome and the immune system in genetically susceptible individuals (19). Genome-wide association studies in humans with Crohn's disease have revealed at least 33 susceptibility genes, with many of these genes associated with defects in innate immunity (e.g., NOD2/CARD15) (20). Therefore, some Crohn's disease patients are unable to effectively clear intracellular commensal or pathogenic bacteria, resulting in robust host immune responses causing excessive epithelial tissue damage. These changes in microbial composition primarily involve a reduction in *Clostridium* clusters XIVa and IV (i.e., *Faecalibacterium, Lachnospiraceae,* and *Clostridiumcoccoides*), with concurrent increases in *Proteobacteria* (*Enterobacteriaceae,* including *Escherichia coli*). Interestingly, many similarities in the dysbiosis of IBD are evident across both humans and companion animals, suggesting that these microbial changes are conserved across animal species (18). The commonly depleted groups in GI disease (i.e., *Firmicutes, Bacteroidetes*) are important producers of SCFA and other beneficial metabolites which help to maintain gut mucosal homeostasis. Depletion of these bacterial groups has been associated with reduced SCFA concentrations (e.g., butyrate, acetate), which exacerbate intestinal inflammation. One important bacterial species is *Faecalibacterium prausnitzii*, which is commonly depleted in humans with IBD. This bacterium has been shown to secrete anti-inflammatory metabolites that downregulate interleukin-12 (IL–12) and interferon-γ but upregulate IL-10 secretions which collectively act to reduce the severity of gut inflammation.

Importance of a Balanced Microbiome for Intestinal Homeostasis

Due to the observed alterations in microbial communities (i.e., dysbiosis) between healthy and diseased individuals, there is increased interest in designing therapeutic approaches aimed at modifying these microbial communities either to induce a beneficial (e.g., anti-inflammatory) effect or to help rebalance the microbiome. The microbiome metabolizes many ingested nutrients but also acts on drugs and other xenobiotics, which are subsequently absorbed by the host. It is now evident that a balanced intestinal microbiota is crucial to the maintenance of intestinal homeostasis and that dysbiosis may alter the physiologic bacterial and/or host metabolic pathways. While the initial focus on probiotic effects was on describing phylogenetic changes within the microbiome (21, 22), more recent studies aim to characterize the functional alterations associated with dysbiosis (23). The use of metagenomics DNA shotgun sequencing performed on feces as well as untargeted metabolomics using mass spectrometry platforms allows the assessment of changes in microbiome gene content and bacterial metabolite profiles which may contribute to the pathophysiology of GI disease. These studies will allow greater understanding of the functional deficiencies in the gut microbiota and help guide selection of the optimal probiotic bacterial species to beneficially modulate the gut microbiome.

A balance in the microbial ecosystem is of benefit to the host through diverse mechanisms, as elegantly demonstrated through work in germ-free mouse models. These animals have altered epithelial architecture (i.e., decreased number of Peyer's patches and lymphoid follicles) and a decreased turnover of epithelial cells compared to conventionally reared mice (24, 25). Exposure to microbes early in life establishes oral tolerance to commensal bacteria and food antigens (26). The resident intestinal microbiota provides "colonization resistance" and therefore protection for the host from invasion by transient enteropathogens. This resistance can be facilitated through competition for nutritional substrates, epithelial adhesion sites, production of antibacterial metabolites (e.g., bacteriocins), and changes in luminal pH. Other important functions of intestinal bacteria are the production of immunomodulatory metabolites such as indole and SCFA, including butyrate, propionate, and acetate) (27). These metabolites are important for epithelial cell proliferation, provide an energy source for the host, and modulate gut inflammation.

PROBIOTICS

Because of the recent advances in understanding the importance of the intestinal microbiome for health and disease, there is renewed interest in modulation of the intestinal microbiome through the use of probiotics, prebiotics, or a combination of them (synbiotics). Probiotics offer a promising approach in the therapy of specific bacterial infections, but also for dysbiosis as it occurs in IBD. Furthermore, it has been shown that administration of antibiotics leads to major perturbations in the intestinal microbiota, independent of the presence of antibiotic-associated diarrhea (28–30). Finally, the potentially deleterious effects of nonsteroidal anti-inflammatory drug–associated enteropathies are now recognized as being microbiome driven (31). Therefore, correction of dysbiosis to prevent antibiotic- or nonsteroidal anti-inflammatory drug–associated diarrhea seems a reasonable therapeutic goal for the use of probiotics.

Probiotics are used clinically in human and veterinary patients to treat certain diseases, but they are also used in livestock and poultry to augment health and growth. Probiotics are defined by the Food and Agriculture Organization of the United Nations and the World Health Organization as "live microorganisms which when administered in adequate amounts confer a health benefit on the host." In contrast, prebiotics are not live bacteria, but rather are nondigestible food ingredients that are added to diets to stimulate the growth/activity of resident beneficial microorganisms within the gut. Prebiotics are fermentable carbohydrates such as inulin, fructooligosaccharides, mannanoligosaccharides, xylooligosaccharides, polydextrose, and galactooligosaccha-

rides. The theoretical advantage of prebiotics over probiotics is that they promote the growth of the already present beneficial bacteria in the gut. However, some of the resident bacteria that utilize prebiotics might not have the therapeutic efficacy of exogenous probiotics. Synbiotics are often sold as commercial products, and they are a combination of probiotics and prebiotics. They are often administered together to provide a growth substrate for the administered probiotic.

Probiotics, also known as direct-fed microbials, are often derived from the normal gut microbiota and are widely used as dietary supplements, food ingredients, or medical food. In the United States, probiotics are typically marketed as dietary supplements or as food additives. Probiotics labelled as medical foods are defined by the FDA as "a food which is formulated to be consumed or administered enterally under the supervision of a physician, and which is intended for the specific dietary management of a disease or condition for which distinctive nutritional requirements, based on recognized scientific principles, are established by medical evaluation" (32). For probiotics sold as dietary supplements or food additives, their product labels are not scrutinized by the FDA and approval is not needed for their use. Commercial marketing for these products can only claim that the probiotic affects the structure or function of the host. Even if clinical data is available for some probiotic strains demonstrating efficacy in treatment or prevention of a specific disease, this claim can only be made when the product is licensed as a drug by the FDA. To the authors' knowledge, no probiotic product currently available in the United States is labelled as a drug. Hence, many claims for the beneficial effects of probiotics are anecdotal, both in humans and in animals.

Mechanisms of Action of Probiotics

There is ample evidence that probiotics can be useful in certain diseases. Yet the exact mechanisms by which they affect the host gut are still poorly understood, at both a molecular and metabolic level. The microorganisms found most frequently in probiotics are lactic acid bacteria (i.e., *Lactobacillus*, *Enterococcus*, *Streptococcus*, and *Bifidobacterium* spp.), although these products feature a range of other bacteria and yeasts (e.g., *E. coli* strain Nissle 1917, *Bacillus coagulans*, *Saccharomyces boulardii*). Every bacterial strain, even if it is derived from the same bacterial species, can differ significantly in its phenotypic, functional, and immunological properties. This is one reason why clinical reports can sometimes be confusing, because one study may report that a specific bacterial species caused clinical disease, while a separate study suggests that this bacterial species may have beneficial properties. Therefore, the reader should be aware of the strain designations reported in those studies. Probiotic strains are named by genus and species using standard microbial taxonomy with an alpha numeric designation (e.g., ATCC strain designation) to define the probiotic at the strain level. Ideally, every strain should be examined for its specific mechanism of action and chosen for a specific clinical application, and the clinical efficacy should be verified in a proper clinical trial (33). Various probiotic products are designed as a mixture of different strains, with the goal being to provide complementary functions within a single product. An example of a well-studied mixture of probiotic strains is the commercially available product VSL#3, which has been studied in clinical trials investigating maintenance of remission for pouchitis and ulcerative colitis in human as well as in canine IBD (34–36).

Probiotic strains can exert a beneficial effect on the host that is highly strain specific (Fig. 1). For example, some probiotic strains have a high affinity to adhere to the intestinal epithelium and are able to displace commensal bacteria (such as *Bacteroides*, *Clostridium*, *Staphylococcus*, and *Enterobacter*) by inhibiting their adherence and growth on the mucosa (37). These same strains differed in their ability to displace and inhibit already adherent bacterial pathogens, emphasizing the strain-specific properties of probiotics (37). Furthermore, the combination of two probiotic strains (i.e., *Bifidobacterium lactis* Bb12 and *Lactobacillus rhamnosus* LGG) had greater synergistic ability to inhibit pathogen

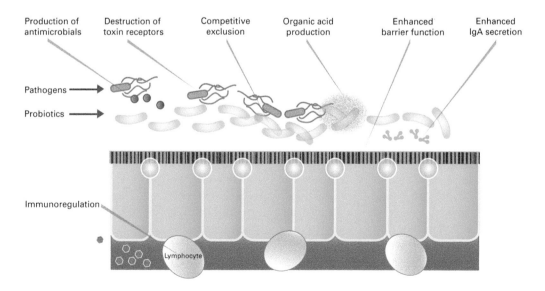

FIGURE 1 **Potential mechanisms for probiotic activity.**

adherence than when strains were administered individually (38). Similarly, while several *Lactobacillus* spp. can inhibit pathogenic strains of *E. coli* and *Salmonella*, the displacement abilities of the probiotic strains differ substantially from each other (39).

Another important probiotic mechanism is the production of immunomodulatory metabolites. This can happen through the formation of biofilms that suppress tumor-necrosis factor alpha (TNF-α) production and that also confer effects on the host to secrete beneficial metabolites such as reuterin (40) or mucosal alkaline sphingomyelinase (35). Some probiotic bacteria can also produce various antimicrobial substances (e.g., butyrate, lactate, and acetate). These fatty acids have immunomodulatory effects and can potentially serve as so-called postbiotics (i.e., bacterial metabolites), because their sole administration has been shown to protect the host from enterohemorrhagic *E. coli* O157:H7 (41). In this instance, the administration of live acetate producing *Bifidobacterium* strains or acetate devoid of bacteria produced protective effects (41). Similarly, indole, the metabolic product of microbial-driven tryptophan degradation, has been shown to be a highly abundant bacterial metabolite in the intestinal lumen. Indole is considered an immunomodulatory metabolite, because *in vitro* studies have shown that indole decreased TNF-α-mediated activation of NF-κB, expression of proinflammatory chemokine IL-8, and the attachment of pathogenic *E. coli* to HCT-8 cells, while it upregulated anti-inflammatory cytokine IL-10 expression (27). Similarly, microbiome exploration using metagenomic sequencing has revealed new bacterial strains as potential probiotics, such as *F. prausnitzii*. This bacterial species has been shown to be an important bacterium that downregulates inflammation through its SCFA production. *F. prausnitzii* is commonly depleted in chronic GI inflammation, and both *in vitro* and *in vivo* studies have demonstrated that the oral administration of live *F. prausnitzii* or its supernatant reduced

the severity of TNBS-induced colitis in mice (17). Also, some probiotic strains within the genus *Lactobacillus* (e.g., *Lactobacillus reuteri* ATCC PTA 6475) inhibit lipopolysaccharide-induced TNFα production, which contributes to mucosal inflammation (42).

While intact, viable bacteria may be responsible for the probiotic effect in some instances, their immunomodulatory effects may also be mediated through their bacterial DNA alone (43). Pure DNA, especially bacterial CpG motifs, from probiotic bacteria as well as fecal DNA obtained after probiotic administration with VSL#3 strains have been shown to modulate the immune response in peripheral blood mononuclear cell (PBMC) cells through inhibition of IL-1β and increased IL-10 (43).

Another mechanism of some probiotic strains is to improve gut barrier function. Probiotic VSL#3 and *Lactobacillus paracasei* B21060 were shown to induce tight junction protein occludin expression, thereby increasing the stability of tight junction protein and intestinal barrier function in animal models of IBD (34, 44, 45).

Another important mechanism of some probiotic strains is their activity against virulence factors of enteropathogens. Bioactive molecules of *Bifidobacterium bifidum* inhibit the expression of virulence genes needed for attachment of *Salmonella enterica* serovar Typhimurium and enterohemorrhagic *E. coli* to a HeLa cell line (46). Molecules secreted by *Lactobacillus acidophilus* La-5 can inhibit the transcription of *E. coli* O157:H7 (EHEC O157) genes that are important for attachment to intestinal epithelial cells. The mechanisms involve either inhibition of quorum sensing or the direct interaction with bacterial transcriptional regulators (47). *Lactobacillus fermentum* strain 104R was shown to silence the beta2-toxin production by *C. perfringens*, most likely due to a decrease in intestinal pH (48). Finally, the nonpathogenic yeast *S. boulardii* produces a 54-kDa protease, which digests the *C. difficile* toxin A molecule and its brush border membrane receptor, causing proteolytic digestion of *C. difficile* toxin B (49).

Probiotic-Host Interactions

The most common site for interactions between probiotics and host cells occurs in the intestinal epithelia and dendritic cells. This requires specific interactions between ligands from probiotic cells and the host receptors termed pattern recognition receptors (PRRs). These PRRs are then the ligands for the microorganism-associated molecular patterns (MAMPs) found on the bacteria. The most common location of MAMPs is on the surface of the probiotic bacteria, but some MAMPS are secreted into the gut lumen. It is important to emphasize that MAMPs are not a particular characteristic of probiotic strains but rather can be expressed by any bacterial species including enteropathogens. Some examples of MAMPs include flagella, fimbriae, secreted protein p40, surface-layer protein A, cell wall-associated polysaccharides, lipoteichoic acid, lipopolysaccharide, and peptidoglycans. The most studied PRRs in mammals are the Toll-like receptors (TLRs). Bacteria may interact with 5 of the 11 characterized TLRs, namely TLR1, TLR2, TLR4, TLR5, and TLR9 (50). How host cells are able to distinguish between ligands from probiotic species and ligands from pathogens is not well understood. Most likely, the cellular localization of the MAMP is one of the most important factors determining the nature of the host-probiotic interaction. After MAMPs are activated, the PRRs induce intracellular signaling through NF-κB and mitogen-activated protein kinase pathways to evoke a specific response. This process then turns on transcription of various genes, for example, those involved in host defense such as defensins (51), proinflammatory cytokines such asIL-8 (52), and TNF-α (53). Other mechanisms induced through these pathways are mucus secretion (54) and the inhibition of cytokine-induced apoptosis (55). Another important family of pattern recognition receptors is the intracellular (cytosolic) nucleotide-binding oligomerization domain (NOD) family of proteins, NOD-1 and NOD-2. Activation of NODs by bacterial peptidoglycans initiates signaling pathways similar to TLRs. As mentioned previously, the interactions between host and bacterial components is mediated similarly by both pathogenic and probiotic bacteria. The defined immune response to these interactions is influenced by both host and probiotic factors, and the mechanisms are still unclear.

Host Responses from Probiotic Administration

To better understand the probiotic responses within a host, several studies have employed transcriptomics to characterize host gene expression using microarray technology, RNA-seq, or reverse transcription polymerase chain reaction (RT-PCR). These studies have shown different responses to probiotic exposure. This is not surprising, given that probiotic strains have unique properties and different strains may up- or downregulate various host genes which control RNA transcription/processing, protein synthesis/transport, metabolism, cell proliferation, cell adhesion, and protein degradation via ubiquitination. While detailed transcriptomic studies have been carried out in humans, mice, and some production animals (e.g., poultry), it is likely that some of the observed transcriptomic changes are similar across various host species. For example, the probiotic strains *Lactobacillus casei* strain Shirota or *Bifidobacterium breve* strain Yakult were administered as single strains to gnotobiotic BALB/c mice, and gene expression of ileal and colonic epithelia was evaluated (56). Probiotic differences in host gene expression were observed and were tissue specific, with *L. casei* Shirota upregulating more genes in the small intestine compared to the *B. breve* Yakult strain. However, both probiotic species attenuated a similar number of genes. Upregulated genes included those involved in pathogen defense mechanisms, growth and development, metabolism, and transport. In the large intestine, more genes were modulated by *B. breve* Yakult than by *L. casei* Shirota. The upregulated genes included those that modulate cell-to-cell contact, cellular growth and cellular development, and general metabolism. Still other studies have explored host transcriptomics and shown that host gene expression is influenced by both the bacterial strain and the bacterial component itself. In one study, transcriptomic analysis of lymphocytes harvested from chicken cecal tonsils treated either with the peptidoglycan-enriched cell envelope extract, bacterial DNA, or cell envelope fractions of *L. acidophilus* revealed treatment-specific upregulation of different numbers of genes (57). Bacterial DNA was the most robust stimulus, which enhanced expression of immune system genes including β2-microglobulin, major histocompatibility complex class I heavy chain, caspase 3, CD25, CD44, CD45, c-myc, IL-2 alpha receptor (CD25), invariant chain, STAT2, and STAT4 (57).

While many studies have evaluated single-strain probiotic-host interactions, there is increased interest in evaluating multiple probiotic strains. Results of transcriptomic studies involving multiple probiotic strains indicate that a combination of bacteria alters host gene expression, which differs from expression induced by a single bacterial species. This suggests that for clinical trials, probiotic mixtures need to be evaluated rather than individual probiotic components. For example, treatment of Caco-2 cells with the probiotic *E. coli* strain 6-1, upregulated 155 genes and downregulated 177 genes (58). When the same cells were incubated with *Lactobacillus plantarum*, only 45 genes and 36 genes were upregulated and downregulated, respectively. However, when the cells were incubated with both *E. coli* strain 6-1 and *L. plantarum* together, different sets of genes were modulated (58). In another study, the cocolonization of *Bacteroides thetaiotaomicron* and *Bifidobacterium longum*

induced higher expression of interferon-γ-responsive genes. The set of modulated genes depended on the cocolonization with both strains since mono-association with *B. thetaiotaomicron* alone produced low levels of gene expression (59), which were also influenced by murine genetic background (59).

The Probiotic Side of Probiotic-Host Interactions

Recent studies indicate that there are differences in gene expression profiles of probiotic strains when compared *in vitro* versus *in vivo*. This suggests that host factors influence gene modulation of probiotic bacteria. This is not surprising since genes induced *in vivo* during colonization are responsible for probiotic survival, adaptation, and growth in the intestinal ecosystem. This microecology also includes host cells and other intestinal resident bacteria. Subsequently, many of these genes are also upregulated in enteropathogens, suggesting the presence of shared survival mechanisms between beneficial and deleterious bacteria. In one study, specific genes responsible for nutrient acquisition and stress responses were highly expressed when mice were colonized with *L. reuteri* 100-23 (60). Another study showed upregulation of genes involving sugar transport, acquisition and biosynthesis of non-sugar compounds, and stress within the genome of *L. plantarum* WCFS1 after a probiotic strain was added to a mouse gut (61). A separate study has shown that the number of bacterial genes modulated may depend upon where the probiotic was introduced, with the stomach, cecum, jejunum, and colon showing substantially different numbers of genes that were differentially expressed (62).

EFFECTS OF PROBIOTICS ON THE RESIDENT GUT MICROBIOTA

Probiotic strains interact with the host on various levels. As described above, colonization with probiotic bacteria modulates gene expression within the host and also affects the immune system. Within the gut lumen, probiotic strains have direct interactions with commensal bacteria to mediate GI health. Probiotics can help break down complex nutrients in the diet, releasing metabolites that are taken up by other bacteria to promote their growth. Conversely, probiotics can also act as growth inhibitors for other bacteria. This can be accomplished through competition for specific nutrients and mucosal adhesion sites, production of acids and antimicrobials, and stimulation of intestinal immune responses. The impact of probiotics on the composition of the gut microbiota was thought to be one of the major mechanisms of their beneficial action. Various studies have evaluated the composition of the gut microbiota using traditional cultivation methods, molecular tools of PCR or fluorescence *in situ* hybridization (FISH) for specific bacterial groups, and most recently, high-throughput sequencing of 16S rRNA genes and metagenomics. The observed changes in the microbiota depend on the methodology used and the gut location.

Generally, studies using metagenomics approaches have illustrated that probiotics can induce some microbiota changes in the large intestine, but these changes typically are minor and transient, persisting only a few days after the end of administration. In one study, seven probiotic species of lactic acid bacteria were administered to 12 healthy dogs, with microbiota composition in fecal samples assessed by 16S rRNA gene sequencing. Probiotic species were detectable in 11/12 dogs during product administration but not before or 4 days following administration. While the abundances of *Enterococcus* and *Streptococcus* spp. were significantly increased during probiotic administration, 454-pyrosequencing did not indicate any changes in the major bacterial phyla (22). Similarly, the administration of *L. acidophilus* NCFM and *B. lactis* Bi-07 led to increases in the abundance of these species in fecal samples; no major changes in gut microbiota

structure were noted via metagenomic sequencing (21). Other studies evaluating cecal or fecal microbial populations using FISH or other molecular tools (denaturing gradient gel electrophoresis or terminal-restriction fragment length polymorphism) resulted in similar minor changes in some bacterial groups but no major effect on the overall composition of the microbiota (63, 64).

Other studies have looked at mucosa-adherent microbiota and identified major changes following probiotic administration. For example, after administration of VSL#3 to colitic mice, major changes in the ileal mucosal microbiota were observed using FISH analysis (65). Probiotic VSL#3 also increased beneficial mucosal bacteria when administered for 8 weeks to dogs with chronic enteropathy (IBD) (Fig. 2) (66).

Still other studies have identified some changes in gut microbiota in response to probiotic administration. A probiotic cocktail composed of *L. reuteri*, *Enterococcus faecium*, *Bifidobacterium animalis*, *Pediococcus acidilactici*, and *Lactobacillus salivarius* led to increases in *Bifidobacterium* spp., *Lactobacillus* spp., and Gram-positive cocci counts in 1-day-old chickens (67). The commonly used strain *E. faecium* NCIMB10415 caused a significant reduction in *Enterococcus* spp., specifically *E. faecalis*, in 2-week-old piglets (68). *Lactobacillus murinus* DPC6003 significantly reduced the number of *Enterobacteriaceae* in fecal samples of healthy pigs (69).

Another focus has been to evaluate the effect of probiotics on the reduction of pathogen counts. One study found a significant reduction in numbers of *S. enterica* serovar Typhimurium PT12 in fecal samples of pigs after 15 days of treatment with a probiotic cocktail composed of five probiotic strains (*L. murinus* DPC6002 and DPC6003, *Lactobacillus pentosus* DPC6004, *Lactobacillus salivarius* DPC6005, and *Pediococcus pentosaceus*) (70). Other studies have evaluated the effect of probiotics to prevent or reduce shedding of Shiga toxin–producing *E. coli* including strain O157:H7 in feedlot cattle

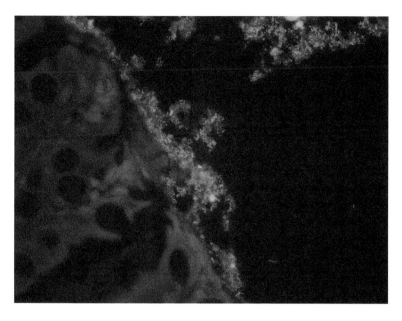

FIGURE 2 **Three-color FISH identifies mucosal bacteria adherent to the colonic mucosa in a dog receiving probiotic VSL #3 as therapy for IBD.** *Clostridia* **spp. appear orange (Erec482-Cy3 probe) against green (Eub338-FITC probe) and blue (DAPI stain) backgrounds.**

to reduce carcass contamination during slaughter. A directly fed probiotic composed of *Streptococcus bovis* LCB6 and *Lactobacillus gallinarum* LCB 12 was successful in inhibiting fecal shedding of *E. coli* O157 in Holstein calves. The reported mechanism was through increased production of volatile fatty acids, especially acetate (71).

Cattle supplemented with *L. acidophilus* strains NP51, NP28, and NP-51-NP35 had an approximately 35% reduction in the shedding of *E. coli* O157 in feces when compared to control cattle not given probiotic bacteria (72). In contrast, a number of other studies using various other probiotic strains have shown no effect on fecal shedding of *E. coli* O157. Young pigs may suffer from diarrhea induced by enterotoxigenic *E. coli*, leading to severe economic losses. The oral administration of *Bacillus subtilis* significantly decreased fecal scores and mortality in pigs (73). Similar results were obtained in piglets fed with *Lactobacillus sobrius* (74), *E. faecium* EK13 (75), and *E. faecium* NCIMB10415 (76).

Another major area of interest for using probiotics is to help mitigate stress responses. This is especially true of piglets at the time of weaning, when various environmental factors (e.g., nutrition, transport) contribute to stress, which increases susceptibility to enteric infections. Various probiotic studies have been performed to evaluate improvement in the porcine stress response. Administration of *L. plantarum* Lq80 alone or in combination with *Megasphaera elsdenii* iNP-001 increased the villous heights of the small intestine in piglets (77), as did administration of *P. acidilactici* when compared to placebo (78).

FECAL BACTERIOTHERAPY (TRANSPLANT)

Overview

Fecal microbiota transplantation (FMT) has emerged as an innovative microbiota target therapy that is effective for recurrent

C. difficile infection (RCDI) and may play a role in treating other GI and non-GI diseases (79–81). FMT is the "infusion of a fecal suspension from a healthy individual into the GI tract of an individual with colonic disease" (79). The goal of FMT is to treat disease by restoring phylogenetic diversity and microbiota reflective of a healthy person. Presumably, the potential health benefits of FMT might also include treatment of small intestinal GI disorders in humans, as has been demonstrated in dogs (34). Interestingly, FMT has existed for decades and has been used successfully in veterinary practice for cattle, horses, sheep, and other animals suffering from rumination disorders and colitis. The first published case of FMT in humans dates back to 1958, when Eiseman et al. reported successful treatment of four patients with severe pseudomembranous colitis (CDI) using fecal enemas (82). Since this time, numerous reports have shown the benefit of FMT in patients with severe or recurrent CDI, with cure rates as high as 100% and a mean cure rate of approximately 90% for the >500 cases reported in the literature to date (83). While FMT is best known for its efficacy in RCDI, it has also been used successfully for IBD, irritable bowel syndrome, idiopathic constipation, and other non-GI diseases.

FMT for GI Diseases

The current literature on FMT for RCDI comprises several single-center case series, case reports, a meta-analysis, systematic reviews, and randomized controlled trials all realizing similar results: astounding success, with ~92% of patients cured of their RCDI. FMT has even been proposed as a first-line therapy for patients with CDI instead of antibiotics because of its rapid effect, minimal risk, relatively low cost, ability to avoid exposure to antibiotics, and re-establishment of a more balanced and healthy microbiota (84). Long-term restoration of the disrupted gut microbiota with CDI

TABLE 1 Clinical disorders associated with altered intestinal microbiota[a]

Gastrointestinal disorders	Nongastrointestinal disorders
Colorectal cancer	Arthritis
Hepatic encephalopathy	Autism[b]
Idiopathic constipation[b]	Autoimmune disease
Irritable bowel syndrome[b]	Chronic fatigue syndrome[b]
Inflammatory bowel disease[b]	Diabetes mellitus/ metabolic syndrome[b]
Recurrent *Clostridium difficile* infection[b]	Fibromyalgia[b]
Cholelithiasis	Multiple sclerosis[b]
	Parkinson's disease[b]

[a]Modified from reference 81.
[b]Clinical improvement or cure noted following fecal microbiota transplantation.

is achievable in most patients with a single FMT procedure.

FMT has also been used to treat a variety of other chronic enteropathies including IBD, irritable bowel syndrome, and constipation, and there is emerging data on altered intestinal microbiota associated with these and other disorders (Table 1). In one large case series of 55 patients with diarrhea, constipation, abdominal pain, or IBD treated with FMT, 36% showed cure, 16% had decreased symptoms, and 47% showed no response (79). A systematic review comprising 41 patients with ulcerative colitis or Crohn's disease showed partial or complete remission in 76% of patients treated with FMT (85). One recent review summarizing data from multiple publications and comprising nine cases of IBD (eight ulcerative colitis and one Crohn's disease) treated with FMT reported remission of clinical disease in all nine patients for a period ranging from 3 months to 13 years. In another series, 45 patients with chronic constipation treated with colonoscopic FMT reported relief of defecation, bloating, and abdominal pain immediately postprocedure (81).

FMT for Extraintestinal Disorders

The pathogenesis of gut microbiota in non-GI diseases has prompted the use of FMT as a

TABLE 2 Practical considerations for FMT[a]

Parameter	Consideration
Donor selection	History of intrinsic GI disease: IBD, IBS, CRC, obesity, metabolic syndrome Past history of food or drug allergy? Diagnostic screening for infectious agents Recent history of antibiotic use
Recipient preparation	Role of diet? Perform bowel lavage? Perform antibiotic trial prior to FMT?
Donor sample storage	Fresh versus frozen feces
Type of diluent	Saline versus water versus milk
Volume of stool required	~60 g feces in 250–300 ml diluent
Route of administration	Nasogastric/enteric versus colonoscopy

[a]Abbreviations: FMT, fecal microbiota transplantation; IBD, inflammatory bowel disease; IBS, irritable bowel syndrome; CRC, colorectal cancer.

primary intervention for Parkinson's disease, chronic fatigue syndrome, multiple sclerosis (MS), obesity, insulin resistance and metabolic syndrome, and childhood regressive autism (Table 2) (79–81, 86). The beneficial effect of FMT was a serendipitous observation, underscored by the salient clinical observation of three patients with multiple sclerosis who underwent FMT for chronic constipation, in whom normal defecation and improved motor function was subsequently observed (87). Changes in the gut microbiota have also been observed in obese humans, where increased levels of bacteria and/or their products (i.e., lipopolysaccharide) were found in the plasma of these individuals, possibly due to increased intestinal permeability (88). Further discussion of the role of FMT in these and other non-GI disorders may be found in several recent comprehensive reviews (79, 80, 86).

FMT: Methodology

Formal treatment guidelines for performing FMT are currently being designed but should include (i) the clinical indications of FMT, (ii) proper donor screening procedures, (iii) fecal material preparation, and (iv) the possible routes of FMT administration (Table 2). The primary indications for FMT in humans are RCDI, especially cases that have failed to respond to a pulse/tapered regimen of vancomycin.

Donor selection

The donor may be an intimate, long-time partner, friend, or unrelated healthy volunteer. Since FMT carries potential risk for transmission of infectious agents, rigorous screening tests are recommended to reduce the risk of donor stool containing *C. difficile* toxin, bacterial pathogens and parasites, and viruses (i.e., hepatitis A/B/C, HIV). Donors should be excluded if they have received antibiotics in the past 3 months since antimicrobial perturbations of the microbiota might persist for 3 months or more. Avoid donors with suspicious histories of chronic diarrhea, constipation, IBD, irritable bowel syndrome, and/or colorectal polyps or cancer (79–81, 86).

Stool preparation

Stool preparation should ideally be performed under a hood since feces is rated as a level 2 biohazard. A stool specimen weighing ~50 to 60 g is added to 250 ml of diluent, usually saline. The mixture is then suspended by hand stirring or a blender and filtered through a coffee filter or gauze pad to remove large particulates. The suspension is then drawn up into a 60-ml catheter-tipped syringe and readied for instillation.

Method of administration

There is no clear consensus on the best method of administration: either upper GI (via endoscopy, nasogastric/nasoenteric, or ingestion of capsules), the proximal colon by colonoscopy, or the distal colon by retention enema (79). Administration of donor feces via the nasogastric/nasoenteric route is quick, convenient, inexpensive, technically simple, and does not require GI endoscopy. With upper endoscopy, 50 to 75 ml of fecal suspension is slowly infused into the duodenum. Many clinicians prefer the colonoscopic route over upper GI administration and fecal enema for RCDI, since the entire colon can be infused with stool and the mucosa assessed during endoscopic examination. FMT is reported to be largely successful by all of these routes, and the preferred method of delivery may vary with the clinical situation and experience of the physician.

Safety of FMT

FMT appears to be relatively safe as a short-term interventional procedure for RDCI; however, only limited data are available. More robust clinical trials are needed to better understand the mechanisms by which FMT is effective and the potential risks (short-term and long-term) to patients receiving these infusions.

CONCLUSION

FMT is a highly effective intervention for RCDI. It has now emerged as an important therapeutic technique in the manipulation of altered intestinal microbiota in different GI diseases, with the indications of FMT now expanded to include a variety of non-GI conditions.

ACKNOWLEDGMENTS

Dr. Suchodolski and Dr. Jergens are scientific consultants to ExeGi Pharma.

CITATION

Suchodolski JS, Jergens AE. 2016. Recent advances and understanding of using probiotic-based interventions to restore homeostasis of the microbiome for the prevention/therapy of bacterial diseases. Microbiol Spectrum 4(2):VMBF-0025-2015.

REFERENCES

1. **Swanson KS, Dowd SE, Suchodolski JS, Middelbos IS, Vester BM, Barry KA, Nelson KE, Torralba M, Henrissat B, Coutinho PM, Cann IK, White BA, Fahey GC Jr.** 2011. Phylogenetic and gene-centric metagenomics of the canine intestinal microbiome reveals similarities with humans and mice. *ISME J* **5:**639–649.

2. **Barry KA, Middelbos IS, Vester Boler BM, Dowd SE, Suchodolski JS, Henrissat B, Coutinho PM, White BA, Fahey GC Jr, Swanson KS.** 2012. Effects of dietary fiber on the feline gastrointestinal metagenome. *J Proteome Res* **11:**5924–5933.

3. **Yatsunenko T, Rey FE, Manary MJ, Trehan I, Dominguez-Bello MG, Contreras M, Magris M, Hidalgo G, Baldassano RN, Anokhin AP, Heath AC, Warner B, Reeder J, Kuczynski J, Caporaso JG, Lozupone CA, Lauber C, Clemente JC, Knights D, Knight R, Gordon JI.** 2012. Human gut microbiome viewed across age and geography. *Nature* **486:**222–227.

4. **Lederberg JM.** 2001. 'Ome sweet 'omics: a genealogical treasury of words. *Scientist* **15:**8–10.

5. **Suchodolski JS.** 2011. Companion animals symposium: microbes and gastrointestinal health of dogs and cats. *J Anim Sci* **89:**1520–1530.

6. **Human Microbiome Project C.** 2012. Structure, function and diversity of the healthy human microbiome. *Nature* **486:**207–214.

7. **Dunn WB, Ellis DI.** 2005. Metabolomics: current analytical platforms and methodologies. *Trends Anal Chem* **24:**285–294.

8. **Minamoto Y, Otoni CC, Steelman SM, Buyukleblebici O, Steiner JM, Jergens AE, Suchodolski JS.** 2015. Alteration of the fecal microbiota and serum metabolite profiles in dogs with idiopathic inflammatory bowel disease. *Gut Microbes* **6:**33–47.

9. **Wishart D.** 2007. Metabolomics in humans and other mammals, p 253–288. *In* Villas-Boas SG, Roessner U, Hansen AEH, Smedsgaard J, Nielsen J (ed), *Metabolome Analysis: An Introduction,* **vol 1**. John Wiley & Sons, Hoboken, NJ.

10. **Langille MG, Zaneveld J, Caporaso JG, McDonald D, Knights D, Reyes JA, Clemente JC, Burkepile DE, Vega Thurber RL, Knight R, Beiko RG, Huttenhower C.** 2013. Predictive functional profiling of microbial communities using 16S rRNA marker gene sequences. *Nat Biotechnol* **31:**814–821.

11. **Arumugam M, Raes J, Pelletier E, Le Paslier D, Yamada T, Mende DR, Fernandes GR, Tap J, Bruls T, Batto JM, Bertalan M, Borruel N, Casellas F, Fernandez L, Gautier L, Hansen T,**

Hattori M, Hayashi T, Kleerebezem M, Kurokawa K, Leclerc M, Levenez F, Manichanh C, Nielsen HB, Nielsen T, Pons N, Poulain J, Qin J, Sicheritz-Ponten T, Tims S, Torrents D, Ugarte E, Zoetendal EG, Wang J, Guarner F, Pedersen O, de Vos WM, Brunak S, Dore J, Antolin M, Artiguenave F, Blottiere HM, Almeida M, Brechot C, Cara C, Chervaux C, Cultrone A, Delorme C, Denariaz G, Dervyn R, Foerstner KU, Friss C, van de Guchte M, Guedon E, Haimet F, Huber W, van Hylckama-Vlieg J, Jamet A, Juste C, Kaci G, Knol J, Lakhdari O, Layec S, Le Roux K, Maguin E, Mérieux A, Melo Minardi R, M'rini C, Muller J, Oozeer R, Parkhill J, Renault P, Rescigno M, Sanchez N, Sunagawa S, Torrejon A, Turner K, Vandemeulebrouck G, Varela E, Winogradsky Y, Zeller G, Weissenbach J, Ehrlich SD, Bork P. 2011. Enterotypes of the human gut microbiome. *Nature* **473:**174–180.

12. **Jeffery IB, Claesson MJ, O'Toole PW, Shanahan F.** 2012. Categorization of the gut microbiota: enterotypes or gradients? *Nat Rev Microbiol* **10:**591–592.

13. **Aagaard K, Petrosino J, Keitel W, Watson M, Katancik J, Garcia N, Patel S, Cutting M, Madden T, Hamilton H, Harris E, Gevers D, Simone G, McInnes P, Versalovic J.** 2013. The Human Microbiome Project strategy for comprehensive sampling of the human microbiome and why it matters. *FASEB J* **27:**1012–1022.

14. **Suchodolski JS, Markel ME, Garcia-Mazcorro JF, Unterer S, Heilmann RM, Dowd SE, Kachroo P, Ivanov I, Minamoto Y, Dillman EM, Steiner JM, Cook AK, Toresson L.** 2012. The fecal microbiome in dogs with acute diarrhea and idiopathic inflammatory bowel disease. *Plos One* **7:**e51907. doi:10.1371/journal.pone.0051907.

15. **Duboc H, Rajca S, Rainteau D, Benarous D, Maubert MA, Quervain E, Thomas G, Barbu V, Humbert L, Despras G, Bridonneau C, Dumetz F, Grill JP, Masliah J, Beaugerie L, Cosnes J, Chazouilleres O, Poupon R, Wolf C, Mallet JM, Langella P, Trugnan G, Sokol H, Seksik P.** 2013. Connecting dysbiosis, bile-acid dysmetabolism and gut inflammation in inflammatory bowel diseases. *Gut* **62:**531–539.

16. **Frank DN, Amand ALS, Feldman RA, Boedeker EC, Harpaz N, Pace NR.** 2007. Molecular-phylogenetic characterization of microbial community imbalances in human inflammatory bowel diseases. *Proc Natl Acad Sci USA* **104:**13780–13785.

17. **Sokol H, Pigneur B, Watterlot L, Lakhdari O, Bermudez-Humaran LG, Gratadoux JJ, Blugeon S, Bridonneau C, Furet JP, Corthier G, Grangette C, Vasquez N, Pochart P, Trugnan G, Thomas G, Blottiere HM, Dore J, Marteau P, Seksik P, Langella P.** 2008. *Faecalibacterium prausnitzii* is an anti-inflammatory commensal bacterium identified by gut microbiota analysis of Crohn disease patients. *Proc Natl Acad Sci USA* **105:**16731–16736.

18. **Honneffer JB, Minamoto Y, Suchodolski JS.** 2014. Microbiota alterations in acute and chronic gastrointestinal inflammation of cats and dogs. *World J Gastroenterol* **20:**16489–16497.

19. **Packey CD, Sartor RB.** 2009. Commensal bacteria, traditional and opportunistic pathogens, dysbiosis and bacterial killing in inflammatory bowel diseases. *Curr Opin Infect Dis* **22:**292–301.

20. **Barrett JC, Hansoul S, Nicolae DL, Cho JH, Duerr RH, Rioux JD, Brant SR, Silverberg MS, Taylor KD, Barmada MM, Bitton A, Dassopoulos T, Datta LW, Green T, Griffiths AM, Kistner EO, Murtha MT, Regueiro MD, Rotter JI, Schumm LP, Steinhart AH, Targan SR, Xavier RJ, Libioulle C, Sandor C, Lathrop M, Belaiche J, Dewit O, Gut I, Heath S, Laukens D, Mni M, Rutgeerts P, Van Gossum A, Zelenika D, Franchimont D, Hugot JP, de Vos M, Vermeire S, Louis E, Cardon LR, Anderson CA, Drummond H, Nimmo E, Ahmad T, Prescott NJ, Onnie CM, Fisher SA, Marchini J, Ghori J, Bumpstead S, Gwilliam R, Tremelling M, Deloukas P, Mansfield J, Jewell D, Satsangi J, Mathew CG, Parkes M, Georges M, Daly MJ.** 2008. Genome-wide association defines more than 30 distinct susceptibility loci for Crohn's disease. *Nat Genet* **40:**955–962.

21. **Larsen N, Vogensen FK, Gobel R, Michaelsen KF, Abu Al-Soud W, Sorensen SJ, Hansen LH, Jakobsen M.** 2011. Predominant genera of fecal microbiota in children with atopic dermatitis are not altered by intake of probiotic bacteria *Lactobacillus acidophilus* NCFM and *Bifidobacterium animalis* subsp. lactis Bi-07. *FEMS Microbiol Ecol* **75:**482–496.

22. **Garcia-Mazcorro JF, Lanerie DJ, Dowd SE, Paddock CG, Grutzner N, Steiner JM, Ivanek R, Suchodolski JS.** 2011. Effect of a multi-species synbiotic formulation on fecal bacterial microbiota of healthy cats and dogs as evaluated by pyrosequencing. *FEMS Microbiol Ecol* **78:**542–554.

23. **McNulty NP, Yatsunenko T, Hsiao A, Faith JJ, Muegge BD, Goodman AL, Henrissat B, Oozeer R, Cools-Portier S, Gobert G, Chervaux C, Knights D, Lozupone CA, Knight R, Duncan AE, Bain JR, Muehlbauer MJ, Newgard CB,**

Heath AC, Gordon JI. 2011. The impact of a consortium of fermented milk strains on the gut microbiome of gnotobiotic mice and monozygotic twins. *Sci Transl Med* **3**:106ra106.

24. **Sellon RK, Tonkonogy S, Schultz M, Dieleman LA, Grenther W, Balish E, Rennick DM, Sartor RB.** 1998. Resident enteric bacteria are necessary for development of spontaneous colitis and immune system activation in interleukin-10-deficient mice. *Infect Immun* **66**:5224–5231.

25. **Imaoka A, Matsumoto S, Setoyama H, Okada Y, Umesaki Y.** 1996. Proliferative recruitment of intestinal intraepithelial lymphocytes after microbial colonization of germ-free mice. *Eur J Immunol* **26**:945–948.

26. **Bauer E, Williams BA, Smidt H, Verstegen MW, Mosenthin R.** 2006. Influence of the gastrointestinal microbiota on development of the immune system in young animals. *Curr Issues Intest Microbiol* **7**:35–51.

27. **Bansal T, Alaniz RC, Wood TK, Jayaraman A.** 2010. The bacterial signal indole increases epithelial-cell tight-junction resistance and attenuates indicators of inflammation. *Proc Natl Acad Sci USA* **107**:228–233.

28. **Shahinas D, Silverman M, Sittler T, Chiu C, Kim P, Allen-Vercoe E, Weese S, Wong A, Low DE, Pillai DR.** 2012. Toward an understanding of changes in diversity associated with fecal microbiome transplantation based on 16S rRNA gene deep sequencing. *MBio* **3**:e00338-12. doi:10.1128/mBio.00338-12.

29. **Suchodolski JS, Dowd SE, Westermarck E, Steiner JM, Wolcott RD, Spillmann T, Harmoinen JA.** 2009. The effect of the macrolide antibiotic tylosin on microbial diversity in the canine small intestine as demonstrated by massive parallel 16S rRNA gene sequencing. *BMC Microbiol* **9**:210.

30. **Dethlefsen L, Huse S, Sogin ML, Relman DA.** 2008. The pervasive effects of an antibiotic on the human gut microbiota, as revealed by deep 16S rRNA sequencing. *PloS Biol* **6**:e280. doi:10.1371/journal.pbio.0060280.

31. **Syer SD, Wallace JL.** 2014. Environmental and NSAID-enteropathy: dysbiosis as a common factor. *Curr Gastroenterol Rep* **16**:377.

32. **US Food and Drug Administration.** 2011. Medical Foods. Guidance for industry: frequently asked questions about medical foods. http://www.fda.gov/Food/GuidanceCompliance RegulatoryInformation/GuidanceDocuments/MedicalFoods/ucm054048htm.

33. **Prakash S, Rodes L, Coussa-Charley M, Tomaro-Duchesneau C.** 2011. Gut microbiota: next frontier in understanding human health and development of biotherapeutics. *Biologics* **5**:71–86.

34. **Rossi G, Pengo G, Caldin M, Palumbo Piccionello A, Steiner JM, Cohen ND, Jergens AE, Suchodolski JS.** 2014. Comparison of microbiological, histological, and immunomodulatory parameters in response to treatment with either combination therapy with prednisone and metronidazole or probiotic VSL#3 strains in dogs with idiopathic inflammatory bowel disease. *Plos One* **9**:e94699. doi:10.1371/journal.pone.0094699.

35. **Soo I, Madsen KL, Tejpar Q, Sydora BC, Sherbaniuk R, Cinque B, Di Marzio L, Cifone MG, Desimone C, Fedorak RN.** 2008. VSL#3 probiotic upregulates intestinal mucosal alkaline sphingomyelinase and reduces inflammation. *Can J Gastroenterol* **22**:237–242.

36. **Mardini HE, Grigorian AY.** 2014. Probiotic mix VSL#3 is effective adjunctive therapy for mild to moderately active ulcerative colitis: a meta-analysis. *Inflamm Bowel Dis* **20**:1562–1567.

37. **Collado MC, Meriluoto J, Salminen S.** 2007. Role of commercial probiotic strains against human pathogen adhesion to intestinal mucus. *Lett Appl Microbiol* **45**:454–460.

38. **Collado MC, Grzeskowiak L, Salminen S.** 2007. Probiotic strains and their combination inhibit *in vitro* adhesion of pathogens to pig intestinal mucosa. *Curr Microbiol* **55**:260–265.

39. **Lee YK, Puong KY, Ouwehand AC, Salminen S.** 2003. Displacement of bacterial pathogens from mucus and Caco-2 cell surface by lactobacilli. *J Med Microbiol* **52**:925–930.

40. **Jones SE, Versalovic J.** 2009. Probiotic *Lactobacillus reuteri* biofilms produce antimicrobial and anti-inflammatory factors. *BMC Microbiol* **9**:35.

41. **Fukuda S, Toh H, Taylor TD, Ohno H, Hattori M.** 2012. Acetate-producing bifidobacteria protect the host from enteropathogenic infection via carbohydrate transporters. *Gut Microbes* **3**:449–454.

42. **Lin PW, Myers LE, Ray L, Song SC, Nasr TR, Berardinelli AJ, Kundu K, Murthy N, Hansen JM, Neish AS.** 2009. *Lactobacillus rhamnosus* blocks inflammatory signaling *in vivo* via reactive oxygen species generation. *Free Radic Biol Med* **47**:1205–1211.

43. **Lammers KM, Brigidi P, Vitali B, Gionchetti P, Rizzello F, Caramelli E, Matteuzzi D, Campieri M.** 2003. Immunomodulatory effects of probiotic bacteria DNA: IL-1 and IL-10 response in human peripheral blood mononuclear cells. *FEMS Immunol Med Microbiol* **38**:165–172.

44. **Shen TY, Qin HL, Gao ZG, Fan XB, Hang XM, Jiang YQ.** 2006. Influences of enteral nutrition

combined with probiotics on gut microflora and barrier function of rats with abdominal infection. *World J Gastroenterol* **12:**4352–4358.

45. **Simeoli R, Mattace Raso G, Lama A, Pirozzi C, Santoro A, Di Guida F, Sanges M, Aksoy E, Calignano A, D'Arienzo A, Meli R.** 2015. Preventive and therapeutic effects of *Lactobacillus paracasei* B21060-based synbiotic treatment on gut inflammation and barrier integrity in colitic mice. *J Nutr* **145:**1202–1210.

46. **Bayoumi MA, Griffiths MW.** 2012. *In vitro* inhibition of expression of virulence genes responsible for colonization and systemic spread of enteric pathogens using *Bifidobacterium bifidum* secreted molecules. *Int J Food Microbiol* **156:**255–263.

47. **Medellin-Pena MJ, Wang H, Johnson R, Anand S, Griffiths MW.** 2007. Probiotics affect virulence-related gene expression in *Escherichia coli* O157:H7. *Appl Environ Microbiol* **73:**4259–4267.

48. **Allaart JG, van Asten AJ, Vernooij JC, Grone A.** 2011. Effect of *Lactobacillus fermentum* on beta2 toxin production by *Clostridium perfringens*. *Appl Environ Microbiol* **77:**4406–4411.

49. **Castagliuolo I, Riegler MF, Valenick L, LaMont JT, Pothoulakis C.** 1999. *Saccharomyces boulardii* protease inhibits the effects of *Clostridium difficile* toxins A and B in human colonic mucosa. *Infect Immun* **67:**302–307.

50. **Takeda K, Kaisho T, Akira S.** 2003. Toll-like receptors. *Annu Rev Immunol* **21:**335–376.

51. **Schlee M, Wehkamp J, Altenhoefer A, Oelschlaeger TA, Stange EF, Fellermann K.** 2007. Induction of human beta-defensin 2 by the probiotic *Escherichia coli* Nissle 1917 is mediated through flagellin. *Infect Immun* **75:**2399–2407.

52. **Granato D, Bergonzelli GE, Pridmore RD, Marvin L, Rouvet M, Corthesy-Theulaz IE.** 2004. Cell surface-associated elongation factor Tu mediates the attachment of *Lactobacillus johnsonii* NCC533 (La1) to human intestinal cells and mucins. *Infect Immun* **72:**2160–2169.

53. **Matsuguchi T, Takagi A, Matsuzaki T, Nagaoka M, Ishikawa K, Yokokura T, Yoshikai Y.** 2003. Lipoteichoic acids from *Lactobacillus* strains elicit strong tumor necrosis factor alpha-inducing activitives in macrophages through toll-like receptor 2. *Clin Diagn Lab Immunol* **10:**259–266.

54. **Mack DR, Ahrne S, Hyde L, Wei S, Hollingsworth MA.** 2003. Extracellular MUC3 mucin secretion follows adherence of *Lactobacillus* strains to intestinal epithelial cells *in vitro*. *Gut* **52:**827–833.

55. **Yan F, Cao HW, Cover TL, Whitehead R, Washington MK, Polk DB.** 2007. Soluble proteins produced by probiotic bacteria regulate intestinal epithelial cell survival and growth. *Gastroenterology* **132:**562–575.

56. **Shima T, Fukushima K, Setoyama H, Imaoka A, Matsumoto S, Hara T, Suda K, Umesaki Y.** 2008. Differential effects of two probiotic strains with different bacteriological properties on intestinal gene expression, with special reference to indigenous bacteria. *FEMS Immunol Med Microbiol* **52:**69–77.

57. **Brisbin JT, Zhou H, Gong J, Sabour P, Akbari MR, Haghighi HR, Yu H, Clarke A, Sarson AJ, Sharif S.** 2008. Gene expression profiling of chicken lymphoid cells after treatment with *Lactobacillus acidophilus* cellular components. *Dev Comp Immunol* **32:**563–574.

58. **Panigrahi P, Braileanu GT, Chen H, Stine OC.** 2007. Probiotic bacteria change *Escherichia coli*-induced gene expression in cultured colonocytes: implications in intestinal pathophysiology. *World J Gastroenterol* **13:**6370–6378.

59. **Sonnenburg JL, Chen CT, Gordon JI.** 2006. Genomic and metabolic studies of the impact of probiotics on a model gut symbiont and host. *PLoS Biol* **4:**e413. doi:10.1371/journal.pbio.0040413.

60. **Walter J, Heng NC, Hammes WP, Loach DM, Tannock GW, Hertel C.** 2003. Identification of *Lactobacillus reuteri* genes specifically induced in the mouse gastrointestinal tract. *Appl Environ Microbiol* **69:**2044–2051.

61. **Bron PA, Grangette C, Mercenier A, de Vos WM, Kleerebezem M.** 2004. Identification of *Lactobacillus plantarum* genes that are induced in the gastrointestinal tract of mice. *J Bacteriol* **186:**5721–5729.

62. **Denou E, Berger B, Barretto C, Panoff JM, Arigoni F, Brussow H.** 2007. Gene expression of commensal *Lactobacillus johnsonii* strain NCC533 during *in vitro* growth and in the murine gut. *J Bacteriol* **189:**8109–8119.

63. **Gerard P, Brezillon C, Quere F, Salmon A, Rabot S.** 2008. Characterization of cecal microbiota and response to an orally administered *Lactobacillus* probiotic strain in the broiler chicken. *J Mol Microbiol Biotechnol* **14:**115–122.

64. **Fuentes S, Egert M, Jimenez-Valera M, Ramos-Cormenzana A, Ruiz-Bravo A, Smidt H, Monteoliva-Sanchez M.** 2008. Administration of *Lactobacillus casei* and *Lactobacillus plantarum* affects the diversity of murine intestinal lactobacilli, but not the overall bacterial community structure. *Res Microbiol* **159:**237–243.

65. **Mar JS, Nagalingam NA, Song Y, Onizawa M, Lee JW, Lynch SV.** 2014. Amelioration of DSS-induced murine colitis by VSL#3 supplementation is primarily associated with changes in ileal

microbiota composition. *Gut Microbes* **5**:494–503.

66. **White RSR, G, Atherly T, Webb C, Hill S, Steiner JM, Suchodolski JS, Jergens AE.** 2015. Effect of VSL#3 probiotic strains on the intestinal microbiota in canine inflammatory bowel disease. *J Vet Intern Med* **9**:423–483. doi:10.1111/jvim.12491.

67. **Mountzouris KC, Tsirtsikos P, Kalamara E, Nitsch S, Schatzmayr G, Fegeros K.** 2007. Evaluation of the efficacy of a probiotic containing *Lactobacillus, Bifidobacterium, Enterococcus,* and *Pediococcus* strains in promoting broiler performance and modulating cecal microflora composition and metabolic activities. *Poult Sci* **86**:309–317.

68. **Vahjen W, Taras D, Simon O.** 2007. Effect of the probiotic *Enterococcus faecium* NCIMB10415 on cell numbers of total *Enterococcus* spp., *E. faecium* and *E. faecalis* in the intestine of piglets. *Curr Issues Intest Microbiol* **8**:1–7.

69. **Gardiner GE, Casey PG, Casey G, Lynch PB, Lawlor PG, Hill C, Fitzgerald GF, Stanton C, Ross RP.** 2004. Relative ability of orally administered *Lactobacillus murinus* to predominate and persist in the porcine gastrointestinal tract. *Appl Environ Microbiol* **70**:1895–1906.

70. **Casey PG, Gardiner GE, Casey G, Bradshaw B, Lawlor PG, Lynch PB, Leonard FC, Stanton C, Ross RP, Fitzgerald GF, Hill C.** 2007. A five-strain probiotic combination reduces pathogen shedding and alleviates disease signs in pigs challenged with *Salmonella enterica* serovar *Typhimurium. Appl Environ Microbiol* **73**:1858–1863.

71. **Ohya T, Marubashi T, Ito H.** 2000. Significance of fecal volatile fatty acids in shedding of *Escherichia coli* O157 from calves: experimental infection and preliminary use of a probiotic product. *J Vet Med Sci* **62**:1151–1155.

72. **Stephens TP, Loneragan GH, Chichester LM, Brashears MM.** 2007. Prevalence and enumeration of *Escherichia coli* O157 in steers receiving various strains of *Lactobacillus*-based direct-fed microbials. *J Food Prot* **70**:1252–1255.

73. **Bhandari SK, Xu B, Nyachoti CM, Giesting DW, Krause DO.** 2008. Evaluation of alternatives to antibiotics using an *Escherichia coli* K88+ model of piglet diarrhea: effects on gut microbial ecology. *J Anim Sci* **86**:836–847.

74. **Konstantinov SR, Smidt H, Akkermans AD, Casini L, Trevisi P, Mazzoni M, De Filippi S, Bosi P, de Vos WM.** 2008. Feeding of *Lactobacillus sobrius* reduces *Escherichia coli* F4 levels in the gut and promotes growth of infected piglets. *FEMS Microbiol Ecol* **66**:599–607.

75. **Strompfova V, Marcinakova M, Simonova M, Gancarcikova S, Jonecova Z, Scirankova L, Koscova J, Buleca V, Cobanova K, Laukova A.** 2006. *Enterococcus faecium* EK13: an enterocin a-producing strain with probiotic character and its effect in piglets. *Anaerobe* **12**:242–248.

76. **Taras D, Vahjen W, Macha M, Simon O.** 2006. Performance, diarrhea incidence, and occurrence of *Escherichia coli* virulence genes during long-term administration of a probiotic *Enterococcus faecium* strain to sows and piglets. *J Anim Sci* **84**:608–617.

77. **Yoshida Y, Tsukahara T, Ushida K.** 2009. Oral administration of *Lactobacillus plantarum* Lq80 and *Megasphaera elsdenii* iNP-001 induces efficient recovery from mucosal atrophy in the small and the large intestines of weaning piglets. *Anim Sci J* **80**:709–715.

78. **Di Giancamillo A, Vitari F, Savoini G, Bontempo V, Bersani C, Dell'Orto V, Domeneghini C.** 2008. Effects of orally administered probiotic *Pediococcus acidilactici* on the small and large intestine of weaning piglets. A qualitative and quantitative micro-anatomical study. *Histol Histopathol* **23**:651–664.

79. **Borody TJ, Paramsothy S, Agrawal G.** 2013. Fecal microbiota transplantation: indications, methods, evidence, and future directions. *Curr Gastroenterol Rep* **15**:337.

80. **Kelly CR, Kahn S, Kashyap P, Laine L, Rubin D, Atreja A, Moore T, Wu G.** 2015. Update on fecal microbiota transplantation 2015: indications, methodologies, mechanisms, and outlook. *Gastroenterology* **149**:223–237.

81. **Brandt LJ, Aroniadis OC.** 2013. An overview of fecal microbiota transplantation: techniques, indications, and outcomes. *Gastrointest Endosc* **78**:240–249.

82. **Eiseman B, Silen W, Bascom GS, Kauvar AJ.** 1958. Fecal enema as an adjunct in the treatment of pseudomembranous enterocolitis. *Surgery* **44**:854–859.

83. **Cammarota G, Ianiro G, Gasbarrini A.** 2014. Fecal microbiota transplantation for the treatment of *Clostridium difficile* infection: a systematic review. *J Clin Gastroenterol* **48**: 693–702.

84. **Brandt LJ, Borody TJ, Campbell J.** 2011. Endoscopic fecal microbiota transplantation: "first-line" treatment for severe *Clostridium difficile* infection? *J Clin Gastroenterol* **45**:655–657.

85. **Anderson JL, Edney RJ, Whelan K.** 2012. Systematic review: faecal microbiota transplantation in the management of inflammatory bowel disease. *Aliment Pharmacol Ther* **36**:503–516.

86. **Xu MQ, Cao HL, Wang WQ, Wang S, Cao XC, Yan F, Wang BM.** 2015. Fecal microbiota transplantation broadening its application beyond intestinal disorders. *World J Gastroenterol* **21:**102–111.

87. **Smits LP, Bouter KE, de Vos WM, Borody TJ, Nieuwdorp M.** 2013. Therapeutic poten-tial of fecal microbiota transplantation. *Gastroenterology* **145:**946–953.

88. **Teixeira TF, Collado MC, Ferreira CL, Bressan J, Peluzio Mdo C.** 2012. Potential mechanisms for the emerging link between obesity and increased intestinal permeability. *Nutr Res* **32:**637–647.

Index